MASTERING
Endovascular Techniques

A Guide to Excellence

MASTERING
Endovascular
Techniques

A Guide to Excellence

PETER LANZER, MD

Hospitals and Clinics Bitterfeld-Wolfen
Department of Internal Medicine
Bitterfeld, Germany
Concept 21 Consulting
Heart Center Coswig
Department of Cardiology and Angiology
Coswig/Anhalt, Germany

Lippincott Williams & Wilkins
a Wolters Kluwer business

Philadelphia • Baltimore • New York • London
Buenos Aires • Hong Kong • Sydney • Tokyo

Acquisitions Editor: Frances R. DeStefano
Developmental Editor: Louise Bierig
Managing Editor: Joanne Bersin
Marketing Manager: Angela Panetta
Project Manager: Nicole Walz
Senior Manufacturing Manager: Ben Rivera
Creative Director: Doug Smock
Cover Designer: Mike Pottman
Production Services: GGS Book Services
Printer: Maple-Vail

© 2007 by LIPPINCOTT WILLIAMS & WILKINS, a Wolters Kluwer business
530 Walnut Street
Philadelphia, PA 19106 USA
LWW.com

Library of Congress Cataloging-in-Publication Data

Mastering endovascular techniques : a guide to excellence / [edited by] Peter Lanzer.
    p. ; cm.
  Includes bibliographical references.
  ISBN-13: 978-1-58255-967-4
  ISBN-10: 1-58255-967-8
  1. Blood-vessels—Surgery. 2. Blood-vessels—Endoscopic surgery. 3. Arterial catheterization. I. Lanzer, P. (Peter), 1950-
  [DNLM: 1. Vascular Surgical Procedures—methods. 2. Catheterization—methods. 3. Vascular Diseases—
radiography. 4. Vascular Diseases—surgery. WG 170 M4225 2006]
  RC598.5.M37 2006
  617.4'1–dc22

              2006019720

Care has been taken to confirm the accuracy of the information presented and to describe generally accepted practices. However, the authors, editors, and publisher are not responsible for errors or omissions or for any consequences from application of the information in this book and make no warranty, expressed or implied, with respect to the currency, completeness, or accuracy of the contents of the publication. Application of the information in a particular situation remains the professional responsibility of the practitioner.

The authors, editors, and publisher have exerted every effort to ensure that drug selection and dosage set forth in this text are in accordance with current recommendations and practice at the time of publication. However, in view of ongoing research, changes in government regulations, and the constant flow of information relating to drug therapy and drug reactions, the reader is urged to check the package insert for each drug for any change in indications and dosage and for added warnings and precautions. This is particularly important when the recommended agent is a new or infrequently employed drug.

Some drugs and medical devices presented in the publication have Food and Drug Administration (FDA) clearance for limited use in restricted research settings. It is the responsibility of the health care provider to ascertain the FDA status of each drug or device planned for use in their clinical practice.

To purchase additional copies of this book, call our customer service department at (800) 638-3030 or fax orders to (301) 223-2320. International customers should call (301) 223-2300.

Visit Lippincott Williams & Wilkins on the Internet: at LWW.com. Lippincott Williams & Wilkins customer service representatives are available from 8:30 am to 6 pm, EST.

10 9 8 7 6 5 4 3 2 1

To those impatient with mediocrity and waste.

CONTRIBUTORS

Wilbert Aarnoudse, MD
Fellow in Interventional Cardiology
Department of Cardiology
Catharina Hospital
Eindhoven, The Netherlands

Dietrich Baumgart, MD
Head/Professor of Cardiology
Preventicum-Klinik für Diagnostik
Essen, Germany

Cees-joost Botman, MD
Interventional Cardiologist
Department of Cardiology
Catharina Hospital
Eindhoven, The Netherlands

Ivo Buschmann, MD
Head/Professor of Physiology
Division of Arteriogenesis Research
Charité CC15 Centre for Cardiology and
Centre for Cardiovascular Research (CCR)
Free University Berlin
Berlin, Germany

Stephen C. Davies, M.Sc.
Manager, Transducer Engineering
Research and Development
VOLCANO Corporation
Rancho Cordova, California

Thomas Egelhof, MD
Chief Radiologist
Preventicum–Klinik für Diagnostik
Essen, Germany

Aloke V. Finn, MD
Fellow in Internal Medicine and Cardiology
Harvard Medical School
Massachusetts General Hospital
Boston, Massachusetts

Herman K. Gold, MD
Associate Professor of Internal Medicine
and Cardiology
Harvard Medical School
Massachusetts General Hospital
Boston, Massachusetts

Helmut Hebazettl, MD, PhD
Professor of Physiology
Charité CC2 Centre for Basic Medical Sciences
Free University Berlin
Berlin, Germany

Hans Henkes, MD
Professor of Interventional Neuroradiology
Department of Radiology and Neuroradiology
Alfried Krupp Hospitals and Clinics
Essen, Germany
Department of Neuroradiology and Radiology

Robert Janker Hospital
Bonn, Germany

Hüseyin Ince, MD

Consultant Physician
Cardiology/Internal Medicine
Rostock University Hospital
Rostock, Germany

Zubin Irani, MD

Clinical Instructor
Interventional Radiologist
Dotter Interventional Institute
Oregon Health & Science University
Portland, Oregon

Michael Joner, MD

Research Fellow in Cardiology
CVPath
Gaithersburg, Maryland
Consultant Physician
Interventional Cardiology
German Heart Center
University of Munich
Munich, Germany

John A. Kaufman, MD

Professor of Interventional Radiology and Surgery
Chief of Vascular and Interventional Radiology
Dotter Interventional Institute
Oregon Health & Science University
Portland, Oregon

Stephan Kische, MD

Fellow in Cardiology and Internal Medicine
Rostock University Hospital
Rostock, Germany

Martin Köcher, MD, PhD

Chief of Interventional Radiology
Associate Professor of Radiology
University Hospital
Palacky University
Olomouc, Czech Republic

Frank Kolodgie, PhD

CVPath
Gaithersburg, Maryland

Dietmar Kühne, MD

Head/Professor of Interventional Neuroradiology
Alfried Krupp Hospitals and Clinics
Essen, Germany

Robert J. Kutys, MS, PA (ASCP)

Pathologist Assistant
Cardiovascular Pathology
CVPath
Gaithersburg, Maryland

Elena Ladich, MD

Staff Pathologist
CVPath
Gaithersburg, Maryland

Peter Lanzer, MD

Chief of Medical Services
European Centre for Endovascular Therapy and
Department of Internal Medicine
Hospitals and Clinics Bitterfeld-Wolfen
Bitterfeld, Germany

Steven Lowens, MD

Staff Radiologist
Department of Neuroradiology
Robert Janker Hospital
Bonn, Germany

M. Pauliina Margolis, MD, PhD

Medical Director
VOLCANO Corporation
Rancho Cordova, California

Haresh G. Mehta, MD, DNB

Consultant Cardiologist
Department of Cardiology
P.D. Hinduja National Hospital and Medical
Research Center
Mahim Mumbai, India

Bernhard Meier, MD

Chairman/Professor of Cardiology
University Hospital Bern
Bern, Switzerland

Elina Miloslavski, MD

Resident in Radiology
Department of Neuroradiology
and Radiology
Robert Janker Hospital
Bonn, Germany

Anuja Nair, PhD

Adjunct Staff
Biomedical Engineering
Cleveland Clinic
Senior Scientist
Research and Development

VOLCANO Corporation
Cleveland, Ohio

Christoph A. Nienaber, MD

Professor of Medicine and Cardiology
Director
Cardiology/Internal Medicine
Rostock University Hospital
Rostock, Germany

Nico H.J. Pijls, MD, PhD

Professor of Interventional Cardiology
Catharina Hospital
Eindhoven, The Netherlands

Lutz Prechelt, PhD

Professor of Informatics
Institute of Informatics
Free University Berlin
Berlin, Germany

Axel R. Pries, MD, FESC

Professor of Physiology
Charité CC 2 Centrum für Grundlagenmedizin
Berlin, Germany

Tim C. Rehders, MD

Consultant Physician
Cardiology/Internal Medicine
Rostock University Hospital
Rostock, Germany

Jörg Reinartz, MD

Consultant Physician
Department of Neuroradiology and Radiology
Robert Janker Hospital
Bonn, Germany

Wolfram Schmidt, PhD

Senior Researcher
Sensors and Biomedical Devices
Institute for Biomedical Engineering
University of Rostock
Rostock, Germany

Klaus-Peter Schmitz, PhD

Director/Professor of Biomedical Sciences
Institute for Biomedical Engineering
University of Rostock
Rostock, Germany

L.D. Timmie Topoleski, PhD

Professor of Mechanical Engineering
University of Maryland, Baltimore County
Professor of Orthopaedic Surgery
University of Maryland Medical Center
Baltimore, Maryland

Petr Utíkal, MD, PhD

Associate Professor of Surgery
University Hospital
Palacky University
Olomouc, Czech Republic

D. Geoffrey Vince, PhD

Adjunct Staff
Biomedical Engineering
Cleveland Clinic
Director
Research and Development
VOLCANO Corporation
Cleveland, Ohio

Renu Virmani, MD

Medical Director/Professor of Pathology
CVPath
Gaithersburg, Maryland

Dierk Vorwerk, MD

Chairman/Professor of Interventional Radiology
Institute for Diagnostic and Interventional Radiology
Hospitals and Clinics
Ingolstadt, Germany
University of Technology Aachen
Aachen, Germany

Ralf Weser, MD

Chief of Interventional Services
Department of Cardiology and Angiology
Heart Centre Coswig
Coswig/Anhalt, Germany

Stephan Windecker, MD

Professor of Cardiology
Head of Invasive Cardiology
University Hospital Bern
Bern, Switzerland

INTRODUCTION

Since Dotter's and Grüntzig's initial attempts at endovascular interventions in the 1960s and 1970s, generations of interventionists have been taught and trained by observing master operators and by imitating their actions. Eventually, in their own clinical practice, some went beyond the skills of their predecessors. This largely empirical process of transferring skills that has been enacted by thousands of physicians has remained virtually unchanged over the years.

More recently, the broad availability of stents and low-profile endovascular instrumentation has created the impression that the expertise and technical skills of interventionists have become less critical. The evidence-based approach to some extent has also seemed to supplant and facilitate interventional rationale. For a number of reasons, however, both the traditional empirical approach to teaching and training endovascular interventions and also the recent trends may be questioned. In fact, it appears that the complexity of interventions and demands on the cognitive and technical skills of interventionists have markedly increased over the years.

First, knowledge transfer based largely on the ability of individual angioplasty professors to communicate their skills appears fragile at best. The very disappearance of many of these professors and the progressively tacit character of their expertise has coincided with the often vague and indeterminate structure of endovascular concepts and strategies. This has successfully curtailed the interventional knowledge base and thrown open the doors for redundant and indiscriminate use of stenting.

Second, better instrumentation has enabled interventionists to address more complex cases that were formerly considered unsuited for interventions. The spectrum of endovascular treatments considered technically feasible now approaches that of open coronary and noncoronary vascular surgery. The endovascular treatment of complex vascular disease is more demanding, necessitating complex strategic planning and high

technical skills, unless the interventionist routinely and indiscriminately resorts to stenting.

Third, interventions are increasingly being performed on elderly and aged patients presenting both with more advanced stages of vascular disease and also with numerous outcome-relevant coexistent morbidities. Endovascular treatments of this vulnerable population may rapidly cross the line at which the benefit to patients is unambiguous, particularly if accompanied by potentially avoidable iatrogenic complications.

Fourth, interventions are increasingly being performed in emergency or ad-hoc settings immediately following diagnostic evaluations. They require quick and sound clinical judgment, frequently unsupported by guidelines, and flawless execution.

Fifth, the huge number of interventions increases the numerical relevance of all complications. Optimistic reporting of results and the needs of marketing and media representation combine to raise public expectations inching ever closer to unrealistic success and zero rates of complications, exposing the interventionists to the risk of perceived personal responsibility in cases of any treatment failure. In addition, the fully digitized documentation of interventional procedures not only allows an instant transfer of data via the electronic highway but can also provide ideal forensic evidence in cases of litigation.

Finally, competing treatment strategies and increasing economic restrictions mandate expert procedural performance in standard settings.

The combination of potentially decreasing interventional skills on the one hand and increasing operational demands on the other could pose a fundamental threat to the future practice of endovascular interventions. Arguably, deeper analysis of the endovascular strategies and principles may be required to improve interventional practices. In addition, broader systemic and bodywide endovascular interventional training may become necessary to fully explore and utilize the benefits of the single-access multiple-target sites catheter-based treatments.

The quality of endovascular interventions may be improved by progress in the state of the art of science and technology and by advances in the quality of interventionists' practice. Improvements resulting from science and technology are typically slower and gradual, while those from better engineering of applied knowledge may be rapid and saltatorial. Therefore, although both better science and technology and better engineered applied knowledge are required to improve the level of skills of interventionists and consequently procedural quality, the latter appears to offer faster prospects of success.

The likelihood of any vascular intervention being successful depends on four factors:

1. The patient's condition, which refers to both the patient's general and vascular status.
2. The technical infrastructure available to the interventionist, which refers to all the facilities associated with the intervention.
3. The interventionist's power of judgment, which comprises all of the interventionist's knowledge about the first two factors and his or her capabilities to arrive quickly and reliably at suitable decisions about strategy. Such decisions depend on the portfolio of possible next interventional steps and the interventionist's ability to select the optimum choices by weighing the expected benefits against foreseeable risks.
4. The interventionist's manual dexterity, which refers to the repertoire of manual skills (or their lack) that allow the interventionist to translate strategy into treatment with accuracy and precision.

Whereas the first two factors may be considered as given and beyond the influence of the interventionist, both power of judgment and technical skills are subject to engineering. Compiling and transferring interventional knowledge require the development of a sound ontology of endovascular interventions, the definition of their constituent parts including the relevant aspects of vascular biology, function, and imaging, endovascular instrumentation, and associated mechanical interactions. Furthermore, the factors that made up the expertise of the masters must be analyzed, understood, and extracted. Then, the acquired knowledge must be implemented in interventional curricula honing both powerful judgment and expert technical skills.

Typically, textbooks on endovascular therapy emphasize guidelines, consensus statements, and recommendations based on evidence data. Less frequently, the practice of endovascular treatments has been defined, mostly by providing how-to-do tips, tricks, and advice by highly skilled and experienced interventionists. More systematic ontology of endovascular interventional practice is still missing.

In this textbook, we attempt to develop ontology of endovascular interventions based on the currently available evidence and the experiences of expert interventionists. In response to the pressing needs to develop interdisciplinary curriculum for mastering systemic endovascular procedures, both coronary and noncoronary interventions are included, although by far the greatest amount of work has been done and reported on coronary artery revascularization.

Formally, the textbook is divided into two parts. In the first part, the general principles of vascular anatomy, function, and diagnostics are reviewed. The reader learns and reviews basic facts about the vascular system and vascular imaging in peri-interventional settings. In the second part, the clinical concepts of endovascular interventional therapy are described for all the major vessels and vascular territories.

In the introductory chapter of Part II, the decision-making process is described with reference to the example of percutaneous coronary interventions, and a theoretical framework based on risk assessment is developed that can be employed and modified for any catheter-based endovascular intervention. To provide a systemic perspective accessible to an analytical approach, the percutaneous interventional process is divided into the basic phases of (1) initialization, (2) the main interventional cycle characterized by diagnostic and interventional stepwise iterations, and (3) termination. In the concluding chapter of the technical section of Part II, the critical importance of the performance characteristics and mechanical properties of endovascular instrumentation are discussed using coronary dilatation catheters and stents as an example.

In the subsequent nine chapters, the state of the art of the practice of endovascular interventions in all the major vascular beds, including the venous system, is reviewed. Discussed are neurovascular interventions, the endovascular treatments applicable to the extracranial carotid arteries, coronary arteries, the thoracic and abdominal aorta, renal arteries, and arteries of the pelvis and lower extremities.

Besides reviewing the current literature, the authors describe practical points of implementation. The term "coronary-like" has been introduced to denote similarities between endovascular interventions performed in coronary and noncoronary vascular beds. These similarities are primarily based on the use of the integrated coaxial telescopic systems consisting of rapid exchange high-technology low-profile instrumentation. By developing and exploring the principal patterns, the textbook unlocks the remarkable synergies and cross-talk inherent to all endovascular interventions. Pattern recognition and individualization consistently applied to endovascular interventions in different patients and different vascular beds enables the reader to acquire professional insights shared by high-class interventionists. In the closing chapter, the basic aspects of foreign body removal are reviewed since damage and embolization of catheter parts can complicate and potentially even mar the outcome of any endovascular intervention.

Who will gain most from reading this textbook? Those professionals challenged by intricacies and tragedy of vascular disease. Those professionals ready to learn, explore, and implement the unique powers of catheter-based techniques to optimize vascular treatments. And those individuals ready to discover the endovascular future by relentlessly pushing back the barriers and limits by endurance and strive for excellence.

This textbook is a team effort. I feel greatly indebted to all colleagues and authors not only for their willingness to share their experience and professional expertise but also for keeping up with the extremely tight time schedule. On an equal base, I wish to express my gratitude to the Lippincott Williams & Wilkins staff associated with this project. In particular, I wish to thank Fran DeStefano, Acquisition Editor, for her enduring encouragement, Angela Panetta, Marketing Manager, for her superb strategic skills, and Nicole Walz, Project Manager, for her ability to deliver on time with excellence.

Peter Lanzer
July 4, 2006

CONTENTS

MASTERING
Endovascular Techniques

A Guide to Excellence

PART 1

GENERAL PRINCIPLES

Frank Kolodgie

Michael Joner

Aloke V. Finn

Elena Ladich

Robert J. Kutys

Herman K. Gold

Renu Virmani

CHAPTER **1**

Key Issues of Vascular Pathoanatomy

Atherosclerotic disease persists as the most frequent cause of death in the Western world and in the 21st century and is predicted to be the primary cause of disability and death worldwide. Cardiovascular disease (CVD) is responsible for nearly half of all deaths in the developed world and for 25% in underdeveloped countries. It is predicted that by the year 2020 CVD will cause 25 million deaths annually and coronary heart disease will surpass infectious disease as the number one killer in the world.[1] In this chapter we will discuss the underlying anatomy and macro- and microanatomy of the coronary arteries, their embryology, and the changes induced by atherosclerosis. The burden of diabetes and its effect on atherosclerosis as well as diabetic angiopathy will also be presented. Final discussion will include the effects of vascular interventions with both bare and drug-eluting stents on the induction and prevention of restenosis.

DEVELOPMENT OF CORONARY VESSELS

The initial step in the development of coronary vessels is the formation of proepicardium (PE), a transient structure that originates from the pericardial serosa in the region of the sinoatrial junction.[2] The proepicardial cells are unique in that they can produce a number of different cell types during heart development. The structure of the PE varies and is dependent on the species in which it is studied. The PE is seen as a promodium. Promodia develop at the ventral midline as bilateral villous projections on the pericardial surface of the septum transversum. Each villus is composed of simple cuboidal epithelium covering a proteoglycan- and hyaluronic-acid-rich extracellular matrix (ECM) core, with occasional clusters of stellate mesenchymal cells embedded within. The villous outgrowth is the source of the epicardial layer, and the proepicardial cells are the progenitors for the coronary arteries and enter the heart around stage 17 or 18. Fate-mapping studies show that PE cells are precursors for the endothelium and smooth muscle cells of the coronary vasculature, and for the connective tissue cells that form the coronary adventitia and interstitial matrix of the myocardium.

The appearance of the epicardium and its evolving coronary vessels correlates with the transition of the heart from a primitive tube with a thin-walled epithelial-type myocardium to the thick-walled, multilayered, pumping heart found in vertebrates. The epicardial layer is closely apposed to the myocardium with a space in between that is composed of abundant extracellular matrix, rich in angiogenic factors, in which the coronary vasculogenesis is carried out. The coronary endothelial cells arise from two sources: One is the angioblasts that form elsewhere and are carried to the heart and the other is the epicardium itself. The subepicardial endothelial cells assemble into a capillarylike vessel network, and these are continuous with the sinus venosus and are considered the forerunners of the coronary venous system. The coronary vessel formation is driven by hypoxia, which is an important stimulus along with the fibroblast growth factor (FGF) and vascular endothelial growth factor (VEGF) families of growth factors. Bogers et al. reported in 1989 that coronary arteries made contact with aortic lumen not by outgrowth from the aorta as was generally accepted but rather by ingrowth of endothelial strands from the peritruncal ring of capillarylike microvessels.[3] It is still poorly understood why only two stable connections are made with the aorta despite the presence of a dense collection of capillaries surrounding the aorta.

BASICS OF GENERAL CLINICAL VASCULAR PATHOANATOMY

The coronary arteries, right and left, arise from the aorta close to the coronary sinus. The ostia are located in the right and left aortic sinuses and arise at the sinotubular junction at the origin of the ascending aorta. Both the coronary arteries supply the vasa vasorum of the ascending aorta. The right coronary artery arises from the right aortic sinus just above the sinotubular junction and runs in the atrioventricular groove, which separates the right atrium from the right ventricle and is surrounded by fat. The first branch of the right, the conus branch, as it arises from the right coronary sinus supplies the anterior wall of the right ventricle. The right coronary artery passes toward the inferior border of the heart and at the right lateral border gives rise to the right marginal branch that runs toward the apex of the heart. The right coronary artery curves around the right border of the heart, running in the posterior right atrioventricular groove, and at the crux of the heart gives rise to the posterior descending artery (PDA). The PDA runs toward the apex in the posterior interventricular sulcus, which separates the right from the left ventricle. At the origin of the PDA the right artery in 85% of cases gives rise to the atrioventricular (AV) nodal artery, whereas the artery to the sinoatrial node arises in 60% of cases from the right coronary artery close to its origin from the aorta. The right artery supplies the right atrium, right ventricle, and posterior portion of the interventricular septum and an adjoining portion of the left ventricular free wall.

The left main coronary artery arises from the left coronary sinus, just below the sinotubular junction, passes behind the right ventricular outflow tract reaching between the left auricle and the pulmonary trunk, and divides into two main branches, the left anterior descending (LAD) artery and the left circumflex (LCx) arteries. Rarely the left main artery is absent and there are two separate ostia for the LAD and LCx. The larger branch is the LAD, which courses along the epicardial surface of the anterior interventricular sulcus to the apex of the heart and is surrounded by fat for most of its course. The LAD branches are the septal and the diagonal branches. The septal branches arise from the LAD at 90-degree angles and pass into the interventricular septum, supplying the anterior interventricular septum of the ventricle. The diagonal branches of the LAD pass over the anterolateral wall of the left ventricle. There is a wide variation in the number and size of the diagonal branches, as most patients have one to three supplying the anterolateral wall of the left ventricle. The LAD supplies the anterior two thirds of the interventricular septum and the anterior wall of the left ventricle. The left circumflex branch follows the left atrioventricular sulcus around the left border of the heart and gives rise to left obtuse marginal branches, which supply the lateral wall of the heart. The LCx also supplies the left atrium and the left surface of the heart. The artery that gives rise to the PDA is said to be the dominant artery with the right artery being the dominant artery in 85% of cases (Fig. 1-1).

In 10% of cases the left circumflex gives rise to the PDA and therefore is the dominant artery; the right is usually a very small artery and terminates at the crux of the heart. In another 5% of cases it is a codominant blood supply with the right giving rise to PDA and the left providing all the lateral branches.

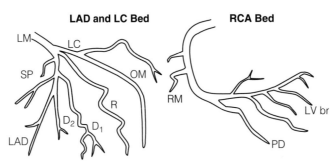

Abbreviations
D = Left diagonal; LAD = Left anterior descending; LCx = Left circumflex; LM = Left main
LV br = Left ventricular branches; OM = Left obtuse marginal; PD = Posterior diagonal
R = Ramus; RCA = Right coronary artery; RM = Right marginal; SP = Septal perforator

FIGURE 1-1.   Coronary artery anatomy. Diagram of the right and left epicardial coronary arteries as they arise from the aorta (right dominance). The four major arteries that must be described in detail are the right (*RCA*), left main (*LM*), left anterior descending (*LAD*), and the left circumflex (*LC*) coronary arteries. Not uncommonly, severe coronary artery disease (>75% cross-sectional area luminal narrowing) affects the smaller branches (*R*, Ramus intermediate; *LD*, left diagonal; *OM*, left obtuse marginal; *PD*, posterior descending; *RM*, right marginal). The proximal LAD extends from the origin of LAD to the D1, the mid LAD extends from the diagonal 1 to 2.5 cm distally, and the remainder of the LAD is distal. The left circumflex is divided into proximal and region proximal to LOM, and the continuation of the LC is the distal segment. The right proximal is the first 2 cm of the artery, the mid extends up to the RM, and the distal extends up to the PDA. Occasionally, the right coronary can extend beyond the PD (so-called hyperdominant right) and provide left ventricular branches (*LV br*). (Reproduced with permission from Virmani R, Burke A, Farb A, et al., eds. *Cardiovascular pathology.* 2nd ed. Major Problems in Pathology. Philadelphia: WB Saunders, 2001:4).

The left main coronary artery is usually 10 to 15 mm in length and varies in diameter from 3 to 6 mm; however, it may be as long as 2.5 cm, although this is seen in <10% of cases. The left anterior coronary artery extends from its origin to the apex of the left ventricle. At the apex the LAD wraps around the apex and supplies the posterior wall of the left ventricle. The left circumflex travels in the atrioventricular groove underneath the left atrial appendage and varies in length depending on the number of left obtuse marginal branches (LOM). Usually after the take-off of the LOM branches, the left circumflex artery tends to suddenly taper and becomes small. The right artery passes along the right atrioventricular groove and gives rise to the PDA near the crux of the heart (the meeting point of the atrioventricular groove and the interventricular sulcus). The first branch of the right artery is usually the conus branch, which arises near the take-off of the right artery in 50% of cases and in the rest arises as a separate ostium in the right coronary sinus. The second branch is usually the sinoatrial node artery, which arises from the right artery in 60% of cases; in 40% of cases it arises from the left circumflex. The posterior papillary muscle is supplied only by the right coronary artery, whereas the anterolateral papillary muscle gets a dual supply from the LAD and LCx.

The coronary arteries vary in size depending on the weight and height of the patient. Anatomic as well as IVUS studies have shown that coronary arteries following their origin from the ostia normally taper until they become intramural.[4–7]

Arterial tapering was determined by measuring the internal elastic lamina (IEL) area in normal arteries with minimal intimal thickening (total intimal cross-sectional area <1 mm²). The normal tapering between serial sections (approximately 10 mm between sections) was 1.20 ± 2.40 mm² per cm for LAD and 1.20 ± 2.15 mm² per cm for circumflex artery.[8] Abnormal tapering between adjacent sections is defined as tapering $>\pm 2$ SD of the expected tapering. Based on the foregoing study, abnormal tapering or negative vessel remodeling is present when a 25% or greater decrease in IEL is present between sections, i.e., every 1 cm. Glagov et al. first introduced the concept of arterial remodeling in the presence of atherosclerosis, in a landmark paper published in 1987; this topic will be addressed with atherosclerosis.[9]

The normal coronary artery is a muscular vessel with a well-defined internal and an external elastic lamina (EEL). In between these structures is the medial wall, composed of organized layers of smooth muscle cells with few interspersed proteoglycans and collagen fibers (Fig. 1-2). The intima exhibits adaptive thickening especially at branch points, consisting of smooth muscle cells, proteoglycan-rich matrix, and type III collagen fibers. Endothelial cells with well-formed junctions line the lumen surface. The outer adventitia juxtaposed to the EEL is composed of type I collagen, and its thickness is almost equivalent to media. Away from the EEL, however, the collagen fibers are loosely arranged, with interspersed mature fat. Further, present in the adventitia are fibroblasts and vasa vasorum that may or may not have surrounding smooth muscle cells (Fig. 1-2). Close to the ostia of the coronary arteries, the medial wall shows presence of multilayered elastic fibers, but these soon disappear within 1 cm of the origin of the artery. The medial wall thickness varies from 150 to 350 μm and varies with the size of the coronary artery, which also varies with the heart weight. The larger the heart, the larger the coronary artery, and as will be discussed, there is positive remodeling of the artery as atherosclerosis advances.

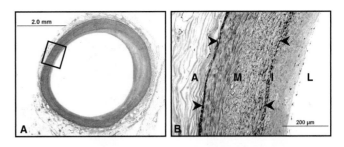

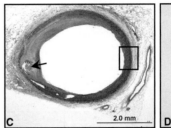

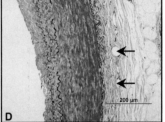

FIGURE 1-2. Coronary artery sections from patients dying a noncardiac death in the absence of any coronary artery disease. **(A)** and **(B)** are low and high power views of the proximal LAD with mild adaptive intimal thickening. Note the high power view in **(B)** of the boxed area in **(A)** showing well demarcated (*arrowheads*) external (EEL) and an internal elastic lamina (IEL) however, in the media (*M*) towards the EEL the smooth muscle cells (SMC) are circularly arranged while those towards the IEL are tranversely arranged and interspersed in between are elastic fibers. The adventitia (*A*) is thin while the intima (*I*) consists of SMCs and proteoglycan matrix. **(C)** and **(D)** are sections from the right coronary artery (RCA) note an eccentric focally calcified neointima (*arrow*) with underlying markedly thinned and destroyed media. The opposite side of the artery shows minimal intimal thickening, which is seen at high power in **(D)**. The media is demarcated by the EEL and IEL (*black*) on either side of the SMC rich medial wall. The intima is mildly thickened and consists of few SMCs interspersed in a proteoglycan matrix. The adventitial wall shows the presence of vasa vasorum (*arrows*) within the collagen rich adventitia.

PROGRESSION OF HUMAN CORONARY ATHEROSCLEROSIS

The cellular and acellular components of atherosclerosis and those leading to plaque rupture reside in the vessel wall and circulating blood (Fig. 1-3). Those integral to the vessel wall include endothelial and smooth muscle cells, together with the extracellular matrix represented by proteoglycans, collagen, and elastic fibers. Proatherogenic circulating factors consist of plasma lipoproteins, fibrinogen, clotting factors, and cells: platelets, red blood cells, monocytes, lymphocytes, mast cells, and neutrophils.[10] The first intimal change observed in human coronary arteries is known as adaptive intimal thickening, characterized by smooth muscle cells and surrounding proteoglycan matrix arranged in a relatively thin layer above the media. These lesions, mostly occurring at branch points, are observed in ~30% of infants at birth, and their distribution and development correlate with the presence of atherosclerotic plaques later in life.[11] Cell replication is generally low at these sites, suggesting that plaques that develop during adulthood may be clonal in origin. Tabas et al. have proposed that the extracellular matrix in early lesions contains enzymes capable of retaining lipids, a step toward early necrotic core formation.[12] There are few published studies, however, on the early evolution and development of intimal mass lesions in

Development of Human Coronary Atherosclerosis

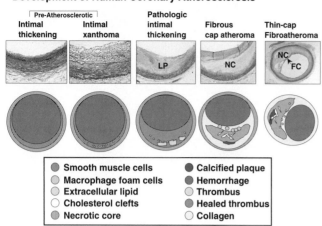

FIGURE 1-3. Development of human coronary atherosclerosis. Coronary lesions are uniformly present in all populations, although intimal xanthomas (so-called fatty streaks) are more prevalent with exposure to a Western diet. Preatherosclerotic lesions (adaptive intimal thickening and intimal xanthoma) occur soon after birth, although the latter are known to regress with age. Adaptive intimal thickening consists mainly of smooth muscle cells (SMCs) in a proteoglycan matrix, whereas intimal xanthomas contain macrophage-derived foam cells, T lymphocytes, and varying amounts of SMCs. Pathologic intimal thickening versus atheroma: Pathological intimal thickening (PIT) is a poorly defined entity, referred to in the literature as "intermediate" lesion. True necrosis is not apparent, as there is no evidence of cellular debris; lipid pools (*LP*) are seen deep in the lesion. The tissue over the lipid pools is rich in SMCs and proteoglycans; scattered macrophages and lymphocytes may also be present. The more definitive lesions, of fibrous cap atheroma, classically shows a true necrotic core (*NC*) containing cholesterol esters, free cholesterol, phospholipids, and triglycerides. The fibrous cap consists of SMCs in a proteoglycan-collagen matrix, with a variable number of macrophages and lymphocytes. The thin-cap fibroatheroma (vulnerable plaque): Thin-cap fibroatheromas are lesions with large necrotic cores containing numerous cholesterol clefts. The overlying fibrous cap (*FC*) is thin (<65 μm) and heavily infiltrated by macrophages; SMCs are rare and microvessels are generally present in the adventitia. (Reproduced with permission from Virmani R, et al. *Arteriosol Thromb Vasc Biol.* 2000;20:1262–1275.) (See Color Fig. 1-3.)

humans, although a clearer understanding of this concept is critical to elucidating the natural progression of the disease process.

The first coronary lesions characterized by inflammatory cells are defined as intimal xanthomas or "fatty streaks" in the AHA classification.[13] In humans, these lesions primarily consist of fat-laden macrophages intermixed with smooth muscle cells and proteoglycan matrix. Intimal xanthomas are commonly found in the thoracic aorta of young individuals, whereas advanced morphologies beyond fatty streaks in the adult thoracic aorta are usually absent.[14] Other typical sites of intimal xanthomas occurring at sites where advanced lesions are usually located are the abdominal aorta and the proximal portion of the left anterior descending coronary artery. Therefore, it is our understanding that fatty streaks may not be part of the atherosclerotic process, because the vast majority regress with age.[15]

Coronary lesion progression from the intimal mass lesion is thought to involve a transitional plaque referred to as pathologic intimal thickening (PIT) or type III lesion in the AHA classification. These plaques are defined as acellular areas containing remnants of smooth muscle cells with extracellular lipid, lipid pools, and extensive proteoglycan matrix.[15] Few viable smooth muscle cells are found among numerous PAS-positive empty

shells, representing the basement membranes of earlier "viable" smooth muscle cells.[16] Attenuated smooth muscle cells contain plasma membrane remnants, and apoptotic bodies are visible by electron microscopy. The lipid pools may also contain free cholesterol appearing as cholesterol clefts in paraffin sections.[17] Specific stains reveal speckled granular calcification, which is underappreciated by hematoxylin and eosin staining in the area of the lipid pools. It is generally believed that smooth muscle apoptosis along with the accumulation of lipids may be responsible for the lipid pools seen in these lesions. The proteoglycan matrix within lipid pools found in PIT is rich in sulfated glycosaminoglycans, which can effectively bind apolipoprotein B. Additional proteoglycans that accumulate during this phase include dermatan sulfate, decorin and biglycan.[18] Other negatively charged proteoglycans such as chondroitin sulfate function in the retention of apo B-100.[19]

The cellular composition above the lipid pool often contains scattered intact lipid-laden macrophages in addition to T lymphocytes.[20] In contrast, B lymphocytes are restricted mostly to the adventitia; only a few are found within the developing plaque.

Similarly, mast cells may also be present, but these cells are far fewer than other cell types.[21] No true necrosis is present at this stage, although these lesions do contain free cholesterol, fatty acid, sphingomyelin, lysolecithin, and triglycerides.[22]

The next stage of lesion development is the fibroatheroma, characterized by distinct layers of superficial fibrous tissue surrounding an area of necrotic core. The fibrous cap consists of smooth muscle cells and proteoglycan-collagen matrix, with varying degrees of inflammatory cells, mostly macrophages and lymphocytes. The fibrous cap thickness primarily distinguishes the fibroatheroma from the thin fibrous cap atheroma (classic "vulnerable" plaque).[15] Moreover, we have recently subtyped fibroatheromas into "early" and "late" depending on the characteristics of the necrotic core (Fig. 1-4).[23] The "early fibroatheroma" is a lesion with a lipid-rich matrix containing

Differential Expression of Hyaluronan and Versican in the Developing Necrotic Core

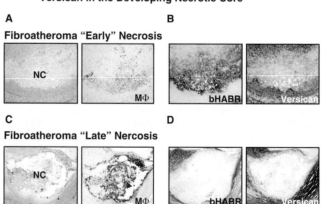

FIGURE 1-4. Fibroatheroma with early (**A,B**) and late (**C,D**) necrosis. **A:** Note that the early core (*NC*) shows an area of acellularity containing proteoglycans (Movat Pentachrome, *blue-green*) and small cholesterol clefts interspersed with CD68+ macrophages (*MΦ*). **B:** This same area shows intense staining for hyaluronan with moderate expression of versican. **C:** The late necrotic core consists of a well-defined area of cellular and acellular debris surrounded by CD68+ macrophages. **D:** The late core shows a virtual absence of hyaluronan and versican. (Matrix staining courtesy of Dr. Tom Wight, Hope Heart Institute, WA.)

proteoglycans, versican, hyaluronan, and type III collagen interspersed with intact foamy macrophages. Early necrotic cores are recognized by special proteoglycan and macrophage stains. In contrast, necrotic cores with late necrosis show numerous cholesterol clefts, cellular debris, and an absence of extracellular matrix (especially versican and hyaluronan).[23] Within the center and perimeter of necrosis, ghosts of macrophages identified by anti-CD68 staining with ill-defined cell membranes are found, and picrosirius red staining within the necrotic core is negative for collagen. The thin-cap fibroatheroma (TCFA) is identified based on the finding of a necrotic core that has a fibrous cap <65 µm thick, is rich in type I collagen, and is heavily infiltrated by macrophages; lymphocytes and smooth muscle cells are rare (Fig. 1-5).[24,25] It is important to classify this lesion as a distinct entity from plaque rupture, because its early diagnosis as a precursor lesion to rupture and its identification and treatment in life may help reduce the incidence of sudden coronary death and the morbidity associated with coronary heart disease.

LESIONS WITH THROMBI

The most frequent cause of thrombosis is plaque rupture (Fig. 1-6), occurring in 60% of cases of sudden coronary death with thrombi. Acute plaque rupture consists of a luminal platelet-fibrin thrombus continuous with an underlying necrotic core.[15] The connection between the thrombus and the lipid core is through a disrupted thin fibrous cap infiltrated by macrophages. The fibrous cap is composed of type I collagen and has few or no smooth muscle cells. The second most frequent cause of coronary thrombosis is plaque erosion, which occurs in 35% of cases of sudden death with a thrombus (Fig. 1-7).[15,26] Plaque erosion is defined as an acute thrombus in direct contact with the intimal plaque without rupture of a lipid core as demonstrated by serial

Causes of Coronary Thrombosis

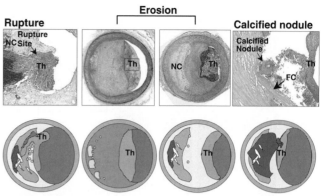

FIGURE 1-6. Atherosclerotic lesion with luminal thrombi. Ruptured plaques are thin fibrous cap atheromas with luminal thrombi (*Th*). These lesions usually have an extensive necrotic core (*NC*) containing large numbers of cholesterol crystals and a thin fibrous cap (<65 µm) infiltrated by foamy macrophages and a paucity of T lymphocytes. The fibrous cap is thinnest at the site of rupture and consists of a few collagen bundles and rare smooth muscle cells. The luminal thrombus is in direct communication with the lipid-rich core. Erosions occur over lesions rich in smooth muscle cells and proteoglycans. Luminal thrombi overlie areas lacking surface endothelium. The deep intima of the eroded plaque often shows extracellular lipid pools, but necrotic cores are not uncommon; when present, the necrotic core does not communicate with the luminal thrombus. Inflammatory infiltrate is usually absent, but if present, is sparse and consists of macrophages and lymphocytes. Calcified nodules are plaques with luminal thrombi showing calcific nodules protruding into the lumen through a disrupted thin fibrous cap (*FC*). There is absence of an endothelium at the site of the thrombus, and inflammatory cells (macrophages, T lymphocytes) are absent. (Reproduced with permission from Virmani R, et al. *Arterioscl Thromb Vasc Biol.* 2000;20:1262–1275.) (See Color Fig. 1-6.)

sections. Typically, the endothelium is absent at erosion site. The exposed intima consists predominantly of smooth muscle cells and proteoglycans, and surprisingly, the erosion site contains few inflammatory cells. Plaque erosion is the most frequent cause of thrombosis in women <50 years of age, whereas in men <50 years plaque rupture is more frequent (Table 1-1). The least frequent cause of thrombosis is calcified nodule, which is present in 2% to 5% of cases.[15] It is characterized by having an underlying calcified plate that is broken into multiple pieces, and calcified nodules are located on the lumen and are in direct contact with the flowing blood, which leads to platelet-rich luminal thrombus (Fig 1-6).

INTRAPLAQUE HEMORRHAGE

Intraplaque hemorrhage is a frequent event and is most often observed in patients dying from acute plaque rupture. In the early to mid-20th century, several leading pathologists forwarded the hypothesis that intraplaque hemorrhage is a major contributor to the progression of coronary atherosclerosis; however, the precise nature of this relationship was not well understood.[27–29] Recent studies from our laboratory suggest that plaque hemorrhages are more frequent in the coronary vasculature in patients dying from rupture as compared to plaque erosion or stable lesions with >75% cross-sectional area luminal narrowing.[10] In an effort to further understand the influence of intraplaque

A Non-Hemodynamically Limiting Thin-cap Fibroatheroma

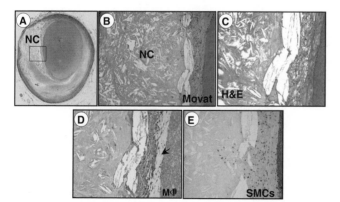

FIGURE 1-5. A non–hemodynamically limiting thin-cap fibroatheroma. **A:** A thin-cap fibroatheroma having a necrotic core (*NC*) and an overlying thin fibrous cap (65 µm). **B:** High-power view of the boxed area in (**A**). Note an advanced necrotic core with large number of cholesterol clefts with a loss of matrix containing numerous cholesterol clefts and cellular debris. The fibrous cap is heavily infiltrated by macrophages, better seen in (**C**) (*H&E*). **D,E:** Macrophage infiltration (CD68 positive) and rare staining of smooth muscle cells (α-actin positive) in the fibrous cap. (Reproduced with permission from Kolodgie FD, et al. *Heart.* 2004;90:1385–1391.)

**Angiographic and Histologic Representation
of Plaque Rupture and Erosion**

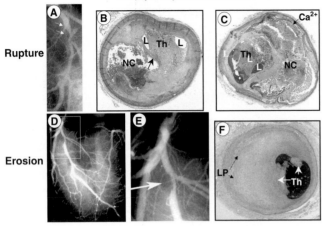

FIGURE 1-7. Angiographic and histologic representation of plaque rupture and erosion. A 43-year-old white man with no known history of risk factors was found unresponsive in the bathroom where he was last seen alive 20 minutes earlier. **A:** Postmortem angiogram shows the LAD at the origin of the left diagonal with a near total occlusion. Sections taken from these sites show a plaque rupture [*arrow*, **(B)**] with an underlying necrotic core (*NC*). The occluded artery shows an organizing thrombus with small lumens (*L*). **C:** The fibrous cap is intact with a large underlying necrotic core with peripheral calcification (Ca^{2+}) and the lumen shows organizing thrombus (*Th*) with small lumens (*L*). At autopsy there was a healing transmural myocardial infarction present in the distribution of the LAD. Postmortem angiogram **(D,E)** and corresponding photomicrograph **(F)** from a 38-year-old man who was last seen alive 8 hours antemortem, died from sudden coronary death. A focal stenosis is present in the left anterior coronary artery (*boxed area*), which is highlighted in **(A),** and an arrow points to the area of narrowing at the take-off of the left diagonal. **F:** Acute nonocclusive luminal thrombus (*Th*) is present on the surface of an erosive plaque rich in proteoglycans (*green*) and the underlying plaque shows pathologic intimal thickening with lipid pools (*LP*). (Reproduced in part from Figure 4, Farb A, et al. *Circulation.* 1995;92:1701–1709.) (See Color Fig. 1-7.)

hemorrhage on lesion progression, we examined various types of human coronary plaques for hemorrhagic events.[23]

In a relatively large series of human coronary plaques from sudden coronary death victims, there was a greater frequency of previous hemorrhages in coronary atherosclerotic lesions prone to rupture (as detected by glycophorin A staining) relative to lesions with early necrotic cores or plaques with pathologic intimal thickening (Fig. 1-8).[23]

Significantly, the degree of reactive glycophorin A staining and the level of iron deposits in the plaque corresponded to the size of the necrotic core, and changes in these variables paralleled an increase in macrophage density, suggesting that hemorrhage itself serves as an inflammatory stimulus (Table 1-2).[23] It is generally accepted that apoptotic macrophages are a likely source of free cholesterol in plaques; however, it is entirely feasible that free cholesterol within the necrotic core could be derived from other sources, including erythrocyte membranes. By contributing to the deposition of free cholesterol, macrophage infiltration, and enlargement of the necrotic core, the accumulation of erythrocyte membranes within an atherosclerotic plaque may represent a potent atherogenic stimulus. These factors may increase the risk of plaque destabilization.

ERYTHROCYTE MEMBRANE-DERIVED FREE CHOLESTEROL AND PLAQUE PROGRESSION

As proof of concept, we developed an animal model of simulated intraplaque hemorrhage to assess the role of erythrocytes in lesion progression.[23] The direct injection of packed erythrocytes (25 μL to 50 μL) into quiescent aortic atherosclerotic plaques produced excessive macrophage infiltration along with free cholesterol crystals, and iron colocalized to areas of red blood cells. In contrast, control (noninjected) lesions showed the characteristics of a regressed lesion with far fewer lesional macrophages and free cholesterol. Neutral lipids identified by Oil Red O were also significantly greater in plaques with injected erythrocytes when compared with controls.

TABLE 1-1. Distribution of Culprit Plaques by Sex and Age in 241 Cases of Sudden Coronary Death

	Acute Thrombi			Organized Thrombi	No Thrombi	Totals
	Rupture	Erosion	Calcified Nodule		Fibrocalcific Plaque	
MEN						
<50 y	45 (46%)	17 (17%)	2 (2%)	15 (15%)	20 (20%)	99
>50 y	19 (23%)	8 (10%)	3 (4%)	27 (33%)	26 (31%)	83
WOMEN						
<50 y	1 (3%)	24 (42%)	0	5 (15%)	13 (40%)	33
>50 y	9 (35%)	6 (23%)	1 (4%)	5 (19%)	5 (19%)	26
TOTALS	74 (31%)	45 (19%)	6 (2%)	52 (22%)[a]	64 (26%)[b]	241

[a]Organized thrombi with healed myocardial infarction (HMI) = 46/52 (89%).

[b]No thrombi (stable plaque) with HMI = 32/64 (50%); thus, 32/241 or (13%) of sudden deaths have stable plaque without HMI or acute myocardial infarction.

Fibrous Cap Atheroma (Late Necrosis)

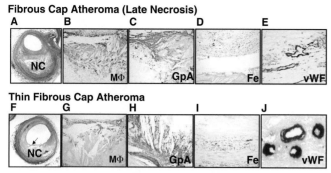

Thin Fibrous Cap Atheroma

FIGURE 1-8. Late core **(A–E)** and thin fibrous cap atheroma **(F–J)** showing intraplaque hemorrhage. **A:** Low-power view of a fibrous cap atheroma with a late necrotic core (*NC*) (Movat Pentachrome × 20). **B:** Intense staining of CD68-positive macrophages is seen within the necrotic core. **C:** Extensive glycophorin A (*GpA*) positive erythrocyte membranes colocalized with numerous cholesterol clefts within the necrotic core (× 200). **D:** Iron deposits (*blue*) are seen within macrophage foam cells (× 200). **E:** Microvessels bordering the necrotic core show perivascular von Willebrand factor (*vWF*) deposition (× 400). **F:** Low-power view of a fibroatheroma with a thin fibrous cap (arrow) overlying a relatively large necrotic core (Movat Pentachrome, × 20). **G:** The fibrous cap is devoid of smooth muscle cells (not shown) and is heavily infiltrated by CD68-positive macrophages (*MΦ*, × 200). **H:** Intense glycophorin (*GpA*) staining of erythrocyte membranes within the necrotic core colocalized with cholesterol clefts (× 100). **I:** Adjacent coronary segment with accumulated iron (*blue pigment*) in a macrophage-rich region deep within the plaque (× 200). **J:** Perivascular diffuse deposits of von Willebrand factor in microvessels; indicates leaky vessels bordering the necrotic core (× 400). (Reproduced with permission from Kolodgie FD, et al., *N Engl J Med.* 2003;349:2316-2325.) (See Color Fig. 1-8.)

Thus the animal studies offer further evidence that episodic hemorrhages in plaques contribute to accumulated free cholesterol and macrophage infiltration.[23] The contribution of erythrocyte membrane cholesterol to necrotic core volume is predicted to be substantial because repeat intraplaque hemorrhages are thought to occur over years. Consistent with this notion, even small bleed volumes of only 0.137 μL per day whole blood (0.068 μL packed red blood cells) over a 2-year period would be sufficient to make a significant contribution to necrotic core size. Since the liquid volume of cholesterol in a single red blood cell is equivalent to 0.378 μm³, approximately 5.2 ×10⁸ RBCs or a single bleed of 100 μL whole blood would contribute at least 0.2 mm³ or 10% of membrane-derived free cholesterol to necrotic core volume, assuming 10% exchange efficiency.[30] As in internal bleeds, the bulk of the erythrocyte would be metabolized over several days, and because cholesterol cannot be metabolized internally, it would be available for absorption into the necrotic core in addition to its uptake by macrophages, which in turn presumably gives up cholesterol to the core by apoptotic cell death. In emerging serial MRI data of carotid plaques over 18 months, evidence of repeat hemorrhages is suggested to contribute significantly to necrotic core volume and lesion bulk.[31] Therefore, RBC-derived cholesterol may represent a critical transition factor promoting the conversion of a stable plaque to an unstable phenotype.

CORONARY PLAQUE MORPHOLOGY IN PATIENTS WITH STABLE AND UNSTABLE ANGINA

Coronary morphology in patients with stable and unstable angina is difficult to assess because most patients with angina do not die from their disease. Patients with unstable angina who come to autopsy most likely have had an acute myocardial infarction (MI) evolving from an angina syndrome. One possible source of data regarding plaque morphology in patients with angina is from autopsy studies in patients who die during or soon after coronary bypass surgery. In the mid-1970s, Guthrie et al. published the earliest work in 35 patients with stable angina who died after coronary bypass.[32] In this study, the extent of severe atherosclerosis in >95% of patients involved two or more vessels, including left main disease in approximately 30%; thrombosis was an infrequent finding. In another study, Han Gartner et al. described substantial plaque variability in the coronary lesions of patients with stable angina who died suddenly within 6 hours of onset of symptoms.[33] They reported that 76% of coronary segments with >75% cross-sectional luminal narrowing showed concentric lesions, 47% were fibrous plaques, and 28% were lipid rich. The remaining 24% of severely narrowed lesions were eccentric and divided equally among fibrous and lipid-rich lesions. Recanalized segments were present in 79% of the hearts. There is no mention of the number of lesions with thrombi.

TABLE 1-2. Morphometric Analysis of Plaque and Hemorrhagic Events in Human Coronary Arteries from Sudden Death Victims

Plaque Type	*GpA Score*	*Iron*	*Necrotic Core (mm²)*	*MΦ (mm²)*
PATHOLOGIC INTIMAL THICKENING, "NO" CORE (*n* = 129)	0.09 ± 0.04	0.07 ± 0.05	0.0	0.002 ± 0.001
FIBROUS CAP ATHEROMAS, "EARLY" CORE (*n* = 79)	0.23 ± 0.07	0.17 ± 0.08	0.06 ± 0.02	0.018 ± 0.004
FIBROUS CAP ATHEROMAS, "LATE" CORE (*n* = 105)	*0.94 ± 0.11	*0.41 ± 0.09	*0.84 ± 0.08	*0.059 ± 0.007
THIN FIBROUS CAP ATHEROMAS (*n* = 52)	*1.60 ± 0.20	*1.24 ± 0.24	*1.95 ± 0.30	*0.142 ± 0.016

Values are reported as the means ±SEM, *p <0.001 versus early core, *n* is the number of lesions examined; total = 365. GpA, glycophorin A; *MΦ*, macrophages.

By coronary angiography, Levin et al. showed smooth borders that impart an "hourglass" configuration correlated histologically with fibrous or fatty uncomplicated plaques.[34] Angiographic irregular borders or intraluminal lucent areas were found primarily in complicated plaques with rupture. In subsequent angiographic studies, Ambrose et al. reported a higher frequency of type II eccentric lesions (asymmetric with a narrow neck, irregular borders, or both) in patients with unstable angina compared with those with stable angina.[35]

The lesion progression in stable angina is greatest at angiographic sites with complex versus smooth stenosis and occurs in 16% of complex lesions but not in smooth lesions at an interval of 9 months (range 3 to 24 months). The annual increase in plaque growth has been shown to be 11.4 ± 28% and 1.5 ± 14% for complex and smooth lesions, respectively ($p < 0.01$).[36] We have shown that plaques with no prior ruptures versus those with ruptures have an increased luminal narrowing, and only 11% of culprit plaques show no prior rupture, thus suggesting that repeated ruptures are the mechanism by which plaques increase in size with eventual severe narrowing.[37] haracterization of culprit lesions by angioscopy in various coronary syndromes reveals the different mechanisms of ischemia. The predominant lesion in acute myocardial infarction is an ulcerated, yellow plaque with thrombus. In unstable angina, different substrates can be seen, from the lipid-rich lesion with thrombus to the fibrous smooth plaque, reflecting a varied physiopathology.[38]

We have reported our findings in 450 cases of sudden coronary death in blacks ($n = 130$) and whites ($n = 320$), mean age 51 ± 12 years. Acute thrombi were observed in 224 (50%), and of these, ruptures were seen in 68% and erosions in 32%. Healed myocardial infarct was present in 40% of cases. Stable plaque in the absence of an acute thrombus in SCD patients was observed in 226 patients (50%), and of these organized thrombi were present in 97 (21%) and another 134 (29%) died with stable plaque in the absence of any acute or chronic total occlusion. Of the 134 patients with stable plaques, healed myocardial infarction in the absence of any thrombus was present in half the patients.

Thus in 69 patients the only cause of death was severe luminal narrowing (>75% cross-sectional area narrowing) in one or more coronary arteries (Figs. 1-9 to 1-11). These stable plaques often show little necrotic core and are predominantly composed of collagen and calcified plaque. The incidence of healed plaque rupture in the stable plaques without healed myocardial infarction is 50%, which is much less than that seen in patients dying with acute plaque rupture, 75%. The highest incidence of healed plaque rupture is observed in patients dying with stable plaque and a healed myocardial infarction (80%).

CORONARY PLAQUES IN ACUTE MYOCARDIAL INFARCTION

The incidence of coronary thrombosis in hospital-based autopsies performed on patients with acute MI is >80%,[39–41] with the exception of the study by Kragel et al., who report a lower 69% incidence of thrombosis.[42] The reported incidence of thrombosis by angiography is as high as 90%. Separate studies by Davies et al. and Falk emphasized plaque rupture as the most important factor in the development of coronary

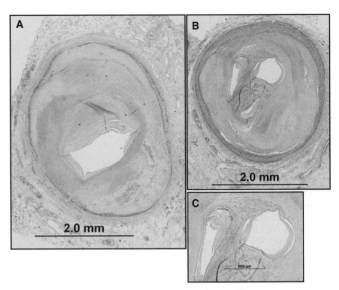

FIGURE 1-9. Histologic sections of stable atherosclerotic plaques with severe narrowing. **A:** The lesion shows a predominantly fibrous plaque with focal calcification and severe luminal narrowing. Note that in this stable lesion the media is extensively destroyed. **B:** A recanalyzed, fully organized thrombus with three centrally located large channels [(two of which are seen in (**C**) in high power)] with severe narrowing. Angiographically it would have appears as a single lumen with >90% diameter stenosis and not as a reanalyzed thrombus.

thrombosis.[40,43] However, Arbustini et al. reported in a series of 300 autopsies in patients with documented ECG proven and enzyme elevation that at least 25% of infarct-related coronary thrombi occurred from plaque erosion, and the incidence was

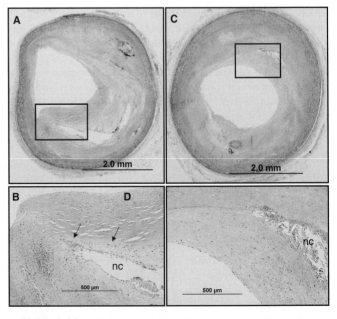

FIGURE 1-10. Photomicrographs of two adjacent sections (**A**) and (**C**) taken 4 mm apart, note presence of necrotic core (*NC*) with a recently organized healed plaque rupture. The boxed areas in (**A**) and (**C**) are shown at high power in (**B**) and (**D**). The area above the necrotic core consists of smooth muscle cells in a proteoglycan-rich matrix (*area above NC outlined by arrows*) representing healed thrombus, and the fibrous cap is attenuated. Note that new neointima has resulted in greater narrowing of the lumen.

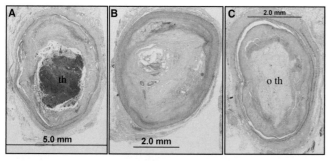

FIGURE 1-11. Three sections of total occlusion of the coronary artery lumen are shown; a fresh thrombus is seen in **(A)**, an organizing thrombus in **(B)**, and a fully organized totally occluded coronary artery is shown in **(C)**. Note, the fresh thrombus (*th*) in **(A)**, fibrin is still present in **(B)** with early organization, and **(C)** loose connective is present with very small vascular channels in the center of the section of the artery.

even higher among women.[44] In our sudden death population at least 21% of patients showed evidence of an acute MI (AMI), and the incidence of thrombosis is 90%. Of these patients with AMI, thrombosis occurs in 70% of cases from plaque rupture and 30% from plaque erosion.[26] In a series of studies by Davies et al., in a sudden coronary death population the incidence of AMI was 41%. Coronary thrombosis was found in 84% with reported chest pain within the week prior to AMI and death. Interestingly, in these AMI cases, 13 showed plaque fissure without a luminal thrombus. Another four of 32 cases (13%) studied without acute coronary events had myocardial infarction. Thus in Davies' series, 13% of cases with AMI did not have any luminal thrombi. In a recent study by us of healed plaque rupture, AMIs were present in only 11% of sudden coronary deaths, whereas 80% had thrombi and 20% had no evidence of an acute event.[37]

In general, intravascular ultrasound (IVUS) studies have shown that positive remodeling is associated with acute coronary syndromes and negative remodeling more frequent with stable angina. The degree of positive remodeling does not correlate with CRP levels.[45] Spotty calcification as identified by IVUS is typically seen in AMI lesions, whereas the highest calcification is seen in stable angina patients.[46] Moreover, at least two sites of rupture can be detected in 15% of patients undergoing PCI for acute coronary syndromes. In a study by Maehara et al., plaque rupture was detected in 46% of patients with unstable angina, 33% with MI and 11% with stable angina or no symptoms.[47] The location of the rupture was identified in the shoulder region of 63% plaques and in lesion center in 37%. IVUS studies have shown that rupture sites are most frequently located in the LAD between 10 mm and 40 mm from the LAD ostium (83%), and in the RCA between 10 mm and 40 mm (48%) and in the segment >70 mm from the ostium (32%); they are least frequently seen in the LCx and are distributed in the entire tree.[48] Our observations in lesions from coronary sudden death victims (Table 1-2) show that the majority of lesions with plaque rupture are localized to the proximal LAD followed by the proximal RCA and LCx coronary arteries.[25] Also, they are most frequent in the proximal and mid portions of the coronary arteries and are only rarely located in the distal arteries.

THE BURDEN OF DIABETES ON ATHEROSCLEROSIS

Diabetes affects more than 100 million individuals worldwide.[49] Of these, 5% to 10% have type I diabetes (juvenile diabetes) and 90% to 95% have type II diabetes, also known as adult-onset diabetes mellitus. Because of increasing obesity due to lifestyle changes in children in the United States, it is expected that the incidence of type II diabetes will increase in the next few decades, and it is predicted to affect as much as 35% to 40% of the population.[50]

Diabetes is associated with the development of accelerated coronary atherosclerotic heart disease, which results in increased morbidity and cardiovascular complications. Angioscopic studies suggest an increased incidence of coronary thrombosis in diabetics.[51] Ultrafast CT studies have shown a greater extent of calcification.[52] Intravascular ultrasound studies have suggested a decrease in adaptive remodeling in diabetics compared to nondiabetics.[53] Pathologic specimens obtained during coronary atherectomy or carotid endarterectomy have shown that there is an increase in macrophage infiltration in diabetics versus nondiabetics.[54]

Diabetes results in a variety of metabolic imbalances with different vascular effects. A combination of hyperglycemia, elevated free fatty acids, and insulin resistance increases oxidative stress, upregulates protein kinase C, and activates receptors for advanced glycosylation end products (RAGE).[55] Within the endothelium, there is increased vasoconstriction, adhesion molecule activation, inflammation, and thrombosis via hypercoagulation and platelet activation.[55] The mechanisms by which diabetes causes differences in coronary plaque morphology are complex and poorly understood, but are likely related to the proinflammatory and prothrombotic diabetic state.

MORPHOLOGIC FINDING FROM THE REGISTRY OF SUDDEN CORONARY DEATH

We have recently reported morphologic findings from our sudden coronary death registry in both type I and type II diabetes and compared these to age- and sex-matched nondiabetic individuals dying suddenly from coronary artery atherosclerotic disease.[56]

The basis for inclusion into the registry of sudden coronary death included either presence of an acute coronary thrombus or severe coronary atherosclerosis (≥1 epicardial artery with ≥75% cross-sectional luminal narrowing) and the absence of noncoronary causes of death at autopsy or prior surgery. The 66 cases of diabetes were selected on the basis of history of type I diabetes mellitus treated with insulin, or the presence of type II diabetes. Type II diabetes was ascertained by history of oral hypoglycemic, or postmortem glycohemoglobin >10% in the absence of type I diabetes. A total of 16 patients had type I diabetes (mean age 50.3 ± 13.2 years) and 50 had type II diabetes (mean age 50.2 ± 11 years); the findings in these were compared with 66 age- and sex-matched nondiabetic individuals dying from severe coronary heart disease. The body mass index was higher in type II diabetes than nondiabetics (30.5 ± 7.5 vs. 26.5 ± 5.4 kg/m² ± SD, $p = 0.001$). The rates of smoking and hypertension were similar in nondiabetics and diabetics (Table 1-3). There was a trend toward higher total cholesterol

TABLE 1-3. Association between Diabetes and Other Risk Factors

	Type I DM	p vs. Nondiabetics	Type II DM	p vs. Nondiabetics	Nondiabetics
GLYCOHEMOGLOBIN	12.2 ± 2.5	0.0001	10.7 ± 2.6	0.0001	6.2 ± 0.6
% SMOKERS	42	0.4	58	0.8	55
% HYPERTENSIVE	29	0.9	35	0.6	30
TOTAL CHOLESTEROL (mg/dL ± SD)	183 ± 52	0.3	227 ± 83	0.3	211 ± 79
HIGH-DENSITY LIPOPROTEIN CHOLESTEROL (mg/dL ± SD)	37 + 14	0.8	33 ± 16	0.1	38 ± 18
TOTAL/HIGH-DENSITY LIPOPROTEIN CHOLESTEROL (mg/dL ± SD)	5.8 ± 2.9	0.7	7.9 ± 3.9	0.02	6.3 ± 3.4

and lower high-density lipoprotein cholesterol in type II diabetics. The ratio of total to high-density lipoprotein cholesterol was significantly higher in type II diabetics compared to nondiabetics.

Acute thrombi due to ruptures or erosions were relatively uncommon in type I diabetics (Table 1-4); in type II diabetics, the proportion of ruptures was similar to that in nondiabetics, but plaque erosions were significantly less frequent. The mean heart weight was significantly increased in type II diabetes; healed infarcts were significantly more frequent in type II diabetics.

The mean percent plaque area composed of necrotic core was greater in type I ($p = 0.05$) and type II ($p = 0.004$) diabetics compared to nondiabetics (Table 1-5). Mean percent calcified area was greatest in type II diabetics and smallest in type I diabetics, but the differences were not significant ($p \geq 0.1$). The mean number of fibrous cap atheromas was greater in type II diabetics as compared to nondiabetics ($p = 0.02$) (Table 1-5).

The numbers of healed plaque ruptures were greatest in type II diabetics (Table 1-5).

By multivariate analysis, there was a positive correlation between mean percent necrotic core size and glycohemoglobin, independent of the ratio of total cholesterol (TC) to high-density lipoprotein (HDL) cholesterol, HDL cholesterol, age, smoking and gender ($p = .005$, $t = 2.9$). There was a similar correlation with body mass index. There was a strong correlation between macrophage area and glycohemoglobin ($p = .004$, $T = 2.9$).

There was a stronger relationship between numbers of fibrous cap atheromas and the ratio of total cholesterol to HDL cholesterol than with other risk factors, including glycohemoglobin.

This study demonstrates that type II diabetics dying suddenly with severe coronary disease have extensive disease, including distal involvement of their coronary arteries, when compared to nondiabetics. Part of the reason for increased plaque burden may be because of the observed high rate of healed plaque ruptures, indicating subclinical ruptures that may participate in

TABLE 1-4. Incidence of Acute Thrombi, Heart Weight, and Healed Infarcts

	Type I DM	p vs. Nondiabetics	Type II DM	p vs. Nondiabetics	Nondiabetics
ACUTE PLAQUE RUPTURES, %	6	0.09	32	0.6	27
EROSIONS, %	6	0.02	12	0.04	29
HEART WEIGHT (g ± SD)	425 ± 119	0.7	524 ± 140	0.004	434 ± 121
CORRECTED HEART WEIGHT[a](g ± SD)	428 ± 94	0.3	508 ± 134	0.03	460 ± 106
HEALED INFARCTS, %	33	0.7	73	0.0001	37

[a]Corrected for body weight.

TABLE 1-5. Plaque Characteristics

	Type I DM	p vs. Nondiabetics	Type II DM	p vs. Nondiabetics	Nondiabetics
NECROTIC CORE, % PLAQUE AREA, MEAN ± SD	12.0 ± 5.7	0.05[a]	11.6 ± 8.4	0.004[a]	9.4 ± 9.3
CALCIFIED MATRIX AREA, % PLAQUE AREA, MEAN ± SD	7.8 ± 9.1	0.9[a]	12.1 ± 11.2	0.05[a]	11.4 ± 13.5
MACROPHAGE PLAQUE AREA, mm ± SD	0.15 ± 0.02	0.03[a]	0.13 ± 0.03	0.03[a]	0.10 ± 0.02[b]
FIBROUS CAP ATHEROMA, n ± SD	7.1 ± 5.0	0.9	8.8 ± 4.3	0.02	6.9 ± 4.7
THIN CAP ATHEROMA, n ± SD	1.0 ± 1.3	0.5	0.8 ± 0.8	0.8	0.7 ± 0.8
HEALED PLAQUE RUPTURES, n ± SD	2.6 ± 2.1	0.2	2.6 ± 1.8	0.04	1.9 ± 1.8
TOTAL PLAQUE BURDEN, % ± SD	275 ± 129	0.04	358 ± 114	0.0001	232 ± 128
DISTAL PLAQUE BURDEN, % ± SD	310 ± 114	0.8	630 ± 263	0.0001	331 ± 199

[a]p value calculated using log normalized data.
[b]p = 0.006 vs. type I and II diabetes combined.

plaque progression.[37] The effect of diabetes on plaque burden has been demonstrated by calcium imaging studies.[57] The implications of these findings are unclear, but suggest a direct atherogenic effect of type II diabetes, probably related to development of lipid-rich cores. The known risk of diabetics following coronary artery bypass graft surgery[58,59] may in part be due to distal disease, as shown in our study, which may impair blood flow distal to graft anastomoses.

REMODELING

In our sudden death registry, the mean internal elastic lamina (IEL) area adjusted for the distance from the coronary ostium was greater in type I and II diabetics compared to nondiabetic subjects (18.2 ± 6.6 mm², 16.5 ± 4.4 mm², and 16.0 ± 4.5 mm², respectively).

The mean IEL was also significantly greater in type I (p = 0.001) and type II diabetic subjects (p = 0.01). By multivariate analysis, there was a correlation between type I diabetes and IEL area independent of heart weight, plaque area, percent necrotic core, and percent plaque calcification (p = 0.0004). This analysis (% necrotic core p = 0.05, plaque area, p < 0.0001, heart weight, p = 0.05) showed a positive correlation with IEL area. Clinical studies have shown that diabetes is associated with positive or a negative/absence of remodeling.[60, 61] Our findings support the notion that diabetics are more likely to show positive remodeling. These data are consistent with previous findings from our laboratory that necrotic core and macrophage infiltrates are associated with expansion of the internal elastic lamina independent of plaque size (see later discussion).[62]

INFLAMMATORY INFILTRATE IN DIABETICS

In our studies from the sudden death registry, the mean percent plaque area composed of necrotic core was greater in type I (p = 0.05) and type II (p = 0.004) diabetics compared to nondiabetics. Macrophage plaque area and T-cell infiltration were also significantly greater in diabetic than nondiabetic patients (p = 0.03) along with HLA-DR expression (Figs. 1-12 and 1-13). The fact that T-cell infiltration was greater in type I diabetics is consistent with the fact that type I diabetes is an autoimmune disease with a common genetic susceptibility to other disorders such as autoimmune thyroiditis, which may also be of pathophysiologic significance in coronary plaques.[63]

Cipollone et al. have shown that carotid plaques from diabetic patients have more macrophages, T lymphocytes, and HLA-DR+ cells (p < 0.0001), more (p < 0.0001) immunoreactivity for RAGE, activated nuclear factor κB (NF-κB), cyclo-oxygenase-2 (COX-2)/membrane-associated prostaglandin E synthase-1 (mPGES-1), and matrix metalloproteins (MMPs); increased (p < 0.0001) gelatinolytic activity; reduced (p < 0.0001) collagen content; and increased (p < 0.0001) lipid and oxidized low-density lipoprotein (oxLDL) content.[64] Interestingly, RAGE, COX-2/mPGES-1, and MMP expression was linearly correlated with plasma level of HbA1c.[64] Therefore, in humans, carotid diabetic plaque RAGE overexpression along with enhanced inflammatory reaction and COX-2/mPGES-1 expression in macrophages may contribute to plaque destabilization by inducing culprit metalloproteinase expression. Moreover,

Identification of MHC Class II in Insulin-Dependent And Independent Diabetics

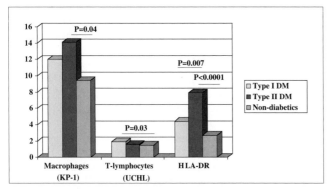

FIGURE 1-12. Inflammation in coronary arteries in patients with diabetes mellitus, comparison to nondiabetics. Shown are coronary lesions (fibroatheromas) illustrating the extent of inflammatory infiltrate [macrophage (*MΦ*) and T-cells (*CD45RO*)] and HLA-DR expression in patients type II (**A–D**) and type I (**E–H**) diabetes mellitus (DM) and in nondiabetic patients (**I–L**). (Reproduced with permission from Burke AP, et al. *Arterioscl Thromb Vasc Biol.* 2004; 24:1266-1271.) (See Color Fig. 1-12.)

experimental studies of murine models of diabetic aortic atherosclerosis have demonstrated that RAGE blockade by soluble RAGE decreases atheroma formation.[65] The same group has also shown again in carotid atherosclerotic plaques that the prostaglandin E2 (PGE2) pathway was significantly prevalent in symptomatic carotid plaques, whereas the prostaglandin D2 (PGD2) pathway was overexpressed in asymptomatic ones, and was associated with NF-κB inactivation and MMP-9 expression.[66] In vitro COX-2 inhibition in monocytes was associated with reduced MMP-9 release only when the PGD2 pathway overcame PGE2. These results suggested to them that COX-2 may have proinflammatory and anti-inflammatory properties as a function of expression of downstream prostaglandin H2 (PGH2) isomerases.[66]

Recently, it has been demonstrated that EN-RAGE (extracellular newly identified RAGE-binding protein, or S100 A12) is a natural ligand for RAGE and is a proinflammatory cytokine expressed especially in macrophages.[67] An association between soluble S100 proteins and human inflammatory bowel disease has been demonstrated.[68] The interactions between S100 Ca^{2+} modulated proteins and RAGE receptors in the fine regulation of leukocyte trafficking and proliferation have been recently reviewed,[69] but the role of EN-RAGE in atherosclerosis-related inflammation has not been studied. We applied immunohistochemical antibodies against RAGE and EN-RAGE (S100 A12) to coronary plaques of diabetics and nondiabetics.[56] Although RAGE was found localized to macrophages, smooth muscle cells, and endothelial cells in both diabetics and nondiabetics, the overall expression of RAGE, as graded semiquantitatively, was significantly greater in diabetics (16.8 ± 6.2 for diabetics, 10.0 ± 6.1 for nondiabetics, $p = 0.004$). Extensive RAGE staining was noted in macrophages and necrotic core of diabetic and nondiabetic patients, but the expression was dependent on the extent of cellular infiltration (Fig. 1-14). Lower smooth muscle cell expression of RAGE was observed, but was greater in type II diabetics. RAGE expression was often associated with apoptotic smooth muscle cells and macrophages, whereas endothelial cells positive for RAGE were generally negative for apoptosis. EN-RAGE expression was most prominent in macrophages and, to a lesser degree in smooth muscle cells, in the core regions of plaques from diabetic patients.

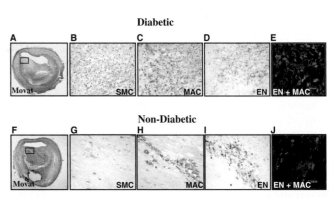

FIGURE 1-14. Expression of S100A12/EN-RAGE (a RAGE binding protein) in human coronary lesions from diabetic (**A–E**) and nondiabetic (**F–J**) sudden coronary death victims. **A:** Lesion from the proximal left circumflex coronary artery stained by Movat Pentachrome. **B–E:** High-magnification micrographs of the black box represented in **A**. **B:** HHF-35 staining for SMCs in the shoulder region of the plaque. **C:** Adjacent section stained for CD68, demonstrating numerous inflammatory macrophages. **D:** The same region, demonstrating intense staining for EN-RAGE. **B–D:** The counterstain is Gill's hematoxylin. **E:** Double-labeled immunofluorescent staining of CD68-positive macrophages (*green*) and EN-RAGE (*red*); nuclei (*blue*) were counterstained with DAPI; areas of overlap appear as yellowish-green. EN-RAGE was primarily found in macrophage-rich areas in macrophages and smooth muscle cells. **F:** A lesion from the proximal left anterior descending coronary artery from a nondiabetic patient stained by Movat Pentachrome. **G–I:** Immunoreactivity to SMC, macrophage, and EN-RAGE, respectively. Overall, macrophage infiltrate was significantly less in nondiabetic patients, corresponding to less immunoreactivity to EN-RAGE. **J:** Double staining for EN-RAGE and macrophages. (Reproduced with permission from Burke AP, et al. *Arterioscl Thromb Vasc Biol.* 2004;24: 1266-1271.) (See Color Fig. 1-14.)

FIGURE 1-13. Bar graph showing a semiquantitative comparison of the extent of macrophage, T-cell infiltration, and HLA-DR expression in coronary arteries from diabetic and nondiabetic patients. Macrophage infiltration is maximal in type II diabetics, whereas T-lymphocyte infiltration was greatest in type I diabetics. In contrast, HLA-DR expression is significantly higher in type I and II diabetics when compared to nondiabetics. (See Color Fig. 1-13.)

Development of Human Coronary Atherosclerosis

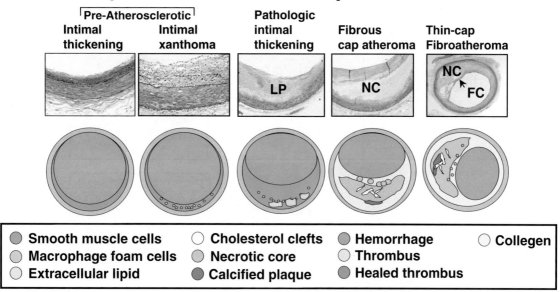

| Pre-Atherosclerotic | | Pathologic | | |
| Intimal thickening | Intimal xanthoma | intimal thickening | Fibrous cap atheroma | Thin-cap Fibroatheroma |

Legend:
- ● Smooth muscle cells
- ● Macrophage foam cells
- ○ Extracellular lipid
- ○ Cholesterol clefts
- ● Necrotic core
- ● Calcified plaque
- ● Hemorrhage
- ○ Thrombus
- ● Healed thrombus
- ○ Collegen

FIGURE 1-3. Development of human coronary atherosclerosis. Coronary lesions are uniformly present in all populations, although intimal xanthomas (so-called fatty streaks) are more prevalent with exposure to a Western diet. Preatherosclerotic lesions (adaptive intimal thickening and intimal xanthoma) occur soon after birth, although the latter are known to regress with age. Adaptive intimal thickening consists mainly of smooth muscle cells (SMCs) in a proteoglycan matrix, whereas intimal xanthomas contain macrophage-derived foam cells, T lymphocytes, and varying amounts of SMCs. Pathologic intimal thickening versus atheroma: Pathological intimal thickening (PIT) is a poorly defined entity, referred to in the literature as "intermediate" lesion. True necrosis is not apparent, as there is no evidence of cellular debris; lipid pools (*LP*) are seen deep in the lesion. The tissue over the lipid pools is rich in SMCs and proteoglycans; scattered macrophages and lymphocytes may also be present. The more definitive lesions, of fibrous cap atheroma, classically shows a true necrotic core (*NC*) containing cholesterol esters, free cholesterol, phospholipids, and triglycerides. The fibrous cap consists of SMCs in a proteoglycan-collagen matrix, with a variable number of macrophages and lymphocytes. The thin-cap fibroatheroma (vulnerable plaque): Thin-cap fibroatheromas are lesions with large necrotic cores containing numerous cholesterol clefts. The overlying fibrous cap (*FC*) is thin (<65 μm) and heavily infiltrated by macrophages; SMCs are rare and microvessels are generally present in the adventitia. (Reproduced with permission from Virmani R, et al. *Arterioscl Thromb Vasc Biol.* 2000;20:1262–1275.) (This figure appears in black and white on page 6.)

Causes of Coronary Thrombosis

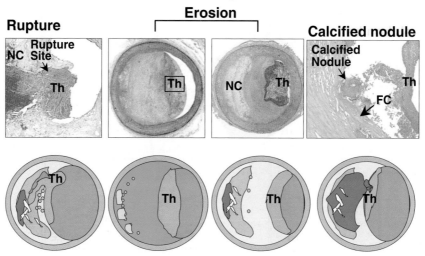

| Rupture | Erosion | | Calcified nodule |

FIGURE 1-6. Atherosclerotic lesion with luminal thrombi. Ruptured plaques are thin fibrous cap atheromas with luminal thrombi (*Th*). These lesions usually have an extensive necrotic core (*NC*) containing large numbers of cholesterol crystals and a thin fibrous cap (<65 μm) infiltrated by foamy macrophages and a paucity of T lymphocytes. The fibrous cap is thinnest at the site of rupture and consists of a few collagen bundles and rare smooth muscle cells. The luminal thrombus is in direct communication with the lipid-rich core. Erosions occur over lesions rich in smooth muscle cells and proteoglycans. Luminal thrombi overlie areas lacking surface endothelium. The deep intima of the eroded plaque often shows extracellular lipid pools, but necrotic cores are not uncommon; when present, the necrotic core does not communicate with the luminal thrombus. Inflammatory infiltrate is usually absent, but if present, is sparse and consists of macrophages and lymphocytes. Calcified nodules are plaques with luminal thrombi showing calcific nodules protruding into the lumen through a disrupted thin fibrous cap (*FC*). There is absence of an endothelium at the site of the thrombus, and inflammatory cells (macrophages, T lymphocytes) are absent. (Reproduced with permission from Virmani R, et al. *Arterioscl Thromb Vasc Biol.* 2000;20:1262–1275.) (This figure appears in black and white on page 7.)

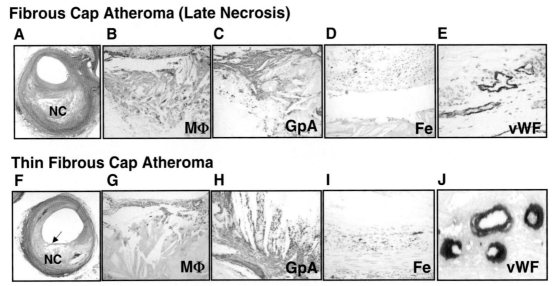

Angiographic and Histologic Representation of Plaque Rupture and Erosion

Rupture

Erosion

FIGURE 1-7. Angiographic and histologic representation of plaque rupture and erosion. A 43-year-old white man with no known history of risk factors was found unresponsive in the bathroom where he was last seen alive 20 minutes earlier. **A:** Postmortem angiogram shows the LAD at the origin of the left diagonal with a near total occlusion. Sections taken from these sites show a plaque rupture [*arrow*, **(B)**] with an underlying necrotic core (*NC*). The occluded artery shows an organizing thrombus with small lumens (*L*). **C:** The fibrous cap is intact with a large underlying necrotic core with peripheral calcification (Ca2+) and the lumen shows organizing thrombus (*Th*) with small lumens (*L*). At autopsy there was a healing transmural myocardial infarction present in the distribution of the LAD. Postmortem angiogram **(D,E)** and corresponding photomicrograph **(F)** from a 38-year-old man who was last seen alive 8 hours antemortem, died from sudden coronary death. A focal stenosis is present in the left anterior coronary artery (*boxed area*), which is highlighted in **(A)**, and an arrow points to the area of narrowing at the take-off of the left diagonal. **F:** Acute nonocclusive luminal thrombus (*Th*) is present on the surface of an erosive plaque rich in proteoglycans (*green*) and the underlying plaque shows pathologic intimal thickening with lipid pools (*LP*). (Reproduced in part from Figure 4, Farb A, et al. *Circulation.* 1995;92:1701–1709.) (This figure appears in black and white on page 8.)

Fibrous Cap Atheroma (Late Necrosis)

Thin Fibrous Cap Atheroma

FIGURE 1-8. Late core **(A–E)** and thin fibrous cap atheroma **(F–J)** showing intraplaque hemorrhage. **A:** Low-power view of a fibrous cap atheroma with a late necrotic core (*NC*) (Movat Pentachrome × 20). **B:** Intense staining of CD68-positive macrophages is seen within the necrotic core. **C:** Extensive glycophorin A (*GpA*) positive erythrocyte membranes colocalized with numerous cholesterol clefts within the necrotic core (× 200). **D:** Iron deposits (*blue*) are seen within macrophage foam cells (× 200). **E:** Microvessels bordering the necrotic core show perivascular von Willebrand factor (*vWF*) deposition (× 400). **F:** Lowpower view of a fibroatheroma with a thin fibrous cap (arrow) overlying a relatively large necrotic core (Movat Pentachrome, × 20). **G:** The fibrous cap is devoid of smooth muscle cells (not shown) and is heavily infiltrated by CD68-positive macrophages (*MΦ*, × 200). **H:** Intense glycophorin (*GpA*) staining of erythrocyte membranes within the necrotic core colocalized with cholesterol clefts (× 100). **I:** Adjacent coronary segment with accumulated iron (*blue pigment*) in a macrophage-rich region deep within the plaque (× 200). **J:** Perivascular diffuse deposits of von Willebrand factor in microvessels; indicates leaky vessels bordering the necrotic core (× 400). (Reproduced with permission from Kolodgie FD, et al., *N Engl J Med.* 2003;349:2316-2325.) (This figure appears in black and white on page 9.)

Identification of MHC Class II in Insulin-Dependent And Independent Diabetics

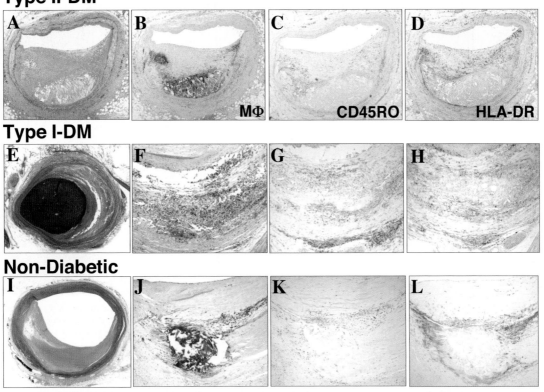

FIGURE 1-12. Inflammation in coronary arteries in patients with diabetes mellitus, comparison to nondiabetics. Shown are coronary lesions (fibroatheromas) illustrating the extent of inflammatory infiltrate [macrophage (*MΦ*) and T-cells (*CD45RO*)] and HLA-DR expression in patients type II **(A–D)** and type I **(E–H)** diabetes mellitus (DM) and in nondiabetic patients **(I–L)**. (Reproduced with permission from Burke AP, et al. *Arterioscl Thromb Vasc Biol.* 2004; 24:1266-1271.) (This figure appears in black and white on page 14.)

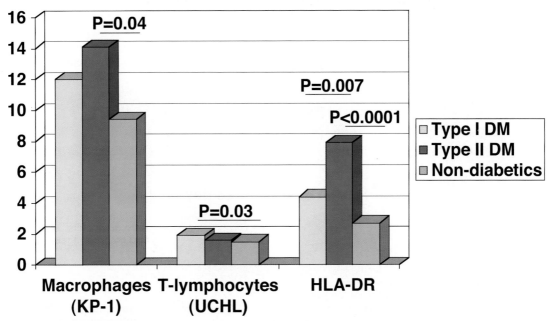

FIGURE 1-13. Bar graph showing a semiquantitative comparison of the extent of macrophage, T-cell infiltration, and HLA-DR expression in coronary arteries from diabetic and nondiabetic patients. Macrophage infiltration is maximal in type II diabetics, whereas Tlymphocyte infiltration was greatest in type I diabetics. In contrast, HLA-DR expression is significantly higher in type I and II diabetics when compared to nondiabetics. (This figure appears in black and white on page 14.)

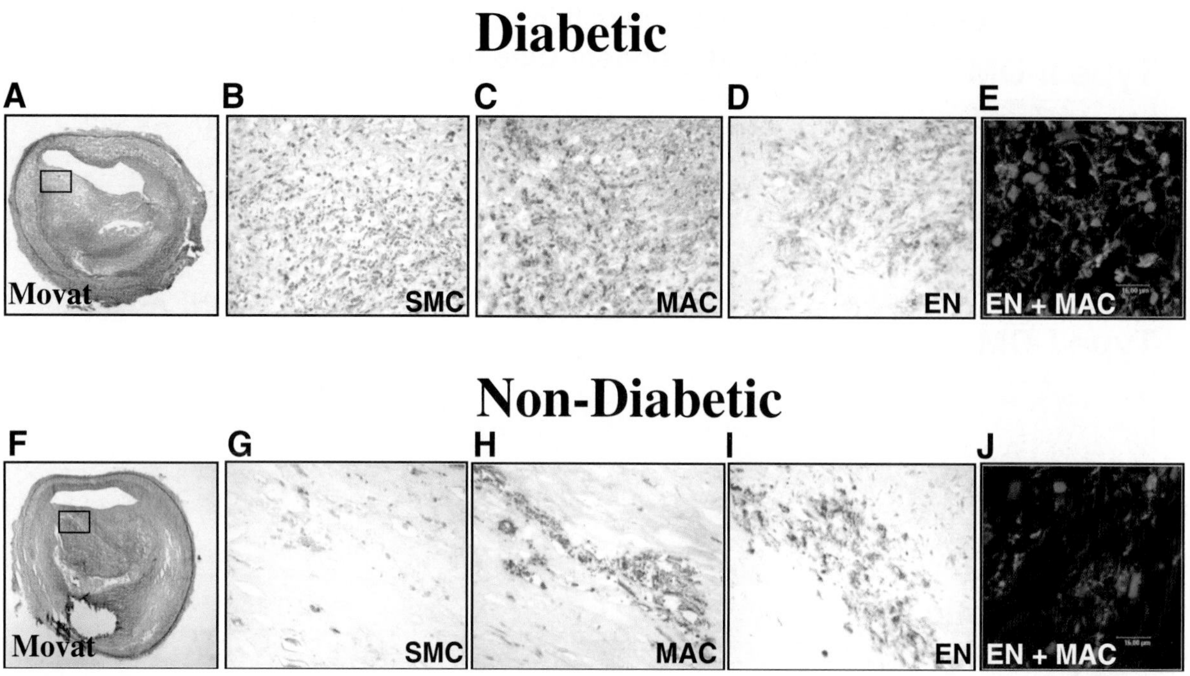

Diabetic

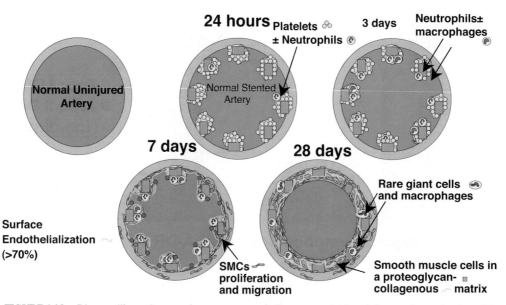

A Movat | **B** SMC | **C** MAC | **D** EN | **E** EN + MAC

Non-Diabetic

F Movat | **G** SMC | **H** MAC | **I** EN | **J** EN + MAC

FIGURE 1-14. Expression of S100A12/EN-RAGE (a RAGE binding protein) in human coronary lesions from diabetic (**A–E**) and nondiabetic (**F–J**) sudden coronary death victims. **A:** Lesion from the proximal left circumflex coronary artery stained by Movat Pentachrome. **B–E:** High-magnification micrographs of the black box represented in **A. B:** HHF-35 staining for SMCs in the shoulder region of the plaque. **C:** Adjacent section stained for CD68, demonstrating numerous inflammatory macrophages. **D:** The same region, demonstrating intense staining for EN-RAGE. **B–D:** The counterstain is Gill's hematoxylin. **E:** Double-labeled immunofluorescent staining of CD68-positive macrophages (*green*) and EN-RAGE (*red*); nuclei (*blue*) were counterstained with DAPI; areas of overlap appear as yellowish-green. EN-RAGE was primarily found in macrophage-rich areas in macrophages and smooth muscle cells. **F:** A lesion from the proximal left anterior descending coronary artery from a nondiabetic patient stained by Movat Pentachrome. **G–I:** Immunoreactivity to SMC, macrophage, and EN-RAGE, respectively. Overall, macrophage infiltrate was significantly less in nondiabetic patients, corresponding to less immunoreactivity to EN-RAGE. **J:** Double staining for EN-RAGE and macrophages. (Reproduced with permission from Burke AP, et al. *Arterioscl Thromb Vasc Biol.* 2004;24: 1266-1271.) (This figure appears in black and white on page 14.)

Diagram Illustrating Vascular Response to Intravascular Stent Placement

Normal Uninjured Artery

24 hours Platelets ± Neutrophils

Normal Stented Artery

3 days Neutrophils± macrophages

7 days
Surface Endothelialization (>70%)

28 days

SMCs proliferation and migration

Rare giant cells and macrophages

Smooth muscle cells in a proteoglycan-collagenous matrix

FIGURE 1-16. Diagram illustrating vascular response to a balloon expandable stainless steel stent implanted in a normal pig coronary or rabbit iliac artery. SMCs, smooth muscle cells. (Reproduced with permission from Virmani R, et al. *Heart.* 2003;89:133–138.) (This figure appears in black and white on page 16.)

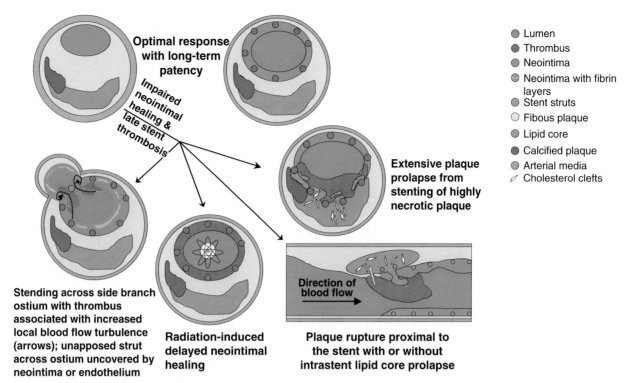

Legend:
- Lumen
- Thrombus
- Neointima
- Neointima with fibrin layers
- Stent struts
- Fibous plaque
- Lipid core
- Calcified plaque
- Arterial media
- Cholesterol clefts

Optimal response with long-term patency

Impaired neointimal healing & late stent thrombosis

Extensive plaque prolapse from stenting of highly necrotic plaque

Stending across side branch ostium with thrombus associated with increased local blood flow turbulence (arrows); unapposed strut across ostium uncovered by neointima or endothelium

Radiation-induced delayed neointimal healing

Direction of blood flow

Plaque rupture proximal to the stent with or without intrastent lipid core prolapse

FIGURE 1-24. Causes of late stent thrombosis for bare metal stents. Diagram of the postulated pathological mechanisms of late stent thrombosis (LST) associated with impaired neointimal healing. (This figure appears in black and white on page 21.)

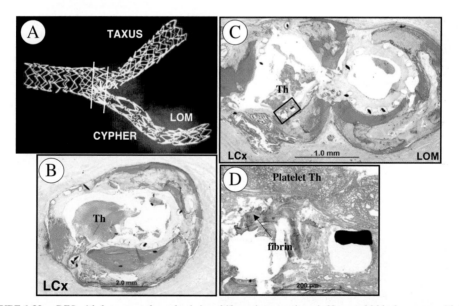

FIGURE 1-29. DES with late stent thrombosis in a bifurcation stenting. A 68-year-old black woman with history of remote coronary artery bypass surgery presented with stable angina pectoris attributed to severe stenosis of the left circumflex (LCx) and left obtuse marginal (LOM) arteries. A long Taxus stent was place in the LCx and a Cypher stent in the LOM 172 days prior to death. The patient presented with an acute myocardial infarction, and angiographic examination showed total occlusion of the LCx at the origin of the LOM secondary to a thrombus. The patient had a balloon angioplasty and the artery was reopened. The individual died 2 days later with severe pump failure. **A:** The radiograph shows well-expanded bifurcating Taxus and Cypher stents in the LCx and LOM, respectively. **B:** Note that just proximal to the bifurcation there is a thrombus in the Taxus LCx stent extending distally beyond the area of the bifurcation **(C)**. **D:** Multiple stent struts are surrounded by a fibrin-rich thrombus while the lumen has a platelet-rich thrombus. Of note, the LOM artery with the Cypher stent **(C)** is 40% narrowed by neointimal tissue (bluish-green on Movat Pentachrome) and lacks a thrombus. (Finn A, et al. Beyond late loss: importance of arterial healing. Submitted for publication.) (This figure appears in black and white on page 24.)

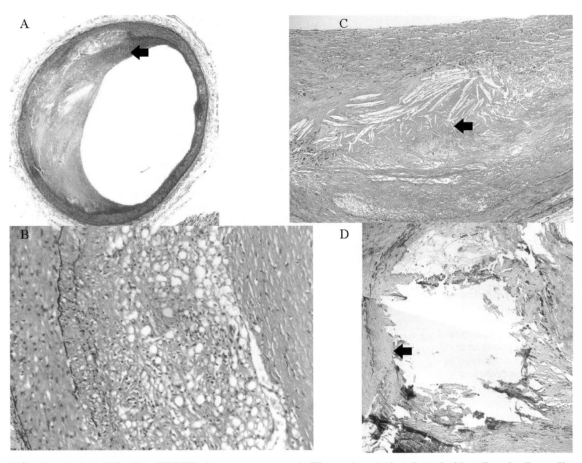

FIGURE 3C-7. Descriptions of the four VH-IVUS plaque components. **A:** Fibrous tissue is densely packed bundles of collagen fibers with no evidence of intrafiber lipid accumulation and no evidence of macrophage infiltration. It appears dark-yellow/green on Movatstained histology sections and dark green on VH-IVUS images. **B:** Fibrofatty tissue is loosely packed bundles of collagen fibers with regions of lipid deposition present. These areas are cellular and have no cholesterol clefts or necrosis present. There is an increase in extracellular matrix, and it appears turquoise on Movat-stained histology sections and light green on VH-IVUS. **C:** Necrotic core is defined as a highly lipidic necrotic region with remnants of foam cells and dead lymphocytes present. No collagen fibers are visible, and mechanical integrity is poor. Cholesterol clefts and microcalcifications are clearly visible. It is red on VH-IVUS images. **D:** Dense calcium is a focal area of calcium deposits. It appears purple or deep blue on Movat-stained histology sections and usually falls out of histology section, but calcium crystals are evident at borders. It is white on VH-IVUS images. (This figure appears in black and white on page 83.)

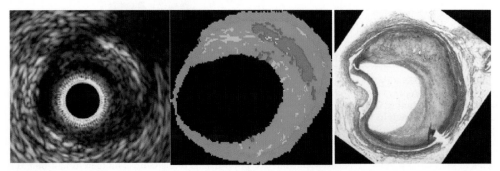

FIGURE 3C-9. Example of an intravascular ultrasound image (*left*) from a human coronary artery imaged ex vivo, and the corresponding VH-IVUS (*middle*) and Movat-stained histology section (right). VHIVUS: (*Dark green*) fibrous tissue; (*light green*) fibrofatty; (*red*) necrotic core; (*white*) dense calcium. (This figure appears in black and white on page 84.)

Example Plot of Plaque Composition Along an Artery

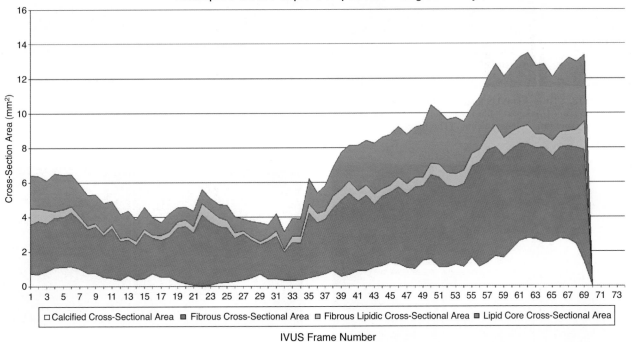

□ Calcified Cross-Sectional Area ■ Fibrous Cross-Sectional Area ☐ Fibrous Lipidic Cross-Sectional Area ■ Lipid Core Cross-Sectional Area

IVUS Frame Number

FIGURE 3C-11. An example output from the VH-IVUS software for quantitative analysis of plaque components along the length of an artery. (This figure appears in black and white on page 84.)

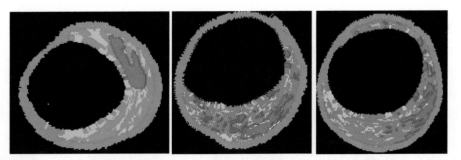

FIGURE 3C-14. Three VH-IVUS fibroatheroma images. (*Dark green*) fibrous tissue; (*light green*) fibrofatty; (*red*) necrotic core; (*white*) dense calcium. (This figure appears in black and white on page 85.)

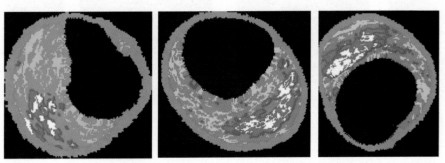

FIGURE 3C-15. Three VH-IVUS fibroatheroma images. (*Dark green*) fibrous tissue; (*light green*) fibrofatty; (*red*) necrotic core; (*white*) dense calcium. (This figure appears in black and white on page 85.)

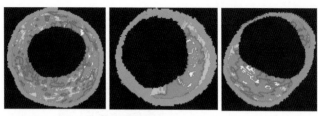

FIGURE 3C-18. Three VH-IVUS images of thin-cap fibroatheromas with necrotic core. (*Dark green*) fibrous tissue; (*light green*) fibrofatty; (*red*) necrotic core; (*white*) dense calcium. (This figure appears in black and white on page 86.)

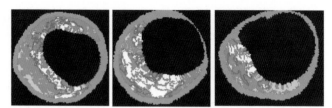

FIGURE 3C-19. Three VH-IVUS images of thin-cap fibroatheromas with dense calcium. (*Dark green*) fibrous tissue; (*light green*) fibrofatty; (*red*) necrotic core; (*white*) dense calcium. (This figure appears in black and white on page 86.)

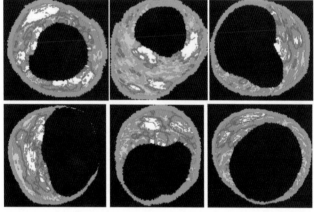

FIGURE 3C-20. Six VH-IVUS images of thin-cap fibroatheromas with multiple foci. (*Dark green*) fibrous tissue; (*light green*) fibrofatty; (*red*) necrotic core; (*white*) dense calcium. (This figure appears in black and white on page 86.)

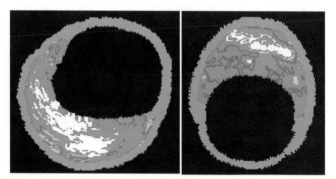

FIGURE 3C-21. Three VH-IVUS images of thin-cap fibroatheromas. (*Dark green*) fibrous tissue; (*light green*) fibrofatty; (*red*) necrotic core; (*white*) dense calcium. (This figure appears in black and white on page 86.)

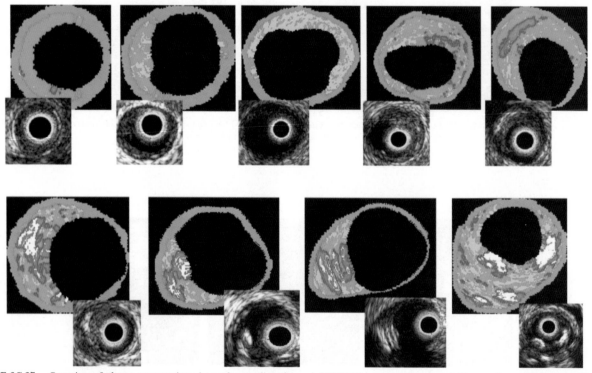

FIGURE 3C-27. Overview of plaque progression. An understanding through VH-IVUS images. (*Dark green*) fibrous tissue; (*light green*) fibrofatty; (*red*) necrotic core; (*white*) dense calcium. (This figure appears in black and white on page 88.)

The role of RAGE/EN-RAGE up-regulation in the atherosclerotic plaque is likely complex and associated with both apoptosis and necrotic cell death; the precise triggers of the inflammatory response that culminate in the formation in some plaques of large necrotic cores, and, in others, in fibrocalcific plaques, remain unknown.

In summary, diabetes is associated with greater inflammatory infiltrate (macrophages and T lymphocytes), larger necrotic core size, and diffuse atherosclerosis in the coronary arteries. The coronary arteries also show positive remodeling. The expression of RAGE and EN-RAGE may further compromise cell survival and promote plaque destabilization. Severe coronary atherosclerosis in diabetics is accompanied by the presence of healed myocardial infarction and cardiomegaly. Further studies are needed to better understand the relationship of hyperglycemia and insulin resistance to the greater induction of inflammation seen in atherosclerotic arteries and whether controlling either or both will result in a decrease in inflammation in atherosclerotic plaques over time.

PERCUTANEOUS CORONARY INTERVENTION PATHOLOGY

Balloon angioplasty was introduced in the 1970s for the treatment of coronary artery disease but was burdened with a high rate of restenosis, 13% to 53%.[70] The mechanisms of balloon angioplasty failure were both acute and chronic. Acute was believed to be secondary to elastic recoil and prolapse of the atherosclerotic plaque into the lumen, along with thrombosis. The late failure was related to negative remodeling, and neointimal growth was responsible to a lesser extent.[4,71] In order to tackle negative remodeling, stents were introduced, which reduced the rate of acute complications as well as late restenosis as compared to balloon angioplasty.[72] The main mechanism of in-stent restenosis in contrast to balloon angioplasty was solely neointimal growth.

NEOINTIMAL RESPONSE IN HUMAN ATHEROSCLEROTIC CORONARY ARTERIES

It is poorly appreciated, however, that neointimal responses are exaggerated and the time course of healing is more prolonged in humans than in animals.[73,74] A comparison of arterial healing after coronary stenting in animals and humans is shown in Fig. 1-15. In a morphometric analysis of more than 40 human stents collected at autopsy, peak neointimal thickness (0.78 ± 0.37 mm) occurs between 6 months and 1 year with approximately 22% regression in neointimal growth >1 year.[75] In contrast, neointimal formation in stented swine coronary arteries is maximal at 1 month (0.33 ± 0.24 mm) with approximately 25% lesion regression taking place over the following 3 to 6 months. Thus, the response to healing after placement of a bare stainless steel stent in a human coronary artery is at least five to six times longer as compared with those in swine or rabbits. This concept is essential in the evaluation of a drug-eluting stent, such that the interval from implantation to the actual data collection becomes crucial to the final outcome of testing. To better understand the differences in stent healing, a brief review of stent pathology in human coronary arteries

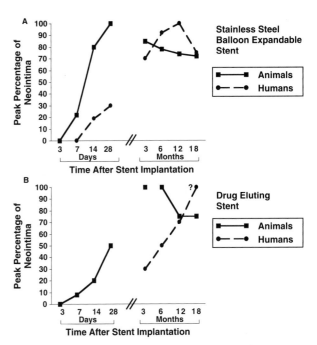

FIGURE 1-15. Line plot showing the temporal relation of peak neointimal growth in animals and humans following the placement of either bare stainless steel (**A**) or drug-loaded sirolimus- or paclitaxel-eluting stents (**B**). The plots are predominantly derived from morphometric analysis of pig and human coronary stents; the drug-eluting stent data in humans are projected from angiographic and recent autopsy results. In animals, peak neointimal growth in stainless steel stents occurs at 28 days, compared with 6 to 12 months in humans. Animal studies of drug-eluting stents show favorable results at 28 days, with a lack of sustained efficacy at 3 and 9 months (Carter AJ, Aggarwal M, Kopia GA, et al. Long-term effects of polymer-based, slow-release, sirolimus-eluting stents in a porcine coronary model. *Cardiovasc Res.* 2004;63:617-624). In contrast, the precise time course of peak neointimal growth in human coronary arteries with drug-eluting stents is unknown (?), although recent autopsy studies show delayed neointimal healing up to 9 months (Joner M, Finn AV, Farb A, et al. Pathology of drug eluting stents: delayed healing and thrombosis. *J Am Coll Cardiol.* 2006. In press). Substantial long-term data in "real-world" patients are as yet unavailable. The generalized delayed arterial healing with drug-eluting stents is thought to occur secondarily from an inhibition of smooth muscle cell proliferation and migration together with suppression of inflammation and endothelialization. (Modified from Virmani R, et al. *Heart.* 2003;89:133-138.) (See Color Fig. 1-15.)

and animals is useful to highlight temporal differences of vascular healing.

HEALING—BARE METAL STENTS

ANIMAL MODELS

Although most tests of stent efficacy are performed at 28 days, there are a surprisingly limited number of long-term morphologic studies on restenosis in swine coronary arteries.[76,77] The early (1 to 3 days) morphologic response to stenting in normal arteries predominantly consists of platelet/fibrin deposition surrounding struts and scattered neutrophils within adherent luminal thrombi. By day 7, organizing mural thrombi extending between stent struts contain smooth muscle cells and macrophages with scattered lymphocytes, red cells, and luminal endothelial cells. At 14 days, fibrin is still present with a few chronic inflammatory cells remaining around stent struts. At this stage, the neointima contains few smooth muscle cells within a proteoglycan-rich matrix.

By 28 days, the neointima contains a larger number of smooth muscle cells, proteoglycans, and type III collagen with rare macrophages and giant cells around stent struts; fibrin is usually absent (Fig. 1-16). The rate of neointimal expansion is greatest between 7 and 14 days, with maximal thickness achieved at 1 month. Over the next 3 to 6 months, the extracellular matrix becomes enriched in collagen type I with neointimal shrinkage and remodeling. Cell proliferation in the neointima peaks at 7 days, is reduced by approximately half at 14 days, and returns to a low baseline level by 1 month. Of note, stented rabbit iliac arteries follow a time course of healing similar to that of swine coronary arteries.

HUMANS

In stented human coronary arteries, platelet and fibrin deposition persists up to 14 and 30 days, respectively.[73] Inflammatory cells, consisting of polymorphonuclear leukocytes and macrophages, are present by 1 to 3 days, and macrophages persist for at least 3 months and in lesions with restenosis even longer. T lymphocytes appear at 2 to 3 weeks and persist beyond 6 months. Collections of smooth muscle cells, the main cellular component of the restenotic lesion, are evident by 14 days following stenting.

The extracellular matrix, composed initially of proteoglycans and type III collagen, is gradually replaced by type I collagen past 18 months (Figs. 1-17 and 1-18). The proteoglycans consist mainly of versican and hyaluronan in stents implanted for up to 18 months, whereas decorin staining and type I collagen deposition is greatest after 18 months. Smooth muscle cell density and neointima tissue are significantly reduced after 18 months.[78]

The time course of intimal smooth muscle cell proliferation in relation to in-stent restenosis in humans is not known. Cell proliferation studies in human restenotic coronary atherectomy tissue retrieved from a few days to just beyond 1 year have thus far generally shown a low proliferation index without the characteristic peak found in existing animal models of angioplasty and stenting.[79] Clearly, significantly more rapid proliferative events appear to occur in animals as distinguished from human restenotic coronary arteries. Further, rather than a simple proliferative response, smooth muscle cell migration from within the plaque or media to the expanding neointima may be the more dominant factor contributing to in-stent restenosis in humans.

We have performed detailed morphologic studies on 116 human stented arteries in place $\geq$90 days in 87 coronary arteries to determine the histologic predictors of restenosis.[74] The mean duration of implant was 10 months. In-stent restenosis was defined as a stent area stenosis of >75%. Lumen area increased as stent area increased ($r^2 = 0.27$, $p = 0.0001$), but there was much stronger correlation between stent area and neointimal area ($r^2 = 0.70$, $p < 0.0001$). Arterial medial fracture was associated with a 29% increase ($p < 0.01$) in neointimal thickness compared with arteries with an intact media. Neointimal thickness ($p = 0.0001$), inflammatory cell density ($p < 0.0001$), and

Balloon Expandable Stainless Steel Stent Healing in Man

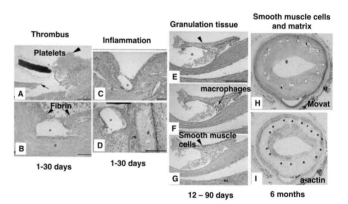

FIGURE 1-17. Arterial healing in a human coronary stainless steel balloon expandable stent. **A:** Platelet-rich thrombus (*arrowhead*) is associated with strut from Gianturco-Roubin II coronary artery stent implanted 1 day antemortem. Numerous acute inflammatory cells are present within the thrombus. Focal fibrous cap disruption is seen (*arrow*). **B:** Fibrin-rich thrombus (*arrowheads*) is focally present around a stent strut (*asterisk*) 1 day after placement of a Palmaz-Schatz stent. Fibrous plaque (*p*) is present below the strut. [Hematoxylin-eosin; **(A)** bar = 0.16 mm; **(B)** bar = 0.12 mm.] **C,D:** Arterial inflammation in coronary arteries with stents placed $\leq$3 days antemortem: Movat Pentachrome stain. **C:** Increased numbers of inflammatory cells are associated with Palmaz-Schatz stent (*asterisk*) that penetrates into necrotic core (*c*). **D:** A Palmaz-Schatz strut (*asterisk*) is in contact with damaged media (*m*) with dissection (*d*) and associated inflammatory cells. [**(C),** bar = 0.10 mm; **(D)** bar = 0.14 mm.] **E-G:** Early neointima present 12 days after Gianturco-Roubin coronary artery stent placement. **E:** Intimal cells within extracellular matrix (*arrowhead*) are seen above the stent strut. **F:** KP-1 immunostaining identifies macrophages adjacent to the strut at base of neointima (*arrow*). **G:** Actin staining shows smooth muscle cells close to luminal surface of neointima (*arrowhead*), within the plaque close to the media, and within the media (*m*). [**(E),** Movat Pentachrome, bar = 0.18 mm; **(F)** KP-1 immunostain; **(G)** smooth muscle actin immunostain.] **H,I:** Restenosis tissue by 6 months is predominantly characterized by α-actin positive smooth muscle cells. (Modified from Farb A, et al. *Circulation.* 1999;99:44-52.)

Diagram Illustrating Vascular Response to Intravascular Stent Placement

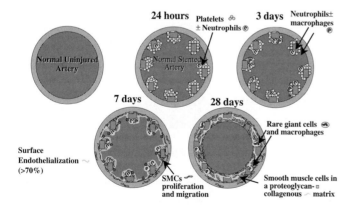

FIGURE 1-16. Diagram illustrating vascular response to a balloon expandable stainless steel stent implanted in a normal pig coronary or rabbit iliac artery. SMCs, smooth muscle cells. (Reproduced with permission from Virmani R, et al. *Heart.* 2003;89:133-138.) (See Color Fig. 1-16.)

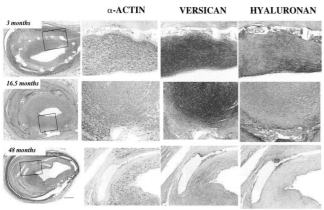

α-ACTIN   VERSICAN   HYALURONAN

3 months

16.5 months

48 months

Immunohistochemical Staining for α-Actin, Versican and Hyaluronan

FIGURE 1-18. Distribution of immunostaining at various time points following bare metal stent implantation. Strong neointimal versican and hyaluronan staining is present in stents in place 3 months (group 1) and 16.5 months (group 2) with colocalization with α-actin-positive SMCs. Versican and hyaluronan staining is reduced in 48-month-old stent (group 3) associated with reduced neointimal SMC density. (*Left*) Movat Pentachrome stain. Scale bar, 0.82 mm in left, 0.14 mm others. (Reproduced with permission from Farb A, et al. *Circulation.* 2004;110:940-947.)

neointimal vascular channel density (*p* <0.0001) were greater when stent struts were in contact with ruptured media compared with fibrous plaque or intact fibrous cap. Stent strut penetration into a lipid core was associated with increased neointimal thickness and inflammatory cell density. Inflammatory cell density was 2.4-fold greater in stents with restenosis versus no restenosis; the percentage of the neointima occupied by macrophages was three-fold higher in restenosis versus no restenosis (Fig. 1-19), and inflammation correlated with increased angiogenesis.

TEMPORAL DIFFERENCES IN ARTERIAL HEALING IN HUMANS AND ANIMALS

One obvious explanation for the delayed arterial healing in humans is contingent on the underlying atherosclerotic process, which usually manifests in the fifth to sixth decade of life. Arterial interventions in animals are usually performed in young adults, and stents are typically placed in apposition to a normal smooth muscle-rich medial wall without inflammation. The absence of atherosclerotic disease likely contributes to a more predictable healing response in animals. In contrast, in diseased human coronary arteries, at least 70% of the stent is in direct contact with the underlying atherosclerotic plaque.[73,74] The physical components of the lesion relative to the position of the stent also affects the local response to healing. For example, stent struts in proximity to a necrotic core are exposed to only a paucity of smooth muscle cells and thus, heal more slowly than stents in direct contact with areas of adaptive intimal thickening, which contain an abundance of smooth muscle cells.[73] Similarly, stents overlying calcified and densely fibrotic plaques also take longer to develop neointima, because these plaques are also relatively hypocellular and must recruit smooth muscle cells from other remote areas of the arterial wall to cover bare struts. In a rabbit model of balloon injury and

atherosclerosis, we have seen a three- to fourfold increase in neointimal growth following stenting as compared to balloon injury and normal diet (RV, unpublished data).

The differential rate of healing between animals and humans may also be proportional to the longevity of the species. The typical life span of a human is >70 years; in contrast, pigs have a life span of 16 years, and rabbits 5 to 6 years. The biological differences in rate of healing are age dependent and are exemplified in animal models of cutaneous wounds. This analogy may be appropriate to in-stent restenosis because the developing neointima is similarly considered a response to traumatic injury (Fig. 1-15). In the swine, the extent of cutaneous re-epithelialization declines with age partly because of a decrease in the expression of growth factors.[80] Further, wound contraction "remodeling" is accelerated in juvenile as compared with adult pigs. The type of injury is another consideration; wound healing is delayed in traumatic as compared to surgically induced injury and if the injury site is large rather than small.[81,82] Human coronary stenting is often associated with extensive local trauma characterized by plaque splitting and medial disruption. Conversely, most stents in animals are deployed in normal arteries with 1.1:1 stent to artery ratio, resulting in only mild arterial injury.[83]

MOLECULAR MECHANISMS OF RESTENOSIS

Injury of the arterial wall is associated with endothelial denudation with immediate adherence of platelets, surface thrombosis and recruitment of inflammatory cells consisting of neutrophils, monocytes or macrophages, and T lymphocytes. Leukocyte

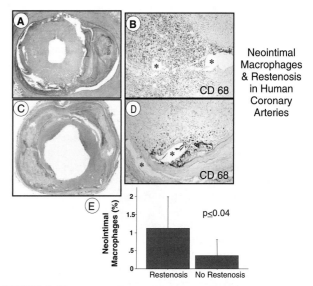

Neointimal Macrophages & Restenosis in Human Coronary Arteries

FIGURE 1-19. Macrophages infiltration and neointimal growth. **A:** In-stent restenosis of a left circumflex artery stent placed 6 months antemortem. **B:** CD68 immunohistochemistry identifies numerous brown-staining macrophages near stent struts (*asterisks*). Fewer intimal macrophages are associated with the widely patent left anterior coronary artery stent deployed 4 months antemortem **(C,D). E:** Bar graph showing the relationship of restenosis with increased neointimal macrophage content. **(A)** and **(C),** Movat Pentachrome stain; **(B)** and **(D)** anti-CD68 immunostain. (Modified from Farb A, et al. *Circulation.* 2002;105:2974-2980.)

recruitment is mediated by multiple adherence and signaling events including selectin-mediated attachment and rolling, intercellular adhesion molecules (ICAM), and integrin-mediated firm adhesion and diapedesis that result in the infiltration of inflammatory cells into the vascular wall. The firm attachment of inflammatory cells is mediated by members of the β_2-integrin family, LFA-1 ($\alpha L\beta_2$, CD11a/CD18), Mac-1 ($\alpha M\beta_2$, CD11b/CD18) and others that bind to endothelial counterligands (ICAM-1), or endothelium-associated matrix proteins. Also, the expression of chemoattractant monocyte chemotactic protein (MCP)-1 and interleukin (IL)-8 plays a critical role in the recruitment of leukocytes to areas of vascular injury.[84] These molecular events result in the liberation of growth factors, which are produced not only by inflammatory cells but also by smooth muscle and endothelial cells. The growth factors that are involved include platelet-derived growth factor (PDGF), basic fibroblast growth factor (bFGF), transforming growth factor (TGF)-beta, insulinlike growth factor (IGF), vascular endothelial growth factor (VEGF), and angiotensin II (ATII). Thrombin not only is involved in homeostasis and chemotaxis of leukocytes, but also acts as a potent stimulator of smooth muscle cell (SMC) proliferation, thus playing an important role in tissue repair.[85,86]

Growth factors stimulate SMC proliferation and migration as well as production of extracellular matrix constituents. Vascular repair, like any other wound repair, requires that a complex network of molecular signals be regulated within the cytoplasm and nucleus of the endothelial and smooth muscle cells. Resting sacs are maintained in a nonproliferative phase (G0); activated SMCs enter a gap period (G1), during which the cell assembles the factors necessary for DNA replication in the subsequent synthetic (S) phase. After DNA replication is completed, the cells again enter a gap period (G2), when proteins are synthesized in preparation for mitosis (M). The molecules that regulate the cell cycle are the cyclins and their cognate enzymes, the cyclin-dependent kinases (CDKs), which are positive regulators of these events. The cyclin-dependent kinase inhibitors (CDKIs) are also critical negative regulators of the cell cycle. The activities of cyclin-CDK complexes depend on the phosphorylation status of the CDKs and the steady-state levels of cyclins. Regulation of cell-cycle machinery is a final step for proliferative response. As has been shown in humans, control of the focus of cell-cycle regulators, such as with macrolide antibiotics (rapamycin, also called sirolimus, SRL), and of microtubular assembly (paclitaxel) has provided a logical site for intervention, and these drugs have been shown clinically to be successful when applied to stent surfaces. Rapamycin inhibits the progression of the cell cycle at the transition from G1-S phase. Following SRL binding to its intracellular receptor FKBP12, it inhibits the mammalian target of rapamycin (mTOR) and ultimately inhibits degradation of p27Kip1, a cyclin-dependent kinase inhibitor, which regulates cell cycle proliferation. On the other hand, paclitaxel (PTX) blocks cell-cycle progression through centrosomal impairment, induction of abnormal spindles, and suppression of spindle microtubule dynamics. As a result, cell replication is inhibited predominantly in the G0/G1 and G2/M phases of the cell cycle. Similarly because paclitaxel acts on the cytoskeleton it also inhibits migration.

Matrix metalloproteins (MMPs) and their inhibitors, called tissue inhibitors of MMPs (TIMPs), play an important role in remodeling of the extracellular matrix.[87] MMPs play an important role in SMC migration and along with TIMPs have been shown to be involved in restenosis.[88] Up-regulation of plasminogen activators such as urokinase plasminogen activator (uPA) or tissue plasminogen activator (tPA) or a decrease in plasminogen activator inhibitor (PAI) leads to plasmin activation, which leads to an increase in latent intracellular MMPs, which are involved in matrix degradation, angiogenesis, growth factor bioavailability, cytokine modulation, receptor shedding, enhanced cell migration, proliferation, invasion, and apoptosis.[89,90]

TREATMENT MODALITIES TO PREVENT RESTENOSIS

In the last decade brachytherapy in animal models, catheter (β or γ radiation) or stent (β radiation) based, inhibits neointimal formation with evidence of incomplete healing at 1 to 3 months.[91–93] Continued healing, however, is accompanied by neointimal growth, and 6-month brachytherapy studies in animals fail to show a benefit. For example, Coussement et al., using ^{186}Re β-radiation (20-Gy dose) delivered via a balloon at 6 months in pig balloon injured coronary arteries, showed a significant decrease in lumen size with a reciprocal greater neointimal area than control nonradiated balloon injured arteries.[92] Persistent fibrin deposition within the neointima was a notable finding in the radiated arteries. Complete endothelialization was absent, a potential mechanism of late subacute thrombosis in animals and humans.[92, 94–96]

The lack of sustained efficacy after brachytherapy in animals stands in direct contrast to early clinical trials, in which reduced arterial stenosis is evident at 6 months.

A likely explanation is that healing occurs more rapidly in normal animal arteries since eventually there is a progressive arterial stenosis between 6 months and 3 years as reported in patients receiving brachytherapy.[97] The longest term human coronary brachytherapy data available (5 years) shows a mean arterial stenosis of $50.5\% \pm 22.9\%$ (range 19.4% to 100%) accompanied by positive remodeling, excessive adventitial fibrosis, and intimal calcification (unpublished results, Ron Waksman, Washington Hospital Center, 2001). Lumen loss and neointimal growth are more dramatic in radioactive stents analyzed between 6 months and 1 year.[98] Taken together, these findings give strong supportive evidence of late lumen loss in radiated arteries in humans and closely parallel the negative results in animal studies. The pathology of delayed healing with radiation is not unlike that of drug-eluting stents, showing persistent intimal fibrin deposition, inflammation, a paucity of smooth muscle cells in a proteoglycan-rich matrix, and incomplete endothelialization. The similarity in histology raises the possibility that as with brachytherapy, neointimal growth with drug-eluting stents will only be delayed rather than prevented.

DRUG-ELUTING STENTS: CLINICAL RESULTS

Clinical results of recent head-to-head comparison of drug-eluting stents (DESs) with bare metal stents have almost all uniformly shown a reduction in-stent restenosis, varying from 80%

to 62%.[99, 100] However, comparison of target vessel revascularization, angiographic restenosis, and late loss following deployment of sirolimus and paclitaxel drug-eluting stents have shown a benefit for sirolimus stents, with greater late loss observed as compared to paclitaxel stents. However, no differences in thrombosis, death, or acute myocardial infarction were observed between the two stents in this study.[101]

In contrast, 9-month follow-up in "real-world" patients suggests that there is a higher rate of stent thrombosis (1.3%) in DES and that there is a trend toward greater thrombosis in the paclitaxel (1.7%) than in the sirolimus (0.8%, $p = 0.09$) group. It is therefore important to understand both in animals and man if there are differences in the morphologic parameters following DES stent implantation.

ANIMAL STUDIES WITH DRUG-ELUTING STENTS

Most of the published studies in animals have been performed following implantation of sirolimus-eluting stents, and these have shown a consistent suppression in neointimal formation at 28 days.[102, 103] Both DESs use nonerodible polymers, which in Cypher consist of a mixture of polyethylene-co-vinyl acetate (PEVA) and poly(*n*-butyl methacrylate) (PBMA), and in Taxus, SIBS [poly(styrene-β-isobutylene-β-styrene)].

SIROLIMUS-ELUTING STENTS

In a study by Klugherz et al., little evidence of increased inflammation or delayed endothelialization was noted with 28-day sirolimus-eluting stents (64 μg or 196 μg per stent) compared with polymer-coated or bare metal stents in rabbit iliac arteries.[102] Our experience in single 28-day stent implants in the rabbit is very similar, with persistence of fibrin and focal mild lack of stent coverage by endothelial cells (Fig. 1-20). In another 28-day study, Suzuki et al. reported higher amounts of accumulated fibrin with sirolimus-eluting stents (180 μg per stent) compared with bare metal stents in porcine coronary arteries, although the degree of endothelialization was similar among groups.[103] More recently, Carter et al. described the long-term effects of Cypher stents, again in porcine coronary

arteries.[104] Arterial inflammation characterized by giant cells gradually progressed from 90 to180 days with a corresponding increase in neointimal formation. However, none of the foregoing reports mentions eosinophilic reactions to sirolimus-eluting stents, and collectively, they emphasize the wide therapeutic index for sirolimus in normal vessels.

PACLITAXEL-ELUTING STENTS

Paclitaxel is a cytotoxic drug known to suppress neointimal formation accompanied by persistent fibrin deposition, macrophage infiltration, and overall decrease in smooth muscle cells at both 28 (Fig. 1-20) and 180 days following implantation in rabbit iliac and porcine coronary arteries.[105–107] Results of overlapping moderate release Taxus stents (1 μg/mm^2) in swine demonstrated a moderate inflammatory response without evidence of eosinophils and increased amount of fibrin deposition with partially complete endothelialization; unfortunately, no results for the neointimal area were reported in this study.[108]

OVERLAPPING DES PATHOLOGY IN RABBIT ILIAC ARTERIES

We have recently reported our findings in the rabbit iliac arteries of overlapping drug-eluting stents, Cypher and Taxus and compared to Bx Velocity and Express bare metal stents.[109] Both DESs showed signs of delayed arterial healing at nonoverlapping sites, which is in agreement with other published reports of sirolimus- and paclitaxel-eluting stents. In contrast to nonoverlapped sites, delayed healing was pronounced at overlapped stent sites. The inflammatory response to either DES was selective such that overlapping Taxus stents induced more fibrin and eosinophils as compared to Cypher (Fig. 1-21). Moreover, although both DESs evoked a giant-cell reaction near stent struts, the response was greater with Cypher. Luminal endothelialization was significantly more incomplete in overlapping 28-day Taxus than Cypher stents when visualized by scanning electron microscopy (Fig. 1-22). Arterial healing was generally more complete in DESs harvested at 90 days; however, Taxus stents failed to provide sustained neointimal suppression. Incomplete healing in both DESs was mostly characterized by persistent fibrin and inflammation cell infiltrate characterized by eosinophils for Taxus stents and giant cells for Cypher stents. Although no differences were found in cell proliferation or intimal cell density, medial cell density at or near stent struts was significantly lower in both 28- and 90-day Taxus stents.

Notably, the relative delay in healing found in overlapping segments of bare stainless steel stents was not nearly to the degree found with DESs and was possibly related to the finishing processes in the final preparation of the stent.[110] This reaction, however, might have affected neointimal growth in overlapping segments, because neointimal thickness measurements of Cypher compared to Bx Velocity and Taxus compared to Express, although lower, were not significantly different. Drug-eluting stents further delay arterial healing and promote inflammation at sites of overlap, compared with bare metal stents. Taxus stents induced greater fibrin deposition, medial cell loss, eosinophils, and late neointimal hyperplasia.

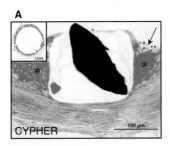
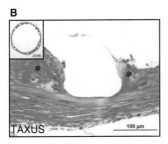

FIGURE 1-20. Histologic sections of rabbit iliac arteries at 28 days following deployment of single Cypher and Taxus stents in two different animals. The image from the Cypher stent shows fibrin deposition (*asterisks*) and a few scattered heterophils/eosinophils (*arrow*) close to the stent struts, whereas Taxus stents are characterized by a predominance of fibrin, with little inflammatory response. There were no significant differences observed in neointimal growth between the two commercially available drug-eluting stents at 28 days.

Inflammatory infiltrate

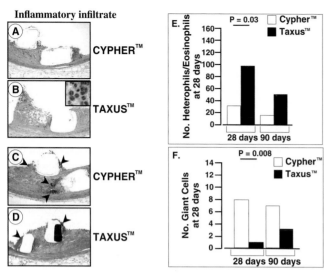

FIGURE 1-21. Digital images showing heterophils/eosinophils **(A,B)** and peristrut giant cells **(C,D)** in overlapping 28-day Cypher or Taxus stents. Greater numbers of heterophils/eosinophils are seen on luminal surface of Taxus stents [*inset in* **(B)**, 1000 × magnification], whereas Cypher stents show more peristrut giant cells (*arrowheads*). Hematoxylin and eosin stain (200 × magnification). **E,F:** Bar graphs representing the number of heterophils/eosinophils and giant cells, respectively, in 28- and 90-day Cypher and Taxus stents. (Reproduced with permission from Finn AV, Kolodgie FD, et al. *Circulation.* 2005;112:270–278.)

PATHOLOGY OF DRUG-ELUTING STENTS IN HUMANS

We have previously reported incidence of late stent thrombosis (LST, ≥30 days) in bare metal stents in the era of brachytherapy. LST was 9.8% (13 of 168 stents) at autopsy, which is significantly higher than that reported clinically; however, with brachytherapy at 2 to 15 months clinically there was a 6.6% incidence of arterial occlusion.[111] At autopsy the pathologic mechanisms of LST were (a) stent across ostia of major coronary arterial branches (five cases); (b) exposure to radiation therapy (three cases); (c) plaque disruption in the nonstented arterial segment within 2 mm of the stent margin (two cases); (d) stenting of marked necrotic, lipid-rich plaques with extensive plaque prolapse (two cases) (Fig. 1-23); and (e) diffuse in-stent restenosis (one case) (Fig. 1-24). Twelve cases failed to form a completely healed neointimal layer overlaying stent struts (range 33 to 270 days, mean 73 ± 23 days).

Drug-eluting stents demonstrate persistence of fibrin beyond 30 days, often with absence of smooth muscle and endothelial cells. Beyond the 30-day period there appears to be difference in the response to Cypher and Taxus stents. With the Cypher stent there appears to be a giant-cell and chronic inflammatory response including macrophages, lymphocytes, and eosinophils at 2 to 3 months. In Taxus one usually sees mostly fibrin deposition with or without acute inflammation; however, with time, usually by 3 to 4 months, there is a chronic inflammation, again consisting of macrophages, lymphocytes, eosinophils, and rare giant cells. In Taxus stents the amount of fibrin deposition is

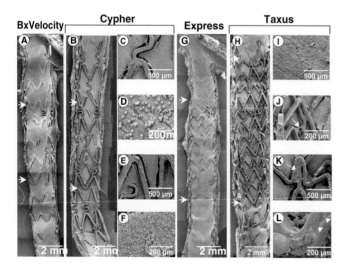

FIGURE 1-22. SEM of overlapping 28-day Bx Velocity **(A)**, Cypher **(B–F)**, Express **(G)**, and Taxus **(H–L)** stents. Regions of overlap are within horizontal arrows. Overall, there is less surface coverage by endothelial cells in Taxus and Cypher stents, specifically in segments with overlap. Overlapping segments within Bx Velocity and Express stents showed far greater endothelialization than DES. Higher-power views of Cypher stents **(C–F)** from segment of overlap show adherent platelets and inflammatory cells on stent struts and adjoining neointima. Higher-power images from overlapping segments of Taxus stents **(I–L)** show greater inflammatory infiltrate **(I)**, polymer sticking and stretching across stent struts [**(J)**, *arrow*], unexpanded struts [**(K)**, *arrow*] and irregular distribution of the polymer over stent strut surface [**(L)**, *arrowheads*]. (Reproduced with permission from Finn AV, Kolodgie FD, et al. *Circulation.* 2005;112:270–278.)

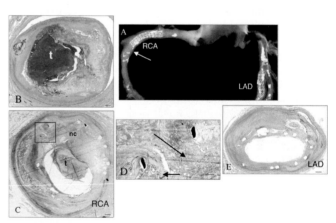

FIGURE 1-23. A 61-year-old man with post–myocardial infarction angina underwent stenting of 90% lesions in the mid-right (*RCA*) and mid-LAD coronary arteries. He presented with asymptomatic ventricular tachycardia and died suddenly 1 day later (32 days after stenting). **A:** The mid-RCA Bx Velocity stent. **B:** Plaque rupture and acute thrombosis of the RCA were present in a lipid-rich plaque just distal to the RCA stent [*arrow* in **(A)**]. **C:** A subocclusive thrombus (*t*) in the RCA stent; the underlying plaque is markedly necrotic with stent struts deeply embedded into the necrotic core (*nc*). The intimal surface remained unhealed; stent struts were covered by a fibrin-rich thrombus, and a confluent smooth muscle cell-rich extracellular matrix had not formed. **D:** High power [of inset in **(C)**] shows fibrous cap rupture (*short arrow*) and plaque prolapse (*long arrow*) covered by fibrin thrombus. The LAD stent (implanted in a stable plaque) was widely patent with a healing neointima overlying stent struts [**(A)** and **(E)**, Movat Pentachrome; scale bars 0.25 mm in **(B)**, **(C)**, and **(E)**, 0.13 mm in **(D)**.] (Modified with permission from Farb A, et al. *Circulation.* 2003;108: 1701–1706.)

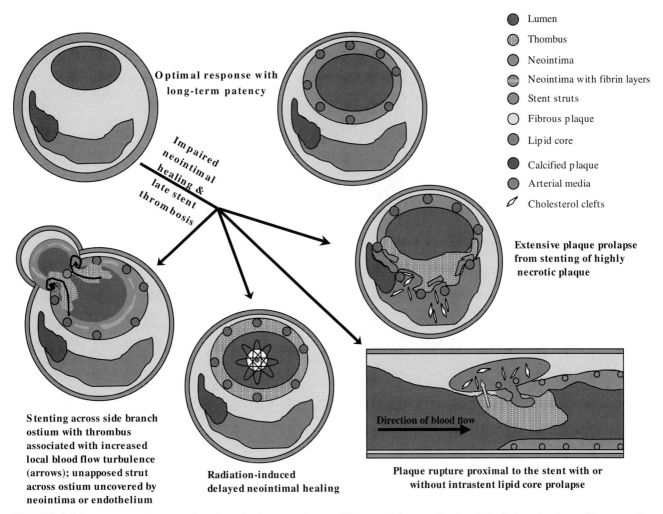

FIGURE 1-24. Causes of late stent thrombosis for bare metal stents. Diagram of the postulated pathological mechanisms of late stent thrombosis (LST) associated with impaired neointimal healing. (See Color Fig. 1-24.)

excessive, whereas in Cypher stents there is usually greater inflammation than fibrin deposition (Figs. 1-25 and 1-26).[111]

"Real-world" studies in humans have shown an increase in the rate of late stent thrombosis, especially ≥30 days following DES placement. We have observed a similar increase in thrombosis at autopsy following deployment of DESs. To investigate the incidence of stent thrombosis (ST), we performed an autopsy study on 35 consecutive human DES cases, with a total number of 39 DESs and seven bare metal stents (BMSs) deployed. Subacute ST (SAT) was defined as development of an acute thrombus within <30 days of stent placement, whereas late ST (LST) occurred at ≥30 days. Incidence of ST was 49% in 35 cases (19 of 39). Fourteen stents showed occlusive thrombi (73%) and five were subocclusive (26%). SAT occurred in eight of 39 stents (21%) and was divided equally between Cypher and Taxus stents. LST occurred in 11 of 39 stents (28%) and was more frequent in Taxus (64%) compared to Cypher (36%) stents (Fig. 1-27). The pathological risk factors of ST were (a) strut penetration of the necrotic core (three cases); (b) hypersensitivity reaction (four cases) (Fig. 1-28); (c) focal delayed nonhealing (absence of neointima) (six cases); (d) malapposition of at least three stent struts (three cases); and (e) stenting across branch ostia of major arterial branches

or bifurcation stenting (three cases) (Fig. 1-29). Of the 19 cases with thrombi, focal absence of endothelium was observed in 13 (68%) with a mean implantation duration of 87 days (1 day minimum, 504 days maximum). Stent length was an independent predictor of ST ($r^2 = 0.21$; $p < 0.08$).[112]

The most important morphologic characteristic that defined the likelihood of presence of thrombus is delayed healing, which is common to all current FDA-approved DESs and consists of persistence of fibrin, poor coverage by endothelial cells (Fig. 1-30), and near-complete absence of smooth muscle cells at multiple stent strut sites; SMCs are usually observed at 3 to 4 months following BMS implantation. There are likely differences in healing from patient to patient, which may be determined by the extent of injury, the type of underlying plaque, and the age of the patient, and by inherent differences in healing between patients. Further, presence of nonerodible polymers and individual sensitivity to the polymer may influence the type and extent of inflammatory reaction, which may delay healing and the amount of neointimal growth. Similarly, individual sensitivity to the drug dose and type of drug will vary from patient to patient and is likely to influence healing and endothelialization. If the stent is over a plaque highly rich in lipids, this will also influence healing, as further delay is likely to occur because the drugs currently

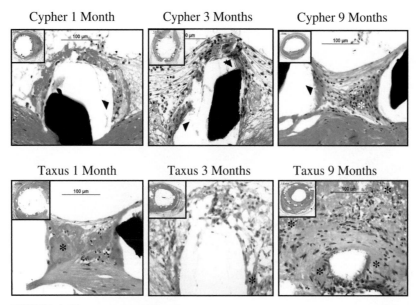

FIGURE 1-25. Photomicrographs of human coronary arteries with patent drug-eluting stents (Cypher and Taxus) removed at autopsy at various time points. The upper row shows Cypher stents and the lower row, Taxus stents at 1, 3, and 9 months following DES stent placement. The Cypher stent at 1 month shows a fibrin-rich thrombus surrounding stent struts with a few inflammatory cells, where as the Taxus stent shows a greater amount of fibrin (*asterisk*) and fewer inflammatory cells. However, at 3 months the Cypher stent shows greater giant cell (*arrowheads*) reaction but less persistence of fibrin than the Taxus stent. The Taxus stent is also surrounded by inflammatory cells; however, the thrombus is greater than with Cypher stent. Both stents show focal eosinophilic infiltrate. By 9 months both stents remain unhealed and there is persistence of fibrin (*asterisks*), which is significantly greater in the Taxus stent than in the Cypher, and there is also greater neointimal formation consisting of smooth muscle cells in a proteoglycan matrix. Both stents show focal areas of lack of endothelium over stent struts. (Finn A, et al. Beyond late loss: importance of arterial healing. Submitted for publication.)

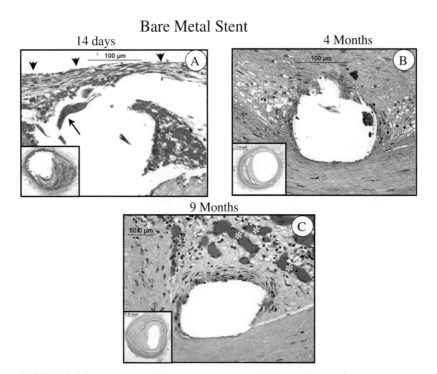

FIGURE 1-26. Digital images of bare metal stents implanted in human atherosclerotic coronary arteries at 14 days and 4 and 9 months. **A:** At 14 days the stent is surrounded by an organizing fibrin (*asterisks*) thrombus with mild inflammation (giant cell, *arrow*) and the luminal smooth muscle cells in a proteoglycan matrix (*arrowheads*). **B:** At 4 months, stent struts are fully covered by smooth muscle cells and the lumen is fully endothelialized. There is absence of fibrin, and few inflammatory cells are seen surrounding the stent struts. **C:** By 9 months, the lumen is 40% narrowed in diameter by smooth muscle cells in a proteoglycan matrix; the stent struts are surrounded by chronic inflammatory cells with extensive angiogenesis (*asterisks*). (Finn A, et al. Beyond late loss: importance of arterial healing. Submitted for publication.)

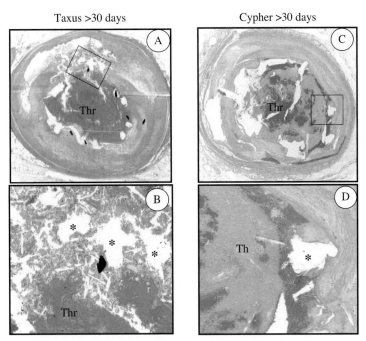

FIGURE 1-27. Late stent thrombosis attributed to drug-eluting Cypher and Taxus stents. Low-power **(A,B)** and higher power **(C,D)** views of Taxus and Cypher stents, respectively, from separate patients who came to autopsy. **A:** The Taxus stent in the left panel is from a 47-year-old man with DES deployed in the left anterior descending (LAD) coronary artery for acute myocardial infarction (AMI). The individual died 41 days postimplantation with an occlusive thrombus (*Thr*) localized to the stented segment. **B:** A higher power represented by the region in the black box in **(A)** Note prolapsed necrotic core material in the central lumen intermingled with the occlusive thrombus. **C:** An occlusive thrombus in a Cypher stent deployed for 38 days for an AMI. The patient presented with a stroke while on anticoagulants (aspirin and clopidogrel) 33 days following stenting and died 5 days later. **D:** The higher power of the thrombus (*Thr*) from the boxed area in **(C)** shows the underlying stent strut (*asterisk*) with surrounding fibrin. Note the complete absence of inflammatory infiltrate. (Finn A, et al. Beyond late loss: importance of arterial healing. Submitted for publication.)

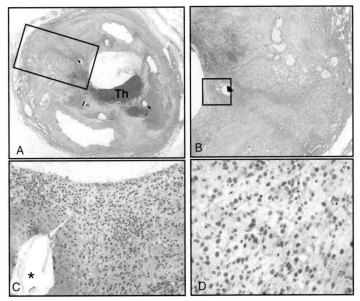

FIGURE 1-28. Localized hypersensitivity and late coronary thrombosis. Low- and high-power views of stented artery from the distal end of a Cypher stent implanted in the left circumflex coronary artery of a 58-year-old man who died of late stent thrombosis at 18 months. **A:** Focal strut malapposition with aneurismal dilatation and a nonocclusive luminal thrombosis. **B:** Higher power view of the black box in **(A),** showing marked inflammation in the intima, media, and adventitia. **C:** Extensive inflammation consisting primarily of eosinophils and lymphocytes, with focal giant-cell reaction around stent struts (*asterisk*) and surrounding polymer from boxed area in **(B).** **D:** Luna stain showing numerous eosinophils within the arterial wall. (Modified and reproduced with permission from Virmani R. *Circulation.* 2004;109:701–705.)

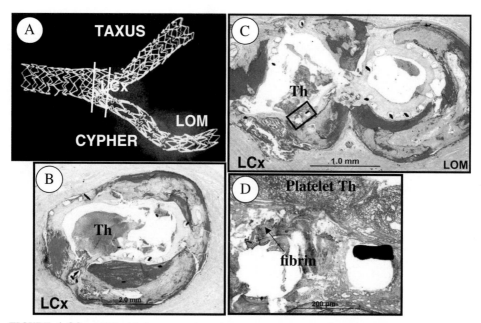

FIGURE 1-29. DES with late stent thrombosis in a bifurcation stenting. A 68-year-old black woman with history of remote coronary artery bypass surgery presented with stable angina pectoris attributed to severe stenosis of the left circumflex (LCx) and left obtuse marginal (LOM) arteries. A long Taxus stent was place in the LCx and a Cypher stent in the LOM 172 days prior to death. The patient presented with an acute myocardial infarction, and angiographic examination showed total occlusion of the LCx at the origin of the LOM secondary to a thrombus. The patient had a balloon angioplasty and the artery was reopened. The individual died 2 days later with severe pump failure. **A:** The radiograph shows well-expanded bifurcating Taxus and Cypher stents in the LCx and LOM, respectively. **B:** Note that just proximal to the bifurcation there is a thrombus in the Taxus LCx stent extending distally beyond the area of the bifurcation **(C). D:** Multiple stent struts are surrounded by a fibrin-rich thrombus while the lumen has a platelet-rich thrombus. Of note, the LOM artery with the Cypher stent **(C)** is 40% narrowed by neointimal tissue (bluish-green on Movat Pentachrome) and lacks a thrombus. (Finn A, et al. Beyond late loss: importance of arterial healing. Submitted for publication.) (See Color Fig. 1-29.)

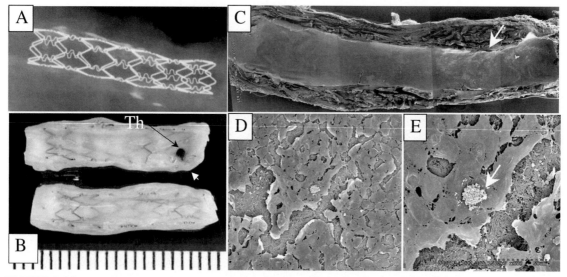

FIGURE 1-30. Human coronary pathology of a 16-month sirolimus-eluting stent. The 71-year-old woman was enrolled in a randomized study with the sirolimus (SRL)-eluting Bx Velocity balloon-expandable stent (RAVEL) Trial. **A:** Radiograph of the proximal LAD containing a well-expanded Cypher stent near a branching artery. The longitudinally cut Bx Velocity stent **(B)** has a translucent neointima and a small thrombus (*arrow*) at the distal end (at the ostium of a small side branch [*white arrowhead*]). Scanning electron microscopy of the stent surface **(C)** shows .80% endothelial coverage while focal areas lacking endothelium are seen at the distal end of the stent (*arrow*). **D,E:** endothelial cells are pavement shaped with poorly formed cell junctions and a small surface platelet aggregate [*arrow* in **(E)**]. (Modified and reproduced with permission from Guagliumi G, et al. *Circulation.* 2003; 107:1340–1341.)

in use are highly lipophilic and will be retained in tissues longer than the known release pharmacokinetics performed in normal nonatherosclerotic vessels in animals. Operator, type of stent, plaque calcification, and apposition of the stent to the arterial wall also influence blood flow turbulence and the induction of thrombosis. It is currently not possible to predict which patient is likely to develop a thrombus following DES deployment. However, in clinical studies it has been shown that withdrawal of platelet therapy is significantly associated with late stent thrombosis. Also, stent length, diabetes, renal failure, bifurcation lesions, and low ejection fraction were identified as predictors of thrombosis.[113] From our autopsy cases we have seen at least four cases of thrombosis occurring as a result of withdrawal of antiplatelet therapy. It is clear that the current recommended practice of administration of antiplatelet drugs 3 months for Cypher and 6 months for Taxus is not sufficient in all cases. To prevent stent thrombosis it is possible that prolonged antiplatelet therapy, beyond 6 months, is needed in patients at higher risk for thrombosis.

REFERENCES

1. Ganziano MJ. General considerations of cardiovascular disease. In: Zipes DP, Libby P, Bonow RO, et al., eds. *Heart Disease. A Textbook of Cardiovascular Medicine.* 7th ed. Philadelphia: Elsevier Saunders, 2005:1–19.
2. Majesky MW. Development of coronary vessels. In: Schatten GP, ed. *Developmental Vascular Biology.* San Diego: Elsevier, 2004:225–259. *Current Topics in Developmental Biology;* vol 62.
3. Bogers AJ, Gittenberger-de Groot AC, Poelmann RE, et al. Development of the origin of the coronary arteries, a matter of ingrowth or outgrowth? *Anat Embryol (Berl).* 1989;180:437–441.
4. Mintz GS, Kent KM, Pichard AD, et al. Contribution of inadequate arterial remodeling to the development of focal coronary artery stenoses. An intravascular ultrasound study. *Circulation.* 1997;95:1791–1798.
5. Nishimura RA, Edwards WD, Warnes CA, et al. Intravascular ultrasound imaging: in vitro validation and pathologic correlation. *J Am Coll Cardiol.* 1990;16:145–154.
6. Nishioka T, Amanullah AM, Luo H, et al. Clinical validation of intravascular ultrasound imaging for assessment of coronary stenosis severity: comparison with stress myocardial perfusion imaging. *J Am Coll Cardiol.* 1999;33:1870–1878.
7. Pasterkamp G, Wensing PJ, Post MJ, et al. Paradoxical arterial wall shrinkage may contribute to luminal narrowing of human atherosclerotic femoral arteries. *Circulation.* 1995;91:1444–1449.
8. Taylor AJ, Burke AP, Farb A, et al. Arterial remodeling in the left coronary system: the role of high-density lipoprotein cholesterol. *J Am Coll Cardiol.* 1999;34:760–767.
9. Glagov S, Weisenberg E, Zarins CK, et al. Compensatory enlargement of human atherosclerotic coronary arteries. *N Engl J Med.* 1987;316:1371–1375.
10. Burke AP, Virmani R, Galis Z, et al. 34th Bethesda Conference: Task force #2—What is the pathologic basis for new atherosclerosis imaging techniques? *J Am Coll Cardiol.* 2003;41:1874–1886.
11. Schwartz SM, deBlois D, O'Brien ER. The intima. Soil for atherosclerosis and restenosis. *Circ Res.* 1995;77:445–465.
12. Tabas I, Marathe S, Keesler GA, et al. Evidence that the initial up-regulation of phosphatidylcholine biosynthesis in free cholesterol-loaded macrophages is an adaptive response that prevents cholesterol-induced cellular necrosis. Proposed role of an eventual failure of this response in foam cell necrosis in advanced atherosclerosis. *J Biol Chem.* 1996;271:22773–22781.
13. Stary HC, Chandler AB, Glagov S, et al. A definition of initial, fatty streak, and intermediate lesions of atherosclerosis. A report from the Committee on Vascular Lesions of the Council on Arteriosclerosis, American Heart Association. *Circulation.* 1994;89:2462–2478.
14. McGill HC, Jr., McMahan CA, Herderick EE, et al. Origin of atherosclerosis in childhood and adolescence. *Am J Clin Nutr.* 2000;72:1307S–1315S.
15. Virmani R, Kolodgie FD, Burke AP, et al. Lessons from sudden coronary death: a comprehensive morphological classification scheme for atherosclerotic lesions. *Arterioscl Thromb Vasc Biol.* 2000;20:1262–1275.
16. Kockx MM, De Meyer GR, Bortier H, et al. Luminal foam cell accumulation is associated with smooth muscle cell death in the intimal thickening of human saphenous vein grafts. *Circulation.* 1996;94:1255–1262.
17. Tanimura A, McGregor DH, Anderson HC. Calcification in atherosclerosis. I. Human studies. *J Exp Pathol.* 1986;2:261–273.
18. Hoff HF, Heideman CL, Gaubatz JW, et al. Correlation of apolipoprotein B retention with the structure of atherosclerotic plaques from human aortas. Apolipoprotein B retention in the grossly normal and atherosclerotic human aorta. *Lab Invest.* 1978;38:560–567.
19. Radhakrishnamurthy B, Tracy RE, Dalferes ER, Jr., et al. Proteoglycans in human coronary arteriosclerotic lesions. *Exp Mol Pathol.* 1998;65:1–8.
20. Hansson GK. Immune mechanisms in atherosclerosis. *Arterioscl Thromb Vasc Biol.* 2001;21:1876–1890.
21. Libby P, Hansson GK, Schonbeck U, et al. Inflammation in atherosclerosis. *Nature.* 2002;420:868–874.
22. Felton CV, Crook D, Davies MJ, et al. Relation of plaque lipid composition and morphology to the stability of human aortic plaques. *Arterioscl Thromb Vasc Biol.* 1997;17:1337–1345.
23. Kolodgie FD, Gold HK, Burke AP, et al. Intraplaque hemorrhage and progression of coronary atheroma. *N Engl J Med.* 2003;349:2316–2325.
24. Burke AP, Farb A, Malcom GT, et al. Coronary risk factors and plaque morphology in men with coronary disease who died suddenly. *N Engl J Med.* 1997;336:1276–1282.
25. Kolodgie FD, Burke AP, Farb A, et al. The thin-cap fibroatheroma: a type of vulnerable plaque: the major precursor lesion to acute coronary syndromes. *Curr Opin Cardiol.* 2001;16:285–292.
26. Farb A, Burke AP, Tang AL, et al. Coronary plaque erosion without rupture into a lipid core. A frequent cause of coronary thrombosis in sudden coronary death. *Circulation.* 1996;93:1354–1363.
27. Patterson JC. The reaction of the arterial wall to intramural hemorrhage. Paper presented at: Symposium of Atherosclerosis, 1954; Washington, DC.
28. Wartman WB. Occlusion of the coronary arteries by hemorrhage into their walls. *Am Heart J.* 1938;15:459–470.
29. Winternitz MC, Thomas RM, Le Compte PM. Thrombosis. In: Thomas CC, ed. *The Biology of Atherosclerosis.* Springfield, IL: 1938:94–103.
30. Virmani R, Kolodgie FD, Burke AP, et al. Atherosclerotic plaque progression and vulnerability to rupture: angiogenesis as a source of intraplaque hemorrhage. *Arterioscl Thromb Vasc Biol.* 2005;25:2054–2061.
31. Chu B, Kampschulte A, Ferguson MS, et al. Hemorrhage in the atherosclerotic carotid plaque: a high-resolution MRI study. *Stroke.* 2004;35:1079–1084.
32. Guthrie RB, Vlodaver Z, Nicoloff DM, et al. Pathology of stable and unstable angina pectoris. *Circulation.* 1975;51:1059–1063.
33. Hangartner JR, Charleston AJ, Davies MJ, et al. Morphological characteristics of clinically significant coronary artery stenosis in stable angina. *Br Heart J.* 1986;56:501–508.
34. Levin DC, Fallon JT. Significance of the angiographic morphology of localized coronary stenoses: histopathologic correlations. *Circulation.* 1982;66:316–320.
35. Ambrose JA, Winters SL, Stern A, et al. Angiographic morphology and the pathogenesis of unstable angina pectoris. *J Am Coll Cardiol.* 1985;5:609–616.
36. Chester MR, Chen L, Tousoulis D, et al. Differential progression of complex and smooth stenoses within the same coronary tree in men with stable coronary artery disease. *J Am Coll Cardiol.* 1995;25:837–842.
37. Burke AP, Kolodgie FD, Farb A, et al. Healed plaque ruptures and sudden coronary death: evidence that subclinical rupture has a role in plaque progression. *Circulation.* 2001;103:934–940.
38. Saltzman AJ, Waxman S. Angioscopy and ischemic heart disease. *Curr Opin Cardiol.* 2002;17:633–637.
39. Davies MJ, Fulton WF, Robertson WB. The relation of coronary thrombosis to ischaemic myocardial necrosis. *J Pathol.* 1979;127:99–110.
40. Falk E. Plaque rupture with severe pre-existing stenosis precipitating coronary thrombosis. Characteristics of coronary atherosclerotic plaques underlying fatal occlusive thrombi. *Br Heart J.* 1983;50:127–134.
41. Falk E, Fernandez-Ortiz A. Role of thrombosis in atherosclerosis and its complications. *Am J Cardiol.* 1995;75:3B–11B.
42. Kragel AH, Gertz SD, Roberts WC. Morphologic comparison of frequency and types of acute lesions in the major epicardial coronary arteries in unstable angina pectoris, sudden coronary death and acute myocardial infarction. *J Am Coll Cardiol.* 1991;18:801–808.
43. Davies MJ, Bland JM, Hangartner JR, et al. Factors influencing the presence or absence of acute coronary artery thrombi in sudden ischaemic death. *Eur Heart J.* 1989;10:203–208.
44. Arbustini E, Dal Bello B, Morbini P, et al. Plaque erosion is a major substrate for coronary thrombosis in acute myocardial infarction. *Heart.* 1999;82:269–272.
45. Hong MK, Park SW, Lee CW, et al. Prospective comparison of coronary artery remodeling between acute coronary syndrome and stable angina in single-vessel disease: correlation between C-reactive protein and extent of arterial remodeling. *Clin Cardiol.* 2003;26:169–172.
46. Ehara S, Kobayashi Y, Yoshiyama M, et al. Spotty calcification typifies the culprit plaque in patients with acute myocardial infarction: an intravascular ultrasound study. *Circulation.* 2004;110:3424-3429.
47. Maehara A, Mintz GS, Bui AB, et al. Morphologic and angiographic features of coronary plaque rupture detected by intravascular ultrasound. *J Am Coll Cardiol.* 2002;40:904–910.
48. Hong MK, Mintz GS, Lee CW, et al. The site of plaque rupture in native coronary arteries: a three-vessel intravascular ultrasound analysis. *J Am Coll Cardiol.* 2005;46:261–265.
49. Amos AF, McCarty DJ, Zimmet P. The rising global burden of diabetes and its complications: estimates and projections to the year 2010. *Diabet Med.* 1997;14(suppl 5):S1–85.
50. Mokdad AH, Bowman BA, Ford ES, et al. The continuing epidemics of obesity and diabetes in the United States. *JAMA.* 2001;286:1195–1200.
51. Silva JA, Escobar A, Collins TJ, et al. Unstable angina. A comparison of angioscopic findings between diabetic and nondiabetic patients. *Circulation.* 1995;92:1731–1736.
52. Schurgin S, Rich S, Mazzone T. Increased prevalence of significant coronary artery calcification in patients with diabetes. *Diabetes Care.* 2001;24:335–338.
53. Kornowski R, Mintz GS, Lansky AJ, et al. Paradoxic decreases in atherosclerotic plaque mass in insulin-treated diabetic patients. *Am J Cardiol.* 1998;81:1298–1304.
54. Moreno PR, Murcia AM, Palacios IF, et al. Coronary composition and macrophage infiltration in atherectomy specimens from patients with diabetes mellitus. *Circulation.* 2000;102:2180–2184.
55. Creager MA, Luscher TF, Cosentino F, et al. Diabetes and vascular disease: pathophysiology, clinical consequences, and medical therapy: Part I. *Circulation.* 2003;108:1527–1532.
56. Burke AP, Kolodgie FD, Zieske A, et al. Morphologic findings of coronary atherosclerotic plaques in diabetics: a postmortem study. *Arterioscl Thromb Vasc Biol.* 2004;24:1266–1271.

57. Mielke CH, Shields JP, Broemeling LD. Coronary artery calcium, coronary artery disease, and diabetes. *Diabetes Res Clin Pract.* 2001;53:55–61.

58. Takazawa K, Hosoda Y, Yamamoto T, et al. Coronary artery bypass grafting. Late result of actual 10-years follow-up in 376 patients. *Jpn J Thorac Cardiovasc Surg.* 1999;47:110–115.

59. van Brussel BL, Plokker HW, Voors AA, et al. Multivariate risk factor analysis of clinical outcome 15 years after venous coronary artery bypass graft surgery. *Eur Heart J.* 1995;16:1200–1206.

60. Gyongyosi M, Yang P, Hassan A, et al. Coronary risk factors influence plaque morphology in patients with unstable angina. *Coron Artery Dis.* 1999;10:211–219.

61. Weissman NJ, Sheris SJ, Chari R, et al. Intravascular ultrasonic analysis of plaque characteristics associated with coronary artery remodeling. *Am J Cardiol.* 1999;84:37–40.

62. Burke AP, Kolodgie FD, Farb A, et al. Morphological predictors of arterial remodeling in coronary atherosclerosis. *Circulation.* 2002;105:297–303.

63. Levin L, Tomer Y. The etiology of autoimmune diabetes and thyroiditis: evidence for common genetic susceptibility. *Autoimmun Rev.* 2003;2:377–386.

64. Cipollone F, Iezzi A, Fazia M, et al. The receptor RAGE as a progression factor amplifying arachidonate-dependent inflammatory and proteolytic response in human atherosclerotic plaques: role of glycemic control. *Circulation.* 2003;108:1070–1077.

65. Bucciarelli LG, Wendt T, Qu W, et al. RAGE blockade stabilizes established atherosclerosis in diabetic apolipoprotein E-null mice. *Circulation.* 2002;106:2827–2835.

66. Cipollone F, Fazia M, Iezzi A, et al. Balance between PGD synthase and PGE synthase is a major determinant of atherosclerotic plaque instability in humans. *Arterioscl Thromb Vasc Biol.* 2004;24:1259–1265.

67. Hofmann MA, Drury S, Fu C, et al. RAGE mediates a novel proinflammatory axis: a central cell surface receptor for S100/calgranulin polypeptides. *Cell.* 1999;97:889–901.

68. Lugering N, Stoll R, Schmid KW, et al. The myeloic related protein MRP8/14 (27E10 antigen)—usefulness as a potential marker for disease activity in ulcerative colitis and putative biological function. *Eur J Clin Invest.* 1995;25:659–664.

69. Donato R. S100: a multigenic family of calcium-modulated proteins of the Efhand type with intracellular and extracellular functional roles. *Int J Biochem Cell Biol.* 2001;33:637–668.

70. Nobuyoshi M, Kimura T, Nosaka H, et al. Restenosis after successful percutaneous transluminal coronary angioplasty: serial angiographic follow-up of 229 patients. *J Am Coll Cardiol.* 1988;12:616–623.

71. Sangiorgi G, Taylor AJ, Farb A, et al. Histopathology of postpercutaneous transluminal coronary angioplasty remodeling in human coronary arteries. *Am Heart J.* 1999;138:681–687.

72. Serruys PW, de Jaegere P, Kiemeneij F, et al. A comparison of balloon-expandable-stent implantation with balloon angioplasty in patients with coronary artery disease. Benestent Study Group. *N Engl J Med.* 1994;331:489–495.

73. Farb A, Sangiorgi G, Carter AJ, et al. Pathology of acute and chronic coronary stenting in humans. *Circulation.* 1999;99:44–52.

74. Farb A, Weber DK, Kolodgie FD, et al. Morphological predictors of restenosis after coronary stenting in humans. *Circulation.* 2002;105:2974–2980.

75. Kuroda N, Kobayashi Y, Nameki M, et al. Intimal hyperplasia regression from 6 to 12 months after stenting. *Am J Cardiol.* 2002;89:869–872.

76. Carter AJ, Laird JR, Farb A, et al. Morphologic characteristics of lesion formation and time course of smooth muscle cell proliferation in a porcine proliferative restenosis model. *J Am Coll Cardiol.* 1994;24:1398–1405.

77. Taylor AJ, Gorman PD, Kenwood B, et al. A comparison of four stent designs on arterial injury, cellular proliferation, neointima formation, and arterial dimensions in an experimental porcine model. *Catheter Cardiovasc Intervent.* 2001;53:420–425.

78. Farb A, Kolodgie FD, Hwang JY, et al. Extracellular matrix changes in stented human coronary arteries. *Circulation.* 2004;110:940–947.

79. O'Brien ER, Alpers CE, Stewart DK, et al. Proliferation in primary and restenotic coronary atherectomy tissue. Implications for antiproliferative therapy. *Circ Res.* 1993;73:223–231.

80. Yao F, Visovatti S, Johnson CS, et al. Age and growth factors in porcine full-thickness wound healing. *Wound Repair Regen.* 2001;9:371–377.

81. Forrester JS, Fishbein M, Helfant R, et al. A paradigm for restenosis based on cell biology: clues for the development of new preventive therapies. *J Am Coll Cardiol.* 1991;17:758–769.

82. Schwartz RS, Huber KC, Murphy JG, et al. Restenosis and the proportional neointimal response to coronary artery injury: results in a porcine model. *J Am Coll Cardiol.* 1992;19:267–274.

83. Carter AJ, Laird JR, Kufs WM, et al. Coronary stenting with a novel stainless steel balloon-expandable stent: determinants of neointimal formation and changes in arterial geometry after placement in an atherosclerotic model. *J Am Coll Cardiol.* 1996;27:1270–1277.

84. Welt FG, Rogers C. Inflammation and restenosis in the stent era. *Arterioscl Thromb Vasc Biol.* 2002;22:1769–1776.

85. Donners MM, Daemen MJ, Cleutjens KB, et al. Inflammation and restenosis: implications for therapy. *Ann Med.* 2003;35:523–531.

86. Patterson C, Stouffer GA, Madamanchi N, et al. New tricks for old dogs: nonthrombotic effects of thrombin in vessel wall biology. *Circ Res.* 2001;88:987–997.

87. Galis ZS, Khatri JJ. Matrix metalloproteinases in vascular remodeling and atherogenesis: the good, the bad, and the ugly. *Circ Res.* 2002;90:251–262.

88. Baker AH, Edwards DR, Murphy G. Metalloproteinase inhibitors: biological actions and therapeutic opportunities. *J Cell Sci.* 2002;115:3719–3727.

89. Fay WP. Plasminogen activator inhibitor 1, fibrin, and the vascular response to injury. *Trends Cardiovasc Med.* 2004;14:196–202.

90. Garcia-Touchard A, Henry TD, Sangiorgi G, et al. Extracellular proteases in atherosclerosis and restenosis. *Arterioscl Thromb Vasc Biol.* 2005;25:1119–1127.

91. Carter AJ, Scott D, Bailey L, et al. Dose-response effects of ^{32}P radioactive stents in an atherosclerotic porcine coronary model. *Circulation.* 1999;100:1548–1554.

92. Coussement PK, Stella P, Vanbilloen H, et al. Intracoronary beta-radiation of de novo coronary lesions using a ^{186}Re liquid-filled balloon system: six-month results from a clinical feasibility study. *Catheter Cardiovasc Intervent.* 2002;55:28–36.

93. Farb A, Shroff S, John M, et al. Late arterial responses (6 and 12 months) after ^{32}P beta-emitting stent placement: sustained intimal suppression with incomplete healing. *Circulation.* 2001;103:1912–1919.

94. Costa MA, Sabate M, van der Giessen WJ, et al. Late coronary occlusion after intracoronary brachytherapy. *Circulation.* 1999;100:789–792.

95. Kaluza GL, Raizner AE, Mazur W, et al. Long-term effects of intracoronary beta radiation in balloon- and stent-injured porcine coronary arteries. *Circulation.* 2001;103:2108–2113.

96. Waksman R, Bhargava B, Mintz GS, et al. Late total occlusion after intracoronary brachytherapy for patients with in-stent restenosis. *J Am Coll Cardiol.* 2000;36:65–68.

97. Teirstein PS. Living the dream of no restenosis. *Circulation.* 2001;104:1996–1998.

98. Kay IP, Wardeh AJ, Kozuma K, et al. Radioactive stents delay but do not prevent in-stent neointimal hyperplasia. *Circulation.* 2001;103:14–17.

99. Moses JW, Leon MB, Popma JJ, et al. Sirolimus-eluting stents versus standard stents in patients with stenosis in a native coronary artery. *N Engl J Med.* 2003;349:1315–1323.

100. Stone GW, Ellis SG, Cox DA, et al. One-year clinical results with the slow-release, polymer-based, paclitaxel-eluting TAXUS stent: the TAXUS-IV trial. *Circulation.* 2004;109:1942–1947.

101. Kastrati A, Dibra A, Eberle S, et al. Sirolimus-eluting stents vs. paclitaxel-eluting stents in patients with coronary artery disease: meta-analysis of randomized trials. *JAMA.* 2005;294:819–825.

102. Klugherz BD, Llanos G, Lieuallen W, et al. Twenty-eight-day efficacy and pharmacokinetics of the sirolimus-eluting stent. *Coron Artery Dis.* 2002;13:183–188.

103. Suzuki T, Kopia G, Hayashi S, et al. Stent-based delivery of sirolimus reduces neointimal formation in a porcine coronary model. *Circulation.* 2001;104:1188–1193.

104. Carter AJ, Aggarwal M, Kopia GA, et al. Long-term effects of polymer-based, slow-release, sirolimus-eluting stents in a porcine coronary model. *Cardiovasc Res.* 2004;63:617–624.

105. Drachman DE, Edelman ER, Seifert P, et al. Neointimal thickening after stent delivery of paclitaxel: change in composition and arrest of growth over six months. *J Am Coll Cardiol.* 2000;36:2325–2332.

106. Farb A, Heller PF, Shroff S, et al. Pathological analysis of local delivery of paclitaxel via a polymer-coated stent. *Circulation.* 2001;104:473–479.

107. Heldman AW, Cheng L, Jenkins GM, et al. Paclitaxel stent coating inhibits neointimal hyperplasia at 4 weeks in a porcine model of coronary restenosis. *Circulation.* 2001;103:2289–2295.

108. Goode J. *FDA Summary: Taxus Express Paclitaxel-Eluting Monorail and Over-the-Wire Coronary Stent Systems: PMA for Marking Approval.* Washington, DC: US Food and Drug Administration; 2003:1–43.

109. Finn AV, Kolodgie FD, Harnek J, et al. Differential response of delayed healing and persistent inflammation at sites of overlapping sirolimus- or paclitaxel-eluting stents. *Circulation.* 2005;112:270–278.

110. Bayes-Genis A, Camrud AR, Jorgenson M, et al. Pressure rinsing of coronary stents immediately before implantation reduces inflammation and neointimal hyperplasia. *J Am Coll Cardiol.* 2001;38:562–568.

111. Farb A, Burke AP, Kolodgie FD, et al. Pathological mechanisms of fatal late coronary stent thrombosis in humans. *Circulation.* 2003;108:1701–1706.

112. Joner M, Finn AV, Farb A, et al. Pathology of drug eluting stents: delayed healing and thrombosis. *J Am Coll Cardiol.* 2006. In press.

113. Iakovou I, Schmidt T, Bonizzoni E, et al. Incidence, predictors, and outcome of thrombosis after successful implantation of drug-eluting stents. *JAMA.* 2005;293:2126–2130.

Axel R. Pries
Ivo Buschmann
Helmut Habazettl

CHAPTER **2**

Key Issues of Vascular Pathophysiology

HEMODYNAMIC RELEVANCE OF STENOSES

HEMODYNAMIC RELATIONS

Atherosclerotic lesions in conduit arteries may lead to a significant reduction in tissue perfusion, and consequently in the availability of oxygen. However, for ischemia to occur, the reduction in vessel diameter must be quite substantial.[1-3]

The hemodynamic consequences of vascular stenoses can be predicted using the laws of Hagen-Poiseuille (also called Poiseuille's law) and Kirchhoff. According to Hagen and Poiseuille, the flow (Q) through a tube with a given length is proportional to the fourth power of the tube radius (r):

$$Q = r^4/l \times \Delta P/\eta \times \pi/8$$

where l is the tube length, ΔP the driving pressure drop across the tube, and η the viscosity of the fluid. Equivalent is a consideration of flow resistance $R = \Delta P/Q$:

$$R = l/r^4 \times \eta \times 8/\pi$$

Thus, a decrease in radius or diameter by 50% will lead to flow reduction of nearly 94% (to 1/16) or an increase in flow resistance by 1500%. However, in contrast to vascular tone, stenoses usually only affect shorter sections of conductance vessels. For serial arrangements of vessels or vascular sections, Kirchoff's second law indicates that the summed resistance of the serial segments (R_i) gives the total resistance of the respective flow pathway (R_Σ):

$$R_\Sigma = R_1 + R_2 + \cdots + R_i$$

The pressure drop across a given section of such a flow pathway (relative to the overall pressure drop) correlates to the share of flow resistance in the respective section:

$$\Delta P_i/\Delta P \sim R_i/R_\Sigma$$

The changes in flow resistance and perfusion due to arterial stenoses are accompanied by changes in intraluminal pressure (Fig. 2-1). In healthy vascular beds, the majority of the flow resistance and thus the main pressure drop resides in the smallest arteries and arterioles (see Fig. 2-2). During development of a severe stenosis, the resistance of the affected section and the pressure drop across it (transstenotic pressure gradient) may become significant. In healthy normal vasculature, the pressure drop from large central arteries to organ arteries is very low, irrespective of the distances traveled to the particular organ. The same is true for the venous drainage with an inverse pressure gradient. As first reported by Poiseuille,[4,5] the main pressure drop and flow resistance reside in the vessels of the terminal vascular beds.[6,7] Here they are located predominantly in small arteries and arterioles. For the coronary circulation, the pressure drop based on in vivo measurements is shown in Figure 2-2 for the resting state and after pharmacological dilatation.[8,9]

On maximal loading or maximal dilatation, the flow resistance in the microcirculation decreases, substantially increasing the relative importance of flow resistance in the larger feeding and draining vessels. This interplay between increasing conduit vessel resistance with increasing severity of a stenosis and concomitantly decreasing peripheral resistance is evidenced by corresponding pressure changes along the vascular bed toward the periphery.

27

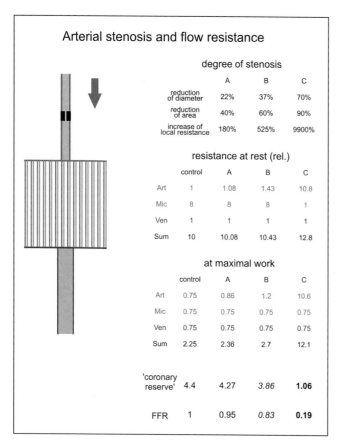

FIGURE 2-1. Distribution of resistance to blood flow for a simplified vascular bed (*left*) which may represent, for example, the coronary vascular bed. An artery (*Art*) supplies the terminal vascular bed and microcirculation (*Mic*), which is drained into a vein (*Ven*). Three different stages (*A,B,C*) of a single arterial stenosis, extending over 10% of the arterial length, are considered (*upper right table*). The tables give the relative flow resistance for the different vascular compartments for control conditions and for maximal loading. At rest, an increase in arterial resistance due to stenosis can be compensated by vasodilatation in the smaller vessels. Thus only severe stenoses lead to an increase in overall resistance. In this condition, no further dilation of the peripheral vascular bed during loading is possible, and the flow at maximal loading (or during pharmacological dilatation) is not significantly higher than in the resting state. This is reflected in the coronary reserve (flow at maximal loading/resting flow or resting resistance/resistance at maximal loading) which is close to 1, and the low values of fractional flow reserve (FFR, the ratio of the flow at maximal loading with stenosis to the flow at maximal loading without stenosis).

The presence of an arterial stenosis affects the local pressure and pressure profile along the vascular bed well before significant changes in perfusion are observed. Because of the compensatory dilatation in the peripheral small arteries and arterioles, overall resistance of the subtended vascular bed can be maintained at a near normal level for a prolonged period of time. However, this compensation is associated with a shift in the relative contribution to resistance and thus of local pressure drop from the microcirculation to the stenotic region. This leads to lower poststenotic pressure levels, even at resting conditions.

SEVERITY OF STENOSES

According to the hemodynamic relations described earlier, pressure measurements exhibit a higher sensitivity than meas-

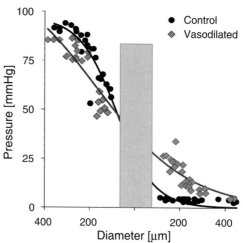

FIGURE 2-2. Intraluminal pressure drops along the vascular tree most prominently in small-resistance arteries <200 μm in diameter and in arterioles. In this example, the pressure distribution was measured in the coronary circulation during control conditions and after maximal vasodilatation with dipyridamole. Vasodilatation redistributes relative resistance away from small-resistance arteries and arterioles, resulting in pressure increase in precapillary arterioles, capillaries, and venules. The *shaded area* represents the segment of smallest vessels where little direct evidence is available, because of methodological difficulties in investigating this segment of the coronary microcirculation. (Adapted from Chilian WM, Layne SM, Klausner EC, et al. Redistribution of coronary microvascular resistance produced by dipyridamole. *Am J Physiol.* 1989;256: H383–H390.)

urements of perfusion in determining stenoses, especially those of low to medium severity (Fig. 2-3). Accordingly, the pressure gradient across a stenosis measured in the catheterization laboratory with a pressure wire may be used to assess the hemodynamic severity of a stenosis. In clinical practice, this relation is utilized, for instance, in the determination of fractional flow reserve (FFR)[10,11] By definition, the FFR represents the ratio of maximal myocardial flow in a patient with a suspected stenosis to the hypothetical maximal myocardial flow in the absence of a stenosis. FFR is estimated as the ratio of distal coronary pressure to aortic pressure obtained simultaneously during maximal vasodilatation. This calculation assumes that the vessel section investigated does not exhibit a significant pressure drop if no stenosis is present and that the venous outflow pressure is about zero.

If, for example, the pressure across a stenotic segment declines by 50% of the aortic pressure (e.g., pressure distal to the stenosis would equal 50 mm Hg at an aortic pressure of 100 mm Hg), this segment would contribute 50% to the total resistance, R_{Σ}. Thus, without the stenosis, R_{Σ} would be halved and flow would be doubled, and the corresponding FFR is resulting in FFR of 0.5 (50 mm Hg/100 mm Hg). It has been shown that for a normal myocardial function, an FFR value of 0.75 represents a valid cutoff between stenoses without (FFR >0.75) and those associated with (FFR <0.75) myocardial ischemia.

For clinical use, determination of FFR can be complemented by the measurement of the coronary flow reserve (CFR, or "flow reserve" in other organs), which is calculated by dividing the antegrade flow at maximal loading or on maximal dilatation by the antegrade flow under baseline resting conditions.

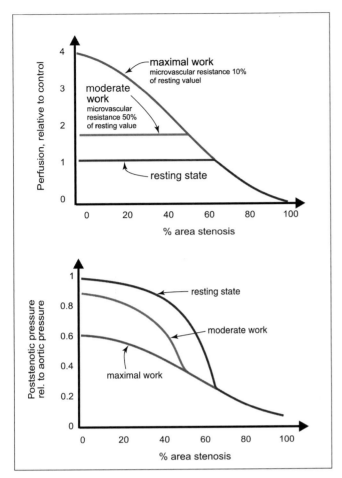

FIGURE 2-3. Perfusion and poststenotic pressure estimated for a hypothetical coronary vascular bed for resting control conditions (*lower line*), and for moderate (*upper line*) and maximal (*oblique line*) loading. At rest, the effect of a stenosis on perfusion (*upper panel*) is counteracted by a vasodilatation of small-resistance arteries and arterioles distal to the stenosis. Above a certain level of stenosis (here, reduction of vessel cross section by ~63%), vasodilatation is maximal and resting blood flow is compromised. During loading, the decrease of peripheral resistance allows a maximal increase in perfusion to about 4 times the resting value in the absence of stenosis (coronary flow reserve). In the presence of stenosis, the dilatory capacity is (to varying degrees) already used under control conditions at the expense of the possible blood flow increase during loading. Thus, the effect of stenosis on perfusion may be masked by compensatory distal dilatation and can be uncovered during loading. In contrast, the presence of a stenosis even of lower grades is evidenced by a decline in poststenotic pressure levels (*lower panel*). The pressure drop across the stenosis and thus the poststenotic pressure reflects the increase in proximal resistance due to the stenosis as well as the decrease of distal resistance due to compensatory dilatation.

Whereas FFR is specific to the hemodynamic effects of a stenosis, CFR includes effects of flow resistance in all sections of the vascular bed, including the microvascular bed. Therefore, a successful endovascular intervention should return FFR to near 1, and the measurement of FFR allows the effect of individual measures to be judged. On the other hand, FFR is insensitive to problems downstream from the investigated section of the vasculature. Abnormal CFR may be caused, in part or in total, by increased flow resistance in the microvascular compartment. The microvascular contribution would not be addressed by the

intervention and, even at normalized FFR values, symptoms may remain.

Because of the fourth-power relation between diameter and flow resistance or pressure drop, measurement errors in diameter may lead to much larger errors in estimating the hemodynamic relevance of a stenosis from vascular images. Thus, such estimates bear a much higher degree of uncertainty than direct measurement of FFR and CFR. The possibility of substantial errors is especially high if vessel projections in only one direction are considered for calculations, assuming a circular cross-sectional vessel area. Better results may be expected from tomographic techniques, which allow a 3D reconstruction of the target vessel section. This spatial target vessel reconstruction may then serve as a template for flow resistance estimation using fluid dynamic simulation software.

Figure 2-4 schematically shows the dependence of functional impairment with respect to relative perfusion reserve on the severity of arterial stenoses.[12] Two parameters are given, the relative perfusion reserve, that is, the flow reserve in the presence of a stenosis divided by that in the absence of the stenosis of the same vessel or in a different vascular bed used as a healthy unaffected control region,[12] and the FFR.[11] Significant reductions in relative perfusion reserve are observed if vessel diameter is decreased by more than about 40% or cross-sectional luminal area by more than about 60% in this model.

MICROVASCULAR COMPENSATION

As shown in Figure 2-1, the decrease in cross-sectional luminal area caused by an arterial stenosis must be about 90% for it to result in the amount of increase in flow resistance necessary to cause reduced perfusion at rest. The main explanation for this long latency before a stenosis becomes hemodynamically significant at rest is the relatively low contribution of larger conduit arteries to overall flow resistance. Depending on the respective organ, about 5% to 15% of overall flow resistance may reside in arterial vessels with diameters ≥ 500 μm. Therefore, only severe narrowing of the conduit vessels will significantly increase the overall organ resistance to eventually reduce the flow.

In addition, compensatory vasodilatation in the terminal vascular bed, and specifically in the microcirculation, may mask the hemodynamic effects of a stenosis at rest. For the highest degree of stenosis in Figure 2-1, dilatation in the microvascular compartment can almost compensate even a 90% reduction in cross-sectional area in the supplying artery. Obviously, whether dilatation of small arteries and arterioles can provide this compensation depends on the resting tone in the specific vascular bed. Therefore, the impact of an arterial stenosis of a given degree will vary in different organs. Organs with a high flow reserve, such as the heart and skeletal muscle, have a high resting vascular tone. Thus, in these organs, even severe stenoses may not lead to symptoms at rest because the range for compensation is large, due to the ability of the resistance vessels to reduce the tone, that is, vasodilate. In contrast, perfusion in the kidney is near maximal at rest, indicating a low vascular tone, and the possibility for vascular compensation in the resistance compartment very limited. Typically, the flow reserve range is about 4 to 5 in the heart, up to 20 in the skeletal muscle, but only about 2 in the kidney.

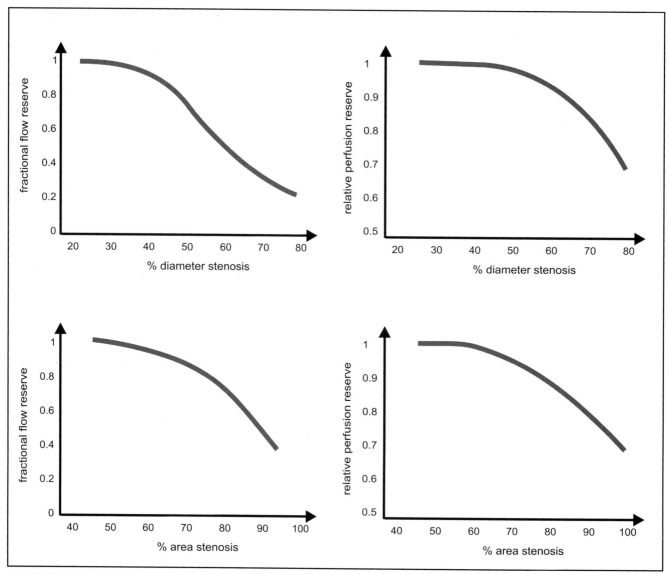

FIGURE 2-4. Fractional flow reserve, that is, the ratio of flow at maximal loading with stenosis to the flow at maximal loading without stenosis, and relative perfusion reserve, which is the ratio of blood flow at maximal loading or dilatation in regions affected by a stenosis to blood flow in unaffected control region, as a function of severity of an arterial stenosis according to results of angiographic (*upper left panel;* Bartunek J, Sys SU, Heyndrickx GR, et al. Quantitative coronary angiography in predicting functional significance of stenoses in an unselected patient cohort. *J Am Coll Cardiol.* 1995;26:328–334.), intravascular ultrasound (*lower left panel;* Briguori C, Anzuini A, Airoldi F, et al. Intravascular ultrasound criteria for the assessment of the functional significance of intermediate coronary artery stenoses and comparison with fractional flow reserve. *Am J Cardiol.* 2001;87:136–141.) and PET (*right panels;* Goldstein RA, Kirkeeide RL, Demer LL, et al. Relation between geometric dimensions of coronary artery stenoses and myocardial perfusion reserve in man. *J Clin Invest.* 1987;79:1473–1478) studies.

During exertion, the regulatory vessels of the terminal vascular bed and microcirculation are already dilated under normal physiological conditions without arterial stenosis. Therefore, if a stenosis is present, only limited compensatory dilation is possible and the maximal perfusion during exertion (or on pharmacological dilatation) is consequently reduced. In the presence of an extremely high-grade stenosis, the compensatory peripheral dilatation in the microcirculation may be complete. A similar effect is seen with a reduction in systemic pressure. The local regulatory mechanisms, e.g., the myogenic response (see the later section entitled "Microcirculation") lead to a compensatory decrease in tone and flow resistance aimed at maintaining resting perfusion. If a prevailing stenosis

has already led to peripheral dilatation, the tolerance for an additional reduction in systemic pressure is reduced.

COLLATERAL CIRCULATION (ARTERIOGENESIS)

A NATURAL RESCUE MECHANISM PROVIDING PROTECTION FROM PERIPHERAL HYPOPERFUSION

Besides depending on differences in the dilatory reserve of resistance vessels in different organs, the effects of arterial stenoses also depend on the availability of alternative flow pathways to the tissue supplied. In most organs, only peripheral regions of an area supplied by a stenosed artery may be supplied by neighboring arteries (Fig. 2-5). However, it has been shown that small arteriolar connections may develop into larger vessels, able to provide substantial blood flow. The transstenotic pressure gradient and pressure differences between arteries in the poststenotic regions and neighboring unaffected vessels has also been postulated as the main mechanism initializing growth of such collateral vessels.

The stenosis or occlusion of an arterial vessel—as described in the previous sections—was a key issue in vascular medicine in the last century and continues to be one today. Coronary heart disease and other vascular diseases such as cerebrovascular and peripheral artery disease are likely to become even more prominent as demographic shifts and progressively unhealthy lifestyles occur in the future. From the evolutionary point of view, the massive increase in atherosclerosis, resulting from a mismatch between calorie intake and consumption, simply overeating, and aggravated by risk factors such as lack of physical exercise, smoking, or diabetes, has taken place rather recently. This might explain why evolutionary pressure has been too short to provide compensation mechanisms to cope with this disease and its devastating human costs.

One important protective endogenous mechanism against the downstream effects of arterial stenosis is the recruitment of collateral arteries and their transformation from resistance arteries into conductance arteries (arteriogenesis).[13,14] However, the time course required to enlarge pre-existing collateral vessels might be too slow in many cases to allow hemodynamic compensation of rapidly evolving stenoses, resulting in perfusion deficits, ischemic endorgan damage, and—in extreme cases—peripheral tissue infarctions. Nevertheless, arteriogenesis is an important natural endogenous rescue mechanism to compensate for the reduction in arterial inflow and is briefly discussed in this section. Several experimental studies in recent years have contributed to a better understanding of the basic physiological and molecular principles of arteriogenesis.

In this context it is important to distinguish between arteriogenesis and angiogenesis. Arteriogenesis, the mechanism responsible for collateralization, represents the enlargement and remodeling of pre-existing small arteriolar collaterals between the perfusion territories of functional endarteries into conduit arteries. The major stimuli for this remodeling are mechanical forces such as shear stress and mechanical stretch. Angiogenesis describes the de novo formation of capillaries by sprouting or intussusception. The major stimuli for angiogenesis are hypoxia, such as occurs in tumor growth, or inflammation in wound healing.

The existence of collateral arteries has been controversially discussed for many years. Several investigators have described myocardial arteries as functional endarteries, while others have provided convincing data about the presence of arteriolar vessels that interconnect adjacent vascular territories in the form of networks or arcades.[13,15,16]

In 1956, Baroldi et al.[17] demonstrated the presence from birth of mostly corkscrew-shaped collateral arteries in normal human hearts, with a luminal diameter of 20 to 350 μm and lengths ranging from 1 to 5 cm. In the hearts of patients suffering from coronary artery disease, autopsy showed that the number of coronary collaterals was increased, notably in cases with a long history of slowly evolving coronary obstructions,

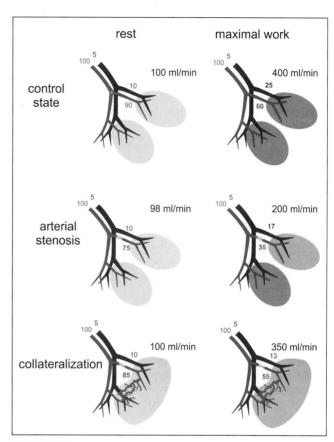

FIGURE 2-5. Schematic representation of pressure and flow distribution in a coronary vascular bed at rest and during maximal loading. Shown are typical values for normal conditions, on arterial stenosis, and after collateralization.

whereas barely any collateral vessels were found following acute myocardial infarcts. Baroldi et al. suggested that functional coronary collateral circulation results from the remodeling of vessels present in normal hearts. Indeed, in 1964, Fulton[13] was able to show at a postmortem examination that the number of large coronary collaterals increased with the duration of the history of angina. When the sum of luminal diameters measured was translated into the capacity of these vessels to transport blood, it could be shown that the functional importance of a few large channels was much greater than that of a large number of small collateral channels. These observations served as an important point of departure for Schaper's experimental studies in dogs and rabbits,[14,18,19] heralding a new era of "arteriogenesis," the positive remodeling of pre-existing collateral pathways and channels. Following convincing research data, the concept of arteriogenesis has been generally accepted.

Under normal conditions, collateral arteries function as a means of efficient blood flow distribution, acting as capacitors for blood displacement in nonsynchronously contracting muscles. Stenosis of a conduit artery induces a pressure fall in the poststenotic downstream vascular bed due to the pressure drop across the stenosis and compensating vasodilatation of poststenotic resistance arterioles, as indicated in Fig. 2-5. Pressure in adjacent vascular beds perfused by nonstenotic arteries remains unchanged and, thus, a pressure gradient develops along pre-existing small collateral vessels connecting the unaffected and the poststenotic vascular territories. This pressure gradient increases flow through the collateral vessels and thus shear stress and mechanical stretch, the initial stimuli of arteriogenesis.

Taken together, the following key pathogenetic steps are important during early phases of arteriogenesis:

1. The pressure drop across an arterial stenosis and the recruitment of collateral pathways with a consecutive increase in shear forces across these collaterals
2. The up-regulation of cell-adhesion molecules on the collateral arterial endothelium (in particular intercellular adhesion molecule 1, ICAM-1)
3. The invasion of circulating mononuclear cells into the perivascular tissue of collateral arteries
4. The proliferation of smooth muscle cells (SMCs) and adventitial cells in the vessel wall, resulting in a positive outward remodeling of pre-existing collaterals (arteriogenesis)

THE ROLE OF MECHANICAL FORCES

The mechanical forces acting on the endothelium within newly recruited collateral arteries (see previous section) trigger a cascade resulting in endothelial activation and vessel growth. As a result of increased levels of shear forces, endothelial cells (ECs) open their chloride channels, which results in a swelling and a volume increase secondary to an influx of free water.[20] Cell-to-cell contacts within the coherent endothelium of the arteriolar structures are partially damaged. At this point, inflammatory cells adhere to the endothelium and transmigrate into the walls of the collateral channels.[21] Currently it is believed that the endothelium is an important source for the cytokine production necessary to recruit further mononuclear cells to the site of vascular growth and proliferation by forming colony-stimulating factors, vascular endothelial growth factors, and transforming growth factors. In this context, Hoefer et al.[22,23] could show that monocytes do indeed appear to play a crucial role during arteriogenesis. In their study, New Zealand White rabbits received phosphate-buffered saline (PBS), monocyte chemoattractant protein-1 (MCP-1), interleukin-8 (IL-8), neutrophil-activating protein-2 (NAP-2), or lymphotactin (Ltn) using osmotic minipumps after unilateral femoral artery ligation. Arteriogenesis was evaluated by angiography and collateral conductance measurements using fluorescent microspheres. Quantitative immunohistology was used to quantify transmigrated leukocyte subtypes after infusion of the factors. The data provided clear evidence that MCP-1 infusion attracted monocytes and granulocytes, whereas IL-8 attracted all three cell types, although monocytes were attracted to a significantly lower degree than by MCP-1. NAP-2 and Ltn selectively attracted granulocytes and lymphocytes, respectively. Importantly, among the tested cytokines, only MCP-1 stimulated arteriogenesis, as assessed by collateral conductance measurements, whereas IL-8, NAP-2, and Ltn had no significant effect on arteriogenic growth.

In a second set of experiments, in vivo treatment with monoclonal antibodies against ICAM-1 completely abolished the stimulatory effect of MCP-1 on collateral arterial growth, suggesting that the mechanism of the MCP-1-induced arteriogenesis proceeded via the attraction of monocytes to the endothelial sites,

rather than by the action of the MCP-1 molecule itself. Furthermore, mice with defective selectin interactions (FT4/7-/-) did not show any significant difference in arteriogenesis, whereas ICAM-1 and Mac-1 double-knockout mice had significantly less arteriogenesis than matched controls. These results seem to indicate that ICAM-1/Mac-1-mediated monocyte adhesion to the endothelium of the preformed collateral arteries represents an essential step for arteriogenesis proceeding via selectin interaction independent mechanisms. However, further studies are needed to explore fully the molecular and cellular biology of collateral vessels' growth.

REMODELING OF RESISTANCE ARTERIOLES INTO CONDUCTANCE VESSELS

The influx of circulating monocytes into the walls of the pre-existing collateral vessels leads to a cascade of molecular events resulting in a marked increase in proliferative activity and growth. Pre-existing arteriolar collaterals have a diameter of ~ 50 μm. They present with one to two layers of SMCs and are morphologically indistinguishable from normal arterioles. The stages of arteriogenesis consist of (a) arteriolar thinning and (b) transformation of SMCs from the contractile into the proliferative and synthetic phenotype, followed by (c) EC and SMC proliferation, SMC migration, and formation of a neointima. Early in this process, the production of ICAM-1 and vascular cell adhesion molecule (VCAM-1) is up-regulated in ECs, and this is accompanied by accumulation of blood-derived macrophages. Moreover, an activation of gelatinase A associated with increased tissue plasminogen activator (tPA) expression and induction of gelatinase B, matrix metallopeptidase-1 (MMP-1), extracellular matrix (ECM) elastin, collagen, and proteoglycans as well as suppression of tissue inhibitors of metalloproteinases (TIMP) levels are also observed.[24]

In short, these multiple cellular and molecular activities during the remodeling phase of collateral artery growth are necessary to loosen up the "old" structure of the vessel including the lamina elastica and to create space for the growth of the vessels. Increased mitotic and secretory activities associated with arteriogenesis result in outward remodeling of an arteriole into an artery, which increases the original diameter of the arteriole up to 12-fold. Hence these vessels are predestined for collateral blood flow bypassing the stenosis or occlusion and providing the required oxygen and nutrition to the endangered peripheral tissue.

THERAPEUTIC ARTERIOGENESIS

In studies of peripheral circulation in an animal model, our group could show that certain cytokines accelerate the speed of arteriogenesis. The design of these studies was derived from Schaper's observation identifying increased levels of monocytes on the surface of dog coronary collateral endothelium.[19] In our model, ligation of the femoral artery in New Zealand White rabbits under normal conditions leads to the development of natural adaptive arteriogenesis. After 1 week of ligation, collaterals are indeed detectable, although the degree of maturation is rather low in this model. Infusing proarteriogenic factors into the collateral circulation (intra-arterially), however, leads

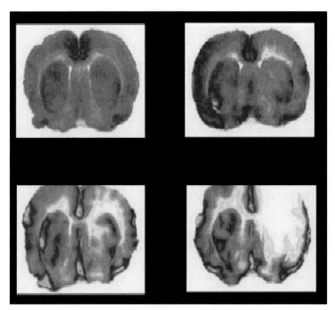

FIGURE 2-6. Protection of brain tissue by therapeutic stimulation of angiogenesis with granulocyte-macrophage colony-stimulating factor (GM-CSF). Shown is the situation under control (*upper panels*) and after induction of hypoxic stroke (*lower panels*) with (*left*) and without (*right*) application of GM-CSF. The infarct size is substantially reduced on GM-CSF treatment.

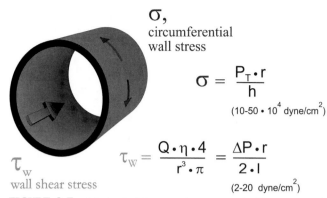

FIGURE 2-7. Mechanical forces acting on vessels (P_T, transmural pressure; r, vessel radius; h, vessel wall thickness; Q, volume flow rate; η, apparent viscosity; ΔP, driving pressure difference along a vessel segment; l, length of vessel segment). Typical ranges for shear stress and circumferential wall stress (hub stress) in the microcirculation are given.

to a dramatic increase in collateral diameter and hence peripheral perfusion. Granulocyte macrophage colony-stimulating factor (GM-CSF) and MCP-1 in particular have been shown to be strong arteriogenesis-enhancing factors,[14,25–28] in an ischemic brain model as well (Fig. 2-6). This observation has led to several experimental strategies to therapeutically enhance the collateral circulation using proarteriogenic compounds. A variety of physiological molecules have been identified that appear to promote angio- and arteriogenesis. Most act by stimulating migration and proliferation of ECs or SMCs, such as the family of fibroblast growth factors (FGF) and vascular endothelial growth factors (VEGF). Both cause vasodilatation by stimulating the release of nitric oxide (NO). The dilatory effect of these growth factors makes it, therefore, important in both animal and clinical studies to differentiate between improved perfusion caused merely by vasodilatation and true collateral growth.

Meanwhile several compounds have been tested experimentally and clinically to promote the growth of collateral arteries; however, the final verdict on their clinical relevance is still awaited at the time of writing.

MATERIAL PROPERTIES OF VASCULAR WALLS

In the circulation, vessels are subjected to mechanical stresses originating from blood flow and blood pressure (cf. Fig. 2-7) as well as from mechanical deformation of the vessel walls due to bending, twisting, and outside compression. The composition of the vessel wall and its mechanical properties adapt to withstand these forces. They also strongly affect the functional properties of vessels.

VESSEL WALL COMPOSITION

The smallest vessels, the capillaries, are composed of a layer of ECs, which in some tissues with a particularly active exchange of molecules may exhibit fenestrations or openings. The single layer of ECs is attached to a basal membrane containing mostly collagen-IV and some pericytes (see next section). Even in small arterioles and venules, the wall exhibits the typical vascular structure with three tissue layers, namely, intima, media, and adventitia. In arterioles and venules, the intima is represented by a single layer of ECs and a more or less continuous basal membrane. The media contains one to five layers of SMCs in arterioles and a sparsely developed adventitia; venules have a very thin media with fewer layers of SMCs, but a thicker adventitia containing more collagen-rich connective tissue. In larger vessels, the intimal and medial layers are thicker and more complex. In arteries, the intima exhibits a layer of connective tissue and is separated from the media by the fenestrated internal elastic membrane. Elastic membranes are also found within the media, which in addition to SMCs also contains fibroblasts and some collagen fibers. Veins again exhibit a lower amount of SMCs but more passive structural elements, mainly collagen and some elastic fibers.

In a given location within the vascular tree, veins exhibit a diameter that is approximately 1.5 to three times greater than that of the corresponding arterioles, lower wall thickness with lower relative shares of smooth muscle and elastin, but a higher collagen content. Thus, the wall-to-lumen ratio is much lower on the venular side (Fig. 2-8). For both arteries and veins the wall-to-lumen ratio decreases from small to large vessels. Typical values for normal human coronary arteries[29] and carotid arteries,[30,31] ranging from about 0.16 to 0.2, have been reported. As a consequence of different wall composition and different thickness, venous vessels will collapse more easily than their counterparts on the arterial side of the circulation if the transmural pressure gradient becomes negative.

FORCES AND STRESSES

Our understanding of the mechanical properties of arterial vessels far exceeds that for veins; however, some of the general concepts may apply for both vessel classes. In situ, arteries are

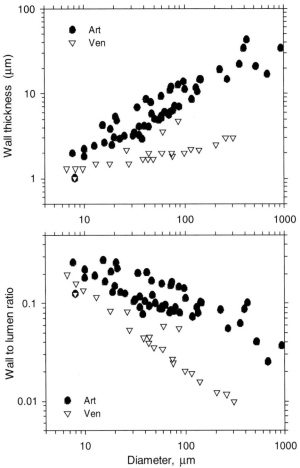

FIGURE 2-8. Relationship between wall thickness (*D*, *top*) and wall-to-lumen ratio (*h/D*, *bottom*) and vessel diameter for relaxed vessels in small laboratory animals. Wall thickness shows a relatively weak increase with vessel size, leading to a substantial decrease in the relation of wall thickness to radius. In addition, both quantities are substantially lower in venous than in arterial vessels. (Data according to Pries AR, Reglin B, Secomb TW. Structural adaptation of vascular networks: role of the pressure response. *Hypertension*. 2001;38:1476–1479, and Pries AR, Reglin B, Secomb TW. Remodeling of blood vessels: responses of diameter and wall thickness to hemodynamic and metabolic stimuli. *Hypertension*. 2005;46:726–731.)

under significant longitudinal tension. On detachment from the tissue and at zero pressure, they shorten by up to 40% in young experimental animals, down to ~10% in old ones.[32,33] Their unstretched length depends on transmural pressure (*P*). If an artery is subjected to increasing transmural pressure, a parallel increase in length and diameter is observed. However, the percentage increase in length is substantially lower than that in diameter. In experimental studies with rat arteries using a pressure increase from 50 to 150 mm Hg, percentage increases of about 80% in diameter and 30% in length have been found.[32]

The most important mechanical factor acting on the vessel wall is the circumferential tension (*T*, newtons per meter) calculated according to Laplace's law for cylindrical tubes as

$$T = P_T r$$

where *r* is the vessel radius and P_T is the distending pressure. For a given structural element in the vessel wall, the tension per unit thickness (*h*) of the vessel wall, the circumferential wall stress or hub stress (σ; $\tilde{N}/m^2$ = Pa, dyne/cm²) represents the most relevant functional parameter:

$$\sigma = P_T r/h$$

(Fig. 2-1). The wall stress in situ increases markedly with vessel diameter, reaching values up to 100 kPa (or 10⁶ dyne/cm²). For human carotid and radial arteries, values in the range of 50 to 75 kPa (or 50 × 10⁴ dyne/cm²) have been reported.[31]

MECHANICAL PROPERTIES

Mechanical properties of the vessel wall[34,35] dictate the relative increase in circumferential length (and thus diameter) or strain ϵ of a vessel for a given increase in circumferential wall stress. This behavior can be described by the incremental Young's elastic modulus (*E*, pascals)

$$E_{inc} = \sigma/\varepsilon$$

With increasing *E*, the vessel gets stiffer. A number of parameters are used to describe such changes in vascular mechanical properties:

- Compliance (*C*; m⁵/N, mL/mm Hg), i.e., the change in volume, ΔV, for a given change in pressure, ΔP:

$$C = \Delta V/\Delta P$$

- The cross-sectional compliance (*Ccs*; m⁴/N, mm²/mm Hg), where *Acs* is the cross-sectional area:

$$Ccs = \Delta Acs/\Delta P$$

- The distensibility (*D*; Pa⁻¹, 1/mm Hg), where *V* is the vessel volume:

$$D = C/V$$

- The cross-sectional distensibility coefficient (*DcsC* or *DC*; Pa⁻¹, 1/mm Hg):

$$DcsC = [\Delta A/\Delta P]/A$$

The development of techniques of measurement based on high-resolution ultrasound (≥10 MHz) combined with measurement of instantaneous blood pressure, for example, using applanation tonometry, allows the measurement of E_{inc}, *Ccs*, and *DcsC* in a clinical setting. Typical values of E_{inc} for human arteries range from about 200 kPa (carotid artery) to 2000 kPa (radial artery).[31] Values for *Ccs* of about 0.07 mm²/mm Hg (carotid), and for *DcsC* in the range of 40 kPa⁻¹ × 10⁻³ (~300 mm Hg⁻¹ × 10⁻³) (carotid) and 6 kPa⁻¹ × 10⁻³ (~45 mm Hg⁻¹ × 10⁻³) (radial) have been reported.[31,36] It is well established, that distensibility and compliance decrease with age and with certain chronic disease conditions, including diabetes.[37]

Pulse Wave

A functionally and clinically relevant circulatory parameter influenced by vascular distensibility is the pulse wave velocity (PWV, meters per second).[38–40] PWV is related to the elastic modulus

$$PWV = [E \times h/D \times 1/\rho]^{0.5}$$

and, with some restrictions, to the inverse of compliance

$$PWV = [1/C \times V/\rho]^{0.5}$$

(where ρ is the specific mass of the blood), which shows that PWV increases with increasing vascular stiffness or decreasing compliance. Arterial stiffening is observed with increasing age and blood pressure, leading to a corresponding increase in PWV. For a pressure level of 100 mm Hg, PVW increases from about 6 m/sec at an age of 20 years to about 10 m/sec at 75 years. For a pressure level of 180 mm Hg, the corresponding values are 9 and 14 m/sec.

Higher values of PWV lead to an earlier impact of the reflected wave on the aortic pulse pressure curve, increasing the pulse pressure amplitude (Fig. 2-9). This in turn causes increased mechanical stress on the arterial vessels and the heart. Arterial stiffness, PWV, and pulse pressure have been established as independent cardiovascular risk factors.[38,39,41,42] A number of methods have been developed for waveform analysis based on noninvasive recordings on peripheral arteries (e.g., radial artery) or in peripheral vascular beds (e.g., finger) to infer aortic pressure waveforms, PVW, and additional relevant parameters of vascular mechanics.[43,44] These techniques are slowly gaining a greater acceptance in clinical vascular medicine, such as for risk assessment, control of treatment, and epidemiologic evaluations.

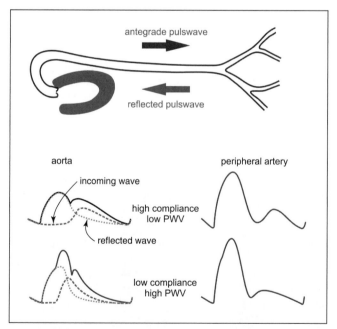

FIGURE 2-9. Pulse-wave velocity (PWV) and arterial pressure pulse. The pulse wave initiated during the ejection phase of the left heart (*dotted line*) travels antegrade toward the peripheral vascular beds. Here, the pulse wave is partially reflected at points of sudden impedance changes in the microcirculation (mostly vascular branch points). In persons with high vascular compliance, PWV is low, and the reflected wave (*interrupted line*) reaches the aorta only after closure of the aortic valve. The resulting integrative pulse pressure curve in the aorta (*continuous line*) consequently exhibits a secondary maximum but a relatively low maximal amplitude (pulse pressure). In contrast, with high PWV, the reflected wave hits the aorta and the left ventricle before ejection has ceased, augmenting the initial peak of the pulse curve and strongly increasing the pulse pressure amplitude. PWV also affects pulse pressure in peripheral arteries, which, because of multiple wave reflections, exhibit high pulse pressure amplitudes.

INTRAVASCULAR INTERVENTIONS

The increasing number of endovascular interventions has stimulated the investigation and analysis of mechanical properties of vessels and vascular lesions.[45–47] It has been suggested that knowledge of the mechanical properties of vessel walls and plaques may be of clinical value in the diagnosis and treatment of vascular occlusive disease. This assumption is based on the observations that composition and morphology of atherosclerotic lesions likely determine the probability of acute vascular occlusion and ischemic syndromes, as well as the responses of vascular walls and plaques, better than simple assessments of degrees of stenoses. Unstable lesions are prone to rupture followed by coagulation and thrombosis. Such lesions, in turn, exhibit a specific histological makeup demonstrating specific mechanical properties. The main histological features of unstable plaques are thought to be a large lipid pool covered by a thin fibrous cap exposed to increased stress with decreasing thickness and increasing vulnerability.

A number of techniques using both invasive (e.g., intravascular ultrasound elastography)[48,49] and noninvasive (e.g., ultrasound tissue Doppler imaging of arterial wall motion)[50] approaches have been used to assess the mechanical properties of defined vascular segments.

Elastography assesses local mechanical properties of tissue by applying an intraluminal pressure to which the vessel section investigated responds according to its mechanical properties. The resulting deformation of the tissue is determined using ultrasound. Using this technique, it was shown that the strain in the arterial vessel wall and in the fibrous cap of atherosclerotic lesions of various plaque types was significantly different (no plaque, fatty, fibrous, or calcified plaque).[51] However, because of cumbersome measurements and calibrations, elastography has not been widely applied in clinical studies.

In the future, developments in the area of molecular medicine may lead to approaches that allow us to influence the mechanical and biological properties of vessels. Intravascular catheter interventions are an option to deliver therapeutic substances to target sections of pathologically altered vessels. Furthermore, improved knowledge of molecular mechanisms supports the development of imaging modalities, helping to locate and characterize vascular lesions.

MICROCIRCULATION

Endovascular interventions are usually directed at large to middle-sized supplying arteries, and it is not immediately clear why we should consider the microcirculation in this context. However, the reduced poststenotic pressure from upstream stenoses also affects regulatory mechanisms in the downstream microvessels. In addition, the underlying diseases that most commonly cause stenoses in the supplying arteries, such as diabetic angiopathy or atherosclerosis, are often accompanied by profound microvascular dysfunction. Also, many endovascular interventions performed to recanalize occluded or stenotic arteries to salvage ischemic tissue result in ischemia-reperfusion injury, which has long been recognized to affect downstream microvessels. Furthermore, thromboembolic complications associated with up to 30% of revascularization procedures primarily involve the downstream microvascular beds. And last, but not least, endovascular interventions induce repetitive brief periods of ischemia and subsequent reperfusion that, if prolonged, may also affect the downstream microvessels. This section, therefore, briefly reviews the morphology and physiology of the microcirculation and its involvement in vascular disease. We focus on the microvasculature of the organs most frequently targeted by endovascular interventions, namely, heart, brain, and skeletal muscle.

MORPHOLOGY, ANGIOARCHITECTURE, AND TOPOLOGY

Whereas it is easy to agree that arterioles, capillaries, and venules belong to the microvascular segment of the vascular systems, their transitions and boundaries are less well defined.[52] There are neither any strict morphological features nor any functional ones that allow a clear definition of the transition points from small arteries to arterioles or from venules to small veins. These transitions appear rather gradual and differ in specific vascular beds. For example, the thickness of the tunica media gradually decreases toward smaller arterial vessels until it is composed of a single layer of SMCs that terminates with the so-called precapillary sphincter in the terminal arteriole.[53,54] More sophisticated approaches to assess transitions, such as the double-logarithmic plot of vessel radius versus wall thickness[55] or wall stress versus vessel diameter plots,[56–58] including large conduit vessels as well as small arterioles, each resulted in data points clustering about a single straight regression line and defying identification of a cutoff feature separating arteries from arterioles. For the purpose of this section, the microvascular segment will be considered to include all arterial vessels that contribute to blood flow control, that is, small arteries from about 200 μm in diameter to terminal arterioles. The major pressure drop has been shown to occur within this range of vessels in most tissues, including skeletal muscle, mesentery, intestinal wall, or pia mater[6,7] and more recently coronary circulation.[8,9,59] On the venous side, too, venules as well as small veins involved in inflammatory processes including leukocyte adhesion and migration will be included.

Arterial microvessels generally are composed of three distinct layers: the tunica intima, with ECs, a basal lamina, subendothelial matrix, and internal elastica; the tunica media of one to several circumferentially arranged layers of SMCs; and the tunica adventitia of fibrous elements, fibroblasts, and sympathetic nerve fibers. The wall of capillaries (internal diameters of 5 to 10 μm) consists of endothelium, basal lamina, and a few pericytes. Thus, distinction between terminal arterioles and capillaries is possible on the basis of the disappearance of SMCs. In contrast, the transition from capillaries to venules is less well defined and lacks any distinct anatomical features. Thus, the smallest postcapillary venules (luminal diameter 10 to 50 μm) lack SMCs, but feature numerous pericytes that may form an almost continuous layer. In this segment of the venous vascular bed, the interendothelial cell contacts are weak, rendering it sensitive to the effects of inflammatory mediators such as histamine, serotonin, or bradykinin and subsequent plasma extravasation. Postcapillary venules turn into muscular venules (inner diameters 50 to 200 μm) with a single to double layer of often discontinuous SMCs, which are thinner than their counterparts in arterioles.[60]

The main arteries give rise to numerous smaller arterial branches, gradually decrease in size, and eventually end as terminal arterioles, which then divide into capillaries. Likewise, on the venous side, smaller venules usually converge stepwise to larger vessels, which finally drain into the main veins (Fig. 2-10). However, this general pattern varies considerably in different organs. Dichotomous branching patterns that result in functional endarteries with well-defined perfusion territories and small interterritorial collateral pathways prevail in the heart and brain, whereas arcading structures that allow for collateral blood flow through large anastomoses are found in the mesentery/gut, skeletal muscle, and skin.[61] Also, the architecture of the capillary network may be fundamentally different in various tissues. Skeletal, myocardial, and intestinal smooth muscle, for example, present with parallel alignment, but capillaries in the cerebral cortex form a polygonal network, and hepatic sinusoids converge radially toward the central venules.

Vessel formation or vasculogenesis occurs early during embryogenesis and starts with differentiation of mesenchymal cells into hemangioblasts, which migrate to the periphery of the embryo and further differentiate into endothelial and hematopoietic cells to form evenly distributed blood islands. These blood islands then connect to form the primary capillary plexus, which is still devoid of blood flow. Simultaneously, the embryonic heart and the central blood vessels, which later develop into the aorta and the caval veins, are generated. This initial vasculogenesis is predetermined by a genetic building plan and results in a uniform pattern of the central vascular tree among healthy individuals. After connection of the primary capillary plexus to the aorta, blood flow is initiated, and the further maturation of the vasculature and outgrowth of vessel trees into the developing organs (angiogenesis) is governed by feedback mechanisms that include vessel

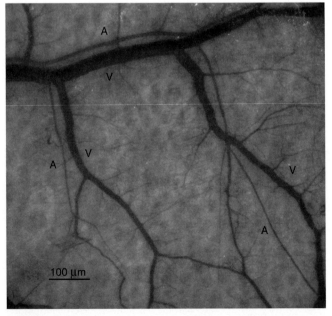

FIGURE 2-10. Example of microvascular branching patterns in the mouse skinfold chamber. Venules (*V*) show considerably more branches and a greater diameter than the accompanying arterioles (*A*). (Image provided by Sabrina Piloth and Axel Sckell, Charité Berlin.)

responses to flow, pressure, and humoral guiding cues provided by metabolic and angiogenic factors such as VEGF and FGF. High-flow pathways in the primary capillary plexus are remodeled by outward growth, increasing vessel diameter, and mature into arteries, while small side branches with low flow are disconnected from these arteries and connect to the emerging venous vasculature. Transmural pressure seems to determine the thickness of the medial smooth muscle layer. At the front of vessel growth into growing tissues, new vessels are formed by sprouting angiogenesis, which is controlled by growth factor gradients in the tissue. Endothelial tip cells at the end of these sprouts extend filopodia, which express growth factor receptors and explore the local extracellular environment for the respective guiding cues. New vessels may also be formed by intussusception, a process where an existing vessel is split into two parallel vessels by transluminal ingrowth of endothelial pillars. Maturation of the emerging capillary networks into functional arterial and venous vascular trees is then mainly controlled by feedback responses to flow and pressure as described earlier (for review, see references 61 and 62).

The stochastic principles of this feedback-controlled peripheral vessel growth result in the high interindividual variability of organ vascular trees. The coronary circulation with the different perfusion territories of the major coronary arteries and the variability in the numbers, positions, and diameters of arterial branches—such as the diagonal and septal arteries rising from the left anterior descending artery—exemplify this general principle.

ANGIOARCHITECTURE AND ANGIOADAPTATION

Microvascular networks have to fulfill a number of functional and structural requirements. They have to transport the blood into the vicinity of all parenchymal cells in all organs and to provide a large surface area for substrate and gas exchange. Microvascular networks have to adapt in response to changes in the function and structure of the supplied tissues by changes in vascular smooth muscle tone and by changes in number of vessels, vessel spatial arrangement, and vessel diameter. The processes that generate, maintain, and adapt the extremely complex vascular networks include the formation of new vessels by vasculogenesis and angiogenesis, but also pruning and remodeling of existent vessels ("angioadaptation").[63] Some of the relevant stimuli for vascular adaptation include blood pressure, blood flow, and the related physical forces such as circumferential wall stress and wall shear stress as well as parameters reflecting the metabolic state of the tissue such as partial oxygen pressure (PO_2).[64–69] The resulting structure of microvascular networks (and vascular beds at large) is usually able to maintain supply of tissues with required substrates including oxygen, but exhibits a great degree of heterogeneity in all functional parameters among tissues.[70]

Structural and functional features of mature vascular beds result from continuous vascular angioadaptive processes that reflect their local environment. The main hemodynamic forces acting on vessels are the wall shear stress resulting from the friction between the flowing blood and the endothelial surface, and the circumferential stress within the vessel wall due to the transmural pressure difference (Fig. 2-7). Despite the fact that the shear stress is smaller by a factor of about 10,000 than the circumferential wall stress, it represents a key component in regulation of vascular integrity and function.[71,72]

Direct observations of vascular responses to acute or chronic changes in hemodynamic or functional loading have revealed a number of stereotypical vascular reaction patterns. For example, an increase in blood flow or shear stress (Fig. 2-11) at the endothelial surface (as well as increased metabolic demand from the tissue) is associated with a positive remodeling of the vessel in terms of enlargement of the vessel lumen and thinning of the vessel wall, whereas an increase in transmural pressure or circumferential wall stress evokes the opposite response.[73,74] On the network level, increased pressure leads to rarefaction of vessels[75–77] associated with a reduced exchange surface and a higher flow resistance.

A complex interplay exists among functional, hemodynamic, and structural parameters in microvascular networks, reflecting their specific functions. For example, wall shear stress, intravascular pressure, and circumferential wall stress ("hub" stress;

Cells

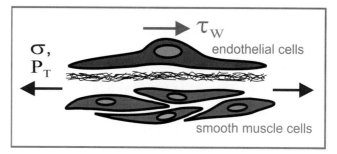

Vessels

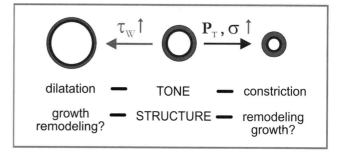

Vascular Beds

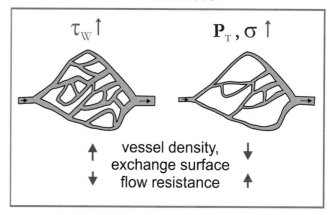

FIGURE 2-11. Schematic representation of the effect of hemodynamic forces (i_w: wall shear stress; σ, circumferential wall tension; P_T, transmural pressure difference) on vascular cells (*top panel*), vessels (*middle panel*), and vascular networks (*bottom panel*).

formula given in Fig. 2-7) and vessel diameter are highly correlated (Fig. 2-12).[6,56] The reduction in shear stress from the high arterial to the low venous pressure level corresponds to the higher flow resistance and higher pressure drop on the arterial side and the larger vascular cross sections on the venous side (cf. pressure profile given in Fig. 2-2). Precise control of perfusion pressure also appears to be critically important for maintaining low levels of capillary pressure to allow balanced fluid exchange between vessels and tissues. Using a logarithmic graph, an almost linear relation between vessel diameter and wall stress is observed, with data for arterial and venous vessels falling on a single line (Fig. 2-12). This observation relates to the presence of the complex mechanisms of structural adaptation of vessels to hemodynamic and metabolic stimuli that control vessel diameter and wall thickness.[78] The increasing force bearing on individual components of the vessel wall with growing vessel size indicates that structural elements able to withstand greater mechanical stresses, such as collagen, seem to play an increasingly important role in determining vascular mechanical properties. This is especially obvious in hypertension, which also leads to a general thickening of vessel walls.[79–84]

RHEOLOGY AND THE ENDOTHELIAL SURFACE LAYER

Mechanical Properties of Red Cells

The basic mechanical properties of human red blood cells are well established.[85] Their cytoplasm is an incompressible Newtonian fluid surrounded by a thin viscoelastic membrane, which consists of a lipid bilayer surrounding a protein cytoskeleton. The membrane shears and bends easily but resists changes in size of surface area and volume. As a consequence of these properties, red cells are highly deformable, as long as changes in surface area or volume are not required, and can pass through capillaries with diameters much smaller than the diameter of an unstressed cell (~8 μm).

Blood of many species, including human blood, can aggregate. Unless fluid flow forces are sufficient to keep them apart, red cells tend to clump because of the presence of bridging plasma proteins.[86] In blood samples studied in viscometers or in larger vessels or tubes, red-cell aggregation at low shear can lead to a marked increase in apparent viscosity.[86,87] As the shear rate increases, the progressive breakup of aggregates leads to a decrease in viscosity ("shear thinning"). Increasing deformation of red cells with increasing shear rate also contributes to a reduction in viscosity, which is observed over a wide range of shear rates. Interestingly, aggregation at very low shear rates was observed to reduce flow resistance in small tubes (or microvessels).[88] This phenomenon is attributed to the aggregation of red cells in the central regions of the vessel, leaving a relatively large lubricating layer of plasma close to the vessel wall. Because red cells have a higher density than plasma, the effects of sedimentation will further influence flow resistance at very low shear rates.[89,90]

Blood Viscosity

Distribution of blood flow through the many parallel, small vessels of the microcirculation is of vital importance. For a given vascular architecture, flow resistance is determined by the rheological behavior of the blood flowing through microvessels. The rheological properties of blood have been intensively studied in vitro. The most stimulating concept was based on the experiments by Fahraeus and Lundquist[91] These authors reported a decline in apparent blood viscosity with decreasing tube diameter: When they perfused blood through glass tubes with diameters below 1000 μm, the observed pressure drop at a given perfusion rate was lower than predicted from the bulk viscosity of blood ("relative viscosity"—relative to that of the suspending plasma—e.g., about 3.2 for a hematocrit of 45%) and Poiseuille's law. To reconcile the data with Poiseuille's law, a lower "apparent" viscosity had to be assumed. This phenomenon has been termed the Fahraeus-Lundquist effect.

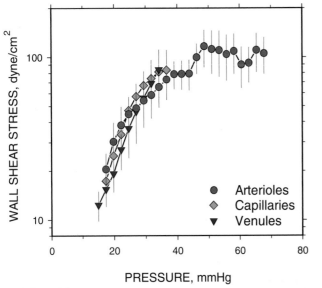

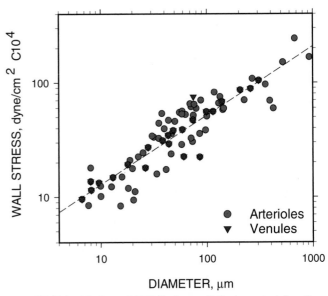

FIGURE 2-12. Relations between wall shear stress and intravascular pressure (*left*) (Pries AR, Secomb TW, Gaehtgens P. Design principles of vascular beds. *Circ Res.* 1995;77:1017-1023) and between circumferential wall stress and vessel diameter (*right*) (Pries AR, Reglin B, Secomb TW. Structural adaptation of vascular networks: role of the pressure response. *Hypertension.* 2001;38:1476-1479.

In the following decades, similar experiments were performed by many researchers[92] testing different hematocrits and extending the diameter range to 3.3 μm. Minimal viscosities were found in tubes with diameters between 5 and 7 μm, corresponding to the size of capillaries. In this diameter range, apparent viscosity is increased by only about 30% if blood with a hematocrit of 0.45 is used for perfusion instead of plasma. In tubes with diameters above 1000 μm, the corresponding increase would be about 220%. This astonishing behavior of blood is explained by the alignment of red cells with the capillary tube (single-file flow) leaving a lubricating sleeve of plasma in the zone between the red cell and the wall where the shear forces are maximal.[93] Thus, in these small tubes (below about 10 μm), apparent viscosity increases more or less linearly and very mildly with vessel diameter.

If tube (or vessel) diameter increases, red cells travel on different streamlines with different velocities (multifile flow). As a consequence, the amount of internal friction between red cells and energy dissipation increases. Also, a more irregular movement of red cells occurs, displacing some red cells much closer to the vessel wall and thus increasing the apparent viscosity at a given hematocrit value. The intensified "cell-to-cell" and "cell-to-wall" interactions also lead to a nonlinear (almost exponential) increase of viscosity with increasing hematocrit. The behavior of blood with different hematocrits perfused through glass tubes of different diameters can be described by empirical equations[92] (Fig. 2-13) to predict apparent viscosity ($\eta_{0.45}$) and flow resistance in vessels in vitro:

$$\eta_{\text{vitro}} = 1 + (\eta_{0.45} - 1) \cdot \frac{(1 - H_{\text{D}})^{C} - 1}{(1 - 0.45)^{C} - 1}$$

where $\eta_{0.45}$, the relative apparent blood viscosity for a fixed discharge hematocrit of 0.45, is given by

$$\eta_{0.45} = 220 \cdot \exp(-1.3D) + 3.2 - 2.44 \cdot \exp(-0.06D^{0.645})$$

The factor C describes the shape of the viscosity dependence on hematocrit

$$C = (0.8 + e^{-0.075D}) \cdot \left(-1 + \frac{1}{1 + 10^{-11} \cdot D^{12}} \right) + \frac{1}{1 + 10^{-11} \cdot D^{12}}$$

In order to extrapolate from the rheological behavior of blood in glass tubes in vitro to the situation in vivo, the presence of the thick stationary layer on the endothelial surface (see the following subsection) has to be taken into account.[78] With a thickness of about 0.5 to 1 μm, this layer leads to an up to fourfold increase in flow resistance in precapillary vessels.

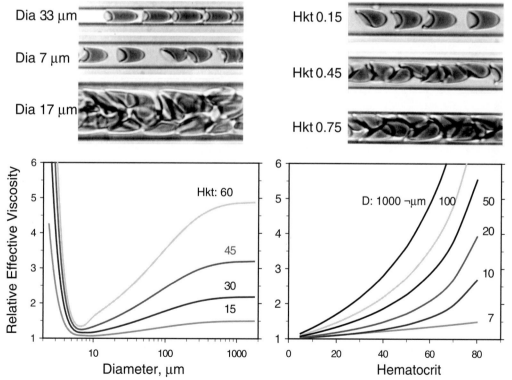

FIGURE 2-13. Relative apparent viscosity for tube flow of blood with discharge hematocrits (H_{D}, flow fraction of red blood cells) of 15%, 30%, 45%, and 60% as a function of vessel diameter (*left*), and for tube diameters of 7, 10, 20, 50, 100, and 1000 μm as a function of hematocrit (*right*). Data represent parametric descriptions based on a large number of literature studies (see Pries AR, Neuhaus D, Gaehtgens P. Blood viscosity in tube flow: dependence on diameter and hematocrit. *Am J Physiol.* 1992;263:H1770-H1778). The micrographs show the flow (from left to right) of human blood through glass tubes.

The Endothelial Surface Layer

It has been shown that the endothelial surfaces are covered with a thick layer (endothelial surface layer, ESL) which restricts the free flow of plasma.[94] Evidence for the presence of such a layer was obtained by analysis of the flow distribution in microvascular networks,[95] by measuring flow resistance in different segments of vascular beds,[96] by showing that the average hematocrit in muscle capillaries is much lower than bulk hematocrit,[97] and by visualizing a zone next to the endothelial surface to which labeled macromolecules have restricted access.[98] These methods led to estimations of the thickness of ESL as ranging between ~0.3 μm and ~1 μm in microvessels and up to 2.6 μm in small arteries of 150 μm in diameter.[99] Based on these measurements, ESL is much thicker than the glycocalyx (~50 nm = 50 $\times$ 10^{-9} m) seen in electron micrographs. Therefore, most of the ESL thickness must be made up by additional components such as plasma proteins or hyaluronan that are adsorbed to the cell-bound molecules of the glycocalyx proper (Fig. 2-14).[94,100,101] However, the mechanical properties of the layer also indicate that its concentration of molecular components is not much higher than that in free-flowing plasma.

The presence of such a layer has obvious consequences for the hemodynamic properties of the microcirculation.[101–104] However, other functional effects may be even more relevant and affect the entire vascular system. These effects include the modulation of oxygen transport, vascular barrier function, and vascular sensing of shear stress,[105–108] inflammation,[109–112] atherosclerosis,[112] and red-cell integrity.[104]

It is of clinical significance that the integrity and thickness of the ESL appear to be altered not only by a number of pathophysiological processes including inflammation and oxidative stress,[111] but also by endovascular interventions, resulting in direct mechanical impairment, or by infusion of artificial plasma replacement fluids.[101] Plasma components adsorbed to the cell-bound glycocalyx make up the majority of the ESL thickness. The macromolecules in this layer are in dynamic equilibrium with the free-flowing plasma and may be washed out by artificial fluids not containing the relevant components (e.g., albumin). This, in turn, will influence all functions of the ESL, most notably those involved in controlling fluid exchange with the tissue.[113]

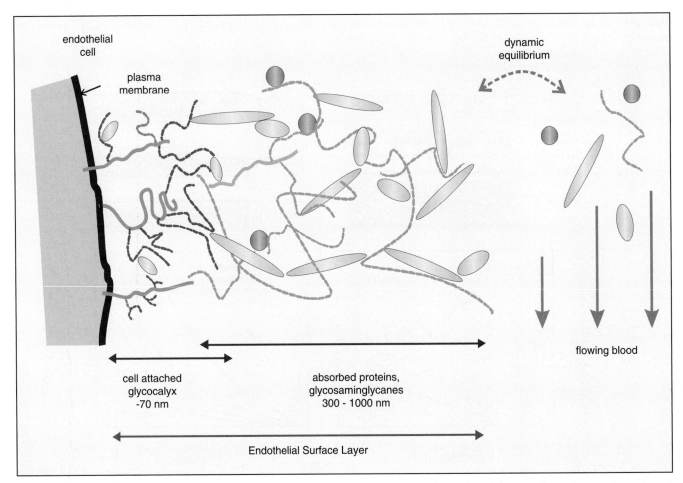

FIGURE 2-14.   Composition of the endothelial surface layer: A thin (50 to 100 nm) glycocalyx consists of glycoproteins and proteoglycans bound directly to the plasma membrane. The main part of the endothelial surface layer (~0.5 μm) is made up by a cluster of soluble plasma components, possibly including a variety of proteins, solubilized glycosaminoglycans, and hyaluronan. This layer is in a dynamic equilibrium with the flowing plasma and stabilized by osmotic forces. The surface layer may be degraded by mechanisms targeting the glycocalyx proper (e.g., enzymes, inflammatory mediators) or by changing the plasma composition (e.g., by infusion of artificial plasma-replacement fluids).

REGULATION OF PERFUSION

Regulation of tissue perfusion is predominantly achieved by controlling the vascular tone in small-resistance arteries and arterioles. However, vascular tone control is employed not only for the maintenance of adequate local tissue perfusion, but also for the regulation of the systemic hemodynamics (blood pressure) and thermoregulation. Accordingly, systemic neuronal and humoral mechanisms interact with local vascular, paracrine, and metabolic mechanisms to form a complex network of agonistic and antagonistic effects on vascular tone (Fig. 2-15). These mechanisms are explored in the following section with special emphasis on the heart and brain as examples.

Systemic Mechanisms

Short-term regulation of blood pressure is achieved by variation of sympathetic nervous system efferent activity to the heart and peripheral vascular beds. Although muscarinic acetylcholine receptors are abundant on endothelial and vascular SMCs, parasympathetic innervation is virtually absent in the vessel wall, and parasympathetic activation has no direct effect on vascular tone. Norepinephrine released from sympathetic synapses induces vasoconstriction of resistance vessels via α-adrenoceptors present in the majority of organs, yet most pronounced in the skin, splanchnic vasculature, and kidneys. Under physiologic conditions, the microvasculature of the brain and the heart are exempt from sympathetic α-receptor-mediated vasoconstriction. In cerebral vessels, α-adrenoceptors are virtually absent and in the coronary vasculature, β_2-adrenoceptor mediated vasodilatation usually overrides potential α-adrenoceptor-induced constriction. Using specific α-adrenoceptor agonists, Chilian et al. demonstrated α_1-adrenoceptor mediated constriction in small coronary arteries and arterioles, but α_2-adrenoceptor induced constriction was limited to smaller arterioles.[114] These data exemplify that vascular responses to a single stimulus may differ not only in different vascular beds, but also in different vessel segments within the same vascular tree. An overview of sympathetic effects on different organ systems is given in Table 2-1.

Mid- and long-term blood pressure control is mainly achieved by humoral mechanisms, which control both blood volume and vascular tone. The humoral mechanisms include the renin-angiotensin-aldosterone system (RAAS), the hypothalamic-hypophysic antidiuretic hormone (ADH, vasopressin),[115,116] and the natriuretic peptides (ANP and BNP),[117–119] which are mainly released from cardiac myocytes. Details on the site of production, release stimuli, receptors, target organs, and effects of these potent hormones are listed in Table 2-2. Whereas angiotensin II and ADH are potent vasoconstrictors, natriuretic peptides antagonize these effects by inducing vasodilatation. In addition, these humoral systems form a complex network of mutual interactions with each other and with the sympathetic system. For example, the plasma levels of angiotensin II and natriuretic peptides correlate inversely with each other in physiologic situations, but are both augmented during pathologic conditions such as heart failure.[117] Angiotensin II not only acts synergistically with vasopressin in inducing vasoconstriction but also stimulates the release of vasopressin. The RAAS is stimulated during sympathetic activation by β_1-receptor-mediated release of renin and, vice versa, angiotensin II augments the effects of sympathetic stimulation by increasing the rate of norepinephrine synthesis, facilitating its synaptic release, and inhibiting its reuptake.

Intrinsic Vascular Mechanisms

Vascular mechanisms of vasomotor tone control include myogenic and endothelial responses to mechanical forces exerted by intraluminal blood pressure via circumferential wall tension and blood flow via longitudinal wall shear stress, as discussed in the previous sections (Fig. 2-7). Myogenic activity is an intrinsic property of the vascular SMCs. Thus, vascular SMCs contract in response to increased transmural pressure and resulting increased circumferential wall tension. Consequently, any

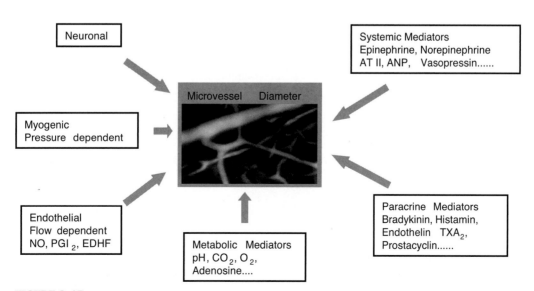

FIGURE 2-15. A multitude of different factors act simultaneously on microvascular tone control. Effects may be synergistic as well as antagonistic.

TABLE 2-1. Organ Distribution of Vascular Responses to Sympathetic Stimulation

Organ	Innervation Density	Receptor Density	Prevailing Effect
BRAIN	—	—	—
HEART	Intermediate	$\beta_2 > \alpha$	Dilation
KIDNEY	High	$\alpha > \beta_2$	Constriction
INTESTINE	High	$\alpha > \beta_2$	Constriction
SKELETAL MUSCLE	Intermediate	$\alpha > \beta_2$	Constriction, but metabolic override during loading
SKIN	Intermediate	$\alpha > \beta_2$	Constriction, but thermoregulatory override

distension of the vessel wall is followed within 20 to 60 seconds by a sustained constriction. The extent of this contraction may result in vessel constriction to a final diameter that is considerably smaller then the baseline diameter. Conversely, decreased transmural pressure results in vessel dilation. This mechanism has been observed in most vascular beds of the systemic circulation and is generally considered to be most pronounced in kidney, cerebral, and coronary resistance vessels. Myogenic activity stabilizes organ perfusion during alterations in systemic arterial pressure and protects the capillaries from excessive

TABLE 2-2. Humoral Factors Regulating Blood Pressure by Affecting Vessel Tone and/or Blood Volume

Mediator	Site of Production	Release Stimuli	Receptors	Targets	Effects
RENIN	Macula densa Extrarenal tissue (e.g., myocardium)	Afferent arteriole blood pressure Tubuloglomerular feedback Sympathetic stimulation		Angiotensinogen	Generation of AT-I
AT-II	Endothelial cells	Constitutively expressed ACE	AT_1	Smooth muscle cells	Constriction, proliferation
			AT_1	Adrenal gland	Release of aldosterone
			AT_2	Endothelial cells	Dilation, antiproliferation
ALDOSTERONE	Adrenal gland	AT-II	Mineral ocorticoid receptors	Tubular cells	Na^+ retention H_2O retention K^+ excretion
VASOPRESSIN/ ADH	Hypothalamus (release from pituitary gland)	Increased plasma osmolarity Decreased blood volume AT-II	V_1	Smooth muscle cells	Constriction, proliferation
			OT	Endothelial cells	Dilation, antiproliferation
			V_2	Collecting duct	Aquaporin-2 expression, H_2O retention
ANP/BNP	Atrial cardiomyocytes	Atrial stretch	NPR-A	Smooth muscle cells	Dilation, antiproliferation
	Ventricular cardiomyocytes	Ventricular stretch	NPR-B	Tubular cells	Na^+/H_2O excretion

Abbreviations: AT-I, angiotensin-I; AT-II, angiotensin-II; AT_1, AT-II receptor type 1; AT_2, AT-II receptor type 2; ACE, angiotensin-converting enzyme; ADH, antidiuretic hormone; ANP/BNP, type A and type B natriuretic peptides; V_1, vasopressin receptor type 1; OT, oxytocin receptor; V_2, vasopressin receptor type 2; NPR-A, natriuretic peptide receptor type A; NPR-B, natriuretic peptide receptor type B.

changes in transmural pressure and consequently fluid filtration. According to the Starling equation

$$Jv = L_p \times S \times \{(P_k - P_i) - \sigma \times (\pi_p - \pi_i)\}$$

the rate of fluid filtration Jv depends on the hydraulic conductivity L_p and surface area S of the capillary wall, the difference of capillary hydraulic transmural pressure $P_k - P_i$, and the transmural colloid-osmotic pressure gradient $\pi_p - \pi_i$ corrected by the reflection coefficient σ. Any increase in capillary pressure P_k would thus also increase fluid filtration until the resulting increase in interstitial pressure P_i would counterbalance this effect.

However, the magnitude of myogenic responses may vary not only in different organs but also along the vascular tree within the same organ. In a comprehensive study on isolated skeletal muscle arterioles from the hamster cheek pouch, Davis demonstrated that myogenic responsiveness increased with decreasing vessel size from small arteries (mean diameter 94.1 μm) to smaller arterioles, reaching a maximum in vessels of 29.9 and 13.0 μm diameter and then decreasing again in terminal arterioles (diameter 7.3 μm).[120] In the same study, the pressure range over which myogenic responsiveness was observed progressively decreased from between 40 and 200 mm Hg in small arteries to between 10 and 80 mm Hg in terminal arterioles. Because pressure decreases in a downstream direction of the arteriolar tree, as shown in Figure 2-2 for the example of the coronary microcirculation, each vessel segment seems to be most myogenically active and operates most efficiently within the pressure range that is considered normal at that level of the vascular tree.

A longitudinal gradient of myogenic responses was also described in the coronary circulation, with myogenic activity increasing from arteries to midsize arterioles and then falling off toward terminal arterioles.[121,122] By observing the changes in perfusion pressure of isolated hearts using fluorescence microscopy of terminal arterioles and mathematical modeling, we recently confirmed that considerable myogenic activity was present in terminal coronary arterioles, but was limited to a low range of transmural pressure of about 10 to 40 mm Hg (Fig. 2-16). The mechanisms of myogenic responses seem to include activation of stretch-activated unspecific cation channels in the sarcolemma, inducing depolarization and calcium influx via voltage-sensitive calcium channels. This response may be enhanced by concomitant release of inositol trisphosphate and diacylglyceride from the phospholipids of the cell membranes, which further increases cytosolic calcium concentration by release from intracellular stores, and by activating protein kinase C, which increases the sensitivity of the smooth muscle contractile apparatus to calcium (for review, see reference 122).

At the molecular level, vessel responses to flow and thus to longitudinal shear stress, are mediated by endothelial production and release of vasodilating substances including NO, prostacyclin (PGI$_2$), and an endothelium-derived hyperpolarizing factor (EDHF).[123] Sudden onset or a step increase in flow activates stretch-sensitive unspecific cation channels, allowing for calcium influx and calcium release from inositol 1,4,5-trisphosphate sensitive calcium stores, followed by hyperpolarization via activation of calcium-sensitive potassium channels (for review, see reference 124). Increased cytosolic calcium then activates, among

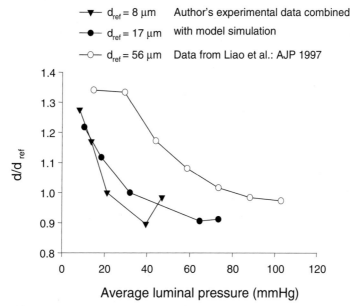

FIGURE 2-16. Diameter changes of precapillary arterioles in response to step changes in perfusion pressure were assessed in isolated perfused rat hearts. The respective luminal pressures were estimated using a computer model of the coronary microcirculation. The slopes of the curves represent myogenic sensitivity, which is at least as strong in the smallest arterioles as previously found in larger vessels (Liao JC, Kuo L. Interaction between adenosine and flow-induced dilation in coronary microvascular network. *Am J Physiol.* 1997;272:H1571–H1581). The main difference is the pressure range at which myogenic sensitivity is present. Precapillary arterioles exhibit myogenic sensitivity at the very low pressures that would normally occur in these vessels.

others, endothelial NO synthase (eNOS). In contrast, basal eNOS activity during constant shear stress seems to be regulated via calcium-independent mechanisms.[125,126] In addition, endothelial release of vasodilators is induced by a number of mediators, which bind to specific receptors on the endothelial surface such as acetylcholine, bradykinin, or serotonin.

Endothelium-mediated vasodilatation in response to flow can be observed throughout the systemic and pulmonary circulation, in large arteries, in arterioles, muscular venules, and veins. Yet, the magnitude of the dilatory response may vary along the vascular tree. In the coronary circulation, endothelium-mediated vasodilatation seems to be more prominent in larger arterioles of 80 to 150 μm in diameter than in upstream larger vessels or downstream smaller ones.[122]

Matching perfusion to metabolic demand is thought to be mainly mediated by locally acting mechanisms including hypoxia, decreased pH, increased carbon dioxide, potassium, or adenosine, all of which induce vasodilatation of microvessels.[122] In the coronary circulation, perfusion is particularly well matched to metabolism such that coronary venous oxygen tension remains unchanged, even during marked changes of myocardial oxygen demand and consumption. Along the arteriolar tree, the dilatory response increases with decreasing vessel size, which is due not only to closer proximity of terminal arterioles to the tissue site of oxygen consumption or metabolite release, but also to a higher sensitivity of the smaller vessels to metabolic dilators such as adenosine.[127]

A comprehensive overview of the differential responsiveness of different microvascular segments to local mechanisms of tone control in the coronary circulation has been proposed by Jones et al.[122] (Fig. 2-17), and similar patterns have been described for other tissues as well.[128] The most potent local mechanism of resistance control in the heart is metabolic dilation. However, the action of the vasoactive metabolites is confined to the site of their production and mainly affects the smallest terminal arterioles. To elicit the full blood flow response to increased metabolic demand, dilation of larger upstream arterioles is induced by three different mechanisms: (a) a hyperpolarizing signal is conducted upstream through endothelial gap junctions and induces remote vasodilatation[129]; (b) metabolic dilation of terminal arterioles decreases pressure in upstream midsize arterioles, which respond by myogenic relaxation; and (c) the increased flow toward the metabolically active tissue induces shear stress-mediated endothelium-dependent additional vasodilatation throughout the supplying vascular tree. The importance of this scheme is that even vessels far upstream from the initial metabolic dilatory stimulus can participate in the overall response and contribute to adaptation of perfusion.[122,128]

PATHOPHYSIOLOGY OF PERFUSION CONTROL

Endothelial Dysfunction

The hallmark of impaired microvascular function is endothelial dysfunction, resulting in insufficient endothelially mediated vasodilatation. The underlying cause of endothelial dysfunction is an imbalance between the underproduction or reduced bioavailability of endothelially produced dilating agents such as prostacyclin, EDHF, and NO on one side and

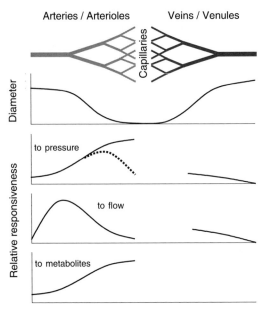

FIGURE 2-17.   Schematic drawing of the relative sensitivity of coronary microvascular segments to different local stimuli such as myogenic responses to luminal pressure, endothelially mediated responses to flow, and responses to local metabolites. In the segment of the smallest vessels, the proposed course of the different curves partly relies on projections from larger vessels or from other tissues. Little is known about coronary capillary and small venular responses. (Adapted from Jones CJ, Kuo L, Davis MJ, et al. Regulation of coronary blood flow: coordination of heterogeneous control mechanisms in vascular microdomains. *Cardiovasc Res.* 1995;29:585–596.)

overproduction of the potent vasoconstrictor endothelin on the other side. Because of the intricate crosstalk among the intracellular pathways of these endothelial mediator systems, reduction of, for example, NO production may also reduce synthesis of the other endothelial dilatory mediators while paradoxically increasing endothelin synthesis[130,131]. A variety of cardiovascular diseases and lifestyle-related risk factors have been associated with endothelial dysfunction, including atherosclerosis, hypertension, congestive heart failure, renal failure, diabetes, smoking, inflammation, dyslipidemia, and obesity.[132,133] The underlying mechanisms are complex and may differ in different disease states. Reduced bioavailability of NO is thought to be one of the central, common factors leading to endothelial dysfunction. This may be due either to inhibition of eNOS expression or activity or to enhanced scavenging of NO by highly reactive oxygen species (ROS).[134]

Recently, a number of polymorphic variations of eNOS have been identified that may affect the enzyme expression and function, but their relevance to pathophysiology of cardiovascular disease remains inconclusive.[134] However, more data are available on the regulation of eNOS activity. Endogenously circulating inhibitors of eNOS such as asymmetric dimethylarginine (ADMA) have been associated with vascular disorders such as hypercholesterolemia and hypertension and may predict cardiovascular risk.[134] An essential cofactor of eNOS, tetrahydrobiopterin (BH_4), is also thought to be of key importance to normal endothelial function. Reduced availability of BH_4 results in uncoupling of eNOS, leading to the production of superoxide anion and H_2O_2 instead of NO, and supplementation of BH_4 in patients with vascular disease seems to improve endothelial function.[134] The most important factor, however, in reducing bioavailability of NO seems to be scavenging by ROS. The foremost mechanism for the loss of NO is thought to be the reaction with superoxide anions. The major sources of endothelial superoxide production are the mitochondrial respiratory chain, NAD(P)H oxidases, and, as mentioned earlier, uncoupled NOS. Normally, superoxide dismutase (SOD) activity is sufficient to detoxify most of the generated superoxide and prevents it from interacting with NO. With excess superoxide production or diminished SOD activity, the superoxide anion reacts with NO, thereby not only scavenging NO and reducing its availability for, as an example, vasodilatation but also producing the potent oxidant peroxynitrite. Superoxide as well as peroxynitrite and their secondary and tertiary oxidants can react with numerous protein and lipid compounds in the cytosol and in cell membranes and thus further compromise EC function.[134]

For diagnosis of endothelial dysfunction in clinical settings, a number of invasive and noninvasive techniques have been developed. For example, changes in diameter of a conduit artery, usually the brachial artery, in response to increased flow, typically induced by reactive hyperemia after 5 minutes of total forearm vessel occlusion, can be measured using high-resolution ultrasound imaging and Doppler techniques. Whereas peripheral vasodilatation is induced by metabolic stimuli, upstream flow-mediated dilation of larger resistance vessels and conduit arteries depends on the intact function of their endothelium. The vasodilatory response is blunted or even abolished in pathological states associated with endothelial dysfunction. As endothelial dysfunction is considered to be present throughout the entire vascular tree of the patient, insufficient flow-mediated relaxation of a conduit artery appears to be also indicative of endothelial dysfunction in the microvasculature. When ultrasound imaging is combined with blood flow velocity measurements using Doppler ultrasound, hyperemic blood flow can be calculated. Reduction of total hyperemic blood flow may also indicate endothelial dysfunction, because blood flow mediated endothelium-dependent relaxation of upstream resistance vessels that are not directly affected by the metabolic mediators is necessary to elicit the full hyperemic flow response.[135] Direct assessment of endothelial dysfunction in humans is difficult to achieve. The closest approximation to in vivo states has been accomplished by studying subcutaneous microvessels removed via biopsies and examined ex vivo in perfusion-pressure or wire micromyographs. However, these experimental conditions might not be fully representative of in vivo states or of the vasculature of other organs. Ongoing research is addressing these important issues.

Besides inducing ischemia, clinical diagnostics of endothelial dysfunction involve the application of agonists (and antagonists) of endothelium-mediated dilation such as acetylcholine. Application of vasoactive agents has been most widely used in the forearm arteries with drug application via cannulated radial artery and blood flow measurements using strain-gauge venous plethysmography. Again, the endothelium of a peripheral organ serves as a surrogate for the microvasculature of more vital organs such as heart and brain, but numerous studies have seemed to confirm a close association between endothelial dysfunction measured using the aforementioned techniques and cardiovascular risk factors and future adverse cardiovascular events.[133,135] Using the same principle, endothelial function of the coronary arteries can also be assessed. Using Doppler wire positioned in a target coronary artery, changes in pressure and flow velocity can be monitored during infusion of vasoactive agents such as acetylcholine for endothelium-dependent and adenosine and nitroglycerin for endothelium-independent vasodilatory responses. In healthy patients, maximum achievable downstream vasodilatation during an intracoronary administration of adenosine increases coronary flow at least 2.5-fold. Lesser responses are indicative of microcirculatory dysfunction. Using acetylcholine, endothelium-dependent vasodilatation and a concomitant increase in blood flow velocity can be observed in healthy patients. Endothelial dysfunction attenuates or abolishes this flow increase and in severe cases may even induce vasoconstriction mediated by muscarinic acetylcholine receptors of vascular SMCs.

In clinical practice, the presence of endothelial dysfunction has been considered an early indicator of cardiovascular disease because it may be present long before any clinical manifestation of atherosclerotic disease. In the presence of hemodynamically critical stenoses in a large vessel, diminution or even lack of flow-mediated relaxation of downstream resistance vessels may further aggravate the ischemic symptoms. However, endothelial dysfunction may well induce transient ischemic symptoms even in the absence of significant stenoses, as documented in patients suffering from cardiac syndrome X, also termed microvascular angina. In these patients, during certain conditions such as mental stress, the microvascular endothelial dysfunction seems to shift the balance between dilatory and constrictive mechanisms toward vasoconstriction associated with malperfusion of the myocardium and clinical signs of ischemia.[136,137]

Inflammation

Activation of the immune system, by autoimmune processes, infectious agents, or transplanted organs, as well as tissue injury by toxic substances, trauma, or ischemia all result in the release of proinflammatory cytokines and chemokines, which then induce quite a uniform inflammatory response in microvascular postcapillary venules, the leukocyte adhesion and emigration cascade[138–140] (Fig. 2-18). Tumor necrosis factor-alpha (TNFα) or interleukin-2, for example, activate ECs to express preformed P-selectin from Weibel-Palade bodies and membrane-bound cytokines within seconds or minutes on their luminal surface. Circulating leukocytes, which are marginated by hemodynamic forces toward the vessel wall, briefly interact with the endothelial surfaces via constitutively expressed L-selectin and its endothelial glycoprotein ligands, which results in their capture by tethering or rolling. In venules with healthy endothelium, most of these cells quickly detach from the vessel wall and return into the bloodstream. In vessels with activated or damaged endothelium, this initial tethering allows for more intensive interactions between endothelial P- or E-selectin and leukocyte ligands, resulting in a slower and more sustained leukocyte rolling.[140] In the course of these interactions the leukocytes become activated, mainly by the endothelially expressed cytokines, shed L-selectin, and increase their avidity and affinity by increased expression and by clustering and activation of β_2 integrins, mostly MAC-1 (CD11b/CD18), on their surface.[141]

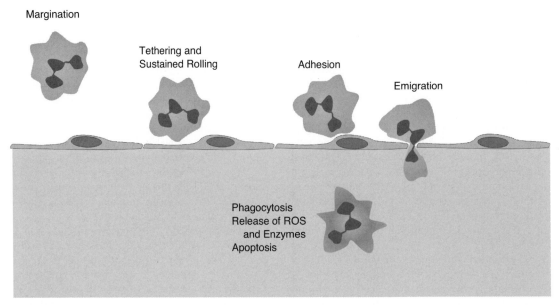

FIGURE 2-18.   The emigration cascade of polymorphonuclear leukocytes (PMN) starts with margination of the cells by rheological forces. Once in contact with the vessel wall, PMN can interact with ECs via constitutively expressed L-selectin on the PMN. In case of endothelial activation, this transient tethering or rolling is slowed down via interaction of endothelial P-selectin or E-selectin with their respective ligands on PMNs. Firm adhesion of PMN requires their activation by endothelially expressed cytokines and is mainly achieved by the PMN integrin MAC-1 (CD11b/CD18) with its endothelial counterpart ICAM-1. Emigration then involves further adhesion molecules and enzymes that destroy extracellular matrix proteins. In the tissue, the PMN will exert its program of phagocytosis and release of reactive oxygen species (oxidative burst) and further enzymes such as elastase. Eventually the PMN undergoes apoptosis, and this program may already be initiated by outside-in signaling of MAC-1 engagement with its ligand.

Interaction of activated MAC-1 with endothelial ligands, the constitutively expressed intercellular adhesion molecules (ICAM-1 and -2), allows for firm adhesion of the leukocyte to the vessel wall and for eventual penetration into the tissue, where it becomes an important source of cytokine production perpetrating inflammation. Once in the tissue, the leukocyte phagocytizes microorganisms, tissue particles, and debris and releases destructive proteases and highly reactive oxygen species (oxidative burst), responsible for peroxidation of lipoproteins and other biochemical species. Activated leukocytes also produce a variety of paracrine mediators. Following emigration, the leukocyte dies within a few hours. Its fate seems to be determined already at the point of its firm integrin-mediated adhesion to the vessel wall by triggering an apoptotic cascade.[142]

Shortly after its initiation, the efficiency of this adhesion and emigration cascade is further enhanced, and activation of nuclear transcription factor κB (NFκB) in ECs seems to be of particular importance in this process. NFκB is a redox-sensitive transcription factor that regulates the expression of a variety of proinflammatory gene products including a number of cytokines, growth factors, adhesion molecules, and enzymes.[143,144] In its nonactivated state, NFκB is associated with its inhibitor subunit IκB. In response to activating stimuli, for example, certain cytokines such as TNFα or oxidative stress, this complex disassociates. IκB is then degraded by proteolytic enzymes. NFκB translocates into the nucleus and binds to its target DNA in the promoter regions of the respective genes. Among the genes expressed in ECs within hours after the initial inflammatory stimulus are E-selectin, which promotes slow leukocyte rolling, and ICAM-1, for firm leukocyte adhesion, both further trigger-

ing the inflammatory cascade. Whereas some of the aforementioned cellular processes may also occur in arterial and capillary ECs, the leukocyte adhesion and emigration cascade is usually confined to venules. Conduit arteries may, however, be affected during inflammatory processes such as atherosclerosis by leukocyte emigration from venular vasa vasorum within the arterial wall.

Although this inflammatory cascade is essential for host defense and tissue repair mechanisms, it may also become a major player in tissue injury associated with ischemia and reperfusion. Therefore, leukocyte migration is tightly controlled, and, under physiological conditions, healthy ECs inhibit leukocyte activation and adhesion mainly by basal luminal release of NO and prostacyclin. Also, NO inhibits the expression of adhesion molecules by ECs by directly stabilizing IκB, thus further attenuating the inflammatory responses. In conclusion, endothelial dysfunction not only is associated with impaired vasodilatation, but also produces a latent proinflammatory state of the ECs.

Ischemia-Reperfusion

Following a brief period of ischemia due to obstruction of the supplying artery, reperfusion results in reactive hyperemia, defined as a transient increase of flow well beyond the baseline preischemic states. Hyperemia appears to be caused by metabolically mediated arteriolar vasodilatation within the ischemic tissue and by upstream flow-mediated endothelium-dependent vasodilatation, as has been already discussed. However, after prolonged periods of ischemia, this reactive hyperperfusion may be blunted, and reflow may remain impaired or even absent despite complete removal of the initial obstruction, a phenomenon termed no-reflow.[145] Thus, successful opening and recanalization of a target lesion associated with TIMI III° antegrade coronary flow in patients with acute coronary syndromes may still be accompanied by impaired myocardial tissue perfusion in ~25% of patients when myocardial perfusion is assessed using contrast echocardiography or other quantitative imaging techniques.[146]

Although the exact pathogenetic mechanism of no-reflow remains obscure, capillary or precapillary vessel wall damage associated with initially functional and later permanent obstruction of the respective microcirculatory bed is generally believed to cause this phenomenon. Pathogenetic mechanisms suggested to cause obstruction of the microcirculation include microemboli released from upstream thrombi, capillary plugging by activated leukocytes, deposition of platelets and fibrin on the capillary wall, rouleau formation of erythrocytes, compression of capillaries by tissue swelling, EC swelling, and formation of endothelial blebs.[147,148] All of these have been observed in different experimental models or tissue specimens from patients, but the actual contribution of each of these mechanisms to the no-reflow phenomenon in clinical settings of ischemia and reperfusion still remains uncertain.

Another important aspect of ischemia and reperfusion in the microcirculation is the participation of inflammatory responses. As discussed earlier, postcapillary venules play a major role in leukocyte recruitment into the tissue and in inflammatory responses. During reperfusion, endothelial activation is triggered by cytokines released from the tissue, possibly by resident macrophages, with the consequent adhesion of leukocytes to the vascular wall, penetration into the reperfused tissue, and induction of inflammatory responses, leading to further aggravation of tissue injury associated with postischemic tissue dysfunction such as transient myocardial stunning, hibernation, or cell death.[149] This concept of secondary tissue injury due to leukocyte-triggered inflammation is supported by numerous studies showing that anti-inflammatory measures may, under experimental conditions, limit infarct size. These measures include anti-inflammatory drugs such as ibuprofen, neutrophil depletion using antineutrophil antisera or leukocyte filters, monoclonal antibodies to endothelial and neutrophil adhesion molecules, or other inhibitors of neutrophil adhesion such as sialyl Lewis^x analogs, adenosine, or prostacyclin (for review, see reference 150). However, there are also studies showing negative results, and as yet none of these experimental treatments has been successfully introduced into clinical practice. In fact, clinical studies aiming to reduce infarct size following recanalization failed to document any beneficial effect of these treatments on infarct size or outcome. Although the reason for the discrepancy between the experimental and clinical findings remains undetermined, it has prompted some investigators to challenge the concept of leukocyte-mediated secondary inflammatory tissue injury.[150]

One possible explanation for the discrepant results in clinical and experimental studies is that treatment in the clinical studies was mostly limited to the acute reperfusion period. Yet, endothelial activation following ischemia and reperfusion may be more prolonged and more sustained, inducing not only acute expression and activation of preformed adhesion molecules and cytokines on the luminal cell membranes but also an increased de novo synthesis of these inflammatory mediators

occurring several hours or possibly days later. The transcription factor NFκB, which controls the expression of numerous proinflammatory gene products, seems to play a key role in this process. In myocardial ischemia and reperfusion the initially released cytokines, in addition to inducing acute leukocyte recruitment, also seem to activate NFκB, which then stimulates increased ICAM synthesis and expression in the EC membrane, rendering the coronary microvasculature more susceptible to other inflammatory stimuli.[149] Consequently, in a pig model, combined treatment with an antibody to the leukocyte adhesion molecule MAC-1 and an anti-NFκB decoy oligopeptide was indeed more effective in preventing reperfusion injury than acute antibody treatment alone.[151] However, whether similar results may be expected in humans remains unknown.

Inflammatory responses after ischemia and reperfusion may be also mediated by adherent platelets. Although platelet adhesion to sites of vascular injury appears essential for thrombus formation, platelets may also attach to intact but activated ECs via the same adhesion molecules that also mediate leukocyte adhesion. The respective ligands on the platelets are PSGL-1, binding to P-selectin, and GP IIb/IIIa, binding to ICAM-1 by forming fibrinogen bridges.[152] In addition, von Willebrand factor and the integrin $\alpha_v\beta_3$ may be involved.[153] These adherent platelets may then recruit further platelets to form microthrombi within the microvessels or serve as a matrix for leukocytes to adhere. The adhesion molecules mediating platelet-leukocyte interaction include P-selectin, ICAM-2, GP Ib, and GP IIb/IIIa on platelets, and PSGL-1 and MAC-1 on leukocytes[153,154] (Fig. 2-19). In a myocardial ischemia and reperfusion model, microvascular deposition of numerous heterotypic aggregates containing platelets as well as leukocytes,[155] and the inhibition of platelet-leukocyte interaction by tirofiban[154] or abciximab[155] has been observed using in situ fluorescence microscopy. Attenuated leukocyte adhesion in microvessels and improved postischemic myocardial function following administration of GPIIb/IIIa inhibitors support the assumption of an essential role of the platelet fibrinogen receptor GP IIb/IIIa in this process. In patients with acute myocardial infarction and successful percutaneous target lesion recanalization, administration of abciximab together with standard anticoagulation and antiplatelet therapy improved myocardial perfusion and recovery of contractile function.[156] Thus, platelets seem to play a critical role in the development of reperfusion-associated inflammatory responses by endothelium-platelet-leukocyte interactions, and initial clinical data suggest that attenuation of this process by administration of GP IIb/IIIa inhibitors may indeed be beneficial in clinical settings.

The duration of ischemia determines the extent of parenchymal and microvascular injury. In the heart and brain, periods of up to 5 minutes of ischemia—even when applied repetitively, as often occurs during endovascular interventions—may actually protect the tissue as well as the microvasculature from injury during a subsequent prolonged ischemic challenge.[157] The protection achieved by such ischemic preconditioning occurs in two time windows. The early or acute phase develops within ~10 minutes and persists for 1 to 3 hours. The delayed phase of preconditioning occurs after 12 to 24 hours and may be sustained for up to 3 days. By preconditioning, the endothelium is thought to acquire a protected phenotype, which attenuates the microvascular consequences of the sustained ischemia including endothelial dysfunction, leukocyte

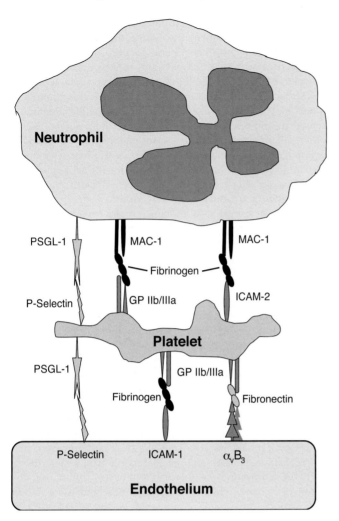

FIGURE 2-19. Platelets may adhere to activated endothelial cells and then serve as a highly adhesive matrix to which neutrophils can bind. The platelet fibrinogen receptor GP IIb/IIIa seems to mediate platelet adhesion to endothelial cells as well as neutrophil adhesion to platelets. This may, in part, explain the beneficial effects of GP IIb/IIIa antagonists such as abciximab or tirofiban on myocardial perfusion and function as well as patient outcome after recanalization of infarcted coronary arteries.

adhesion, and no-reflow phenomenon. The duration after which an ischemic challenge shifts from inducing protective preconditioning to causing sustained tissue and microvascular injury is not well defined. In the heart and brain, this shift seems to occur after anywhere between 5 and 15 minutes of vessel occlusion. In other tissues with less basal oxygen demand and greater ischemic tolerance such as skeletal muscle, much longer periods of up to 40 minutes of preconditioning ischemia have been reported to protect microvascular functional integrity during a subsequent, sustained ischemia.[158]

Hypertension

As already stated, chronic elevation of blood pressure is often associated with microvascular endothelial dysfunction. Although it has not yet been clearly established whether endothelial dysfunction is the cause or a sequel of hypertension, it appears nevertheless to contribute to the progression of the vascular disease and hypertension-related endorgan damage.[52,159–161] Thus, increased peripheral vascular resistance is one of the hallmark features of hypertension. Structural alterations in small-resistance arteries and arterioles are regularly

observed in animal models of hypertension and in hypertensive patients, including concentric hypertrophic remodeling of the vessel walls associated with an increase of the media cross-sectional area and the media-to-lumen diameter ratio. The balance between endothelial dilatory factors such as NO and prostacyclin and constrictive factors such as endothelin and angiotensin II seems to be disturbed in hypertension (Fig. 2-20), determining not only the arterial tone but also vascular remodeling through modulation of vascular SCM growth and ECM production.

In conclusion, microvascular dilatory mechanisms may compensate for the effects of upstream stenoses.[162,163] However, in most patients endothelial and thus microvascular dysfunction limits this compensatory microvascular response. In addition, endothelial dysfunction may further promote atherosclerotic processes and aggravate the inflammatory response after ischemia and reperfusion. New treatments will have to specifically target microvascular endothelial dysfunction to enhance the long-term benefits of endovascular interventions. The beneficial effects of statins that improve patient outcome beyond their cholesterol-lowering effects by rescuing endothelial function exemplify this principle.

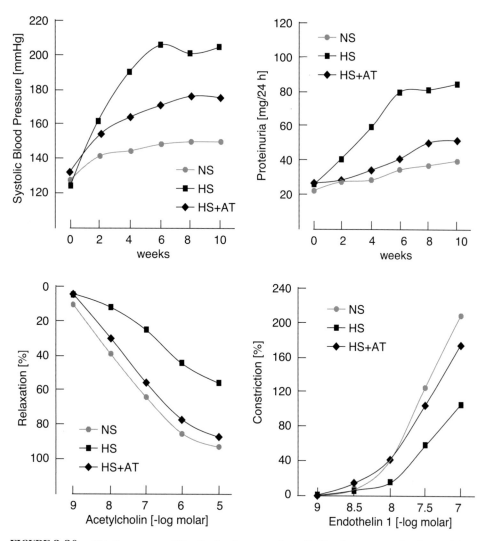

FIGURE 2-20. This figure exemplifies the development of systolic blood pressure and endorgan injury represented by proteinuria in Dahl salt-sensitive rats during 10 weeks of high-salt (*HS*) diet as compared to normal-salt (*NS*) diet. The *two lower panels* represent the blunted responses of aortic ring preparations to acetylcholine-induced endothelium-dependent relaxation (*left*) and to endothelin-induced vasoconstriction (*right*) in the rats fed the HS diet and developing hypertension. Treatment with atorvastatin markedly attenuated the observed vascular dysfunction, exemplifying the pleiotropic action of this class of cholesterol-lowering drugs. (Adapted from Zhou MS, Jaimes EA, Raij L. Atorvastatin prevents end-organ injury in salt-sensitive hypertension: role of eNOS and oxidant stress. *Hypertension*. 2004;44:186-190.)

REFERENCES

1. Gould KL, Lipscomb K. Effects of coronary stenoses on coronary flow reserve and resistance. *Am J Cardiol*. 1974;34:48–55.

2. Gould KL, Kirkeeide RL, Buchi M. Coronary flow reserve as a physiologic measure of stenosis severity. *J Am Coll Cardiol*. 1990;15:459–474.

3. Siebes M, Chamuleau SA, Meuwissen M, et al. Influence of hemodynamic conditions on fractional flow reserve: parametric analysis of underlying model. *Am J Physiol Heart Circ Physiol*. 2002;283:H1462–H1470.

4. Poiseuille JLM. Recherches sur la force du coeur aortique. Dissertation, École Polytechnique 1828.

5. Poiseuille JLM. Recherches sur les causes du mouvement du sang dans les veins. *J Physiol Exp Pathol*. 1830;10:277–295.

6. Pries AR, Secomb TW, Gaehtgens P. Design principles of vascular beds. *Circ Res*. 1995;77:1017–1023.

7. Renkin EM. Control of microcirculation and blood-tissue exchange. In: Renkin EM, Michel CC, eds. *Handbook of Physiology*, section 2: *The Cardiovascular System*, vol IV, *Microcirculation*, part 2. Bethesda, MD: American Physiological Society, 1984:627–687.

8. Chilian WM, Eastham CL, Marcus ML. Microvascular distribution of coronary vascular resistance in beating left ventricle. *Am J Physiol*. 1986;251:H779–H788.

9. Chilian WM, Layne SM, Klausner EC, et al. Redistribution of coronary microvascular resistance produced by dipyridamole. *Am J Physiol*. 1989;256:H383–H390.

10. Bech GJ, de Bruyne B, Akasaka T, et al. Coronary pressure and FFR predict long-term outcome after PTCA. *Int J Cardiovasc Intervent*. 2001:4:67–76.

11. Pijls NH. Is it time to measure fractional flow reserve in all patients? *J Am Coll Cardiol*. 2003;41:1122–1124.

12. Goldstein RA, Kirkeeide RL, Demer LL, et al. Relation between geometric dimensions of coronary artery stenoses and myocardial perfusion reserve in man. *J Clin Invest*. 1987;79:1473–1478.

13. Fulton WF. The time factor in the enlargement of anastomoses in coronary artery disease. *Scott Med J*. 1964;37:18–23.

14. Schaper W, Buschmann I. Arteriogenesis, the good and bad of it. *Cardiovasc Res*. 1999;43:835–837.

15. Scholz D, Ito W, Fleming I, et al. Ultrastructure and molecular histology of rabbit hind-limb collateral artery growth (arteriogenesis). *Virchows Arch*. 2000;436:257–270.

16. Koerselman J, van der Graaf Y, de Jaegere PP, et al. Coronary collaterals: an important and underexposed aspect of coronary artery disease. *Circulation*. 2003;107:2507–2511.

17. Baroldi G, Mantero O, Scomazzoni G. The collaterals of the coronary arteries in normal and pathologic hearts. *Circ Res*. 1956;4:223–229.

18. Flameng W, Schwarz F, Schaper W. Coronary collaterals in the canine heart: development and functional significance. *Am Heart J*. 1979;97:70–77.

19. Schaper W, Jageneau A, Xhonneux R. The development of collateral circulation in the pig and dog heart. *Cardiology*. 1967;51:321–335.

20. Nilius B, Eggermont J, Voets T, et al. Volume-activated Cl- channels. *Gen Pharmacol.* 27:1131–1140, 1996.

21. Arras M, Ito WD, Scholz D, et al. Monocyte activation in angiogenesis and collateral growth in the rabbit hindlimb. *J Clin Invest* 101:40–50, 1998.

22. Hoefer IE, Grundmann S, van Royen N, et al. Leukocyte subpopulations and arteriogenesis: specific role of monocytes, lymphocytes and granulocytes. *Atherosclerosis.* 2005;181:285–293.

23. Hoefer IE, van Royen N, Rectenwald JE, et al. Arteriogenesis proceeds via ICAM-1/Mac-1-mediated mechanisms. *Circ Res.* 2004;94:1179–1185.

24. Tyagi SC, Kumar S, Cassatt S, et al. Temporal expression of extracellular matrix metalloproteinases and tissue plasminogen activator in the development of collateral vessels in the canine model of coronary occlusion. *Can J Physiol Pharmacol.* 1996;74:983–995.

25. Schirmer SH, Buschmann IR, Jost MM, et al. Differential effects of MCP-1 and leptin on collateral flow and arteriogenesis. *Cardiovasc Res.* 2004; 64(2):356–364.

26. Carmeliet P. Mechanisms of angiogenesis and arteriogenesis. *Nat Med.* 2000;6:389–395.

27. Buschmann I, Schaper W. The pathophysiology of the collateral circulation (arteriogenesis). *J Pathol.* 2000;190:338–342.

28. Jung O, Schreiber JG, Geiger H, et al. gp91phox-containing NADPH oxidase mediates endothelial dysfunction in renovascular hypertension. *Circulation.* 2004;109:1795–1801.

29. Ono Y, Ono H, Matsuoka H, et al. Apoptosis, coronary arterial remodeling, and myocardial infarction after nitric oxide inhibition in SHR. *Hypertension.* 1999;34:609–616.

30. Scuteri A, Manolio TA, Marino EK, et al. Prevalence of specific variant carotid geometric patterns and incidence of cardiovascular events in older persons. The Cardiovascular Health Study (CHS E-131). *J Am Coll Cardiol.* 2004;43:187–193.

31. Boutouyrie P, Germain DP, Fiessinger JN, et al. Increased carotid wall stress in vascular Ehlers-Danlos syndrome. *Circulation.* 2004;109:1530–1535.

32. Levy BI, Tedgui A. *Biology of the Arterial Wall.* Dordrecht, The Netherlands: Kluwer Academic Publishers, 1999.

33. Levy BI. Mechanics of the large artery vascular wall. *Pathol Biol (Paris).* 1999;47:634–640.

34. Lee RT, Kamm RD. Vascular mechanics for the cardiologist. *J Am Coll Cardiol.* 1994;23:1289–1295.

35. O'Rourke MF, Adji A. An updated clinical primer on large artery mechanics: implications of pulse waveform analysis and arterial tonometry. *Curr Opin Cardiol.* 2005;20:275–281.

36. van den Berkmortel FW, van der Steen M, Hoogenboom H, et al. Progressive arterial wall stiffening in patients with increasing diastolic blood pressure. *J Hum Hypertens.* 2001;15:685–691.

37. Tajaddini A, Kilpatrick DL, Schoenhagen P, et al. Impact of age and hyperglycemia on the mechanical behavior of intact human coronary arteries: an ex vivo intravascular ultrasound study. *Am J Physiol Heart Circ Physiol.* 2005;288:H250–H255.

38. Asmar R, Rudnichi A, Blacher J, et al. Pulse pressure and aortic pulse wave are markers of cardiovascular risk in hypertensive populations. *Am J Hypertens.* 2001;14:91–97.

39. Safar ME, Henry O, Meaume S. Aortic pulse wave velocity: an independent marker of cardiovascular risk. *Am J Geriatr Cardiol.* 2002;11:295–298.

40. Safar ME, Levy BI, Struijker-Boudier H. Current perspectives on arterial stiffness and pulse pressure in hypertension and cardiovascular diseases. *Circulation.* 2003;107:2864–2869.

41. Laurent S, Boutouyrie P, Asmar R, et al. Aortic stiffness is an independent predictor of all-cause and cardiovascular mortality in hypertensive patients. *Hypertension.* 2001;37:1236–1241.

42. Laurent S. Arterial stiffness: intermediate or surrogate endpoint for cardiovascular events? *Eur Heart J.* 2005;26:1152–1154.

43. Adji A, O'Rourke MF. Determination of central aortic systolic and pulse pressure from the radial artery pressure waveform. *Blood Press Monit.* 2004;9:115–121.

44. Gallagher D, Adji A, O'Rourke MF. Validation of the transfer function technique for generating central from peripheral upper limb pressure waveform. *Am J Hypertens.* 2004;17:1059–1067.

45. Giannattasio C, Failla M, Emanuelli G, et al. Local effects of atherosclerotic plaque on arterial distensibility. *Hypertension.* 2001;38:1177–1180.

46. Shaw JA, Kingwell BA, Walton AS, et al. Determinants of coronary artery compliance in subjects with and without angiographic coronary artery disease. *J Am Coll Cardiol.* 2002;39:1637–1643.

47. Holzapfel GA, Sommer G, Regitnig P. Anisotropic mechanical properties of tissue components in human atherosclerotic plaques. *J Biomech Eng.* 2004;126:657–665.

48. de Korte CL, van der Steen AF. Intravascular ultrasound elastography: an overview. *Ultrasonics.* 2002;40:859–865.

49. de Korte CL, Schaar JA, Mastik F, et al. Intravascular elastography: from bench to bedside. *J Intervent Cardiol.* 2003;16:253–259.

50. Ramnarine KV, Hartshorne T, Sensier Y, et al. Tissue Doppler imaging of carotid plaque wall motion: a pilot study. *Cardiovasc Ultrasound.* 2003;1:17.

51. Baldewsing RA, Schaar JA, de Korte CL, et al. Intravascular ultrasound elastography: a clinician's tool for assessing vulnerability and material composition of plaques. *Stud Health Technol Inform.* 2005;113:75–96.

52. Levy BI, Ambrosio G, Pries AR, et al. Microcirculation in hypertension: a new target for treatment? *Circulation.* 2001;104:735–740.

53. Wiedeman MP, Tuma RF, Mayrovitz HN. Defining the precapillary sphincter. *Microvasc Res.* 1976;12:71–75.

54. Wiedeman MP. Architecture. In: Renkin EM, Michel CC, eds. *Handbook of Physiology*, section 2: *The Cardiovascular System*, vol IV, *Microcirculation*, part 2. Bethesda, MD: American Physiological Society, 1984:11–40.

55. Podesser BK, Neumann F, Neumann M, et al. Outer radius-wall thickness ratio, a postmortem quantitative histology in human coronary arteries. *Acta Anat (Basel).* 1998;163:63–68.

56. Pries AR, Reglin B, Secomb TW. Structural adaptation of vascular networks: role of the pressure response. *Hypertension.* 2001;38:1476–1479.

57. Pries AR, Secomb TW. Structural adaptation of microvascular networks and development of hypertension. *Microcirculation.* 2002;9:305–314.

58. Pries AR, Reglin B, Secomb TW. Remodeling of blood vessels: responses of diameter and wall thickness to hemodynamic and metabolic stimuli. *Hypertension.* 2005;46:726–731.

59. Muller JM, Davis MJ, Chilian WM. Integrated regulation of pressure and flow in the coronary microcirculation. *Cardiovasc Res.* 1996;32:668–678.

60. Simionescu M, Simionescu N. Ultrastructure of the microvascular wall: functional correlations. In: Renkin EM, Michel CC, eds. *Handbook of Physiology*, section 2: *The Cardiovascular System*, vol IV, *Microcirculation*, part 2. Bethesda, MD: American Physiological Society, 1984:41–101.

61. le Noble F, Fleury V, Pries A, et al. Control of arterial branching morphogenesis in embryogenesis: go with the flow. *Cardiovasc Res.* 2005;65:619–628.

62. Eichmann A, Yuan L, Moyon D, et al. Vascular development: from precursor cells to branched arterial and venous networks. *Int J Dev Biol.* 2005;49:259–267.

63. Zakrzewicz A, Secomb TW, Pries AR. Angioadaptation: keeping the vascular system in shape. *News Physiol Sci.* 2002;17:197–201.

64. Pries AR, Reglin B, Secomb TW. Structural adaptation of microvascular networks: functional roles of adaptive responses. *Am J Physiol.* 2001;281:H1015–H1025.

65. Bongrazio M, Baumann C, Zakrzewicz A, et al. Evidence for modulation of genes involved in vascular adaptation by prolonged exposure of endothelial cells to shear stress. *Cardiovasc Res.* 2000;47:384–393.

66. Sun D, Huang A, Koller A, et al. Adaptation of flow-induced dilation of arterioles to daily exercise. *Microvasc Res.* 1998;56:54–61.

67. Monos E, Lorant M, Feher E. Mechanisms of vascular adaptation to long-term orthostatic gravitational loading. *J Gravit Physiol.* 1997;4:39–40.

68. Unthank JL, Nixon JC, Lash JM. Early adaptations in collateral and microvascular resistances after ligation of the rat femoral artery. *J Appl Physiol.* 1995;79:73–82.

69. Fillinger MF, Cronenwett JL, Besso S, et al. Vein adaptation to the hemodynamic environment of infrainguinal grafts. *J Vasc Surg.* 1994;19:970–978.

70. Pries AR, Secomb TW, Gaehtgens P. Structure and hemodynamics of microvascular networks: heterogeneity and correlations. *Am J Physiol.* 1995;269:H1713–H1722.

71. Bevan JA. Shear stress, the endothelium and the balance between flow-induced contraction and dilation in animals and man. *Int J Microcirc Clin Exp.* 1997;17:248–256.

72. Papadaki M, Eskin SG. Effects of fluid shear stress on gene regulation of vascular cells. *Biotechnol Prog.* 1997;13:209–221.

73. Mulvany MJ. Small artery remodeling and significance in the development of hypertension. *News Physiol Sci.* 2002;i17:105–109.

74. Buus CL, Pourageaud F, Fazzi GE, et al. Smooth muscle cell changes during flow-related remodeling of rat mesenteric resistance arteries. *Circ Res.* 2001;89:180–186.

75. Greene AS, Tonellato PJ, Lui J, et al. Microvascular rarefaction and tissue vascular resistance in hypertension. *Am J Physiol.* 1989;256:H126–H131.

76. Prasad A, Dunnill GS, Mortimer PS, et al. Capillary rarefaction in the forearm skin in essential hypertension. *J Hypertens.* 1995;13:265–268.

77. Price RJ, Skalak TC. Circumferential wall stress as a mechanism for arteriolar rarefaction and proliferation in a network model. *Microvasc Res.* 1994;47:188–202.

78. Pries AR, Secomb TW. Microvascular blood viscosity in vivo and the endothelial surface layer. *Am J Physiol Heart Circ Physiol.* 2005;289(6):H2657–H2664.

79. Baumbach GL, Dobrin PB, Hart MN, et al. Mechanics of cerebral arterioles in hypertensive rats. *Circ Res.* 1988;61:56–64.

80. Baumbach GL, Heistad DD. Remodeling of cerebral arterioles in chronic hypertension. *Hypertension.* 1989;13:968–972.

81. Baumbach GL, Ghoneim S. Vascular remodeling in hypertension. *Scanning Microsc.* 1993;7:137–143.

82. Baumbach GL, Hajdu MA. Mechanics and composition of cerebral arterioles in renal and spontaneously hypertensive rats. *Hypertension.* 1993;21:816–826.

83. Baumbach GL, Sigmund CD, Faraci FM. Cerebral arteriolar structure in mice overexpressing human renin and angiotensinogen. *Hypertension.* 2003;41:50–55.

84. Hajdu MA, Baumbach GL. Mechanics of large and small cerebral arteries in chronic hypertension. *Am J Physiol.* 1994;266:H1027–H1033.

85. Skalak R, Chen PH, Chien S. Effect of hematocrit and rouleaux on apparent viscosity in capillaries. *Biorheology.* 1972;9:67–82.

86. Chien S. Biophysical behaviour of red cells in suspensions. In: Surgenor DMN, ed. *The Red Blood Cell.* Vol II. New York: Academic Press, 1975:1031–1133.

87. Cokelet GR. The rheology of human blood. In: Fung YC, Perrone N, Anliker M, eds. *Biomechanics: Its Foundations and Objectives.* Englewood Cliffs, NJ: Prentice-Hall, 1972:64–103.

88. Cokelet GR, Goldsmith HL. Decreased hydrodynamic resistance in the two-phase flow of blood through small vertical tubes at low flow rates. *Circ Res.* 1991;68:1–17.

89. Alonso C, Pries AR, Gaehtgens P. Time-dependent rheological behaviour of blood flow at low shear in narrow horizontal tubes. *Biorheology.* 1989;26:229–246.

90. Alonso C, Pries AR, Gaehtgens P. Time-dependent rheological behaviour of blood at low shear in narrow vertical tubes. *Am J Physiol.* 1993;265:H553–H561.

91. Fahraeus R, Lindqvist T. The viscosity of the blood in narrow capillary tubes. *Am J Physiol.* 1931;96:562–568.

92. Pries AR, Neuhaus D, Gaehtgens P. Blood viscosity in tube flow: dependence on diameter and hematocrit. *Am J Physiol.* 1992;263:H1770–H1778.

93. Secomb TW, Skalak R, Özkaya N, et al. Flow of axisymmetric red blood cells in narrow capillaries. *J Fluid Mech.* 1986;163:405–423.

94. Pries AR, Secomb TW, Gaehtgens P. The endothelial surface layer. *Pflugers Arch.* 2000;440:653–666.

95. Pries AR, Secomb TW, Gessner T, et al. Resistance to blood flow in microvessels *in vivo. Circ Res.* 1994;75:904–915.

96. Pries AR, Secomb TW, Jacobs H, et al. Microvascular blood flow resistance: role of endothelial surface layer. *Am J Physiol.* 1997;273:H2272–H2279.

97. Duling BR, Desjardins C. Capillary hematocrit—what does it mean? *News Physiol Sci.* 1987;2:66–69.

98. Vink H, Duling BR. Identification of distinct luminal domains for macromolecules, erythrocytes, and leukocytes within mammalian capillaries. *Circ Res.* 1996;79:581–589.

99. van Haaren PM, VanBavel E, Vink H, et al. Localization of the permeability barrier to solutes in isolated arteries by confocal microscopy. *Am J Physiol Heart Circ Physiol.* 2003;285:H2848–H2856.

100. Henry, CBS, Duling, BR. Hyaluronidase treatment suggests a role for cell surface hyaluronan in determining vascular permeability [abstract]. *FASEB J.* 1998;12(4, pt 1):no.139.

101. Pries AR, Secomb TW, Sperandio M, et al. Blood flow resistance during hemodilution: effect of plasma composition. *Cardiovasc Res.* 1998;37:225–235.

102. Damiano ER. The effect of the endothelial-cell glycocalyx on the motion of red blood cells through capillaries. *Microvasc Res.* 1998;55:77–91.

103. Secomb TW, Hsu R, Pries AR. A model for red blood cell motion in glycocalyx-lined capillaries. *Am J Physiol.* 1998;274:H1016–H1022.

104. Secomb TW, Hsu R, Pries AR. Motion of red blood cells in a capillary with an endothelial surface layer: effect of flow velocity. *Am J Physiol.* 2001;281:H629–H636.

105. Secomb TW, Hsu R, Pries AR. Effect of endothelial glycocalyx on oxygen transport from capillaries to tissue: a theoretical model [abstract]. *FASEB J.* 1999;13:A25.

106. Secomb TW, Hsu R, Pries AR. Effect of the endothelial surface layer on transmission of fluid shear stress to endothelial cells. *Biorheology.* 2001;38:143–150.

107. Vogel J, Sperandio M, Pries AR, et al. Influence of the endothelial glycocalyx on cerebral blood flow in mice. *J Cereb Blood Flow Metab.* 2000;20:1571–1578.

108. Thi MM, Tarbell JM, Weinbaum S, et al. The role of the glycocalyx in reorganization of the actin cytoskeleton under fluid shear stress: a "bumper-car" model. *Proc Natl Acad Sci U S A.* 2004;101:16483–16488.

109. Henry CB, Duling BR. TNF-alpha increases entry of macromolecules into luminal endothelial cell glycocalyx. *Am J Physiol Heart Circ Physiol.* 2000;279:H2815–H2823.

110. Zhao Y, Chien S, Weinbaum S. Dynamic contact forces on leukocyte microvilli and their penetration of the endothelial glycocalyx. *Biophys J.* 2001;80:1124–1140.

111. Constantinescu AA, Vink H, Spaan JA. Elevated capillary tube hematocrit reflects degradation of endothelial cell glycocalyx by oxidized LDL. *Am J Physiol.* 2001;280:H1051–H1057.

112. Vink H, Constantinescu AA, Spaan JA. Oxidized lipoproteins degrade the endothelial surface layer : implications for platelet-endothelial cell adhesion. *Circulation.* 2000;101:1500–1502.

113. Rehm M, Zahler S, Lotsch M, et al. Endothelial glycocalyx as an additional barrier determining extravasation of 6% hydroxyethyl starch or 5% albumin solutions in the coronary vascular bed. *Anesthesiology.* 2004;100:1211–1223.

114. Chilian WM, Layne SM, Eastham CL, et al. Heterogeneous microvascular coronary alpha-adrenergic vasoconstriction. *Mol Cell.* 1989;64:376–388.

115. Holmes CL, Landry DW, Granton JT. Science Review: Vasopressin and the cardiovascular system, part 2—clinical physiology. *Crit Care.* 2004;8:15–23.

116. Holmes CL, Landry DW, Granton JT. Science review: Vasopressin and the cardiovascular system, part 1—receptor physiology. *Crit Care.* 2003;7:427–434.

117. Houben AJ, van der Zander K, de Leeuw PW. Vascular and renal actions of brain natriuretic peptide in man: physiology and pharmacology. *Fundam Clin Pharmacol.* 2005;19:411–419.

118. Suttner SW, Boldt J. Natriuretic peptide system: physiology and clinical utility. *Curr Opin Crit Care.* 2004;10:336–341.

119. Ahluwalia A, Hobbs AJ. Endothelium-derived C-type natriuretic peptide: more than just a hyperpolarizing factor. *Trends Pharmacol Sci.* 2005;26:162–167.

120. Davis MJ. Myogenic response gradient in an arteriolar network. *Am J Physiol.* 1993;264:H2168–H2179.

121. Liao JC, Kuo L. Interaction between adenosine and flow-induced dilation in coronary microvascular network. *Am J Physiol.* 1997;272:H1571–H1581.

122. Jones CJ, Kuo L, Davis MJ, et al. Regulation of coronary blood flow: coordination of heterogeneous control mechanisms in vascular microdomains. *Cardiovasc Res.* 1995;29:585–596.

123. de Wit C, Bolz SS, Pohl U. Interaction of endothelial autacoids in microvascular control. *Z Kardiol.* 2000;89(suppl 9):IX/113–IX/116.

124. Nilius B, Droogmans G. Ion channels and their functional role in vascular endothelium. *Physiol Rev.* 2001;81:1415–1459.

125. Fulton D, Gratton JP, Sessa WC. Post-translational control of endothelial nitric oxide synthase: why isn't calcium/calmodulin enough? *J Pharmacol Exp Ther.* 2001;299:818–824.

126. Boo YC, Jo H. Flow-dependent regulation of endothelial nitric oxide synthase: role of protein kinases. *Am J Physiol Cell Physiol.* 2003;285:C499–C508.

127. Habazettl H, Vollmar B, Christ M, et al. Heterogeneous microvascular coronary vasodilation by adenosine and nitroglycerin in dogs. *J Appl Physiol.* 1994;76:1951–1960.

128. Pohl U, de Wit C, Gloe T. Large arterioles in the control of blood flow: role of endothelium-dependent dilation. *Acta Physiol Scand.* 2000;168:505–510.

129. de Wit C, Roos F, Bolz SS, et al. Impaired conduction of vasodilation along arterioles in connexin40- deficient mice. *Circ Res.* 2000;86:649–655.

130. Galley HF, Webster NR. Physiology of the endothelium. *Br J Anaesth.* 2004;93:105–113.

131. Lavallee M, Takamura M, Parent R, et al. Crosstalk between endothelin and nitric oxide in the control of vascular tone. *Heart Fail Rev.* 2001;6:265–276.

132. Kawashima S. The two faces of endothelial nitric oxide synthase in the pathophysiology of atherosclerosis. *Endothelium.* 2004;11:99–107.

133. Brunner H, Cockcroft JR, Deanfield J, et al. Endothelial function and dysfunction. Part II: Association with cardiovascular risk factors and diseases. A statement by the Working

134. Group on Endothelins and Endothelial Factors of the European Society of Hypertension. *J Hypertens.* 2005;23:233–246.

134. Naseem KM. The role of nitric oxide in cardiovascular diseases. *Mol Aspects Med.* 2005;26:33–65.

135. Deanfield J, Donald A, Ferri C, et al. Endothelial function and dysfunction. Part I: Methodological issues for assessment in the different vascular beds: a statement by the Working Group on Endothelin and Endothelial Factors of the European Society of Hypertension. *J Hypertens.* 2005;23:7–17.

136. Kaski JC. Pathophysiology and management of patients with chest pain and normal coronary arteriograms (cardiac syndrome X). *Circulation.* 2004;109:568–572.

137. Kaski JC, Aldama G, Cosin-Sales J. Cardiac syndrome X. Diagnosis, pathogenesis and management. *Am J Cardiovasc Drugs.* 2004;4:179–194.

138. Kubes P, Kerfoot SM. Leukocyte recruitment in the microcirculation: the rolling paradigm revisited. *News Physiol Sci.* 2001;16:76–80.

139. Kubes P. The complexities of leukocyte recruitment. *Semin Immunol.* 2002;14:65–72.

140. Ley K. The role of selectins in inflammation and disease. *Trends Mol Med.* 2003;9: 263–268.

141. Springer TA, Wang JH. The three-dimensional structure of integrins and their ligands, and conformational regulation of cell adhesion. *Adv Protein Chem.* 2004;68:29–63.

142. Weinmann P, Scharffetter-Kochanek K, Forlow SB, et al. A role for apoptosis in the control of neutrophil homeostasis in the circulation: insights from CD18-deficient mice. *Blood.* 2003;101:739–746.

143. Paterson RL, Galley HF, Webster NR. The effect of N-acetylcysteine on nuclear factor-kappa B activation, interleukin-6, interleukin-8, and intercellular adhesion molecule-1 expression in patients with sepsis. *Crit Care Med.* 2003;31:2574–2578.

144. Macdonald J, Galley HF, Webster NR. Oxidative stress and gene expression in sepsis. *Br J Anaesth.* 2003;90:221–232.

145. Rezkalla SH, Kloner RA. Coronary No-reflow Phenomenon. *Curr Treat Options Cardiovasc Med.* 2005;7:75–80.

146. Roe MT, Ohman EM, Maas AC, et al. Shifting the open-artery hypothesis downstream: the quest for optimal reperfusion. *J Am Coll Cardiol.* 2001;37:9–18.

147. Reffelmann T, Kloner RA. Microvascular alterations after temporary coronary artery occlusion: the no-reflow phenomenon. *J Cardiovasc Pharmacol Ther.* 2004;9:163–172.

148. Reffelmann T, Kloner RA. The "no-reflow" phenomenon: basic science and clinical correlates. *Heart.* 2002;87:162–168.

149. Kupatt C, Habazettl H, Goedecke A, et al. Tumor necrosis factor-alpha contributes to ischemia- and reperfusion-induced endothelial activation in isolated hearts. *Circ Res.* 1999;84:392–400.

150. Baxter GF. The neutrophil as a mediator of myocardial ischemia-reperfusion injury: time to move on. *Basic Res Cardiol.* 2002;97:268–275.

151. Kupatt C, Wichels R, Deiss M, et al. Retroinfusion of NFkappaB decoy oligonucleotide extends cardioprotection achieved by CD18 inhibition in a preclinical study of myocardial ischemia and retroinfusion in pigs. *Gene Ther.* 2002;9:518–526.

152. Habazettl H, Hanusch P, Kupatt C. Effects of endothelium/leukocytes/platelet interaction on myocardial ischemia–reperfusion injury. *Z Kardiol.* 2000:89(suppl 9): IX/92-IX/95.

153. Gawaz M. Role of platelets in coronary thrombosis and reperfusion of ischemic myocardium. *Cardiovasc Res.* 2004;61:498–511.

154. Kupatt C, Wichels R, Horstkotte J, et al. Molecular mechanisms of platelet-mediated leukocyte recruitment during myocardial reperfusion. *J Leukoc Biol.* 2002;72:455–461.

155. Kupatt C, Habazettl H, Hanusch P, et al. c7E3Fab reduces postischemic leukocyte-thrombocyte interaction mediated by fibrinogen. Implications for myocardial reperfusion injury. *Arterioscler Thromb Vasc Biol.* 2000;20:2226–2232.

156. Neumann FJ, Blasini R, Schmitt C, et al. Effect of glycoprotein IIb/IIIa receptor blockade on recovery of coronary flow and left ventricular function after the placement of coronary-artery stents in acute myocardial infarction. *Circulation.* 1998;98:2695–2701.

157. Dayton C, Yamaguchi T, Warren A, et al. Ischemic preconditioning prevents postischemic arteriolar, capillary, and postcapillary venular dysfunction: signaling pathways mediating the adaptive metamorphosis to a protected phenotype in preconditioned endothelium. *Microcirculation.* 2002;9:73–89.

158. Wang WZ, Fang XH, Stepheson LL, et al. NOS upregulation attenuates vascular endothelial dysfunction in the late phase of ischemic preconditioning in skeletal muscle. *J Orthop Res.* 2004;22:578–585.

159. Nadar S, Blann AD, Lip GY. Endothelial dysfunction: methods of assessment and application to hypertension. *Curr Pharm Des.* 2004;10:3591–3605.

160. Budhiraja R, Tuder RM, Hassoun PM. Endothelial dysfunction in pulmonary hypertension. *Circulation.* 2004;109:159–165.

161. Zhou MS, Jaimes EA, Raij L. Atorvastatin prevents end-organ injury in salt-sensitive hypertension: role of eNOS and oxidant stress. *Hypertension.* 2004;44:186–190.

162. Bartunek J, Sys SU, Heyndrickx GR, et al. Quantitative coronary angiography in predicting functional significance of stenoses in an unselected patient cohort. *J Am Coll Cardiol.* 1995;26:328–334.

163. Briguori C, Anzuini A, Airoldi F, et al. Intravascular ultrasound criteria for the assessment of the functional significance of intermediate coronary artery stenoses and comparison with fractional flow reserve. *Am J Cardiol.* 2001;87:136–141.

Dietrich Baumgart
Thomas Egelhof

CHAPTER **3A**

Magnetic Resonance Imaging

Magnetic resonance (MR) imaging has emerged as a key imaging technique in medical diagnostics in the past 20 years. The dramatic improvement in detailed body organ imaging has been recognized by the Nobel prize granted to Paul Lauterbur and Sir Peter Mansfield in 2003. MR imaging is characterized by its unsurpassed soft tissue contrast with high accuracy. In addition, it allows functional imaging of moving structures, such as the beating heart, or quantification of blood flow. The absence of x-ray exposure is a further substantial advantage and makes MR imaging attractive for repetitive investigations as well as screening purposes. Consequently, the combination of MR imaging (MRI) and MR angiography (MRA) allows simultaneous evaluation of the vessels and of the dependent end-organ function. MR imaging is mainly limited by its costs and availability.

MAGNETIC RESONANCE IMAGING: BRAIN, HEART/LUNGS, AND ABDOMINAL ORGANS (BRIEF OVERVIEW)

BRAIN

Magnetic Resonance Imaging in Ischemic and Hemorrhagic Stroke

MRA/MRI imaging allows evaluation of cerebral circulation and brain parenchyma to allow therapeutic decision making in stroke patients.[1] Multimodal MRI can be implemented safely in the process of emergency stroke diagnostics and treatment.[2] It offers fast and reliable information with respect to the arterial and functional status of the brain. Basis of imaging studies in stroke patients is diffusion-weighted imaging (DWI), which is the most sensitive method for stroke detection, and, combined with perfusion-weighted imaging (PWI), provides information on the functional status of the ischemic brain.[1] Additionally MRA then offers information on stroke mechanism and pathophysiology that can guide interventional and medical management.[2] Typical protocols of DWI and PWI brain imaging vary according to the individual type of scanners and field strength. On average image acquisition takes <20 to 30 minutes. Figure 3A-1 shows examples of both imaging techniques.

MRA finally provides assessment of intra- and extracranial vascular status in stroke. Extracranial vessels are preferably visualized using 3D gadolinium-contrast techniques. Images are usually acquired in coronal planes with 3D reconstruction.[3] On average, image acquisition takes <5 minutes. Alternatively, time-of-flight (TOF) MRA techniques can be used allowing visualization of the cerebral vessels without use of contrast medium. 3D-TOF is preferred over two-dimensional 2D-TOF because of better resolution and lower sensitivity for flow voids. Axial images are reconstructed rendering maximum-intensity projections (MIPs), algorithms to subtract background and to highlight arteries. To assess the target pathology, source images may also be reformatted at different angles and displayed as rotating 3D vascular structures. Figure 3A-2 shows an example of an intracranial TOF.

Intracranial vessels are typically visualized using 2D and 3D TOF imaging sequences. Whereas 2D methods are highly sensitive to slow flow, 3D acquisition allows better sensitivity to a wide range of flows and therefore better visualization of intraluminal flow phenomena. Drawbacks of 3D TOF are longer acquisition time and greater sensitivity to motion artifacts. On average image acquisition takes <5 minutes.

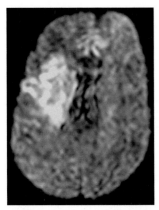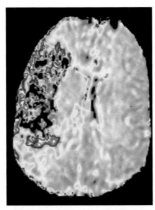

FIGURE 3A-1. Diffusion-weighted (DWI, *left panel*) and perfusion-weighted (PWI, *right panel*) images with acute infarct of the medial cerebral artery on the right side. The area with impaired diffusion and the bright signal corresponds to the infarcted area. This area is somewhat smaller than the area with impaired perfusion. Cerebral tissue with impaired perfusion but without impaired diffusion is called penumbra and will most likely profit from interventional recanalization procedures.

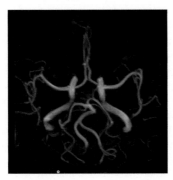

FIGURE 3A-2. Time-of-flight angiography of cerebral vessels without contrast enhancement.

Magnetic Resonance Imaging in Cerebral Angiopathy

There is neuropathological evidence that confluent white matter lesions in the elderly reflect brain damage due to microangiopathy. Cerebral small-vessel alterations are responsible for subcortical lesions associated with cognitive impairments. Small-vessel diseases are classified according to pathology. The most important cerebral microangiopathies are related to long-lasting hypertension. Resulting small-vessel changes may cause ischemic damage to the brain parenchyma and are associated with blood–brain-barrier alterations. Both mechanisms are thought to contribute to the occurrence of white-matter alterations and lacunar infarcts. Modern MR techniques such as fluid-attenuated inversion recovery (FLAIR) and DWI sequences allow noninvasive detection and progress of white-matter lesions (WMLs). There is evidence for an association between long-standing hypertension and WMLs. In the Ansan Study on suboptimally controlled hypertension, despite a multimodal antihypertensive medication, isolated systolic hypertension before medication and untreated systolic and diastolic hypertension were all significantly and independently correlated with the presence and severity of WMLs.[4]

Magnetic Resonance Imaging in Intracranial Aneurysm

Intracranial aneurysms are common. Autopsy studies have shown that the overall frequency in the general population ranges from 0.8% to 10%.[5] Management of intracranial aneurysms has improved significantly during recent years because of major advances in endovascular techniques and microsurgery.[5,6] Digital subtraction angiography is still the gold standard for diagnosing cerebral vessel disease, but MRI and MRA are offering complementary data essential for treatment decisions: size and anatomic localization in respect to surrounding tissue or intraluminal thrombus. TOF MRA is basically a fast gradient-echo technique that makes it possible to visualize the arterial lumen. A second technique, contrast-enhanced MRA (CE-MRA), is less affected by flow artifacts and uses gadolinium-containing contrast medium to enhance vessel contrast. Figure 3A-3 shows typical MRA/MRI findings in a patient with intracranial aneurysm.

HEART/LUNGS

Cardiac imaging of the beating heart by magnetic resonance technology has long been hampered by the lack of technical solutions to overcome motional artifacts. However, the advent of rapid gradients and fast sequences, as well as multidetection array coils, has now made cardiac magnetic resonance tomography (cMRT) an important tool in the cardiovascular diagnostic workup. Advantages of cMRT include comprehensive and operator-independent visualization of cardiac structures and function free from ionizing radiation. However, as yet, multislice computed tomography (MSCT) and coronary angiography render an up to 10-fold higher resolution of cardiac structures and especially the coronary arteries.

Nevertheless, MRT is best suited to precisely answer a number of questions concerning cardiac anatomy, function, and viability.[7] Both acute myocardial infarction and myocardial scar tissue can be detected using T2 weighed sequences and late enhancement techniques. cMRT is the best volumetric technique for quantification of both ventricles and atria. Dissections as well as aneurysms can be diagnosed noninvasively with great precision. Thus far, coronary arteries cannot

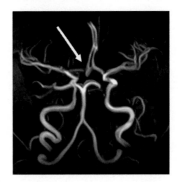

FIGURE 3A-3. Intracranial aneurysm (*arrow*).

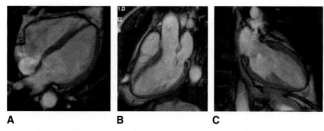

A   **B**   **C**

FIGURE 3A-4. Cardiac MR imaging: view of four chambers (**A**), outflow tract (**B**), and long axis (**C**).

be visualized with satisfactory accuracy. However, the refinement of cMRT using navigator sequences as well as the development of intra-arterial contrast media raises hopes for a direct visualization of proximal coronary arteries and stenoses in the future. Figure 3A-4 illustrates typical cardiac MR images.

MRT of the lungs has improved over the years but still is lacking in precision compared to CT images. The imaging of the lungs by MRT is complicated by motion artifacts of the heart and respiration. With ECG triggering and breath-hold techniques it is, however, possible to acquire artifact reduced images. Further improvements have been achieved by navigator echo sequences. Nevertheless, CT imaging techniques represent the gold standard in diagnostic imaging of the lungs. In addition, CT imaging techniques are less time consuming compared to MRT.[8]

On the other hand, MRT images render a much better soft-tissue contrast for diagnostic purposes. At present, the indications for lung or mediastinal MRT are the diagnosis of tumors of the thorax organs and the thorax wall, abscess, retrosternal or mediastinal mass, or thyroid tumors. Although contrast-enhanced x-ray angiography is still considered the gold standard for evaluation of pulmonary vascular pathology, recent years have seen exciting developments in CT and MR angiography of the pulmonary vasculature. With development of parallel imaging and navigator echo techniques, MR image quality has improved substantially. With similar imaging quality, CT techniques still have the advantage of shorter examination times.[9]

ABDOMINAL ORGANS

Abdominal ultrasound is the mostly widely available and cost-effective noninvasive imaging technique for diagnosis of abdominal pathologies. However, image quality decreases with increasing body dimensions and the presence of intra-abdominal air.

The acquisition of CT images can be achieved within a short time frame, at reasonable costs, with high spatial resolution, but at the expense of radiation exposure. MR imaging has the advantage of providing the highest accuracy of all available imaging modalities with excellent postprocessing options.[3]

To diagnose abdominal tumors or metastases and to differentiate malignant from benign lesions requires mostly contrast medium. Body array coils and breathing straps will improve image quality and help to avoid artifacts. Liver, pancreas, kidney, adrenal glands, and retroperitoneal space are the preferably targeted sites for MRT imaging. With maximum-intensity projections it is possible to acquire accurate three-dimensional

noninvasive images of the biliary and pancreatic ducts. These techniques represent an adequate alternative to conventional endoscopic retrograde cholangiopancreatographic (ERCP) imaging.[3]

MAGNETIC RESONANCE PANVASCULAR ANGIOGRAPHY

TECHNICAL ASPECTS

Basically there are native MRA techniques and MRA techniques using contrast agents for the visualization of vascular structures.

The inflow or time of flight, TOF techniques do not use any contrast medium. In short T1 gradient echo sequences, the relaxation of resting tissue is low associated with a decreased signal whereas the flowing blood provides high signals. This method of contrast enhancement is, however, dependent on the fact that flow is perpendicular to the scanning plane and that flow is sufficiently fast to refresh spins and to enhance the signal. The contrast is further influenced by the flip angle, which can be modified (for review, see reference 3).

The technique is best suited for small vessels in stationary organs. The acquisition time is relatively long, approximately 5 to 9 minutes, making this technique suitable primarily for brain vessel imaging. Turbulent flow reduces the signal, accounting for signal attenuation or signal voids in the vicinity of stenoses. Consequently, stenoses might be overestimated with this imaging technique. TOF angiography can be used with two- and three-dimensional sequences (for review, see reference 9).

Phase-contrast angiography relies on a unique pixel coding based on frequency and phase encoding and does not utilize any contrast agents. Reversing the polarity of the gradient will rephase the spins of the stationary tissues. In contrast, spins of the moving blood experience a phase delay in proportion to flow velocity allowing reliable flow velocity measurements. Phase-contrast angiography is mostly used to image brain veins. Flow measurements are primarily performed during cardiac imaging. The technique is also suited as a fast "angio-localizer" for subsequent contrast enhanced angiography.

MR angiography of the thorax, abdomen, or iliac vasculature cannot reliably be performed with native MR-angiographic techniques because the acquisition times are too long and breathing and pulsation artifacts will disturb image quality. Only fast 3D-gradient echo sequences with short TR and TE can achieve the necessary acquisition times of 15 to 30 seconds. The strong T1 weight allows imaging only of tissue with a very short T1-relaxation time. Fat tissue has the shortest T1-relaxation time (150 msec). With the help of intravenous contrast medium, the T1-relaxation time of blood can be reduced to 50 msec. Hence, blood gives the brightest signal as long as the contrast bolus is not diluted. Therefore, a successful angiographic imaging can only be performed shortly after the contrast bolus was injected. As the acquisition times are short, measurements should not be performed too early before the contrast bolus has reached the region of interest. Optimal timing is thus crucial for perfect image acquisition. In clinical practice, a small test bolus is given prior to the actual MR angiography and a dynamic sequence registers the advent of the contrast agent in the region of interest. Subsequently, acquisition of the angiography can be timed exactly to the bolus appearance (for review, see reference 9). Table 3A-1 gives sequence parameters for whole-body MRA.

CONTRAST AGENT

Paramagnetic contrast agents are pivotal for imaging of the vascular system using fast three-dimensional gradient echo sequences (Table 3A-1). Images acquired with these sequences and without contrast medium are void of any intravascular contrast and are therefore nondiagnostic.

Contrast enhancement is achieved by paramagnetic contrast agents through shortening T1-relaxation time of blood. A principal advantage of contrast-enhanced magnetic resonance angiography (CE-MRA) is that the signal of flowing blood is no longer flow dependent. Hence, flow-induced artifacts seen with time-of-flight or phase-contrast MRA are largely eliminated, and images can be acquired in the plane of the vessels of interest. This, in turn, permits the coverage of large vascular territories in short imaging times, which facilitates the generation of images that are similar in appearance to conventional angiography[10] (Fig. 3A-5).

CE-MRA is comparable to spiral CT angiography with respect to resolution and diagnostic accuracy. In addition to the absence of ionizing radiation and the ability to depict large vascular territories in 3D imaging volumes, side effects of the paramagnetic contrast agents are rare. The minor nephrotoxicity of these contrast agents and low incidence of allergic reactions makes the CE-MRA an attractive alternative to conventional angiography even in patients with renal insufficiency. Table 3A-2 summarizes the recommended evidence based indications for MRA.

WHOLE-BODY ANGIOGRAPHY

MRA has broadened the spectrum of magnetic resonance imaging applications, enabling morphological and functional assessment of the entire vascular system including quantitative measurements of blood flow.

Whole-body angiography has been limited due to the large amount of contrast agent required to visualize the entire vascular system. Initially, the examination was restricted to the display

TABLE 3A-1. Sequence Parameters for Whole-Body MR Angiography

True FISP Moving Scout

TR	4.45 msec
TE	2.22 msec
FOV	400 mm
Flip angle	70 degrees
Slice thickness	10 mm
Number of slices	6
Acquisition time	9 sec
Spatial resolution	$3.1 \times 1.6 \times 10$ mm^3
Matrix	256

TEST BOLUS

TR	1,000 msec
TE	1.58 msec
FOV	400 mm
Plane orientation	Coronal
Flip angle	8 degrees
Slice thickness	10 mm
Number of slices	60
Acquisition time	60 sec
Spatial resolution	$3.0 \times 1.6 \times 10$ mm^3
Matrix	256
Contrast injection	Test bolus, 1 mL Gd-BOPTA, flow, 1.3 mL/sec+30 mL NaCl; flow, 1.3 mL/sec; scan, proximal third descending aorta

CONTRAST-ENHANCED 3D FLASH

TR	2.2 msec
TE	0.74 msec
FOV	390 mm
Plane orientation	Coronal
Flip angle	20 degrees
Slice thickness	1.5
Number of slices	64
Acquisition time	12 sec
Spatial resolution	$1.8 \times 1.5 \times 1.5$ mm^3
Matrix	256
Contrast injection	0.2 mmol/kg bw Gd-BOPTA, diluted with NaCl to 60 mL; biphasic injection protocol, 1.3 mL/sec for the first half, 0.7 mL/sec for the second half of the bolus+30 mL NaCl; flow, 1.3 mL/sec

TABLE 3A-2. Indications for Magnetic Resonance Imaging in Acquired Diseases of the Vessels According to Evidence-based Classification[a]

Indication	Class
1. Diagnosis and follow-up of thoracic aortic aneurysm including Marfan disease	I
2. Diagnosis and planning of stent treatment for abdominal aortic aneurysm	II
3. Aortic dissection	
Diagnosis of acute aortic dissection	II
Diagnosis and follow-up of chronic aortic dissection	I
4. Diagnosis of aortic intramural hemorrhage	I
5. Diagnosis of penetrating ulcers of the aorta	I
6. Pulmonary artery anatomy and flow	I
7. Pulmonary emboli	
Diagnosis of central pulmonary emboli	III
Diagnosis of peripheral pulmonary emboli	Inv
8. Assessment of thoracic, abdominal and pelvic veins	I
9. Assessment of leg veins	II
10. Assessment of renal arteries	I
11. Assessment of mesenteric arteries	II
12. Assessment of iliac, femoral and lower leg arteries	I
13. Assessment of thoracic great vessel origins	I
14. Assessment of cervical carotid arteries	I
15. Assessment of atherosclerotic plaque in carotid artery/aorta	III
16. Assessment of pulmonary veins	I
17. Endothelial function	Inv

Inv = invalid

[a]Pennell DJ, Sechtem UP, Higgins CB, et al. Clinical indications for cardiovascular magnetic resonance (CMR): Consensus Panel report. *Eur Heart J.* 2004;25(21):1940–1965.

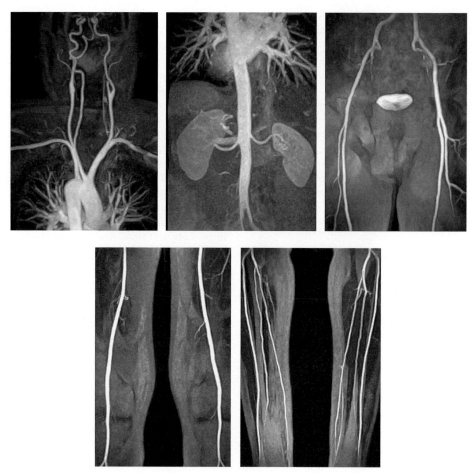

FIGURE 3A-5. Whole-body angiography using the AngioSURF technique. Angiographic images are displayed in reconstructed format by maximum-intensity projections (MIPs).

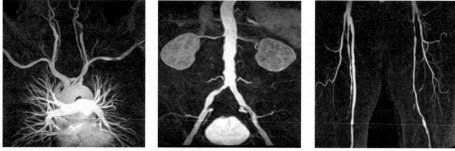

FIGURE 3A-6. Generalized atherosclerosis in a diabetic patient (MIP).

of vessels contained in a single field of view. The advent of bolus chase techniques later extended its use to examinations of two or even three vascular territories in one setting. The bolus chase technique requires a table platform that can be moved manually or electronically. After a single bolus of contrast medium, the table platform rapidly follows the contrast bolus throughout the body.[11] Atherosclerosis, however, affects the whole vascular tree; thus, imaging of the entire vasculature from the supra-aortic arteries to the distal runoff vessels is desirable (Fig. 3A-6).

The first step toward panvascular whole-body angiography was made with the development of new gradient hardware and a five-station moving table strategy otherwise known as the AngioSURF

(System for Unlimited Rolling Field-of-view) technique. This hardware allowed the acquisition of five 3D data sets in only 72 seconds. The actual data acquisition for each field of view is accomplished in 12 seconds, separated by four 3-second intervals for table motion. The data acquisition is carried out during a continuous infusion of contrast medium lasting 60 seconds.[12]

The rolling table platform with integrated surface coil was developed in cooperation with Siemens, Erlangen, Germany and can be mounted on top of the original patient table of a Siemens Symphony System. Data acquisition is performed with a standard body array surface coil. The system was first tested on three volunteers and one patient with angiographically documented vascular pathology. Data acquisition was performed with a 3D-FLASH-sequence (TR/TE 2.1/0.7 msec, flip angle: 20 degrees, FOV 40 × 40 cm, 80 partitions, matrix 512 × 420 with zero interpolation). Five data sets were collected in immediate succession during continuous injection of a paramagnetic contrast agent. Time of acquisition per data set was 10 seconds. Table repositioning was performed manually within 3 seconds. Thus, the total acquisition time amounted to 72 seconds. No problems with handling occurred in any of the four cases. The excellent image quality enabled detailed assessment of the displayed vascular territories and prompted further clinical studies.[13]

Further developments using the parallel imaging technique (PAT) refined the technique of whole-body MR angiogram in order to increase the spatial resolution of the 3D MRA data sets resulting in a more detailed MR angiogram. In a clinical study a standard imaging protocol was compared to a modified high-resolution protocol employing PAT using the generalized auto-calibrating partially parallel acquisitions (GRAPPA) algorithm with an acceleration factor of 3. For an intraindividual comparison of the two MR examinations, the arterial vasculature was divided into 30 segments. Signal-to-noise ratios (SNRs) and contrast-to-noise ratios (CNRs) were calculated for all 30 arterial segments of each subject. Vessel segment depiction was qualitatively assessed applying a five-point scale to each of the segments. Image reconstruction times were recorded for the standard as well as the PAT protocol. PAT allowed for increased spatial resolution through a threefold reduction in mean voxel size for each of the five stations. Mean SNR and CNR values over all specified vessel segments decreased by factors of 1.58 and 1.56, respectively, when the modified protocol was used. Despite the reduced SNR and CNR, the depiction of all specified vessel segments increased in PAT images, reflecting the increased spatial resolution. Qualitative comparison of standard and PAT images showed an increase in vessel segment conspicuity with more detailed depiction of intramuscular arterial branches in all volunteers. The time for image data reconstruction of all five stations was, however, significantly increased from about 10 minutes to 40 minutes when using the PAT acquisition.[14]

Additional studies demonstrated that MR angiography is well comparable to conventional DSA techniques with respect to diagnostic accuracy. In preliminary studies five volunteers and six patients with angiographically documented peripheral vascular disease were examined using 0.3 mmol/kg bodyweight Gd-BOPTA. Compared with conventional DSA, sensitivities and specificities of MR angiography for the detection of critical vascular disease ranged between 91 and 94%.[12] Furthermore, interobserver agreement excellent with a kappa value of 0.94 indicating that the approach was accurate and robust for morphologic vascular screening.

More recent studies determined the optimal dose of gadobenate dimeglumine for diagnostic high-resolution whole-body 3D-MR angiography. Ten healthy volunteers were examined three times with an ascending dose of Gd-BOPTA (0.1/0.2/0.3 mmol/kg BW) using the AngioSURF system. Signal-to-noise ratio (SNR)- and contrast-to-noise ratio (CNR)-values were calculated for 30 segments per patient. While significantly higher signal-to-noise values and CNR values were determined for Gd-BOPTA at a dose of 0.2 and 0.3 mmol/kg compared with 0.1 mmol/kg, qualitative and quantitative assessment failed to demonstrate a statistically significant difference between 0.2 and 0.3 mmol/kg BW. Consequently, a dose of

0.2 mmol/kg BW Gd-BOPTA appears sufficient to render adequate diagnostic image quality in all vascular segments.[15]

A more complete evaluation of both the imaging procedure and contrast agent was performed in 102 consecutive patients with peripheral vascular disease. Using 3D CE-MRA as described earlier, the study confirmed that the whole-body approach is a quick and risk-free approach that allows a comprehensive evaluation of the arterial system in patients with atherosclerosis.[16]

Using the AngioSURF technology, it is possible to visualize the whole vascular tree during a single investigation. However, the vascular tree can only be imaged in different sections depending on the field of view size and not in a continuous fashion.

Further technical developments using a total imaging matrix (TIM) technology by Siemens, which was first implemented in the AVANTO Magnetom, allow full and continuous assessment of the whole vascular tree. A full-body scan from head to toe can be achieved in 12 minutes (Fig. 3A-7).

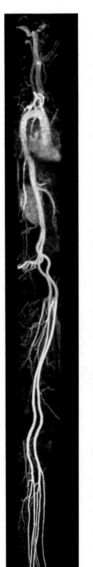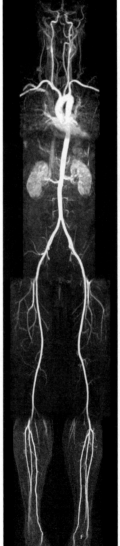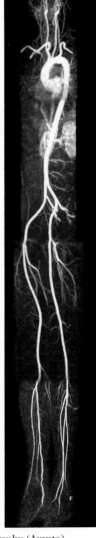

FIGURE 3A-7. Continuous total-body angiography (Avanto).

The revolutionary matrix-coil concept combines 76 coil elements with up to 32 high-frequency channels, which improves image quality and speeds up acquisition time. A further advantage of the system lies in parallel imaging and parallel acquisition techniques. A disadvantage of the system is the fact that the whole body is covered with coil elements, which aggravate the stress associated with the examination in patients with claustrophobia.

Other providers aimed at the elimination of claustrophobic anxiety by a unique comfort patient zone. The integration of a high-quality body coil can reduce the need for surface coils and further enhance patient comfort. The SENSE parallel imaging system (Philips, Eindhoven, The Netherlands) is integrated into the MobiFlex system, which provides the speed for dynamic angiography with increased resolution in morphological and vascular imaging (Fig. 3A-8). The system is based on the FreeWave data acquisition system with scalable 32-channel architecture. Scanning parameters for contrast enhanced MRA at 1.5 tesla for specific vendors are given in Table 3A-3.

In general, MR angiography independent of the respective arterial territory is suitable for detection of stenoses, dissection, aneurysm, vascular malformations and periarterial pathology, such as tumor or extra-arterial compression (Fig. 3A-9). At present MR angiography is not recommended for venous disease.

Peripheral vascular disease, especially of the lower extremities, represents a frequent finding in smokers and diabetic patients and may require repeated vascular imaging. Available MR imaging technology provides a noninvasive alternative to conventional invasive x-ray digital subtraction angiography (DSA). In one of the first patient series diagnostic performance of whole-body 3D contrast-enhanced MR angiography was assessed in comparison with DSA of the lower extremities in patients with peripheral arterial occlusive disease. Fifty-one patients with clinically documented peripheral arterial occlusive disease referred for DSA of the lower extremity arterial system underwent whole-body MR angiography on a 1.5-T MR scanner. Paramagnetic gadobutrol was administered and five contiguous stations were acquired with 3D T1-weighted gradient-echo sequences in a total scanning time of 72 seconds. DSA was available as a reference standard for the peripheral vasculature in all patients. Separate blinded data analyses were performed by two radiologists. Additional vascular disease detected by whole-body MR angiography was subsequently assessed on sonography, dedicated MR angiography, or both. All whole-body MR angiography examinations were feasible and well tolerated. AngioSURF-based whole-body MR angiography had overall sensitivities of 92.3% and 93.1% (both 95% confidence intervals [CIs], 78% to 100%) with specificities of 89.2% and 87.6% (both CIs, 84% to 98%) and excellent interobserver agreement (kappa = 0.82) for the detection of

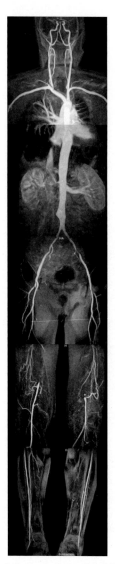

FIGURE 3A-8. Whole-body angiography (MobiFlex system).

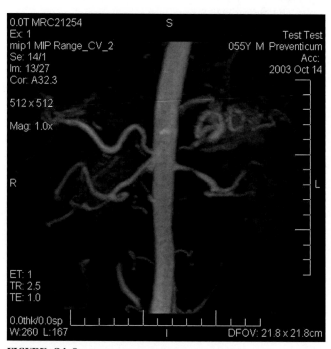

FIGURE 3A-9. Left-sided renal artery stenoses in a hypertensive patient (MIP).

TABLE 3A-3. Typical Scanning Parameters for CE 3D MRA at 1.5 Tesla for Specific Vendors

Imaging Parameter	General Electric	Philips	Siemens
Pulse sequence	**3D FSPGR**	**3D FFE**	**3D FLASH**
Imaging options	Fast, GX	Contrast enhancement-T1	—
Repetition time (TR)	Minimum (e.g., 4 to 6 msec)	Minimum (e.g., 4 to 6 msec)	Minimum (e.g., 3 to 5 msec)
Echo time (TE)	Minimum (e.g., 1 to 2 msec)	Minimum (e.g., 1 to 2 msec)	Minimum (e.g., 1 to 2 msec)
Flip angle (FA)	45 degrees	40 degrees	25 degrees
Bandwidth	± 32.25 kHz (option: ± 62.5 kHz)	WFS = 0.9 (@448 matrix = ± 57kHz)	Variable (± 590 Hz/pixel)
Field of view (FOV)	30 to 40 cm (option: 0.8 FOV)	400 mm, RFOV = 0.75	400 mm
Matrix	256 or 512 × 192–256	448 × 258	256–512 × 192–384
Number of partitions	40 to 60	40 to 60	60 to 80
Partition thickness (true)	1.0 to 2.5 mm	1.0 to 2.5 mm	1.0 to 2.5 mm
K-space	Elliptical centric	CENTRA	Elliptical centric
	Centric	Low to high	± partial Fourier
	Reverse	Linear	—
	Sequential (with partial Fourier or 0.5 NEX)	Half scan (= partial Fourier)	—
Number of excitations (NEX or NSA)	1 (option: 0.5)	1 (option: 0.5)	1 (option: 0.5
Timing	SMARTPREP Fluoro Trigger or test bolus	Bolus Trak or test bolus	Care bolus or test bolus
Misc. options	ZIP × 2 ZIP 512 ASSET	Overcontiguous slices Reconstruct 256, 512,1024 SENSE	Reconstruct 256, 512, 1024 SENSE, GRAPPA

high-grade stenoses. Additional vascular disease was detected in 12 patients (23%). Based on these investigations, whole-body MR angiography permits a rapid, noninvasive, and accurate evaluation of the lower peripheral arterial system in patients with peripheral arterial occlusive disease, and it may allow identification of additional relevant vascular disease that was previously undetected[17] (Figs. 3A-10 to 3A-14). Also, larger studies including other vascular provinces, such as carotid, renal, or subclavian arteries, confirmed the accuracy of whole-body MRA without false positive or negative findings.[11] Certainly, the principle of overestimation of peripheral stenoses by MR imaging techniques, as described earlier, has to be taken into account

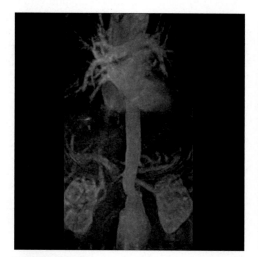
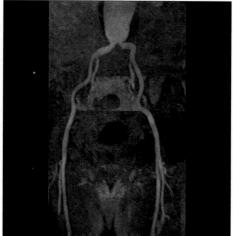

FIGURE 3A-10. Aneurysm of the abdominal aorta in a patient with long-lasting coronary artery disease (MIP).

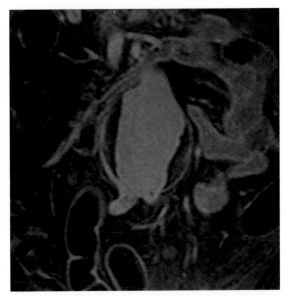

FIGURE 3A-11.   The partial thrombosis of the aneurysm from the patient in Figure 3A-10 can only be detected in the original 2D source plane images and not in the reconstructed images.

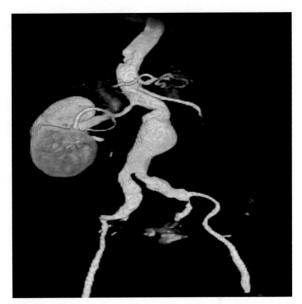

FIGURE 3A-13.   Peripheral vascular disease with abdominal aortic aneurysm.

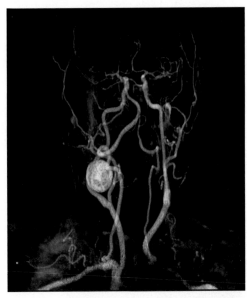

FIGURE 3A-12.   Angiography of the head and neck arteries with a glomus tumor.

during the clinical interpretation of the results. Nevertheless, MR imaging allows sequential and longitudinal studies in chronically ill patients without radiation exposure.

CORONARY ARTERIES

At present MR imaging does not yield sufficient resolution to allow reliable diagnostics of coronary artery disease. Clearly, MR coronary angiography remains experimental tool at this stage and cannot be considered a competitor for radiographic

coronary angiography in clinical settings at this time. In contrast, CT coronary angiography provides at present clinically relevant image quality allowing diagnostic evaluation of proximal segments of coronary arteries in selected subsets of patients. CT coronary angiography is, however, limited to coronary arteries (for review see reference 18).

However, with increasing experience and further technical developments, diagnostic MR coronary imaging appears feasible in the future. In the early 1990s, breath-hold techniques in expiration with ECG triggering using true FISP (fast imaging with steady-state precession) sequences reached only sensitivities and specificities ranging from 50% to 90%.[19,20]

The introduction of navigator techniques compensating for cranio-caudal as well as anterior-posterior shifts improved the accuracy of the method substantially, reaching sensitivities and specificities over 80% to 90%.[21,22] The current development of MR imaging technology in conjunction with intravascular contrast media will allow the visualization of the proximal and thus, relevant segments of the coronary arterial tree with a sufficient accuracy to diagnose coronary artery disease correctly or rule out relevant disease. MR coronary imaging is not limited by calcifications and radiation exposure.

CONCLUSIONS

Magnetic resonance tomographic imaging and angiography has emerged as a noninvasive tool to assess vascular pathology in all vascular territories and can achieve high-quality angiography not only for screening purpose but also for accurate diagnosis of all peripheral arterial vessels. At present the image quality of coronary arteries is not sufficiently adequate for reliable stenosis detection.

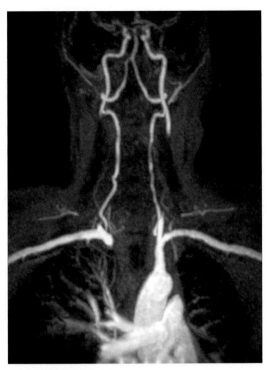

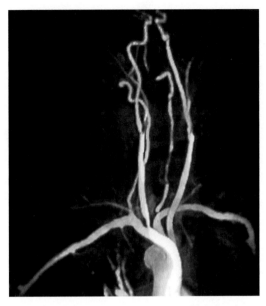

FIGURE 3A-14. Peripheral vascular disease with multiple obstructions and severe stenoses of head and neck arteries.

REFERENCES

1. Schellinger PD, Fiebach JB, Jansen O, et al. Stroke magnetic resonance imaging within 6 hours after onset of hyperacute cerebral ischemia. *Ann Neurol.* 2001;49(4):460–469.
2. Schellinger PD, Fiebach JB, Hacke W. Imaging-based decision making in thrombolytic therapy for ischemic stroke: present status. *Stroke.* 2003;34(2):575–583.
3. Edelman RR, Hessellink JR, Zlatkin MB. *Clinical Magnetic Resonance Imaging.* Philadelphia: WB Saunders; 1996.
4. Park MK, Jo I, Park MH, et al. Cerebral white matter lesions and hypertension status in the elderly Korean: the Ansan Study. *Arch Gerontol Geriatr.* 2005;40(3):265–273.
5. Wanke I, Egelhof T, Dorfler A, et al. Intracranial aneurysms: pathogenesis, rupture risk, treatment options [in German]. *RoFo* 2003;175(8):1064–1070.
6. Wanke I, Doerfler A, Dietrich U, et al. Endovascular treatment of unruptured intracranial aneurysms. *AJNR Am J Neuroradiol.* 2002;23(5):756–761.
7. Manning WJ, Pennell DJ. *Cardiovascular Magnetic Resonance.* Philadelphia: Churchill Livingstone; 2002.
8. Fink C, Plathow C, Klopp M, et al. MRT of bronchial carcinomas [in German]. *Radiologie* 2004;44(5):435–443.
9. Schneider G, Prince MR, Meaney JFM, et al. *Magnetic Resonance Angiography.* New York: Springer-Verlag; 2004.
10. Goyen M, Debatin JF. Gadobenate dimeglumine (MultiHance) for magnetic resonance angiography: review of the literature. *Eur Radiol.* 2003;13(suppl):N19-N27.
11. Ruehm SG, Goehde SC, Goyen M. Whole body MR angiography screening. *Int J Cardiovasc Imaging.* 2004;20:587–591.
12. Ruehm SG, Goyen M, Barkhausen J, et al. Rapid magnetic resonance angiography for detection of atherosclerosis. *Lancet.* 2001;357(9262):1086–1091.
13. Ruehm SG, Goyen M, Quick HH, et al. Whole-body MRA on a rolling table platform (AngioSURF). *RoFo.* 2000;172:670–674.
14. Quick HH, Vogt FM, Maderwald S, et al. High spatial resolution whole-body MR angiography featuring parallel imaging: initial experience. *RoFo.* 2004;176:163–169.
15. Goyen M, Herborn CU, Lauenstein TC, et al. Optimization of contrast dosage for gadobenate dimeglumine-enhanced high-resolution whole-body 3D magnetic resonance angiography. *Invest Radiol.* 2002;37:263–268.
16. Goyen M, Herborn CU, Kroger K, et al. Detection of atherosclerosis: systemic imaging for systemic disease with whole-body three-dimensional MR angiography—initial experience. *Radiology.* 2003;227(1):277–282.
17. Herborn CU, Goyen M, Quick HH, et al. Whole-body 3D MR angiography of patients with peripheral arterial occlusive disease. *AJR Am J Roentgenol.* 2004;182(6):1427–1434.
18. Cury RC, Pomerantsev EV, Ferencik M, et al. Comparison of the degree of coronary stenoses by multidetector computed tomography versus by quantitative coronary angiography. *Am J Cardiol.* 2005;96(6):784–787.
19. Manning WJ, Li W, Edelman RR. A preliminary report comparing magnetic resonance coronary angiography with conventional angiography. *N Engl J Med.* 1993;328(12):828–832.
20. Pennell DJ, Bogren HG, Keegan J, et al. Assessment of coronary artery stenosis by magnetic resonance imaging. *Heart.* 1996;75(2):127–133.
21. Jahnke C, Paetsch I, Nehrke K, et al. Rapid and complete coronary arterial tree visualization with magnetic resonance imaging: feasibility and diagnostic performance. *Eur Heart J.* 2005;26:2313–2319.
22. Sandstede JJ, Pabst T, Beer M, et al. Three-dimensional MR coronary angiography using the navigator technique compared with conventional coronary angiography. *AJR Am J Roentgenol.* 1999;172(1):135–139.

Peter Lanzer

CHAPTER **3B**

X-ray Coronary Angiography

X-ray angiography, despite its limitations, is the sole means of guidance used in the vast majority of coronary interventions. Intracoronary ultrasound imaging (Chapter 3C) and flow/pressure wire measurements (Chapter 3D) are additionally employed in <5% of procedures. The limitations of x-ray coronary angiography have been discussed extensively (for review, see reference 1). The luminographic and projectional character of the technique that is associated with the inability to visualize arterial walls, the actual seat of coronary atherosclerosis, and the inability to accurately visualize lesions, the actual target of interventions, are considered the two major drawbacks. However, the high image resolution, the robustness of image acquisition, and the on-line availability of images combined with instant fluoroscopic imaging make x-ray angiography seem indispensable as a first-line imaging tool in peri-interventional settings.

Because the operator is unable to view the interventional site directly, he must rely entirely on interpretation of angiographic images throughout the entire percutaneous coronary intervention (PCI) process. The diagnostic quality of periprocedural coronary imaging depends on operator-independent factors (e.g., the quality of the available imaging equipment) and operator-dependent ones (e.g., the ability to acquire optimal projections, image interpretation). Operator-independent factors have been described elsewhere (for review, see reference 2) and are not reviewed in the context of this chapter. Here, selected, critical, operator-dependent factors relevant to diagnostic quality of coronary images are reviewed.

PERIPROCEDURAL CORONARY ANGIOGRAPHY AND FLUOROSCOPY

It is assumed that the reader is familiar with the established standards concerning the operation of an interventional catheter-ization laboratory[3] and radiation safety.[4] In PCI settings, diagnostic x-ray coronary angiographic images are critical for establishing the indication, for determining revascularization strategy, for the real-time monitoring of the interventional site throughout the intervention, and for documentation of the results. During the main interventional cycle, fluoroscopic images and cine angiograms are acquired after each interventional step. On the basis of image interpretation, each subsequent procedural step is planned or the procedure terminated (see chapter 4). To fully assess the interventional site using angiography, there must be complete visualization of the target lesion, adjacent segments and side branches, proximal and distal target vessel, dependent microcirculation, and nontarget ("bystander") coronary arteries. Optimum visualization and consistent image interpretation allow successful interventions. Suboptimal image quality and interpretation set the stage for impending disasters. Table 3B-1 summarizes the individual components required to fully assess the PCI site.

TARGET VESSELS AND TARGET SEGMENTS

Despite numerous attempts to date,[5–9] no standard nomenclature of coronary arteries and coronary artery segments is available. To avoid confusion, only a basic terminology reflecting the major patterns of coronary artery ramifications will be used in this chapter (Table 3B-2).[10] To optimally visualize coronary arteries, typical projections ("coronary views") should be employed in diagnostic coronary angiography.[11,12] To unequivocally identify individual projections, side (left and right) and angulation (degrees) are given. Angulation of the x-ray beam in craniocaudal and left-to-right directions is indicated by referring to the position of the image intensifier with respect to the patient. All positions of the image intensifier toward the head of the patient (headward from the transverse planes) are termed

TABLE 3B-1. Targets of Cine Coronary Angiography and Fluoroscopy in PCI and the Corresponding Types of Information to be Acquired and Stages of the Procedure Affected

Target	Information to be Acquired	Stage of Procedure Affected
Target lesion	Quantification (severity, length) Morphology (plaque burden, distribution, redistribution, calcification; dissection; perforation, de novo lesion)	Indication, initiation, main cycle (sizing!), termination
Balloon, stent	Position, apposition, integrity	Main cycle
Adjacent segments	Morphology (plaque burden, distribution, redistribution; initial and de novo lesion; dissection; perforation)	Main cycle, termination
Side branches	Quantification (diameter ≥2 mm; initial stenosis present: severity, length)	Initiation, main cycle
Target vessel	Angle of take-off, ostium, morphology (plaque burden, distribution, calcification; initial and de novo lesion; dissection; perforation), flow	Indication, initiation, main cycle, termination
Dependent microcirculation	Open, altered, closed	Termination
"Bystander" coronary arteries	Initial lesions: number, severity, length; morphology and flow before and after intervention	Indication, termination

PCI, percutaneous coronary intervention.

TABLE 3B-2. Ramification Patterns and Basic Nomenclature of Coronary Arteries

Coronary Artery	Primary Branches	Secondary and Terminal Branches
Left coronary artery (LM)	Left anterior descending artery (LAD)	Right ventricular branches Left ventricular (diagonal) branches Septal branches
	Left circumflex artery (LCx)	Three atrial branches (superior, medium, inferior)
		One or more ventricular (lateral) branches
Right coronary artery (RCA)	—	Three atrial branches (superior, medium, inferior), of which the superior is the sinus node artery
		Three kinds of right ventricular branches (anterior, marginal, inferior)
		Two terminal branches: posterior descending branch and posterior left ventricular branch

Modified from Cabrol C, Christides C. *Usual arrangement and nomenclature of the coronary arteries. Bull Assoc Anat (Nancy).* 1976;60:645–649.

cranial; all positions of the image intensifier toward the feet of the patient are termed caudal. All positions of the image intensifier between frontal and lateral positions are termed anterior oblique, and the specification "right" or "left" is added depending on the side. Table 3B-3 shows an example of the recommended diagnostic coronary angiography projections. However, the recommended "coronary views" frequently need modifications to permit optimal definition of target sites in individual patients. During interventions, recommended views are even less useful, and individual angulations for each target lesion must be individually sought and identified. These views are then maintained throughout the intervention. To allow consistent documentation of the initial findings, all the relevant intermediary steps, and the final results, it is

TABLE 3B-3. Suggested Coronary Artery Projections for Diagnostic Angiography

Coronary Artery	Projection
Left coronary artery (LM)	45 degree and 60 degree straight left anterior oblique (LAO), left lateral with shallow cranial angulation, 30 degree straight right anterior oblique (RAO), 30 degree RAO with 25 degree caudal angulation and 30 degree RAO with 20 degree cranial angulation
Right coronary artery (RCA)	60 degree straight LAO, 30 degree RAO with shallow cranial angulation

recommended that a standard imaging protocol be adopted. Table 3B-4 provides an example of the suggested coronary artery projections for angiography-guided PCI. Table 3B-5 provides an example of a standard angiography protocol to document PCI results. In Figure 3B-1, coronary artery segmentation is presented according to the American Heart Association nomenclature. Figure 3B-2 is an example of standard coronary angiographic projections.

TABLE 3B-4.   Suggested Coronary Artery Projections for Angiography-guided PCI

Coronary Artery	Projection
Left main (LM)	Ostium—10 degree RAO with steep cranial angulation, AP with shallow caudal angulation
	Body—30 degree RAO with 20 degree cranial angulation, 15 degree LAO with steep cranial angulation
	Distal—LAO caudal, LAO cranial, caudal
	Full length—10 degree LAO with steep caudal angulation ("spider" view)
LAD	Take-off—10° LAO with steep caudal angulation ("spider" view)
	Proximal—15 degree LAO with steep cranial angulation
	Middle to distal—15 degree RAO with shallow caudal angulation
	Full length—left lateral
LCx	Take-off—10 degree LAO with steep caudal angulation ("spider" view), 20 degree RAO with shallow caudal angulation
	Body—20 degree RAO with shallow caudal angulation, straight 30 degree LAO
	Full length—10 degree LAO with steep caudal angulation ("spider" view), 20 degree RAO with shallow caudal angulation
RCA	Ostium—20 degree LAO with shallow cranial angulation
	Body—Straight 20 degree LAO, straight 30 degree RAO
	Distal—20 degree LAO with shallow cranial angulation, 30 degree RAO with shallow cranial angulation
Internal mammary graft (IMA)	Ostium—Straight AP
	Body—Straight AP, 15 degree RAO with shallow caudal angulation
	Distal/native LAD—Left lateral, 15 degree RAO with shallow caudal angulation
RCA: venous and radial grafts (proximal)	Ostium—20 degree LAO with shallow cranial angulation
	Body—Straight 20 degree LAO, straight 30 degree RAO
	Distal—20 degree LAO with shallow cranial angulation, 30 degree RAO with shallow cranial angulation
LAD: venous and radial grafts (second from proximal)	Ostium—45 degree straight LAO
	Body—Straight 45 degree LAO, 30 degree straight RAO, left lateral Distal—30 degree RAO with shallow caudal angulation, 15 degree RAO with shallow caudal angulation
Rd: venous and radial grafts (third from proximal)	Ostium—45 degree straight LAO Body—30 degree LAO with 30 degree cranial angulation, 45 degree RAO with 15 degree cranial angulation
LCx: venous and radial grafts (fourth from proximal)	Ostium—45 degree straight LAO Body—Straight 45 degree LAO, straight 20 degree RAO

LM, left main coronary artery; LAD, left anterior descending artery; LCx, left circumflex artery; RCA, right coronary artery; RAO, right anterior oblique; LAO, left anterior oblique.

TABLE 3B-5. Example of a Standard Angiography Protocol for Documentation of PCI Results

Timing Documentation	Target Lesion	Target Vessel	Interventional Site
Before intervention	3. Cine, two best projections orthogonal to the long axis of the lesion, high magnification (14 cm)	2. Cine, two best projections, medium magnification (17 cm)	1. Cine, one overview projection, low magnification (23 cm)
During intervention	Cine, one best projection optional after each interventional step, additional projections as needed, high magnification (14 cm)	If needed, cine, best projections, medium magnification (17 cm)	
	Fluoroscopy for continuous visualization of target lesion, target vessel, target ostium, and guidewire tip		
After intervention	1. Cine, two best projections orthogonal to the long axis of the lesion, guidewire in place;	3. Cine, two best projections, guidewire retracted, medium magnification (17 cm)	4. Cine, one overview projection, low magnification (23 cm)
	2. Cine, two best projections orthogonal to the long axis of the lesion, guidewire retracted to proximal segment of lesion or stent; high magnification (14 cm)		

PCI, percutaneous coronary intervention.

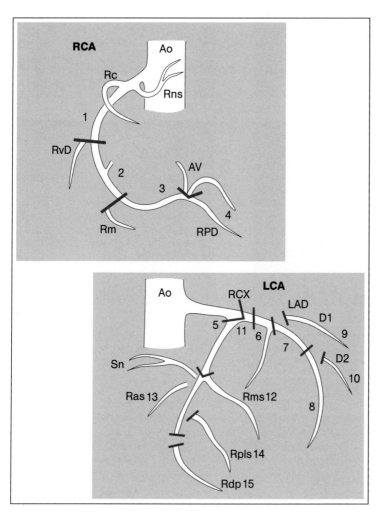

FIGURE 3B-1. American Heart Association nomenclature of coronary artery segments. (Modified from Erbel R, et al. Richtlinien der interventionellen Koronartherapie. www.dgk.org/leitlinien, accessed August 12, 2005.)

TARGET LESIONS

Target PCI lesions are located in the epicardial segments of the coronary arteries that are >2 mm in diameter. Predilection sites include the proximal third,[13,14] bifurcations,[15] and inner sides of curved segments.[16] Besides major cardiovascular risk factors, regional flow disturbances are thought to be a cause of

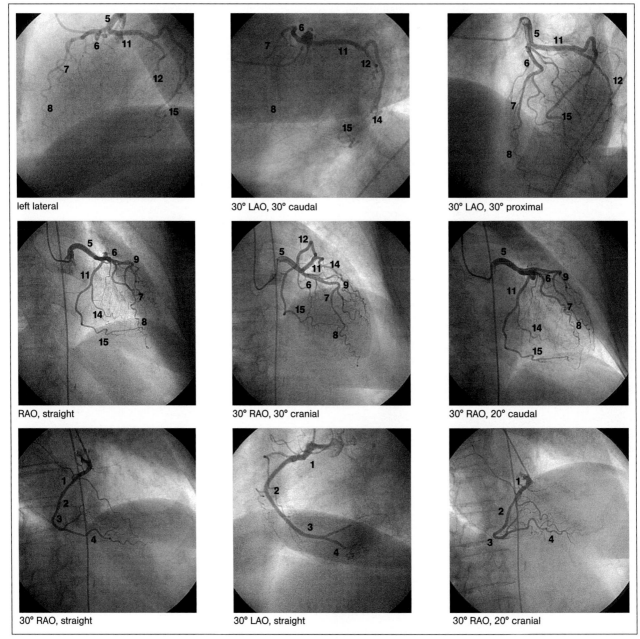

left lateral

30° LAO, 30° caudal

30° LAO, 30° proximal

RAO, straight

30° RAO, 30° cranial

30° RAO, 20° caudal

30° RAO, straight

30° LAO, straight

30° RAO, 20° cranial

FIGURE 3B-2.   Example of typical angiographic coronary artery projections. Typical projections of the left and right coronary arteries are shown. The numbers correspond to the American Heart Association coronary artery segment classification. (See Fig. 3B-1.)

coronary atherosclerosis at predilection sites.[17] Because of the diffuse character of coronary atherosclerosis, several potential target lesions may be present at different coronary sites. Furthermore, multiple plaque ruptures may be documented in individual patients.[18]

Quantitative Assessment

The initiation, continuation, and termination of PCI depend on the angiographic and/or physiologic definition of the hemodynamic significance of target lesions. The hemodynamic significance of lesions depends on the magnitude of coronary flow and is determined by a number of factors including the severity, length, geometric shape, dynamic behavior of the stenosis and interactions with the microcirculations.[19,20] The hemodynamic impact of fixed stenoses is proportional to the transstenotic pressure gradients ΔP at different coronary flow (CF) levels. Ex vivo measurements showed that $\Delta P/\Delta CF$ [mm Hg/cm^3 per minute] begins to rise steeply for stenoses whose diameter is >60% of the diameter, whereas resting blood flow begins to fall at stenoses >80% in diameter.[21] Clinically, estimates of the hemodynamic severity of coronary lesions have been primarily based on measurements of the degree of maximum narrowing visualized by angiography. However, these estimates are inaccurate because of the geometric complexity and variable dynamic behavior of in vivo stenoses, which frequently

leads to under- or overestimation of the true hemodynamic severity.[22] In addition to the degree of narrowing, the length of the stenosis is another important determinant of its hemodynamic relevance. However, in clinical practice, measuring the length of the stenosis has primarily been used to size dilatation devices such as balloons and stents not to determine the hemodynamic relevance of lesions.

The severity of a stenosis can be determined angiographically by means of visual estimations or quantitative measurements using computer-assisted analysis. Visual estimation is associated with high intra- and interobserver variability.[23,24] Quantitative, edge detection, or video-densitometry-based coronary angiography (QCA) provides consistent and highly reproducible results.[25,26] To facilitate QCA measurements during PCI, on-line modules allowing the direct measurement of the severity, length, and geometric profile of lesions are available. In lesions with angiographically indeterminate hemodynamic relevance, added flow/pressure and/or intravascular ultrasound (IVUS) measurements may be performed.[27]

The severity of coronary stenoses is measured as a percentage reduction in the nominal diameter of the target vessel (%D) using the formula $\%D = Ds/Dn \times 100$, where Ds designates the minimum diameter of the stenosis, measured as the shortest distance between opposing endoluminal edges at the narrowest point (neck) of the lesion, and Dn designates the nominal diameter of a reference segment that is adjacent, usually proximal, and unobstructed. Lesions in which the coronary stenosis represents at least 70% of the vessel diameter are usually considered significant and represent a target for revascularization. Lesions with <50% diameter stenosis are considered insignificant and are treated medically. Intermediate lesions with 50% to 70% diameter stenosis are considered "borderline," and additional means are required to determine their hemodynamic significance. However, in the literature stenoses >50% diameter are also sometimes called significant, particularly when the left main coronary artery and bifurcation lesions are concerned. Lesions with >95% diameter stenosis are termed subtotal occlusions. In the left main coronary artery and in bifurcation lesions, critical stenoses are considered to be present where the reduction in diameter exceeds 50%. The presence of lesions with >50% diameter stenosis in one or more major coronary arteries determines whether the status of coronary artery disease is defined as one-, two-, three-, or multiple-vessel disease.[28] The length of a stenosis is determined angiographically as the distance between the points of transition between the luminal irregularity of the lesion and the smooth endothelial interface of the healthy adjacent segment. Lesions <5 mm in diameter are considered focal; those >20 mm are considered diffuse.

Qualitative Assessment

Since the impact of the morphology of coronary lesions on outcome was recognized, attempts were made to classify lesions systematically on the basis of their angiographic appearance. The most frequently employed classification, proposed by the American College of Cardiology and the American Heart Association,[29] was subsequently evaluated in clinical trials, and the prognostic value of different types of lesions validated (Table 3B-6).[28] Although the morphologic characteristics of coronary lesions are still important determinants of outcome,

TABLE 3B-6. ACC/AHA Classification System of Coronary Artery Lesions

TYPE A (LOW RISK, EXPECTED SUCCESS >85%)

Discrete (length <10 mm)

Concentric

Readily accessible

Nonangulated segment (<45 degrees)

Smooth contour

Little or no calcification

Less than totally occlusive

Not ostial in location

No major side branch involvement

Absence of thrombus

TYPE B (MODERATE RISK, EXPECTED SUCCESS 60–85%)

Tubular (length 10 to 20 mm)

Eccentric

Moderate tortuosity of proximal segment

Moderately angulated segment (>45 degrees, <90 degrees)

Irregular contour

Moderate or heavy calcification

Total occlusions <3 months old

Ostial in location

Bifurcation lesions requiring double guidewires

Some thrombus present

TYPE C (HIGH RISK, EXPECTED SUCCESS <60%)

Diffuse (length >20 mm)

Excessive tortuosity of proximal segment

Extremely angulated segments > 90 degrees

Total occlusions >3 months old and/or bridging collaterals

Inability to protect major side branches

Degenerated vein grafts with friable lesions

Modified from Ryan TJ, Faxon DP, Gunnar RM, et al. Guidelines for percutaneous transluminal coronary angioplasty: A report of the American College of Cardiology/American Heart Association Task Force on Assessment of Diagnostic and Therapeutic Cardiovascular Procedures. *J Am Coll Cardiol.* 1988;12:529–545.

their impact has diminished with the advent of stents. Additional descriptors of targets for coronary interventions have been defined that allow better risk assessment and improve standards of communication. Unfortunately, most of these descriptive terms are at present used rather loosely, thus leaving considerable room for inaccuracy and semantic confusion. Table 3B-7 provides a selection of angiographic definitions proposed by the National Heart, Lung, and Blood Institute Bypass Angioplasty Revascularization Investigation (BARI) in their unpublished BARI Central Radiographic Laboratory Operations Manual. These definitions still appear useful today and allow unequivocal image interpretation and communication. The clinical importance of bifurcation lesions has more recently prompted several classification attempts based on morphologic plaque distribution within the bifurcation segments.[30,31] Figure 3B-3 shows an classification of bifurcation lesions proposed by Lefevre. The nomenclature of coronary

TABLE 3B-7.   Angiographic Coronary Lesion Definitions Based on National Heart, Lung, and Blood Institute Bypass Angioplasty Revascularization Investigation (BARI) from an Unpublished BARI Central Radiographic Laboratory Operations Manual

Angiographic Lesion Morphology	Definition
Bifurcation stenosis	Branch vessel of medium or large size originating from within the stenosis and completely surrounded by a significant portion of the lesion to be dilated
Calcification	Readily apparent densities within the apparent vascular wall of the artery at the site of the stenosis
Chronic total occlusion	TIMI flow grade 0 judged to be ≥3 months duration on the basis of clinical and angiographic findings
Eccentric stenosis	(Angiographic) lumen in the outer quarter of the diameter of the apparently normal lumen
High-grade stenosis	80% to 99% narrowing relative to the adjacent normal coronary artery dimension
Irregular contour	Rough or "sawtooth" appearance of the vascular margin
Lesion length	Distance from the proximal to distal shoulder of the lesion in the projection that displays the stenosis at its greatest length; 10 to 20 mm tubular stenosis, >20 mm diffuse stenosis
Modified ACC/AHA score	B1—one adverse characteristic
	B2—two adverse characteristics
Multivessel disease	Presence of ≥50% diameter stenosis in two of the three major epicardial vessels or their surgically bypassable branches. In nondominant RCA failing to supply the LV myocardium, the first two moderately or large-sized LCx were considered to supply one vascular territory, and the distal obtuse marginal branches and the posterior descending coronary artery were said to supply a different vascular territory
Ostial stenosis	Involving the origin of the proximal LAD, LCx, or RCA
Target lesion associated with other stenoses	Presence of ≥50% stenoses in the same or adjacent (BARI classification) coronary segment
Primary target stenosis	Identified based on severity and morphologic characteristics, their jeopardized (myocardial) territories, presumed viability of subserved myocardium, and clinical data, if available
Stenosis angle	Formed by a center line through the lumen proximal to the stenosis extending beyond it and a second center line in the straight portion of the artery distal to stenosis in a nonforeshortened view at end-diastole
	(Bending graded as mild or absent [<45 degrees], moderate [45 degrees–60 degrees], or excessive [>60 degrees])
Successful dilatation	Final result <50% diameter stenosis associated with no major adverse clinical sequelae (death, myocardial infarction, or emergency bypass surgery)
Thrombus	Intraluminal, clearly definable filling defect largely separated from the adjacent vessel wall
Tortuosity	Moderate—stenosis distal to two bends
	Excessive—stenosis distal to ≥3 bends
Abrupt proximal face	Present if in any angiographic projection its proximal face formed an angle with a contiguous proximal lumen of <135 degrees
Active kink point	Present if in any angiographic projection the lesion was located in a portion of the vessel that was bent by >15 degrees between end-diastole and end-systole
Branch point	Present if any part of the lesion was adjacent to a branch vessel of diameter ≥25% of the diameter of the nondiseased native (target) vessel
Bend point	Present if in any angiographic projection the balloon in position to dilate was located in a portion of the vessel that had a ≥45 degree angulation at end-diastole. Fixed bent point was present if angulation between end-diastole and end-systole was <15 degrees in any angiographic projection.
Collaterals	Present if any degree of collateral filling beyond the site to be dilated was noted on predilatation angiograms
Diffuse disease	Three or more 50% narrowings in the target vessel or luminal irregularities present in one-third of the target vessel
Eccentricity	Stenosis asymmetrically positioned in the vessel in any angiographic projection
Distal ectasia	Present if dilatation of the vessel beyond the normal luminal diameter immediately distal to the target stenosis was present

(*Continued*)

TABLE 3B-7   (*Continued*)

Angiographic Lesion Morphology	Definition
Ulceration	Present if a discrete luminal widening of the area of the stenosis in the form of a "crater" was visualized. If the widening exceeded the diameter of the normal lumen, it was judged to be an area of ectasia.
Intimal tear or dissection	Present if after PTCA a curvilinear intraluminal filling defect or widening with contrast staining at the site of dilatation was visualized
Roughened lumen	Present if the luminal edge at the site of the dilatation was irregular or had a "sawtooth" component
Successful angioplasty	Procedure in which a ≥20% change in luminal diameter is achieved, with the final diameter stenosis <50% and without death, acute myocardial infarction, or the need for emergency bypass

PTCA, percutaneous transluminal coronary angioplasty.

Modified from Ellis SG, Vandormael MG, Cowley MJ, et al. Coronary morphologic and clinical determinants of procedural outcome with angioplasty for multivessel coronary disease; Implications for patient selection. *Circulation.* 1990;82:1193–1202.

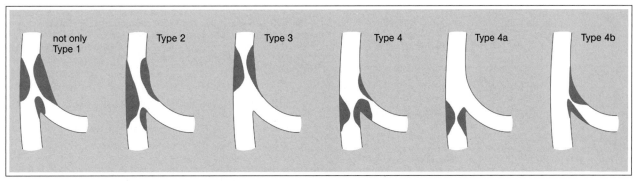

FIGURE 3B-3.   Classification of coronary artery bifurcation lesions proposed by Lefevre et al. (Modified from Lefevre T, Louvard Y, Morice M-C, et al. Stenting of bifurcation lesions: classification, treatment and results. *Cathet Cardiovasc Intervent.* 2000;49:274–283.

occlusions differentiates between functional and total occlusions. Functional occlusions are present when antegrade coronary flow graded Thrombolysis In Myocardial Infarction-1 (TIMI-1) has been documented, and total occlusions when no antegrade flow (TIMI-0) has been detected (for TIMI grades, see next section).

Lesions that appear ambiguous on angiography include the following: intermediate lesions of uncertain hemodynamic relevance ("borderline lesions"), lesions with post- and prestenotic or congenital aneurysms, a number of lesions located at the aortocoronary ostia (particularly that of the left main coronary artery), branching sites, angiographically obscured locations (particularly within tortuous vessels), and lesions with focal spasms. Other sites that are difficult to interpret on angiography include ruptured plaques, postinterventional sites, intraluminal filling defects, and lesions with haziness and locally disturbed flow. IVUS may be used to clarify these ambiguous angiographic findings. However, although IVUS images allow clarification of angiographically ambiguous lesions in many instances, they do not provide any information on their physiological relevance.[32] The important drawbacks of

IVUS include problems with access to anatomically or topographically difficult sites. The considerable stiffness of the ultrasound transducer presents in some cases the passage of the probe into the coronary target site.

Following interventions, the angiographic appearance of lesions may change dramatically as a result of plaque redistribution, fissuring, dissections, and hemorrhage. Plaque shifts occur mainly in an axial direction.[32] They are seen on angiography as de novo irregularities or de novo proximal or distal stenoses. Major plaque shift may result in abrupt target vessel closure. Dissections are seen as haziness, radiolucent areas, parallel tracks, spiral luminal filling defects, persistent filling defects within the coronary lumen, or extraluminal contrast depots. In severe cases, complete disintegration of angiographic vessel anatomy, acute vessel closure, or perforation may occur. The classification of dissections proposed by BARI in an unpublished BARI Central Radiographic Laboratory Operations Manual (shown in Fig. 3B-4) includes:

- Type A: small radiolucent area within the lumen of the vessel
- Type B: linear, nonpersisting extravasations of contrast

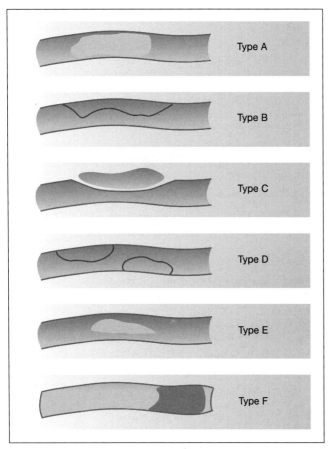

FIGURE 3B-4. Classification of dissections proposed by National Heart, Lung, and Blood Institute Bypass Angioplasty Revascularization Investigation (BARI). (Modified from Erbel R, et al. Richtlinien der interventionellen Koronartherapie. www.dgk.org/leitlinien, accessed August 12, 2005.)

- Type C: extraluminal, persisting extravasations of contrast
- Type D: spiral-shaped filling defect with delayed but complete distal flow
- Type E: persistent filling defect with delayed antegrade flow and incomplete distal flow
- Type F: filling defect with total occlusion

Measuring the end-to-end length of the dissection and the degree of persistence of contrast within the dissection compared with the downstream segment of the vessel may also be helpful in evaluating the severity of the dissection.[33]

Coronary artery perforations and ruptures are associated with persistent contrast agent extravasations. Three types have been proposed by Ellis et al.[33] on the basis of angiographic severity (Fig. 3B-5):

- Type I: extraluminal crater without (visible) extravasation
- Type II: pericardial and myocardial blush without contrast jet extravasation
- Type III: extravasation through a frank (>1 mm) perforation

In a simplified classification, Ajluni et al. suggested two types of perforations, contained (Ellis types I and II) and free (Ellis type III).[34]

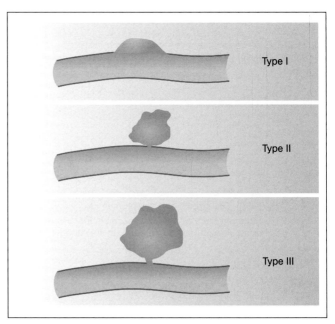

FIGURE 3B-5. Classification of coronary artery perforation proposed by Ellis et al. (Modified from Ajluni SC, Glazier S, Blankenship L, et al. Perforations after percutaneous coronary interventions: clinical, angiographic, and therapeutic observations. *Cathet Cardiovasc Diagn.* 1994;32:206–212).

Morphology and topographic distribution of in-stent restenoses has also been recently classified[35] (Fig. 3B-6).

CORONARY FLOW

Coronary artery flow is visualized as progressive opacification of the vessel lumen, as typically follows selective intracoronary injection of 4 to 10 mL contrast agent. On simple visual examination the flow appears normal, sluggish, or absent. Based on the recognition of the prognostic significance of coronary reflow following revascularization, the investigators behind the TIMI study have proposed a qualitative grading system for unequivocal definition and comparisons.[36] Table 3B-8 shows a summary of TIMI flow grades. More recently, a more detailed assessment of coronary flow, termed "corrected TIMI frame count" (CTFC), has been introduced.[37] However, reproducible assessments of CTFC are cumbersome and not widely used in clinical practice. Ambiguous flow patterns may also provide insights into the status of the site of intervention (Table 3B-9).

MYOCARDIAL ANGIOGRAPHY OF MYOCARDIAL PERFUSION

Successful PCI is defined as removal of a stenosis in the epicardial segment of the coronary artery and restoration of blood flow and myocardial perfusion to the normal state. Following a number of early brilliant observations,[38–40] it has taken us a long time to understand the clinical significance of a successful epicardial stenosis revascularization without myocardial reperfusion. The paper published by Topol and Yadav in *Circulation* in 2000 was truly felt as a revelation. It extended the paradigm broadening our perspective and, eventually, giving us a full

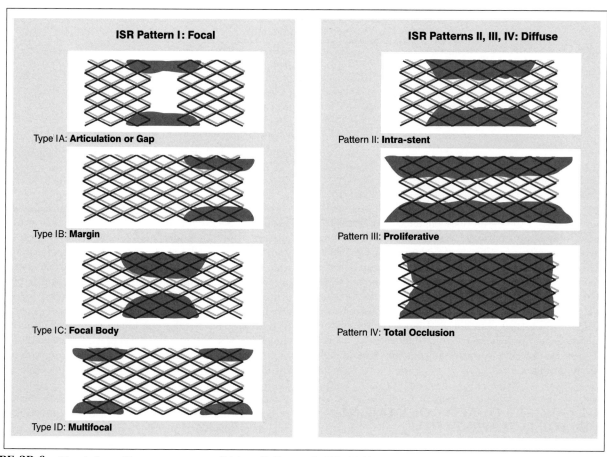

FIGURE 3B-6.   Morphology of in-stent restenoses. (Mehran R, Dangas G, Abizaid AS, et al. Angiographic pattern of in-stent restenosis: classification and implications for long-term outcome. *Circulation.* 1999;100:1872–1878.)

TABLE 3B-8.   Thrombolysis In Myocardial Infarction (TIMI) Flow Grades

TIMI Grade	State of Flow	Description
0	No perfusion	Antegrade flow is present to the lesion; no flow distal to the lesion
I	Penetration of contrast media with only minimal perfusion	Contrast media passes beyond lesion but fails to opacify distal vessel during cine run
II	Partial perfusion	Contrast media passes beyond lesion and fills distal vessel. Rate of filling and/or washout is slower than for nondependent coronary arteries.
III	Complete perfusion	Contrast media washin and washout is similar to that of unaffected coronary arteries.

picture to assess the outcome of the endocoronary revascularization interventions.[41] Subsequently, peripheral distal embolizations and myocardial malperfusion have become recognized as a frequent potential complication of virtually any endovascular intervention, and the concept of a distal embolization protection has been developed.[42]

X-ray coronary angiography visualizes the passage of contrast media through the microcirculation as a brief flush of opacification of the subtended myocardium followed by venous filling. In an attempt to assess perfusion, the intensity and duration of contrast following the epicardial flow phase has been graded and termed the myocardial blush grades (MBG).[43] A similar grading

TABLE 3B-9.   Angiographic Ambiguous Coronary Flow Patterns

Coronary Artery Flow Patterns	*Potential Causes*
Competitive flow	Secondary feeding artery or graft
"To and fro" flow	Aortic regurgitation, high pulse pressure
Disturbed (turbulent) flow	Protruding coronary artery lesions, distorted stents, intraluminal obstructions
Accentuated normal systolic–diastolic flow pattern	Myocardial bridging
Sluggish antegrade flow	Endothelial dysfunction, low blood pressure
"No flow," "no reflow"	Downstream embolization, mechanical obstruction, endothelial dysfunction

scale for the same purpose, termed the TIMI Myocardial Perfusion Grade (TMPG), provides an alternative means of assessment.[44] Table 3B-10 provides a summary of both grading systems. However, despite encouraging initial clinical experience,[45,46] technical complexity may limit the use of this new tool to research. There is an obvious need for a simple and reproducible tool for estimating myocardial perfusion in the interventional laboratory following PCI. The challenges posed by the complexity of myocardial perfusion and the technical costs of real-time assessment may, however, prove difficult to overcome. Yet, the new CT-like x-ray coronary angiography systems hold some future promise.

IMAGE QUALITY, QUALITY OF IMAGING, AND IMAGE INTERPRETATION

Expert image interpretation requires optimum image quality and optimum quality of imaging. Radiographic image quality, as defined in laboratory settings, primarily means the measurement of two parameters of spatial contrast resolution, namely, *modulation transfer function* (MTF), defined as the ability of the x-ray imaging system to measure the contrast of an object as a function of object detail, and *signal-to-noise ratio* (SNR), defined as the ratio of the information-containing signal to the random, unuseful signal. More recently, a third important parameter has been added, namely, *detected quantum efficiency* (DQE), defined as the integrated expression in percent of the overall efficiency of the imaging system to transfer signal and reduce noise from the input to the output of the entire imaging chain. Other parameters include *limiting spatial resolution* (LSR), defined as the spatial frequency at which the observer can no longer discern high-contrast test patterns under optimum viewing conditions, and *contrast resolution*, which indicates the number of shades of gray detectable.[2,47] In coronary angiography and fluoroscopy, the absence of motion artifacts is an important determinant of image quality. The absence is due to the rapid and complex intrathoracic motion of the coronary arteries resulting from the contractile cycle, the pendular motion of the heart at its suspension at the roots of the aortic and pulmonary arteries, and respiration based on the high temporal resolution. These parameters are independent of the PCI operator.

Operator-dependent factors include selection of the "best" projections, including correct size of the field of view (FOV), degree of magnification, degree of filtering, and resolution mode to optimally visualize the interventional site. Typical values for the FOV in coronary angiography are 14 cm (smallest FOV, highest resolution), 17 cm, and 23 cm (largest FOV, lowest resolution). The geometric magnification factor—see Figure 3B-7 for an illustration of the principles of geometric image magnification—is calculated by dividing the source-to-image distance (SID) by the source-to-object distance (SOD). Thus, for a fixed SID, the magnification factor increases with decreasing SOD.[2] The clinical usefulness of geometric magnification is greatly limited, however, because the skin dose increases with SOD and radiation exposure increases with SID and the difference $\Delta = SID - SOD$.

To permit reproducible projections during the intervention, voluntary movements by the patient should be avoided. Breath

TABLE 3B-10.   Grading Systems of Myocardial Blush Grades (MBG) and TIMI Myocardial Perfusion Grade (TMPG) for Qualitative Myocardial Perfusion Assessment

Grade	*MBG[a]*	*TMPG*
0	No blush	Minimal or no myocardial blush (no contrast penetration into microcirculation)
1	Minimal blush	Contrast agent stains the myocardium and persists on the next injection (slow entry and slow or no exit into microvasculature)
2	Moderate blush	Contrast agent stains the myocardium but washes out slowly and persists at the end of injection (delayed entry and exit into microvasculature)
3	Normal blush	Contrast agent stains and exits rapidly (rapid entry and exit into microvasculature)

[a] Comparable with that obtained during angiography of a contralateral or ipsilateral non-infarct-related coronary artery.
Modified from van't Hof AW, Liem A, Suryapranata H, et al. Angiographic assessment of myocardial reperfusion in patients treated with primary angioplasty for acute myocardial infarction. *Circulation.* 1998;97:2302–2306 and Gibson CM, Cannon CP, Murphy SA, et al. Relationship of TIMI myocardial perfusion grade to mortality after administration of thrombolytic drugs. *Circulation.* 2000;101:125–130.

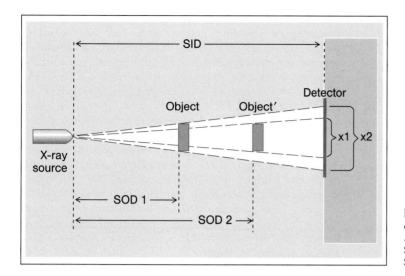

FIGURE 3B-7. Principles of geometrical magnification in coronary x-ray angiography. *SID*, source-to-image distance; *SOD*, source-to-object distance. At a given SID, decreasing SOD increases the magnification factor (defined as SID/SOD).

holds should be limited to the acquisition of critical views because of the considerable discomfort to the patient in return for a relatively small benefit of some reduction of motional artefacts since the imaging frame rate (25 images/sec in Europe and 30 images/sec in the United States) is high in comparison with the low frequency of respirations (typically 12 breaths per minute). In some cases, repositioning the patient on the table and altering the position of the shoulders or arms might improve the quality of projections, particularly when coronary bypasses are imaged.

Coronary image quality is also influenced by luminal contrast. The magnitude of the resulting contrast enhancement is determined by the rate of iodine delivery into the vascular system, which in turn is governed by the concentration of iodine in the contrast medium, the rate of injection, and the injection volume. At a given rate of delivery, attenuation of the x-ray beam corresponds to the mass attenuation coefficient (μ) of iodine concentration. Excellent contrast is achieved at 33 keV photon energy because of the sharp increase in the mass attenuation coefficient of iodine ($I\mu$) at that energy level compared with the surrounding tissues. With an increasing energy of radiation (photon keV), $I\mu$ decreases more rapidly compared with μ of the surrounding soft tissues, which results in lower contrast. There are basically four different types of vascular iodine contrast agents (Table 3B-11), all with the basic structure of a benzene ring with symmetrically coupled iodine atoms. Vascular iodine contrast agents differ in important properties including:

- *Water solubility*, which determines the maximum concentration of iodine that can be achieved and, therefore, the maximum x-ray absorption, which itself generates coronary artery image contrast
- *Osmolality*, i.e., the osmotic pressure of the solution, determining the magnitude of water shifts between vascular and extravascular spaces
- *Viscosity*, which determines the force required for intracoronary injections (warming contrast media to 37°C before administration sharply reduces viscosity!)
- *Chemotoxicity*, determined by hydro- and lipophilicity, protein binding and electrical charge, and histamine release, factors responsible for biological incompatibility and adverse effects

Dimeric ionic and nonionic contrast media contain ~320 mg iodine per milliliter, and monomeric nonionic ones, ~370 to 400 mg iodine per milliliter. In terms of osmolality, high and low osmolality contrast agents (HOCM and LOCM) can be distinguished: HOCM have ~1.500 mosmol/L, and LOCM typically ~500 to 800 mosmol/L. "Isotonicity," i.e., osmolality of human plasma (290 mosmol/L) has been nearly achieved

TABLE 3B-11. Iodine Contrast Agents Applicable to Coronary Angiography

Contrast Agent Generic (Product)			
Ionic		Nonionic	
Monomer	Dimer	Monomer	Dimer
Diatrozate (Renografin)	Ioxaglate	Iopromide	Iotrolan (Isovist)
Iothalamate (Conray)	Ioxaglate (Hexabrix) (low osmolality)	Iohexol (Omnipaque)	Iodixanol (Visipaque)
		Iopamidol (Isovue)	
		Ioversol (Optiray)	
		Iopromide (Ultravist) (all low osmolality)	

(~300 mosmol/L) in some nonionic dimeric contrast agents, such as iotralan and iodixanol.[48] Vascular contrast agents are generally safe, and severe responses (such as hypotensive shock, laryngeal edema, or cardiac arrest) are exceedingly rare (~<0.1%). Because of their better tolerance, nonionic LOCM are preferably used in PCI. Despite voluminous literature on the differential effects of modern contrast agents on various body systems, no clear advantages of individual agents in the sum of their efficacy and biological tolerance has been unequivocally documented.[49,50] The total volume of contrast agent required for PCI varies; in the author's laboratory, it is 70 ± 40 mL. To avoid dose-dependent adverse effects, contrast agents should be used judiciously, and the total volume kept low. Manual injections are almost always used for PCI.

The importance of the intensity and homogeneity of opacification for *quantitative* coronary image analysis[26] and clinical interpretation[50] has been clearly recognized. In contrast, the image criteria relevant for *qualitative* image analysis, e.g., for the identification of morphologic details such as intimal flaps, dissections, plaque shifts, and thrombi, are less well known. Although some initial research seems to address this question,[51] in the absence of established criteria the amount and rate of contrast agent coronary injection remain a matter of individual preference.

Important determinants of the quality of imaging are safety and radiation exposure. Operator-independent vendor-determined factors include the energy spectrum of the x-ray beam, collimation, and filtering. Operator-dependent factors include:

- Total fluoroscopy and cine time
- Fluoroscopy pulse rate (e.g., rates available in the United States are 30, 15, and 7.5 pulses per second)
- Distance between the image intensifier/flat panel and the patient
- Use of the high, normal, and low resolution modes
- Use of high magnification
- Use of semitransparent filters with each image acquisition
- Changes in the direction of projections for the same target

Judicious use of these imaging variables, all of which are contained in the ALARA (as low as reasonably achievable) principle,[4] need to be considered for optimum image acquisition and low radiation exposure.

The rapid sequence of coronary angiograms during PCI requires high-quality images and real-time reading. Interpretations of poor-quality images by an inexperienced operator are invitations for disaster. Furthermore, standard terminology is required in order to avoid "reading signs in the sand" and to permit consistent reading, image interpretation, and documentation.

PCI results are reported in terms of angiographic, procedural, and clinical outcome. Angiographic outcome is usually defined by the status of the target lesions and the interventional site recorded on the final angiograms, whereas procedural and clinical outcomes are defined by the overall short-term (e.g., inpatient) and long-term results (e.g., 6 months). Table 3B-12 presents the definitions of procedure-related outcomes as defined by the BARI investigators.[28] At present, the frequently reported quantitative parameters of stenosis outcome include:

- Reference vessel diameter (RVD). RVD is the luminal diameter of a comparable segment. Usually used for reference is either the closest side branch or an angiographically normal appearing segment of the target vessel, either proximal or distal to the target lesion and typically 5 mm from it. The RVD is measured in millimeters as a sum of the diameters in one left anterior oblique (LAO) and one right anterior oblique (RAO) projection divided by 2.
- Minimal luminal diameter (MLD). MLD is the smallest measured luminal diameter across the site of the target lesion at which it is most severe. It is measured before and after an intervention and on follow-up and reported in millimeters.
- Diameter stenosis (DS). DS is calculated as MLD/RVD $\times$ 100; the result is a percentage (%).
- Restenosis is defined as DS <50% on follow-up analysis.
- Binary restenosis rate (BRR). BRR indicates the percentage of patients with DS >50% on follow-up.
- Acute gain/acute loss/late loss indicate the percentage change in the diameter of the stenosis after intervention compared to its baseline value.

The TIMI flow grade on the final angiograms should also be reported. A sample standard protocol and documentation

TABLE 3B-12.   Procedural Outcome Based on National Heart, Lung, and Blood Institute Bypass Angioplasty Revascularization Investigation (BARI) from an Unpublished BARI Central Radiographic Laboratory Operations Manual

Procedural Outcome	Definition
Procedural success	Reduction in diameter of stenosis in one or more stenosis to <50% stenosis associated with no major ischemic complications during hospitalization
Procedure-related myocardial infarction	Changes in cardiac enzymes or ECG resulting from procedure-related ischemia
Procedure-related death	Death resulting from attempted PTCA
Procedure-related complications	Death, emergency bypass surgery, or myocardial infarction resulting from attempted PTCA.

PTCA, percutaneous transluminal coronary angioplasty.

Modified from Ellis SG, Vandormael MG, Cowley MJ, et al. Coronary morphologic and clinical determinants of procedural outcome with angioplasty for multivessel coronary disease; Implications for patient selection. *Circulation.* 1990;82:1193–1202.

form for PCI is available on the Internet from the American College of Cardiology National Cardiovascular Data Registry.[52]

In summary, coronary angiography and fluoroscopy are employed to guide and to document the results of coronary interventions. Image quality, quality of imaging, and image interpretations are fundamental for the initiation, performance, and termination of PCI. A diligent imaging technique and interpretative skills are key factors in successfully guiding coronary procedures. To avoid oversights and complications, the PCI operator needs to retain a critical attitude toward angiographic documentation of the intermediate and final results. To achieve optimum results, the operator must select the "worst" views for PCI guidance, not the "best" ones. It is only this critical attitude that allows the operator to recognize impending complications early and to respond optimally. Attaining and maintaining this critical professional attitude represents one of the most critical steps in mastering coronary interventions. This fact is all the more important in the increasingly competitive environment of modern, busy, catheterization laboratories.

FUTURE PERSPECTIVES

X-ray coronary angiography has been a standard means for guiding coronary interventions since the beginnings of percutaneous transluminal coronary angioplasty (PTCA) three decades ago. Recent developments in angiographic CT and MRI technology hold some promise for the development of noninvasive coronary angiography in the future. At least in the foreseeable future, however, it is highly unlikely that they will replace x-ray angiography and fluoroscopy in peri-interventional settings. A more liberal use of flow and pressure measurements and intracoronary ultrasound imaging is required to improve the quality of diagnosis of "borderline" coronary states and outcomes. Yet despite all these technical improvements, expert cognitive skills, manual dexterity, and the high professional ethics of the PCI operators will remain the primary determinants of outcome.

REFERENCES

1. Topol EJ, Nissen SE. Our preoccupation with coronary luminology. The dissociation between clinical and angiographic findings in ischemic heart disease. *Circulation.* 1995;92:2333–2342.
2. Kamm K-F, Onnasch DGW. X-ray radiography. In: Lanzer P, Lipton M, eds. *Diagnostics of Vascular Diseases; Principles and Technology.* Berlin: Springer Verlag, 1997:63–98.
3. ACC/SCA & I Expert Consensus Document: American College of Cardiology/Society for Cardiac Angiography and Interventions clinical expert consensus document on cardiac catheterization laboratory standards. *J Am Coll Cardiol.* 2001;37:2172–2214.
4. ACCF/AHA/HRS/SCAI fluoroscopy clinical competence statement. ACCF/AHA/HRS/SCAI clinical competence statement on physician knowledge to optimize patient safety and image quality in fluoroscopically guided invasive cardiovascular procedures. *J Am Coll Cardiol.* 2004;44:2260–2281.
5. Gensini GG, Esente P. International angiographic nomenclature for the human coronary circulation. *Giornale Ital Cardiol.* 1975;5:913–918.
6. James TN, Bruschke AVG, Böthig S, et al. Report of WHO/ISFC Task Force on nomenclature of coronary arteriograms. *Circulation.* 186;74:451a–455a.
7. v. Ludinghausen M. *The Clinical Anatomy of the Coronary Arteries.* Berlin: Springer Verlag, 2003.
8. Principal Investigators of CASS and Associates. National Heart, Lung, and Blood Institute Coronary Artery Surgery Study. *Circulation.* 1981;63(suppl I):I-1-I-139.
9. Dodge JT, Brown BG, Bolson EL, et al. Intrathoracic spatial location of specified coronary segments of the normal human heart; application of quantitative arteriography,

10. Cabrol C, Christides C. Usual arrangement and nomenclature of the coronary arteries. *Bull Assoc Anat (Nancy).* 1976;60:645–649.
11. Bruschke AVG, Reiber JHC, Relik-van Wely L, van Wesemael JWJ. Coronary arteriography—I. Available at: www.nhj.nl/cardiologie.nl/2/pagecontent/main_richtlijnen/richtlijnen/1991_coronaryarteriography.pd. Accessed August 12, 2005.
12. King SB III, Douglas JS Jr., Morris DC. New angiographic views for coronary arteriography. In: Hurst JW, ed. *Update IV: The Heart.* New York: McGraw-Hill, 1981:193.
13. Wang JC, Normand S-LT, Mauri L, et al. Coronary artery spatial distribution of acute myocardial infarction occlusions. *Circulation.* 2004;110:278–284.
14. Gibson CM, Kirtane AJ, Murphy SA, et al. Distance from the coronary ostium to the culprit lesion in acute ST-elevation myocardial infarction and its implications regarding the potential prevention of proximal plaque rupture. *J Thromb Thrombol.* 2003;15:189–196.
15. Endoh R, Homma T, Furihata Y, et al. A morphometric study of the distribution of early coronary atherosclerosis using arteriography. *Artery.* 1988;15:192–202.
16. Tsutsui H, Yamagashi M, Uematsu M, et al. Intravascular ultrasound evaluation of plaque distribution at curved coronary segments. *Am J Cardiol.* 1998;81:977–981.
17. Schettler G, Nerem RM, Schmid-Schönbein H, et al., eds. *Fluid Dynamics as a Localizing Factor for Atherosclerosis.* Berlin: SpringerVerlag, 1983.
18. Rioufol G, Finet G, Ginon I, et al. Multiple atherosclerotic plaque rupture in acute coronary syndrome: a three-vessel intravascular ultrasound study. *Circulation.* 2002; 106:804–808.
19. Gould KL. Quantitative coronary arteriography. In: Gould KL, ed. *Coronary Artery Stenosis and Reversing Atherosclerosis.* 2nd edition. London: Arnold, 1998:107–121.
20. Gould KL, Lipscomb K, Calvert C. Compensatory changes of the distal coronary vascular bed during progressive coronary constriction. *Circulation.* 1975;51:1085–1094.
21. Gould KL. Phasic pressure-flow and arteriographic geometry. In: Gould KL, ed. *Coronary Artery Stenosis and Reversing Atherosclerosis.* 2nd edition. London: Arnold, 1998:67–78
22. Pijls HJ, De Bruyne B, eds. *Coronary Pressure.* 2nd edition. Dordrecht, The Netherlands: Kluwer Academic Publishers, 2000: 163–165.
23. Zir L, Miller S, Dinsmore R, et al. Interobserver variability in coronary angiography. *Circulation.* 1976;53:627–632.
24. DeRouen TA, Murray JA, Owen W. Variability in the analysis of coronary arteriograms. *Circulation.* 1977;55:324–331.
25. Serruys PW, Booman E, Troost J, et al. Computerized quantitative coronary arteriography applied to percutaneous transluminal coronary angioplasty: advantages and limitations. In: Kaltenbach M, Grüntzig A, Rentrop K, et al., eds. *Transluminal Coronary Angioplasty and Intracoronary Thrombolysis—Heart Disease IV.* Berlin: Springer Verlag, 1982:110–121.
26. Reiber JHC, Serruys PW, Kooijman CJ, et al. Assessment of short-, medium-, and long-term variations in arterial dimensions from computer-assisted quantitation of coronary cineangiograms. *Circulation.* 1985;71:280–288.
27. ACC Clinical Expert Consensus Document. American College of Cardiology Clinical Expert Consensus Document on standards for acquisition, measurement and reporting of intravascular ultrasound studies (IVUS). *J Am Coll Cardiol.* 2001;37:1480–1492.
28. Ellis SG, Vandormael MG, Cowley MJ, et al. Coronary morphologic and clinical determinants of procedural outcome with angioplasty for multivessel coronary disease; implications for patient selection. *Circulation.* 1990;82:1193–1202.
29. Ryan TJ, Faxon DP, Gunnar RM, et al. Guidelines for percutaneous transluminal coronary angioplasty: A report of the American College of Cardiology/American Heart Association Task Force on Assessment of Diagnostic and Therapeutic Cardiovascular Procedures. *J Am Coll Cardiol.* 1988;12:529–545.
30. Lefevre T, Louvard Y, Morice M-C, et al. Stenting of bifurcation lesions: classification, treatment and results. *Cathet Cardiovasc Intervent.* 2000;49:274–283.
31. Pompa J, Bashore T. Qualitative and quantitative angiography—Bifurcation lesions. In: Topol E, ed. *Textbook of Interventional Cardiology.* Philadelphia: WB Saunders, 1994: 1055–1058.
32. Mintz GS, Popma JJ, Pichard AD, et al. Limitations of angiography in the assessment of plaque distribution in coronary artery disease. *Circulation.* 1996;93:924–931.
33. Ellis SG, Ajluni S, Arnold SZ, et al. Increased coronary perforation in the new device era. Incidence, classification, management, and outcome. *Circulation.* 1994;90:2725–2730.
34. Ajluni SC, Glazier S, Blankenship L, et al. Perforations after percutaneous coronary interventions: clinical, angiographic, and therapeutic observations. *Cathet Cardiovasc Diagn.* 1994;32:206–212.
35. Mehran R, Dangas G, Abizaid AS, et al. Angiographic pattern of in-stent restenosis: classification and implications for long-term outcome. *Circulation.* 1999;100:1872–1878.
36. The TIMI Study Group. The thrombolysis in myocardial infarction (TIMI) trial. *N Engl J Med.* 1985;312:932–941.
37. Gibson CM, Cannon CP, Daley WL, et al. TIMI frame count: a quantitative method of assessing coronary artery flow. *Circulation.* 1996;93:879–888.
38. Ito H, Tomooka T, Sakai N, et al. Lack of myocardial perfusion immediately after successful thrombolysis. A predictor of poor recovery of left ventricular function in anterior myocardial infarction. *Circulation.* 1992;85:1699–1705.
39. Ito H, Murayama A, Iwakura K, et al. Clinical applications of the 'no-reflow' phenomenon: a predictor of complications and left ventricular remodelling in reperfused anterior wall myocardial infarction. *Circulation.* 1996;93:223–228.
40. Lefkovitz J, Holmes DR, Califf RM, et al., for the CAVEAT II Investigators. Predictors and sequelae of distal embolization during saphenous vein graft intervention from the CAVEAT II trial. *Circulation.* 1995;92:734–740.
41. Topol EJ, Yadav JS. Recognition of the importance of embolization in atherosclerotic vascular disease. *Circulation.* 2000;101:570–580.
42. Grube E, Gerckens U, Yeung AC, et al. Prevention of distal embolization during coronary angioplasty in saphenous venous grafts and native vessels using porous filter protection. *Circulation.* 2001;104:2436–2441.

43. van't Hof AW, Liem A, Suryapranata H, et al. Angiographic assessment of myocardial reperfusion in patients treated with primary angioplasty for acute myocardial infarction. *Circulation.* 1998;97:2302–2306.

44. Gibson CM, Cannon CP, Murphy SA, et al. Relationship of TIMI myocardial perfusion grade to mortality after administration of thrombolytic drugs. *Circulation.* 2000;101:125–130.

45. Gibson DM, Murphy SA, Daley WL, et al. Relationship of the TIMI myocardial perfusion grades, flow grades, frame count, and percutaneous coronary intervention to long-term outcomes after thrombolytic administration in acute myocardial infarction. *Circulation.* 2002;105:1909–1913.

46. Henriques JPS, Zijlstra F, van't Hof AWJ, et al. Angiographic assessment of reperfusion in acute myocardial infarction by myocardial blush grade. *Circulation.* 2003;107:2115–2119.

47. Bushberg JT, Seibert JA, Leidholdt, Jr., et al. The Essential Physics of Medical Imaging. 2nd edition. Philadelphia: Lippincott Williams & Wilkins, 2002.

48. Krause W. X-ray contrast agents. In: Lanzer P, Lipton M, eds. *Diagnostics of Vascular Diseases: Principles and Technology.* Berlin: Springer Verlag, 1997:99–113.

49. Schrader R, Esch I, Fach WA, et al. A randomized trial comparing the impact of nonionic (iomeprol) vs ionic (ixoglate) low osmolar contrast medium on abrupt vessel closure and ischemic complications after angioplasty. *J Am Coll Cardiol.* 1999;33:395–402.

50. Himi KH, Takermoto A, Hirni S, et al. Clinical usefulness of iomeprol 400mg/ml in cardioangiography evaluation of patient discomfort and hemodynamic and ECG effects. *Acad Radiol.* 1998;5(Suppl):54–57.

51. Harrison JK. Image quality and coronary blood flow assessment: The influence of radiographic contrast. *J Clin Basic Cardiol.* 2001;4:249–251.

52. American College of Cardiology. National Cardiovascular Data Registry (catheter laboratory module, version 3.04 [status August 2005 version]. Available at: http://www.accncdr.com/WebNCDR/COMMON/DEFAULT.ASPX.

Anuja Nair

M. Pauliina Margolis

Stephen C. Davies

D. Geoffrey Vince

CHAPTER **3C**

Intracoronary Ultrasound

The ideal in vivo imaging technique for atherosclerosis and guiding interventions should be safe, relatively inexpensive, and portable, and it should provide high-resolution images in real time. In addition, the image data should provide information that is comparable to the microanatomical and histological gold standard to allow appropriate clinical decisions in the course of vascular catheter-based interventions. Whereas contrast angiography has been the traditional mode of viewing coronary arteries in interventional settings, clinical intravascular ultrasound (IVUS) represents a relatively recent development in the field that has already gained significant acceptance over the past decade (for review, see reference 1).

This chapter aims to explain the principles of IVUS technology and image acquisition and the valuable information that can be obtained from ultrasound signal backscatter. Analysis of ultrasound signal backscatter can be used to create color-coded tissue maps of a plaque or VH-IVUS images, which provide crucial knowledge of the vascular disease at a target lesion or target artery.

PRINCIPLES OF ULTRASOUND

The term *ultrasound* indicates sound of frequency higher than the extent of human hearing range, which is 20 Hz to 20 kHz. Barring bats, dolphins, whales, and certain rodents, most animals can hear up to only approximately 45 to 50 kHz. Any sound of frequency higher than the human range of hearing (usually >20 kHz) is considered to be ultrasound. Sound energy moves through media like a wave and is therefore subject to laws of wave motion. Since the propagation is also dependent on the medium the sound energy transverses, any changes to the original wave are indicative of the properties of that medium. Therefore, by studying these changes to the ultrasound waves, one can reasonably derive conclusions about composition of any such media. However, it is important to understand the underlying principles of ultrasound waves to extract information from them.

The first instance of cardiac imaging with ultrasound was perhaps the development of echocardiography by Elder in the early 1950s (for review, see reference 2). Like other ultrasound research in that period, medical diagnosis suffered from poor ultrasound transducer design and primitive algorithms for image display. As a result, the images could be interpreted to detect major tissue outlines but lacked information about detailed tissue texture. With the pulse-echo mode of operation, a single ultrasound beam is transmitted in tissue, and the resulting echoes that "bounce" off the different tissue interfaces are acquired by the ultrasound console. The distance between these echoes is indicative of the dimensions of the tissue structures. Their amplitudes and frequency content can be further analyzed to determine the type of tissue or its composition. The usage of medical ultrasound and its development increased tremendously following improvements in image processing techniques.[3,4] Currently, a major characteristic of the typical gray-scale IVUS images is that they are a result of envelope-detection and log compression of the backscattered data. Briefly, envelope detection is a technique where the amplitude of a signal is noted along distance or time. All the highs and lows are then log compressed and the amplitudes are mapped to a value between 0 and 255, resulting in 8-bit resolution or 256 gray-scale levels in one image (see Fig. 3C-1 for schematic). Thus, IVUS images are only representative of the amplitude or strength of signals and they do not represent the frequency content of the signals. Subsequent subsections of this chapter explain why both signal strength and frequency are important in interpreting ultrasound data.

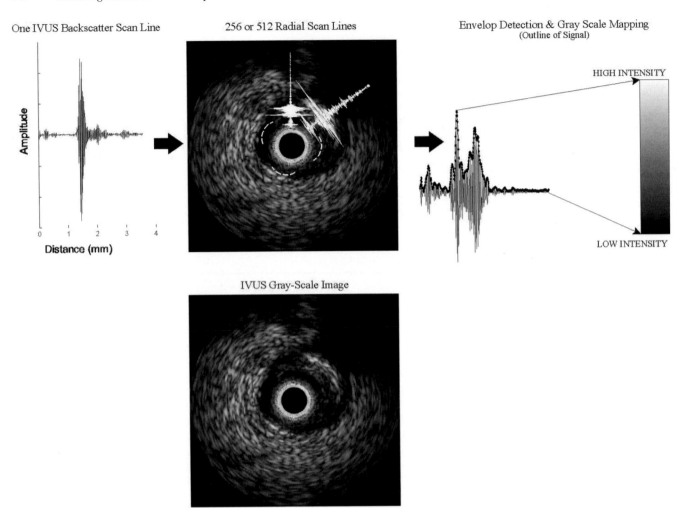

One IVUS Backscatter Scan Line

256 or 512 Radial Scan Lines

Envelop Detection & Gray Scale Mapping
(Outline of Signal)

HIGH INTENSITY

LOW INTENSITY

IVUS Gray-Scale Image

FIGURE 3C-1.   Conventional intravascular ultrasound (IVUS) images are reconstructed from 256 or 512 single backscatter scan lines that span 360 degrees for one cross-sectional image. The "peaks" and "valleys" of these backscatter signals are identified by a technique called envelope detection. The lowest value of this signal is assigned black, and the highest value is assigned white. All signals in between are various shades of gray, resulting in a gray-scale cross-section IVUS image.

ULTRASOUND PROPAGATION IN TISSUE

In the pulse-echo mode of operation, the ultrasound transducer is excited with a certain voltage, which makes it oscillate and produce an ultrasound pulse. This is characteristic of piezoelectric materials, which are commonly chosen as ultrasound transducers. The reflected or scattered echoes of the original ultrasound are converted to an electrical signal and called the backscatter. With IVUS, an ultrasound pulse or wave is sent out into the vessel wall to be imaged in the radial direction. In the clinically available consoles, the backscatter is acquired by the transducer, with typically 256 or 512 such A-scans (backscattered signals) forming one IVUS arterial cross-sectional image (Fig. 3C-1). Analysis of these A-scans holds potential for tissue characterization.

Ultrasound propagation is generally approximated as a compression or longitudinal wave. For simplicity, this propagation can be approximated in one dimension using equations of wave motion where the speed of sound, c, in the medium is:

$$c = \sqrt{\frac{1}{\kappa\rho}} = \lambda f$$

with κ being the compressibility of the surrounding medium and ρ its density; λ is the wavelength and f is the frequency of ultrasound.[2,3] This simple representation of sound-wave propagation demonstrates how backscattered signals acquired with ultrasound medical systems are attributed to the tissue properties they are reflected from, namely density and compressibility, both contained in the amplitude and frequency spectrum of the ultrasound backscatter. The backscattered signals are composed of two types of signal echoes that are visible in IVUS gray-scale images. These are specular reflections and diffuse scattering.[4,5] The specular echoes are a result of strong ultrasound reflections and refractions from an interface and are governed by a relationship between the angles of incidence, reflection, and refraction and the acoustic impedances of the two tissues at the interface. Such reflections are obvious in major tissue transitions, such as the blood-plaque or the media-adventitia wall interface (see Fig. 3C-2). In addition, in ultrasound systems where the same transducer is also the receiver for the backscatter (e.g., the current IVUS catheters), detection of specular echoes are highly dependent on the angle of incidence. If the angle is large, the reflected wave will not be detected; only

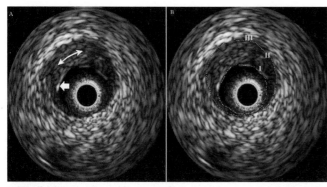

FIGURE 3C-2. **A:** Intravascular ultrasound (IVUS) image with specular reflection (*block arrow*) and diffuse scattering (*double-headed arrow*). **B:** Same image with segmented plaque illustrating the three-layer appearance of IVUS images. *I*, echogenic lumen-plaque boundary; *II*, echolucent media; *III*, echogenic adventitia.

reflections off perpendicular interfaces and those with small angles are received by the IVUS catheter and hence displayed in an image. Studies have been conducted to examine the effect of angle of incidence of ultrasound with respect to the plaque, and results have indicated some dependency to tissue characterization.[6,7] The second type of ultrasound scattering, called diffuse scattering, is from tissue microstructure at cellular or subcellular levels. Diffuse scatter is due to a phenomenon of scattering from structures smaller in dimension than the ultrasound wavelength, often called Rayleigh scattering.[8] These reflections are independent of the angle of incidence and they result in the speckled appearance of tissue in IVUS gray-scale images.[4,9] Since the ultrasound scattering is in many directions, only a small portion of the signal is reflected back to the ultrasound transducer. Given the low intensities observed with diffuse scattering, in comparison to specular reflections, diffuse scatter is often attributed to noise in the signals. Detailed studies have demonstrated that ultrasound attenuation due to diffuse scattering is small. However, this phenomenon is considered important for discerning soft tissue detail.[10,11] It is observed as "speckle" in the log compressed gray-scale ultrasound images. IVUS images of atherosclerotic plaques constitute mostly diffuse scattering, except for the specular reflections off the vessel-wall boundaries or in plaques with large areas of dense calcium (as shown in Fig. 3C-2).

ULTRASOUND-TISSUE INTERACTIONS

Ultrasound energy propagates through tissue during imaging and is also reflected from various tissue interfaces based on differences in acoustic impedance.[4] Besides the phenomena of propagation and reflection, there are other effects on the ultrasound signals caused by tissue type. These are absorption and scattering, both resulting in weakening of the signals as a function of the ultrasound frequency.[4] Hence, an IVUS transducer operating at a lower frequency, for example 20 MHz, produces signals that are less attenuated and is useful in viewing small or larger arteries (range about 2 to 9 mm diameter). Conversely, IVUS at higher frequencies, at about 45 to 50 MHz, causes increased attenuation and is well suited to imaging smaller coronary arteries (see later discussion).

The dominant part of ultrasound attenuation in tissue results from absorption of ultrasound energy. The specific absorption

due to different macromolecules varies significantly and is related to the structure of the biological macromolecule and its hydration level, and it can also vary with heat denaturation and pH.[11] Energy is lost through absorption mainly due to viscosity of the medium.[4] Absorption is almost linearly dependent on the frequency of ultrasound. Ultrasound scattering, on the other hand, has been researched extensively by many groups[5,8,9,13,14] and is dependent on the following:

- Density of tissue
- Size and spacing of tissue components
- The homogeneity or heterogeneity of the plaque/tissue components
- Acoustic impedance differences between them
- Water content and distribution
- The frequency of ultrasound

Spectral analysis techniques (see later discussion) can be used to calculate certain acoustic properties of tissues, such as relative acoustic impedance or the attenuation coefficient. Prior knowledge of such tissue properties is a tremendous help in classification of ultrasound backscatter. To date, no detailed studies have been performed for atherosclerosis; however, many studies have documented the trends in acoustic attenuation and speed of sound in various gross human organs and tissues.[11,15] An important aspect that was highlighted in these studies is that there is significant overlap in acoustic properties of gross human tissues, indicating the difficulty of tissue characterization at the molecular level for small structures such as vascular tissue. A few studies performed with scanning acoustic microscopy (SAM) determined key properties of vascular tissues, since SAM entails very high frequency evaluation of tissue microstructure (100 to 2,000 MHz).[12,16] These studies reported the range of speed of sound in vascular wall to be between 1,500 and 1,760 meters per second. The speed of sound was found to be 1,568 meters per second in normal intima, 1,760 meters per second in calcified plaques, 1,677 meters per second in fibrous or stable plaques, and 1,526 meters per second in lipidic regions. Current IVUS systems do not allow speed of sound calculations with high precision, therefore limiting such detailed evaluation to ex vivo analysis with equipment capable of very high frequencies, such as SAM. Results from similar studies and the theoretical aspects of acoustics emphasize the importance of frequency-based analysis in ultrasonic tissue characterization and interpretation of images with current commercially available IVUS systems.

INTRAVASCULAR ULTRASOUND

The potential of IVUS to quantify the structure and geometry of normal and atherosclerotic coronary arteries is well documented.[1,17–20] In IVUS images, the three-layer appearance of the normal muscular-artery wall is formed by (I) the echogenic lumen/intimal interface; (II) the echolucent zone that represents the media, and (III) the echogenic outer adventitial region of connective and adipose tissue, as illustrated in Figure 3C-2. Current IVUS catheters, which are as small as 0.9 mm in diameter, permit the interrogation of most areas of the human coronary vasculature. In addition, spatial resolution is on the order of 80 to 120 μm radially (axial resolution) and 160 to 250 μm around the circumference (lateral resolution).[21,22] IVUS clinical systems are designed to be portable; the procedure is relatively inexpensive, and the images are acquired in real time at the rate of 30 frames per second. Several studies have compared geometric parameters (i.e., plaque area and thickness of gross features) measured by histological evaluation or by angiography to IVUS images.[19,23,24] These studies dispelled much of the initial skepticism toward the accuracy and reliability of IVUS images. At the same time, these studies caused the clinical field to take a more critical look at the traditional imaging modality of angiography. Many investigations have indicated difficulty in obtaining consistent agreement between the data from IVUS and angiography. Of those studies that did obtain good correlations, the data produced regression fits with slopes far from unity, indicating that angiography and IVUS are correlated, but do not provide quantitatively identical results. A large number of researchers contend that IVUS is, in fact, the more accurate of the two coronary imaging modalities.[25-27]

INTRAVASCULAR ULTRASOUND DEVICES

IVUS devices work using the same principles as conventional external B-mode ultrasound scanners. The salient differences between intravascular devices and external devices are the size of the probe, 360-degree radial imaging, and the operating frequency. As mentioned in the section on "Principles of Ultrasound," ultrasound imaging utilizes variations in the acoustic properties of the tissue to generate a map of backscatter intensity with respect to time. A backscatter echo is generated when ultrasound is reflected at interfaces where there is a change in the acoustic properties of the tissues on either side of the interface. The strength of the echo is proportional to the differences in the acoustic properties of the materials. For example, differences between acoustic properties of blood and plaque are large, leading to a clearly defined blood-plaque border. In contrast, differences in properties of atherosclerotic tissues (fibrous, fibrofatty, necrotic core, or dense calcium) within a heterogeneous plaque are subtle, leading to speckle in gray-scale images and no clear boundaries between plaque components (Fig. 3C-2).

Ultrasound imaging devices utilize piezoelectric materials to generate and receive the ultrasound energy. A material commonly used in such devices is lead zirconate titanate (PZT). Piezoelectric materials possess specific electrical properties that cause the material to change in dimension when subjected to an electric field of a specific orientation. Conversely, when the material is stretched or compressed it generates an electric field or voltage across opposite surfaces. This electromechanical phenomenon is used to both generate and receive ultrasound

energy in imaging applications. The PZT is subjected to a very short pulse of electrical energy, leading to a rapid change in its thickness that subsequently results in the generation of an ultrasound pulse. Sound energy is simply the propagation of regions of compression and expansion through any material: solid, liquid, or gas. As the pulse of ultrasonic energy passes through the tissue, a portion of it is reflected at all incident interfaces. The resultant reflected energy or echoes propagate back toward the PZT, causing it to contract and expand resulting in the generation of electrical energy and a signal or backscatter that can be interpreted by the imaging console. As mentioned earlier, IVUS systems do not allow precise measurement of speed of sound through various tissues. In fact, all ultrasound imaging systems assume constant speed of sound in all tissue types. This being the case, the elapsed time between the generation of an ultrasound pulse and the reception of the resultant echoes is directly proportional to the distance between the PZT and the tissue interface generating the echo. It is this relationship that makes it possible to generate a spatial ultrasound intensity map or a gray-scale IVUS image from the backscatter signals (Fig. 3C-1 shows a schematic).

INTRAVASCULAR ULTRASOUND MODE OF OPERATION

The ultrasonic field generated by a single piece of piezoelectric material is strongly directional. Therefore, it is necessary to scan the ultrasonic field through 360 degrees to generate a full cross-sectional image. Commercially available IVUS devices achieve this in two ways, either by mechanical scanning (rotation) of a single PZT transducer or by electrical scanning of a solid-state cylindrical array of multiple PZT transducers (see Fig. 3C-3).

Intravascular Ultrasound Catheters

MECHANICAL DEVICES. Mechanically scanned IVUS devices typically comprise a single PZT transducer that is located at the distal end of a length of the drive cable, all of which is surrounded by a flexible catheter sheath along its length. The drive cable enables the transducer to be rotated using a drive unit that is external to the patient. The desired refresh rate of current IVUS systems for real-time imaging is approximately 30 frames per second. The speed of rotation of the transducer and drive cable necessitate the need for a sheath that prevents direct contact between the moving parts and the patient. For the sheath to work effectively it must have the mechanical durability and strength to accommodate the drive cable for running durations of up to 1 hour. It must also be transparent to acoustic energy so as not to impede the ultrasound and compromise the IVUS data.

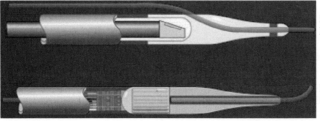

Single Element
Mechanically Rotating

Multiple Element
Solid State

FIGURE 3C-3. Diagrams of typical single-element mechanically rotated and solid-state multiple transducer intravascular ultrasound catheters.

In addition, it should be flexible enough to reach the target site(s). The material properties necessary to achieve all of these requirements are not available in any single material. As a consequence, sheaths typically comprise a number of different materials. This presents a unique problem for mechanical IVUS devices. In order for the PZT transducer to be able to rotate freely within the catheter sheath, it is necessary that both components be free to move with respect to each other, resulting in a gap between the transducer and the catheter sheath (Fig. 3C-3). If the gap were to be occupied by air, this would represent a layer of significantly different acoustic properties compared to the materials on either side. Consequently, image quality could be severely compromised. However, this problem is overcome by flushing the lumen of the catheter sheath with saline immediately prior to imaging. In most cases it is also necessary to flush the device periodically throughout the procedure, as air trapped within the drive cable becomes mobile and travels toward the distal end of the catheter.

Most commercially available mechanically rotating IVUS catheters operate at frequencies between 30 and 45 MHz with high axial resolution (80 to 100 μm).[21,22] One of the main drawbacks of these devices currently is the lack of range dynamic focusing due to the single transducer element.[22] The fixed-focus ultrasound imaging does not enable use of these devices with large peripheral vessels, which require a greater imaging depth.

CYLINDRICAL ARRAY DEVICES. Solid-state cylindrical transducer array devices comprise an array of PZT transducers that are mounted circumferentially around the distal end of a catheter body. Typical commercially available catheters have an array comprising 64 transducer elements (Fig. 3C-3). The individual transducer elements are operated sequentially to scan the ultrasound energy around the device. After each element or groups of elements have operated in "transmit mode," they are then operated in "receive mode" to obtain backscatter information. The adjacent element or groups of elements then perform the same operation until the process has been completed through 360 degrees for the entire artery cross-section. A full scan of 360 degrees occurs approximately 30 times per second, resulting in a real-time image refresh rate similar to that of the mechanical IVUS devices.

The solid-state devices do not have any moving parts. As such, the construction of phased array devices does not include any air-filled voids, and therefore, their usage does not require saline flushing prior to or during usage. This aspect of the cylindrical array device operation greatly reduces the preparation time required prior to a procedure compared with that of the mechanical devices. The currently available solid-state devices operate at lower frequency compared to the mechanical devices. Hence, the axial resolution is somewhat compromised with the solid-state devices. However, electronic focusing is implemented with these devices, and the ultrasound energy can be focused at varying depths, favoring the array devices for imaging of both large and small vessels.

Operating Frequency

A key feature that sets IVUS devices aside from conventional noninvasive ultrasound devices is the operating frequency. Most external ultrasound imaging devices operate within 3 to 12 MHz. IVUS devices operate in the range of 12 to 50 MHz. The

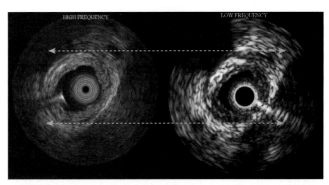

FIGURE 3C-4. Two intravascular ultrasound (IVUS) images of the same plaque (ex vivo) with IVUS catheters operating at high (*left*) and low (*right*) frequencies. The higher frequency image displays better resolution but lacks in depth of penetration, whereas the lower frequency image displays less resolution but one can observe information further out into the surrounding tissue.

operating frequency has a major impact on two aspects of the IVUS images: (a) resolution, and (b) image depth. The resolving power of the IVUS system increases with the frequency of operation. The trade-off with increasing frequency is the depth of penetration in the vessel wall (see Fig. 3C-4). Therefore, the higher the frequency of ultrasound, the faster the backscatter is weakened as it propagates through tissue. The effect of this phenomenon is that high-frequency IVUS cannot penetrate far into the vessel wall and surrounding adventitia. The lack of penetration is usually not an issue in coronary arteries, since IVUS is used to visualize tissue that is relatively close to the transducer. However, this trade-off is apparent in instances where it is desirable to image very large peripheral arteries.

ATHEROSCLEROTIC TISSUE CHARACTERIZATION WITH INTRAVASCULAR ULTRASOUND

Many studies have recognized the importance of IVUS in clinical assessment of atherosclerosis.[1,25,28–31] Multiple efforts are underway to employ IVUS for gaining better understanding of:

- Plaque composition[32–36]
- Three-dimensional (3D) visualization of arteries in real time[37–39]
- Plaque/arterial wall mechanical properties (for review, see reference 40 or recent work by Tajaddini et al.[41]).

This chapter focuses mainly on techniques for determining plaque composition. Over approximately the past 15 years, extensive research has been conducted on image- and signal-based analysis methods for plaque characterization. The following sections describe some of these approaches, including their pros and cons. Finally, a description of the novel VH-IVUS technique is provided.

IMAGE ANALYSIS

Fibrous or "hard" plaques are generally advanced lesions that contain dense fibrous tissue, collagen and elastin fibers, and proteoglycans. Similar to calcified regions of plaque, dense fibrous plaque components reflect ultrasound energy well and

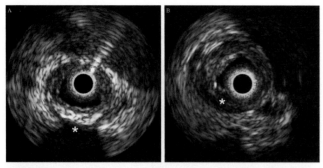

FIGURE 3C-5. Intravascular ultrasound images of diseased human coronary arteries, ex vivo. **A:** Calcified plaque distinguished by high echogenicity followed by a shadow (*asterisk*). **B:** (*Asterisk*) An echolucent region considered to be representative of a lipid-laden necrotic core.

thus appear bright and homogeneous on IVUS images (see Fig. 3C-5).[42] One of the major problems with many of the image-based studies is their dependence on plaque brightness as a discriminator of fibrous tissue content. This parameter is highly dependent on the gain setting of the IVUS console and its transmit power. Therefore, direct comparison of brightness in IVUS images acquired at different times may not be possible. In an attempt to overcome this problem, Hodgson et al. suggested comparing the echo reflectance of the plaque with that of the adventitial reflectance.[28] Unfortunately, the signal produced by the adventitia may be significantly attenuated by the intervening tissue and consequently produce a dimmer image.

Lipidic or "soft" plaques have been implicated in acute ischemic syndromes such as plaque rupture. In IVUS images, regions of low echo reflectance are usually labeled soft plaque (Fig. 3C-5).[28,43] Echolucent regions believed to be lipid pools were first reported by Mallery et al.[44] and later by Potkin et al.[42] In a similar study comparing ex vivo IVUS images to histology sections using 40-MHz transducers, IVUS detection of lipid deposits was shown to have a sensitivity of 88.9% and a specificity of 100%.[45] However, this study did not demonstrate data comparing the size of lipid deposits in IVUS images with those in histology, nor was the vessel pressurized during pullback, making comparisons between the data sets difficult. In addition, this study utilized paraffin-embedded tissue, which requires dehydration and "clearing" stages that dissolve and elute lipid. In another study by Zhang et al., automated image processing techniques were applied to IVUS images captured from video in an attempt to classify lesions as soft plaque, hard plaque, or hard plaque with shadow (i.e., calcified).[46] The technique's performance was assessed by comparing the results with those determined by manual interpretation. Other IVUS image analysis studies with high-order, statistical texture-based algorithms have been shown to perform well in determining plaque.[46–49] However, image-based analysis techniques are slow, and they are limited to offline processing.[49]

BACKSCATTER SIGNAL ANALYSIS

Analysis of the ultrasound backscatter signals eliminates the need to postprocess the IVUS images and affords an entry to the important frequency information contained in the backscatter. Studies have shown that differentiation between vessel layers and tissue types is possible ex vivo.[11,33,36,50–52] To date, two different approaches have been examined for characterization of

atherosclerotic plaque components by IVUS backscattered signals: time-domain analysis and frequency-domain analysis. Frequency-domain analysis or spectral analysis has demonstrated the ability to characterize tissue.[33,34,36,51–54] In the past, studies were mainly limited to the use of classic Fourier techniques to extract spectral parameters from IVUS backscatter. Although the fast Fourier transform (FFT) is an efficient mathematical approach, it does not perform well with high-resolution biological data (such as IVUS backscatter).[55,56] The Welch periodogram, another classic spectral technique, is a modified FFT algorithm calculated by windowing data in a certain number of segments and overlapping those segments by a specified number of samples.[55] It aims to stabilize the spectrum to some extent by statistical averaging but requires additional mathematical operations which suffer from a trade-off between resolution and accuracy. In contrast, autoregressive (AR) modeling can produce high resolution in spectra without compromising accuracy or resolution.[56,57] Therefore, assuming an AR mathematical model for the IVUS backscatter could improve accuracy in estimation of spectral parameters.[58,59]

Spectral Analysis: VH-IVUS

As noted earlier, the amplitude of the RF backscatter of ultrasound systems is dependent on the density, concentration, size, and spacing of scatterers, the homogeneity or heterogeneity of the scatterer type, their acoustic impedance differences, water content, and distribution, and the frequency of ultrasound. In early 1980s, Lizzi et al. and O'Donnell et al. documented some of the early spectral analysis approach with B-mode ultrasound backscatter analysis.[60–62] The work that followed with IVUS adopted the analysis laid out by these groups, but utilized a higher frequency range and unfocused mechanical transducers.[33,51,54] The results from these studies, of analyzing spectral parameters (Fig. 3C-6), indicated that the slope, y-intercept, and midband fit are representative of different tissue structures, sizes, and intervening attenuation. Y-intercept and midband fit are also indicative of the ultrasound scatterer concentration.[63] Previously, midband fit had not been extensively studied for IVUS data, although its potential was evaluated for ultrasonic tissue characterization for other tissues.[64,65] Another parameter that has been examined extensively is integrated backscatter, and it aims to provide a crude estimation of the backscatter coefficient, similar to the midband fit parameter.[13,66]

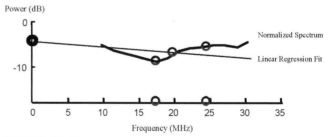

FIGURE 3C-6. Spectral parameters are calculated using the normalized spectra and the linear regression fit within a certain frequency bandwidth. Some of the parameters that are marked (*circles*) are the y-intercept, the minimum power and its corresponding frequency, the midband fit, and the maximum power and its corresponding frequency. Others are slope of the regression line and integrated backscatter (not shown).

In the Cleveland Clinic Foundation's (Cleveland, OH, USA) spectral analysis technique for plaque characterization (licensed to Volcano Corporation, Rancho Cordova, CA, USA and called "VH-IVUS"), eight such spectral parameters are calculated by estimating the backscatter with AR models.[36,67] In brief, ex vivo IVUS data were used with corresponding digitized histology as the gold standard to build a database of homogenous regions of interest (ROI). ROI areas were selected on the Movat Pentachrome stained and morphed histology images[52] and represented one of the four VH-IVUS plaque components (Fig. 3C-7)—fibrous tissue, fibrofatty, necrotic core, and dense calcium. The corresponding regions were highlighted on the reconstructed IVUS gray-scale images, and the original ultrasound backscatter radiofrequency samples representing those ROI areas were retrieved (Fig. 3C-8). Since these ROI areas represent one of four homogeneous plaque components, the IVUS backscatter from each such ROI was further examined for "spectral signatures" of that tissue component. Furthermore, statistical analysis was used to devise classification rules with an extensive database of spectral signatures of representative plaque components.[36] Tree-based modeling or classification is an exploratory technique of data mining for discovering structure in data and can be used to formulate prediction rules from multivariate data. Classification trees comprise a collection of such prediction rules that are determined by a procedure called recursive partitioning. At each node in a tree, unclassified data are separated based on one variable (spectral parameter) that displays maximum separation at the 95%

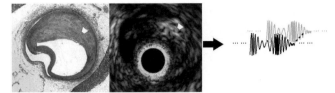

FIGURE 3C-8. Selection of regions of interest (ROIs) for VH-IVUS development. Movat Pentachrome stained histology section (*left*) and the corresponding intravascular ultrasound image (*middle*) with ultrasound signal backscatter data (*right*). A representative homogenous ROI is indicated by the white box marked on each image. Spectral analysis of the backscatter data from such regions was used to build the database of spectral parameters for VH-IVUS tissue classification.

confidence level. Various criteria may be used for the split at each node.[68] The Classification and Regression Trees (CART) procedure was described initially by Breiman et al.[69] and has been used significantly since then.[68] The classification trees are typically built with 75% of the data and then cross-validated by resolving the type of plaque in the remaining 25% of the test data. The outcomes of these predictions are compared to the known pathologies for each ROI to obtain the corresponding sensitivity and specificity of the classification.

Recently, classification results were reported for a database of 88 plaque sections from 51 ex vivo human left anterior descending coronary arteries imaged with 30-MHz IVUS.[36] In that database, ROIs were selected from corresponding histology sections for fibrous tissue ($n = 101$), fibrofatty ($n = 56$), necrotic-core ($n = 70$), and dense-calcium ($n = 50$) areas. The tree calculated from the AR tissue spectra classified fibrous, fibrofatty, necrotic-core, and dense-calcium regions with high predictive accuracies of 90.4%, 92.8%, 89.5%, and 90.9%, respectively, for the training data and 79.7%, 81.2%, 85.5%, and 92.8%, respectively, for the test data. Predictive accuracy can be calculated by combining the sensitivity and specificity for a test outcome. It is the sum of all correct decisions divided by the total number of decisions.[70] In another study, the AR models were optimized by regularizing the estimates so that the "virtual-histology" tissue maps (or VH-IVUS images) were of increased spatial accuracy.[67] A brief outline of the VH-IVUS development procedure is:

- Acquire ex vivo IVUS radiofrequency data and the corresponding histology, which is the gold standard
- Select multiple homogeneous ROI on digitized histology images representing a particular plaque component and find the matching backscatter from those ROI areas in the IVUS data (software was developed for quantitative and accurate ROI selection)[52]
- Calculate and normalize the spectra from the ROIs with appropriate AR models followed by automated data normalization by a technique called blind deconvolution and the estimation of eight spectral parameters.[67,71]
- Develop nonlinear regression (or classification) tree with multiple spectral and depth-related parameters
- Finally, implement the classification tree in software for automated tissue characterization of in vivo data. Figure 3C-9 displays an example IVUS image with corresponding histology and the calculated color tissue-map or VH-IVUS image with the four colors representing fibrous tissue (dark green), fibrofatty (light green), necrotic core (red), and dense calcium (white).

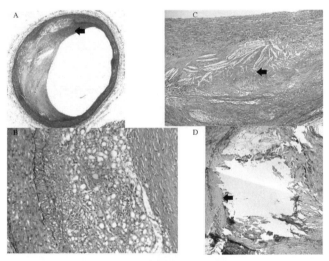

FIGURE 3C-7. Descriptions of the four VH-IVUS plaque components. **A:** Fibrous tissue is densely packed bundles of collagen fibers with no evidence of intrafiber lipid accumulation and no evidence of macrophage infiltration. It appears dark-yellow/green on Movat-stained histology sections and dark green on VH-IVUS images. **B:** Fibrofatty tissue is loosely packed bundles of collagen fibers with regions of lipid deposition present. These areas are cellular and have no cholesterol clefts or necrosis present. There is an increase in extracellular matrix, and it appears turquoise on Movat-stained histology sections and light green on VH-IVUS. **C:** Necrotic core is defined as a highly lipidic necrotic region with remnants of foam cells and dead lymphocytes present. No collagen fibers are visible, and mechanical integrity is poor. Cholesterol clefts and microcalcifications are clearly visible. It is red on VH-IVUS images. **D:** Dense calcium is a focal area of calcium deposits. It appears purple or deep blue on Movat-stained histology sections and usually falls out of histology section, but calcium crystals are evident at borders. It is white on VH-IVUS images. (See Color Fig. 3C-7.)

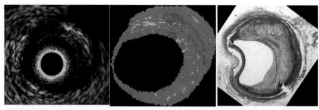

FIGURE 3C-9.   Example of an intravascular ultrasound image (*left*) from a human coronary artery imaged ex vivo, and the corresponding VH-IVUS (*middle*) and Movat-stained histology section (right). VH-IVUS: (*Dark green*) fibrous tissue; (*light green*) fibrofatty; (*red*) necrotic core; (*white*) dense calcium. (See Color Fig. 3C-9.)

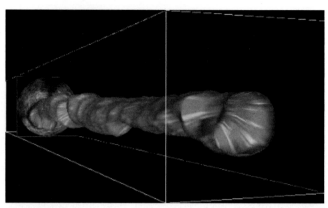

FIGURE 3C-10.   Three-dimensional surface rendering of VH-IVUS images with intravascular ultrasound (IVUS) pullback data in a human coronary artery. The plaque composition is depicted in color on the lumen surface of a human left anterior descending coronary artery, over a length of 56 mm. VH-IVUS: (*Dark green*) fibrous tissue; (*light green*) fibrofatty; (*red*) necrotic core; (*white*) dense calcium.

The VH-IVUS plaque characterization software is currently in use at various clinical sites. A custom-designed ECG-gated IVUS backscatter data acquisition system is used for acquiring clinical IVUS pullback data. The electronics monitor the patient's ECG signal and trigger the analog-to-digital converter card to acquire scan lines representing an IVUS image when the peak of an R-wave is detected.[72] The software also incorporates semiautomated three-dimensional segmentation of the lumen-plaque and media-adventitia interfaces after IVUS image reconstruction. These techniques involve a combination of spectral parameters and active contour models and have been extensively validated on clinical data.[73,74] A volumetric data set of histology composition is hence available by applying the foregoing principles to the IVUS backscatter from each end-diastolic image in the sequences resulting from the ECG-gated pullbacks. After plaque segmentation, the lumen surface can be color coded according to the histology components, allowing a unique fly-through visualization of the inside of the coronary lumen, where the color of the inside of the arterial wall denotes the most superficial histology feature (Fig. 3C-10). The volumetric data set also provides quantitative assessment of both arterial geometry and composition. Plots of lumen, vessel, and plaque cross-sectional area versus image

slice number can be created for geometric assessment and identification of positive remodeling. Also, the characterized plaques can be subdivided into areas of the four plaque components and plotted versus image slice number, creating a panarterial assessment of plaque composition that was previously unavailable (Fig. 3C-11).

CLINICAL UTILITY OF INTRAVASCULAR ULTRASOUND

CURRENT PRACTICE

Coronary angiography is most widely used to guide percutaneous coronary interventions (PCIs), but its limitations are well documented.[1] In current catheterization laboratories, IVUS is

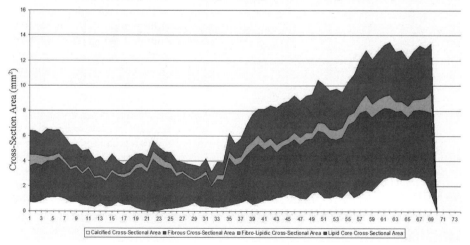

Example Plot of Plaque Composition Along an Artery

IVUS Frame Number

FIGURE 3C-11.   An example output from the VH-IVUS software for quantitative analysis of plaque components along the length of an artery. (See Color Fig. 3C-11.)

definitely leading the new and upcoming pack of imaging modalities in earning a "gold-standard" status for itself. Its usage has increased tremendously over the past 15 years as the interpretation of gray-scale images steadily improved.[75,76] IVUS is currently used broadly for clinical and research applications.

IVUS is typically used in preinterventional assessment of the arteries, and it is routinely used in guidance for various PCI procedures ranging from balloon angioplasty, stent deployment, atherectomy, brachytherapy, and treatment and understanding mechanisms of in-stent restenosis.[1,77] Specifically, in preinterventional settings, IVUS is frequently employed to size endovascular devices based on precise measurements of the nominal size of the target vessel and relevant dimensions of the target lesions, to assess ambiguous angiographic findings such as "borderline" lesions and, frequently, left main disease, and to guide interventions in selected complex cases. Established standards for performance, interpretation, and reporting of findings allow for quality-assured routine clinical IVUS applications essentially in any clinical setting.[78] In fact, IVUS is now an indispensable clinical tool in the majority of catheterization centers. Furthermore, IVUS is now the gold standard in assessing plaque burden and hence has found a well-placed application in serial drug therapy studies with or without assessment of positive remodeling[1,76,79,80] in addition to providing an increased understanding of atherosclerosis.[81,82] Current assessment of plaque vulnerability from IVUS gray-scale images is limited to evaluation of plaque remodeling (quantitative)[79] and studying the shape of plaque (qualitative).[83] Addition of tissue characterization based on spectral analysis holds immense potential to add to the long list of usage IVUS currently enjoys in the catheterization laboratories, including the possibility of detecting rupture-prone atheroma in real time.

PLAQUE CLASSIFICATION BY VH-IVUS

VH-IVUS has shown high accuracy (>85%) both in vitro and in vivo in characterizing plaques.[36,84,85] In addition, VH-IVUS is being assessed to classify different plaque types in similar categories as described by pathologists. Specifically, adaptive intimal thickening (AIT), pathological intimal thickening (PIT), fibroatheroma (FA), thin-cap fibroatheroma (TCFA), and fibrocalcific plaque[86] are being assessed. Furthermore, these different plaque types are currently being evaluated in clinical studies with invasive follow-up to assess plaque progression, regression, stabilization, and activity. In addition, a "vulnerability index" (VI) has been created to describe the typical features seen postmortem in patients with a history of sudden coronary death.

1. Adaptive intimal thickening (AIT): Plaque comprised of mainly fibrous tissue (<5% of fibrofatty, calcification and/or necrotic core plaque components) (Fig. 3C-12).
2. Pathological Intimal Thickening (PIT): Mainly mixture of fibrous, fibrofatty (>5%), and necrotic core including minimal calcified tissue <5% (Fig. 3C-13).
3. Fibroatheroma (FA): This is defined as a plaque with a thick fibrous cap and significant necrotic core (confluent necrotic core >5% of total plaque volume) in fibrous and/or fibrofatty tissue. For purposes of risk assessment, FA can be further subdivided as:
   3.1. This subclassification contains minor amount of dense calcium (<5% of plaque volume) (Fig. 3C-14).

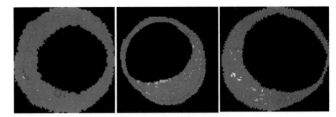

FIGURE 3C-12. Three VH-IVUS images representing adaptive intimal thickening. (*Dark green*) fibrous tissue; (*light green*) fibrofatty; (*red*) necrotic core; (*white*) dense calcium.

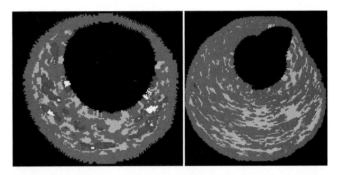

FIGURE 3C-13. Two VH-IVUS images depicting pathological intimal thickening. (*Dark green*) fibrous tissue; (*light green*) fibrofatty; (*red*) necrotic core; (*white*) dense calcium.

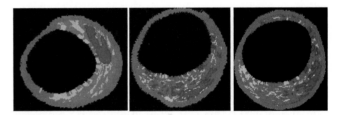

FIGURE 3C-14. Three VH-IVUS fibroatheroma images. (*Dark green*) fibrous tissue; (*light green*) fibrofatty; (*red*) necrotic core; (*white*) dense calcium. (See Color Fig. 3C-14.)

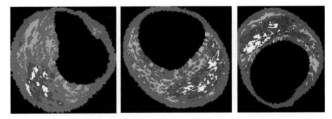

FIGURE 3C-15. Three VH-IVUS fibroatheroma images. (*Dark green*) fibrous tissue; (*light green*) fibrofatty; (*red*) necrotic core; (*white*) dense calcium. (See Color Fig. 3C-15.)

   3.2. FA with significant dense calcium >5% of plaque volume. This is generally viewed as more dangerous than FA without any dense calcium (Fig. 3C-15).
4. This next type of plaque is defined as FA without evidence of fibrous cap, and necrotic core within 5% to 10% of plaque volume (more advanced), with two subclasses.
   4.1. With minor amount of dense calcium (≤5%) (Fig. 3C-16). This type of plaque could be focal (<2 mm of necrotic core) or diffuse (>2 mm of necrotic core).

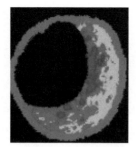

FIGURE 3C-16. One VH-IVUS fibroatheroma. (*Dark green*) fibrous tissue; (*light green*) fibrofatty; (*red*) necrotic core; (*white*) dense calcium.

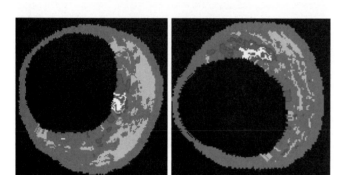

FIGURE 3C-17. Two VH-IVUS fibroatheroma images. (*Dark green*) fibrous tissue; (*light green*) fibrofatty; (*red*) necrotic core; (*white*) dense calcium.

4.2. With increase in dense calcium >5% and, as above, can be further divided as focal or diffuse based on length of the necrotic core (Fig. 3C-17).

5. IVUS defined thin-cap fibroatheroma (ID-TCFA): Such plaque has necrotic core >10%, without IVUS evidence of fibrous cap, and can be further subdivided into four types of plaques.

   5.1. With minor amount of dense calcium (<5%). This has a vulnerability index of 1 (VI 1) (Fig. 3C-18).

   5.2. With increased dense calcium >5% of plaque volume and a vulnerability index of 2 (VI 2) (Fig. 3C-19).

   5.3. ID-TICFA, with multiple foci, confluent necrotic cores (at least one necrotic core without evidence of fibrous cap), suggesting underlying previous rupture(s) with calcification (Fig. 3C-20). This has a vulnerability index of 3 (VI 3).

   5.4. This is ID-TICFA, with high risk. It is most often found as a cause of sudden coronary death and has a vulnerability index of 4 (VI 4) (Fig. 3C-21}. This type of plaque is defined to have confluent necrotic core >20%, with no evidence of fibrous cap, dense calcium >5%, a remodeling index >1.05, and significant (>50%) cross-sectional area luminal narrowing as observed from gray-scale IVUS.

6. Fibrocalcific plaque: This type of plaque is defined to be mainly fibrous with increased dense calcium (>5% of plaque volume). Any presence of necrotic core is <5% of entire plaque volume, and single or multiple layers of calcium are present with or without severe narrowing (in form of deep or superficial sheets of calcium) (Fig. 3C-22). This type could signify plaque stabilization.

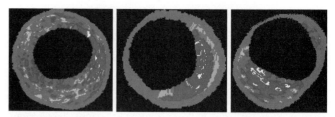

FIGURE 3C-18. Three VH-IVUS images of thin-cap fibroatheromas with necrotic core. (*Dark green*) fibrous tissue; (*light green*) fibrofatty; (*red*) necrotic core; (*white*) dense calcium. (See Color Fig. 3C-18.)

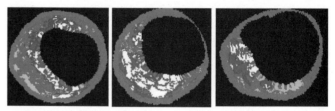

FIGURE 3C-19. Three VH-IVUS images of thin-cap fibroatheromas with dense calcium. (*Dark green*) fibrous tissue; (*light green*) fibrofatty; (*red*) necrotic core; (*white*) dense calcium. (See Color Fig. 3C-19.)

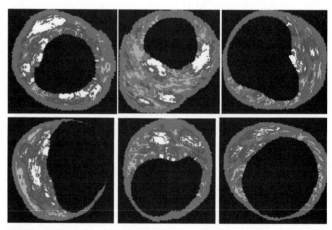

FIGURE 3C-20. Six VH-IVUS images of thin-cap fibroatheromas with multiple foci. (*Dark green*) fibrous tissue; (*light green*) fibrofatty; (*red*) necrotic core; (*white*) dense calcium. (See Color Fig. 3C-20.)

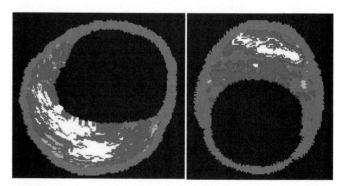

FIGURE 3C-21. Three VH-IVUS images of thin-cap fibroatheromas. (*Dark green*) fibrous tissue; (*light green*) fibrofatty; (*red*) necrotic core; (*white*) dense calcium. (See Color Fig. 3C-21.)

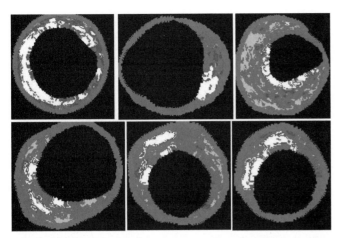

FIGURE 3C-22. Six VH-IVUS images of fibrocalcific plaques. (*Dark green*) fibrous tissue; (*light green*) fibrofatty; (*red*) necrotic core; (*white*) dense calcium.

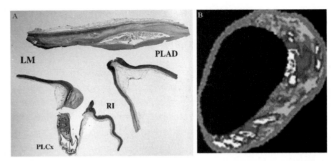

FIGURE 3C-23. **A:** Histology image from a bifurcation (courtesy of Dr. R. Virmani). **B:** VH-IVUS at a bifurcation. VH-IVUS: (*Dark green*) fibrous tissue; (*light green*) fibrofatty; (*red*) necrotic core; (*white*) dense calcium.

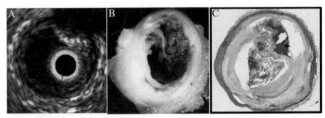

FIGURE 3C-24. Gray-scale IVUS (**A**), tissue sample (**B**) and histology (**C**) illustrating acute rupture of a fibroatheroma. Images courtesy of Dr. R. Virmani.

VH-IVUS and the Location of Plaque Growth

Most of the lesions responsible for acute occlusions are located in the proximal third of the LAD and LCX and in the proximal and mid part of the RCA.[87] There is also a strong body of evidence that the growth of fibroatheromatous plaque is related to the level of shear stress.[88] Normal shear stress is vasculoprotective, whereas low shear stress is atherogenic and high shear stress is thrombogenic.[89] As the plaque grows, the region of the vessel enlarges and becomes positively remodeled (the so-called Glagowian effect).[90] Positive remodeling is typically related to fibroatheromas, TCFA, acute plaque ruptures, plaque hemorrhage, and healed plaque ruptures.[91] As the plaque begins to compromise the lumen, the shear stress conditions change, and at high shear stress the plaque becomes thrombogenic. Erosive, thrombogenic lesions without plaque rupture are typically negatively remodeled and composed mainly of fibrous tissue.[91]

Supporting the previous literature, VH-IVUS has shown in vivo that ID-TCFA plaques are typically located at the proximal part of the coronary tree[92] and that positive remodeling is strongly associated with fibroatheromas and TCFA.[93] In addition, regions of the coronary tree or "coronary river," known typically as low shear stress areas, have been shown by VH-IVUS to have significantly more necrotic core (red color on VH-IVUS). Such regions are typically the inner curvature of nonbranching artery segments and across the flow divider at bifurcations (Fig. 3C-23).[88,94] In addition, these areas have larger plaque burden, more eccentric plaques, higher maximum plaque thickness, and more calcium (white color on VH-IVUS).[94]

VH-IVUS and the Role of Thrombus in Plaque Progression and Sudden Coronary Death

Intravascular thrombosis is due to plaque rupture, dissection, fissure, or plaque erosion. It is typically the final cause of cerebral and myocardial infarcts and rapid plaque progression.[81] After a plaque rupture, the organization of both intramural hemorrhage and intraluminal thrombus can lead to a higher plaque burden as seen before the rupture (Fig. 3C-24).

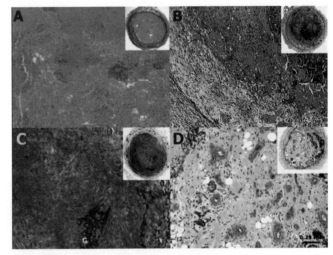

FIGURE 3C-25. Organization of intraluminal thrombus from histology sections of thrombotic rabbit carotid arteries. **A:** Acute thrombus (≤6 hours). Red blood cell rich thrombus with platelets, inflammatory cells, and fibrin meshes. **B:** One-week-old thrombus. Beginning of organization, with neointimal proliferation, showing a mixture of fibrin and collagen fibers. **C:** Six-week-old thrombus. Dense fibrocellular matrix with myointimal cells and elastic fibril dissolution. **D:** Eight-week-old thrombus. Revascularization of the thrombus with extensive macrovascular proliferation and adipocytes (Sirol M, Fuster V, Badimon JJ, et al. Chronic thrombus detection with in vivo magnetic resonance imaging and a fibrin-targeted contrast agent. *Circulation.* 2005;112:1594-1600).

Furthermore, this can be angiographically silent because of positive remodeling.

Intraluminal thrombus becomes mainly fibrous tissue as it organizes (Fig. 3C-25),[95] whereas intraluminal hemorrhage serves as a nidus for another fibroatheroma and later on, through proteolysis, leads to tissue calcification. Seventy-five percent of plaques that cause a sudden coronary death have ruptured at the site of the same plaque more than two times, and 50% of plaques have ruptured at the same site more than three times (Fig. 3C-26).[86]

With VH-IVUS, the layers of fibroatheroma with or without calcium can be seen as layers of necrotic core (red) mixed with calcium (white). Typically a fibrous/fibrofatty layer is seen between the necrotic-core layers. Figure 3C-27 displays an overview of plaque progression with VH-IVUS, based on our understanding from postmortem data.

VH-IVUS is currently used as a primary end point in several clinical trials to improve our understanding of plaque progression and the features of high-risk plaques prone to rupture. These studies combine and compare data from VH-IVUS images with multiple risk factors and blood-borne markers in order to maximize our ability to identify the factors or a combination of factors that most often lead to another coronary or cerebral event in the future. In addition, VH-IVUS makes it possible to

study the effect of systemic therapy on plaque composition. The first results of ongoing clinical trials are expected in 1 to 2 years.

Detection of Vulnerable Plaques

A recent study by Glasser et al. determined that as many as 5.8% of PCI patients will undergo nonculprit lesion progression requiring further PCI on the nontarget lesion within the first year after the initial procedure, indicating new lesion instability.[96] Hence, potentially unstable but nonculprit lesions should also be identified and treated during initial PCI or with more efficient systemic therapy to prevent future events. The lesions that harbor these plaques are frequently only mildly stenotic on angiographic examination. Identification of plaques that have a high likelihood of causing clinical events will undoubtedly create new opportunities for treatment before the onset of acute ischemic syndromes. Systemic stabilization of arteries is increasingly becoming the theme in interventions even for patients with acute myocardial infarction,[97] and VH-IVUS allows assessment of the disease in the entire artery with volumetric data of the individual plaque components. This unique facet could also enable plaque regression or progression studies and facilitate the evaluation of systemic therapies.

The identification of the at-risk noncritical lesions is dependent on the interpretation of each VH-IVUS image. The current perspective of experts on vulnerable plaques suggests that plaques prone to rupture are not the only vulnerable plaques.[98] These could vary in description and be identified as the typical large lipid-necrotic core and thin fibrous cap, or the subocclusive thrombus with early organization, or the proteoglycan matrix in smooth muscle cell-rich plaque, or intraplaque hemorrhage, or the calcified nodule close to the lumen, and finally the chronically stenotic plaque with dense calcium, organized thrombus, and an eccentric lumen.[98] All of these plaque types can be recognized by an interventional

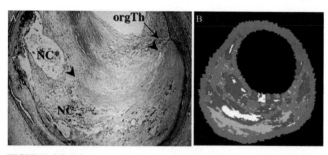

FIGURE 3C-26. **A:** Histopathology of a lesion with multiple previous rupture sites (Virmani R, Kolodgie FD, Burke AP, et al. Lessons from sudden coronary death: a comprehensive morphological classification scheme for atherosclerotic lesions. *Arterioscler Thromb Vasc Biol.* 2000;20:1262–1275). **B:** VH-IVUS with several layers of calcified necrotic core. (*Dark green*) fibrous tissue; (*light green*) fibrofatty; (*red*) necrotic core; (*white*) dense calcium.

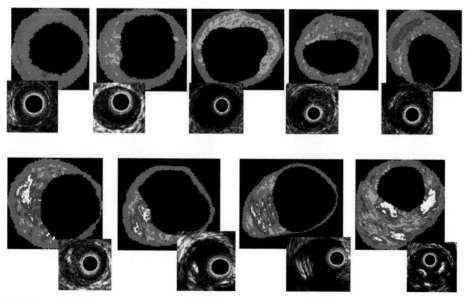

FIGURE 3C-27. Overview of plaque progression. An understanding through VH-IVUS images. (*Dark green*) fibrous tissue; (*light green*) fibrofatty; (*red*) necrotic core; (*white*) dense calcium. (See Color Fig. 3C-27.)

cardiologist viewing VH-IVUS images with the four plaque components and their relevant location within the plaques (an exception is the detection of early or organizing thrombus, which is currently excluded). The foregoing definition of VH-IVUS images based on plaque classification can further aid in this diagnosis.

The VH-IVUS system also has the ability to provide volumetric plaque composition (Fig. 3C-11). Increasing evidence has shown that positive remodeling and plaque composition are two factors related to the likelihood of acute coronary syndromes,[79] both of which can be detected by the VH-IVUS software. Also, ex vivo studies on human coronary arteries have demonstrated that positively remodeled plaques have greater lipid content, inflammation, and macrophage count than plaques that do not exhibit positive remodeling.[99] Hence, the analysis of three-dimensional plaque composition and geometry has the unique potential for identification of vulnerable plaques. Further, these tools could help elucidate relationship of plaque vulnerability with geometry in vivo, potentially providing insights into plaque rupture that were previously unavailable, in addition to the potential usage in the clinical monitoring of plaque burden over time.

Current Limitations

The window size currently applied for selection of ROIs and eventual color tissue map or VH-IVUS image reconstructions is approximately 246 μm in the axial direction. Therefore, detection of a thin fibrous cap <65 μm in thickness[86,100] is below the resolution of IVUS, and detection by VH-IVUS is compromised. This may restrict the identification of some vulnerable atheromas. However, the predictive accuracy of detecting necrotic core is 86% to 94%,[36,85] which bodes well for detection of TCFA since its definition includes a necrotic core >40% of the total plaque volume in addition to the thin fibrous cap.[100] Efforts are underway to improve this and make full use of resolutions possible with commercially available IVUS systems (100 to 150 μm) by advanced mathematical techniques. Similarly, in vessel-wall sections with a low extent of disease, plaque classification depends on analysis of backscatter data spanning <246 μm and could cause minor errors in the predictions. However, results from a recent study by Rodriguez-Granillo et al. are encouraging where TCFAs identified with VH-IVUS were well correlated to positive remodeling.[93] Another limitation of the current VH-IVUS algorithm is the lack of identification of early or organized thrombus, which also limits the recognition of certain at-risk plaques. However, the high accuracy observed with VH-IVUS with the four plaque components has established the value of spectral analysis and statistical classification trees. Endeavors are being made to study thrombus formation for subsequent inclusion in the VH-IVUS family of plaque components. Also, the previous sections aid in understanding plaque progression, vulnerability index, and appearance of thrombus in current VH-IVUS images given the foregoing limitations.

FUTURE OF INTRAVASCULAR ULTRASOUND

The role of gray-scale IVUS is well established in the catheterization laboratories and clinical research studies conducted in the past 15 years. IVUS is a powerful tool that aids in real-time assessment of target lesions. However, because of current limitations of resolution with commercially available IVUS systems, its usage is somewhat restricted due to difficulty in interpretation of gray-scale images. The color-coded VH-IVUS could provide additional information based on the foregoing plaque classification system and, with improvements, could also help identify thrombus and nature of in-stent restenosis. In addition, IVUS could provide increased knowledge of plaques in combination to other emerging catheter-based techniques. Optical coherence tomography (OCT), thermography, and near-infrared spectroscopy are all emerging intravascular technologies that are catheter based and may or may not require physical contact with the plaque surface to acquire information. A study by Yabushita et al. has demonstrated results with OCT for characterizing atherosclerosis with high resolution.[101] However, because of a number of drawbacks, this technique is currently limited to ex vivo studies. The most detrimental of these drawbacks are the impermeability through blood and the lower depth of penetration through plaque not allowing a full view of the artery wall (when the extent of stenosis is >500 to 600 μm, very common with atheromas). Thermography aims at identifying "hot" plaques that are indicative of plaque vulnerability.[102,103] Both OCT and thermography are not yet available in the clinical setting but are promising, especially since OCT can attain a high axial resolution of about 10 μm.[101,104,105] Similarly, near-infrared spectroscopy is in the embryonic stages of development. It provides information on tissue chemical composition and can thus be used to detect vulnerable plaques.[106,107] However, near-infrared spectroscopy has to be combined with another imaging technique to first detect the plaque. Furthermore, the catheter has to be in contact with the tissue, which could lead to complications, particularly if the plaque is unstable with a thin fibrous cap. A combination catheter, for example of IVUS and OCT, would thus provide sufficient additional data to cardiologists for accurately identifying plaque prone to rupture and the thin fibrous cap. In addition to combining different imaging modalities with IVUS, adding functionality to the IVUS catheter could also increase and improve the usage of this important technology. For example, a catheter that could assist in balloon deployment with simultaneous imaging would be a valuable tool for an interventional cardiologist. Finally, future improvements to the VH-IVUS algorithm will also improve and increase the utility of IVUS:

- Very good frequency resolution is attained with AR spectral analysis. However, this might result in poor distance or time-domain information in the tissue characterization outcomes. Hence, a joint time-frequency approach, such as wavelet analysis, could provide a detailed investigation of IVUS backscatter signals.
- Another technique that could be investigated is the calculation of spatial impedance profiles, which has been shown in non-IVUS applications to significantly increase spatial resolution.[108] Previous research using B-mode ultrasound for the determination of plaque composition was limited by low-frequency transducers, availability of fresh tissue, and inefficient ultrasound-histological correlation.[108,109] Despite these limitations, Tobocman et al. reported encouraging results for the determination of aortic plaque

composition. With a 4-MHz transducer, they achieved resolution comparable to that of a 30-MHz catheter using the plane-wave Born approximation.

- Further development of the VH-IVUS algorithm to include effects of blood scatter at various frequencies and the angle of incidence of the IVUS catheter to the vessel wall would also enhance the images in addition to inclusion of fresh or organized thrombus detection.

With constant improvement in IVUS clinical systems, and development of some of the techniques mentioned earlier, a clinical system adjunct to current VH-IVUS software can be envisioned that performs real-time plaque characterization and aids in PCI as well as detection of rupture-prone plaques. These improvements will add to the utility of VH-IVUS, which is already a plaque characterization technique that provides accurate panarterial information on atherosclerosis. It has considerable potential for assessment of plaque vulnerability by interrogating the entire length of the artery. It can assist in stent deployment, and evaluation of systemic therapies, and it can provide crucial information on target lesions in real time. This technique finally enables prospective patient outcome studies, thus far impossible because of the lack of commercially available plaque characterization techniques.

REFERENCES

1. Nissen SE, Yock P. Intravascular ultrasound: novel pathophysiological insights and current clinical applications. *Circulation.* 2001;103:604-616.
2. Morse PM, Ingard KU. *Theoretical Acoustics.* Princeton, NJ: Princeton University Press, 1968.
3. Kino GS. *Acoustic Waves: Devices, Imaging, and Analog Signal Processing.* Englewood Cliffs, NJ: Prentice-Hall, 1987.
4. Shung KK, Thieme GA. Chapters 1–3. In: Shung KK, Thieme GA, eds. *Ultrasonic Scattering in Biological Tissues.* Boca Raton, FL: CRC Press, 1993.
5. Lyons ME, Parker KJ. Absorption and attenuation in soft tissues ii—experimental results. *IEEE Transact Ultrason Ferroelect Freq Control.* 1988;35:511–521.
6. Picano E, Landini L, Distante A, et al. Angle dependence of ultrasonic backscatter in arterial tissues: A study in vitro. *Circulation.* 1985;72:572–576.
7. Hiro T, Leung CY, Karimi H, et al. Angle dependence of intravascular ultrasound imaging and its feasibility in tissue characterization of human atherosclerotic tissue. *Am Heart J.* 1999;137:476–481.
8. Senapati N, Lele PP, Woodin A. A study of the scattering of sub-millimeter ultrasound from tissue and organs. *IEEE Ultrason Symp Proc.* 1972;59–63.
9. Pauly H, Schwan HP. Mechanism of absorption of ultrasound in liver tissue. *J Acoust Soc Am.* 1970;50:692–699.
10. Goss SA, Johnston RL, Dunn F. Compilation of empirical ultrasonic properties of mammalian tissues ii. *J Acoust Soc Am.* 1980;68:93–108.
11. Lockwood GR, Ryan LK, Hunt JW, et al. Measurement of the ultrasonic properties of vascular tissues and blood from 35–65 MHz. *Ultrasound Med Biol.* 1991;17:653–666.
12. Saijo Y, Hidehiko S, Okawai H, et al. Acoustic properties of atherosclerosis of human aorta obtained with high-frequency ultrasound. *Ultrasound Med Biol.* 1998;24:1061–1064.
13. Bridal SL, Fornes P, Bruneval P, et al. Parametric (integrated backscatter and attenuation) images constructed using backscattered radio frequency signals (25–56 MHz) from human aortae in vitro. *Ultrasound Med Biol.* 1997;23:215–229.
14. Teh B-G, Cloutier G. Modeling and analysis of ultrasound backscattering by spherical aggregates and rouleaux of red blood cells. *IEEE Transact Ultrason Ferroelect Freq Control.* 2000;47:1025–1035.
15. Bridal SL, Fornes P, Bruneval P, et al. Correlation of ultrasonic attenuation (30 to 50 MHz) and constituents of atherosclerotic plaque. *Ultrasound Med Biol.* 1997;23:691–703.
16. Lizzi FL, Rorke MC, King DL, et al. Simulation studies of ultrasonic backscattering and b-mode images of liver using acoustic microscopy data. *IEEE Transact Ultrason Ferroelect Freq Control.* 1992;39:212–226.
17. Nissen SE, Gurley JC, Grines CL, et al. Intravascular ultrasound assessment of lumen size and wall morphology in normal subjects and patients with coronary artery disease. *Circulation.* 1991;84:1087–1099.
18. Cavaye DM, White RA, Kopchok GE, et al. Three-dimensional intravascular ultrasound imaging of normal and diseased canine and human arteries. *J Vasc Surg.* 1992;16:509–517; discussion 518–509.
19. De Scheerder I, De Man F, Herregods MC, et al. The use of intracoronary ultrasound for quantitative assessment of coronary artery lumen diameter and for on-line evaluation of angioplasty results. *Acta Cardiol.* 1993;48:171–181.

20. Stahr P, Honda Y, Fitzgerald PJ, et al. Coronary intravascular ultrasonography. In: Lanzer P, Topol EJ, eds. *Pan Vascular Medicine: Integrated Clinical Management.* Berlin: Springer Verlag, 2002:667–677.
21. Foster FS, Knapik DA, Machado JC, et al. High-frequency intracoronary ultrasound imaging. *Semin Intervent Cardiol.* 1997;2:33–41.
22. Teo TJ. High frequency IVUS. In: Saijo Y, Van der Steen AFW, eds. *Vascular Ultrasound.* Tokyo: Springer-Verlag, 2003:66–78.
23. Cavaye DM, Tabbara MR, Kopchok GE, et al. Three dimensional vascular ultrasound imaging. *Am Surg.* 1991;57:751–755.
24. Siegel RJ, Ariani M, Fishbein MC, et al. Histopathologic validation of angioscopy and intravascular ultrasound. *Circulation.* 1991;84:109–117.
25. Gussenhoven EJ, Frietman PA, The SH, et al. Assessment of medial thinning in atherosclerosis by intravascular ultrasound. *Am J Cardiol.* 1991;68:1625–1632.
26. Yoshida K, Yoshikawa J, Akasaka T, et al. Intravascular ultrasound imaging—in vitro and vivo validation. *Jpn Circ J.* 1992;56:572–577.
27. Ng KH, Evans JL, Vonesh MJ, et al. Arterial imaging with a new forward-viewing intravascular ultrasound catheter, ii. Three-dimensional reconstruction and display of data. *Circulation.* 1994;89:718–723.
28. Hodgson J, Reddy K, Suneja R, et al. Intracoronary ultrasound imaging: correlation of plaque morphology with angiography, clinical syndrome and procedural results in patients undergoing coronary angioplasty. *J Am Coll Cardiol.* 1993;21:35–44.
29. Mintz GS, Kent KM, Pichard AD, et al. Contribution of inadequate arterial remodeling to the development of focal coronary artery stenoses. An intravascular ultrasound study [see comments]. *Circulation.* 1997;95:1791–1798.
30. Tuzcu EM, Kapadia SR, Tutar E, et al. High prevalence of coronary atherosclerosis in asymptomatic teenagers and young adults: evidence from intravascular ultrasound. *Circulation.* 2001;103:2705–2710.
31. Serruys PW, Degertekin M, Tanabe K, et al. Intravascular ultrasound findings in the multicenter, randomized, double-blind ravel (randomized study with the sirolimus-eluting velocity balloon-expandable stent in the treatment of patients with de novo native coronary artery lesions) trial. *Circulation.* 2002;106:798–803.
32. Wilson L, Neale M. Characterization of arterial plaque using intravascular ultrasound: in vitro and in vivo results. *Int J Imaging Syst Technol.* 1997;8:52–60.
33. Moore MP, Spencer T, Salter DM, et al. Characterization of coronary atherosclerotic morphology by spectral analysis of radiofrequency signal: in vitro intravascular ultrasound study with histological and radiological validation. *Heart.* 1998;79:459–467.
34. Watson RJ, McLean CC, Moore MP, et al. Classification of arterial plaque by spectral analysis of in vitro radio frequency intravascular ultrasound data. *Ultrasound Med Biol.* 2000;26:73–80.
35. de Korte CL, Pasterkamp G, van der Steen AF, et al. Characterization of plaque components with intravascular ultrasound elastography in human femoral and coronary arteries in vitro. *Circulation.* 2000;102:617–623.
36. Nair A, Kuban BD, Tuzcu EM, et al. Coronary plaque classification using intravascular ultrasound radiofrequency data analysis. *Circulation.* 2002;106:2200–2206.
37. Sonka M, Liang W, Zhang X, et al. Three-dimensional automated segmentation of coronary wall and plaque from intravascular ultrasound pullback sequences. *Comput Cardiol.* 1995;637–640.
38. von Birgelen C, de Vrey EA, Mintz GS, et al. ECG-gated three-dimensional intravascular ultrasound: feasibility and reproducibility of the automated analysis of coronary lumen and atherosclerotic plaque dimensions in humans. *Circulation.* 1997;96:2944–2952.
39. Klingensmith JD, Schoenhagen P, Tajaddini A, et al. Automated three-dimensional assessment of coronary artery anatomy using intravascular ultrasound [review]. *Am Heart J.* 2003;145:795–805.
40. Humphrey JD. Mechanics of the arterial wall: review and directions. *Crit Rev Biomed Eng.* 1995;23:1–162.
41. Tajaddini A, Kilpatrick DL, Schoenhagen P, et al. Impact of age and hyperglycemia on the mechanical behavior of intact human coronary arteries: an ex vivo intravascular ultrasound study. *Am J Physiol Heart Circ Physiol.* 2005;288:H250–H255.
42. Potkin BN, Bartorelli AL, Gessert JM, et al. Coronary artery imaging with intravascular high-frequency ultrasound. *Circulation.* 1990;81:1575–1585.
43. Gussenhoven EJ, Essed CE, Frietman P, et al. Intravascular ultrasonic imaging: Histologic and echographic correlation. *Eur J Vasc Surg.* 1989;3:571–576.
44. Mallery JA, Tobis JM, Griffith J, et al. Assessment of normal and atherosclerotic arterial wall thickness with an intravascular ultrasound imaging catheter. *Am Heart J.* 1990;119:1392–1400.
45. Di Mario C, The SH, Madretsma S, et al. Detection and characterization of vascular lesions by intravascular ultrasound: an in vitro study correlated with histology. *J Am Soc Echocardiogr.* 1992;5:135–146.
46. Zhang X, McKay C, Sonka M. Tissue characterization in intravascular ultrasound images. *IEEE Trans Med Imaging.* 1998;17:889–899.
47. Zhang XM, DeJong SC, McKay CR, et al. Automated characterization of plaque composition from intravascular ultrasound images. Proceedings of Computers in Cardiology, 1996;649–652.
48. Dixon KJ, Vince DG, Cothren RM, et al. Characterization of coronary plaque in intravascular ultrasound using histological correlation. *Annu Int Conf IEEE Eng Med Biol Proc.* 1997;2:530–533.
49. Vince DG, Dixon KJ, Cothren RM, et al. Comparison of texture analysis methods for the characterization of coronary plaques in intravascular ultrasound images. *Comp Med Imaging Graphics.* 2000;24:221–229.
50. Wilson LS, Neale ML, Talhami HE, et al. Preliminary results from attenuation-slope mapping of plaque using intravascular ultrasound. *Ultrasound Med Biol.* 1994;20:529–542.
51. Spencer T, Ramo MP, Salter DM, et al. Characterization of atherosclerotic plaque by spectral analysis of intravascular ultrasound: an in vitro methodology. *Ultrasound Med Biol.* 1997;23:191–203.

52. Nair A, Kuban BD, Obuchowski N, et al. Assessing spectral algorithms to predict atherosclerotic plaque composition with normalized and raw intravascular ultrasound data. *Ultrasound Med Biol.* 2001;27:1319–1331.

53. Lee DJ, Sigel B, Swami VK, et al. Determination of carotid plaque risk by ultrasonic tissue characterization. *Ultrasound Med Biol.* 1998;24:1291–1299.

54. Jeremias A, Kolz ML, Ikonen TS, et al. Feasibility of in vivo intravascular ultrasound tissue characterization in the detection of early vascular transplant rejection. *Circulation.* 1999;100:2127–2130.

55. Welch PD. The use of fast Fourier transform for the estimation of power spectra: a method based on time averaging over short, modified periodograms. *IEEE Trans Audio Electroacoust.* 1967;15:70–73.

56. Marple SL, Jr. *Digital Spectral Analysis with Applications.* Englewood Cliffs, NJ: Prentice-Hall, 1987.

57. Wear KA, Wagner RF, Garra BS. Comparison of autoregressive spectral estimation algorithms and order determination methods in ultrasonic tissue characterization. *IEEE Transact Ultrason Ferroelect Freq Control.* 1995;42:709–716.

58. Wear KA, Wagner RF, Garra BS. High-resolution ultrasonic backscatter coefficient estimation based on autoregressive spectral estimation using burg algorithm. *IEEE Trans Med Imaging.* 1994;13:500–507.

59. Baldeweck T, Laugier P, Herment A, et al. Application of autoregressive spectral analysis for ultrasound attenuation estimation: interest in highly attenuating medium. *IEEE Transact Ultrason Ferroelect Freq Control.* 1995;42:99–110.

60. Mimbs JW, Bauwens D, Cohen RD, et al. Effects of myocardial ischemia on quantitative ultrasonic backscatter and identification of responsible determinants. *Circ Res.* 1981;49:89–96.

61. O'Donnell M, Miller JG. Quantitative broad-band ultrasonic backscatter—an approach to non-destructive evaluation in acoustically inhomogeneous materials. *J Appl Phys.* 1981;52:1056–1065.

62. Lizzi FL, Greenebaum M, Feleppa EJ, et al. Theoretical framework for spectrum analysis in ultrasonic tissue characterization. *J Acoust Soc Am.* 1983;73:1366–1373.

63. Lizzi FL, Ostromogilsky M, Feleppa EJ, et al. Relationship of ultrasonic spectral parameters to features of tissue microstructure. *IEEE Transact Ultrason Ferroelect Freq Control.* 1987;33:319–328.

64. van der Steen AFW, Thijssen JM, van der Laak AWM, et al. Correlation of histology and acoustic parameters of liver tissue on a microscopic scale. *Ultrasound Med Biol.* 1994;20:177–186.

65. Lizzi FL, Astor M, Feleppa EJ, et al. Statistical framework for ultrasonic spectral parameter imaging. *Ultrasound Med Biol.* 1997;23:1371–1382.

66. Thomas LJI, Barzilai B, Perez JE, et al. Quantitative real-time imaging of myocardium based on ultrasonic integrated backscatter. *IEEE Transact Ultrason Ferroelect Freq Control.* 1989;36:466–470.

67. Nair A, Calvetti D, Vince DG. Regularized autoregressive analysis of intravascular ultrasound backscatter: Improvement in spatial accuracy of tissue maps. *IEEE Transact Ultrason Ferroelect Freq Control.* 2004a51:420–431.

68. Mola F, Siciliano R. A fast splitting procedure for classification trees. *Stat Comput.* 1997;7:209–216.

69. Breiman L, Friedman JH, Olshen RA, et al. Classification and regression trees. New York, NY: Chapman and Hall/ CRC, 1993.

70. Metz CE. Basic principles of roc analysis. Seminars in Nuclear Medicine 1978;VIII:283–298.

71. Nair A, Calvetti D, Kuban BD, et al. Novel technique for normalization of intravascular ultrasound backscatter data: Toward automated and real-time plaque characterization. *Am J Cardiol. Suppl. S* 2004;94:123E.

72. Klingensmith JD, Nair A, Kuban BD, et al. Volumetric coronary plaque composition using intravascular ultrasound: Three-dimensional segmentation and spectral analysis. *Proc Comput Cardiol.* 2002;29:113–116.

73. Klingensmith J, Vince D, Kuban B, et al. Assessment of coronary compensatory enlargement by three-dimensional intravascular ultrasound. *Int J Cardiac Imaging.* 2000;16:87–98.

74. Klingensmith JD, Tuzcu EM, Nissen SE, et al. Validation of an automated system for luminal and medial-adventitial border detection in three-dimensional intravascular ultrasound. *Int J Cardiovasc Imaging.* 2003;19:93–104.

75. Gussenhoven EJ, Essed CE, Lancee CT, et al. Arterial wall characteristics determined by intravascular ultrasound imaging: an in vitro study. *J Am Coll Cardiol.* 1989;14:947–952.

76. Mintz GS, Painter JA, Pichard AD, et al. Atherosclerosis in angiographically "Normal" Coronary artery reference segments: an intravascular ultrasound study with clinical correlations. *J Am Coll Cardiol.* 1995;25:1479–1485.

77. Ligthart J, de Feyter PJ. Intra-coronary ultrasound to guide percutaneous coronary intervention. In: Saijo Y, Van der Steen AFW, eds. *Vascular Ultrasound.* Tokyo: Springer-Verlag, 2003:184–198.

78. Mintz GS, Nissen SE, Anderson WD, et al. American College of Cardiology clinical expert consensus document on standards for acquisition, measurement and reporting of intravascular ultrasound studies (IVUS). A report of the American College of Cardiology task force on clinical expert consensus documents. *J Am Coll Cardiol.* 2001;37:1478–1492.

79. Schoenhagen P, Ziada KM, Kapadia SR, et al. Extent and direction of arterial remodeling in stable versus unstable coronary syndromes. *Circulation.* 2000;101:598–603.

80. Schoenhagen P, Ziada KM, Vince DG, et al. Arterial remodeling and coronary artery disease. The concept of "dilated" versus "obstructive" coronary atherosclerosis. *J Am Coll Cardiol.* 2001. In press.

81. Yokoya K, Takatsu H, Suzuki T, et al. Process of progression of coronary artery lesions from mild or moderate stenosis to moderate or severe stenosis: a study based on four serial coronary arteriograms per year. *Circulation.* 1999;100:903–909.

82. Schmermund A, Erbel R. Unstable coronary plaque and its relation to coronary calcium. *Circulation.* 2001;104:1682–1687.

83. Fitzgerald PJ, St. Goar FG, Connolly AJ, et al. Intravascular ultrasound imaging of coronary arteries. Is three layers the norm? *Circulation.* 1992;86:154–158.

84. Nair A, Calvetti D, Kuban BD, et al. Intravascular ultrasound plaque characterization: spectral analysis and tissue maps. *J Am Coll Cardiol. Supplement A* 2003;41:59A.

85. Nasu K, Tsuchikane E, Katoh O, et al. Correlation of in vivo intravascular ultrasound radiofrequency data analysis with in vitro histopathology in human coronary atherosclerotic plaques (VH-DCA Japan trial). Paper presented at: European Society of Cardiology Congress; 2005; Stockholm, Sweden. Abstract 3679.

86. Virmani R, Kolodgie FD, Burke AP, et al. Lessons from sudden coronary death: a comprehensive morphological classification scheme for atherosclerotic lesions. *Arterioscler Thromb Vasc Biol.* 2000;20:1262–1275.

87. Wang JC, Normand S-LT, Mauri L, et al. Coronary arterial spatial distribution of acute myocardial infarction occlusions. *Circulation.* 2004;110:278–284.

88. Kimura BJ, Russo RJ, Bhargava V, et al. Atheroma morphology and distribution in proximal left anterior descending coronary artery: in vivo observations. *J Am Coll Cardiol.* 1996;27:825–831.

89. Malek A, Alper S, Izumo S. Hemodynamic shear stress and its role in atherosclerosis. *JAMA* 1999;282:2035–2042.

90. Glagov S, Weisenberg E, Zarins CK, et al. Compensatory enlargement of human atherosclerotic coronary arteries. *New Engl J Med.* 1987;316:1371–1375.

91. Burke AP, Kolodgie FD, Farb A, et al. Morphological predictors of arterial remodeling in coronary atherosclerosis. *Circulation.* 2002;105:297–303.

92. Rodriguez-Granillo GA, Garcia-Garcia HM, Mc Fadden EP, et al. In vivo intravascular ultrasound-derived thin-cap fibroatheroma detection using ultrasound radiofrequency data analysis. *J Am Coll Cardiol.* 2005;46:2038–2042.

93. Rodriguez-Granillo GA, Serruys PW, Garcia-Garcia HM, et al. Coronary artery remodeling is related to plaque composition. *Heart.* 2006;92:388–391.

94. Rodriguez-Granillo G, Garcia-Garcia HM, Wentzel JJ, et al. Plaque composition and its relationship with acknowledged shear stress patterns in coronary arteries. *J Am Coll Cardiol.* 2005. In press.

95. Sirol M, Fuster V, Badimon JJ, et al. Chronic thrombus detection with in vivo magnetic resonance imaging and a fibrin-targeted contrast agent. *Circulation.* 2005;112:1594–1600.

96. Glasser R, Selzer F, Faxon DP, et al. Clinical progression of incidental, asymptomatic lesions discovered during culprit vessel coronary intervention. *Circulation.* 2005;111:143–149.

97. Tanaka A, Shimada K, Sano T, et al. Multiple plaque rupture and C-reactive protein in acute myocardial infarction. *J Am Coll Cardiol.* 2005;45:1594–1599.

98. Naghavi M, Libby P, Falk E, et al. From vulnerable plaque to vulnerable patient: a call for new definitions and risk assessment strategies: part I. *Circulation.* 2003;108:1664–1672.

99. Varnava AM, Mills PG, Davies MJ. Relationship between coronary artery remodeling and plaque vulnerability. *Circulation.* 2002;105:939–943.

100. Kolodgie FD, Burke AP, Farb A, et al. The thin-cap fibroatheroma: a type of vulnerable plaque: the major precursor lesion to acute coronary syndromes. *Curr Opin Cardiol.* 2001;16:285–292.

101. Yabushita H, Bouma BE, Houser SL, et al. Characterization of human atherosclerosis by optical coherence tomography. *Circulation.* 2002;106:1640–1645.

102. David M, Hathorn B, McAllister HAH, et al. Atherosclerotic plaque thermography—a new approach to the diagnosis of unstable plaques. *Circulation.* 1996;94:4154.

103. Naghavi M, Siadaty S, Willerson JT, et al. Thermosensor catheter: a nitinol shape memory basket catheter to measure temperature of vessel wall with continuous blood flow. *Am J Cardiol.* 1999;84:94P.

104. Brezinski ME, Tearney GJ, Weissman NJ, et al. Assessing atherosclerotic plaque morphology: comparison of optical coherence tomography and high frequency intravascular ultrasound. *Heart.* 1997;77:397–403.

105. Fujimoto JG, Boppart SA, Tearney GJ, et al. High resolution in vivo intra-arterial imaging with optical coherence tomography. *Heart.* 1999;82:128–133.

106. Moreno PR, Lodder RA, Purushothaman KR, et al. Detection of lipid pool, thin fibrous cap, and inflammatory cells in human aortic atherosclerotic plaques by near-infrared spectroscopy. *Circulation.* 2002;105:923–927.

107. Wang J, Geng Y-J, Guo B, et al. Near-infrared spectroscopic characterization of human advanced atherosclerotic plaques. *J Am Coll Cardiol.* 2002;39:1305–1313.

108. Tobocman W, Santosh K, Carter JR, et al. Tissue characterization of arteries with 4 MHz ultrasound. *Ultrasonics.* 1995;33:331–339.

109. Santosh K, Tobocman W, Haacke EM, et al. In vivo biomicroscopy with ultrasound. *Ultrasonics.* 1987;25:274-282.

Wilbert Aarnoudse

Cees-Joost Botman

Nico H.J. Pijls

CHAPTER **3D**

Pressure Wire

For more than 40 years the technique of coronary arteriography has played a pivotal role in the diagnosis and treatment of patients with ischemic heart disease.[1,2] However, coronary arteriography has several well-recognized limitations. A number of studies have reported both severe underestimation and overestimation of stenosis severity as assessed from the angiogram as compared to pathologic findings at autopsy.[3–5] Furthermore, a high intraobserver and interobserver variability has been reported.[6] But, most important, the pathophysiological significance of a stenosis cannot be judged reliably from the angiogram alone, whereas both for quality of life and prognosis of a patient, the functional significance is most important.[7] In this respect it is important to define that a stenosis is called functionally significant, hemodynamically significant, or physiologically significant if it is able to limit maximum achievable blood flow to such a degree that ischemia of the myocardium supplied by that particular stenotic artery can be induced if the patient is sufficiently stressed.

A number of studies confirmed a poor correlation between anatomic estimation of coronary narrowings and physiologic measures of coronary function, especially in ranges of 50% to 90% diameter stenosis.[8] It was shown repeatedly that in patients with angiographically significant coronary disease, outcome was clearly related to the extent of inducible ischemia and not to the anatomic degree of narrowing.[9,10]

In that respect, it is important to realize that the physiological impact of a coronary artery stenosis on blood flow is determined by interaction with several other factors such as aortic pressure, central venous pressure, collateral flow, and resistance and size of the depending myocardial bed.[11,12] To overcome these limitations of coronary arteriography, and to obtain more information on blood flow and to improve clinical decision making, additional techniques have been developed such

as intracoronary Doppler flow velocity measurements and intracoronary pressure measurements.

CONCEPT AND PRACTICAL SETUP

The exercise tolerance of patients with stable coronary artery disease is determined by maximum achievable myocardial blood flow. In the presence of a stenosis, the exercise level at which ischemia will occur is directly related to the maximum coronary blood flow that is still achievable by the stenotic vessel. Therefore, not *resting flow* but only *maximum achievable blood flow* to the myocardium at risk is the best parameter to determine the functional capacity of the patient. Expressing myocardial blood flow in absolute dimensions, however, has some disadvantages because this is dependent on the size of the distribution area, which is unknown, and will differ among patients, vessels, and distribution areas. It is therefore better to express maximum achievable (stenotic) blood flow in relation to normal maximum blood flow. Therefore, the ratio between maximum achievable stenotic blood flow and maximum achievable normal blood flow was introduced, and this index was called fractional flow reserve (FFR).[13–15] Fractional flow reserve is defined as the maximum achievable blood flow to a distribution area in the presence of a stenosis as a ratio to the normal maximum achievable blood flow to that distribution area in the hypothetical situation that the supplying vessel was completely normal. In other words, fractional flow reserve expresses maximal blood flow in the presence of a stenosis as a fraction of normal maximum blood flow. This index is not dependent on resting flow and is therefore not subject to many of the limitations related to the concept of coronary flow reserve.

HOW TO DETERMINE FRACTIONAL FLOW RESERVE

Under circumstances generally present in the coronary catheterization laboratory, it is impossible to determine the ratio of maximum flow in the presence of a stenosis in relation to normal maximum coronary blood flow directly. However, by using a pressure-monitoring guidewire at maximum hyperemia, it is possible to calculate this ratio of flows by a ratio of pressures. This is explained in Figures 3D-1 and 3D-2. Figure 3D-1A represents a normal coronary artery and its dependent myocardium. Suppose that this system is studied at maximum vasodilation. In this situation, myocardial resistance is minimal and constant, and maximum myocardial hyperemia is present, as is the case at maximum exercise. In this situation, as can be seen in Figure 3D-2, the relation between myocardial perfusion pressure and myocardial flow is linearly proportional, and a change in myocardial perfusion pressure results in a proportional change in myocardial flow. In the case of a normal coronary artery (Fig. 3D-1A), the epicardial artery does not have any resistance to flow, and the pressure in the distal coronary artery is equal to aortic pressure. In the example, therefore, myocardial perfusion pressure (defined as distal coronary pressure P_d minus venous pressure P_v) equals 100 mm Hg. In case of a stenosis, however (Fig. 3D-1B), because of this stenosis there will be resistance to blood flow, and distal coronary pressure will be lower than aortic pressure: a pressure gradient

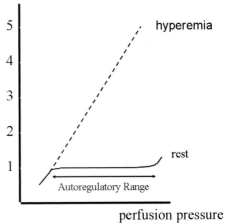

Pressure-flow relation at rest and during hyperemia

FIGURE 3D-2. As opposed to the resting situation, at maximum hyperemia, myocardial perfusion pressure is linearly proportional to myocardial flow.

across the stenosis exists (in the example $P_a - P_d = 30$ mm Hg) and myocardial perfusion pressure will be diminished (in the example $P_d - P_v = 70$ mm Hg). In the example, therefore (Fig. 3D-1B), myocardial perfusion pressure has decreased to 70 mm Hg. Because during maximum hyperemia, myocardial perfusion pressure is directly proportional to myocardial flow, the ratio of maximum stenotic and normal maximum flow can be expressed as the ratio of distal coronary pressure and aortic pressure at hyperemia.

Therefore,

$$FFR_{myo} = \frac{\text{Maximum myocardial blood flow in the presence of a stenosis}}{\text{Normal maximum myocardial blood flow}}$$

can be expressed as

$$FFR_{myo} = \frac{(P_d - P_v)}{(P_a - P_v)}$$

Because generally, central venous pressure is close to zero, the equation can be further simplified to

$$FFR_{myo} = \frac{P_d}{P_a}$$

As P_a can be measured in a regular way by the coronary or guiding catheter, and P_d is easily obtainable by crossing the stenosis with a sensor-tipped guidewire, it is clear that FFR_{myo} can be simply obtained, both during diagnostic and interventional procedures, by measuring the respective pressures. From the foregoing equations it is also obvious that FFR_{myo} for a normal coronary artery will equal 1.0 (Fig. 3D-3).

Numerous studies have convincingly shown that treating a coronary stenosis in patients with a fractional flow reserve below 0.75 to 0.80 improves functional class and prognosis, whereas treating stenoses above that threshold does not improve prognosis and therefore is not recommended.[15–17] More specifically, FFR <0.75 has 100% specificity for indicating

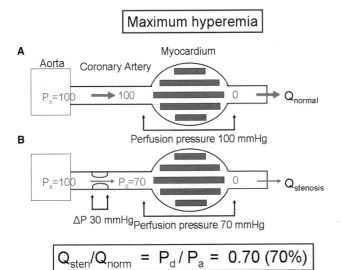

Maximum hyperemia

FIGURE 3D-1. **A:** Schematic representation of a normal coronary artery and its dependent myocardium, studied at hyperemia. In this normal situation, the (conductive) coronary artery gives no resistance to flow, and thus distal coronary pressure is equal to aortic pressure. Assuming that venous pressure is zero, perfusion pressure across the myocardium is 100 mm Hg. **B:** The same coronary artery, now in the presence of a stenosis. In this situation, the stenosis will impede blood flow and thus a pressure gradient across the stenosis will arise ($\Delta P = 30$ mm Hg). Distal coronary pressure is no longer equal to aortic pressure, but will be lower ($P_d = 70$ mm Hg). Consequently, the perfusion pressure across the myocardium will be lower than in the situation that no stenosis was present (perfusion pressure is now $100 - 30 = 70$ mm Hg). Because during maximum hyperemia, myocardial perfusion pressure and myocardial blood flow are linearly proportional (Fig. 3D-2), the ratio of maximum stenotic and normal maximal flow can be expressed as the ratio of distal coronary pressure and aortic pressure at hyperemia: FFR = $P_d/P_a = 70$ mm Hg. Importantly, it is distal coronary pressure at hyperemia that determines myocardial flow, and not the pressure gradient across the stenosis.

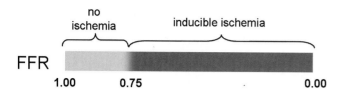

FIGURE 3D-3. Schematic representation of the threshold values of FFR. It has been convincingly shown that if FFR is <0.75, ischemia in this myocardial territory will be inducible, and that in this situation by treating a focal stenosis, the prognosis as well as the complaints of the patient will improve. If FFR is >0.80, on the other hand, it is almost certain that treating an angiographically visible stenosis will not alter the patient's complaints or prognosis. If FFR is in the small "gray zone" between 0.75 and 0.80, close attention should be paid to the individual patient's characteristics (such as site and extent of perfusion abnormalities on noninvasive testing, and typical or atypical complaints) to guide sound clinical decision making.

inducible ischemia,[14,15,17] whereas >FFR 0.80 has a sensitivity of >90% for excluding inducible ischemia.

PRACTICAL SETUP

In practice, to measure coronary pressure in the catheterization laboratory, no major technical adaptations are needed as compared with a regular diagnostic procedure. A regular pressure transducer is necessary for aortic pressure (P_a), recorded through the guiding catheter as usual. Furthermore, a micromanometer-tipped guidewire (PressureWire, Radi Medical Systems, Sweden) is needed. This is a 0.014-in. floppy guidewire with a micromanometer at 3 cm from its floppy tip (at the junction of the radiopaque distal tip and the radiolucent part of the wire), so that the sensor can be moved back and forth across a stenosis while the tip of the wire remains distal. The wire is connected to an interface with dedicated software for measurements. The handling characteristics of this wire permit its use as a first-line guidewire in case an intervention should be performed. In general, pressure wires can be advanced through 6F diagnostic catheters. However, the use of a 6F (or larger) angioplasty guiding catheter is strongly recommended, because the better inner coating of these catheters allow for better torque control of the wire in the coronary tree. In addition, angioplasty can be performed when indicated by the measurements, without pulling back the wire.

Heparin should be administered according to local routine as during angioplasty. Intracoronary nitrates should always be given before the pressure wire enters the coronary artery. First, the sensor of the wire is positioned at the same location as the tip of the guiding catheter, that is, at the ostium of the coronary artery. At this location, P_a and "P_d" should be equal. If a slight drift is present, the signals are electronically equalized. Next, the pressure guidewire is positioned with the sensor distal to the stenosis (and ideally as far distal in the vessel as possible),

and hyperemia is induced. As hyperemic stimulus, we prefer adenosine as a continuous infusion through a central venous line, because it causes true and sustained hyperemia. For dosages of adenosine and alternative hyperemic stimuli, see the later section "Important Considerations." Before administering IV adenosine, the patient should be informed and reassured regarding side effects: Almost every patient will experience mild chest discomfort or dyspnea during infusion. Other possible side effects are a mild lowering of arterial blood pressure and occasional second-degree heart block.

If steady-state hyperemia is established (usually this occurs within 2 minutes and is obvious from the screen of the analyzer if the P_d/P_a ratio is minimal and constant), FFR is registered, and if necessary, a pull-back maneuver is performed to exactly localize pressure drops.

PITFALLS, LIMITATIONS, AND SAFETY

As with every new technique, the cardiologist starting to perform coronary pressure measurements by wire technology will face some potential pitfalls. Most of these pitfalls are easily recognized; a few are more tricky. However, once having mastered the technique (which will be done easily and rapidly), and having encountered these pitfalls at least once, it is easy to avoid them. Some of these pitfalls and precautions to be taken are discussed here.

Guiding catheters with side holes should be avoided, because the pressure signal recorded through such a catheter does not necessarily correspond to the pressure at its tip, but may be determined in part by aortic pressure (measured through the side holes), leading to erroneous conclusions. Also, an intracoronary hyperemic stimulus cannot be administered through a side-hole catheter. If a side-hole catheter has to be used, the catheter should be slightly pulled back out of the ostium during the measurements (leaving the wire distal to the stenosis), and an intravenous infusion of a hyperemic stimulus is mandatory.

The fluid-filled pressure transducer should be at the correct height. When coronary pressure is measured by a sensor-tipped guidewire, its value is compared to aortic pressure, measured by the fluid-filled guiding catheter. The pressure transducer of this catheter is generally fixed to the table at a height of 5 cm below the sternum, which is estimated to be the location of the aortic root. If the sensor is close to the tip of the guiding catheter, it should be realized that adjusting the height of the pressure transducer will lead to small differences between both signals. If the signals are more than 1 or 2 mm Hg apart, the level of the fluid-filled pressure transducer should be adjusted, to correct this difference. Alternatively, both pressures can be electronically equalized before advancing the pressure wire into the coronary artery.

A reversed or paradoxical gradient can occur if the sensor is advanced distally into a normal coronary artery. In such a case, P_d will exceed P_a by a few millimeters of mercury. This is due to the fact that the atmospheric level of the ascending aorta (where P_a is measured) may be different from that of the distal coronary artery. The opposite can also be the case, but mostly will not be realized as such because the small extra gradient is ascribed to pressure decline along the coronary artery. Generally, these differences are small and do not confound clinical decision making.

Damping of pressure by the guiding catheter sometimes occurs, especially in normal right coronary arteries. The guiding catheter in these situations can be considered as an additional proximal stenosis. This does not preclude accurate calculation of FFR, unless blood pressure in the coronary artery falls below the threshold of the autoregulatory range. Therefore, if significant damping is noted, it is recommended to pull back the guiding catheter during the measurements, leaving the wire distal to the stenosis, and to use an intravenous hyperemic stimulus.

The risk of being below the autoregulatory range can also be present in general when measurements are performed in severely hypotensive patients. Therefore, when P_a has a mean value of <60 mm Hg in the presence of a stenosis, we generally increase mean blood pressure by volume expansion to at least 70 or 80 mm Hg before measuring FFR.

Drift of the pressure signal is minimal with current equipment. It is detected by comparing the pressure recorded by the wire to the pressure recorded by the catheter, after withdrawal of the sensor to the tip of the catheter at the end of the procedure. This emphasizes the critical importance of verifying equal pressures at that location both at the start and at the end of the evert procedure.

Safety of obtaining FFR at a diagnostic procedure is related to the introduction of a floppy guidewire into the coronary artery. It has been repeatedly demonstrated that introduction of such wires can be safely performed by well-trained operators and that the very small risk is counterbalanced by the valuable information obtained in case of ambiguity about the functional significance of a stenosis.[14,15] In interventional procedures, the question is trivial because introduction of a wire into the coronary artery is mandatory in those cases anyway and the technical manipulations are exactly the same as in routine percutaneous transluminal coronary angioplasty.

UTILITY OF CORONARY PRESSURE MEASUREMENT DURING CORONARY INTERVENTIONS

In clear-cut cases of typical chest pain, positive noninvasive testing and single vessel stenosis, it is not necessary to use any physiologic method to justify a coronary intervention. However, complaints of patients are often not very typical, and noninvasive testing is often equivocal or just not performed. Moreover, coronary disease is often diffuse and complex, affecting multiple coronary arteries, and it is often unclear if and to what extent a particular stenosis contributes to ischemia. In such cases, FFR measurements can reliably identify culprit lesions and thus avoid unnecessary interventions that may increase risk without any benefit for the patient. Furthermore, as discussed later, FFR measurements can be used to evaluate the result of an intervention and subsequent prognosis. In almost all specific patient groups, the threshold values just described are universally usable, including in case of multivessel disease and previous myocardial infarction. The only situations where FFR should not be used is in the setting of acute coronary syndromes and severe left ventricular hypertrophy.

In other words, FFR accurately distinguishes which coronary stenoses or segments need to be treated and which do not.

MULTIVESSEL INTERVENTIONS

The majority of patients in the catheterization laboratory have multivessel disease. Several trials, though performed in the pre-DES era, favor CABG over PCI in multivessel coronary artery disease.[18,19] However with the expansion of possibilities in interventional cardiology, such as the evolution of drug-eluting stents with lower restenosis rates, it can be expected that more and more patients will qualify for interventional treatment, and it will become increasingly important to determine which lesions should be stented and which not. It is unwise to implant an undefined number of stents in these patients, for several reasons. First, the advantage of reducing the reintervention rate using drug-eluting stents will disappear with an increasing number and length of implanted stents. The risk of subacute stent thrombosis is 3% to 5% in the first year, and also for that reason, unnecessary stents should be avoided. Second, making a metal cast of a coronary artery will disturb flow, will affect perforating branches, and will have a negative influence on normal physiology. Third, the treatment will become expensive and future bypass surgery becomes very difficult. Moreover, as was demonstrated extensively by several studies, only hemodynamically significant lesions need to be treated, and dilation of functionally nonsignificant lesions should be avoided.[10,16]

It is the presence and extent of inducible ischemia that determines the prognosis in these patients, not the angiographic extent of disease. Therefore, for an optimum benefit from drug-eluting stents in patients with complex disease and multiple abnormalities, it is mandatory to make a strategic selection of those arteries or locations where stenting will be the most effective. This means that detailed spatial, focal, and segmental information about the functional impact of all the abnormalities is required. Coronary pressure measurements give a detailed answer to all these questions. For a typical example of the usefulness of FFR in these patients, see Figure 3D-4.

SEQUENTIAL STENOSIS AND THE PRESSURE PULL-BACK CURVE

A situation that is frequently encountered in the catheterization laboratory is the patient with multiple stenoses within a single vessel. Coronary pressure measurement, and especially the so-called hyperemic pressure pull-back curve, is an elegant and straightforward method to evaluate the individual contribution of each of the multiple stenoses to the extent of disease in the myocardial tissue supplied by that artery.[20,21]

To record a pressure pull-back curve, the pressure wire is positioned distally in the coronary artery. After that, sustained maximum hyperemia is induced (by adenosine in a central vein, 140 µg/kg/min, or papaverine intracoronary bolus in a dose of 15 mg in the RCA or 20 mg in the LAD). After steady-state hyperemia is reached, the sensor is slowly and manually pulled back under fluoroscopy, while the pressure tracing is observed. Studying the pressure tracing makes clear the location of each flow-limiting spot and segment and, moreover, quantifies the extent of ischemia caused by each spot. Providing such detailed spatial resolution is a unique feature of coronary pressure measurements. It should be realized that treating one of a series of stenoses can change the hemodynamic significance of the other stenoses. For a detailed

67 y/o male with stable angina and positive exercise test

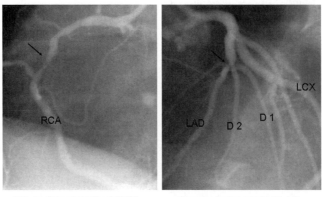

Intermediate stenosis mid RCA   Complex lesion proximal LAD

A

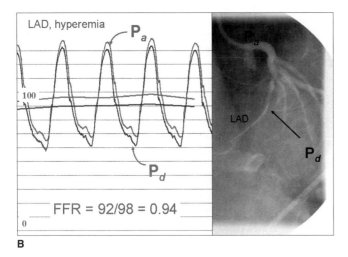

B

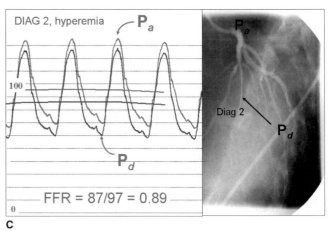

C

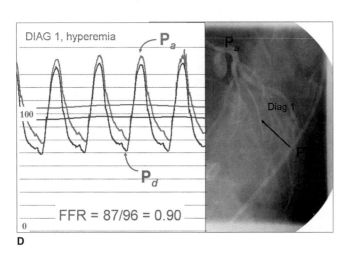

D

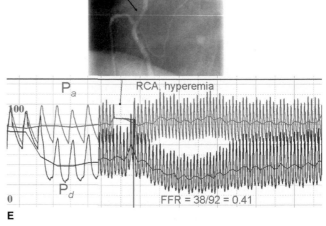

E

FIGURE 3D-4. Example of the usefulness of FFR in a patient with multivessel abnormalities. This 67-year-old patient had typical angina and a positive exercise test. At angiography, a complex lesion at the proximal LAD was found, as well as an intermediate stenosis in the mid-RCA (**A**). To guide clinical decision making, FFR was measured in the LAD and in both diagonals, as well as in the RCA. As the pressure tracings show, the complex and angiographically severe lesion in the proximal LAD (**B**) was not hemodynamically significant, as opposed to the angiographically mild RCA lesion. The RCA lesion was treated percutaneously and thus an unnecessary CABG or hazardous PCI of the LAD was avoided. The patient did well after 4 years of follow-up.

theoretical background, the reader is referred to dedicated papers.[20,21] For practical purposes, however, it is recommended that, after having identified one or several focal pressure drops, the spot with the largest pressure drop should be treated first, after which FFR measurement can be repeated and, if necessary, a second spot with a focal pressure drop can be treated.

It is important that the pressure pull-back curve be made during sustained maximum hyperemia, because pressure drops are easily visible in such a hyperemic state. In the case of diffuse disease or when evaluating stents, the pressure pull-back curve can also be very helpful, as indicated next.

DIFFUSE EPICARDIAL DISEASE

Ischemia in a myocardial territory can be the result of a focal stenosis, and in this case it makes sense to perform PCI. On the other hand, myocardial ischemia can also be the result of a diffusely atherosclerotic coronary artery, without a demonstrable focal lesion. In the case of a diffusely diseased vessel, stenting certain segments or spots will not be beneficial to the patient, unless focal obstruction to flow exists. The pressure pull-back curve is a helpful instrument for assessing the presence and the extent of such diffuse disease. As can be seen in the example in Figure 3D-5, the FFR measured distally in the LAD is 0.71, which means that myocardial ischemia is certainly inducible in this region. When making the hyperemic pull-back curve, it can be clearly seen that the pressure decline in the artery is gradual, and there is no sudden pressure drop corresponding to a focal stenosis. This means that this patient cannot be helped with PCI and should be managed medically. On the other hand, in other patients with similar diffuse disease, coronary pressure measurement may indicate a particular location where a pressure drop occurs. In such cases, stenting the respective spot or segment is recommended.

FRACTIONAL FLOW RESERVE AFTER MYOCARDIAL INFARCTION

It is important to realize that in the acute setting of a myocardial infarction or unstable angina, FFR should not be used for clinical decision making. This is due to the fact that rapidly changing conditions of both the microvasculature (e.g., distal embolization, stunning) and the coronary artery itself may cause dynamically changing physiological conditions, in which, for example, stable and true hyperemia is difficult to obtain. Fortunately, in most acute situations, there is also no need for pressure measurements, because complaints and ECG changes can mostly guide the clinician to make the optimal treatment decisions. However, from 5 days after the acute event, when almost all patients have stabilized, FFR measurement can be very useful. In many cases, patients are then referred to the catheterization laboratory without any functional assessment of residual ischemia, and if one ore more stenoses are seen on angiography, the question arises whether the (residual) stenosis is hemodynamically significant or not. It is important to keep in mind, regarding these decisions, that because of the myocardial infarction, the perfused myocardial territory will be decreased, and a stenosis that was functionally significant beforehand can become insignificant after myocardial infarction, though the anatomical appearance stays exactly the same.

As De Bruyne et al. elegantly showed,[22] in case of a previous myocardial infarction, the threshold value of 0.75 to 0.80 accurately distinguishes patients in which residual ischemia is present and the infarcted area can be expected to be viable, so that PCI

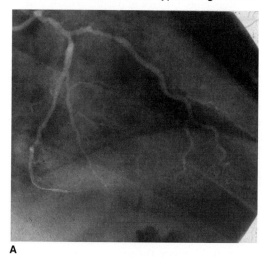

FIGURE 3D-5. Example of the use of FFR and the pressure pull-back curve to demonstrate diffuse disease. **A:** On the angiogram, severe and diffuse atherosclerosis is present. To fully investigate the LAD, the pressure wire was placed distally in the vessel and was manually pulled back towards the guiding catheter under fluoroscopy and steady-state maximum hyperemia. **B:** As can be clearly seen from the pressure tracings, FFR is <0.75, indicating that inducible ischemia is present, and the patient will be likely to have ischemic complaints. However, no local pressure drop exists, but a gradual increase in distal coronary pressure is seen across the full length of the vessel. This implies that a PCI in any segment of the vessel will not be beneficial, and conservative treatment is indicated.

of a residual stenosis will benefit the patient. In that study, the relations among stenosis severity, coronary blood flow, myocardial viability and ischemic threshold were clearly evaluated. Similar notes can be made with respect to unstable angina: The ECG will guide the operator to stent the culprit lesion; the pressure wire can be used for decision making about other lesions.

LEFT MAIN DISEASE

The presence of left main disease has important prognostic and therapeutic implications. Many intermediate left main lesions are discovered "accidentally" in patients who have concomitant peripheral coronary artery disease or in older patients who undergo angiography before major noncardiac surgery. In these patients, noninvasive testing is often inconclusive. Because of the major implications of significant left main disease, definite information regarding the hemodynamic significance of the lesion is mandatory. Therefore, we investigated whether coronary pressure measurements in such patients could be helpful in decision making.[23] In this study, 60 patients were included with an intermediate left main (LM) stenosis of 40% to 60% by visual estimation. If FFR was <0.75, bypass surgery was performed, and if FFR was >0.75, medical treatment was chosen. The conservatively managed group had a favorable outcome, and therefore it can be concluded that in this type of patients, with an intermediate, often "accidentally" discovered left main stenosis, conservative treatment is justified if FFR is >0.75. Several other prospective studies[24] have confirmed that such a policy is accompanied by a good prognosis, also in the long term. Using FFR as a gold standard, Jasti et al.[24] demonstrated a close correlation between certain intravascular ultrasound (IVUS) criteria and FFR <0.75 in determining the hemodynamic significance of an LM stenosis, indicating that both modalities could probably be used. However, IVUS, like angiography, is another "anatomic modality," whereas the advantage of FFR is that it is a "functional/physiological modality" (see the first paragraphs of this chapter).

EVALUATION OF CORONARY INTERVENTIONS

Coronary pressure measurement can be helpful in the evaluation of coronary interventions by analyzing the immediate result after balloon angioplasty or stenting, but has also prognostic importance regarding long-term outcome and restenosis.

Bech et al.[25] have shown that, after plain balloon angioplasty with a good angiographic result, FFR of <0.90 indicates an excellent long-term clinical outcome: The restenosis rate in this group was 16% in contrast to patients with a similar angiographic result but FFR <0.90, in which restenosis rate was 38%. However, in the present era, determining the effect and prognosis after stenting is more important. Using coronary pressure measurements, evidently the FFR poststenting can be determined immediately after stenting, and the gain can be expressed quantitatively (for example, "by placing the stent, FFR was increased from 0.64 to 0.88"). Of course, if there is diffuse disease or multiple stenoses or wall irregularities, FFR after stenting will not become 1.0 as in the ideal situation. The aim of coronary stenting should therefore be at least to normalize the conductance of the stented segment, which means that after optimal stent deployment, no detectable hyperemic gradient across the stent should remain. It has been shown that this correlates very well with optimum stent deployment by IVUS criteria. Using the pressure pull-back curve as described earlier, the pressure gradient across the stent can be easily determined in these situations, and if a significant pressure drop still exists, stent deployment can be optimized. FFR after stenting is strongly inversely correlated with the chance to develop restenosis and the need for repeated revascularization or occurrence of other events during follow-up. In a large multicenter registry,[26] FFR measurement immediately after angiographically successful stent deployment was correlated with major adverse cardiac events and the need for repeated revascularization in the next 6 months. A strong inverse correlation was found: The restenosis rate in the group of patients with FFR between 0.96 and 1.00 was 4%, compared to a restenosis rate of 40% in the group of patients with FFR <0.80. Furthermore, this study indicated that a FFR of >0.90 can be achieved in 75% of patients, and that in such patients the restenosis rate at follow-up and the event and repeated revascularization rate are three to four times lower than in patients with FFR <0.90. Note that the angiographic result of stenting was similar in all patients and could not be used for this type of risk stratification.

COST-EFFECTIVENESS

In case of typical or atypical complaints and one or more coronary artery stenoses of intermediate significance, many physicians will use stress perfusion scintigraphy in conjunction with angiography to facilitate clinical decision making. However, this policy has several disadvantages. It can delay hospital discharge and thereby increase the cost of hospitalization. Also, it will often imply that two catheterizations have to be performed in a short time span: one for diagnosis and one for PCI. Using FFR is a very elegant way to shorten the duration and cost of hospitalization.[27] In a recent study, Leesar et al.[28] demonstrated that in a subset of patients with recent unstable angina or myocardial infarction and an intermediate stenosis and single-vessel disease, measurement of FFR can be safely performed in the same setting as coronary angiography and that this approach shortens the duration of hospitalization significantly (by 77%) compared with stress perfusion scintigraphy, resulting in a decrease in the costs of hospital admission. Measuring FFR was not associated with an increase in procedure time, radiation exposure time, or amount of contrast media used during the procedure. Furthermore, they found no differences with respect to event rates in patients in whom PCI was deferred because the FFR was >0.75 compared with those in whom it was deferred because the perfusion scan was negative for ischemia. The increased costs incurred in the catheterization laboratory because of the use of a pressure guidewire were offset by the reduction in hospitalization costs.

It should be noted that apart from being more cost effective, FFR measurement is also more patient-friendly because of the avoidance of repeated catheterizations and the reduction in hospital stay.

PART 2

PRINCIPLES OF ENDOVASCULAR INTERVENTIONS

Lutz Prechelt
Peter Lanzer

CHAPTER **4**

The Decision-Making Process in Percutaneous Coronary Interventions

INTRODUCTION

As the range and quality of endovascular instruments improve, the industry supplying these tools is increasingly trying to create the impression that percutaneous coronary intervention (PCI) is a simple and straightforward procedure. It is nothing of the sort. In PCI, in fact, an operator performs high-risk procedures under time pressure, with only indirect and incomplete angiographic information about the interventional site, and is constantly trading off one risk against another. Mastering this complex process requires years of experience and an attitude characterized by the constant willingness to learn and reflect when faced with each unexpected development or new situation. Unfortunately, to the best of our knowledge, the complexity of this repetitive and evolving process, consisting of the triad of angiographic imaging, image interpretation, and interventional action, has not yet been fully described. Furthermore, there are no data on the factors determining the decision trade-offs or their relative weights in various common situations. Consequently, physicians learning PCI today need a gifted teacher or have to gain experience the hard way, by trial and error, which exposes patients to avoidable risks and complications. Existing materials on learning PCI (e.g., references 1–4) describe only formal training requirements and the parameters of institutional and operator competence. They provide no help on how to make hard decisions during an intervention.

The purpose of this chapter is to start filling this void by providing an overview of some important basic factors and how they interact. One obviously cannot fully describe the actual decision-making process because, although each component of the triad and the resulting trade-offs are quantitative in principle, most of these quantities cannot be measured in practice. Therefore, only general decision-making rules can be formulated to facilitate the training and clinical experience necessary for becoming a master PCI operator. We hope that this description will help transform a rather vaguely formulated practical exercise into a conscious process of skill acquisition. The goal is to become capable of successfully handling even unexpected and adverse developments in the course of complex interventions.

The following section describes the basic elements of the PCI decision-making process, whereas the process itself is described in subsequent sections. We assume that the reader has a basic understanding of the PCI process and that the elements therefore need little or no description.

INPUT AND OUTPUT VARIABLES

The PCI decision-making process involves a number of input and output variables. The input variables include:

- Interventional scenario
  - Emergency or elective
- General patient status
  - General health

- Cardiac function
- Cardiovascular risk factors (e.g., type II diabetes)
- History of cardiovascular diseases (e.g., coronary bypass surgery)
- Stability (clinical, hemodynamic, electrical)
- Current physician status
  - Rested or exhausted
  - Skilled in handling unexpected developments or overwhelmed by them
  - Stress resistant or low in morale
- Accumulated time and costs
  - Procedure time
  - Radiation exposure
  - Contrast agent dose
  - Monetary costs (physician, staff, equipment, material)
  - Schedule pressure (availability of physician, staff, and laboratory)
- Current interventional status
  - Presence of single/multiple lesions
  - Presence of single/multiple coronary artery diseases
  - Presence of stents or coronary bypasses
  - Target vessel size and status
  - Location, severity, and complexity of the target lesion
  - Status of the antegrade coronary blood flow
  - Amount of dependent myocardium
  - Availability of required instrumentation
  - Status of deployed instrumentation
      - Guiding catheter
      - Guidewire
      - Balloon catheter
      - Stent
      - Pressure/volume sensor
      - Ultrasonic sensor
  - Performance of deployed instrumentation
      - As expected
      - Suboptimum
      - Malfunctioning
      - Tracking, crossing, pushing abilities
  - Uncertainty about the reliability of all of the above information

The output variables in PCI decision making, that is, the potential actions of the operator, include:

- Initial actions
  - Establishing arterial access
  - Placement of the guiding catheter
- Imaging
  - Image acquisition (cine, fluoroscopy) and visualization of the target vessel and lesion
  - Imaging by ultrasonic sensor
  - Review and interpretation of acquired images
- Initial and subsequent interventions
  - Placement of the guidewire
  - Placement and inflation of the balloon catheter
  - Stent deployment
  - Employment of auxiliary techniques (whether diagnostic or revascularization)
  - Removal of equipment and instrumentation
- Auxiliary acts

- Drug administration
- Addressing and responding to staff
- Addressing and responding to the patient
- Termination of the procedure

RISKS AND BENEFITS

The primary categories used to judge the consequences of each subsequent interventional step are those of *benefit* and *risk*. Benefits are what we would like and expect to achieve in both tactical and strategic terms, whereas risks we would rather avoid, but can never be sure of doing so. The benefits we strive for include remedy or palliation of the coronary artery syndrome and an improved prognosis, or at least preparing the ground for later definitive repair. Since most risks and risk considerations are inherent in the PCI procedure itself, they play a prominent part in the entire decision-making process. They are discussed in the following section.

RISK CONSIDERATIONS

The central consideration in the decision-making process during PCI is risk and how to prevent, evaluate, and control it. A thorough understanding of the character and magnitude of the risks and benefits involved in each interventional step is crucial for effective decision making during a PCI.

Risk can be defined qualitatively or quantitatively. Qualitatively, a risk is just any undesirable event that may or may not occur. If it occurs, the risk is said to *materialize*. Quantitatively, risk is the product of the probability of the event and the damage expected if it happens. Here, we are interested in the quantitative understanding of risk: *Risk* is the extent of damage expected in terms of its probability. It is important to note that we may use this notion of risk even if we understand the probability and the size of the damage only vaguely (high uncertainty). In the context of PCI, we clearly cannot express risk as a number, but the notion will still help to distinguish greater risks from lesser ones.

The task of a PCI operator is to identify the course of action with the lowest overall risk and highest benefit for the individual patient.

We distinguish between two very different kinds of risk, namely, latent and actional risk, and two different ways of dealing with each of them. Actional risk is further subdivided to reflect a possible adverse course of PCI (see Fig. 4-1).

LATENT RISK

Latent risk is risk that is already inherent in the individual situation before any procedure is initiated and which remains there unless removed. The most typical example of latent risk in the context of PCI is myocardial infarction. Latent risk may materialize at any time or, at least in elective cases, it may remain dormant.

There are two ways of dealing with latent risk: One may either *accept* it and not address it, or *mitigate* it by working actively to reduce it.

The two main purposes of PCI are mitigation of the latent risk and reduction of a patient's symptoms.

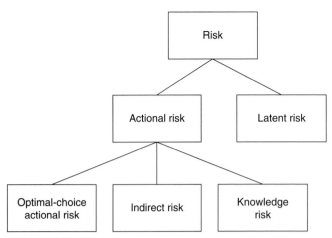

FIGURE 4-1. Types of risk. Upward lines signify a part-of relationship.

ACTIONAL RISK

Actional risk is that risk created by the actions of the operator, whether diagnostic or interventional. PCI involves many different actional risks including vessel closure, dissection and perforation of the target vessel at the target lesion, and vessel wall damage elsewhere in the coronary circulation or along the vascular access path, with ensuing local and/or systemic complications and patient instability.

There are two ways of dealing with actional risk (see Fig. 4-2): One may either *avoid* it by not performing the respective action, or *accept* it and perform the action anyway.

The main issue for PCI is to identify those actions that, given the context of the current procedure, result in the maximum reduction of latent risk with a minimum and acceptable level of actional risk. Much of PCI decision making revolves around the question of what constitutes acceptable actional risk.

In terms of risk management, there is a great difference between emergency and elective PCI. During emergency PCI, the operator will be prepared to accept substantially higher levels of actional risk for two reasons. First, in patients with acute coronary syndromes and hence the high latent risk of permanent myocardial damage or cardiovascular death, there is a lot

to be gained by taking higher actional risks. Second, the need for rapid action conflicts with the lengthy evaluation of risk factors and the consequent risk reduction that might be possible in elective situations.

Actional risk is always accompanied by two other effects. First, the intervention entails concrete financial *costs*, which rise with its duration, the number of steps involved, and the materials required. Second, if successful, the intervention will result in some kind of *benefit*. This benefit, whether a reduction of latent risk or merely the preparation of such a reduction, must be traded off against both actional risk and costs. Furthermore, when looking at the actual PCI decision-making process, it is useful to consider the three additive components of actional risk: optimum-choice actional risk, knowledge risk, and indirect risk.

Optimum-choice Actional Risk

Optimum-choice actional risk refers to that part of actional risk that an ideal operator acting under ideal circumstances would accept, in particular, given perfect information about the current status of the vessels. Optimum-choice actional risk is the actional risk incurred by those interventional steps that are required for optimum success.

Knowledge Risk

Knowledge risk is the part of actional risk incurred only because the operator's information about the vessel and lesion status is incomplete and imprecise (see Chapter 3B for the shortcomings of x-ray coronary angiography in visualizing the interventional site). Incomplete information or incorrect image interpretation may start a chain of inaccurate judgments, possibly leading to a suboptimal or overly dangerous intervention, and which in turn leads to increased actional risk. This *increase* in actional risk we call knowledge risk. There are three ways to reduce knowledge risk: first, by means of optimized image acquisition and evaluation; second, by performing additional diagnostic evaluations such as flow/pressure measurements or intracoronary ultrasonography; and third, by obtaining tactile information if the operator demonstrates advanced manual dexterity and operational skills. Note that extending diagnostic evaluations will always imply actional risk and must be traded off against the reduction in knowledge risk.

Indirect Risk

Indirect risk refers to the part of actional risk incurred by voluntarily giving up existing benefits. This is best explained by an example: Assume we have a guiding catheter in place in a vessel. If the PCI is not yet terminated, this is a benefit. Now, assume we want to exchange this catheter for another one (say, to switch from 5F to 7F). Obviously, this step involves actional risk since we may inflict damage on the patient during catheter exchange. However, even if no damage occurs, it may happen that for some reason the target vessel cannot be accessed because it proves impossible to appropriately position either this new catheter or any other one tried later. Thus, by removing a guiding catheter, we risk losing the benefit of having a well-positioned catheter (even if only 5F) in place. The possibility that this will happen is represented as indirect risk.

The only way to reduce indirect risk is by carefully planning the potential courses of intervention that may lie ahead, and how to proceed without giving up any intermediate benefits.

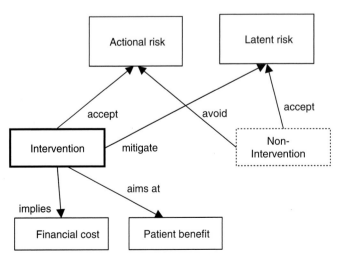

FIGURE 4-2. Relationship of intervention (vs. nonintervention) to the risk types actional risk and latent risk.

Indirect risk can often be reduced at the expense of financial cost by using the equipment best suited for a job rather than the cheapest that is expected to be sufficient.

RISK LEVEL CLASSIFICATION

To roughly classify the level of risks, we propose a five-level ordinal scale with the levels *very low, low, medium, high,* and *very high.* The component aspects *probability of the adverse event* and *expected resulting damage* can be described on the same scale. In principle, it is possible to describe the meaning of the probability levels numerically as a percentage. However, as people are known to estimate probabilities poorly, this is unwise. In any case, no intersubjective scale is available to quantitatively represent the damage incurred. Overall, the classification of both probability and damage (and thus of the total risk) is subjective and difficult. Therefore, a significant aspect of the skill of a master PCI operator consists in the ability to accurately (if not precisely) assess and compare the levels of alternative risks.

It is important to understand that potentially all aspects of PCI entail actional risk, even such apparently innocent acts as considering a decision (because that takes time during which the patient may become unstable) or terminating the procedure by suturing the access site (because that involves removal of the sheath and wound closure, and hence lack of an emergency access in the case of acute complications). Nevertheless, some actions carry an obviously greater risk than others. The most risk-intensive actions during PCI are usually the following:

- Using force in advancing instrumentation
- Inflating a dilatation balloon at high pressures (with or without a stent)
- Inflating an oversized dilatation balloon at any level of pressure (with or without a stent)
- Recanalization of subacutely occluded vessels
- Crossing subtotal occlusions
- Recrossing iatrogenically unstable lesions, iatrogenic coronary artery occlusions, and incomplete stent apposition

For all of these, the actional risk is high because of the large knowledge risk component involved. Knowledge risk is high for several reasons:

1. The information available about the status of the interventional site based on x-ray angiography is incomplete and imprecise.
2. The ensuing damage when an injury is inflicted is usually severe.
3. Access to the vessel may be compromised, making further deployment of instrumentation dangerous or impossible.

VALUE OF OPERATOR EXPERIENCE

The difficulty with minimizing risk during a PCI is obviously the fact that the risk inherent in any situation or step is usually uncertain and can only be estimated. Much of the experience of a master PCI operator is reflected in the precision and accuracy of his or her risk estimates and also the ability to manage unexpected and adverse outcomes.

A PCI beginner will only have a vague understanding that "something may go wrong" at some point, but will have serious difficulties classifying the likelihood of problems or discerning their nature and the limits imposed on their resolution.

A PCI operator with some experience can assess risk with a certain amount of accuracy and can also explain the nature of the risk in terms of which specific set of adverse events is currently to be feared (as opposed to those that are implausible in the given situation); his or her repertoire of technical skills allows the management of standard complications.

A master PCI operator has still greater accuracy in assessing the risks, though his or her knowledge is still imperfect because of deficiencies in the input information and the intricacies of individual cases. More importantly, he or she cannot only enumerate the plausible adverse events, but can also estimate with competence the likelihood of each one of them separately. The intervention strategy can hence be adapted accordingly in order to minimize risk and to be prepared to manage any adversities that occur. It appears that for the majority of master operators, the estimation of risks and adaptation of the process is not a conscious sequence of estimates and decisions. Rather, it is perceived as an intuition that tells them what and what not to do. Only a minority of master operators can easily explain *why* they decide on a specific course of action and *how* they do *what* they do. The details of the decision-making process of a master PCI operator remain largely unexplored at this point.

THE BASIC DECISION-MAKING PROCESS

The decision-making process in PCI consists of three overlapping, but different, stages:

1. Initialization: Considerations and actions before or at the beginning of the intervention. They prestructure the entire interventional process. Changing decisions made here is possible later on, but should be avoided as far as possible.
2. The main cycle of assessment and intervention: Many, if not all, interventions consist of multiple, consecutive interventional steps. The decision in each step is based on an assessment of the situation resulting from the previous step. The primary question is always: Which intervention promises the highest reduction in latent risk per investment of actional risk? Cost considerations may suggest deviations from this ideal path of the intervention. A helpful rule of thumb is to keep the number of interventional steps to a minimum, as these tend to increase both procedural costs and actional risk.
3. Termination: The decision when to terminate the intervention is based on the question of when, considering all available interventional approaches, the required investments in further procedural costs, time, and actional risk actually outweigh the expected resulting reduction in latent risk.

We will discuss each of these stages in a separate subsection.

INITIALIZATION

Initialization produces two consecutive results:

1. Decision whether to intervene
2. Decision how to intervene (decision as to the initial interventional approach, including selection of the access site)

We will discuss each of these in a separate subsection.

Decision for or Against Intervention

The decision whether a PCI should be attempted at all is based on three sets of information:

1. The coronary vascular status of the patient
2. Other data on the patient's health status
3. Technical feasibility and practicability of the intervention

We will not discuss issues of patient consent here.

The patient's **coronary vascular status** is assessed on the basis of existing diagnostic coronary angiography and supporting clinical information such as clinical symptoms and ECGs. The decision to intervene requires that (a) the target coronary lesions are sufficiently critical and sufficiently likely to cause the perceived symptoms to warrant PCI and (b) a suitable balance of latent risk, PCI actional risk, and expected PCI benefit appears to be present. Although the available initial data may be different, the issues to be considered are the same as during the main cycle of PCI and will thus be described there.

The estimate of PCI actional risk must now be modified by taking into account **other patient health status data,** such as the presence of multiple-vessel coronary disease, generalized vascular disease, comorbidities, further major cardiovascular risk factors, and status of the left ventricular function. The presence of any of these additional risk factors increases individual PCI actional risk considerably and may tip the balance toward non-intervention. If intervention appears desirable, one should consider whether it appears technically feasible and operationally practicable.

To decide on the **technical feasibility and practicability** of PCI, the operator typically considers the following aspects:

- Localization and percutaneous accessibility of the target lesion
- Status of vessels constituting the interventional path to the target vessel
- Status of the neighboring segments of the target vessel
- Status of other vessels near the target vessel
- Status of the dependent circulation distal to the target vessel
- Expected ability of the patient to handle the stress imposed by the intervention
- Expected incurred procedural costs

Adverse characteristics may indicate an unacceptable level of actional risk for the given intervention or may make the intervention completely impossible. Positive characteristics serve as indicators for a decision to intervene.

Initial Strategy

The initial strategy to intervene is determined by selection of the access site and initial instrumentation. More specifically:

- Selection of **the vascular access site** is based primarily on the status of the intended vascular path between the access site and the target vessel, and on the experience and personal preference of the operator. Because of its high versatility, right transfemoral access typically is selected. Alternative access sites are the left femoral, left and right brachial, and left and right radial arteries.
- Selection of initial instrumentation consists primarily of decisions as to the **French size, form, and type of the guiding catheter** on the basis of considerations such as required backup, expected need for larger devices such as bifurcation stents or thrombectomy catheters, use of special techniques such as "kissing" balloon dilatations, and the topography and vulnerability of the ostium. Choices regarding the performance requirements of the guidewire and balloon catheter with or without stent complete the selection of the interventional starting set.

The importance of these initial decisions cannot be overemphasized. Any suboptimal choice will make the operation unnecessarily difficult and may even prevent its successful completion. Any initial choice that must be revised during the intervention entails additional actional risk and increases overall procedural costs.

The intervention commences with the placement of the introductory sheath, followed by advancing and positioning the guiding catheter at the ostium over a guidewire (typically 0.035 in.). Optimum positioning and backup of the guiding catheter represents a primary success factor for the subsequent intervention.

It is important to be aware of possible problems at this stage of the procedure and to solve them, if at all possible, before the actual intervention has started; this increases the prospect of positive outcome and keeps indirect risk low. Typical considerations include:

- Selecting a **sheath** of appropriate French size and length that can overcome possible problems such as excessive length, tortuosity, or luminal obstructions in the conduit vessels. If the initial choice does not work well, the operator should consider switching at once to an alternative approach.
- Checking the adequacy of the **guiding catheter** to provide optimum backup and positioning at the ostium. If the initial choice does not work well, the operator should consider switching at once to another catheter.
- Being aware of other unexpected **difficulties** of any kind during the initialization of the intervention, including changes in the patient's clinical status in response to vascular manipulations, and complications in advancing the instrumentation within the target vessel and across the target lesion. If difficulties occur, the operator should reconsider the strategy and the decision to intervene. Stopping the intervention at this point should also be considered if the risk/benefit ratio no longer appears good.

If changes in overall strategy are needed, the operator should not hesitate to make these changes. The intervention will be burdened with significant levels of avoidable indirect risk and may cause adverse outcomes if difficulties that are accepted at this stage make a change in strategy necessary later.

THE MAIN PROCEDURAL CYCLE

Once access to the target vessel has been gained, the intervention enters a repeated cycle of assessment and intervention. More specifically:

- Assessing the status of the target vessel and target lesion by acquiring and interpreting cine or fluoroscopic x-ray coronary artery images
- Deciding how to perform the next interventional step and carrying it out.

Coronary intervention may encompass any number of iterations within the main cycle. In principle, the operator alternates among information gathering, data interpretation, and actual intervention. In practice, however, these phases are closely intertwined because information gathering and interpretation are essentially continuous processes during PCI. It should be noted that subsequent intervention steps can be directed at the same target lesion and vessel, or to different vessels or vessel segments, depending on the results of the evolving intervention.

The process ends when the termination criteria described later are reached.

Assessment of Status

Assessment of the target vessel and target lesion is primarily based on x-ray angiography and less frequently on intravascular ultrasonography or pressure/flow sensor probes. Discussion of the characteristics, limitations, and interpretation of each of these sources of information can be found in Chapters 3B–3D. We will therefore limit the description here to the following:

1. The risk considerations involved in interpreting the available information
2. The lesion characteristics to be considered

In terms of **risk considerations** for a particular target lesion, two issues must be addressed:

1. Objective situation: Is an intervention objectively appropriate for the selected lesion, that is, would an intervention provide a favorable ratio of risk (and cost) to the expected benefit to the patient?
2. Subjective evaluation: Is an intervention appropriate for this lesion in the operator's opinion?

If both answers are no, we have a *true negative*, and the intervention should not be performed.

If both answers are yes, we have a *true positive*, and the selected lesion is correctly considered for intervention as described below.

If the subjective evaluation is no, although objectively it should be yes, a *false negative* results. The intervention does not take place, and an opportunity to benefit the patient is lost.

If the subjective evaluation is yes, although objectively it should be no, a *false positive* results. The subsequent intervention exposes the patient to a substantial risk. Depending on the outcome, the intervention either will be merely fruitless or may cause damage that could have been avoided.

It should be noted that in reality the answers to these questions are usually not yes or no, but somewhere in between. The lesion receiving the most positive answers in the subjective evaluation will become the candidate target for the next interventional step in the evolving scenario of the intervention.

In complex procedures with several candidate lesions, the process of selecting the target lesions and their sequence should consider the following **criteria:**

- Selection criteria from the patient's point of view:
  - Which lesion is likely to be the most critical for myocardial salvage and/or perfusion? Identification and successful removal of this lesion promises to yield the greatest potential benefit in terms of clinical improvement.

- Which lesion is likely to be the most dangerous one? Repairing unstable lesions (or stabilizing them) promises to bring about the greatest reduction in latent risk.
- Selection criteria from the interventionist's point of view:
  - Which lesions provide the best substrate for successful repair? The likelihood of successful repair depends on reasonably well-determined criteria such as length, degree, and complexity of stenosis, but also on characteristics that are rather difficult to assess, such as the tissue composition of the atheroma and overall plaque burden of the adjacent vessel walls.
  - Which lesions carry the highest risk of complications such as vessel wall dissection or rupture on mechanical intervention? The consequences of severe complications may be such that PCI of lesions with a high risk of severe dissections or ruptures (such as high-grade stenosis in diffusely degenerated venous grafts) should be performed only in exceptional cases, if at all.
- Interventional priorities. Generally, the most critical stenosis should be approached first, not only because it promises the greatest benefit, but also to reduce the risks involved in subsequent interventional steps on associated lesions. In lesions of similarly critical status the most distal one is commonly tackled first to avoid recrossing.
- Sequences and staging of intervention. In patients with multiple lesions it is important not only to decide the sequence in which the competing lesions should be revascularized, but also whether single- or multiple-stage revascularization would optimize the risk/benefit trade-off while keeping the indirect risk low. The possibility of surgical or hybrid, that is, combined percutaneous/surgical, revascularization should also be considered.

Performing Interventional Steps

The actual intervention typically consists of five steps, some of which may have to be repeated several times in the course of the procedure:

1. Selecting the guidewire
2. Positioning the guidewire distal to the target lesion and verifying the position
3. Selecting the dilatation balloon or stent catheter
4. Performing dilatation
5. Checking the results

The **guidewire** is selected primarily for its expected ability to track the target vessel up to the lesion, cross the lesion without producing trauma, and reside distal to the lesion with enough support to enable tracking of the endovascular instrumentation. The rigidity of the shaft for optimum support has to be traded off against the greater risk of vessel injury.

While **positioning the guidewire,** which in coronary interventions is typically 0.014 in. in diameter, the operator may experience difficulties in tracking the target vessel, and in reaching, crossing, or advancing beyond the lesion. Several situations are common:

- The guidewire tip is inappropriately shaped for navigating toward and along the target vessel. The usual procedure is then to withdraw the wire, reshape the tip, and try again; the indirect risk from withdrawing the wire is clearly lower than the actional risk from working with a wrongly shaped tip.

- The stiffness of the tip is inappropriate for avoiding or crossing obstacles while avoiding traumatization of vessel walls along its path. The usual procedure is then to withdraw the wire and try a softer or stiffer one. Note that the new wire may need to have a differently shaped tip. The risk consideration is similar to the previous one.
- The guidewire shaft is too stiff to navigate the course of the target vessel or too soft to support tracking of the endovascular instruments. The usual procedure is to withdraw the wire and to try again with the next softer or stiffer option. Again, the risk consideration is as described previously. In difficult cases, switching from rapid-exchange to over-the-wire techniques, employing a second guidewire, or even changing the guiding catheter for extra support may become necessary. In all of these cases, the operator is usually willing to accept the indirect risk involved in withdrawing the current wire, because the actional risk of working with an inappropriate wire (or catheter) is high and the time lost during multiple ineffective positioning attempts increases it further.

In any of the foregoing cases, the decision for or against correction trades the expected tactical benefit against the increased indirect risk associated with making the correction. In a few cases, the indirect risk may be high enough to warrant abstaining from the intended correction, which in turn requires reconsideration of the overall strategy and feasibility of the intervention.

When the lesion has been passed successfully, the operator decides what will be the **final position of the guidewire tip distal to the target lesion.** The common choices are:

- Aggressive approach. The distal segment of the target vessel is selected for optimum control of the target vessel and maximum support. In more forceful interventions, this action runs the risk of damaging the distal vessel wall. It may be inappropriate for guidewires with stiffer shafts or tips.
- Conservative approach. An intermediate distance from the lesion is chosen to avoid distal target vessel wall damage, particularly in diffusely diseased vessels and in interventions requiring the use of greater force. This provides greater clearance for the to-and-fro motion of the guidewire tip, while trading the better support associated with a greater risk of damage in favor of risk reduction.
- Alternative approach. "Parking" the guidewire in functionally less important side branches prevents the guidewire tip from making contact with the distal segment of the target vessel. The aggressive lean-on approach may become more acceptable in this case.

Once the guidewire tip has been securely positioned, it is critical for at least two projections with the guidewire in place to be acquired to **verify** and document unequivocally its correct placement in the target vessel and the lack of trauma along the guidewire passage. Accidental placement in a different vessel that runs parallel to the target vessel must be avoided.

The selection of the **type of dilatation balloon catheter** or stent catheter is based on the overall assessment of the severity of the stenosis, its length, its location with respect to the left main coronary artery or ostium, side branches, and expected plaque burden. In selecting the balloon catheter, it is important to bear in mind that information about the mechanical properties of the target vessel and target lesions is incomplete. The choice of using balloon dilatation or attempting direct stenting depends on a number of criteria discussed in Chapter 4. Regardless of which is chosen, the following parameters should be considered:

- Balloon diameter. Does the balloon diameter match the nominal size of the target vessel at the lesion?
- Balloon length. Does the balloon length match that of the target lesion?
- Mechanical properties of the balloon/stent. Do the mechanical properties of the balloon catheter (pushing and crossing abilities, and noncompliance at high pressures) meet the requirements posed by the status of the target vessel and the stenosis?
- Balloon refolding ability. Will the balloon catheter refold safely to avoid damage during its retraction after successful dilatation?

As with positioning of the guidewire tip, worst-case scenarios should be borne in mind during the selection and use of balloon catheters. Here, the actional risk from choices that are too aggressive should be considered, as well as the disadvantages of choices that are too conservative. There may be actional risk from time lost due to multiple inflation attempts and indirect risk from perhaps having to withdraw more than one balloon.

From the foregoing, it is clear that PCI entails active risk management throughout its entire course, but the phase of balloon inflation is typically associated with the highest actional risk. In contrast to open heart surgery, it may become more difficult to control the consequences of severe vessel damage inflicted by mechanical overexposure during PCI. Careful decision making, including careful and rather conservative sizing of the balloon or stent, is therefore essential. It is at this critical point—removing a stenosis without inflicting uncontrolled damage to a vessel—that the superior power of judgment of an expert PCI operator makes the biggest difference.

Following deflation and removal of the device, a brief contrast flush injection is typically used to check the lesion after the intervention. Subsequently, at least two projections of the interventional site at high resolution must be acquired and thoroughly studied to assess the results. If there are doubts about the results, the operator must look closely at the projections that seem most unfavorable in order to obtain reassurance that the results are acceptable or to evaluate the problems. Evaluating the results of the preceding interventional steps also serves as an indicator for the next iteration with which the procedure will continue, unless it indicates that terminating the procedure is preferable.

TERMINATION

Deciding when to terminate the procedure is relatively simple in patients with single-vessel, single-lesion coronary artery disease, but often difficult in more complex cases. In principle, the criterion is always the same: The procedure should stop as soon as the risk involved in further intervention appears to exceed the expected benefits. It is useful to distinguish among the following major reasons for terminating the procedure:

1. Full procedural success. All target lesions have been successfully repaired, and the patient's condition is stable and asymptomatic.
2. Satisfactory procedural success. Some target lesions have been successfully repaired, the patient's condition is stable and asymptomatic, and any remaining lesions are considered not significant or amenable to later repair.
3. Palliative procedural success. Target lesions have been improved, but not completely removed, and the patient's condition is stable and largely asymptomatic.
4. Intractability. Despite one or more attempts, the goal of the intervention has not been met; the target lesion is unchanged; the patient's condition is stable.
5. Unacceptable risk of complications. Revascularization has to be aborted because of the excessive risk of local or systemic complications. Depending on the general clinical condition and coronary status of the patient, conservative and surgical treatment options will be considered.
6. Failed procedure. The intervention resulted in deterioration of the lesion or of the patient's clinical condition, requiring immediate consideration of alternative emergency therapy options.

In individual cases, procedural success might be interpreted differently by different operators, whereby the degree of freedom in defining procedural success is lowest for case 1 situations and highest for case 5. Additional variability is introduced by other factors, in particular the difference between elective and emergency cases: The level of risk the operator is willing to accept is considerably higher in emergency cases, thus greatly reducing the operator's willingness to terminate the procedure for reasons 4 or 5.

DECISION-MAKING EXAMPLES

In order to illustrate the use of this decision-making approach in practice, this section presents two real intervention scenarios (including patient status, intervention history, and coronary images) with examples of the reasoning behind them (including some discussion of alternatives) and their outcomes. The decisions are discussed in terms of latent risk (or, alternatively, patient benefit), actional risk, and the uncertainty about both.

A STRAIGHTFORWARD ELECTIVE CASE

A 61-year-old male patient (D.F.) with diffuse single-vessel disease had undergone an elective complex stent coronary intervention of the left circumflex coronary artery 14 months prior to the present admission. Although his exercise tolerance had initially improved following that intervention, it had then declined for the past 9 months. At the time of admission, the patient reported exertional angina and shortness of breath at a moderate level of exercise while taking antianginal medication. Elective angiography confirmed the presence of single-vessel disease with a subtotal occlusion of the left circumflex coronary artery. Elective revascularization was indicated.

Given the symptoms and angiographic status (Fig. 4-3), coronary bypass surgery was not considered a primary option for revascularization because of its much higher actional risk and cost. Therefore, PCI was recommended. PCI for a subtotal chronic occlusion older than 3 months, corresponding to a type C lesion on the classification of the American College of Cardiology/American Heart Association, carries a likelihood of procedural success of about 60%. Overall, the expected risk was moderate, while the expected benefits were high.

Based on diagnostic angiograms, a standard guiding catheter (6F Judkins 4.5 left, no side holes) was selected. The subtotal left circumflex (LCx) occlusion was explored using the Boston Scientific Choice PT guidewire. On reaching the site of the subtotal occlusion, the guidewire tip could not be advanced on multiple attempts. To improve the support, an over-the-wire (OTW) system along with Boston Scientific Choice PT^2 guidewire was introduced and slowly advanced under probing pressure past the subtotal occlusion into the periphery; the maximum exerted pressure was small enough that the actional risk incurred by this procedure was clearly warranted by the expected success. At this point "no-flow" was noted and the OTW balloon catheter appeared wedged. Since the lack of a docking wire prevented its replacement by a low-profile monorail balloon, the guidewire tip was used to explore the side-branches guidewire to confirm the intraluminal position of the system in order to minimize the risk from wire-position knowledge. It was felt that the actional risk of perforation or vessel rupture or true lumen compression due to balloon inflation (2/20 mm at 4 bar) within the false lumen was low and justified proceeding with the intervention. After multiple dilatations, the antegrade blood flow was restored. This unmasked a high-grade restenosis at the occlusion site with longitudinal dissection lines corresponding to type D on the National Heart Lung and Blood Institute classification, intermittent thrombus formation, and a hemodynamically significant lesion of the ostial left circumflex coronary artery. Obtaining this information represented another important reduction in knowledge risk. Following both an intracoronary bolus and intravenous infusion of eptifibatide, the OTW system was replaced by a monorail one. Overlapping distal to proximal dilatations with increasing balloon diameters (up to 3.5 mm) and pressures (up to 14 bar) were performed, achieving a complete angiographic revascularization of the proximal-to-middle left circumflex coronary artery. Such lengthy interventions inherently carry a certain amount of actional risk simply due to the time on the table that they require, but the individual dilatations were not dangerous in the given case and there was clearly no better alternative route. Then, several angiographic projections of the ostium plaque were acquired and analyzed. Based on the angiographic plaque distribution within the proximal left circumflex coronary artery, it was felt that plaque repair should be possible without left main intervention. Because the actional risk level of the left main intervention was estimated as low to intermediate, it was decided to stent the left circumflex coronary artery ostial lesion such that the last ring of the stent exactly matched the plane of the left circumflex coronary artery take-off, with the rest of the stent fully covering the lesion. A 3.5/8 mm Biotronik Lekton motion stent was selected and deployed at 12 bar. The final angiogram confirmed that revascularization was complete and the left main artery intact. The patient remained asymptomatic and was discharged on day 3. This case

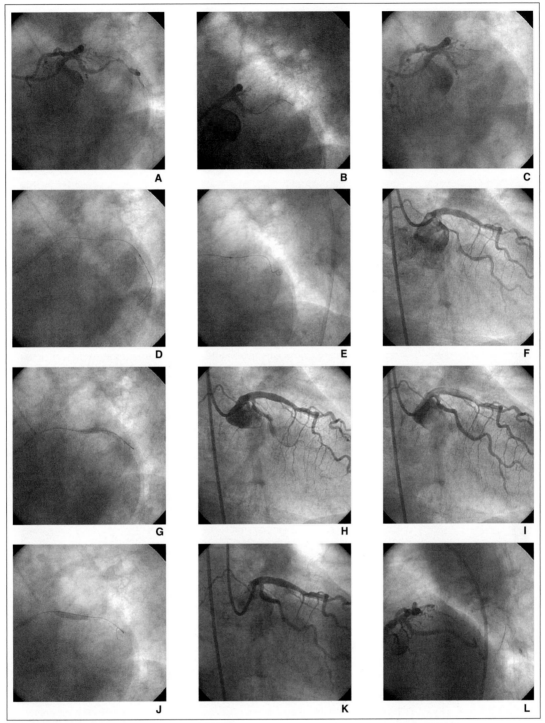

FIGURE 4-3.   Subtotal chronic occlusion, a straightforward elective case. The angiogram revealed subtotal left circumflex coronary artery occlusion in a diffusely diseased vessel **(A)**. Initially, the guidewire could not be advanced beyond the proximal third of the target vessel (American Heart Association classification segment 11) **(B)** and was replaced by the OTW system. On further exploration, no-reflow occurred **(C)**. Following the successful passage of the proximal dissection, the guidewire was advanced into the distal position, and successive distal **(D)** to proximal **(E)** dilatations were performed. Following these dilatations, the antegrade flow was restored and dissecting plaques within the target lesion were documented **(F)**, prompting proximal redilatations **(G)**, which resulted in plaque shifts and intermittent thrombus formation **(H)**. A bolus of intracoronary glycoprotein IIb/IIIa receptor inhibitor and repeated proximal dilatations restored vessel patency with a residual 70% ostial stenosis **(I)**. After stent placement **(J)**, satisfactory revascularization was documented **(K,L)**. OTW, over-the-wire.

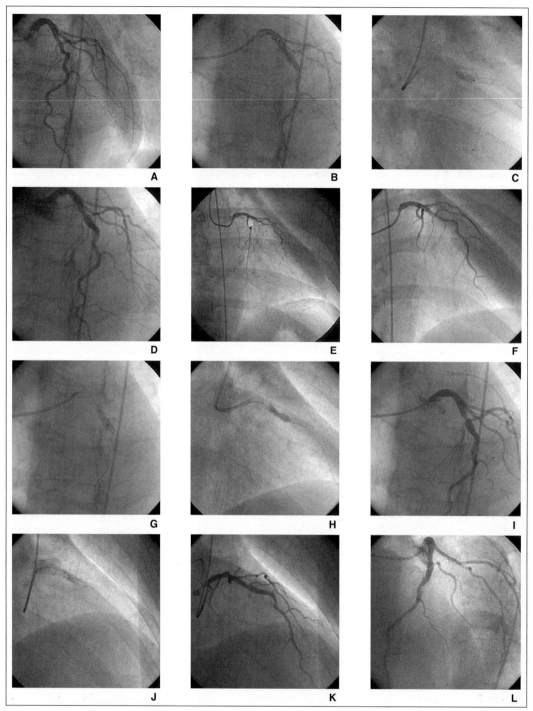

FIGURE 4-4. Failed PCI LAD, nondilatable lesion, an elective case forwarded to surgery. The previously documented proximal LAD stenosis appeared unchanged compared with the previous angiogram ["angiographically stable," **(A)**]. Direct stenting of the lesion, with the distal ring placed just above the diagonal ramus take-off, was performed **(B).** Control angiography revealed distal edge dissection (not shown), prompting implantation of a second stent **(C).** Subsequent multiple dilatation did not produce full stent expansion, resulting in a residual 40% funnel-shaped stenosis **(D).** This intermediate result was accepted, and the intervention terminated. Severe chest pain and a drop in blood pressure called for immediate renewed angiography minutes later; this showed a subtotal LAD occlusion at the stent level **(E),** which resolved spontaneously on a second contrast agent injection **(F).** To clarify the site morphology, an IVUS transducer was introduced, but failed to cross the lesion. To reinforce the proximal LAD, an additional stent was deployed, and multiple dilatations were performed **(G,H).** The stenosis persisted **(I),** so the LAD lesion was considered nondilatable, and the patient was referred to semielective coronary artery bypass grafting (CABG). **J–L:** The site in native and contrast angiograms. PCI, percutaneous coronary intervention; LAD, left anterior descending; IVUS, intravascular ultrasound.

proceeded as expected: No significant risk materialized, yet high patient benefit was attained.

AN ESCALATING ELECTIVE CASE FORWARDED TO SURGERY

A 52-year-old female patient (D.H.) had known two-vessel coronary artery disease and a recent history of an inferior myocardial infarction and emergency PCI on the right coronary artery (RCA). She was readmitted for increasing anxiety and crescendo angina. Ergometry revealed 0.2 mV ST-segment depression in electrocardiographic leads V3 to V6 at 75 W. Diagnostic angiograms in steep left anterior oblique (LAO) and right anterior oblique (RAO) projections with cranial tilt revealed a bifurcation lesion, classified as Type B1 according to the American College of Cardiology/American Heart Association and as Type A according to the Lefevre classification, just proximal to the take-off of the first diagonal branch (Fig. 4-4). The lesion appeared no different from that documented by angiography 2 weeks earlier. The proximal segment was straight, the lesion appeared smooth, and there were no signs of thrombus and no angiographic calcifications. The RCA showed an excellent short-term result. On the basis of history and diagnostic evaluations, left anterior descending artery (LAD) revascularization was indicated. Because of the angiographically benign appearance of the LAD lesion, PCI actional risk appeared modest, and so PCI was selected.

A standard guiding catheter (6F Judkins 4.0 left, without side holes) was selected and seated. A Guidant Whisper M guidewire was placed, and direct stenting was performed using a 3.5/15 mm Medtronic Driver stent at 12 bar such that the distal ring of the stent was positioned just proximally to the bifurcation. The control angiogram revealed a distal edge dissection, requiring placement of a second stent (one ring overlap, 3.0/9 mm Medtronic Driver at 10 bar). Subsequently, multiple dilatations using 3.5/20 mm balloons at up to 20 bars were performed without a full stent expansion. The residual stenosis was 40% diameter. The operator judged that the further benefits expected were insufficient to warrant still more forceful intervention, as that would incur rather significant actional risk. Therefore, the current result was considered adequate, the intervention stopped, and the patient scheduled for renewed angiography the next day.

While being transferred into a monitored bed close to the catheterization laboratory, the patient experienced a sudden crushing chest pain and drop in systolic blood pressure from 120 mm Hg to 60 mm Hg. Immediate repeat angiography revealed slow LAD flow with no other changes at the interventional site compared with the previous film. The next angiographic sequence indicated normal coronary flow (Thrombolysis In Myocardial Infarction, TIMI III°). To reduce knowledge risk, an intravascular ultrasound (IVUS) catheter was employed but failed to pass the site. Because of the intermittent character of the symptoms, a thrombus associated with incomplete stent deployment, strut damage, tissue intussusception, intimal flap, or dissection were considered the most likely cause. On the basis of these hypotheses, it was unclear whether PCI would be able to

help (high benefit uncertainty), but there was also no reason not to try (acceptable actional risk).

To avoid proximal dissection in the course of high-pressure dilatation, the stented segment was first reinforced by an additional proximal stent (3.5/9 mm Medtronic Driver at 14 bar). Then a number of dilatations were performed, using 3.5/20 mm and 4.0/10 mm balloons inflated up to 24 bar. However, the funnel-shaped LAD stenosis persisted. Moreover, slight recoil, corresponding to a partial radial stent collapse, was noted during control angiography. This event is crucial for the course taken. It limits the endovascular treatment options and hence the expectable benefit. Worse, it signals a sharp increase in actional risk. For this reason, the patient was referred to coronary artery bypass surgery the next day. The surgery and the postoperative course were uneventful.

Complete review of all angiograms has not revealed any cause for the nondilatable character of the LAD stenosis. In the absence of angiographic calcifications, the most likely explanation for the unusual rigidity of the lesion appeared to be the presence of a fibrotic or fibrocalcific stricture, or the presence of massive plaque burden with full-circle circumferential distribution associated with negative remodeling. In such a case, the knowledge risk uncertainty is so high that attempts at dilatation beyond those just described appear unjustifiable (at least in an elective situation), so surgery is required instead.

CONCLUSION

This chapter presents an approach to understanding PCI on the basis of the notion of risk. The aim of PCI is to provide benefits that reduce latent risk by means of procedures that entail actional risk. From this point of view, PCI is an iterative process of highly complex decisions that aims to provide low-risk, low-cost, high-benefit endovascular repair of coronary artery lesions. We have provided a description of the PCI intervention process in terms of the risk considerations involved when the available alternatives are selected at each point of the intervention.

To develop a realistic model of PCI and a useful tool for teaching, further practical differentiations and improvements in the strategic and tactical decision-making processes are necessary.

REFERENCES

1. Hirshfeld JW Jr., Banas JS, Cowley M, et al. for the Writing Committee Members. American College of Cardiology training statement on recommendations for the structure of an optimal adult interventional cardiology training program. *J Am Coll Cardiol.* 1999;34:2142-2147.
2. Standards for institutions/organizations offering interventional procedural course training. American College of Cardiology. Available at: http://www.acc.org/education/courses/courses.htm. Accessed August 26, 2005.
3. ACC/AHA guidelines for percutaneous coronary intervention (Revision of the 1993 PTCA Guidelines). A report on the American College of Cardiology/American Heart Association Task Force on Practice Guidelines. *J Am Coll Cardiol.* 2001;37:IV. Institutional and Operator Competency.
4. American Board of Internal Medicine. Policies for added qualifications in interventional cardiology; eligibility for certification and board policies. Available at: http://www.abim.org/cert/policies_aqic.shtm. Accessed August 27, 2005.

Wolfram Schmidt
Klaus-Peter Schmitz

CHAPTER **5**

Devices

Endovascular therapy has a relatively short but rich history, characterized by the work of strong individuals and marked by remarkable events.[1,2]

Today, to the uninitiated, endovascular instrumentation can easily be mistaken for a simple matter-of-course tool of the trade. However, today's facile, lower-risk instruments required years of development, employing the integrated professional expertise of designers, material and production specialists, biologists, and physicians in an increasingly high-tech industrial environment. On the path from an idea to a finished product, efficient design, flawless production, and excellent quality must coincide. And since the quality of a product is never the result of a fortunate coincidence, it can and has to be measured to ensure safe and efficacious medical application.

The sheer number of endovascular devices available prevents us from providing a comprehensive discussion of all of them in this chapter. We have, therefore, selected dilatation balloon catheters and stents for coronary and peripheral vascular applications as representative examples providing insights into the objective performance and quality assessment of endovascular instrumentation. Specifically, we review and discuss:

1. Performance parameters measured by in vitro laboratory tests
2. Methods of measuring these parameters
3. Typical results
4. The impact of specific results on clinical applications

In the past, a number of attempts have been made to measure, validate, and simulate performance parameters, and some of these methods and results have been published.[3–17] It is not our intention to consider all of these tests, but rather to inform the reader why specific properties should be measured and how the results should be interpreted.

DILATATION BALLOON CATHETERS

PERFORMANCE PARAMETERS

High-pressure, dilatation balloon catheters are designed to dilate or to reopen narrowed or occluded vessels by inserting and inflating a balloon within the lesion using internal hydraulic pressure. This simple operating principle determines the main performance characteristics and requirements of any angioplasty balloon catheter, including:

- Low *entry and crossing profile* of the balloon catheter for optimum tracking and crossing
- Short *inflation* and *deflation time* to avoid ischemic complications
- Optimum *refolding characteristics* to avoid traumatization or stent damage
- Predictable and low *balloon compliance* to allow precise diameter sizing
- High *balloon-burst strength* for high-pressure dilatations
- Low *bending stiffness* for easy tracking of curved vessels

These parameters must be integrated into several complex functional parameters such as *trackability (tracking ability), crossability (crossing ability),* and *pushability (pushing ability)* to characterize the clinical performance of the final product.

Rapid exchange (RX) catheters have a guidewire lumen only in their distal part. This means the catheter produces less friction on the guidewire, but also provides less support than the traditional over-the-wire (OTW) systems, which contain a guidewire lumen throughout the entire length of their shaft. A typical RX balloon dilatation catheter design is shown in Figure 5-1.

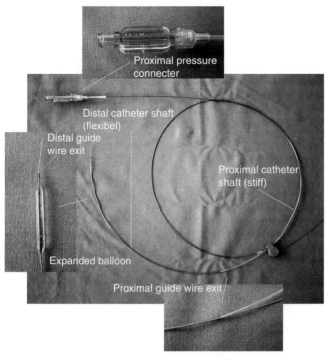

FIGURE 5-1. Typical PTCA balloon catheter system with description of the essential parts of a rapid exchange catheter (Guidant Voyager). PTCA, percutaneous transluminal coronary angioplasty.

TEST METHODS

Profile

Several profiles of a balloon catheter can be measured to characterize its performance, as illustrated in Figure 5-2. The *crossing profile* is the most important of these and is commonly defined as the largest diameter in the balloon region of the dilatation catheter. To position the dilatation balloon safely across tight lesions, the lowest possible profiles are required. To cross extremely tight and long lesions, both the entry and the crossing profiles must be low. Low profiles are also desirable to avoid luminal obstructions, which could potentially result in myocardial ischemia in time-consuming procedures.

The maximum profile of catheters can be measured using a calibrated aperture plate. Using this method, the maximum diameter of the folded balloon can be assessed, as can the compressibility of the balloon material required for insertion into tight lesions, therefore providing a combined measurement of the geometry and compressibility of the dilatation balloon in its deflated and folded state.

The pinhole diameters of the aperture plate used for this measurement are adjusted to the typical dimensions of the balloon catheters. The accuracy of these profile measurements depends on the accuracy of the dimension of the pinholes and on a fine gradation of the diameters. Steps of 0.05 mm appear to provide sufficiently accurate measurements (Fig. 5-3).

To mimic the behavior of the balloons during in vivo vascular applications, it is necessary to conduct the measurement in an aqueous environment at 37°C. Because of the strong dependence of polymer characteristics on temperature, in vivo conditions should be simulated as close as possible. However, no long-term sample conditioning is needed of the kind required in the measurement of mechanical parameters of polymers according to technical standards.[18,19] Device testing is intended to simulate conditions for clinical use rather than to measure physical material constants. Since, in most cases, vascular interventions should be finished within a space of minutes, constant material properties of small devices such as balloon catheters are typically assumed to be achieved within 5 minutes of conditioning.

The measurements are performed by starting with the largest pinhole diameter and continuing with smaller pinhole diameters until the balloon cannot pass through the aperture. Profile data of the distal and proximal balloon shoulders frequently represent the highest profiles of the entire dilatation balloon, thus corresponding to the crossing profile of the balloon catheter.

Current percutaneous transluminal coronary angioplasty (PTCA) catheter balloons usually have maximum diameters of about 1.00 mm, whereas percutaneous transluminal angioplasty (PTA) balloons may be in the order of 2.00 mm, depending on the design for specific vascular regions (e.g., renal, iliacal, carotid). For all vascular applications, there is a trend towards decreasing profiles and smaller sizes to allow less traumatic dilatations of increasingly complex lesions.

A more accurate and user-independent profile measurement can be made using a noncontact diameter measurement. For this application, laser scanner technology provides the most accurate and objective results because mechanical interference can be completely avoided. However, tactile distance sensors may also be used if the conditions of measurements are well defined, in particular the contact force.

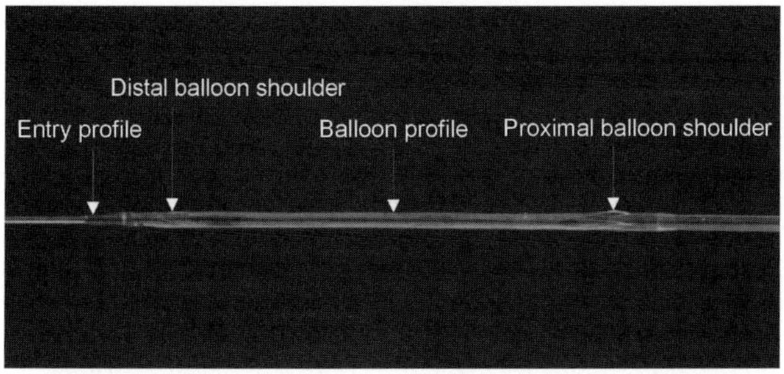

FIGURE 5-2. Folded balloon with relevant profiles as indicated.

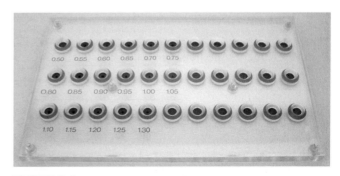

FIGURE 5-3. Aperture plate with 17 pinholes from 0.50 up to 1.30 mm (diameter steps of 0.05 mm).

Figure 5-4 illustrates the operating principle of a two-axis laser scanner. The test specimen is situated in the center of the two-axis laser measurement head. Each axis laser scanner measures the dimension in the *x* or *y* projection of the specimen in the plane of the measurement (dimension *z*). Using this experimental setup the measured diameter values d_x and d_y are recorded and the root mean square (RMS) is calculated, assuming a cylindrical shape of the folded balloon. Deviations from this assumption can be assessed by considering the diameter difference $d_x - d_y$. The profile measurement is repeated automatically for consecutive adjacent *z*-planes to achieve a profile function along the long axis of the catheter.

A laser scanning device of this kind can typically operate at a measurement range of 0.1 to 30 mm with an accuracy of ±0.01 mm and a resolution of ±0.001 mm. The sensitivity in the *z* direction should be high to allow for measurements of changing profiles and structures. A thickness of the effective *z* plane of 0.2 mm can be reached. Additional optical adaptation of the system is required for measuring the specimen in a water bath because of additional refraction and scattering effects.

Typical results of profile measurements can be seen in Table 5-1 and Figure 5-5. Comparing the maximum diameters resulting from the aperture plate measurement with the non-contact laser scanner data, it is clear that most of the tested

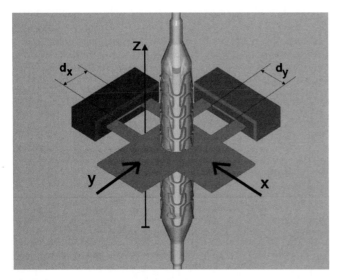

FIGURE 5-4. Schematic drawing of the setup for measuring the diameter of a catheter (here with a mounted stent) using a two-axis laser scanner.

TABLE 5-1. Maximum Profile of PTCA Balloon Catheters, Measured Using an Aperture Plate ($\Delta d = 0.05$ mm)

	Distal profile (mm)	Proximal profile (mm)
Medtronic Sprinter 3.0/20 mm	0.85	1.00
Biotronik Elect 3.0/20 mm	0.85	1.00
Guidant Voyager 3.0/20 mm	0.80	0.95
Boston Scientific Maverick[2] 3.0/20 mm	0.85	0.95
Cordis Aqua$_{T3}$ 3.0/20 mm	0.80	0.95

PTCA, percutaneous transluminal coronary angioplasty.

dilatation balloons can be pushed through smaller pinholes than would be assumed from noncontact measurements. In some cases the balloon shoulders are compressed by nearly 0.2 mm if maximum push is applied. However, the laser measurements are completely free of any manipulation and thus represent an excellent method for objective comparison of devices.

Inflation and Deflation Time

Inflation of a dilatation balloon within a narrowed, but not completely occluded, blood vessel results in ischemia of the dependent tissue. To keep the ischemic time short, the operator must retain full control over the obstruction time of the target vessel, represented by a sum of the time required to transmit the pressure in the hand pump mounted at the proximal side of the catheter to the inside of the balloon, time for balloon inflation, and deflation time.

Physically, the dilatation balloon is expanded by pumping a specific volume of liquid (mixture of normal saline and contrast agent) under pressure into the limited volume of the noncompliant balloon. The liquid flow (volume per unit time) between the pump and the balloon is driven by the pressure difference. The time needed to fill or to fully evacuate this volume, termed the inflation and deflation times, respectively, is commonly used as the relevant parameter to compare dilatation balloons. The flow required to fill or to evacuate the balloon is mainly restricted by the flow resistance *R* of the hypotube of the shaft connecting the hub and the balloon. *R* is determined by the viscosity of the liquid η and the inner radius *r* and length *l* of the hypotube, described by Poiseuille's law applicable to the laminar flow conditions:

$$R \propto \frac{\eta l}{r^4}$$

On the basis of this equation, it is clear that the radius *r* of the tubing is the major determinant of resistance (raised to the fourth power). Low-caliber hypotubes mean long inflation or deflation time, thus placing limits on decreasing catheter shaft profiles. The inflation and deflation times depend, furthermore, on the volume of the balloon. However, because the volume of balloons of comparable sizes is similar, this is not a useful measurement in balloon comparisons.

To measure the inflation and deflation time of the balloon, the pressure and the test liquid must be well defined. It is useful to adjust nominal pressure (NP) conditions, as specified by the manufacturer. Thus, for balloon inflation, a clinically relevant mixture of saline and x-ray contrast agent (e.g., 1:1) should be used. In addition, the end points of balloon filling (inflation) or emptying (deflation) must be exactly defined. In practice, these points are those at which no further changes in the outer balloon shape occur; objective measurements of the outer contour can precisely define these points. These shape measurements can be made by tactile or noncontact sensors (e.g., optical, magnetic, capacitive distance sensors). In Figure 5-6 a setup is shown where the state of the balloon is measured by a capacitive distance sensor. Figure 5-7 shows typical results of deflation time measurements.

Inflation and deflation times, however, do not fully describe the extent of flow obstruction and the risk posed by ischemia. Even if the balloon is folded or refolded after expansion, the

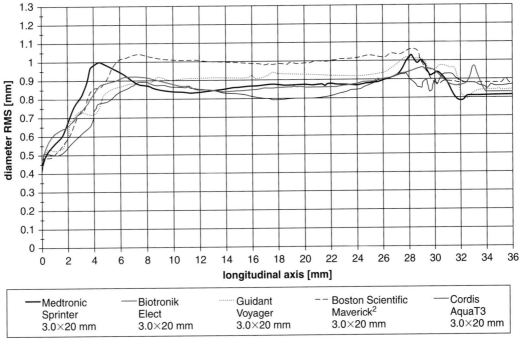

FIGURE 5-5. Distal profile of PTCA balloon catheters, noncontact measurement of RMS values using a two-axis laser scanner (ODAC 32XY, Zumbach Electronic). PTCA, percutaneous transluminal coronary angioplasty; RMS, root mean square.

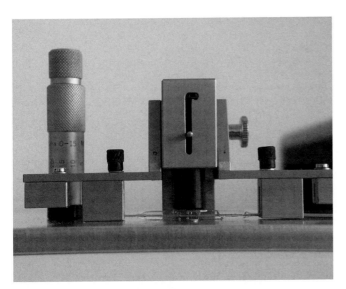

FIGURE 5-6. View of a test setup with inflated balloon; indication of balloon deflation by a tactile sensor.

deflated balloon remains within the lumen and obstructs the blood flow. Therefore, to minimize the residual obstruction and to avoid vessel wall damage by "flaring" of unfolded balloon parts on retraction, the geometric refolding characteristics of a balloon after deployment are also important. The lowest cross-sectional area and smooth profile of the refolded balloon is associated with the least blood-flow obstruction and avoids vessel traumatization and stent damage on withdrawal.

Balloon Compliance

Compliance of balloon catheters C is defined as the change in balloon diameter (Δd) for a given change in balloon pressure (Δp). High-pressure balloons for PTCA/PTA therapy have extremely low compliance compared with low-pressure balloons commonly used for diagnostic purposes. However, even when high-pressure balloons are sometimes termed "noncompliant," measurable diameter compliance always exists. Compliance of a specific balloon can be either indicated as a percentage increase in diameter per bar, or listed as a table of pressures and corresponding balloon diameters. The first is useful for classification of balloons as noncompliant or semicompliant, whereas the latter is usually given by the manufacturer for each device as the compliance chart.

Balloon compliance can be measured using the setup for profile measurement shown above in Figure 5-4. This setup must additionally include the means to adjust and measure balloon pressure up to at least 20 bar. To achieve this, a computer-controlled piston pump and a pressure sensor are added. It is important to use a basin of temperate water (37°C) for this measurement, because the elastic modulus of the polymeric balloon material strongly depends on temperature. The technical setup for compliance measurements is shown in Figure 5-8. Figure 5-9 demonstrates the compliance of five different PTCA dilatation balloons.

To calculate compliance, the average diameters at NP (d_{NP}) and rated burst pressure (d_{RBP}) are typically measured at the corresponding NP and rated burst pressure (RBP):

$$C = \frac{d_{RBP} - d_{NP}}{(RBP - NP) \cdot d_{NP}} \cdot 100\%$$

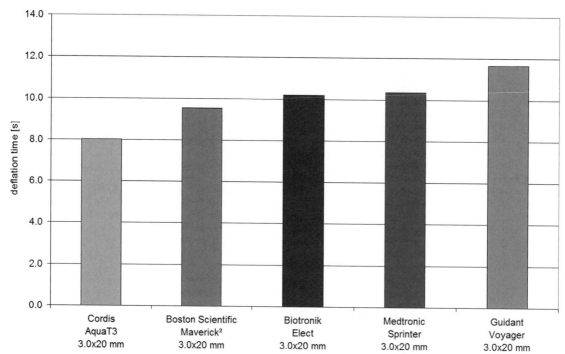

FIGURE 5-7.   Average deflation time of PTCA balloon catheters (saline and contrast liquid Accupaque 300, Amersham Buchler, 50:50). PTCA, percutaneous transluminal coronary angioplasty.

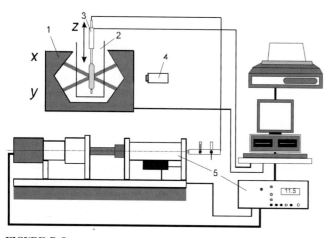

FIGURE 5-8.   Measurement setup for balloon compliance (*1*, laser scanner; *2*, water basin; *3*, linear actuator; *4*, camera; *5*, pressure controller).

Table 5-2 demonstrates that three balloons have a similar compliance, whereas the compliance of the two other balloons (Elect, Biotronik, and Aqua T3, Cordis) is much smaller; this can be seen in Figure 5-9, where the slope of the diameter versus the pressure curve indicates balloon compliance.

Balloon Burst Strength

High-pressure dilatation balloons are exposed to high stresses. The radial and axial stresses (σ_{rad}, σ_{ax}) in the balloon material depend on balloon pressure p, balloon diameter d, and the thickness s of the balloon wall, assuming a simple cylindrical shape. Gross estimation provides[20]:

$$\sigma_{rad} = \frac{pd}{2s}$$

$$\sigma_{ax} = \frac{pd}{4s}$$

The balloon will burst if the stresses exceed the rupture stress of the material. It can be seen that under ideal conditions there is a linear correlation between stress, balloon pressure, and balloon diameter, and an inverse relationship to the balloon thickness. This means that, given the same material, a larger balloon diameter and thin balloon material will result in a lower burst pressure. In addition, the equations show that within the balloon the axial stress is half as big as the radial stress.

The burst strength is measured using a pressure controller, which is preferably computer controlled. The balloon must be stored in temperate water, and the regime of pressurization must be exactly defined. Usually the pressure is increased in steps of 1 bar until the balloon ruptures (burst pressure). This burst pressure is taken as the measure of the burst strength of the balloon.

TABLE 5-2.   Diameter Compliance of Different High-pressure PTCA Balloons

	Diameter compliance (%/bar)
Medtronic Sprinter 3.0/20 mm	9.92
Biotronik Elect 3.0/20 mm	5.50
Guidant Voyager 3.0/20 mm	8.99
Boston Scientific Maverick² 3.0/20 mm	9.88
Cordis Aqua$_{T3}$ 3.0/20 mm	5.88

PTCA, percutaneous transluminal coronary angioplasty.

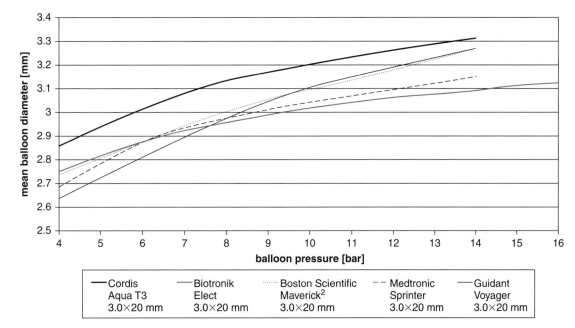

FIGURE 5-9. Measured compliance curves of five different PTCA balloon catheters. All the balloons were 3.0 mm in nominal diameter. PTCA, percutaneous transluminal coronary angioplasty.

The RBP indicated by the manufacturer represents the maximum recommended pressure for safe use of the balloon, and it is calculated from a statistically sufficient number of tests, ensuring that 99.9% of the tested balloons will not fail at RBP with 95% confidence.[21] There is typically only a small pressure difference between RBP (recommended maximum pressure) and balloon rupture (failure), indicating a low margin of safety beyond RBP.

Bending Stiffness

Bending stiffness is an important physical parameter of many interventional devices. When the bending stiffness is low, passage through curved pathways is expected to be easy and nontraumatic, but sufficient axial stiffness is required for the operator to be able to transmit the forces and control catheter movement. Low bending stiffness means high flexibility.

The flexibility of catheters and stents are measured using the setup shown in the Figure 5-10. The test object is fixed by a grip. The free bending length is fixed at 12 mm for practical reasons. The bending deformation *d* is applied automatically using the linear actuator. The resulting force *F* is measured by the load cell, which is contacted by a special device. The load cell has a measurement range of 0 to 100 mN at an accuracy of ±0.5% FS.

The displacement and force information is recorded using a computer, connected via a serial interface. The force-distance curve describes the spring modulus of the test object for bending. The bending stiffness (*EI*) is calculated taking the mean value of *F/d*, indicated by linear regression of the entire force-distance curve using the equation

$$EI = \frac{F \cdot l^3}{3d}$$

based on the theory describing the mechanics of a bent beam (*F*, bending force; *l*, bending length; *d*, bending deflection).[22]

Taking into account possible asymmetric structural properties of the test samples, the bending stiffness is measured in five different directions around the circumference and averaged. Typical results are discussed later, together with measurements of stent delivery systems with and without crimped stents.

Trackability, Crossability, and Pushability

The term *trackability* takes its origin from within the border zone between medicine and engineering. It describes the ability of a system to be advanced to a target lesion affected by several technical parameters such as friction, bending stiffness, and other factors.

The measurement of a vascular system's tracking ability is designed to assess the ability of a stent/balloon system to pass

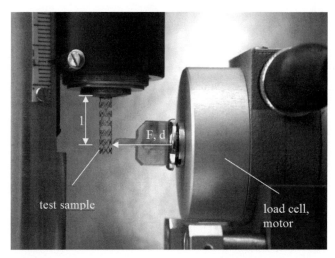

FIGURE 5-10. Test setup for the measurement of the flexibility of a cylindrical device (shown on behalf of an expanded coronary stent).

from a guiding catheter along a predetermined curved path. The results allow objective comparisons between different devices for each predetermined path. Long experience in measuring trackability shows experimental and clinical data to be highly comparable.

The measurements can be performed using a two-channel push device (Fig. 5-11), which allows measurements of proximal and distal forces during the passage of the stent system through the guiding catheter and the vessel model. The test path is adapted to the anatomy of coronary vessels (Fig. 5-12), iliac bifurcation, or renal artery. A guiding catheter and a guidewire complete the simulated test environment. The test path is placed in a water bath at 37°C, to simulate the physiologic conditions important for the mechanical properties of hydrophilic or hydrophobic coatings of the catheters, associated with low-friction gliding, and for the mechanics of polymer devices.

For each dilatation or stent delivery system pushed through the test path, the tracking forces required along the path are measured, and the force-distance curves are recorded. Typical tracking curves are presented in Figure 5-13. From the tracking curves, it is clear that for all dilatation balloon catheters, the required track force increases with the length of the path. This behavior is immanent in the system because friction forces accumulate, and the larger the upfront loading force (indicated by the severity and rigidity of the obstruction at the catheter tip), the greater the pushing force required and the greater the tendency of the tip of balloon catheter to bend. However, the required pushing forces are decreasing as the design of modern balloon and catheter technology improves. Most balloon catheters and stent delivery systems currently used are coated with thin polymer layers to reduce the friction coefficient between the guiding catheter and the dilata-

tion balloon, and between the dilatation balloon and the surrounding endovascular environment. The importance of coating can be measured using track tests and appears significant; yet, systematic comparison tests are difficult to perform because information on the nature of the coating is rarely available.

The *crossability* of a catheter describes its ability to pass stenoses. It is measured as a reactive head force distal to the stenosis. To test crossability, a setup can be used that simulates a vessel path with a stenosis at its end (Fig. 5-14). In this model, the lesion is characterized by an eccentric conical narrowing of the lumen, ranging from 2.5 to 1.2 mm. The model is attached to a load cell to measure the distal reactive force F_{dist}, which is taken as the measure of crossability. The proximal push force F_{prox}, applied by the operator to pass the lesion, is measured in parallel. It can be used to separate friction and bending effects along the whole catheter. The test arrangement of the vessel model with the simulated lesion is shown in Figure 5-14. For the crossability tests, the proximal traverse path of the drive is 60 mm long, starting from the end of the vessel model (point A in the figure). Distal displacement is not measured directly, but is assumed to be a little lower than the proximal traverse path due to catheter bending.

It can be expected that a low (distal) crossing profile, defined as the largest diameter of the folded balloon, will correspond to a low cross force, resulting in high crossability. Although there is no generally accepted definition, it has been suggested that the average distal reaction force F_{dist} should be used as the measure of crossability of the catheter (the lower the force, the better the crossability). In addition to the crossing profile, crossability also depends on balloon folding and compression characteristics.

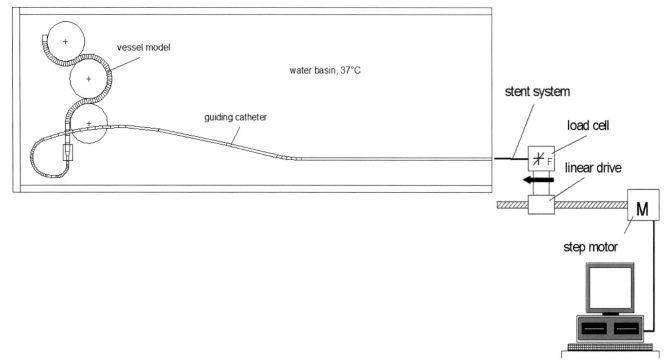

FIGURE 5-11. Schematic drawing of the two-channel push device with test arrangement for crossability investigations on coronary catheter/stent systems.

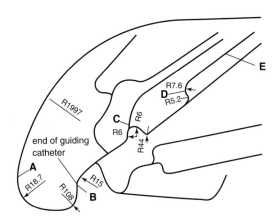

path	distance [mm]
A-B	60
A-C	115
A-D	175
A-E	220

FIGURE 5-12. Tortuous path in the vessel model for trackability measurements of coronary systems.

Pushability characterizes the load transfer from the proximal (interventionist's) end to the distal tip of the catheter. High load transfer allows finer and more direct tactile control of the instrumentation. Even small obstructions that cause only a minor increase in reaction forces at the catheter tip can be felt by the operator, allowing him to tune and finely adjust the pushing force to overcome the obstacle while utilizing the least

injurious maneuver. At the same time, high load transfer, if it is too high, may exceed the tactile abilities of the operator to precisely control and adjust the forces exactly to match the encountered resistance, leading to the transfer of potentially injurious forces to the catheter tip. Pushability is given in percent by:

$$Pushability = \frac{F_{dist}}{F_{prox}} \cdot 100\%$$

where F_{dist} and F_{prox} stand for the maximal measured distal and proximal forces.

The test setup developed to measure pushability is shown in Figure 5-15. It consists of a thrust piece (simulating a total occlusion) with a load cell at its distal end. To measure the distal reaction force, the proximal push force is measured with the second force channel. The push test is stopped in a force-controlled manner when the proximal force exceeds a specified maximum force to avoid catheter damage (e.g., 4.0 N). Before each test, the distal end of the stent delivery system is placed immediately in front of the simulated occlusion (starting point). The results given in Figure 5-16 show that <50% of the proximally applied force is transferred to the distal tip of the balloon catheter. Although the exact percentage may vary depending on specific test arrangements, the general challenge presented by difficult anatomical substrates to catheter technology is evident. The properties required include a low profile and high flexibility, but also high axial stiffness. All solutions are trade-offs with respect to design, material selection, manufacturing process, and tolerances.

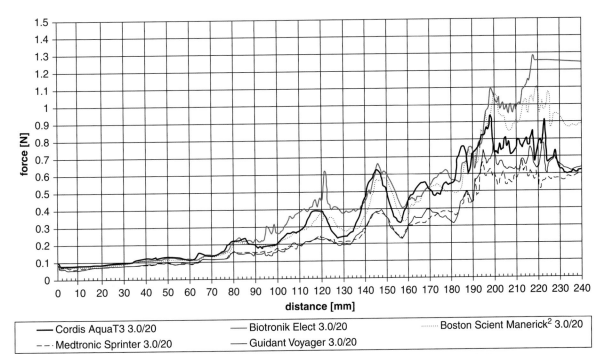

FIGURE 5-13. Force-distance curves of PTCA balloon catheters passing the coronary tortuous path from points *A* to *E*. PTCA, percutaneous transluminal coronary angioplasty.

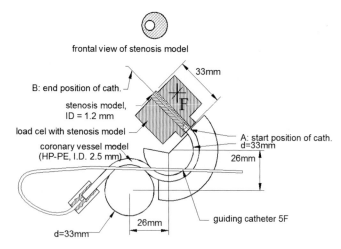

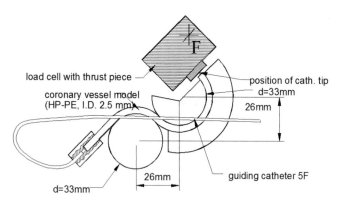

FIGURE 5-14. Test arrangement for the crossability measurements of PTCA balloon catheters or coronary stent systems using a stenosis model. PTCA, percutaneous transluminal coronary angioplasty.

FIGURE 5-15. Total occlusion at the distal end of the test path as used for the pushability tests.

VASCULAR STENTS

PERFORMANCE PARAMETERS

Vascular stents are designed for endovascular implantation and to act as scaffolding for collapsing vessel walls. For implantation, stents are mounted on delivery systems, typically balloon catheters (balloon-expandable stents, Fig. 5-17) or delivery-specific catheters (self-expanding stents).

Within the two groups of balloon-expandable and self-expanding stents, individual stents can be classified into categories based on a number of criteria:

- Stent material (stainless steel, tantalum, cobalt-chromium alloys, nitinol, recently also biodegradable polymers and metals)
- Type of coating to reduce thrombogenicity and the risk of restenosis (passive coatings such as heparin, phosphorylcholine, carbon-based coatings, silicon carbide, and active coatings for local drug release and biologically modified surfaces)
- Technology of stent production (laser-cut and wire-based stents)
- Stent structure

Because the stent structure is of basic importance for stent mechanics,[23–26] it will be discussed in greater detail, starting with the different types of designs:

- *Slotted tube stents* are made just by cutting longitudinal slashes in tubes. This structure provides a rhombuslike geometry of the cells of opened stents. The best known example is the Palmaz-Schatz stent, which was later modified to improve its flexibility.
- *Modular stents* consist of several crown-shaped modules, which may be manufactured from metal wires that are punctually connected to form a tube, or they may be laser cut

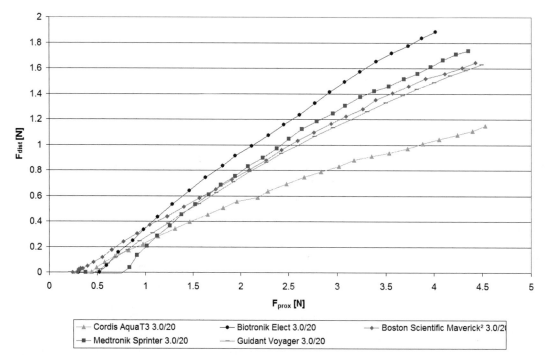

FIGURE 5-16. Distal reactive force as a function of applied proximal push force (test concluded at 3.5 N of proximal force).

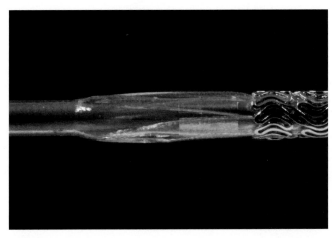

FIGURE 5-17. Detail of a balloon expanding stent system with distal balloon shoulder and distal part of the crimped stent (Boston Scientific Liberté).

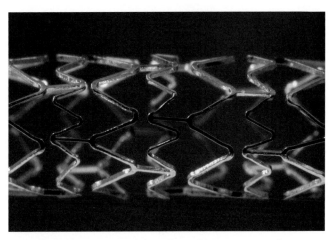

FIGURE 5-18. Modular stent—Boston Scientific Express[2].

from single tubes. Thanks to their modular design, these stents are expected to be highly flexible. Typical examples are the Medtronic-AVE S660/S670 stents (Medtronic, Minneapolis, MN, USA) and the Boston Scientific Express stent (Boston Scientific, Natick, MA, USA; Fig. 5-18).

- *Multicellular stents* have a completely closed cell design where the stent segments are connected by longitudinal connectors. Strictly multicellular stents are less flexible but provide uniform vessel wall coverage preventing tissue prolapse. This design is demonstrated by the Guidant Multi-Link (Guidant, Indianapolis, IN, USA) and Boston Scientific NIR(Boston Scientific, Natick, MA, USA) stents (Fig. 5-19).
- *Modular-multicellular stents* combine modular and multicellular design principles to achieve adapted properties regarding longitudinal and radial flexibility, uniformity of wall coverage, and constant length. Stents of this group, which are sometimes also called hybrid stents, are the BioDivYsio OC/SV/AS (Biocompatibles, Farnham, UK) or the Biotronik Rithron, Lekton Motion, and Pro Kinetic stents (Biotronik, Berlin, Germany) (Fig. 5-20).

Although some stent-specific terms are commonly used to describe stent structures, no standard terminology and nomenclature applicable to stent design and stent geometry have yet been developed. The vocabulary that is consequently available to describe the complex three-dimensional geometrical patterns that determine the performance characteristics of the stents is limited.

- A *strut* is a single element that forms larger structural entities such as cells, rings, or crowns.
- The term *cell* is used for a small but regularly repetitive structure of a stent. Open cells have a more complicated structure than closed cells, which enclose a simpler geometric area. Cells represent the elementary geometrical figure of the stent; they will deform during stent expansion.
- *Rings* and *crowns* comprise a cluster of cells forming a higher-order geometrical pattern of the stent, which may form complete *stent segments* usually coupled by longitudinal *bridges* or *links*.

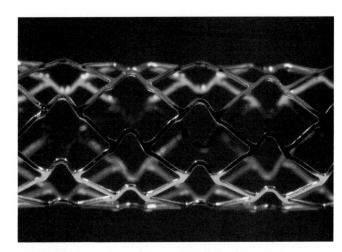

FIGURE 5-19. Multicellular stent—Boston Scientific NIR stent.

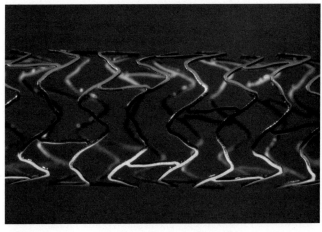

FIGURE 5-20. Modular-multicellular stent—Biotronik Pro Kinetic.

Thus, struts, cells, rings, and segments represent increasingly complex geometrical elements in a hierarchical order, which together form the complex three-dimensional surface geometry of individual stents.

Mechanical function is determined by stent structure. In most cases, however, interactions are still rather complex. Some rules of thumb are:

- Segmented stents with open cells separate radial from longitudinal deformation, with the consequence that radial strength does not have to depend on flexibility
- The higher the number of longitudinal links, the lower the stent's flexibility, but the more regular the wall coverage
- Closed-cell designs provide a less flexible but regular structure
- Modular-multicellular designs try to combine the advantages of multicellular and modular stents.

Most stent designs represent a compromise between the desired functional parameters (for definition, measurement, and discussion, see below), manufacturing limitations, and commercial practicability. And last but not least, typical stent design principles are the subject of many patents protecting the intellectual property and market claims of the owners.

Although the operating principle of self-expanding stents is different from that of balloon-expandable stents, the design principles are similar. A typical, modular, self-expanding stent indicated for use in peripheral vasculature is Precise (Cordis, Warren, NJ, USA) (Fig. 5-21). A summary of stent designs would be incomplete without mentioning of the mesh stent principle represented by the Wallstent (Boston Scientific, Natick, MA, USA; originally marketed by Schneider, Bülach, Switzerland), shown in Figure 5-22. Wallstents are woven from several single wires and provide mechanical properties that are difficult to compare with those of other stent types because they have no cells, or linked segments. The entire structure is a homogeneous unit. Wallstents have an extremely smooth outer contour, are highly flexible if longitudinal displacements are not constricted by the vessel wall, have no longitudinally fixed points, and shorten markedly during expansion. Tissue coverage, including bends, is excellent.

The delivery catheters of balloon-expandable stents have to meet requirements similar to those for regular high-pressure

dilatation balloon catheters. Consequently, the same set of performance parameters must be measured and the same test devices must be used to assess the performance of stent delivery systems for both types of catheters. Additional parameters are derived from interactions of the mounted stent with the catheter as well as from the stent's mechanical properties during and after deployment. Specific stent-related parameters include:

- *Outer contour* of the bent stent in its crimped state to assess the propensity of smooth passage of sharp edges and rough lesions
- *Firmness of crimped stents* to avoid stent dislodgment or loss before expansion
- Mechanics of stent deployment including *length change* (accurate placement), *profile during expansion*, and *elastic recoil* after balloon deflation and removal
- Sufficient *radial strength* to ensure the support function of the stent
- *Radial force* during expansion of self-expanding stents
- *Stent structure* (e.g., cell size, spatial arrangement, stent-free surface area) for optimum scaffolding of the stented vessel and to avoid protrusion of tissue debris
- Low *bending stiffness* (or high flexibility) of expanded stents for optimum anatomical adaptation
- *Radiopacity* of stents for fluoroscopic monitoring of primary success and follow-up
- *Fatigue resistance* of implanted stents during their lifetime while subject to long-term loading

Although this list may be incomplete, it summarizes the most common characteristics of vascular stents that are currently discussed. Other specifications are related to coated and drug-eluting stents (DESs) that recently became state of the art. Most of these new DESs are based, however, on established, conventional, balloon-expandable stent designs, and the identical mechanical considerations also apply. Such DESs consist of a metallic structure, similar to stents based on traditional stent designs, which is responsible for most of the mechanical properties. The eluted drug is linked by a degradable or permanent polymer coating only a few micrometers in thickness. Such coatings are not expected to change the mechanical strength, but may affect surface friction (tribology). Stents may adhere more tightly to the balloon surface, which may result in firmer

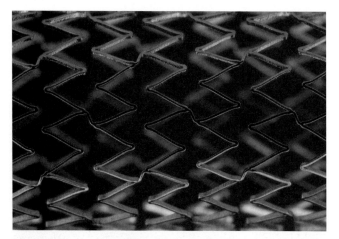

FIGURE 5-21.   Modular peripheral stent—Cordis Precise.

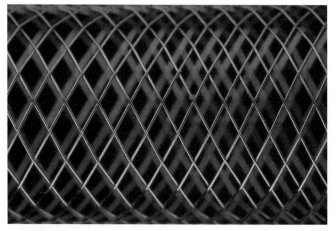

FIGURE 5-22.   Mesh stent—Boston Scientific Wallstent.

crimping. On the other hand, trackability and crossability may be reduced by higher friction coefficients. Both of these effects have to be investigated in systematic studies.

Last but not least, new diagnostic technology, such as magnetic resonance imaging (MRI), creates new requirements on the properties of stent materials to achieve MRI compatibility. This includes MRI safety and efficacy of MRI imaging.[27]

TEST METHODS

Outer Contour of Bent Stents and Stent Systems

Usually, stents are designed to provide a smooth and even outer surface contour when mounted on the balloon catheter. But when bent, this smooth contour may be disturbed depending on the stent structure, size, and thickness of stent struts. Because bending is unavoidable, it is desirable for any kind of kink effects to be avoided.

The outer contour is tested by bending the stent delivery system in the stent-carrying region using a specified bending radius (i.e., $R = 7.5$ mm for coronary stent systems, larger radii for peripheral stents; Fig. 5-23). The outer contour can be documented using an incident light microscope or a video system consisting of a video camera with a PC frame-grabber card.

The stent-delivery system to be analyzed is introduced into the test system over a guidewire according to the specifications of the manufacturer (0.014, 0.018, or 0.035 in.), which fixes the stent region in close contact with the radius of the selected flexion. Photographs of the outer contour are taken, and several parameters are visually assessed. Of special interest are the regions of transition between the stent and the balloon catheter as well as the middle part of the bent stent (Fig. 5-24). Distances by which individual cells deviate from being perfectly

round curvatures, the so-called fish-scale effect, can be measured by a traveling microscope if required by the individual test standard.

Firmness of Crimping (Dislodgment Force)

Under no circumstances should the stent be lost from the delivery catheter before reaching the desired position across the target lesion. A number of delivery conditions may reduce the risk of stent dislodgment, including low friction of the path, optimum support by the guidewire, and predilatation of a severe lesion that facilitates crossing. Sufficiently firm crimping, however, is required in all cases.

The stent-dislodgment force is defined as the force required to move the crimped stent on the evacuated balloon. The test is performed using a universal test machine equipped with a load cell (range ± 50 N, accuracy 0.05% FS; Fig. 5-25).

To measure the stent-dislodgment force, the shaft of the balloon catheter is gripped at one end of the tensile testing fixture. The stent is attached to the other grip with adhesive tape (Fig. 5-25). The distal part of the stent system is supported by a guidewire in the guidewire lumen of the balloon catheter. The balloon is kept under vacuum during the test. The distance between the grips is standardized as is the traverse speed and the travel distance. The force required to pull the grips apart is measured as a function of the grip-separation distance. The force at which the stent first moves relative to the balloon is taken as the stent-dislodgment force. Higher pull forces may occur when the stent is moved over the distal balloon shoulder.

It is useful to measure the dislodgment forces for each type of stent system in its original state and after conclusion of mechanical loading, such as after track, cross, and push tests and additional bending, because most stent systems tend to lose their firm grip as a result of small displacements between

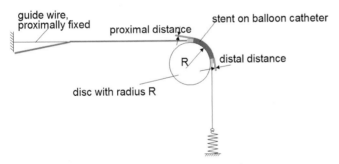

FIGURE 5-23. Test setup for the measurement of the outer contour of curved stents.

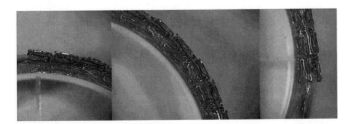

FIGURE 5-24. Guidant Vision 3.0/15, outer contour of bent stent ($R = 7.5$ mm)—proximal end, middle portion, and distal end of the stent (*from left to right*).

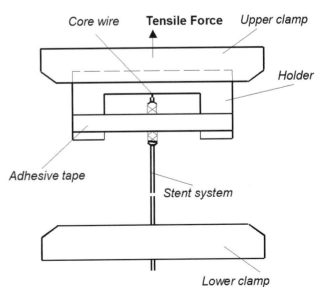

FIGURE 5-25. Test setup for the measurement of dislodgment forces.

stent and balloon. Initial static friction forces, which are always higher than dynamic friction, and an initial form fit between the balloon and the stent struts may be diminished because of these small displacements. In practice, it is recommended that unnecessary flexion of the stent region during the implantation procedure be avoided to reduce the risk of stent loss. Figures 5-26 and 5-27 demonstrate the differences in firmness of crimping both between originally crimped and preloaded stent systems, and between different stent and balloon designs.

Stent Deployment, Profile, Length Change, and Elastic Recoil

Stent deployment is a rather complex process which is influenced not only by the pressure-diameter characteristics of the inflated balloon (see the earlier subsection on "Balloon Compliance"), but also by the structural mechanical properties of the stent, interactions between balloon and stent, and—importantly—between the stent and vessel walls. To document

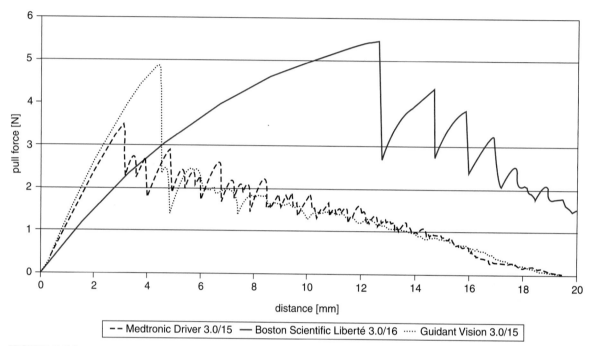

FIGURE 5-26.   Force-distance curves from measurement of stent dislodgment forces (original stent systems without any preloading).

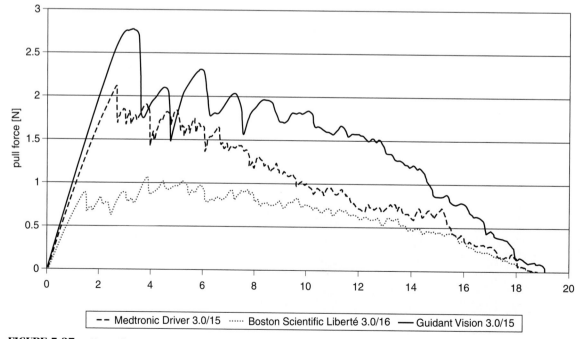

FIGURE 5-27.   Force-distance curves from measurement of stent dislodgment forces (stent systems preloaded by track, cross, and push tests).

stent performance fully, it is recommended that as many parameters as possible be measured and that the entire process of stent expansion be visualized and documented.

To measure and characterize stent deployment, the basic setup described earlier is employed. Using this setup, the profile of the stent system is measured in its original state (crimped stent) and during all subsequent adjusted balloon pressure steps. Figure 5-28 shows that stent expansion starts at the distal and proximal balloon shoulders and stent ends, respectively, which are typical and help the stent to sit and to hold itself inside the stenosis. This characteristic shape has been termed the "dog-bone" effect in the literature. In general, dog boning is thought to potentially damage the target vessel distal or proximal to the target lesion. However, as in the case shown here, the balloon diameter is smaller than the expected final diameter of the fully expanded stent, thus making vessel wall damage by an initial dog-bone effect unlikely. However, the necessity of inflating the balloon at high pressure to achieve full expansion and apposition might be associated with an early full expansion of stent ends, making the dog-bone effect potentially traumatic.

Figure 5-28 further demonstrates the appearance of a fully expanded stent at a balloon pressure of 6 bar, following gradual inflation in steps of 2 bar. The total expansion could have taken place between 4 and 6 bar in this setting. Stent diameter increases with balloon inflation pressure, showing characteristics similar to those observed when measuring balloon compliance.

In the course of the measurement, the stent is deployed with maximum pressure of 9 bar, corresponding to NP (diameter d_{NP}). Subsequently, the balloon is deflated, and the profile measured again. The resulting curve delivers the stent diameter after expansion (d_{recoil}) and contains information on elastic deformation, which is called elastic recoil. Calculation of elastic recoil is performed using the following equation:

$$Recoil = \frac{d_{NP} - d_{recoil}}{d_{NP}} \cdot 100\%$$

The amount of elastic recoil depends on the individual stent structure, the degree of stent expansion, and the deformation characteristics of the stent material. Slotted-tube stainless steel stents usually have recoil values of about 3% to 5%, whereas modern cobalt-chromium stents tend to have slightly larger elastic recoil (around 5%, Fig. 5-29).

The larger recoil of newer stents does not appear to be critical at this level, but should be observed in future developments. In deploying the stent, it must be considered that the stent has to be overdilated at least by the amount of its elastic recoil to achieve full apposition. However, it should also be kept in mind that excessive overdilation carries the risk of uncontrolled vessel wall dissections and ruptures.

Stent length may be measured before and after stent expansion with a digital caliper or measurement microscope. The results demonstrate the influence of stent structure on any shortening or prolongation of the stent. Ideally, the stent should not change its length during expansion, to facilitate exact placement.

Radial Strength

The intended main function of a stent is to provide scaffolding for a vessel wall that is mechanically unstable because of spontaneous or iatrogenic plaque rupture. The loads actually acting on a stent in vivo are not exactly known and may vary considerably as a result of the different mechanical properties of individual vessel walls. Nevertheless, the supporting function must be described, and a minimum radial strength must be guaranteed for each stent.

Radial strength is measured with the pressure controller, pressurizing a test chamber sealed with a cover plate (Fig. 5-30). The

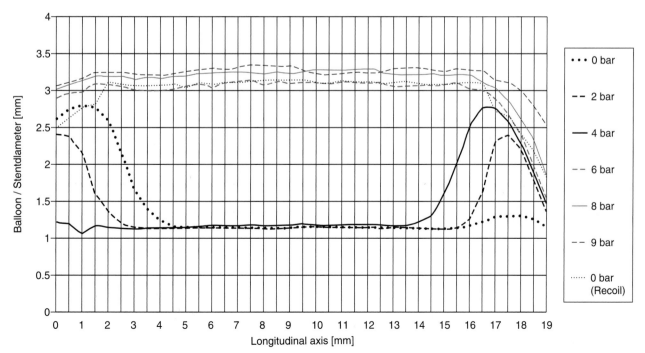

FIGURE 5-28.   Stent system diameter as a function of the balloon pressure (Medtronic AVE Driver 3.0/15).

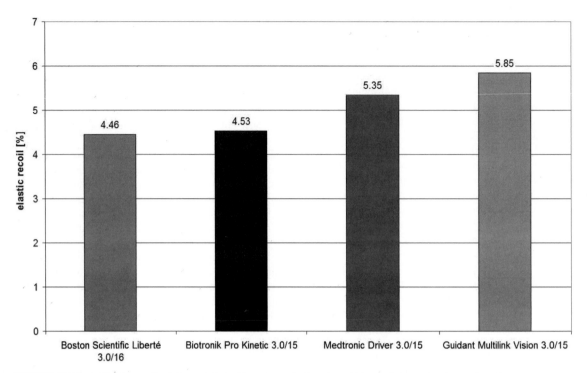

FIGURE 5-29. Elastic recoil of three Cobalt Chromium, CoCr, stents (Biotronik Pro Kinetic, Medtronic Driver, Guidant Multilink Vision) compared to a stainless steel stent (Boston Scientific Liberté).

stent is encased in a tube that simulates the vasculature and at the same time separates the stent from the temperature-controlled (37°C) water bath. The tube that simulates the vasculature is fabricated from polyurethane. It has an internal diameter equal to the nominal diameter of the stent and a typical wall thickness of 0.075 mm. This thin-walled test tube is so flexible that it will not support any outer pressure load. The connection of the stent to atmospheric pressure is accomplished with a pipe and a gland joint.

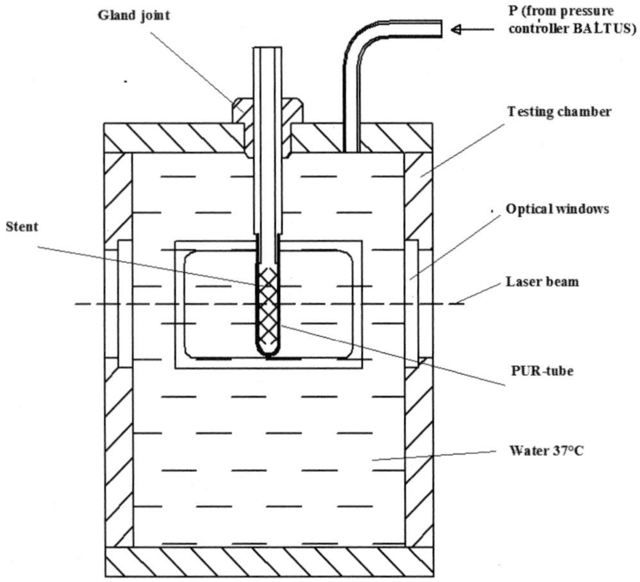

For the measurement, the test chamber is completely filled with temperature-controlled water and connected via a tubing system to the pressure controller. A radial outer load is applied to the stent by increasing the pressure in the test chamber. The use of a pressure load instead of a single force guarantees uniform circumferential loading with forces perpendicular to the outer surface of the test tube and transmitted directly to the stent structure. The pressure at which the stent can no longer bear the loading and collapses is called collapse pressure, which is considered a measure of the stent's radial strength. To generate reproducible pressure versus diameter curves, it is imperative that the stent makes contact with the surrounding polyurethane tube over its entire peripheral length. This is accomplished by placing the stent directly into the testing tube using a balloon delivery catheter. The beam of a laser scanner is focused on the center of the stent to measure the stent diameter at the various pressure steps here.

Current coronary stents are able to withstand an outer pressure of 1.0 to 1.5 bar or even higher, yet 0.5 bar may be sufficient, as measured on commercially available, clinically widely used stents in the 1990s. Stents for peripheral use have larger diameters than coronary devices, and thus a larger mantle surface. Therefore, their radial force is lower and they can withstand only substantially lower pressure before collapsing (Fig. 5-31). In self-expanding stents, the collapse is reversible and of lesser importance provided there is sufficient elasticity and radial strength to hold up against standard outer forces and loads.

FIGURE 5-30. Testing chamber for radial strength determination.

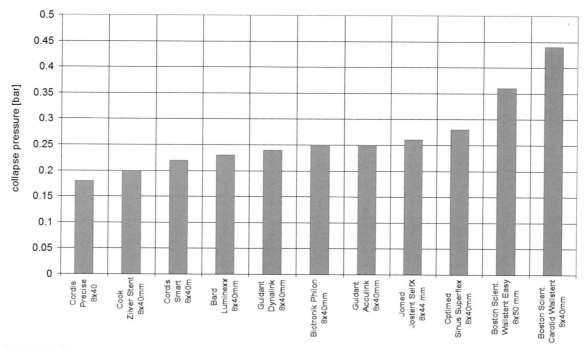

FIGURE 5-31. Collapse pressure values, measured on several self-expanding stents (nominal diameter 8.0 mm).

Radial Force of Self-expanding Stents

Self-expanding stents are implanted by removing a cover sheath from the compressed stent. Since the radial force of the stent initially acts on the vessel wall to reopen the lumen, only a minimum amount of radial force is required for the stent to open. Subsequent balloon dilatation using a larger force may be required to improve stent apposition. On the other hand, self-expanding stents cannot be overexpanded to a size larger than their nominal diameter to achieve intimate contact with the vessel wall and to avoid stent migration. If overexpanded, they would immediately return to their nominal diameter or lower. Thus, to place these stents safely and permanently, their diameter following full expansion should be greater than the diameter of the target vessel at the target segment. The radial force of these stents should only be moderate in order to prevent high stresses from being permanently exerted on the vessel walls.

Radial force can be determined using a divided prismatic setup with d_{min} as the minimum distance of opposite planes (see Fig. 5-32). The distance d_{min} is also the minimum diameter of the stent which is released in the test setup. The resulting force F is measured by a universal test machine. Subsequently, the distance is increased, and F is measured in parallel. Because of the geometry of the test setup, radial force F_R can be represented by the following equation:

$$F_R = \frac{1}{\sqrt{2}} \cdot F$$

Figure 5-33 shows the radial forces measured for several self-expanding stents. They were normalized by the nominal length of the stent for better comparison. Nearly all self-expanding stents are made of nitinol, a memory shape alloy with super-elastic properties; one exception is the Carotid Wallstent, which is made of a so-called drawn-filled tubing alloy.[28]

Bending Stiffness of Expanded Stents

Stent flexibility (or to be technically more precise, bending stiffness, which is inversely proportional to flexibility) has been considered a decisive mechanical parameter responsible for the navigation and tracking of complex and tortuous vascular anatomy. Furthermore, stent flexibility avoids straightening of the vessel, mechanical friction at the transition points between

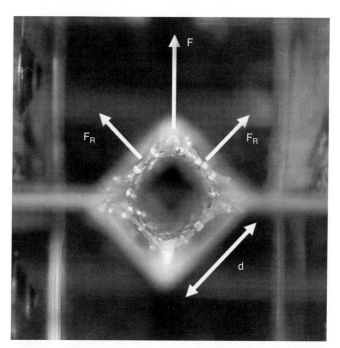

FIGURE 5-32. Arrangement for the measurement of the radial force of stents as a function of their expansion diameter.

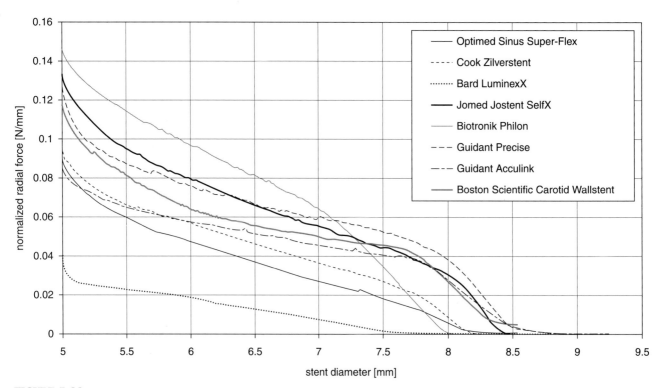

FIGURE 5-33.   Radial forces of different self-expanding stents, normalized by the stent length (nominal expanded diameter 8.0 mm).

stent and native vessel, and blood flow obstructions, thus improving long-term results.

The bending stiffness of a stent can be measured by several means.[6,8,9,17] The most common one was described earlier. This method is based on the idea of measuring the force necessary to achieve a defined deformation. To hold the stent within the grip, it is supported by an inner rod inside the grip. This rod does not affect the bending stiffness of the stent outside the grip.

The bending stiffness of dilatation balloon catheters or stent delivery systems with mounted stents differs significantly from that of expanded stents. Figure 5-34 demonstrates the differences in both parameters measured in self-expanding stents and their delivery systems. The differences may be significant, but they are remarkably lower in the coronary than in carotid delivery systems. Coronary stent systems and coronary stents must be more flexible.

During expansion, the geometrical structure of the stent changes dramatically, which may lead to a completely different bending stiffness. This difference appears particularly great in multicellular stent designs. In modular stents, this effect is reduced by means of a spatial geometrical arrangement that utilizes only a few, very flexible joints between stiffer segments. It has been shown that optimal geometric design of the individual stent components make it possible for high stent flexibility to be successfully combined with sufficient radial stiffness.[29]

In addition to bending stiffness, the geometry of the stent in bends and curves determines the overall clinical performance of the stent delivery system. Partial straightening of parts of the stent on beds, termed fish scaling, may increase resistance and cause vessel wall injury by protruding struts.

Radiopacity (Visibility)

The visibility of balloon catheters, stent systems, and implanted (expanded) stents during transcatheter revascularizations is based on their radiopacity. Because the x-ray attenuation coefficient of most of the polymer components is low, which means that they generally remain invisible on radiography, balloon catheters and stent delivery systems require radiopaque markers for visualization. These markers are made from metals of higher atomic weight (e.g., tantalum, gold, platinum) or other chemical compounds (e.g., barium sulfate), and their inside edges usually indicate the beginning and end of the straight segment of dilatation balloons and/or the full length of mounted stents. The majority of metallic stents are, however, sufficiently visible and do not require any radiopaque markers. Yet some stents that consist of thin struts or less radiopaque stent material (Cobalt Chromium, CoCr, Nickel Titanium, NiTi) may require additional markers.

There is no specific test for the radiopacity of stents and related delivery systems. Other test methods, such as that used for medical plastics, are usually adapted and provide adequate results. An American Society for Testing and Materials (ASTM) standard[30] describes a setup and methodology for devices in the shape of film, sheet, rod, tube, and moldings in order to indicate the likelihood of locating the parts within the human body. The setup consists of a standardized arrangement of x-ray tube, filters, body phantom, and a grid to reduce scattering effects. Most current standards[31,32] are based on film systems that measure and evaluate the resulting optical density (Fig. 5-35).

Modern digital x-ray systems can also be used with a similar arrangement, but they analyze the digital gray-scale values of the test sample and standard test specimen such as an aluminum phantom of different thicknesses.

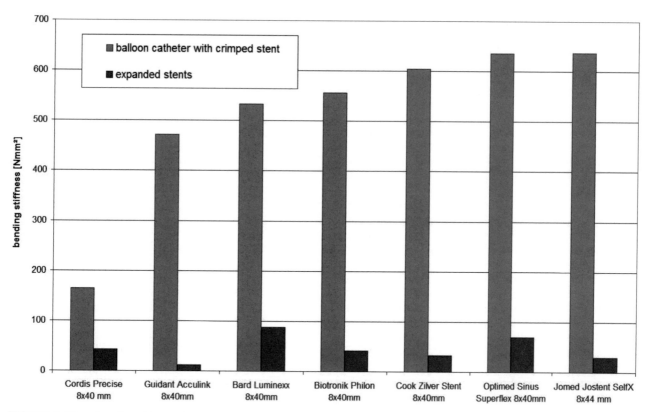

FIGURE 5-34. Bending stiffness of stent delivery systems with mounted stents compared to expanded stents (self-expanding stents).

In Figure 5-36 several self-expanding peripheral stents are shown. Slight differences in the radiopacity of the stent bodies can be seen. Fluoroscopic markers on four of the stents mark the ends and remarkably improve the stent visibility. Usually, the radiopacity of markers on balloon catheters or stent delivery systems is considerably higher than that of stents.

Fatigue Analysis

Vascular stents are permanent implants that are exposed to a variety of loading conditions during their lifetime. Even if they resist the primary loads, long-term cyclic loading may cause

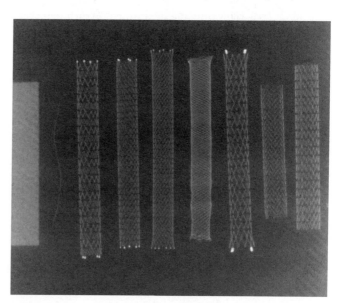

FIGURE 5-36. X-ray image of the expanded peripheral stents. (*Left to right*)—10–mm thick poly(methyl methacrylate) reference; 80 μm tungsten wire; Biotronik Astron; Cook Zilverstent; Cordis Smart Control; Boston Scientific Wallstent RP; Bard Luminexx; Guidant Dynalink; Jomed Jostent SelfX (Siemens Mobilett, 70 kV, 10 mAs).

FIGURE 5-35. Imaging setup for determining x-ray contrast according to DIN 13273–7.

fatigue fractures. Therefore, a detailed, in vitro, fatigue analysis is always required before product approval for marketing. National and international product standards or guidance documents describe the needs for such testing.[21,27,32] All of these tests are designed as nondestructive tests. They are designed to show that the devices will not disintegrate and become dysfunctional while exposed to physiological long-term loading stresses. However, the great variety of testing devices and testing protocols makes direct comparison between individual measurements nearly impossible. However, some of the ongoing discussions concern the kind of loading sufficiently representative to mimic physiological loading relevant to the stent applications.

It is generally accepted that radial loading that arises from the arterial pulse pressure (difference between diastolic and systolic pressures) acts on all arterial stents. Three different test principles for pulsatile loading are known. The first approach, called the *physiological pressure test method*, uses a mock artery with physical parameters similar to native vessels, in which the stent is implanted and loaded by applying physiological static and dynamic hydraulic pressure within the vessel model.[33] The stent load arises from the elastic properties of the mock artery. The *diameter control test method* uses artery models that are stiffer than their physiological counterparts and applies an inner pressure that causes vessel wall displacements related to physiological loading conditions. The pressure-generated change in diameter is controlled externally (i.e., by a laser scanner). Both of these test methods are limited with respect to test loading frequency by the material properties of the test tubes.[36]

In a third method, the *external pressure test method*, physiological loading is applied to the stent by outer hydraulic, static, and dynamic pressure.[37] Additional loading is provided by overexpansion of the stent inserted into the thin-walled polymeric test tube. The degree of overexpansion and the hydraulic loading are adjusted such that the loading is equivalent to targeted physiological pressures (Fig. 5-37). Tests have shown that frequency limitations result only from the stent structure, such that accelerated testing at 100 Hz and above is possible (Fig. 5-38[38]).

Stents for peripheral vasculature may have to bear additional loads, such as flexion, longitudinal tension, and torque. The test methods to simulate such loads are not standardized, but prototypes are being developed. It must be understood that limited stent fatigue resistance will continue to represent a con-

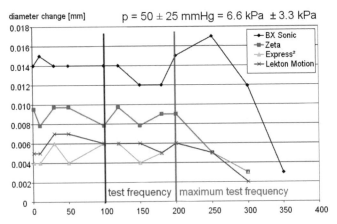

FIGURE 5-38. Pressure-induced stent displacement as a function of test frequency for fatigue testing with the external pressure test method.

siderable challenge for stenting in mechanically exposed regions such as the femoral and infrapopliteal arteries.

Specific Test Requirements for Recent Stent Developments

There are two major developments in the field of stent technology that should be briefly considered from the standpoint of functional parameters, namely, drug-eluting and biodegradable stents. Even the combination of both principles has potential and is under development.

DRUG-ELUTING STENTS. Drug-eluting stents were developed to solve the problem of restenosis by providing local delivery of a drug that would inhibit proliferation and migration of vascular smooth muscle cells. Several methods for the storage and controlled release of drugs have been designed. In the majority of cases a nondegradable or biodegradable polymer matrix is used as a drug carrier. Alternatively, cavities on the stent struts are used as drug depots. Small amounts of drugs have been also applied directly to the stent surface. Reviews of drug-eluting stent designs and selected drugs such as the nondegradable polymers polyurethane,[39] silicone,[40] polyorganophosphazene,[41] polymethacrylate,[42] poly(ethylene terephthalate),[43] and phosphorylcholine[44] are available in the literature. Furthermore, a number of biodegradable polymer matrices have also been investigated, including poly(l-lactide),[45] poly(3–hydroxybutyrate), polycaprolactone, polyorthoester,[40] and fibrin.[46] In order to avoid thrombosis following stent implantation, stents have been coated with the polysaccharide heparin,[47] which is known to inhibit blood coagulation. Among the antiproliferative drugs tested for release, the most important ones include antiphlogistic (i.e., dexamethasone, methylprednisolone),[41,48] cytostatic (paclitaxel, colchicine, actinomycin-D, methotrexate),[49–52] and immune suppressive (sirolimus, tacrolimus, cyclosporin A, mycophenol acid)[53,54] agents. To prevent thrombus formation, antithrombogenic inhibitors such as abciximab or iloprost[55,56] have been incorporated into the polymer matrix.

From the technical point of view, several new aspects of stent testing arise from drug-eluting stent technology. Although it is not expected that the thin polymer coatings will measurably

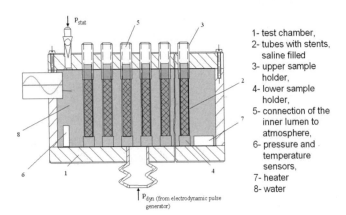

1- test chamber,
2- tubes with stents, saline filled
3- upper sample holder,
4- lower sample holder,
5- connection of the inner lumen to atmosphere,
6- pressure and temperature sensors,
7- heater
8- water

FIGURE 5-37. Fatigue test arrangement for external pressure test method.

change the structural behavior of the stents, such as their radial strength or flexural stiffness, some other differences may be measurable:

- Friction-related changes in trackability and crossability
- Adherence of crimped stents to the delivery balloon
- Structural integrity of the coating, in particular after simulated use in curved vessels and stenosis, after stent expansion, and after durability testing

Investigation of the coating integrity will require scanning electron microscopy and other high-resolution imaging techniques.

BIODEGRADABLE STENTS. Biodegradable stents are intended to support a vessel for just as long as is necessary to complete the healing process and to then disappear after a specified time period. On the basis of this principle, complications resulting from the long-term intravascular presence of a foreign body, including thrombogenicity, permanent mechanical irritation, and prevention of positive remodeling, are eliminated.

Several *polymeric biodegradable stent* designs have been reported, most of them based on poly(L-lactic acid) (PLLA), but some also on poly(D,L-lactic acid) (PDLA), poly(e-caprolactone) (PCL), and poly(glycolic acid) (PGA) materials (Fig. 5-39).[57,58] In addition to consideration of the biological interactions between the implants and the surrounding blood and tissue, polymer-specific properties must be taken into account since these may be affected by the manufacturing and sterilization processes.[58]

According to a summary by Labinaz et al.,[59] the important characteristics of an ideal intravascular stent include a low profile, a flexible design, and a relatively noncompliant balloon. It should be nonthrombogenic, adequately visible, and reliably expandable, with a high ratio between its crimped and expanded diameter. It should achieve complete wall contact. Corrosion resistance and mechanical durability are natural requirements for traditional metal stents, yet are of limited importance in degradable implants. From the technical point of view, a uniform biodegradation process appears critical, while overall biocompatibility combined with nontoxic degradation products represent essential requirements.

With regard to mechanical properties, conventional stents and polymeric stents should be compared using the same performance criteria. Thus, suboptimal deployment characteristics, even if achieved by a special expansion regime (e.g., balloon expansion by means of a heated dye,[60,61] larger profiles in the crimped state, low radial strength, and higher elastic recoil) may become critical for the clinical acceptance of biodegradable stents.[62]

To overcome the technical limitations of polymeric stents, *biodegradable metal stent models* have been developed. These models use corrodable materials such as magnesium alloys (Fig. 5-40)[63] or iron.[64] Following the first animal experiments with magnesium-based, absorbable metal stents,[65] design and material optimization has now led to the first implantation in humans "below the knee," and the clinical outcome after 12 months is promising.[66] A first human coronary clinical trial (PROGRESS) has also started. In this trial, excellent MRI compatibility was demonstrated as an additional benefit of the magnesium-based device.[67]

Biodegradable stents need to conform to the mechanical standards required for the deployment of traditional stents at the time of deployment. Because degradation proceeds as a corrosive process within the bloodstream, in vitro corrosion testing can be performed to determine degradation kinetics. Corrosion testing of biomaterials is known in the context of tests for biostable materials[68] to identify corrosion products. These tests assume low corrosion speed. The methodology has to be adapted to accommodate short-term degradable metals. Special emphasis should be on durability testing. Obviously, biodegradable stents are not required to endure implantation periods of several years, and their shorter lifetime has to be defined. In addition, tests that allow mechanical loading in a physiological corrosive environment will be required. Because of time-dependent degradation and corrosion processes, accelerated testing is limited to low test frequencies. This means that fatigue behavior is accompanied by corrosion or biodegradation during real-time testing at a normal pulse frequency.

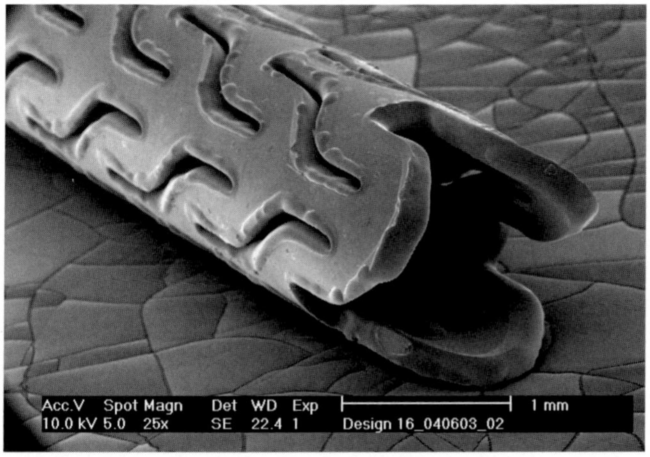

FIGURE 5-39. Scanning electron micrograph of a PLLA stent prototype. PLLA, poly(L-lactic acid). (Reproduced from Grabow N, Schlun M, Sternberg K, et al. Mechanical properties of laser cut poly (L-lactide) micro-specimens: implications for stent design, manufacture, and sterilization. *J Biomech Eng.* 2005;127:25–31, with permission from American Society of Medical Engineers, ASME.)

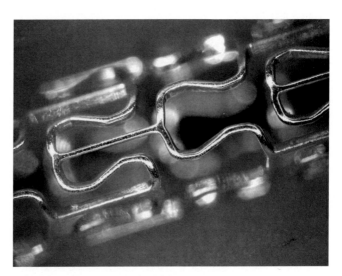

FIGURE 5-40. Biotronik Absorbable Metal Stent (AMS), based on a biocorrodable magnesium alloy.

To allow rigorous performance and quality control, standardized methods that are adapted to the shorter lifespan should be employed to test the mechanical performance of biodegradable stents compared with conventional bare metal stents.

CONCLUSION AND OUTLOOK

Endovascular interventions involve the precise handling of small devices over a distance ranging from several centimeters up to more than a meter in an anatomically difficult environment. Their successful performance depends primarily on the expertise and manual dexterity of the operator and on the suitability and quality of the instrumentation. Overcoming the adversities represented by the tortuosity and rigidity of the target vascular system along with the considerable structural complexity of the pathologically deformed endovascular interfaces represents a considerable challenge for the design and performance of the small devices.

Atraumatic advancing, precise positioning, and overcoming local obstacles at interventional sites impose the highest demands on a number of mechanical and biological device properties. Most of these properties can be measured and used to characterize device performances under standardized and highly reproducible conditions. The properties measured under these strictly controlled and well-defined conditions provide a framework for systematic comparisons between devices, thus permitting the development of more efficient endovascular devices. Furthermore, the objectively measured properties of endovascular instrumentation reflect the tactile experience of the master operators, allowing them a better understanding of their working tools and finer handling in actual clinical situations. New stent developments to prevent restenosis and bioabsorbable devices that allow the vessel to naturally remodel following temporary scaffolding will greatly improve the combined mechanical and biological endovascular repairs.

REFERENCES

1. King III SB, Meier B. Interventional treatment of coronary heart disease and peripheral vascular disease. *Circulation.* 2000;102:IV-81–IV-86.
2. Geddes KA, Geddes LE. *The Catheter Introducers.* Chicago: Mobium Press, 1983.
3. Duda SH, Wiskirchen J, Tepe G, et al. Physical properties of endovascular stents: an experimental comparison. *J Vasc Intervent Radiol.* 2000;11(5):645–654.
4. Dumoulin C, Cochelin B. Mechanical behaviour modelling of balloon-expandable stents. *J Biomech.* 2000;33(11):1461–1470.
5. Dyet JF, Watts WG, Ettles DF, et al. Mechanical properties of metallic stents: How do these properties influence the choice of stent for specific lesions? *Cardiovasc Intervent Radiol.* 2000;23:47–54.
6. Ormiston JA, Dixon SR, Webster MWI, et al. Stent longitudinal flexibility: a comparison of 13 stent designs before and after balloon expansion. *Cathet Cardiovasc Intervent.* 2000;50:120–124.
7. Rieu R, Barragan P, Garitey V, et al. Assessment of the trackability, flexibility, and conformability of coronary stents: a comparative analysis. *Cathet Cardiovasc Intervent.* 2003;59:496–503.
8. Schmidt W, Andresen R, Behrens P, et al. Characteristic mechanical properties of balloon expandable peripheral stent systems. *Fortschr Röntgenstr.* 2002;174:1430–1437.
9. Schmidt W, Behrens P, Behrend D, et al. Measurement of mechanical properties of coronary stents according to the European Standard prEN 12006–3. *Prog Biomed Res.* 1999;4:45–51.
10. Schmidt W, Behrens P, Kaminsky J, et al. Methodenspektrum zur strukturmechanischen Charakterisierung von Kathetern und Stents für arterielle Blutgefäße. *Biomed Technik.* 2003;48:394–395.
11. Schmidt W, Grabow N, Behrens P, et al. Trackability, crossability, and pushability of coronary stent systems—an experimental approach *Biomed. Technik.* 2002;47:124–126.
12. Schmitz K-P, Behrens P, Schmidt W, et al. Quality determining parameters of balloon angioplasty catheters. *J Invasive Cardiol.* 1996;8(4):144–152.
13. Schmitz K-P, Behrend D, Behrens P, et al. Entwicklung von Koronarstents und experimentelle Untersuchungen der strukturmechanischen Eigenschaften. *VDI Ber.* 1999;1463:79–84.
14. Schmitz K-P, Behrend D, Behrens P, et al. Comparative studies of different stent designs. *Prog Biomed Res.* 1999;4:52–58.
15. Schmitz K-P, Schmidt W, Behrens P, et al. In-vitro examination of clinically relevant stent parameters. *Prog Biomed Res.* 2000;5:197–203.
16. Stöckel D, Pelton A, Duerig T. Self-expanding nitinol stents: material and design considerations. *Eur Radiol.* 2004;14:292–301.
17. Wehrmeyer B, Kuhn F-P. Experimental studies of the pressure stability of vascular endoprostheses. *Fortschr Röntgenstr.* 1993;158(3):242–246.
18. ISO 1110: Plastics—Polyamides—Accelerated conditioning of test specimens.
19. ISO 291: Plastics—Standard atmospheres for conditioning and testing.
20. Saab, MA. Applications of high-pressure balloons in the medical device industry. *Med Dev Diagn Ind Mag.* 2000;9:86.
21. FDA, Non-clinical tests and recommended labeling for intravascular stents and associated delivery systems, guidance for industry and FDA staff. U.S. Department of Health and Human Services, Food and Drug Administration, Center for Devices and Radiological Health, January 13, 2005.
22. Young WC, Budynas RG. *Roark's Formulas for Stress and Strain.* 7th ed. New York: McGraw-Hill, 2002. *General Engineering Series.*
23. Wiskirchen J, Pusich B, Kramer U, et al. Stent struts and articulations: their impact on balloon-expandable stents' hoop strength, pushability, and radiopacity in an experimental setting. *Invest Radiol.* 2002;37:356–362.
24. Grewe PH, Machraoui A, Deneke T, et al. Structural analysis of 16 different coronary stent systems. *Z Kardiol.* 1997;86:990–999.
25. Lau KW, Mak KH, Hung JS, et al. Clinical impact of stent construction and design in percutaneous coronary intervention. *Am Heart J.* 2004;147:764–773.
26. Mahr P, Fischer A, Brauer H, et al. Biophysical study of coronary stents: which factors influence the dilatation and recoil behavior? *Z Kardiol.* 2000;89:513–521.
27. EN 14299:2004. Non-active surgical implants—Particular requirements for cardiac and vascular implants—specific requirements for arterial stents and endovascular prostheses.
28. Boston Scientific. Carotid Wallstent Monorail Carotid Endoprosthesis, instructions for use.
29. Schmitz K-P, Behrend D, Behrens P, et al. Interaction of radial strength and flexibility of coronary stents. *Biomed Technik.* 1998;43:376–377.
30. ASTM F640–79(2000). Standard test methods for radiopacity of plastics for medical use.
31. DIN 13273–7:2003–08. Katheter für den medizinischen Bereich—Teil 7: Bestimmung der Röntgenstrahlenschwächung von Kathetern; Anforderungen und Prüfung.
32. EN 12006–3:1998. Non-active surgical implants—Particular requirements for cardiac and vascular implants—Part 3: endovascular devices.
33. High frequency intravascular prosthesis fatigue tester. US patent 5 670 708. 1997.
34. Conti JC, Strope ER, Goldenberg LM, et al. The durability of silicone versus latex mock arteries. *Biomed Sci Instrum.* 2001;37:305–312.
35. Conti JC, Strope ER, Price KS, et al. The high frequency testing of vascular grafts and vascular stents: influence of sample dimensions on maximum allowable frequency. *Biomed Sci Instrum.* 1999;35:339–346.
36. Glenn R, Lee J. Accelerated pulsatile fatigue testing of Ni-Ti coronary stents. Available at: http://www.enduratec.com/techpapers.
37. Arrangement and method for testing of vascular implants. DE 19903476.1.
38. Schmidt W, Behrens P, Behrend D, et al. Fatigue analysis of coronary stents. *J Med Biol Eng Comput.* 1999;37(suppl 2):594–595.
39. Lambert TL, Dev V, Rechavia E, et al. Localized arterial wall drug delivery from a polymer-coated removable metallic stent. Kinetics, distribution, and bioactivity of forskolin. *Circulation.* 1994;90:1003.
40. van der Giessen WJ, Lincoff AM, Schwartz RS, et al. Marked inflammatory sequelae to implantation of biodegradable and nonbiodegradable polymers in porcine coronary arteries. *Circulation.* 1996;94:1690.
41. de Scheerder I, Wang K, Wilczek K, et al. Local methylprednisolone inhibition of foreign body response to coated intracoronary stents. *Coron Artery Dis.* 1996;7:161.
42. Suzuki T, Kopia G, Hayashi S, et al. Stent-based delivery of sirolimus reduces neointimal formation in a porcine coronary model. *Circulation.* 2001;104:1188–1193.
43. Schellhammer F, Walter M, Berlis A, et al. Polyethylene terephthalate and polyurethane coatings for endovascular stents: preliminary results in canine experimental arteriovenous fistulas. *Radiology.* 1999;211:169.
44. Chronos NAF, Robinson KA, Kelly AB, et al. Thromboresistant phosphorylcholine coating for coronary stents. *Circulation.* 1995;92:I-685.
45. Zilberman M, Schwade ND, Meidell RS, et al. Structured drug-loaded bioresorbable films for support structures. *J Biomater Sci.* 2001;12:875.
46. Holmes D, Camrud AR, Jorgenson MA, et al. Polymeric stenting in the porcine coronary artery model: differential outcome of exogenous fibrin sleeves versus polyurethane-coated stents. *J Am Coll Cardiol.* 1994;24:525–531.
47. Beythien C, Gutensohn K, Bau J, et al. Influence of stent length and heparin coating on platelet activation: a flow cytometric analysis in a pulsed floating model. *Thromb Res.* 1999;94:79–86.
48. Lincoff A, Furst JG, Ellis SG, et al. Sustained local delivery of dexamethasone by a novel intravascular eluting stent to prevent restenosis in the porcine coronary injury model. *J Am Coll Cardiol.* 1997;29:808–816
49. Drachman DE, Rogers C. Stent based release of paclitaxel to prevent restenosis. *Z Kardiol.* 2002;91:III/42.
50. Serruys PW, Ormiston JA, Sianos G, et al. Actinomycin-eluting stent for coronary revascularization: a randomized feasibility and safety study: the ACTION trial. *J Am Coll Cardiol.* 2004;44(7): 1363–1367.
51. Tanabe K, Serruys PW, Grube E, et al. TAXUS III Trial: in-stent restenosis treated with stent-based delivery of paclitaxel incorporated in a slow-release polymer formulation. *Circulation.* 2003;107(4):559–564.
52. Huang Y, Salu K, Liu X, et al. Methotrexate loaded SAE coated coronary stents reduce neointimal hyperplasia in a porcine coronary model. *Heart.* 2004;90(2):195–199.

53. Regar E, Sianos G, Serruys PW. Stent development and local drug delivery. *Br Med Bull.* 2001;59:227–248.
54. Mohacsi PJ, Tuller D, Hulliger B, et al. Different inhibitory effects of immunosuppressive drugs on human and rat aortic smooth muscle and endothelial cell proliferation stimulated by platelet-derived growth factor or endothelial cell growth factor. *J Heart Lung Transplant.* 1997;16:484–492.
55. Fontaine AB, Borsa JJ, Dos Passos S, et al. Evaluation of local abciximab delivery from the surface of a polymer-coated covered stent: in vivo canine studies. *J Vasc Intervent Radiol.* 2001;12:487–492.
56. Alt E, Haehnel I, Beilharz C, et al. Inhibition of neointima formation after experimental coronary artery stenting: a new biodegradable stent coating releasing hirudin and the prostacyclin analogue iloprost. *Circulation.* 2000;101:1453–1458.
57. Eberhart RC, Su S-H, Ngyen KT, et al. Bioresorbable polymeric stents: current status and future promise. *J Biomater Sci Polym Ed.* 2003;14(4):299–312.
58. Grabow N, Schlun M, Sternberg K, et al. Mechanical properties of laser cut poly(L-lactide) micro-specimens: implications for stent design, manufacture, and sterilization. *J Biomech Eng.* 2005;127:25–31.
59. Labinaz M, Zidar JP, Stack RS, et al. Biodegradable stents: the future of interventional cardiology? *J Intervent Cardiol.* 1995;8(4):395–405.
60. Tamai H, Igaki K, Kyo E, et al. Initial and 6–month results of biodegradable poly-L-lactic acid coronary stents in humans. *Circulation.* 2000;102:399–404.
61. Tamai H, Igaki K, Tsuji T, et al. A biodegradable poly-L-lactic acid coronary stent in porcine coronary artery. *J Intervent Cardiol.* 1999;12(6):443–450.
62. Venkatraman S, Poh TL, Vinalia T, et al. Collapse pressure of biodegradable stents. *Biomaterials.* 2003;24:2105–2111.
63. Di Mario C, Griffiths H, Goktekin O, et al. Drug-eluting bioabsorbable magnesium stent. *J Intervent Cardiol.* 2004;17(6):391–395.
64. Peuster M, Wohlsein P, Brugmann M, et al. A novel approach to temporary stenting: degradable cardiovascular stents produced from corrodible metal—results 6–18 months after implantation into New Zealand white rabbits. *Heart.* 2001;86(5):563–569.
65. Heublein B, Rohde R, Kaese V, et al. Biocorrosion of magnesium alloys: a new principle in cardiovascular implant technology? *Heart.* 2003; 89:651–656.
66. Peeters P, Bosiers M, Verbist J, et al. Preliminary results after application of absorbable metal stents in patients with critical limb ischemia. *J Endovasc Ther.* 2005;12(1):1–5.
67. Eggebrecht H, Rodermann J, Hunold P, et al. Novel magnetic resonance–compatible coronary stent: the absorbable magnesium-alloy stent. *Circulation.* 2005;112:e303–e304.
68. ISO 10993–15: 2000–12: Biological evaluation of medical devices—Part 15: Identification and quantification of degradation products from metals and alloys.

Hans Henkes

Jörg Reinartz

Elina Miloslavski

Steven Lowens

Dietmar Kühne

CHAPTER **6**

Intracranial Vessels

Catheter-based therapy of neurovascular disorders started in the early 1960s[1] but remained in a rudimentary state until the mid-1980s. Since then the ideas and collaborative efforts of individual physicians and engineers have helped create a completely new technology within <20 years.

The clinical practice of neuroendovascular therapy is today still far from being a standardized process. The indications, concepts and strategies of treatment, techniques, and results still vary widely from center to center and even from one physician to another. This situation is also reflected in this chapter, which summarizes some of the personal experiences of the two senior authors (HH, DK) who have performed or supervised several thousand neuroendovascular procedures. The reader will not find a universal "cookbook" on how to perform neurovascular interventions, but rather our perspective and our representation of the field. Some of our statements are based on scientifically documented evidence, but all of them are justified by our clinical practice, even if some may appear more or less speculative and are only confirmed by our personal observations.

TRAINING REQUIREMENTS AND QUALITY ASSURANCE

Currently, there are no formal criteria or guidelines regarding facility and training requirements, just as there are no quality standards for neurovascular interventions, although several guidelines regarding the performance of specific neurovascular procedures have been advanced.[2] The question of who should be entitled to carry out neuroendovascular procedures is still unanswered. The two major regulatory mechanisms (the medicolegal system and reimbursement policies) and the

efforts of professional societies are only beginning to have an impact. For example, the initiatives of the European Society of Neuroradiology (ESNR) and of the American Society of Neuroradiology (ASNR) are still in their early stages.[3,4]

During the past 15 to 20 years, a number of centers dedicated to neurovascular interventions have been established worldwide. No fewer than 200 intracranial procedures per year should be performed at centers providing formal training, and both the technical success and the clinical outcome of these procedures, including complications, should be documented in standard protocols to permit quality control and assurance.

The technical results and clinical outcome of neuroendovascular procedures depend on a number of factors, including the patient selection criteria, technical equipment, and quality of instrumentation. Most important are, however, the experience and technical skills of the operator and the competence of the entire team.[5] Critical features that are probably beyond the realm of any formal criteria are whether the operator has the cognitive and intellectual skills to analyze clinical and anatomic case scenarios, the abilities to draw proper conclusions, and the ability to implement concepts of endovascular treatments. Given the frequently mutilating or even fatal outcomes of complications from neuroendovascular treatments, physicians performing these procedures should have undergone a minimum of 2 years of full-time supervised training in a dedicated high-volume center. One should keep in mind that this is still a fraction of what is required until a neurosurgeon is able and allowed to operate on an intracranial aneurysm.

There is a broad consensus that emergency endovascular procedures such as selective intra-arterial thrombolysis or coil occlusion of ruptured aneurysms should be offered in neuroradiology departments servicing neurosurgical and neurological clinics. An unresolved issue is how more specialized treatments, such as embolization of brain arteriovenous malformations (AVMs) without acute intracranial hemorrhage, and infrequent procedures, such as stent percutaneous trans-luminal angioplasty (stent PTA) of intracranial atherosclerotic stenoses or the management of newborns with vein of Galen malformations, should be performed. One might expect that clinical results are better in high-volume centers and in those that can refer to their own historical data.[6]

GENERAL CONSIDERATIONS

Most of the endovascular procedures described in this chapter can be standardized up to a certain degree, but some personal aspects and preferences will always remain.

Technical standards facilitate a procedure and make incidental mistakes or errors less likely. These standards may, within limits, apply to individuals and institutions and can later form the basis of our "common sense."

The use of high-resolution digital subtraction angiography (DSA) instead of film-based angiographic technology, manufactured microcatheters instead of self-assembled ones, and detachable coils instead of balloons in the treatment of aneurysms are just a few examples of established technical standards.

The duration of a procedure represents a critical quality factor. Every neuroendovascular treatment should be finished as quickly as reasonably possible, and any voluntary delay should be avoided. Adherence to the principle of simplicity helps to avoid complications. Although the simultaneous use of several microcatheters, balloons, and wires is sometimes required in order to treat challenging lesions, in most cases the use of just a single microcatheter is sufficient for successful treatment. Thorough familiarity with the radiographic equipment, the ability to generate and to interpret high-quality diagnostic angiograms,[7] and the ability to properly handle the endovascular devices employed are preconditions for successful neurovascular interventions. It is important to realize that the fortunate supply of constantly new equipment for neuroendovascular interventions always opens a new learning curve, which only in retrospect can be justified by improved technical and clinical outcomes. The conservative expert use of well-selected and familiar catheters, wires, coils, and embolic agents is probably superior to the habit of immediately pursuing each and every unproven new trend or fashion. The conservative selection of equipment appears to be particularly important during the learning phase of less experienced operators. The meticulous evaluation of clinical and technical results is the best source of knowledge and the most accomplished means of validating and establishing new standards. The teaching value and intellectual yield of follow-up angiograms are frequently more important for education and sharpening cognitive skills than the technical performance of the underlying treatment. The rigorous analysis of complications is the only way to avoid their repetition.

PREINTERVENTIONAL EVALUATION OF PATIENTS

Not all patients referred to our centers are really suitable for endovascular treatment, but sometimes this only becomes evident in retrospect. Meticulous documentation is required in order to understand as much as possible about a patient, his disease, his complete medical history, and his expectations. Speaking to the patient and his family is the key. The patient's file has to include his complete neurological status, comprising handedness, his history of stroke and epilepsy, and also that of his ancestors. Known diseases (family and personal), medication, previous imaging findings, and previous procedures of all kinds (surgery, irradiation, and endovascular) are actively queried. It is not sufficient to just collect what a patient spontaneously reports. Images from previous examinations are sometimes decisive and should be available. The results of laboratory examinations such as serum electrolytes, creatinine, thyroid gland hormones, and standard coagulation tests are updated if necessary. Before undergoing a procedure, the patient is examined by a specialized neurologist or neurosurgeon; examination by a neuroanesthesiologist is very helpful. It is important to emphasize that everything not clearly documented in the patient's file is literally nonexistent, especially from a legal standpoint.

PATIENT CONSENT FOR NEUROENDOVASCULAR TREATMENT

Informed consent is required in all elective procedures, but is sometimes difficult to obtain.[4,8] Whereas in emergency situations the physician does whatever he assumes would be the best for the patient, the opposite attitude is required in elective treatments. The patient should be fully informed about his disorder, all aspects of its natural course, and all the available treatment options with their respective pros and cons. The patient must have sufficient time (minimum 1 day) to consider these options before the initiation of treatment. This is best achieved if the first consultation takes place on an outpatient basis. All explanations have to be kept as simple as possible.

The information provided to the patient as a basis for his informed consent should include a clear statement about the chance for cure or at least improvement, on both a subjective and an objective level. This differentiation is sometimes critical. If we embolize, for instance, an asymptomatic AVM of the occipital lobe that is afterward excised surgically, the patient may regard the anticipated limitation of his visual field to be an impairment of his previous condition despite the fact that the lifelong risk of a potentially devastating hemorrhage has been removed.

Information about the risks of a proposed treatment concept should be as precise as possible. Risks that are common to all neurovascular diagnostic and interventional procedures include:

- Puncture site: bleeding, infection, vascular dissection, and/or occlusion, need for surgical intervention
- Contrast medium application: severe and even fatal allergic reaction, impaired renal function, renal failure, induced hyperthyroidism, toxic effects on the brain including transient severe neurological deficit (e.g., hemiplegia, aphasia, blindness)
- Vessel injury in the groin or to pelvic, abdominal, thoracic, cervical, or intracranial vessels, with occlusion, bleeding, or both as a consequence

- Brain ischemia or intracranial hemorrhage potentially from any procedure involving the intracranial vasculature directly or indirectly
- Direct or induced intracranial vessel occlusions or vessel perforation potentially from any intracranial endovascular procedures
- Ischemic or hemorrhagic stroke that can cause
- Transient or permanent neurological deficits
- The need for temporary or permanent support in the activities of daily life
- Death

Statistical probabilities should be quoted for these risks. For example, for a diagnostic angiography of the supra-aortic and intracranial vessels, the cumulative risk of permanent morbidity and mortality should be 0.1% or less.[9]

The patient and his family should also be told that the success of a neuroendovascular procedure can never be guaranteed. Misfortune always remains a possibility.

Our informed consent catalogue further contains items such as the potential need to extend the procedure in unexpected directions (e.g., open surgery), to administer transiently or permanently any medication (e.g., anti-platelet-aggregation drugs), or to use medical products that are not certified for this specific indication (e.g., polymer tissue glue or coronary stents not approved for neurovascular use).[10]

The potential complications of specific procedures are described later and should as such be integrated into the informed consent list.

The patient's desire for treatment in accordance with the chances and risks that have been explained should be documented by his personal signature. A printed form specific for any disorder with a handwritten supplement is acceptable. The physician who obtains the inform consent and interviews the patient should be the same one who will later perform the procedure.

PRINCIPLES OF NEUROVASCULAR IMAGING

Only high-resolution (i.e., 1024×1024 pixel matrix) DSA units are acceptable for neuroendovascular procedures.[4] In DSA units, the roentgen image is generated from roentgen rays that have been subject to variable attenuation by the penetrated tissue and are measured by an electronic image intensifier. The

signal from the image intensifier is transferred to a computer that generates the angiogram.

High-quality good systems have sufficient memory to store several thousand pictures. The standard picture frequency (frame rate) is 2 per second for at least 40 seconds. For specific purposes (e.g., any kind of pathologic high-flow situation), increased frame rates of 6 to 10 frames per second are useful. A system's contrast setting and spatial resolution may deteriorate over time and should be maintained by experienced company technicians. High magnification is frequently very helpful. The image intensifiers with a nominal diameter of 6.5 cm that are now available allow sufficient visualization of most intracranial vessels relevant to endovascular treatments. The "road map" is an important electronic function of DSA systems.[11] It is an image generated after the injection of contrast medium into the relevant vessel displayed with inverted contrast (i.e., the vessel later appears white). During the subsequent manipulation, this "road map" view is superimposed onto the actual fluoroscopic image. During "road map" and fluoroscopy guided interventions, any movement by the patient or the table must be avoided. It is helpful to store road map images during intermittent DSA runs. Geometric misregistration is sometimes an issue with a high-magnification road map. For the standard projections of neuroangiography and the angiographic vascular anatomy, refer to the existing textbooks.[12,13]

Modern DSA units provide the option of three-dimensional image reconstruction based on rotational angiography. The value of this technology generally seems to be overestimated, but it is clearly useful for the rapid definition of the relationship between an aneurysm, its parent artery, and the adjacent vessels.[14]

THE TYPICAL ANGIOGRAPHIC FINDINGS AND THEIR INTERPRETATION

Intracranial Aneurysm

An aneurysm of an intracranial artery is generally an enlargement (mostly saccular) of the vessel wall. The large majority of aneurysms are located on or adjacent to the circle of Willis. Frequent locations are the origin of the posterior communicating artery from the internal carotid artery, the anterior communicating artery, and the middle cerebral artery bifurcation (Fig. 6-1).

The diameter of an aneurysm sac (fundus) may vary between <2 mm and >20 mm. Equally important for treatment are the

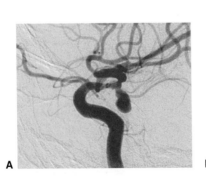 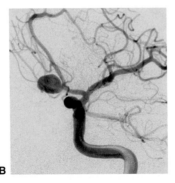 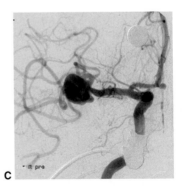

FIGURE 6-1. Aneurysm of the internal carotid artery at the origin of the posterior communicating artery **(A)**, of the anterior communicating artery **(B)**, and of the middle cerebral artery bifurcation **(C)**.

aneurysm neck (i.e., the transition from the sac to the parent artery) and the relation between fundus and neck. A fundus-to-neck ratio of ≤1 or a neck width >4 mm is frequently not ideal for coil occlusion alone. In this case, balloon remodeling or stent deployment prior to coil occlusion may substantially improve the result of endovascular treatment. The rupture site of an aneurysm or the weakest point of its wall can frequently be recognized as a small bleb in the aneurysm contour ("daughter aneurysm"). This site should not be touched by the microcatheter or microguidewire during the catheterization of the aneurysm. The coils inserted into the aneurysm fundus should by all means cover the daughter aneurysm.

Large aneurysms frequently contain an intra-aneurysmal thrombus. Contrast-enhanced computed tomography (CT) and T1- and T2-weighted magnetic resonance imaging (MRI) may show the thrombus as a nonperfused compartment of an aneurysm. Partially thrombosed aneurysms always require several endovascular treatment sessions. Circumscribed narrowing of the parent artery proximal to the aneurysm, possibly in combination with a fusiform instead of a saccular vessel dilatation, indicates that an underlying dissection is the cause of aneurysm formation (Fig. 6-2). Dissecting aneurysms carry a particular risk of hemorrhage, re-hemorrhage, and continued growth after endovascular treatment.

Brain Arteriovenous Malformations

AVMs of the brain are congenital direct connections between pial arteries and the regional draining veins (arteriovenous shunt, AV shunt). The key finding on angiography is the opacification of veins during the early arterial phase (Fig. 6-3). The underlying cause is the absence of capillaries in a brain region of variable volume. An AV shunt is associated with locally decreased blood-flow resistance and increased blood-flow volume. The size of brain AVMs varies from a few millimeters to the size of a complete hemisphere. In the majority of AVMs, the diameters of both the feeding arteries and the draining veins are increased.

The connection between arteries and veins (nidus) may consist of a network of pathological vessels (plexiform nidus). Direct connections of varying caliber are also found (macro- or microfistula) (Fig. 6-4). In many AVMs the nidus shows both components. Further findings of interest are associated aneurysms, which may be found in the standard locations on the circle of Willis (proximal). Aneurysms close to or inside the AVM nidus (perinidal, intranidal) are sometimes less obvious. Peri- and intranidal aneurysms carry a high risk of bleeding and should be prime targets for the embolization.

In addition to the direct supply, leptomeningeal anastomoses may contribute to the AV shunt. This pattern is frequently associated with a proximal occlusion of cortical branches. The leptomeningeal collaterals to an AVM are less suitable for endovascular occlusion but can be obliterated during microsurgical excision of the AVM with relative ease. After partial embolization or incomplete surgical excision, but also independent of prior treatment, transdural feeding arteries may contribute to the AV shunt. These vessels can mostly be obliterated by endovascular means without further difficulty. Analysis of the venous drainage of an AVM sometimes shows stenoses or saccular dilatations (varix) of the draining veins, both of which may indicate an increased risk of bleeding. Since the course of the draining veins is important for the planning of the surgical excision, proper documentation of the phlebogram is mandatory.

Acute Thromboembolic Occlusion of Intracranial Vessels

A thrombus within an intracranial artery obliterates the vessel lumen partially or completely (Fig. 6-5). Angiography, which is almost always carried out as an emergency procedure, will show the site of artery occlusion. If the lumen is completely filled by the embolus, it will be impossible to recognize the length of the thrombus. Complete angiography of all intracranial vessels is required prior to further endovascular considerations. The diagnostic workup should show the available collaterals to the occluded artery and eventually associated lesions (e.g., atherosclerotic occlusions of supra-aortic vessels, intracranial aneurysms). Chronic occlusions, as opposed to acute embolic occlusions, which are not suitable for revascularization, can be recognized by the presence of extensive collaterals. In endovascular treatment, the thrombus can almost always be penetrated with a suitable microcatheter. Gentle injection of contrast medium distal to the thrombus will show the length of vessel occlusion (Fig. 6-5C). Atherosclerotic stenoses proximal to or at the level of the thrombotic vessel occlusion may warrant stent PTA after local fibrinolysis in order to avoid early reocclusion.

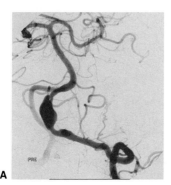
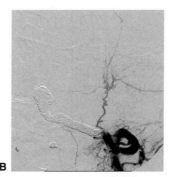
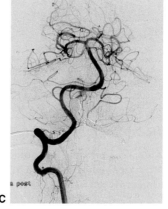

A **B** **C**

FIGURE 6-2.   Fusing dissecting aneurysm of the vertebral artery (**A**), treated by coil occlusion of aneurysm and parent artery (**B**). The contralateral vertebral artery supplies the brain stem and cerebellum (**C**).

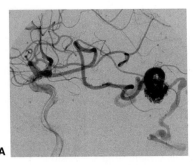
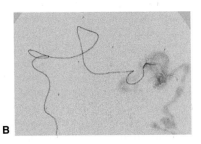
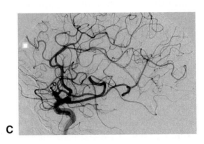

FIGURE 6-3. Brain arteriovenous malformation (AVM) with a plexiform nidus **(A)** and early opacification of the draining vein. The feeding artery was catheterized with a Marathon microcatheter **(B)**. Subsequent injection of polymer glue (Histoacryl/Lipiodol mixture 1:5) resulted in a complete interruption of the arteriovenous shunt **(C)**.

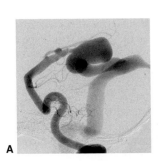
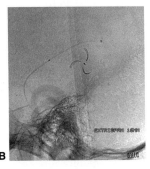
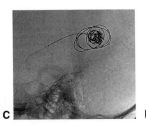
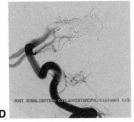

FIGURE 6-4. Macrofistula type of an AVM nidus in a child. Direct, large-caliber connection between the left posterior cerebral artery and the draining vein **(A)**. Two TriSpan coils (16 mm) were detached in the varix (enlarged vein) adjacent to the fistula **(B)**. The TriSpan devices prevented regular coils, which were subsequently inserted, from venous escape **(C)**. The coils within the varix and at the level of the fistulous arteriovenous connection induced a sufficient reduction of the shunt. Complete occlusion of the fistula was achieved by the injection of 0.1 cc Histoacryl/Lipiodol 1:3. AVM, arteriovenous malformation **(D)**.

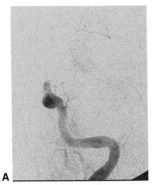
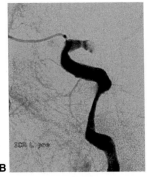
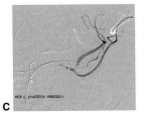
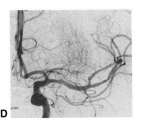

FIGURE 6-5. Internal carotid artery (ICA) and middle cerebral artery (MCA), obliterated by an embolus. Injection of the left internal carotid artery shows embolic occlusion of the vessel distally to the ophthalmic artery [**(A,B)**; posterior and lateral view]. Penetration of the thrombus with a microcatheter was easily possible **(C)**. Disintegration of the thrombus with a Catch device, partial thrombus removal with a 4F aspiration microcatheter (Penumbra device) and dilatation of a proximal M1 stenosis resulted in a complete restoration of the patency of the ICA and MCA **(D)**.

Atherosclerotic Intracranial Arterial Stenosis

Atherosclerotic stenoses relevant for endovascular treatment concern the intracranial internal carotid artery, the proximal middle cerebral artery, the intracranial vertebral artery, and the basilar artery (Fig. 6-6). Angiography should define the degree, the length, and the wall contour of the stenotic vessel segment. It is important to understand the collaterals to the stenosis and the vasculature proximal and distal to it. Extreme vessel tortuosity or a long (>10 mm) and irregular stenosis are arguments against endovascular treatment. Angiographic images that show the stenosis without foreshortening and that are free from superimposed vessels must be obtained. Because of the variability of vessel anatomy, no standard projections can be proposed for this purpose. Exact measurement of the vessel diameter proximal and distal to the stenosis is helpful for

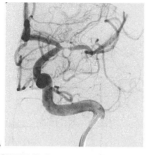
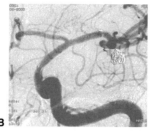

FIGURE 6-6. Stenosis of the left middle cerebral artery, incidentally observed with rapid progression during the angiographic follow-up of a ruptured and subsequently coiled MCA bifurcation aneurysm **(A)**. The stenosis was successfully treated by undersized balloon dilatation, followed by the deployment of a self-expanding Neuroform stent **(B)**. MCA, middle cerebral artery.

balloon and stent sizing. Most DSA units provide integrated measurement software for calibrated vessel diameter determination and quantification of stenoses.

Occipital Dural Arteriovenous Fistula

In so-called occipital dural AV fistulas, angiography of the ipsilateral external carotid artery shows early opacification of the sigmoid/transverse sinus (Fig. 6-7). The potentially supplying branches are the occipital artery (mastoid perforators), the stylomastoid artery, the retroauricular artery, the ascending pharyngeal artery (neuromeningeal branch), the middle and/or posterior meningeal artery, and the marginal tentorial branches of the meningohypophyseal trunk. Further supply from dural branches of the vertebral artery and from pial arteries (e.g., the posterior communicating artery) is frequently found. The occipital sinus can be completely patent and allow drainage of the fistula. Alternatively, sequelae of previous thromboses can be present and may obstruct the sinus to varying degrees. This can cause drainage of the fistula through the sinus in a retrograde direction (i.e., toward the torcular instead of the jugular bulb). The outlet of the arteries supplying the fistula is in the wall of the venous sinus, adjacent to the draining

veins. This neighborhood allows the establishment of a direct AV shunt from the supplying arteries into cortical draining veins. The likelihood of this cortical drainage pattern increases with more prominent thrombotic changes of the sinus. Accelerated perfusion of superficial veins in a retrograde direction (i.e., away from the dural venous sinus) is the key finding of cortical venous drainage and associated with a significant risk of intracranial hemorrhage.

Arteriovenous Fistula Between the Carotid Artery and the Cavernous Sinus

The common feature of fistulas between the carotid artery and the cavernous sinus (carotid cavernous sinus fistula, CCF) is the AV shunt into the cavernous sinus and the afferent veins. Direct fistulas either are related to a head trauma with an injury of the wall of the internal carotid artery or result from the rupture of an aneurysm of the cavernous segment of the internal carotid artery into the cavernous sinus (Fig. 6-8). Dural fistulas are completely different in nature. Their supply may come from dural branches of the internal carotid artery and the external carotid artery of one or both sides. The fistula is generally located on the posterior aspect of the cavernous sinus of one side or on the intercavernous sinus. The shunt volume of dCCFs may vary over a wide range but is mostly only a fraction of the shunt volume of direct CCFs. The drainage runs through the superior and inferior ophthalmic veins, which are perfused in a retrograde direction (i.e., from the cavernous sinus toward the angular vein). Further possible routes of drainage are all veins connected to the cavernous sinus (e.g., superior and inferior petrosal sinus, sphenoparietal sinus) (Fig. 6-9). The CCF drainage via cortical veins implies a risk of intracranial hemorrhage. Postthrombotic changes of the orbital veins are associated with a reduced shunt volume and more severe ocular symptoms.

STANDARD PROCEDURE

Any endovascular procedure starts with a predefined treatment plan, based on the analysis of available CT, MRI/MRA, and DSA examinations. Other decisions concern preprocedural

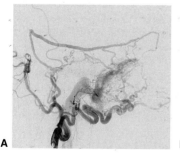
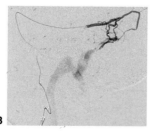
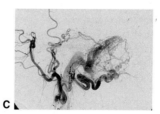
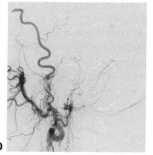

FIGURE 6-7. So-called occipital dural arteriovenous fistula. Injection of the left ECA shows the enlarged middle meningeal and occipital arteries, with multiple branches converging to the sigmoid sinus **(A)**. Within the lumen of the sigmoid sinus, remnants of a previous thrombotic occlusion are still visible as streaky defects in the opacification. The direction of venous drainage is orthograde toward the jugular bulb, without drainage via cortical veins. The arterial supply was reduced by selective catheterization of the middle meningeal and occipital arteries with injection of Histoacryl/Lipiodol **(B,C)**. Complete interruption was achieved by dense filling of the affected sigmoid sinus with electrolytically detachable fibered coils **(D)**. ECA, external carotid artery.

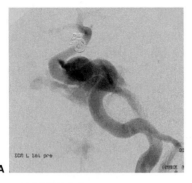
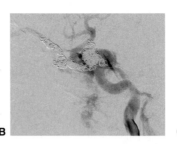
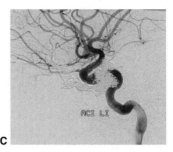

FIGURE 6-8.   Direct carotid-cavernous sinus fistula following a car accident with head injury in a 14-year-old boy, presenting with chemosis and proptosis of the left eye. The injection of the left ICA shows an early opacification of the surrounding cavernous sinus and the inferior petrosal sinus **(A)**. (The coils projecting on the distal ICA are within a dissecting aneurysm of the right ICA.) Via a transvenous access through the inferior petrosal sinus the left superior and inferior ophthalmic veins and the left cavernous sinus were occluded with electrolytically detachable fibered coils **(B)**. Despite dense filling of the veins, complete interruption of the arteriovenous shunt was not achieved during the procedure. Angiographic follow-up 2 weeks later confirmed the patency of the left ICA and occlusion of the pre-existing arteriovenous fistula **(C)**. The ocular symptoms had completely resolved. ICA, internal carotid artery.

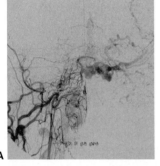
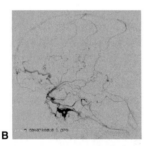

FIGURE 6-9.   Dural carotid-cavernous sinus fistula without ocular but with extensive cortical drainage. Injection of the right ECA (frontal view) shows several dural branches, converging toward the left cavernous sinus, with venous drainage via cortical veins **(A)**. Microcatheter injection of the left cavernous sinus confirms both the complete thrombotic occlusion of the left ophthalmic veins and the drainage via the sphenoparietal sinus and the basal vein of Rosenthal **(B)**. ECA, external carotid artery.

medication (e.g., antiaggregation prior to stent deployment), preparation for treatment under general anesthesia or with local anesthesia, and the size and number of guiding catheters. From the beginning of the treatment, it is usually obvious whether one or several sessions will be required. If more than one session is needed, the most dangerous (part of the) lesion should be addressed first. It may, however, be necessary to deal first with less threatening lesions in order to get a well-controlled access to the main pathology. A typical example for this situation is the stent PTA of a proximal stenosis of the internal carotid artery in order to provide optimized conditions for the catheterization and coil occlusion of an intracranial aneurysm.

The vast majority of procedures can be carried out using standardized access products. They comprise a 6F or 8F sheath (11 cm long; e.g., Cordis), a 6F or 8F guiding catheter (e.g., Guider Softip, Boston Scientific), and a 0.035-in. guidewire (e.g., Radiofocus, Terumo). As steerable microcatheters, we prefer Nautica, Echelon14, and Echelon10 together with SilverSpeed16, -14, or -10 microguidewires (MTI/ev3).

Another good option with a remarkable atraumatic tip is Synchro14 or -10 (Boston Scientific).

The two most frequently used self-expanding stents for intracranial vessels are Neuroform (Boston Scientific) and Leo (Balt). The Neuroform stent has an open cell design, comes premounted in a two-microcatheter set, and is very flexible and atraumatic. A drawback is the need for an inner 0.010-in. or 0.014-in. microguidewire (X-celerator10, MTI/ev3, works best). Distal vessel injury from this wire remains a serious concern. The stent itself is not very stable and can easily be destroyed after deployment by forced catheterization.

The braided Leo stent is introduced through a microcatheter (Vasco, Balt) without an inner guidewire, is quite robust, and has radiopaque markers along two struts. Aneurysm coverage is better with the Leo. The Vasco microcatheter for this stent is less flexible than the Neuroform catheter (Renegade Hi Flo, Boston Scientific), and the Leo stent appears more traumatic and thrombogenic. There are several coil systems available that differ in the mode of detachment and the shape, stiffness, and surface of the implant. Electrolytic detachment is convenient and reliable. The efficacy of so-called bioactive coil surfaces (e.g., Matrix, Boston Scientific) and hydrogel-coated coils (Hydrocoils, Microvention) is questionable. Coils with an imprinted three-dimensional shape are most useful for the treatment of wide-necked aneurysms (e.g., from Micrus or MTI/ev3). Soft coils are provided by several companies (e.g., Boston Scientific, Micrus, MTI/ev3). We have achieved very good results with detachable nylon fibered coils (MTI/ev3).

INTRACRANIAL ANEURYSMS

The incidence of intracranial aneurysms in the general population has been estimated to be 3% to 6%.[15] The frequency of aneurysmal subarachnoid hemorrhage (SAH) is in the range of 6 to 10 per 100,000 persons per year. The mortality from SAH is about 50%.[16,17] Although the frequency and clinical relevance of intracranial hemorrhage secondary to previously unruptured aneurysms have been a matter of debate in recent years, no conclusive recommendations are available at present. Initially, a very low rupture rate was reported for aneurysms

≤10 mm in diameter,[18] but these figures were later updated, and the actual rate of rupture may be higher. The reported rate depends on the site and size of the aneurysm and the patient's specific risk factors.[19]

The presence of an intracranial aneurysm may be confirmed by a contrast-enhanced CT or an MRI examination.[20] CT angiography has been significantly improved and is now frequently employed diagnostically. Final decision making, however, is still mostly based on a selective catheter angiography. Angiography should comprise a series of oblique and magnified views of the aneurysm. Rotational angiography with three-dimensional rendering is sometimes quite useful. A pretreatment angiogram should clearly reveal the size, shape, location, and adjacent vessels of the target aneurysm.

In patients with a ruptured aneurysm, the need for treatment is evident. Empirical data has revealed that the clinical results after endovascular treatment of ruptured aneurysms are better than after surgical clipping.[21] In unruptured aneurysms, the decision regarding treatment has to take several factors into account. Statistical data is of limited help in individual patients. During surgery of unruptured aneurysms, it became evident that among aneurysms with essentially the same angiographic appearance some could have a thick, fibrous wall, insinuating a low tendency to rupture, whereas others have very thin and fragile walls. Because current diagnostic techniques do not allow any reliable distinction between thick- and thin-walled aneurysms, this feature can only be evaluated after surgical preparation. At present, the decision to treat is favored by a majority of patients.

Other important factors to be considered are the patient's age, coexisting illnesses, and the anticipated technical ability to exclude a given aneurysm by either surgical or endovascular means. Ultimately, however, the patient decides which treatment option he or she prefers. In general, we offer patients with an unruptured aneurysm—regardless of its size—either endovascular or surgical treatment whenever it appears technically feasible. The location of the aneurysm is irrelevant for the chances and risks of endovascular treatment. Technical difficulty may be anticipated in the case of very tortuous proximal vessels, in very small (i.e., ≤2 mm diameter) and in giant (>25 mm diameter) aneurysms, in those with a very wide neck (>4 mm), and in the case of a fundus-to-neck ratio <1. Proximal vessels without severe atherosclerosis and aneurysms with a well-circumscribed neck are ideally suitable for endovascular coil occlusion.

Technical Aspects of Coil Occlusion of Intracranial Aneurysms

It is necessary that the guiding catheter has stable, atraumatic, and controlled access to the respective supra-aortic artery. After insertion of the sheath into the right and/or left femoral artery, a standard 5F or 6F diameter guiding catheter (e.g., Guider Softip, Boston Scientific) that is 90 or 100 cm long is positioned using a 0.035-in. guidewire such as Radiofocus (Terumo). A continuous flush with a heparinized saline solution via a rotating hemostatic valve (RHV) is required to prevent formation of thrombi.

Self-mounted coaxial systems are an alternative; examples are a 100-cm-long 6F guiding catheter inside another (90-cm-long 8F), or a 100-cm-long 8F guiding catheter inside a 90-cm-long

10F guiding catheter. Direct puncture of the common carotid artery, using a LeaderCath G14 (Vygon), provides even better support and stability and can be used in the case of difficult peripheral access. Since direct puncture of the common carotid artery may result in vessel dissection and stroke, accurate puncture and gentle insertion of the guidewire and the Teflon sheath under fluoroscopy without increased force are mandatory. Options for alternate access to the posterior circulation are insertion of a 6F sheath into the axillary artery and the use of a 6F internal mammaria artery guiding catheter.

Before beginning treatment, the angiographic images of the target aneurysm must be thoroughly analyzed. Most important is that the appropriate working projections are acquired, showing if possible the aneurysm in its full length, without overlying vessels, and in clear relation to the parent artery and to vessels originating in its proximity. Although rotational angiography with three-dimensional rendering is sometimes helpful for determining the presence, location, and geometry of the aneurysm,[22] its importance appears to be overestimated. Factors that are likely to be more important for successful endovascular aneurysm treatment are high image magnification, low image noise, optimal spatial resolution, and a road-map function with a well-adapted contrast setting.

As soon as a suitable angiographic working projection has been determined, a dual marker microcatheter (i.e., with two radiodense markers, one at the distal tip of the microcatheter and one marker 3 cm proximal to it) will be selected based on the location and geometry of the target aneurysm. The outer diameter (OD) of the microcatheter appears in most cases to be of lesser importance. The microcatheter should, however, be stable in its later position with the tip adjacent to or inside the aneurysm. During insertion of the coils, it may become necessary to pull or to push the microcatheter, which should follow these intended movements as precisely as possible. Inner diameters (IDs) that are too small may restrict the choice of usable devices. These requirements are sufficiently met by microcatheters such as Nautica (OD 2.2F, 0.71 mm; ID 0.018-in., 0.46 mm, MTI/ev3) or Excelsior1018 (OD 2.0F, 0.66 mm; ID 0.019-in., 0.48 mm, Boston Scientific). Preshaped microcatheters such as the Echelon14 (MTI/ev3) with a given tip angulation of 45 degrees or 90 degrees remain quite stable in this position. Vessels with a naturally small caliber or whose lumen is reduced due to vasospasm may require a thinner microcatheter. Echelon10 (OD 1.7F, 0.57 mm; ID 0.017-in., 0.43 mm, MTI/ev3) and Excelsior SL-10 (OD 1.7F, 0.56 mm; ID 0.0165-in., 0.43 mm, Boston Scientific) are among the suitable ones. If a straight microcatheter is used, proper shaping is important. The shape to be imprinted on the catheter tip by steam or dry heat has to anticipate the route the microcatheter has to follow until reaching the aneurysm, as well as the angle at which the microcatheter will enter the aneurysm neck. Wrong shaping can result in failure to coil an aneurysm. Proper shaping relies on skill and experience.

The microguidewire that is used with the microcatheter should be sufficiently radiopaque, should precisely follow applied torque movements, and must not cause significant friction in the microcatheter or the intracranial vessel. An atraumatic tip is most important. The SilverSpeed10 and SilverSpeed14 wires (MTI/ev3) are our standard microguidewires. The Synchro10 and Synchro14 microguidewires (Boston Scientific) follow torque movement in an excellent way, and the tip is very soft. The Synchro wire is recommended for more challenging vessels. All these wires come straight and require individual shaping. A more or less steep curve, similar to the shape that was given to the microcatheter, is usually appropriate.

Catheterization of the aneurysm is then carried out using the just-mentioned working projection under road-map fluoroscopy. Slow advancement of the microcatheter and microguidewire is crucial. Most frequently, the microguidewire is slightly pushed forward, and the microcatheter is then pushed while pulling on the guidewire gently. Perfect control of both movements is the key. The reason for any resistance has to be found and removed. Potential sources of increased resistance include inadvertent proximal looping of the microcatheter, displacement of the tip of the guiding catheter from the internal into the external carotid artery, or vasospasm anywhere in the course of the microcatheter. Under no circumstances should the operator be tempted to overcome the resistance by pushing harder.

The aneurysm is then partly entered by the tip of the microguidewire. Any contact between the aneurysm wall and the tip of the wire should be avoided. Daughter aneurysms (i.e., small additional sacs, bulging out of the contour of the aneurysms) are very fragile and may not be touched with either the wire or the tip of the following microcatheter. In most aneurysms the ideal position for the tip of the microcatheter is at the level of the aneurysm neck. The aneurysm is filled with coils from its neck inward (Fig. 6-10). This again underlines the importance of a stable microcatheter and explains why the diameter of the aneurysms is generally irrelevant in selecting the size of the microcatheter.

The selection of the coils to be inserted has to address several aspects. The most frequently used implants are electrolytically detachable platinum coils (GDC, Boston Scientific; NXT MTI/ev3), in which direct current is used to separate the platinum coil from an insertion wire. The original concept of electrothrombosis, induced by the application of direct current (which is also used for coil detachment), turned out to be non-functional.[23] Mechanically detachable coils (Detach, Cook) are not well suited for aneurysms. These coils are attached to an insertion wire via a winding. Detachment is achieved by turning the insertion wire against the coil with a potential transmission

of this movement to the coil. Two coil systems are based on hydrodynamic detachment (Microvention, Cordis). The coil is attached to a thin tube using a distal valve mechanism. The valve is opened, and the coil is detached by injecting saline solution or diluted contrast medium. The Micrus coil system uses an electrothermal mechanism (i.e., electric heating of a wire with disruption of a polymer fiber) for coil detachment.[24]

The process of filling an aneurysm with coils may start with a regular coil or, in the case of a wide aneurysm neck (≥4 mm), with a coil with an imprinted three-dimensional shape.[25,26] The diameter of the aneurysmal sac and of the first coil should be equal. Subsequent coils are inserted and detached until the aneurysm sac accepts no further coil material. Dense filling is mandatory for the result of treatment to be stable. In the case of wide-neck aneurysms, the parent artery can temporarily be protected by the inflation of a nondetachable compliant balloon (Fig. 6-11).[27] Hyperglide and Hyperform (MTI/ev3) work very well for this purpose.[28] During this "balloon remodeling," parent vessel occlusion should be limited to intervals of <3 minutes, especially if the collaterals to the artery affected are absent or of dubious sufficiency. Balloon remodeling is mostly performed via an 8F guiding catheter. It is sometimes easier if the balloon catheter is first brought in front of the aneurysm and the microcatheter is introduced afterward. Several publications mention that the frequency of complications (thromboembolic or vessel dissection) is increased in balloon remodeling procedures.[29]

The coil treatment of wide-necked aneurysms can also be supported by deploying a self-expanding stent. Neuroform (Boston Scientific) is a very flexible nitinol stent with an open-cell design[30] (Fig. 6-12). The Leo stent (Balt) is a more stable but also a more thrombogenic closed-cell device.[31] The Solo stent is electrolytically detachable and fully retrievable (Fig. 6-13). Before stent deployment, profound medical antiaggregation has to be started. The usual protocol includes loading doses of 500 mg acetylsalicylic acid (ASA) and 300 mg clopidogrel 3 days before the treatment. Medical antiaggregation makes stent-assisted procedures less suitable for treatment in the acute phase after aneurysm rupture. With either device, it is possible to deploy the stent and catheterize the aneurysm afterward with a microcatheter.[32] In this case, it is recommended that coil insertion be delayed for 6 to 8 weeks after stent deployment for unruptured aneurysms. In the meantime the deployed stent will become integrated into the wall of the parent vessel. Alternatively, it is possible to catheterize the aneurysm with a microcatheter, deploy the stent over the aneurysm orifice, and coil the aneurysm afterward ("jailed catheter"). The microcatheter can always be pulled out of the parent artery.

TriSpan (Boston Scientific) is a modified coil with three partly radiopaque nitinol petals[33] (Fig. 6-14). These petals in the shape of a flower blossom are placed and opened in the neck level of the aneurysm. Wide-necked bifurcation aneurysms are frequently well suitable for this treatment strategy. The TriSpan coil is introduced and kept in place via a large-lumen and robust microcatheter (e.g., RapidTransit, Cordis; Excelsior1018, Boston Scientific; Nautica, MTI/ev3). For coil insertion, a second microcatheter is used. Simultaneous insertion of two microcatheters requires an 8F guiding catheter with a double RHV. The TriSpan remains attached to the insertion wire until coil insertion is completed. In order to avoid premature TriSpan detachment, it is required that the detachment zone of the TriSpan remain covered by the

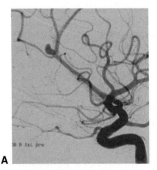 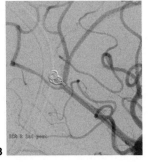

FIGURE 6-10.   Proper position of the tip of a microcatheter for filling an aneurysm with coils from outside. Small aneurysm of the right pericallosal artery **(A)**. The position of the tip of the microcatheter adjacent to the neck but outside the aneurysmal sac was maintained throughout the entire procedure **(B)**. This requires a robust microcatheter, resilient to "kick back" effects, in a stable position.

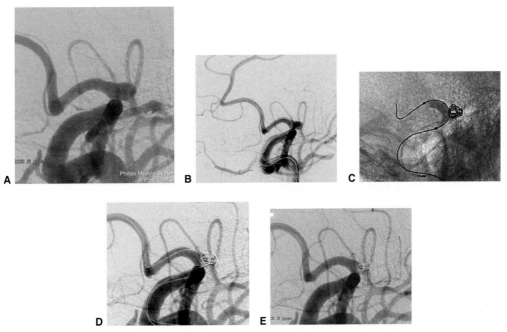

FIGURE 6-11.   Balloon remodeling for the treatment of a wide necked aneurysm. Aneurysm of the proximal A1 segment without a circumscribed neck (**A**). Catheterization of the right ACA with a Hyperglide balloon micro-catheter while the tip of a second microcatheter is already within the aneurysm sac (**B**). Temporary filling of the balloon during insertion of coils into the aneurysm (**C**). The aneurysm is already filled, while balloon-catheter and microcatheter are left in place for several minutes (**D**). Patency of the parent artery and complete occlusion of the aneurysm after gentle withdrawal of both catheters (**E**). ACA, anterior cerebral artery.

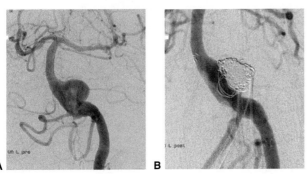

FIGURE 6-12.   Treatment of a wide-necked aneurysm of the proximal basilar artery with stent-assisted coil occlusion. Injection of the left vertebral artery shows a wide-necked aneurysm immediately distal to the vertebral artery junction (**A**). After deployment of a self-expanding Neuroform stent, the aneurysm was filled with platinum coils (**B**).

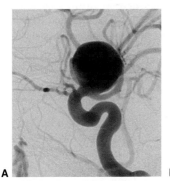

FIGURE 6-13.   Treatment of a wide-necked aneurysm with a Solo stent. Large and wide-necked aneurysm of the right internal carotid artery in paraophthalmic location (**A**). Deployment of a self-expanding stent, followed by complete coil occlusion of the aneurysm (**B**).

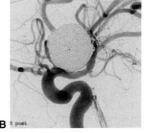

microcatheter until voluntary detachment. We usually open the TriSpan proximal to the final level of occlusion. Via a second microcatheter a slightly undersized three-dimensional coil (e.g., Boston Scientific, Micrus, MTI/ev3) is inserted. As soon as this three-dimensional coil is fully pushed out of the microcatheter, the TriSpan device together with the concerning microcatheter is gently advanced until the three-dimensional coil starts to be compressed. The three-dimensional coil is detached as soon as the TriSpan device achieves stabilization. During the following process of coil insertion, the TriSpan coil can be manipulated in a way that avoids coil displacement out of the aneurysm into the parent vessel. Fibered coils (MTI/ev3) are especially useful for the treatment of these aneurysms. The fibers facilitate fixation of the TriSpan pedals at the coil mesh and prevent major recurrence due to coil compaction.

An underexploited strategy for the treatment of dissecting and fusiform aneurysms is the parent vessel occlusion (PVO) with coils. PVO is feasible whenever a sufficient collateral circulation is available. Even fusiform aneurysm of the trunk of the basilar artery can be treated by PVO if at least one posterior communicating artery and the P1 segment concerned have a significant diameter[34] (Fig. 6-15). Mycotic aneurysms mostly result from infected cardiogenic emboli in brain arteries. A transient embolic occlusion of the parent artery is part of the specific pathogenesis. For these lesions, the appropriate treatment is usually the occlusion of the aneurysm *and* parent vessel with coils or/and polymer glue.[35]

Alternatives to Coil Occlusion

The use of the liquid embolic agent Onyx HD 500 (MTI/ev3) together with temporary balloon protection of the parent vessel, which was advocated by several authors, has now been

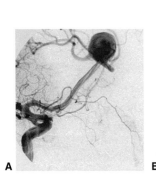
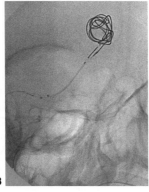
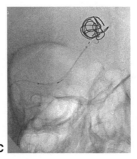
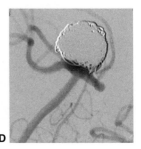

A **B** **C** **D**

FIGURE 6-14. TriSpan procedure for the endovascular treatment of a wide-necked bifurcation aneurysm. Injection of the right ICA shows an unpaired ACA (A2) with an aneurysm, located at the ICA bifurcation **(A)**. The aneurysm is catheterized with two microcatheters. 3D coils are inserted into the aneurysm, held in place and occasionally compressed by a TriSpan coil **(B,C)**. The final injection of the ICA confirms complete filling of the aneurysm with reconstruction of the parent artery bifurcation **(D)**. ICA, internal carotid artery; ACA, anterior cerebral artery.

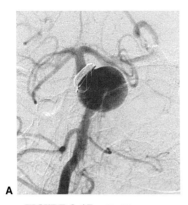
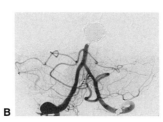
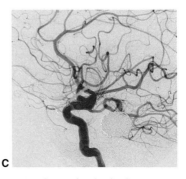

A **B** **C**

FIGURE 6-15. Fusiform aneurysm of the basilar trunk after partial coil treatment in another institution several years before **(A)**. The aneurysm was excluded from circulation by endovascular coil occlusion of parent artery and aneurysm after tolerated balloon test occlusion **(B)**. The upper part of the basilar artery and both superior cerebellar arteries are supplied via the posterior communicating artery **(C)**.

widely abandoned because of unacceptable high complication rates.[36] The available stent grafts (e.g., GraftMaster, Abbott) are not optimized for intracranial purposes. They are too stiff and require excessive inflation pressures (16 atm), and should therefore only be used for intracranial aneurysms if other options have failed.[37] If there is no alternative to using such a stent graft, medical antiaggregation is required (loading dose 500 mg ASA, 300 mg clopidogrel). Sufficient backup has to be provided by the guiding catheter. A coaxial system with a 100-cm-long, 6F catheter inside a 90-cm-long, 8F guide catheter may work. It has proved helpful to make the extracranial internal carotid artery straighter and stiff by preparatory deployment of a self-expanding stent (e.g., a 7 mm/40 mm Protegé, ev3). Direct puncture of the common carotid artery using a 14 G Leader Catheter (Vygon) set provides optimal support but is considered more invasive than a transfemoral approach. Adding nimodipine to the guiding catheter flush (15 mL nimodipine [Nimotop] per 1000 mL saline solution) and the prophylactic injection of glycerin trinitrate (2 mg per injection diluted in 8 mL saline solution) are helpful. A 0.014-in. guidewire has to be inserted far distally into a cortical branch of the middle communicating artery or posterior communicating artery, which always bears the risk of a vessel injury. The

passage of these stent grafts is usually easier through the atlas loop than through the cavernous segment of the internal carotid artery. Short stent grafts (e.g., 9 mm or 12 mm) follow much more easily than longer ones.

The injection of rapidly solidifying polymer glue has great potential for treating intracranial aneurysms. In contrast to the precipitating Onyx HD 500, which remains separated from the aneurysm wall, the polymer glue becomes firmly attached to it. Although occlusion of intracranial aneurysms has been achieved using this technique, unresolved issues are the precise control of the injected glue volume and reproducible avoidance of escape of glue to the distal vessels.[38]

Complications of Endovascular Aneurysm Treatment

Periprocedural aneurysm perforation and thromboembolic parent or distal artery occlusion are the two most frequent complications of the endovascular treatment of intracranial aneurysms.[39]

The incidence of periprocedural aneurysm perforation is in the range of 3% to 4%. Among the many factors that contribute to or result in aneurysm perforation are previous rupture, elongated proximal vessels, irregular aneurysm shape, an unfortunate angle between the longitudinal axes of the parent vessel and the aneurysmal sac, a misleading working projection hiding or foreshortening parts of the aneurysm, an unstable position of the microcatheter, insertion of a microguidewire or coils perpendicular to the aneurysm wall, any impact on the daughter aneurysm, use of a coil that is oversized or too stiff, and coil insertion with too much force.[40,41]

Even under deep general anesthesia, an immediate increase in the heart rate and the systemic blood pressure can be observed. Contrast medium injection through the guiding catheter will confirm the extravasation. Soon after, if the increase of intracranial pressure has reached a critical level, a delay in cerebral circulation will become apparent. If an aneurysm perforation has been confirmed, only a rapid and successfully performed sequence of actions will help to save the patient's life. The anesthesiologist must provide deep anesthesia with complete muscle relaxation, adding barbiturates (1000 mg thiopental [Trapanal]). Hypotension ($\leq$70 mm Hg systolic blood pressure) must be induced immediately. Any heparin that was previously given must be antagonized with 1 mL protamine intravenously for every 1000 U heparin. If the procedure is being carried out after medical antiaggregation, platelet function is restored by the intravenous administration of desmopressin (Minirin, 0.3 μg/kg).[42] The intra-arterial or intravenous administration of nimodipine is started or continued.[43] The neuroradiologist will immediately identify the site of aneurysm perforation. If the microcatheter tip is in the subarachnoid space, a 2-mm helix and a 2- to 6-cm-long nylon fibered detachable coil are introduced. After one or two loops are deployed into the subarachnoid space, the microcatheter can be gently pulled back into the aneurysmal sac, where the rest of the coil will be inserted. If the microcatheter is not in the subarachnoid space, the aneurysmal sac should be filled with fibered coils, starting as close as possible to the rupture site. If the perforation is located at the aneurysm neck, preservation of the patency of the parent vessel is usually not possible, in which case parent artery occlusion with a fibered coil, possibly combined with the injection of a small amount of highly concentrated *n*-butyl cyanoacrylate (nBCA) (Histoacryl, Braun) may be the best choice. As soon as the extravasation is stopped, normal systemic blood pressure must be reestablished. CT examination will show the amount of blood in the cisterns and possibly within the brain parenchyma. External ventricular drainage will generally be required. Craniotomy for removal of a space-occupying intracerebral hematoma is normally not required.

Thromboembolic events and complications will be observed during or after 10% to 20% of endovascular aneurysm treatments.[44] Asymptomatic small lesions are frequently found on postprocedural diffusion- and perfusion-weighted MRI, with some of the published extremely high frequencies probably not representative for skilled endovascular practice.[45] The incidence of symptomatic brain ischemia, including transient symptoms, has to be <5%.[46]

Factors that predispose for thrombosis of the parent artery and emboli to the distal vasculature include atherosclerosis of the vessels proximal to the aneurysm, posthemorrhagic vasospasm, partial thrombosis of the aneurysmal sac, thrombophilia, procedural vessel dissection, use of balloon remodeling, incomplete filling of the aneurysmal sac, displacement of coil loops from the aneurysm into the lumen of the parent artery, and extreme length of the procedure.

Premedication with antiplatelet aggregation may be beneficial, but sealing of the rupture site will certainly be more difficult in the case of procedural vessel injury or aneurysm perforation. The most frequently used precautions to prevent thromboembolic complications include systemic heparinization with a single dose of 5000 U of heparin, supplemented with 1000 U of heparin for every additional hour of the procedure.[47] In unruptured aneurysms, heparin is given as soon as the sheath is introduced. During the treatment of ruptured aneurysms, one might wait until the aneurysm is at least partly filled. The intravenous administration of 500 mg of ASA (Aspisol) in unruptured aneurysms is frequently used in those countries where this drug is available. In the acute phase after an aneurysm rupture, the intravenous administration of ASA may cause bleeding complications if an external ventricular drainage has to be inserted afterward. After the procedure, low-molecular heparin is given in a body-weight-adapted dosage for another 2 days, and frequently 100 mg of ASA orally is added for 10 days. Rapid and simple performance of the procedure and "complete" filling of the aneurysm sac are important. If thrombus formation becomes obvious, countermeasures should be started immediately. If, in a ruptured aneurysm, heparinization is still pending, it can be started if the aneurysm is considered secure from rerupture. The intravenous bolus injection of a body-weight-adapted dosage of abciximab (ReoPro) is quite effective.[48] It remains unclear whether the intra-arterial injection of this drug is more efficient.[49] Another option is local intra-arterial fibrinolysis with urokinase or recombinant tissue plasminogen activator (rtPA).[50] Combinations of these drugs (e.g., heparin and abciximab, or abciximab and urokinase) significantly increase the risk of hemorrhagic complications. Our currently favored agent is abciximab. In case such measures are required while other aneurysms are still untreated, endovascular occlusion of these lesions should be done during the same session. If hemorrhagic complications occur that require surgical intervention, abciximab can be antagonized by platelet transfusion.

If the thrombus formation is apparently independent of the inserted coils and related to the foreign body surface of the microcatheters and guidewires, thrombophilia is probably the underlying cause.[51] In that case, early withdrawal of the microcatheter and systemic administration of abciximab is probably superior to efforts to achieve local recanalization.

Although displacement of entire coils or coil loops from the aneurysm into the parent artery or the distal vasculature is relatively rare, it is sometimes encountered in wide-necked aneurysms. Further circumstances that may cause coil displacement are unstable position of the microcatheter (e.g., deflection into the middle communicating artery–middle cerebral artery during the treatment of aneurysms of the anterior communicating artery), the use of undersized coils, and the insertion of a three-dimensional coil after the detachment of two-dimensional ones. Insertion of a coil into a partly filled aneurysm may displace one of the already detached coils or a coil loop. The preferential use of relatively long coils creates a more stable coil mesh and can thus prevent coil displacement. The attempt to insert coils that are too long may, however, cause other difficulties. The phenomenon that such a coil can neither be fully inserted into nor withdrawn from the aneurysm can force the operator to stretch the coil into the parent artery and maybe fixate it there with a microstent (e.g., Neuroform). Protruding coil loops can sometimes be pushed back into the aneurysm, for instance using a small nonsoft three-dimensional or fibered coil. Deploying a self-expanding stent over the aneurysm is another valid option.[52] If this fails or seems impossible, leaving the loop wherever it is and starting intravenous heparinization or administration of body-weight-adapted subcutaneous low-molecular heparin for 2 weeks is advised, provided the coil is unfibered.

There may be an increase in posthemorrhagic vasospasm. The risk is especially high if the treatment is carried out while vasospasm is already visible on angiography. Sometimes asymptomatic vasospasm is converted into symptomatic vasospasm without much angiographic change. Delaying treatment is an option that carries always the risk of recurrent bleeding. Alternatives are the intra-arterial infusion of nimodipine via the guiding catheter (15 mL of nimodipine in 1000 mL of heparinized saline solution for drip infusion), if necessary together with the intra-arterial injection of glycerin trinitrate in a dosage of 2 mg in 10 mL saline solution per injection (Fig. 6-16). Careful limitation of the amount of contrast medium injected may help to avoid an increase of vasospasm.

Increased mass effect and parenchymal edema around the aneurysm are sometimes observed in large and giant aneurysms.[53,54] Although the edema frequently remains asymptomatic, an increased mass effect can cause or aggravate cranial nerve palsy or symptoms due to brainstem compression. The mass effect may be observed in cavernous, paraophthalmic, and paraclinoid aneurysms of the internal carotid artery and in those of the vertebral artery, the vertebral artery junction, and the basilar artery trunk. Incomplete filling of the aneurysmal sac with much remaining space between the coil loops seems to predispose for an increase in mass effect. In contrast, loose filling of the aneurysm dome and very dense coil occlusion of the aneurysm neck and the adjacent parts of the fundus may prevent postprocedural aneurysm swelling.

Toxic effects of contrast medium are nowadays rare. They are assumed if the patient presents a focal neurological deficit after the procedure without a correlate on diffusion- and perfusion-weighted MRI. These deficits fortunately resolve spontaneously within a few days.

Bleeding of an intracranial aneurysm after coil occlusion is rare, with a reported incidence <1% per year.[55] The prognosis of these bleedings is poor. Related factors are initially incomplete occlusion, recurrent flow, and underlying vessel dissection. The vast majority of these potentially fatal bleedings after coiling are avoidable if aneurysm recurrences are detected in timely fashion and endovascular or surgical treatment is performed.

Follow-up Regimen

Following the treatment with bare platinum coils, about 20% to 30% of intracranial aneurysms show some degree of reperfusion or recurrence and about 10% will require more than one treatment. Coil compaction is the mechanism most frequently underlying aneurysm reperfusion (Fig. 6-17). Other mechanisms are potentially important but sometimes difficult to recognize. This is especially true for aneurysm enlargement (Fig. 6-18). In patients with intracranial aneurysms treated by endovascular coil occlusion, structured follow-up examinations are therefore mandatory. Several authors recommend MRA for noninvasive follow-up.[56,57] We prefer catheter angiography for the majority of patients. The direct comparison of pre- and posttreatment angiograms with the follow-up examinations allows a better understanding of the occlusion rate of the aneurysm initially achieved and maintained thereafter. The timing for follow-up depends on various factors. The standard schedule includes DSA examinations 6 and 24 months after the treatment. In dissecting aneurysms, the first follow-up angiogram has to be obtained within 1 or 2 weeks since very early recurrences are frequently encountered. In large or giant, partially thrombosed aneurysms DSA performed after 4 to 6 weeks may already show a degree of reperfusion that deserves a second treatment session. After retreatment, the follow-up schedule starts again. Individualized follow-up regimens are recommended for patients either with

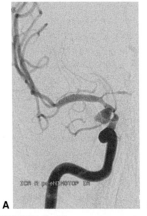 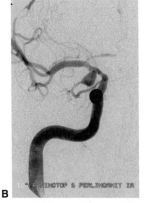 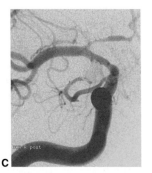

A   **B**   **C**

FIGURE 6-16.   Posthemorrhagic intracranial vasospasm, reduced after intra-arterial infusion of nimodipine and glycerol trinitrate. Ruptured paraclinoid aneurysm of the right internal carotid artery, with severe vasospasm of the adjacent parent vessel (**A**). After intra-arterial injection of nimodipine and glycerol trinitrate, a dramatic increase of the vessel diameter was observed (**B**), which allowed complete and uneventful coil filling of the aneurysm (**C**).

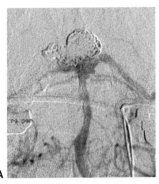
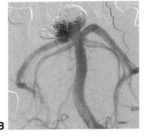

FIGURE 6-17. Aneurysm recurrence due to coil compaction. Wide-necked aneurysm of the basilar tip, treated in the acute phase after bleeding. Vasospasm of the surrounding arteries (**A**). After 5 months, complete resolution of the pre-existing vasospasm. Following coil compaction, <50% of the aneurysmal sac is filled by platinum coils (**B**).

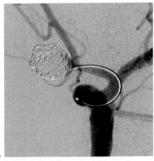
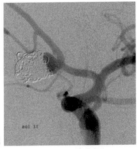

FIGURE 6-18. Aneurysm recurrence due to enlargement of the aneurysmal sac. Ruptured aneurysm of the anterior communicating artery. Coil treatment with subtotal occlusion in the acute phase after aneurysm SAH (**A**). Six months later, recurrent aneurysm perfusion due to aneurysmal sac enlargement (**B**). SAH, subarachnoid hemorrhage.

aneurysms that are complicated in any aspect or after incomplete occlusion. An aneurysm shown to be occluded and unchanged for 2 years can be considered as permanently isolated from circulation.

SELECTED NEUROVASCULAR DISORDERS

BRAIN ARTERIOVENOUS MALFORMATIONS

Brain AVMs are thought to be congenital and relatively infrequent lesions. The exact incidence is not known because of an uncertain number of asymptomatic carriers, but the relation of the numbers of diagnosed brain AVMs to intracranial aneurysms is about 1:10. The two most frequent clinical manifestations are epilepsy and intracranial (mostly intracerebral) hemorrhage. Very large AVMs can cause a progressive neurological deficit and also a progressive decline in intellectual function. Headache in AVM patients is associated with lesions located in the occipital lobe or with those with transdural supply.

The so-called nidus of an AVM is the virtual ensemble of pathological brain vessels where pial arteries and veins are directly connected without intervening capillaries. The hemorrhage originates from the nidus or the draining veins, which are under an elevated, almost "arterial," pressure.[58] Intranidal

aneurysms are associated with an increased rate of bleeding.[59,60] Epilepsy may be induced by glial changes in the surrounding brain tissue, which could be related to the malnutrition due to the AV shunt.[61]

The goal of treatment is customarily the complete interruption of the AV shunt, which is the key to removing the risk of hemorrhage. Epilepsy disappears in about 70% of patients in whom complete cure of the AVM is achieved.[62] Headache in the two just-mentioned subgroups can frequently be improved. In those large lesions that cause progressive hemiparesis and other focal neurological deficits, complete occlusion is generally not possible, but some patients report at least a transient subjective clinical improvement. In general, palliative (i.e., partial) embolization does not always provide a future benefit to the patient.[63]

The interruption of the pial AV shunt can be achieved by microsurgical excision of the vascular malformation, by high-dosage stereotactic radiation, by endovascular vessel occlusion, and by a combination of two or three of these treatment modalities.[64] Surgical results are good in experienced hands if the AVM is small, is located in or adjacent to the surface of the brain, and is in "noneloquent" brain regions.[65–67] If one or several of these criteria are not fulfilled, AVM surgery can become extremely challenging, if not disastrous. Small AVMs in any location can be treated by stereotactic irradiation.[68] If the diameter of the target volume exceeds 2 cm, the obliteration rate decreases to unacceptable low levels. Another drawback is the latency interval between treatment and final effect, which is in the range of 2 to 3 years. The patient is not protected against an AVM bleeding during this time, specifically not until complete obliteration of the AVM vessels.[69] Even under optimal conditions, the failure rate of stereotactic AVM irradiation is around 20%.

Endovascular treatment of brain AVMs can be used to make these lesions more amenable to either microsurgery or radiosurgery.[70] Complete and permanent interruption of the AV shunt by endovascular means is possible. The rates reported for complete endovascular occlusion vary considerably. A realistic estimate of the frequency of curative embolization is 20% to 30%; successes are usually achieved in small single-pedicle AVMs.[71] Success rates >50% are certainly difficult to achieve.

The preoperative embolization of a brain AVM will address the specific needs of the vascular neurosurgeon.[72,73] It is usually helpful to occlude arterial feeders coming from the depth of the brain, large AV connections (macrofistulas), or excessive transdural supply. In contrast, it is better to coagulate leptomeningeal anastomoses during surgery without major damage to the adjacent parenchyma. Under most circumstances, a shunt reduction of an estimated 80–90% will be sufficient to allow a well-controlled surgical AVM excision.

Endovascular preparation of an AVM for subsequent stereotactic irradiation should include the occlusion of peri- and intranidal aneurysms and pseudoaneurysms since these lesions are clearly related to an increased risk of hemorrhage during the latency phase after irradiation (Fig. 6-19). Macrofistulas and leptomeningeal collaterals will generally not obliterate after irradiation and should therefore be occluded by endovascular means before the stereotactic treatment is performed. The key criterion for radiosurgery is the target volume to be exposed. Preradiosurgical endovascular treatment should therefore reduce the cumulative volume of patent AVM vessels

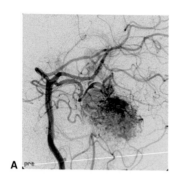
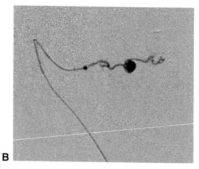
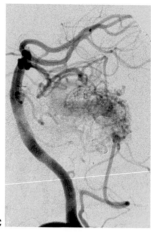

FIGURE 6-19. Endovascular occlusion of an intranidal aneurysm in a large cerebellar AVM adjacent to the brain stem. Midsize AVM nidus of the cerebellum, supplied by the left superior, anterior inferior, and posterior inferior cerebellar arteries (**A**). Catheterization of an intranidal aneurysm via the right AICA (**B**). Significant size reduction after the endovascular treatment (**C**). AVM, arteriovenous malformation; AICA, anterior inferior cerebellar artery.

and nidus. Dividing a solid AVM nidus in several separate compartments is of no value for that purpose.

Curative embolization is generally possible if only one or a few arteries of sufficient caliber supply the AVM. Multiple arteries, especially those of a small caliber or those that reach the nidus through lenticulostriate or perforating vessels, reduce the chance of safely embolizing an AVM totally.

Several methods have been described to embolize brain AVMs. We recommend treatment under general anesthesia or neuroleptic analgesia. A 6F guiding catheter generally suffices, unless the use of several microcatheters is contemplated. The use of heat-shaped flow-dependent microcatheters (e.g., Magic1.5 and Magic1.2, Balt) is fast and atraumatic, but requires sufficient preferential blood flow toward the brain AVM. These microcatheters as well as the others described later are delivered straight and have to be heat shaped. A small, steep curve is generally adequate. The microcatheter with an insertion wire ("stylet") is then introduced into the continuously flushed guiding catheter. The tip of the stylet is sharp and may not touch any vessel wall. As soon as the tip of the microcatheter becomes visible in the guiding catheter, the stylet must be withdrawn. The Magic catheters will then follow the preferential bloodstream, which may take a while. The steerable Ultraflow and Marathon microcatheters (MTI/ev3) are used together with a microguidewire (Mirage 0.008-in., MTI/ev3). These catheters are largely independent of flow differences and allow a well-controlled and fast catheterization distally, even after major shunt reduction.

As soon as a proper position within the feeding artery is reached, selective contrast medium injection of the vessel will help to determine which embolic agent should be used. Macrofistulas are best occluded with thin and very flexible platinum coils (Liquid coils, Boston Scientific). To occlude the AV shunt, the *n*-butyl cyanoacrylate polymer glues Trufill n-BCA (Cordis), Histoacryl (Braun Melsungen), and Glubran2 (GEM), diluted with variable amounts of the oily contrast medium Lipiodol (Guerbet), are available.[74,75] In most situations, concentrations of 1:4 to 6 for Histoacryl and Lipiodol and 1:2 to 3 for Glubran2 and Lipiodol are appropriate. The liquid embolic agent will be mixed under sterile conditions.

Any contact of the liquid or the catheter with blood, contrast medium, or saline solution has to be avoided. A homogeneous solution is achieved by extended shaking both liquids together in a closed, partly filled syringe. Before injection of the liquid embolic agent, the microcatheter including the hub has to be carefully rinsed and flushed with sterile glucose solution (5% or higher concentrations). The injection of the liquid embolic agent is then started under continuous fluoroscopy. A very slow, controlled injection is most important. In the case of venous passage, the speed of injection has to be reduced even more. Slow propagation of the glue column within the microcatheter will form a drop with a solidified surface at the tip of the microcatheter. If this drop has grown enough, it will break at any point and further partially solidified embolic material will fill the vessel lumen. With highly diluted polymer glue (e.g., Histoacryl and Lipiodol 1:6, Glubran2, and Lipiodol 1:3), 1 to 2 cm reflux around the tip of the microcatheter can be accepted without a major risk of getting the microcatheter fixated in the vessel. Limited reflux and partial solidifying of the embolic agent around the tip of the microcatheter will prevent proximal propagation and facilitate a more distal penetration of the embolic agent. Again, avoidance of venous passage of the embolic agent and subsequent occlusion of the draining veins is most important to prevent an induced AVM bleeding.

Onyx (MTI/ev3) is also a liquid embolic agent. It is an ethylene vinyl alcohol copolymer preparation dissolved in dimethyl sulfoxide (DMSO) with added tantalum. It does not polymerize. On contact with blood, it starts to precipitate. Because of the DMSO, only microcatheters resilient to this solvent can be used for the injection of Onyx. The technique described earlier of voluntary reflux around the microcatheter and subsequent injection far distally may allow the filling of large AVM volumes from a single artery.[76] Onyx, despite being relatively new in the market, has achieved wide acceptance as an embolic agent for brain AVMs.

Ethibloc (Ethicon) is used by only a few physicians for AVM treatment and has never gained the general acceptance of polymer glue and Onyx.

In most centers, the policy for AVM embolization is based on the performance of multiple treatment sessions. How much of an AVM is embolized in one session and how far the endovascular treatment should go is difficult to summarize in a standard guideline. In a single session, too much shunt reduction and vessel occlusion can easily cause edema around the nidus. In brain AVMs in an eloquent location, one or two feeders should be occluded per session. In less sensitive brain regions or if a hemorrhage in the past has already caused a fixed neurological deficit, more generous sessions can be performed.

In AVMs supplied by several large-caliber feeding arteries, it can be helpful to catheterize more than one of these vessels at the same time. Simultaneous injection of glue enables a more homogenous penetration of the nidus since the access of native blood will be suppressed.

Large transdural feeding arteries should be embolized if the subsequent treatment is to be radiosurgery or if this step is considered helpful by the neurosurgeon. We prefer glue embolization for transdural feeders because of its permanency.

Intracranial aneurysms are found in 20% or more of AVM patients.[77] The occasional claims that these aneurysms tend to spontaneous thrombosis after obliteration of the AV shunt are unreliable. On the contrary, these aneurysms may rupture and cause significant rates of morbidity and mortality. Aneurysms at or adjacent to the circle of Willis are therefore coiled or clipped. Peri- and intranidal aneurysms are generally occluded together with the parent artery by means of the injection of a liquid embolic agent.[78]

Completely occluded AVMs have to be followed up by angiography. After curative embolization, follow-up examinations are due after 2 and 6 months, at a minimum, since recanalization may occur. After surgical excision with an expected complete removal of the AVM, a first follow-up angiogram should be carried out within 2 weeks of the operation. A second follow-up angiography after 1 year is frequently helpful because the behavior of arteries that were previously feeding and are now stagnant can be quite puzzling, just like the reactive hypervascularization adjacent to the borders of the resection. If the operating neurosurgeon is not certain about the complete resection of the AVM, intraoperative angiography is probably the best choice.[79] After radiosurgery, primary follow-up is done by MRI and MRA examinations. If these examinations no longer show AVM vessels, an angiography is required. If the AVM is apparently not obliterated 3 years after the irradiation, an angiogram is needed to decide on further therapeutic options.

Complications of the endovascular treatment of brain AVMs are related to the technique used and the location of the AVM within the brain.[80] Edema around the nidus is not rare but is mostly asymptomatic. The administration of steroids (e.g., 8 mg dexamethasone [Fortecortin] three to four times a day for 10 days) is generally sufficient to induce regression of symptomatic edema. Symptomatic brain ischemia may occur if the embolic agent has been injected too far from the nidus, or if it entered a nutritive vessel. This happens frequently if a cortical branch divides into two vessels, one reaching the AVM and the other supplying the cerebral cortex ("en passant feeding artery"). After embolization via lenticulostriate and perforating arteries, the risk of an ischemic neurological deficit is significantly increased. Another mechanism for a mostly delayed ischemic deficit is related to the retrograde thrombosis of previously feeding, large-caliber arteries.[81] The most frequent cause of hemorrhage after AVM embolization is venous passage

of the embolic agent and occlusion of the draining vein(s).[82] This occurs more frequently in AVMs with fistulous components and in those drained by only one vein. Such a hemorrhage may occur during the procedure or at any time during the subsequent week. In case a venous occlusion is recognized in an AVM accessible to surgery, immediate resection is probably better than waiting for the hemorrhage to occur. In lesions not suitable for surgery (e.g., those of the basal ganglia), evacuation of the hematoma without major brain damage can be very difficult. Vessel injury is a less frequently encountered cause of periprocedural intracranial bleeding. Perforation with a guidewire and dissection by the proximal rupture of a microcatheter are both possible. Known mechanisms are kinking of the microcatheter or solidification of the embolic agent within the microcatheter with continued injection. The fixation of the microcatheter within the catheterized artery by reflux of the solidifying embolic agent around the tip of the catheter is mainly a technical event. It is neither recommended nor necessary to forcefully pull the proximal catheter shaft. The best way to deal with this situation is to cut off the microcatheter immediately at the exit from the sheath after the guiding catheter has been removed carefully. The microcatheter fragment is then pushed inside the sheath. Weight-adapted low-molecular heparin is given for 10 days. The risk of ischemic sequelae from this procedure is low, and the catheter will be integrated into the vessel wall within 2 months.

INTRACRANIAL THROMBOLYSIS AND MECHANICAL THROMBUS EXTRACTION

Acute thromboembolic occlusion of a large intracranial artery is an emergency situation. The occlusive material may come from the heart as well as from arteries proximal to the occlusion. Depending on the location and diameter of the artery affected, the onset of clinical symptoms is often instantaneous. Some of the brain tissue deprived of perfusion will irrecoverably undergo necrosis within a few minutes. This necrotic compartment may be surrounded by tissue at risk. Because of a critical reduction in blood supply, the function of this brain tissue may have already ceased, although the remaining metabolism may be sufficient to maintain the cell structure for a variable amount of time. This tissue at risk (penumbra) is the subject of all efforts at vessel recanalization. Because orthograde flow is interrupted, the size of the penumbra in the dependent brain area correlates with the extent of leptomeningeal collaterals. Extensive collaterals on the brain surface significantly increase the chance of a good clinical recovery after revascularization, and vice versa.

Recombinant tissue plasminogen activator (rtPA) converts plasminogen to plasmin and is largely fibrin dependent. Urokinase has the same function but does not rely on fibrin.

In selected patients, intravenous injection of 1 mg rtPA per kilogram body weight may be effective in recanalizing an acutely occluded artery if this is started within 3 hours of the clinical manifestation. After that, conservative treatment, secondary prophylaxis, and endovascular attempts are available options. A combination of intravenous rtPA administration followed by local intra-arterial fibrinolysis (LIF) is a promising concept.[83]

Endovascular treatment of acute intracranial thromboembolic arterial occlusions is currently restricted to occlusions of the distal internal carotid artery, the proximal segment of the middle

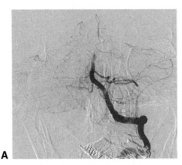
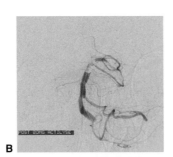
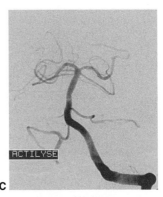

FIGURE 6-20.   Local intra-arterial fibrinolysis of an acute basilar artery thrombosis. Injection of the left vertebral artery shows acute thrombotic occlusion of the distal third of the basilar artery **(A)**. Significant maceration of the thrombus was achieved by local hand injection of 20 mg rtPA **(B)**. After administration of 40 mg rtPA and complete patency of the basilar trunk, both superior cerebellar and posterior cerebral arteries were re-established **(C)**.

cerebral artery or adjacent large vessels, the intracranial vertebral artery, and the trunk and bifurcation of the basilar artery (Fig. 6-20). Parenchymal injury and structural decay start almost simultaneously with the arterial occlusion. Even if the endovascular treatment starts very early (which is hardly within <60 minutes after the onset of vessel occlusion), the fate of the parenchyma relies on the functional effectiveness of the collaterals to the occluded vessel.[84] Endovascular treatment is an option if the patient is referred within given time limits after the onset of clinical symptoms or before major clinical deterioration.

The endovascular treatment with fibrinolytic agents in the anterior circulation should not go beyond 6 hours after clinical onset. In the posterior circulation, there is no fixed time limit, mainly because of the poor prognosis of thromboses of the basilar artery. Coma, however, is considered a contraindication for endovascular stroke therapy. Before starting angiographic workup, a CT examination has to rule out parenchymal hypodensity of more than one-third of the middle communicating artery territory, midline shift, and intracranial hemorrhage. The discrepancy of the size of the lesion between diffusion and perfusion MRI may relate to the penumbra. Other examinations are essentially a waste of time.

As soon as an acute thromboembolic occlusion of one of the vessels just mentioned is confirmed, endovascular treatment should be started. This procedure is best done under general anesthesia, without delaying the initiation of the thrombolysis. First, a complete angiographic examination of all four supraaortic vessels should be performed, which should be completed in <5 minutes. The analysis of collaterals and the site and extent of arterial occlusion are of particular interest. Enzymatic thrombolysis is currently performed with local injection of either urokinase (maximum dosage 1.2 million units) or rtPA (maximum dosage 40 mg) in and around the thrombus.

A 6F guiding catheter and a standard microcatheter (e.g., RapidTransit, Cordis; Nautica, MTI/ev3) with a shallow heatshaped curve are used. The most versatile and atraumatic guidewire is a Synchro14 (Boston Scientific). A SilverSpeed16 (MTI/ev3) is recommended in case a more robust wire is needed. As soon as the sheath is inserted into the femoral artery, 5000 U heparin is given intravenously. Angiography will then show the site of arterial occlusion. The microcatheter should be advanced proximal to the thrombus. Gentle pushing of the

microguidewire will generally allow passage of the thrombus. Injection of the thrombolytic agent starts immediately distal to the thrombus. Continuous machine injection seems to be less efficient than injecting by hand small volumes ("pulse spray") of rtPA or urokinase as repetitive boluses. Further adjunctive options are repeated passages of the thrombus with the microguidewire and/or the microcatheter, use of a retrieval snare, and use of a small PTCA balloon. LIF can be very effective, and complete recanalization is sometimes achieved after an acceptable interval. There is still, however, a significant uncertainty about the success, and many physicians recognize the need for a method with more physical impact on the thrombus. Several devices have recently been introduced or used for this purpose. The efficacy of thrombus aspiration catheters alone (Pronto, Vascular Solutions; Proboscis, Medical Braiding) seems to be low. Concentric Medical achieved FDA clearance for a nitinol wire (MERCI Retriever) that is intended to grasp a thrombus using shape memory properties.[85] The Alligator retrieval device (Chestnut Medical) is constructed for foreign-body removal but might also be usable to pull a firm thrombus out of a brain artery. A modification of the self-expanding Leo stent that is distally closed and proximally attached to an insertion wire is offered by Balt (CATCH). It is currently too early to tell which (if any) of these devices will provide more efficacy for the endovascular treatment of acute ischemic stroke.

If sufficient recanalization is achieved and angiography shows an intracranial atherosclerotic stenosis proximal to the previous occlusion, treatment of this stenosis with stent PTA may be necessary to avoid recurrent vessel occlusion.

Complications during and after LIF are mainly related to intracerebral hemorrhage. Such bleedings are more frequently encountered after a delayed onset of therapy. Their appearance ranges from a diffuse intraparenchymal oozing to a solid intracerebral hematoma. A large hematoma with mass effect or midline shift is always a therapeutic dilemma, and the benefit provided by surgical evacuation is frequently less than expected. The risk of mechanical vessel injury during the manipulation with the microcatheter and microguidewire is increased in very tortuous vessels and may even be higher when the above-mentioned devices are used.

If the patient who was treated with LIF or one of the other methods nevertheless develops a space-occupying infarct, decompressive craniectomy may save his life. The functional outcome, however, is frequently poor.[86]

INTRACRANIAL ATHEROSCLEROTIC ARTERIAL STENOSES

Atherosclerotic stenoses of intracranial arteries are the cause of about 8% to 10% of ischemic strokes. The main pathomechanism is probably a hemodynamically caused insufficient supply of the brain tissue, but repeated emboli may play a role. The natural history of asymptomatic intracranial stenoses is sometimes relatively benign, but untreated symptomatic or progressive lesions are a continuous threat and there is never a guarantee that the first symptom will be a transitory ischemic attack and not a complete stroke. Symptomatic lesions, especially when the symptoms arise despite medical antiaggregation or anticoagulation, and those increasing over time should be treated since the associated risk of stroke is at least 11% per year. Medical therapy with aspirin and perhaps a second compound (e.g., clopidogrel) is sometimes sufficient. In clinical trials, however, the risk of stroke remained high. Anticoagulation with coumarin is more protective, but hemorrhagic complications under effective anticoagulation will in the long-term run outweigh the immediate benefit related to stroke prevention.[87] Surgical creation of an extraintracranial bypass for distal internal carotid artery and proximal middle communicating artery stenoses is an option, but patency rates vary significantly and the surgical procedure itself can be challenging.

In general, endovascular treatment can be contemplated for symptomatic stenoses of the petrous, cavernous, and intradural segments of the internal carotid artery, for the intradural segment of the vertebral artery, and for the basilar artery.[88] Various technical methods are available for the endovascular treatment of these arterial stenoses.

Balloon dilatation has been used in several centers since the mid-1990s.[89] During the past 10 years, mainly in response to cardiologic requirements, balloon profiles have been decreased and the flexibility of balloon catheters improved. These improvements have not, however, overcome the issues of balloon-induced vessel wall dissection and elastic recoiling. Both phenomena may potentially cause (post)procedural vessel occlusion. For the reasons discussed next, we reserve stentless balloon dilatations for those intracranial stenoses that for any reason cannot be reached with a stent.

Balloon-expandable coronary stents were used early for the treatment of intracranial stenoses. These stents are offered premounted on monorail PTCA balloon catheters. Their relative stiffness makes the use of stents longer than 10 mm sometime difficult, especially in the anterior circulation. Even more critical is the proper sizing of balloon-expandable stents. Intracranial vessels are extremely unforgiving to overdilatation because they are thin and not supported by surrounding tissue in the subarachnoid space. Overdilatation may happen with a balloon-expandable stent with an inflation pressure of 6 atm or more. Undersizing of a balloon-expandable stent may result in instability of the deployed stent, which then behaves as a movable foreign body in the vessel lumen. The occurrence of in-stent stenoses due to intimal hyperplasia has led to the use of drug-eluting coronary stents in some centers.[90] Procedural and follow-up benefits have not been confirmed in larger series.

A recently proposed safe and effective endovascular treatment option for intracranial stenoses is the combination of undersized balloon dilatation, followed by the deployment of an oversized self-expanding nitinol stent[91] (Fig. 6-21). We offer this treatment to patients with stenoses in the locations just mentioned if the stenosis is symptomatic despite adequate medical therapy, or if the patient prefers endovascular to medical treatment. In asymptomatic patients, documented progression of the stenosis or an anticipated risk due to anatomic circumstances (e.g., missing collaterals) may be an argument in favor of endovascular treatment.

Preparation of a patient includes the full range of relevant laboratory examinations, including those to rule out vasculitis as a possible cause of the stenosis to be treated. Doppler sonography, MRI, and MRA examinations of the brain are required to define the pretreatment status. Medical pretreatment starts with orally administered loading doses of 500 mg ASA and 300 mg clopidogrel, ideally given 3 days before the procedure, and followed by the administration of 100 mg ASA per day plus 75 mg clopidogrel per day. The treatment is always carried out under general anesthesia with complete muscle relaxation. As soon as a 6F sheath is introduced in one femoral artery, 5000 U heparin is given intravenously. In more time-consuming procedures, heparinization is maintained by an additional 1000 U heparin per hour. Repeated activated clotting time (ACT) measurements are used to confirm sufficient heparinization, which is achieved at duplication of the initial ACT value (if the patient was not previously heparinized).

A diagnostic angiogram with injection of both vertebral and carotid arteries should be obtained either before or at the beginning of the procedure. A 6F guiding catheter is then introduced into the concerning supra-aortic artery (vertebral or internal carotid). Adding nimodipine to the flushing solution will help to prevent mechanically induced vasospasm. If this is not sufficient, slow injection of glycerin trinitrate in doses of 2 mg in 10 mL saline solution can be used. Induced tachycardia and drop in systemic blood pressure has to be covered by the anesthesiologist. The target stenosis is then evaluated by angiography.

Several projections might be necessary until the stenosis is shown without foreshortening or overlying vessels. High magnification is required to clearly understand all the anatomic details. The working projection should ideally show the full

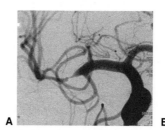 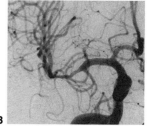

FIGURE 6-21. High-grade, symptomatic stenosis of the right MCA (M1). The stenosis is located between the origin of the lenticulostriate arteries and the temoro-polar branches and the MCA bifurcation. Technical difficulty of Stent-PTA was anticipated because of the irregular tapering of the affected vessel segment **(A)**. The stenosis was dilated with a 1.5 mm/20 mm (8 atm) and a 2 mm/9 mm balloon (4 atm). Subsequently a 2.5 mm/15 mm Neuroform stent was deployed **(B)**. MCA, middle cerebral artery.

length of the stenosis, the distal tip of the guiding catheter, and the vasculature distal to the stenosis. A regular microcatheter (e.g., Echelon10 with 45-degree preshape) with a suitable guidewire (e.g., SilverSpeed10 or Synchro10) is then introduced across the stenosis. For distal positioning, the vessel beyond the stenosis with the largest lumen and the least steep angles is preferable. For stenoses of the internal carotid artery and middle communicating artery, this is mostly the artery of the angular gyrus. For the treatment of V4 and basilar artery stenoses, the posterior communicating artery with the largest P1 segment is preferred. If both posterior communicating arteries are essentially equal, the right one should be chosen since the clinical sequelae of wire-induced ischemia or hemorrhage might be less severe. As soon as a suitable distal position is reached with the microcatheter, the microguidewire is replaced by an X-celerator10 wire (300 cm) (MTI/ev3). With this exchange wire in place, the microcatheter is withdrawn. A balloon catheter is then introduced over the exchange wire. Both the Avion (Invatec) and the Maverick (Boston Scientific) balloon catheter work well. A critical point for the success of the whole procedure is the proper sizing of the balloon. In making this decision, both the normal diameter of the target vessel and the residual lumen of the stenosis have to be taken into account. The "normal" diameter of the cavernous internal carotid artery is about 5 mm, of the intradural internal carotid artery between 3 and 4 mm, of the middle cerebral artery segment around 2.5 mm, and of the basilar trunk around 3.5 mm. The size of the balloon may certainly not be beyond these values and in fact, it has proved safer to purposely underdilate. Because flow is related to vessel diameter by the fourth power, relatively small increases in vessel diameter will result in a significant increase in blood flow. We found 3 to 4 mm for the internal carotid artery, 2 mm for the middle cerebral artery segment, and 3 mm for the basilar artery to be defensive and effective compromises. If there is only a very narrow residual lumen left, the sequential use of two balloons with increasing diameters is recommended. The length of the balloon should cover the stenosis both proximally and distally. Excessive overhang on either side will be of no value and even adds an unnecessary risk of vessel injury. A mixture of equal parts of contrast medium and saline solution is used for manometer-controlled balloon inflation. Balloon inflation has to be done very slowly over 1.5 to 2 minutes. Stepwise inflation and evacuation of the balloon up to gradually increasing maximum pressure values may be helpful. We inflate until the balloon is just entirely straightened but not beyond. After complete vacuum evacuation, the balloon is gently pulled back for several centimeters while keeping the microguidewire in place. Early and very gentle contrast medium injection should be done before the balloon is pulled back into the guiding catheter. If this injection reveals a vessel dissection or perforation, the balloon can be reinserted into the level of the previous dilatation in order to temporarily seal the vessel. If the stenosis if sufficiently dilated and the vessel integrity is confirmed, the balloon catheter can be removed. A self-expanding stent is then introduced. Wingspan and Neuroform (Boston Scientific) are both suitable for this purpose. Wingspan has double the radial force of the Neuroform stent, and the stent catheter is like a miniversion of the Wallstent system. It is not yet clear if one of these two stents will yield better results. The stent length is selected in a way that the previous stenosis is well covered with some overhang proximally and distally (i.e., 15 or 20 mm stent length). The stent diameter will be oversized in relation to the previously used balloon, and nominal stent diameters are mostly in the range of or slightly above the normal vessel diameter (i.e., 4.5 mm for the internal carotid artery, 2.5 to 3 mm for the middle cerebral artery, 3.5 to 4 mm for the basilar trunk). After the self-expanding stent is deployed, an angiogram will be obtained to confirm the result and the integrity of the involved vessels. We either remove both the X-celerator wire and the guiding catheter at this point or decide to wait for another 10 to 15 minutes for a final angiogram.

At the end of the procedure, the sheath is withdrawn and the general anesthesia is terminated. The patient has to be monitored for at least 24 hours. Postprocedural medication includes body-weight-adapted low-molecular heparin for at least 2 days, 100 mg ASA per day permanently, and 75 mg clopidogrel per day for 2 months. Follow-up examinations start with an MRI/MRA examination some days after the treatment, combined with a CT angiography (CTA). If the treated vessel segment is easily accessible to transcranial Doppler sonography, sonographic follow-up examinations are recommended 2 days and 1, 2, 3, and 6 months after the procedure. The angiographic follow-up examinations should be performed 2 months (if no Doppler examination is available), 6 months, and 12 months after the treatment.

CTA seems to be an elegant method for the noninvasive follow-up examination of these patients. In case significant intimal hyperplasia with resulting vessel stenosis is revealed at any point of the follow-up process, redilatation is done better earlier than later. If for any reason the decision to redilate is postponed, frequent follow-up examinations are required. Though quite rare and mostly affecting the anterior circulation, rapidly progressive intimal hyperplasia may cause a vessel occlusion within a few weeks. If detected early enough, intimal hyperplasia within a stent can be removed by balloon redilatation. The repeated passage of the balloon catheter is facilitated by the fact that a Neuroform stent will be integrated into the vessel walls within 8 weeks after deployment.

Complications are rare using the method just described and taking precautions. Vasospasm may occur despite medical pretreatment. In that case, it may be better to stop the initial procedure and give the patient nimodipine intravenously for 2 to 3 days before undertaking the next attempt. Dissection or perforation of a distal vessel with a guidewire or a microcatheter should be treated according to the guidelines just described. Perforation or rupture of the target vessel or stenosis may be sealed temporarily with the balloon catheter used for prior dilatation. Reversal of heparin and antiaggregation drugs has to be started immediately. The anesthesiologist must lower the systemic blood pressure and deepen the narcosis. If the extravasation continues despite these measures, endovascular occlusion of the injured vessel segment distal and proximal to the rupture site has to be contemplated. After the extravasation has stopped, external ventricular drainage may help to reduce the intracranial pressure. If the patient survives the vessel perforation, repeated follow-up examinations starting within the first week after the event are required to address the risk of the patient developing a dissecting aneurysm at the site of the previous vessel wall injury. These aneurysms carry a high risk of rupture and should be treated like any other dissecting intracranial aneurysm.

The frequency of procedural thromboembolic complications using this method is low. Side-branch occlusions are rare. If they occur, little can be done to improve the situation. Thrombus formation in or around the stent is usually avoided by proper premedication. If this occurs nevertheless, the first step could be the intravenous administration of a glycoprotein IIb/IIIa antagonist such as abciximab (ReoPro). An effect should become visible after 10 to 15 minutes. If thrombus formation progresses or if the stent (or vessel) is already occluded, mechanical recanalization should be started. If the guidewire is still in place, passage of the deployed stent with a low-profile balloon and gentle dilatation of the thrombosed vessel segment is a viable option. If the guidewire has already been removed, insertion of a second guidewire beyond the stent would be very helpful. For this maneuver one has to keep in mind that the deployed stent (WingSpan, Neuroform) is quite fragile and that displacement and destruction of the stent can easily take place. The combination of a glycoprotein IIb/IIIa antagonist together with high dosages of heparin or anticoagulants may significantly increase the risk of hemorrhagic complications and should therefore be avoided.

If a long-lasting, significant brain ischemia is reversed to normal conditions, parenchymal hemorrhage may occur. The bleeding can be located a clear distance from the previous stenosis and may affect brain regions that with certainty have not been touched during the procedure. This phenomenon is sometimes explained by the "normal perfusion pressure breakthrough" theory (NPPB).[92] The NPPB concept is based on the idea that in a condition of chronic hypoperfusion, the capillary vessels are maximally dilated in order to compensate for the reduced perfusion pressure. After these capillaries have undergone morphological adaptation to this dilatation, they are no longer able to constrict if exposed to an increased perfusion pressure, which may then rupture these vessels. This theory, appealing as it is, has always been the subject of controversy. NPPB phenomena are rare after intracranial stent PTA, but generally have a poor prognosis. The best way to avoid them is close monitoring of the patients for 1 to 2 days after the procedure with medical treatment of increased arterial systemic blood pressure.

DURAL ARTERIOVENOUS FISTULAS

Dural arteriovenous fistulas (dAVFs) are acquired connections between dural arteries and draining veins, located within the dura mater. Previous sinus vein thrombosis, infection, trauma, or surgery can sometimes be identified as predisposing factors. In the majority of patients, however, none of these circumstances is found.

Clinical signs and symptoms are closely related to the site of the fistula and the pattern of venous drainage, whereas the arterial supply is usually of limited relevance.

dAVFs occur at any location of the cranial dura, but with different frequencies.

The risk of intracranial hemorrhage is related to the drainage of the fistula via cortical veins.[93] Nonhemorrhagic manifestations may result from increased venous pressure, causing disturbance of cerebrospinal fluid (CSF) circulation and congestion in the dependent brain territory (e.g., in the orbit, the temporal lobe, or the spinal cord). Tinnitus or bruit is apparently related to increased blood flow in feeding vessels from the external carotid artery adjacent to the temporal bone (e.g., occipital artery, stylomastoid artery, retroauricular artery).

Tentorial and ethmoidal dAVFs are generally supplied by many small-caliber arteries, making them less accessible to endovascular treatment. Surgical clipping of the draining vein adjacent to the fistula is usually a straightforward approach.[94]

In dAVFs located at the sigmoid sinus (so-called occipital dAVF) or at the cavernous sinus (dural carotid–cavernous sinus fistula, dCCF), endovascular treatment can be offered with good results. For the less frequent dAVFs in other locations, similar treatment principles may apply.

Occipital Dural Arteriovenous Fistula

So-called "occipital" dural AV fistulas are actually located in the wall of the transverse-sigmoid sinus and may extend to the jugular bulb.[95] In many patients, thrombosis of the affected sinus or remnants of a previous sinus thrombosis (such as irregularities of the sinus wall from partial thrombus recanalization) can be found. Patients mostly present with tinnitus synchronous to the heart beat or with an intracranial hemorrhage. Venous drainage of the fistula through cortical veins always carries a risk of bleeding. The arterial supply comes from the occipital artery and further regional branches of the external carotid artery (e.g., stylomastoid artery, retroauricular artery, ascending pharyngeal artery) and from dural branches of the vertebral artery and posterior cerebral artery.

The fistula can be considered as a single pouch or a group of pouches in the wall of the sinus. From there the drainage either follows the sigmoid sinus or uses regional cortical veins. If the sinus is at least partially thrombosed, the probability of cortical venous drainage increases. Treatment may start with a reduction of the AV shunt, achieved by occlusion of supplying branches of the external carotid artery. Poly(vinyl alcohol) (PVA) particles are a suitable embolic agent for nonpermanent vessel occlusion. Both control and permanency are better if polymer glue (Histoacryl, Braun; Glubran2, GEM) diluted with ethiodized oil (Lipiodol, Guerbet) is used.[96] If there is no cortical venous drainage visible and if a bruit was the patient's only complaint, partial embolization with transarterial occlusion of the occipital artery may be sufficient.

In the case of cortical venous drainage or intracranial hemorrhage, complete interruption of the AV shunt is always required. In rare cases with only one or two feeding branches of the external carotid artery, the transarterial injection of polymer glue with a limited amount of venous passage can occlude the fistula. If the fistula is supplied by many branches of the external carotid artery, injection of glue via a single branch will probably fail to occlude the proximal part of the draining vein(s) since native blood from other feeders will dilute the glue or prevent sufficient venous penetration.

The transvenous treatment of occipital dural AV fistulas can follow different strategies. If a meticulous analysis of the arteriograms of the external carotid artery and the vertebral artery clearly shows the segment of the occipital sinus where the fistula is located, transvenous coil occlusion of this sinus segment can obliterate the dural fistula. If the sigmoid sinus is not thrombosed, transvenous catheterization and coil occlusion of the sinus segment are straightforward. This occlusion may, however, not compromise the venous drainage of either the temporal lobe or the cerebellum. Before the acceptable limits of coil occlusion are defined, phlebograms after injection of the internal carotid artery and vertebral artery have to be analyzed. The occlusion of a sinus segment can only be considered safe if the outlets of the drainages from below and above into the sigmoid sinus are identified and left patent.

A more selective strategy, however, may be available. If the sigmoid sinus is widely patent, the pouch of the fistula within the wall of the sinus can sometimes be localized. In that case, transvenous selective catheterization and coil occlusion of the pouch may succeed.[97] Stent deployment within the sigmoid sinus takes advantage of the concept of the fistula as a venous pouch.[98] The normal dimensions of the sigmoid sinus require a large stent. The tortuous passage from the jugular bulb into the sigmoid sinus may be difficult, but we have succeeded several times with a Wallstent (Boston Scientific). The radial force of the available stents is insufficient for the necessary compression of the fistula pouch from inside the sigmoid sinus. It is therefore necessary to dilate the stent with a sufficiently large balloon. If the segment of the sigmoid sinus where the fistula is located is completely thrombosed, transvenous treatment is only possible after endovascular recanalization. As soon as access to the sinus is achieved, the venous pouch with the fistula may be obliterated following the principles described earlier. Stepwise dilatation of the thrombosed sinus using balloons with increasing diameters, thus pressing thrombus material into the pouches, is an alternative though a technically more challenging option.

Follow-up examinations after endovascular occlusion of an occipital dAVF are based on angiography. Invasive follow-up is certainly required if an occipital dAVF with cortical venous drainage has been treated. Clinical follow-up might be considered sufficient if the lesions treated had no cortical drainage, they were completely occluded, and the patient originally presented with a bruit without recurrence.

Transvenous occlusion of the sigmoid sinus with compromise of the outlet of temporal and cerebellar draining veins causes venous congestion and subsequent venous hemorrhage in the affected brain regions. Coils escaping during transvenous occlusion of the sinus may follow the bloodstream and ultimately cause pulmonary artery embolism. Large coil emboli require a foreign-body removal procedure (see later discussion). Transarterial injection of polymer glue with excessive venous passage is dangerous. Inadvertent occlusion of cortical veins can cause venous congestion and hemorrhage. If several cortical veins drain the dural fistula, occlusion of one vein can redirect the drainage blood flow to another vein, eventually resulting in rupture of this vessel.

Dural Carotid Cavernous Sinus Fistula

Spontaneous or dural CCFs (dCCFs) are relatively rare lesions that mainly affect women of advanced age.[99] The pathogenesis remains poorly understood and the history prior to thrombosis of the cavernous sinus is mostly speculative. Clinical signs and symptoms, which are found unilaterally in the majority of cases, include periorbital pain, chemosis, proptosis, increased intraocular pressure, impaired vision, and palsy of the third, fourth, fifth, and sixth cranial nerves with diplopia. Contrast enhanced CT and MRI show the dilated superior ophthalmic vein of the symptomatic eye (Fig. 6-22).[100] Catheter angiography is required to evaluate the pattern of arterial supply and venous drainage. The dural branches of the internal and

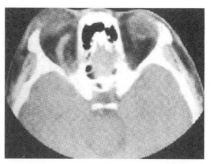

FIGURE 6-22.   CT image of an enlarged superior ophthalmic vein in a patient with a dural carotid cavernous sinus fistula.

external carotid arteries of both sides may contribute to the AV shunt.

The Barrow classification of CCFs refers to the arterial supply discerning direct high-flow shunts between the internal carotid artery and the cavernous sinus (type A), dural shunts between meningeal branches of the internal carotid artery and the cavernous sinus (type B), dural shunts between meningeal branches of the external carotid artery and the cavernous sinus (type C), and dural shunts between meningeal branches of both the internal and external carotid arteries and the cavernous sinus (type D).[101]

The fistula is usually located on the posterior aspect of one cavernous sinus. From there the drainage is through the cavernous sinus itself and then via the superior and inferior ophthalmic veins of one side. An opacification of the inferior and superior petrosal sinus may or may not be visible. Drainage via the sphenoparietal sinus is equivalent to cortical drainage and is associated with the risk of intracranial hemorrhage.[102] The intensity of ocular symptoms is directly related to the extent of venous thrombosis and inversely related to the shunt volume. In fistulas with no or little venous thrombosis (e.g., of the superior ophthalmic vein) and a subsequently large shunt volume with unrestricted venous drainage, the intraocular pressure and the other symptoms mentioned earlier are mostly less pronounced than in fistulas in which thrombosis affects most of the draining veins.

Treatment of dCCFs should be carried out as soon as possible. The chance of either spontaneous thrombosis or thrombosis induced by manual compression of the common carotid artery is very low. Cranial nerve palsy or visual impairment may become permanent if the AV shunt has existed for weeks or months. Unfortunately, many patients are referred for angiographic workup and endovascular treatment after several months of failed attempts at conservative or medical treatment.

If the AV shunt is apparently supplied exclusively by branches of the external carotid artery, endovascular treatment can be started by particulate embolization of these vessels.[103] Depending on the ability of the patient to cooperate, embolization of the external carotid artery branch can be carried out under local anesthesia. Via a 6F guiding catheter, a suitable pre- or self-shaped steerable microcatheter (e.g., Excelsior1018, Boston Scientific, Nautica, MTI/ev3), will be introduced into the affected branch(es) of the external carotid artery. Subselective injection of the vessel is required to confirm the proper position of the microcatheter and the absence of distal collaterals.

For occlusion of the vessel, slow injection of PVA (250 to 350 μm particle size, Contour, Boston Scientific) sufficiently diluted in equal parts of saline solution and contrast medium is suitable. The injection must be monitored continuously using fluoroscopy. Reflux of the PVA particle–carrying liquid column, forceful injection, and injection of inappropriate amounts of particles or of particles that are too small may contribute to the inadvertent occlusion of vessels supplying the brain, cranial nerves, and orbital structures. Any anastomoses between branches of the external carotid artery and intracranial vessels have to be taken into consideration (e.g., middle meningeal artery–ophthalmic artery, internal maxillary artery–middle cerebral artery). If particle embolization via branches of the external carotid artery results in angiographically complete interruption of the AV shunt, close clinical follow-up and angiographic examinations are required since there is always a risk that previously small dural branches of the internal carotid artery, which were not visible before, increase in caliber and maintain the dCCF.

Transvenous coil occlusion is preferable in the majority of dCCFs.[104] This is always the case if the fistula is at least partly supplied by dural branches of the internal carotid artery. These are mostly so many small vessels that a transarterial cure can hardly be achieved. Since transvenous coil occlusion of the cavernous sinus can be both time-consuming and painful, the procedure needs general anesthesia.

A 4F sheath in the right femoral artery is sufficient for intermittent opacification of the arterial supply to the fistula. A 6F sheath will be inserted into the femoral vein of either the ipsilateral or contralateral side. The femoral vein can be punctured 2 cm medial to the palpable femoral artery. We prefer both sheaths in the right groin and have never encountered a postprocedural femoral AV fistula.

Endovascular treatment typically starts with injection of both common carotid arteries. At this point, the location of the fistula and the preferred transvenous approach to it has to be defined. The arterial catheter is then withdrawn. A 6F guiding catheter will be inserted into the venous sheath. The 6F Brite tip guiding catheter with MPA configuration (Cordis) is quite suitable. The entrance of the guiding catheter into the internal jugular vein is sometimes hampered by the venous valves. A Valsalva maneuver, performed by the anesthesiologist manually inflating the patient's lung, is helpful. As soon as the guiding catheter has been introduced into the jugular bulb, the tip of the catheter is positioned opposite to the lower end of the inferior petrosal sinus. This position is achieved when the catheter tip is in the roof of the jugular bulb, pointing to the external auditory channel in the lateral view and pointing 45 degrees medially and up in the posterior-anterior view. In this position, a 0.035-in. guidewire (e.g., Radiofocus 45°, Terumo) is gently inserted into the inferior petrosal sinus (Fig. 6-23). In the majority of cases, it will be possible to even enter the posterior part of the cavernous sinus. With this wire in place, an empty road map can be initiated. Subsequent withdrawal of the guidewire will create a positive road-map image of the inferior petrosal sinus. This will guide the insertion of a robust microcatheter (e.g., Nautica, MTI/ev3; Excelsior1018, Boston Scientific) heat-shaped with a shallow curve. Partial thrombosis and fibrous tissue in the veins can pose significant difficulties to catheterization. Recommended microguidewires for this task are Synchro14, Transend14, Choice PT extra support (Boston Scientific), and SilverSpeed14 or SilverSpeed16 (MTI/ev3).

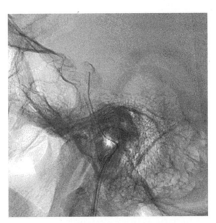

FIGURE 6-23. Lateral view of the skull base. A 6F Brite tip guiding catheter is located adjacent to the orifice of the inferior petrosal sinus (IPS). The IPS is catheterized with a 0.035 in. Terumo Radiofocus guidewire.

In theory, the ideal location for coil occlusion would be the compartment of the cavernous sinus that is immediately adjacent to the fistula. This compartment is, however, frequently not easy to define. Insertion of coils may prevent later navigation within the cavernous sinus and surrounding veins. We therefore prefer to first catheterize the superior ophthalmic vein and then start coil occlusion in the middle of its entire length. The increased thrombogenicity of fibered coils is again beneficial. Starting from the superior ophthalmic vein, the inferior ophthalmic vein and the cavernous sinus should be filled with fibered coils as densely as possible. Leaving nonoccluded compartments has to be carefully avoided. As soon as the posterior aspect of the cavernous sinus is reached and occluded with coils, injection of both common carotid arteries will show if the dCCF is obliterated. At this point of the procedure, separate or previously unrecognized compartments of the cavernous sinus may become visible and should also be occluded with coils. The procedure is continued until early opacification of an ophthalmic or cerebral vein is no longer visible. This requires injection in both common carotid arteries and, if any doubt remains, selective injections in both the internal and external carotid arteries. During the transvenous catheterization, the flushed arterial catheter may remain in the common or internal carotid artery. If the transvenous occlusion of the dCCF has been accomplished, clinical improvement will become evident shortly thereafter. In that case, we do not regularly perform angiographic follow-up examinations. If the patient does not improve within 2 weeks, an angiographic examination is mandatory. Further action depends on the outcome of this examination.

Alternate access routes to the cavernous sinus are via the superior petrosal sinus,[105] the superior ophthalmic vein,[106] and the pterygoid plexus.[107]

Complications of this procedure are rare. The attempt to catheterize the cavernous sinus may fail and requires some level of practice and experience. After the occlusion of a dCCF, a paradoxical aggravation of the ocular symptoms may be observed. This usually resolves within 1 to 2 weeks. During catheterization of the cavernous sinus and the superior ophthalmic vein, venous perforation is possible. Intraorbital venous injury will cause a hematoma, which in our experience has never caused persistent clinical symptoms. Perforation of an intradural vein causes a venous subarachnoid hemorrhage, which is usually a much more serious event. If the coil occlusion of the cavernous sinus fails to occlude the dCCF and the microcatheter has already been withdrawn, it may simply be impossible to recatheterize the cavernous sinus. The situation becomes even worse if the inserted coils redirect the venous drainage from the superior ophthalmic vein to the sphenoparietal sinus with the associated risk of an intracranial hemorrhage. In that case, direct puncture of the cavernous sinus through the foramen ovale may be a final option. The sheath in the femoral vein for venous access may become a source of venous thrombosis and subsequent pulmonary artery embolism. Although we usually do not use heparin during the treatment itself, postprocedural heparinization for 2 days with body-weight-adapted low-molecular heparin is therefore recommended.

DIRECT CAROTID CAVERNOUS SINUS FISTULAS

Direct AV connections between the cavernous segment of the internal carotid artery and the surrounding cavernous sinus result either from the rupture of an aneurysm located at the cavernous internal carotid artery or from a head trauma, mechanically causing this pathological AV connection.[108,109] The size of the rupture in the wall of the internal carotid artery and thus the shunt volume can differ considerably. The clinical sequelae can be due to ischemia of the dependent hemisphere, but more frequently the arterial pressure inside the venous vessels of the cavernous sinus will cause dysfunction of the third, fourth, fifth, and sixth cranial nerves, chemosis, proptosis, and increased intraocular pressure.

These clinical signs and symptoms together with the medical history and a subjectively and objectively audible pulse-synchronous bruit are highly suggestive of this diagnosis. Contrast-enhanced CT and MRI will show an enlarged superior ophthalmic vein. DSA invariably verifies the AV shunt and shows the pattern of venous drainage. In the case of a large fistula and patent collaterals through the circle of Willis, the affected internal carotid artery may only supply the AV shunt. Runs with an increased frame rate (e.g., 6 frames per second) are sometimes helpful to identify the site of the fistula precisely. Manual compression of the affected common carotid artery and injection in a vertebral artery or in the contralateral internal carotid artery may result in an opacification of the fistula through the posterior or anterior communicating artery with a reduced volume of blood, which again can help to better locate the connecting hole. The diagnostic workup can usually be carried out under local anesthesia.

Endovascular treatment is the only therapeutic option for this disorder. The procedure can be technically demanding and time-consuming and should therefore be done under general anesthesia. Preparatory antiaggregation is only necessary if the deployment of a stent or stent graft is contemplated; otherwise, it might prevent the necessary thrombotic occlusion of the fistula. A 6F guiding catheter is generally sufficient, but an 8F guiding catheter may open more technical options. A second 4F sheath via the contralateral femoral artery is sometimes helpful for angiographic monitoring of possible collaterals.

In the past, the great majority of direct CCFs were treated by transarterial balloon occlusion.[110] A silicone or latex balloon with an in-built valve was mounted on the distal tip of a microcatheter that was filled with contrast medium and stiffened by a regular microguidewire. After the balloon had been brought into the cavernous segment of the internal carotid artery adjacent to the fistula, the microguidewire was withdrawn and the balloon was gently filled with small amounts of contrast medium. If the hole in the wall of the internal carotid artery was large enough and the AV shunt flow of sufficient strength, the partially filled balloon drifted from the lumen of the internal carotid artery into the cavernous sinus. Once there, slow or stepwise filling of the balloon with an isotonic contrast medium and intermittent contrast medium injection in the internal carotid artery were used to achieve occlusion of the fistula without compromising the internal carotid artery.[111] The balloon was detached by abrupt or slow pulling on the microcatheter. It was hoped that the balloon would stay in place within the cavernous sinus, held by the wall of the internal carotid artery.

At this point, displacement of the balloon either into the lumen of the internal carotid artery or deeper into the cavernous sinus was sometimes difficult to avoid. Other possible complications were premature detachment of the balloon within the lumen of the internal carotid artery and subsequent passage to the middle communicating artery, compression of the cranial nerves in the wall of the cavernous sinus by the inflated balloon, or early deflation of the detached balloon (e.g., induced by bone fragments jutting into the cavernous sinus) with recurrence of the fistula.[112,113] Because the production of detachable silicone balloons has been abandoned (Boston Scientific), only latex balloons are now available.

A covered stent or stent graft would be the ideal device for the occlusion of a direct CCF. The only stent graft currently available is a balloon-expandable double stent with a PTFE membrane between the two stent tubes (GraftMaster, Abbott). This stent is very stiff, and the required expansion pressure of 16 atm may be beyond the safety limits of intracranial vessels. The use of this stent graft is only recommended if the other options fail or are expected to fail.[37] The technical aspects of the use of this device are described in the aneurysm section.

A technically much easier and better controllable approach to the treatment of a direct CCF is transarterial and/or transvenous coil occlusion of the cavernous sinus.[114,115] In order to avoid inadvertent occlusion of the internal carotid artery, it is mandatory to obtain a DSA run that clearly shows the course of the internal carotid artery, the AV connection, and the borders of the cavernous sinus. If this is not possible, for instance because the cavernous sinus overlaps the lumen of the internal carotid artery in all possible angiographic projections, we recommend that the lumen of the internal carotid artery be protected either by a balloon catheter (e.g., Hyperglide, MTI) or by initial deployment of a porous self-expanding stent (e.g., Neuroform, Boston Scientific; Leo, Balt). The cavernous sinus is then catheterized with a regular dual marker microcatheter of any type and brand. Since the occlusion of the cavernous sinus has to be very dense to seal the CCF, bare coils are less suitable for this purpose because of their low thrombogenicity. Nylon-fibered electrolytically detachable coils have proved very effective. Since the space of the cavernous sinus can be very large, especially if the CCF has existed for some time, it may take a large number of coils to completely fill it. It is frequently necessary to perform two or more treatment sessions within 1 to 2 weeks to achieve a complete interruption of the AV shunt. Early coil compaction is frequent and should be compensated by additional coil insertion.

After interruption of the AV shunt, the ocular symptoms usually improve within a few days. Regression of a pre-existing chemosis can sometimes be observed immediately after the procedure. Cranial nerve palsies sometimes persist longer, and recovery of function may only be incomplete, especially if the symptoms existed for several weeks or months before the treatment.

Follow-up examinations after the endovascular occlusion of a direct CCF are mainly clinical. Angiography should only be performed if the patient does not improve or if the signs and symptoms recur after a transient improvement.

Complications of the coil occlusion of the cavernous sinus are rare. Inadvertent occlusion of the internal carotid artery or displacement of a detached coil from the cavernous sinus into the distal arterial vasculature is possible. New or worsened cranial nerve palsies induced by the insertion of coils into the cavernous sinus have not been encountered by us. Paradox aggravation of symptoms is apparently less frequent than in dCCFs.

FOREIGN-BODY REMOVAL

Microguidewires, microcatheter fragments, and coils may become "foreign bodies." Unintentional electrolytic detachment of microguidewire tips has been reported. After the deployment of a self-expanding open-cell-design nitinol stent (Neuroform), the microguidewire may become firmly attached to the stent struts, probably by intermingling of a part of the wire with the strut angles. If a wire fragment lies free in a vessel, it should be possible to remove it with a microsnare or a microforceps (see later discussion). The anatomic circumstances will help to determine if the effort is appropriate. Very tortuous or thin vessels or those very liable to suffer vasospasm are always discouraging. A wire snared by a deployed Neuroform stent would be better left in place instead of risking vessel dissection, stent displacement, or stent destruction.[116] In that case, the microcatheter is gently pulled from the microguidewire. The microguidewire is then brought under slight tension and cut just at the level of the sheath membrane. The sheath dilatators filled with a 0.035-in. guidewire can be used to help push the remaining microguidewire into the sheath and from there into the external iliac or femoral artery. During the following weeks or months, the wire will break anywhere in its course from the head to the groin and the free fragment will leave the vessel lumen. When it reaches the skin, the loose fragment can be pulled out under sterile conditions. The remaining part will undergo endothelialization.

The issue of microcatheters fixed by the reflux of a solidifying embolic agent has been addressed in the section on AVM.[117] Free fragments from broken microcatheters can be pulled out (see later discussion).

Displaced coils and coil loops are now probably the most frequently encountered intracranial foreign body. If one or several coils have left their proper position, they may easily occlude the vessel in which they became trapped. Several devices may be considered to remove the coils.

The Attractor (Target Therapeutics/Boston Scientific) was essentially a nondetachable coil with attached long fibers. This device did not work well and is no longer offered. The In-Time Retrieval Device (Target Therapeutics/Boston Scientific), a nitinol double basket, is too stiff and passage of the carotid siphon is very difficult. The Retriever microcatheter (Target Therapeutics/Boston Scientific) is a mechanically fixed combination of a microguidewire and a microcatheter. Its function is basically that of a snare, but access to distal target vessels is easier if microcatheter and retrieval device are independent of each other. The Microvena snare (ev3) is made of a steel wire with a radiopaque nitinol loop at its distal end.[118] Under unrestricted conditions, the loop assumes a 90-degree angle in relation to the wire. Two loop sizes, 2 mm and 4 mm, are suitable for intracranial purposes. The device works best with a separate 0.021-in. ID microcatheter (e.g., RapidTransit, Cordis). After the target object has been brought within the open loop, gentle pulling on the wire will close the loop at the distal end of the microcatheter, thus fixating the object.

The use of this microsnare can be straightforward if the target object is sufficiently radiopaque and if the proximal or distal end is accessible. However, it is difficult if not impossible to use it to retrieve, for instance, coils. In small vessels the available lumen may be insufficient to open the snare. If pulled through vessel curves, the loop always has a tendency to turn away from the foreign body. The Alligator Retrieval Device (Chestnut Medical) is made of a 0.016-in. stainless steel insertion wire with microfabricated precision grasping arms attached to its tip.[119] Arms 2 mm or 4 mm in length are preferred for intracranial applications (Fig. 6-24). The grasping arms are radiopaque and easily visible under fluoroscopy. The microforcep is introduced through a microcatheter with a 0.021-in. inner diameter. When 3 mm in front of the target object, the grasping arms are advanced beyond the distal tip of the microcatheter until they are fully open. Further advancement of microcatheter and Alligator will bring the grasping arms adjacent to the target. The grasping arms are then closed by holding the Alligator in an unchanged position and slightly advancing the microcatheter. Keeping the Alligator wire under tension will allow withdrawal of the target object. This device is suitable for the well-controlled removal of metallic foreign bodies from intracranial vessels.

FINAL REMARKS

The successful performance of endovascular treatment of cerebral and spinal vessel disorders requires a minimum of 2 years of dedicated and supervised training in a specialized high-volume center.

Interventionists must find the narrow path between rigid conservatism and unethical experimentation.

Interventional neuroradiologists rely on a sufficient number of referring hospitals, a trained and knowledgeable interdisciplinary team, a rational relationship to the medical device companies, and reliable mid- and long-term follow-up.

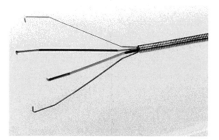

FIGURE 6-24. Alligator Retrieval Device, suitable for foreign body removal from intracranial arteries.

Note

Off-Label Use: Several of the products mentioned in this text have neither a CE mark nor FDA approval for the described applications.

REFERENCES

1. Luessenhop AJ, Kachman R, Shevlin W, et al. Clinical evaluation of artificial embolization in the management of large cerebral arteriovenous malformations. *J Neurosurg.* 1965;23:400–417.
2. Barr JD, Connors JJ III, Sacks D et al. Quality improvement guidelines for the performance of cervical carotid angioplasty and stent placement. *J Vasc Intervent Radiol.* 2003;14:321–335.
3. Higashida RT, Hopkins LN, Berenstein A, et al. Program requirements for residency/fellowship education in neuroendovascular surgery/interventional neuroradiology: a special report on graduate medical education. *AJNR Am J Neuroradiol.* 2000;21:1153–1159.
4. American Society of Interventional and Therapeutic Neuroradiology (ASITN). General considerations for endovascular surgical neuroradiologic procedures. *AJNR Am J Neuroradiol.* 2001;22:1–3.
5. Singh V, Gress DR, Higashida RT, et al. The learning curve for coil embolization of unruptured intracranial aneurysms. *AJNR Am J Neuroradiol.* 2002;23:768–771.
6. Turjman F, Massoud TF, Sayre J, et al. Predictors of aneurysmal occlusion in the period immediately after endovascular treatment with detachable coils: a multivariate analysis. *AJNR Am J Neuroradiol.* 1998;19:1645–1651.
7. Citron SJ, Wallace RC, Lewis CA, et al. Quality improvement guidelines for adult diagnostic neuroangiography; cooperative study between ASITN, ASNR, and SIR. *J Vasc Intervent Radiol.* 2003;14:257–262.
8. Picard L. Medicolegal aspects in neuroradiologic emergencies. *J Neuroradiol.* 2004;31:340–346.
9. Grzyska U, Freitag J, Zeumer H. Selective cerebral intraarterial DSA. Complication rate and control of risk factors. *Neuroradiology.* 1990;32:296–299.
10. Smith JJ, Jensen ME, Dion JE. FDA medical device regulation and informed consent. *Am J Neuroradiol.* 1998;19:1815–1817.
11. Turski PA, Stieghorst MF, Strother CM, et al. Digital subtraction angiography "road map." *AJR Am J Roentgenol.* 1982;139:1233–1234.
12. Krayenbühl H, Yasargil MG, Huber P. *Cerebral Angiography.* Thieme Medical Publishers, 1982.
13. Osborn AG. *Diagnostic Cerebral Angiography.* Lippincott Williams & Wilkins, 1998.
14. Anxionnat R, Bracard S, Ducrocq X, et al. Intracranial aneurysms: clinical value of 3D digital subtraction angiography in the therapeutic decision and endovascular treatment. *Radiology.* 2001;218:799–808.
15. Wardlaw JM, White PM. The detection and management of unruptured intracranial aneurysms. *Brain.* 2000;123:205–221.
16. ACROSS Australasian Cooperative Research on Subarachnoid Hemorrhage Study: epidemiology of aneurysmal subarachnoid hemorrhage in Australia and New Zealand: incidence and case fatality from the Australasian Cooperative Research on Subarachnoid Hemorrhage Study (ACROSS). *Stroke.* 2000;31:1843–1850.
17. Keris V, Buks M, Macane I, et al. Aneurysmal subarachnoid hemorrhage in Baltic population: experience from Latvia (1996–2000). *Eur J Neurol.* 2002;9:601–607.
18. Anonymous. Unruptured intracranial aneurysms—risk of rupture and risks of surgical intervention. International Study of Unruptured Intracranial Aneurysms Investigators. *N Engl J Med.* 1998;339:1725–1733.
19. Wiebers DO, Whisnant JP, Huston J 3rd, et al. International Study of Unruptured Intracranial Aneurysms Investigators. Unruptured intracranial aneurysms: natural history, clinical outcome, and risks of surgical and endovascular treatment. *Lancet.* 2003;362:103–110.
20. Villablanca JP, Martin N, Jahan R, et al. Volume-rendered helical computerized tomography angiography in the detection and characterization of intracranial aneurysms. *J Neurosurg.* 2000;93:254–264.
21. Molyneux AJ, Kerr RS, Yu LM, et al. International Subarachnoid Aneurysm Trial (ISAT) Collaborative Group. International subarachnoid aneurysm trial (ISAT) of neurosurgical clipping versus endovascular coiling in 2143 patients with ruptured intracranial aneurysms: a randomised comparison of effects on survival, dependency, seizures, rebleeding, subgroups, and aneurysm occlusion. *Lancet.* 2005;366:809–817.
22. Hochmuth A, Spetzger U, Schumacher M. Comparison of three-dimensional rotational angiography with digital subtraction angiography in the assessment of ruptured cerebral aneurysms. *AJNR Am J Neuroradiol.* 2002;23:1199–1205.
23. Henkes H, Brew S, Felber S, et al. In vitro and in vivo studies of the extent of electrothrombotic deposition of blood elements on the surface of electrolytically detachable coils. *Intervent Neuroradiol.* 2004;10:189–201.
24. Pierot L, Flandroy P, Turman F, et al. Selective endovascular treatment of intracranial aneurysms using micrus microcoils: preliminary results in a series of 78 patients. *J Neuroradiol.* 2002;29:114–121.
25. Cloft HJ, Joseph GJ, Tong FC, et al. Use of three-dimensional Guglielmi detachable coils in the treatment of wide-necked cerebral aneurysms. *AJNR Am J Neuroradiol.* 2000;21:1312–1314.
26. Vallee JN, Pierot L, Bonafe A, et al. Endovascular treatment of intracranial wide-necked aneurysms using three-dimensional coils: predictors of immediate anatomic and clinical results. *AJNR Am J Neuroradiol.* 2004;25:298–306.
27. Moret J, Cognard C, Weill A, et al. Reconstruction technique in the treatment of wide-neck intracranial aneurysms. Long-term angiographic and clinical results. Apropos of 56 cases. *J Neuroradiol.* 1997;24:30–44.

28. Lubicz B, Leclerc X, Gauvrit JY, et al. HyperForm remodeling-balloon for endovascular treatment of wide-neck intracranial aneurysms. *AJNR Am J Neuroradiol.* 2004;25:1381–1383.
29. Malek AM, Halbach VV, Phatouros CC, et al. Balloon-assist technique for endovascular coil embolization of geometrically difficult intracranial aneurysms. *Neurosurgery.* 2000;46:1397–1407.
30. Henkes H, Bose A, Felber S, et al. Endovascular coil occlusion of intracranial aneurysms assisted by a novel self-expandable nitinol microstent (Neuroform). *Intervent Neuroradiol.* 2002;8:107–119.
31. Pumar JM, Blanco M, Vazquez F, et al. Preliminary experience with LEO self-expanding stent for the treatment of intracranial aneurysms. *AJNR Am J Neuroradiol.* 2005;26:2573–2577.
32. Fiorella D, Albuquerque FC, Deshmukh VR, et al. Usefulness of the Neuroform stent for the treatment of cerebral aneurysms: results at initial (3–6-mo) follow-up. *Neurosurgery.* 2005;56(6):1191–1201.
33. Raymond J, Guilbert F, Roy D. Neck-bridge device for endovascular treatment of wide-neck bifurcation aneurysms: initial experience. *Radiology.* 2001;221:318–326.
34. Henkes H, Liebig T, Reinartz J, et al. Endovascular occlusion of the basilar artery for the treatment of dissecting and dysplastic fusiform aneurysms. *Nervenarzt.* 2005;77(2):194–196;198–200.
35. Chapot R, Houdart E, Saint-Maurice JP, et al. Endovascular treatment of cerebral mycotic aneurysms. *Radiology.* 2002;222:389–396.
36. Molyneux AJ, Cekirge S, Saatci I, et al. Cerebral Aneurysm Multicenter European Onyx (CAMEO) trial: results of a prospective observational study in 20 European centers. *AJNR Am J Neuroradiol.* 2004;25:39–51.
37. Felber S, Henkes H, Weber W, et al. Treatment of extracranial and intracranial aneurysms and arteriovenous fistulae using stent grafts. *Neurosurgery.* 2004;55:631–638.
38. Henkes H, Reinartz J, Preiss H, et al. Endovascular treatment of small intracranial aneurysms: three alternatives to coil occlusion. *Minim Invasive Neurosurg.* 2006. In press.
39. Henkes H, Fischer S, Weber W, et al. Endovascular coil occlusion of 1811 intracranial aneurysms: early angiographic and clinical results. *Neurosurgery.* 2004;54:268–280.
40. Cloft HJ, Kallmes DF. Cerebral aneurysm perforations complicating therapy with Guglielmi detachable coils: a meta-analysis. *AJNR Am J Neuroradiol.* 2002;23:1706–1709.
41. Peltier J, Nowtash A, Toussaint P, et al. Aneurysmal rupture during embolization with Guglielmi detachable coils. *Neurochirurgie.* 2004;50(4):454–460.
42. Lethagen S. Desmopressin (DDAVP) and hemostasis. *Ann Hematol.* 1994;69:173–180.
43. Biondi A, Ricciardi GK, Puybasset L, et al. Intra-arterial nimodipine for the treatment of symptomatic cerebral vasospasm after aneurysmal subarachnoid hemorrhage: preliminary results. *AJNR Am J Neuroradiol.* 2004;25:1067–1076.
44. Ross IB, Dhillon GS. Complications of endovascular treatment of cerebral aneurysms. *Surg Neurol.* 2005;64:12–18.
45. Soeda A, Sakai N, Sakai H, et al. Thromboembolic events associated with Guglielmi detachable coil embolization of asymptomatic cerebral aneurysms: evaluation of 66 consecutive cases with use of diffusion-weighted MR imaging. *AJNR Am J Neuroradiol.* 2003;24(1):127–132.
46. Brilstra EH, Rinkel GJ, van der Graaf Y, et al. Treatment of intracranial aneurysms by embolization with coils: a systematic review. *Stroke.* 1999;30:470–476.
47. Batista LL, Mahadevan J, Sachet M, et al. 5-year angiographic and clinical follow-up of coil-embolised intradural saccular aneurysms. A single center experience. *Intervent Neuroradiol.* 2002;8:349–366.
48. Bendok BR, Padalino DJ, Levy EI, et al. Intravenous abciximab for parent vessel thrombus during basilar apex aneurysm coil embolization: case report and literature review. *Surg Neurol.* 2004;62:304–311.
49. Mounayer C, Piotin M, Baldi S, et al. Intraarterial administration of abciximab for thromboembolic events occurring during aneurysm coil placement. *AJNR Am J Neuroradiol.* 2003;24:2039–2043.
50. Cronqvist M, Pierot L, Boulin A, et al. Local intraarterial fibrinolysis of thromboemboli occurring during endovascular treatment of intracerebral aneurysm: a comparison of anatomic results and clinical outcome. *AJNR Am J Neuroradiol.* 1998;19:157–165.
51. Berg-Dammer E, Henkes H, Trobisch H, et al. Sticky platelet syndrome: a cause of neurovascular thrombosis and thrombo-embolism. *Intervent Neuroradiol.* 1997;3:145–154.
52. Fessler RD, Ringer AJ, Qureshi AI. Intracranial stent placement to trap an extruded coil during endovascular aneurysm treatment: technical note. *Neurosurgery.* 2000;46:248–251.
53. Blanc R, Weill A, Piotin M, et al. Delayed stroke secondary to increasing mass effect after endovascular treatment of a giant aneurysm by parent vessel occlusion. *AJNR Am J Neuroradiol.* 2001;22:1841–1843.
54. Russell SM, Nelson PK, Jafar JJ. Neurological deterioration after coil embolization of a giant basilar apex aneurysm with resolution following parent artery clip ligation. Case report and review of the literature. *J Neurosurg.* 2002;97:705–708.
55. Byrne JV, Sohn MJ, Molyneux AJ. Five-year experience in using coil embolization for ruptured intracranial aneurysms: outcomes and incidence of late rebleeding. *J Neurosurg.* 1999;90:656–663.
56. Derdeyn CP, Graves VB, Turski PA, et al. MR angiography of saccular aneurysms after treatment with Guglielmi detachable coils: preliminary experience. *AJNR Am J Neuroradiol.* 1997;18:279–286.
57. Anzalone N, Righi C, Simionato F, et al. Three-dimensional time-of-flight MR angiography in the evaluation of intracranial aneurysms treated with Guglielmi detachable coils. *AJNR Am J Neuroradiol.* 2000;21:746–752.
58. Duong DH, Young WL, Vang MC, et al. Feeding artery pressure and venous drainage pattern are primary determinants of hemorrhage from cerebral arteriovenous malformations. *Stroke.* 1998;29:1167–1176.
59. Redekop G, TerBrugge K, Montanera W, et al. Arterial aneurysms associated with cerebral arteriovenous malformations: classification, incidence, and risk of hemorrhage. *J Neurosurg.* 1998;89:539–546.

60. Hirai S, Mine S, Yamakami I, et al. Angioarchitecture related to hemorrhage in cerebral arteriovenous malformations. *Neurol Med Chir (Tokyo)*. 1998;38(suppl):165–170.

61. Yeh HS, Kashiwagi S, Tew JM Jr, et al. Surgical management of epilepsy associated with cerebral arteriovenous malformations. *J Neurosurg*. 1990;72:216–223.

62. Piepgras DG, Sundt TM Jr, Ragoowansi AT, et al. Seizure outcome in patients with surgically treated cerebral arteriovenous malformations. *J Neurosurg*. 1993;78:5–11.

63. Kwon OK, Han DH, Han MH, et al. Palliatively treated cerebral arteriovenous malformations: follow-up results. *J Clin Neurosci*. 2000;7(suppl 1):69–72.

64. Henkes H. Endovaskuläre Behandlung zerebraler arteriovenöser Malformationen. Konzepte und Ergebnisse: Landsberg, Germany. *Ecomed*. 2000.

65. Schaller C, Pavlidis C, Schramm J. Differential therapy of cerebral arteriovenous malformations. An analysis with reference to personal microsurgery experiences. *Nervenarzt*. 1996;67:860–869.

66. Hassler W, Hejazi N. Complications of angioma surgery—personal experience in 191 patients with cerebral angiomas. *Neurol Med Chir (Tokyo)*. 1998;38(suppl):238–244.

67. Han PP, Ponce FA, Spetzler RF. Intention-to-treat analysis of Spetzler-Martin grades IV and V arteriovenous malformations: natural history and treatment paradigm. *J Neurosurg*. 2003;98:3–7.

68. Karlsson B, Lindquist C, Steiner L. Prediction of obliteration after gamma knife surgery for cerebral arteriovenous malformations. *Neurosurgery*. 1997;40:425–430.

69. Maruyama K, Kawahara N, Shin M, et al. The risk of hemorrhage after radiosurgery for cerebral arteriovenous malformations. *N Engl J Med*. 2005;352:146–153.

70. Henkes H, Nahser HC, Berg-Dammer E, et al. Endovascular therapy of brain AVMs prior to radiosurgery. *Neurol Res*. 1998;20:479–492.

71. Yu SC, Chan MS, Lam JM, et al. Complete obliteration of intracranial arteriovenous malformation with endovascular cyanoacrylate embolization: initial success and rate of permanent cure. *AJNR Am J Neuroradiol*. 2004;25:1139–1143.

72. Vinuela F, Dion JE, Duckwiler G, et al. Combined endovascular embolization and surgery in the management of cerebral arteriovenous malformations: experience with 101 cases. *J Neurosurg*. 1991;75:856–864.

73. Jafar JJ, Davis AJ, Berenstein A, et al. The effect of embolization with N-butyl cyanoacrylate prior to surgical resection of cerebral arteriovenous malformations. *J Neurosurg*. 1993;78:60–69.

74. n-BCA Trail Investigators. *N*-Butyl cyanoacrylate embolization of cerebral arteriovenous malformations: results of a prospective, randomized, multi-center trial. *AJNR Am J Neuroradiol*. 2002;23:748–755.

75. Leonardi M, Barbara C, Simonetti L, et al. Glubran2: A new acrylic glue for neuroradiological endovascular use. Experimental study on animals. *Intervent Neuroradiol*. 2002; 8:245.

76. Jahan R, Murayama Y, Gobin YP, et al. Embolization of arteriovenous malformations with Onyx: clinicopathological experience in 23 patients. *Neurosurgery*. 2001;48:984–995.

77. Kim EJ, Halim AX, Dowd CF, et al. The relationship of coexisting extranidal aneurysms to intracranial hemorrhage in patients harboring brain arteriovenous malformations. *Neurosurgery*. 2004;54:1349–1357.

78. Ezura M, Takahashi A, Jokura H, et al. Endovascular treatment of aneurysms associated with cerebral arteriovenous malformations: experiences after the introduction of Guglielmi detachable coils. *J Clin Neurosci*. 2000;7(suppl 1):14–18.

79. Pietilä TA, Stendel R, Jansons J, et al. The value of intraoperative angiography for surgical treatment of cerebral arteriovenous malformations in eloquent brain areas. *Acta Neurochir (Wien)*. 1998;140:1161–1165.

80. Taylor CL, Dutton K, Rappard G, et al. Complications of preoperative embolization of cerebral arteriovenous malformations. *J Neurosurg*. 2004;100:810–812.

81. Miyasaka Y, Kurata A, Tanaka R, et al. The significance of retrograde thrombosis following removal of arteriovenous malformations in elderly patients. *Surg Neurol*. 1998;49:399–405.

82. Keller E, Yonekawa Y, Imhof HG, et al. Intensive care management of patients with severe intracerebral haemorrhage after endovascular treatment of brain arteriovenous malformations. *Neuroradiology*. 2002;44:513–521.

83. Lee KY, Kim DI, Kim SH, et al. Sequential combination of intravenous recombinant tissue plasminogen activator and intra-arterial urokinase in acute ischemic stroke. *AJNR Am J Neuroradiol*. 2004;25:1470–1475.

84. Brekenfeld C, Remonda L, Nedeltchev K, et al. Endovascular neuroradiological treatment of acute ischemic stroke: techniques and results in 350 patients. *Neurol Res*. 2005;27(suppl 1):S29–35.

85. Smith WS, Sung G, Starkman S, et al. MERCI Trial Investigators. Safety and efficacy of mechanical embolectomy in acute ischemic stroke: results of the MERCI trial. *Stroke*. 2005;36:1432–1438.

86. Kilincer C, Asil T, Utku U, et al. Factors affecting the outcome of decompressive craniectomy for large hemispheric infarctions: a prospective cohort study. *Acta Neurochir (Wien)*. 2005;147:587–594.

87. Chimowitz MI, Lynn MJ, Howlett-Smith H, et al. Warfarin-Aspirin Symptomatic Intracranial Disease Trial Investigators. Comparison of warfarin and aspirin for symptomatic intracranial arterial stenosis. *N Engl J Med*. 2005;352:1305–1316.

88. Higashida RT, Meyers PM, Connors JJ 3rd, et al. American Society of Interventional and Therapeutic Neuroradiology; Society of Interventional Radiology; American Society of Neuroradiology. Intracranial angioplasty and stenting for cerebral atherosclerosis: a position statement of the American Society of Interventional and Therapeutic Neuroradiology, Society of Interventional Radiology, and the American Society of Neuroradiology. *AJNR Am J Neuroradiol*. 2005;26:2323–2327.

89. Berg-Dammer E, Henkes H, Weber B., et al. Percutaneous transluminal angioplasty of intracranial artery stenosis: clinical results in 24 patients. *Neurosurg Focus*. 1998;5: Article 13.

90. Abou-Chebl A, Bashir Q, Yadav JS. Drug-eluting stents for the treatment of intracranial atherosclerosis. Initial experience and midterm angiographic follow-up. *Stroke*. 2005;36(12):e165–168.

91. Henkes H, Miloslavski E, Lowens S, et al. Treatment of intracranial atherosclerotic stenoses with balloon dilatation and self-expanding stent deployment (WingSpan). *Neuroradiology*. 2005;47:222–228.

92. Spetzler RF, Wilson CB, Weinstein P, et al. Normal perfusion pressure breakthrough theory. *Clin Neurosurg*. 1978;25:651–672.

93. Sarma D, ter Brugge K. Management of intracranial dural arteriovenous shunts in adults. *Eur J Radiol*. 2003;46:206–220.

94. Tomak PR, Cloft HJ, Kaga A, et al. Evolution of the management of tentorial dural arteriovenous malformations. *Neurosurgery*. 2003;52:750–760.

95. Naito I, Iwai T, Shimaguchi H, et al. Percutaneous transvenous embolisation through the occluded sinus for transverse-sigmoid dural arteriovenous fistulas with sinus occlusion. *Neuroradiology*. 2001;43:672–676.

96. Nelson PK, Russell SM, Woo HH, et al. Use of a wedged microcatheter for curative transarterial embolization of complex intracranial dural arteriovenous fistulas: indications, endovascular technique, and outcome in 21 patients. *J Neurosurg*. 2003;98:498–506.

97. Mironov A. Selective transvenous embolization of dural arteriovenous fistulas without occlusion of the dural sinus. *AJNR Am J Neuroradiol*. 1998;19:389–391.

98. Liebig T, Henkes H, Brew S, et al. Reconstructive treatment of dural arteriovenous fistulas of the transverse and sigmoid sinus: transvenous angioplasty and stent deployment. *Neuroradiology*. 2005;47:543–551.

99. Phatouros CC, Meyers PM, Dowd CF, et al. Carotid artery cavernous fistulas. *Neurosurg Clin N Am*. 2000;11:67–84.

100. Wei R, Cai J, Ma X, et al. Imaging diagnosis of enlarged superior ophthalmic vein. *Zhonghua Yan Ke Za Zhi*. 2002;38:402–404.

101. Barrow DL, Spector RH, Braun IF, et al. Classification and treatment of spontaneous carotid-cavernous sinus fistulas. *J Neurosurg*. 1985;62:248–256.

102. Brown RD Jr, Wiebers DO, Nichols DA. Intracranial dural arteriovenous fistulae: angiographic predictors of intracranial hemorrhage and clinical outcome in nonsurgical patients. *J Neurosurg*. 1994;81:531–538.

103. Liu HM, Wang YH, Chen YF, et al. Long-term clinical outcome of spontaneous carotid cavernous sinus fistulae supplied by dural branches of the internal carotid artery. *Neuroradiology*. 2001;43:1007–1014.

104. Meyers PM, Halbach VV, Dowd CF, et al. Dural carotid cavernous fistula: definitive endovascular management and long-term follow-up. *Am J Ophthalmol*. 2002;134:85–92.

105. Mounayer C, Piotin M, Spelle L, et al. Superior petrosal sinus catheterization for transvenous embolization of a dural carotid cavernous sinus fistula. *AJNR Am J Neuroradiol*. 2002;23:1153–1155.

106. Miller NR, Monsein LH, Debrun GM, et al. Treatment of carotid-cavernous sinus fistulas using a superior ophthalmic vein approach. *J Neurosurg*. 1995;83:838–842.

107. Jahan R, Gobin YP, Glenn B, et al. Transvenous embolization of a dural arteriovenous fistula of the cavernous sinus through the contralateral pterygoid plexus. *Neuroradiology*. 1998;40:189–193.

108. Debrun GM. Angiographic workup of a carotid cavernous sinus fistula (CCF) or what information does the interventionalist need for treatment? *Surg Neurol*. 1995;44:75–79.

109. Kobayashi N, Miyachi S, Negoro M, et al. Endovascular treatment strategy for direct carotid-cavernous fistulas resulting from rupture of intracavernous carotid aneurysms. *AJNR Am J Neuroradiol*. 2003;24:1789–1796.

110. Kwon BJ, Han MH, Kang HS, et al. Endovascular occlusion of direct carotid cavernous fistula with detachable balloons: usefulness of 3D angiography. *Neuroradiology*. 2005; 47:271–281.

111. Weber W, Henkes H, Berg-Dammer E, et al. Cure of a direct carotid cavernous fistula by endovascular stent deployment. *Cerebrovasc Dis*. 2001;12:272–275.

112. Kendall B. Results of treatment of arteriovenous fistulae with the Debrun technique. *AJNR Am J Neuroradiol*. 1983;4:405–408.

113. Lewis AI, Tomsick TA, Tew JM Jr. Management of 100 consecutive direct carotid-cavernous fistulas: results of treatment with detachable balloons. *Neurosurgery*. 1995;36:239–244.

114. Nishio A, Nishijima Y, Tsuruno T, et al. Direct carotid-cavernous sinus fistula due to ruptured intracavernous aneurysm treated with electrodetachable coils—case report. *Neurol Med Chir (Tokyo)*. 1999;39:681–684.

115. Chun GF, Tomsick TA. Transvenous embolization of a direct carotid cavernous fistula through the pterygoid plexus. *AJNR Am J Neuroradiol*. 2002;23:1156–1159.

116. Henkes H, Kirsch M, Mariushi W, et al. Coil treatment of a fusiform upper basilar trunk aneurysm with a combination of "kissing" neuroform stents, TriSpan-, 3D- and fibered coils, and permanent implantation of the microguidewires. *Neuroradiology*. 2004; 46:464–468.

117. Debrun GM, Aletich V, Ausman JI, et al. Embolization of the nidus of brain arteriovenous malformations with *n*-butyl cyanoacrylate. *Neurosurgery*. 1997;40:112–120.

118. Prestigiacomo CJ, Fidlow K, Pile-Spellman J. Retrieval of a fractured Guglielmi detachable coil with use of the Goose Neck snare "twist" technique. *J Vasc Intervent Radiol*. 1999;10:1243–1247.

119. Henkes H, Lowens S, Preiss H, et al. A new device for endovascular coil retrieval from intracranial vessels (Alligator Retrieval Device, ARD). Technical note. *AJNR Am J Neuroradiol*. 2006. In press.

Peter Lanzer
Ralf Weser

CHAPTER **7**

Internal Carotid Artery

CAROTID ARTERY DISEASE AND STROKE

Stroke, the destruction of brain tissue, may be related to focal or global ischemia (approximately 80%) or hemorrhage (approximately 20%). Ischemic strokes are caused mostly by focal arterial occlusions due to thrombosis or embolization, and less frequently by global hypoperfusion or coagulation disorders; hemorrhagic strokes are due to intracerebral hemorrhage (rupture of small intracerebral vessels) or subarachnoid hemorrhage (rupture of arterial aneurysms).

The majority of ischemic strokes are due to atherothrombotic and thromboembolic extracranial carotid artery disease; other less frequent vascular pathologies include spontaneous dissections, arteritides, fibromuscular dysplasia, arterial kinking, aneurysms, and complications of head and neck neoplasias. In small intracranial vessels, other vasculopathies may be also responsible such as noninflammatory degenerative disorders, Moyamoya disease, and persistent vasospasms.

Embolic occlusions are mostly thrombogenic, related to known cardiac sources including the left atrium in patients with atrial fibrillation or left atrial myxoma, the left ventricle in patients with acute myocardial infarction or severe left ventricular dysfunction, and aortic or mitral valves in patients with endocarditis or degenerative valvular disorders. Other potential sources of thrombogenic emboli include deep peripheral veins in patients with patent foramen ovale or interventricular septum defects, and ascending aortic atherothrombotic disease in patients with advanced generalized atherosclerosis. Nonthrombogenic emboli such as atherosclerotic debris, air, nitrogen bubbles, fat emboli, septic emboli, or tumor tissue are less frequent and mostly associated with specific situations such as cardiac surgery, major trauma, and cases of sudden decompression (e.g., Caisson's disease).

Global brain hypoperfusion is related to states associated with major circulatory compromise such as cardiac arrest, cardiogenic shock, or severe arrhythmias (for a review of stroke etiologies, see references 1 and 2). Furthermore, a number of genetic loci associated with stroke have been identified (for review, see reference 3).

In a recent study conducted by the American Stroke Association and American Heart Association in the United States in 2002, of 700,000 strokes, of which 500,000 were new and 200,000 recurrent; 88% were ischemic and 12% were hemorrhagic (9% intracerebral and 3% subarachnoid hemorrhages). The age-adjusted stroke incidence rates per 100,000 for the first stroke were 167 for white male patients, 138 for white female patients, 323 for black male patients, and 260 for black female patients.[4]

Major nonmodifiable risk factors for stroke include age, gender, race, ethnicity, and heredity; major potentially modifiable risk factors for ischemic stroke include hypertension, heart disease (mainly atrial fibrillation, left ventricular dysfunction, and valvular diseases), diabetes mellitus, lipoprotein disorders, smoking, alcohol, and drug abuse, adverse lifestyle habits, contraceptives, and—importantly—asymptomatic carotid artery disease and transitory ischemic attack. Major risk factors of intracerebral hemorrhage include hypertension, smoking, and heavy alcohol abuse (for review, see reference 5).

Carotid artery disease was recognized as a cause of stroke during the second half of the 19th century by a number of eminent pathologists and clinicians; however, it appears that in clinical medicine "the prevailing notion held by most physicians was that strokes were caused by intracranial vascular disease" lasted well into the 20th century (for review, see reference 6). Among those who provided major contributions to understanding the extracranial pathogenesis of stroke, one should perhaps at least mention the name of J. Ramsay Hunt (1872–1937), who clearly established the link between ipsilateral partial or total occlusion of a carotid artery and contralateral clinical symptoms.[7] In a more recent era, C. Miller Fisher (b. 1913) is credited with providing a major contribution to our present understanding of the principal role of the atherosclerotic carotid artery disease in the pathogenesis of stroke (for review, see reference 8).

Besides the traditional and new risk factors for stroke, local factors such as unsteady flow conditions at the carotid flow divider[9] associated with low shear stress[10] and cyclic mechanical strain[11,12] are important factors in the localization, development, and progression of extracranial carotid atherosclerosis.

The pathogenetic and clinical significance of carotid artery disease is based on its propensity to reduce the blood flow locally because of atherothrombosis, or peripherally because of embolization. Whereas in the early days, the severity of the local disease was considered the most critical factor in stroke etiology, the importance of the embolization potential of internal carotid lesions in addition to their severity has increasingly been recognized. Thus, on the basis of ultrasound with integrated backscatter, echolucent atherosclerotic plaques with low integrated backscatter can be visualized as vulnerable, lipid-and macrophage-rich carotid plaques.[13,14] The embolization potential of plaque ulcerations has also been determined.[15] More recently, the irregularity of the plaque surface seen on angiography has been recognized as a predictive risk factor for ipsilateral ischemic stroke in all degrees of stenosis; the predictive power increases with increasing severity of stenosis.[16] However, while the angiographic severity of stenosis can be measured, and criteria for making measurements comparable have been established,[17,18] morphologic criteria are more difficult to identify objectively. In fact, the degree of concurrence between carotid angiography and surgical observation in detecting carotid plaque ulcerations has been found to be low (Table 7-1) (for review, see reference 19). Nevertheless, a strong association between histology and angiographic carotid artery surface morphology has been reported in a recent study. Here, four different morphologies of carotid artery ulcerations (ulcer types 1 to 4) and two different types of carotid artery surface irregularities (a, b) are described as distinct markers of plaque instability (Fig. 7-1).[20]

Total or subtotal occlusions of the internal carotid artery or occlusions of its branches may remain clinically silent, or they may produce specific and usually sudden clinical neurological syndromes that are characteristic of the site of the brain ischemia or infarction. In approximately 50% of cases, stroke may be preceded by transient ischemic attacks. In patients with carotid artery disease, middle cerebral artery syndromes are characterized by motoric and sensory impairments of the contralateral face, arm, and leg, vision disturbances, usually homonymous hemianopsia or homonymous quadrantonopsia, or paralysis of conjugate gaze to the opposite side (patient looks toward the

TABLE 7-1. Studies Comparing Angiographic Carotid Plaque Surface Morphology with Pathology

	Number of Plaques	Number with Angiographic Ulceration (%)	Blinding Stated	Pathological Features	Results	
					Sensitivity	Specificity
STUDIES OF HISTOLOGICAL APPEARANCE						
Estol, 1991	36	12 (33)	Yes	Rupture	56%	89%
Kim, 2000	55	46 (84)	Yes	Rupture	86%	33%
Croft, 1980	64	2 (3)	Yes	Rupture	Not given	
Endo, 1996	40	6 (15)	No	Rupture, thrombus, and hemorrhage	4 of 6 ulcers were found in plaque with rupture, hemorrhage, and localized thrombus	
STUDIES OF GROSS MACROSCOPIC APPEARANCE ONLY						
Maddison, 1969	45	38 (84)	No	Macroscopic ulceration	88%	0%
Houser, 1974	349	139 (40)	No	Macroscopic ulceration	Not given	100%
Blaisdell, 1974	50	38 (76)	No	Macroscopic ulceration	100%	63%
Edwards, 1979	50	29 (58)	No	Macroscopic ulceration	60%	43%
O'Donnell, 1985	79	30 (38)	Yes	Macroscopic ulceration	59%	73%
Eikelboom, 1983	155	84 (54)	No	Macroscopic ulceration	73%	62%
Ricotta, 1986	84	54 (64)	Yes	Macroscopic ulceration	78%	56%
Comerota, 1990	126	44 (35)	No	Macroscopic ulceration	53%	92%
Streifler, 1994	480	181 (38)	No	Macroscopic ulceration	46%	74%
Kagawa, 1996	48	24 (50)	No	Macroscopic ulceration	57%	73%
Liberopoulos, 1996	52	25 (48) small ulcers 16 (30) large ulcers	No	Macroscopic ulceration	93% small ulcers 100% large ulcers	Not given
Rothwell, 2000	1671	1066 (63.8) Irregular or ulcerated	No	Macroscopic ulceration Macroscopic thrombus	69% (ulcer) 72% (thrombus)	47% (ulcer) 40% (thrombus)

From Streifler JY, Eliasziw M, Fox AJ, et al. Angiographic detection of carotid plaque ulceration. Comparison with surgical observations in multicenter study. *Stroke.* 1994;25:1130–1132.

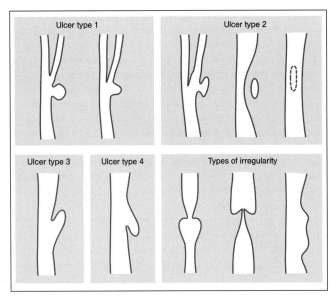

FIGURE 7-1. Examples of angiographic carotid plaque surface ulceration (*types 1–4*) and surface irregularities (*a*, pre- and poststenotic dilatation; *b*, wall irregularities) associated with plaque instability. (Redrawn from Lovett JK, Gallagher PJ, Hands LJ, et al. Histological correlates of carotid plaque surface morphology on lumen contrast imaging. *Circulation.* 2004;110:2190–2197.)

infarcted side). If the lesion is on the dominant side of the brain, aphasia may be present; conversely, if the nondominant side is involved, unilateral neglect and agnosia or anterior cerebral artery syndromes associated with motoric and sensory impairment of the contralateral lower extremity with impaired gait and stance might be present. In addition to the hemispheric syndromes (rarely bilateral syndromes), monocular visual disturbances due to impaired blood flow through the ophthalmic artery may be present. Ischemic syndromes of the posterior cerebral circulation secondary to carotid artery disease are rare (for a review of neurological syndromes associated with carotid artery disease, see reference 2). Interventionists performing carotid artery procedures must be thoroughly familiar with the major neurological manifestations potentially associated with thromboembolic complications of extracranial carotid disease in peri-interventional settings.

DIAGNOSTIC EVALUATIONS

In addition to the patient's clinical history and a physical examination, the diagnosis of carotid artery disease should also be based on direct visualization of the carotid arteries using one of the available imaging modalities. Carotid artery ultrasound, magnetic resonance (MR) and computed tomography (CT) angiography may be used for primary diagnostic purposes; however, in patients considered for revascularization and in peri-interventional settings only conventional and digital subtraction angiography, DSA, are applicable.

Duplex ultrasound (Doppler flow measurement plus B-mode image) allows functional and morphologic assessment of the carotid artery stenosis on the basis of measurements of the peak systolic and end-diastolic velocity, spectral dispersion, and the carotid index (defined as a ratio of peak systolic velocities

of the poststenotic internal carotid artery and common carotid artery),[21] and visual assessment of the entire common carotid and, to a certain extent, the extracranial segments of the internal and external carotid arteries. The opportunity to define potentially unstable echolucent (as opposed to echogenic) atherosclerotic plaques via B-mode ultrasound is of particular clinical interest.[13,22] Importantly, a carotid index of >4.0 has been shown to be a highly accurate predictor of high-grade (70% to 99%) stenosis according to the North American Carotid Endarterectomy Trial (NASCET) criteria.[23] The limitations of duplex ultrasound include high operator dependence, low sensitivity in low-grade lesions, and a tendency to overestimate severity (for review, see reference 24). Transcranial Doppler using transtemporal, orbital, transforaminal, and submandibular windows may be used in conjunction with duplex ultrasound to evaluate the impact of the extracranial artery disease on intracranial hemodynamics, including assessment of collateral flow in the circle of Willis, reversal of flow in the ophthalmic and anterior cerebral arteries, absence of ophthalmic or carotid siphon flow, and reduced middle cerebral artery flow velocity and pulsatility.[25] In addition, transcranial Doppler is useful in a more comprehensive evaluation of pathophysiology of cerebrovascular disease, including the detection of microemboli (for review, see reference 26). Three-dimensional and compound ultrasound imaging techniques might further improve the definition of carotid artery atherosclerotic plaque morphology, and clinical utility of MR angiography and CT angiography in the assessment of carotid artery disease in conjunction with neuroimaging using MR and CT are summarized in references 24 and 27.

Despite its numerous shortcomings, x-ray carotid artery angiography, which was introduced in 1927[28] and became popular after the percutaneous technique of establishing arterial access,[29] dedicated catheterization instrumentation,[30] and digital imaging technology[31] had become available, continues to represents the gold standard in neurovascular imaging and is the only angiographic technique available as a guide during interventional therapy on the carotid artery.

Neuroangiography is used to evaluate intracranial and extracranial head and neck circulation following selective catheterization of the target arteries. The recommended indications for neuroangiography are summarized in Table 7-2.[32] Technique and interpretation of diagnostic neuroangiography has been extensively reviewed in the literature.[33–35]

To evaluate patients for extracranial carotid artery revascularization, standard imaging protocols are implemented that include angiography of the aortic arch and the main thoracocervical vessels and selective bilateral extracranial and intracranial carotid angiograms in at least two, preferably orthogonal, projections. In patients with complex cerebrovascular anatomy and multiple collateral pathways, all four neck arteries, carotids and vertebrals, must be selectively visualized to fully assess the intracranial blood supply.

To evaluate patients for carotid artery stenting (CAS), a suitable femoral artery access must be available, and the technical ability to reach and to cross the target vessel must be ensured. To determine whether the target internal carotid artery lesion is accessible using either one of the common femoral arteries access sites, the course and the morphology of the ipsilateral iliac artery, descending aorta, aortic arch, brachiocephalic trunk, and the common carotid arteries should be evaluated.

TABLE 7-2. Indications for Diagnostic Neuroangiography

Define presence/extent of vascular occlusive disease and thromboembolic phenomena.

1. Define etiology of hemorrhage (subarachnoid, intraventricular, parenchymal, craniofacial).
2. Define presence, location, and anatomy of intracranial aneurysms and vascular malformations.
3. Evaluate vasospasm related to subarachnoid hemorrhage.
4. Define presence/extent of trauma to cervicocerebral vessels (e.g., dissection, pseudoaneurysm).
5. Define vascular supply to tumors.
6. Define presence/extent of vasculitis (infectious, inflammatory, drug-induced).
7. Diagnose and/or define congenital or anatomic anomaly (e.g., vein of Galen fistula).
8. Define presence of venous occlusive disease (e.g., dural sinus, cortical, deep).
9. Outline vascular anatomy for planning and determining the effect of therapeutic measures.
10. Perform physiologic testing of brain function

From Citron SJ, Wallace RC, Lewis CA, et al., for the Joint Standards of Practice Task Force of the Society of Interventional Radiology, the American Society of Interventional and Therapeutic Neuroradiology. Quality improvement guidelines for adult diagnostic neuroradiography. Cooperative study between ASITN, ASNR, and SIR. *J Vasc Intervent Radiol.* 2003;14:S257–S262.

Specifically, the aortic arch must be assessed to define its form and elongation and the angle of the take-off of the target common carotid artery. Particularly in patients with elevated diaphragm and arterial elongation, the entire aortic arch may be shifted upward, usually displacing the ascending limb of the thoracic aorta laterally and thereby often creating a steep up-sloping shoulder. This aortic arch configuration is indicative of greater technical difficulty in approaching the target vessel. In addition, the presence of associated disease of the aortic arch and of the nontarget cerebrovascular vessels should be noted.

The target common carotid artery must be assessed to determine the angle of the take-off, level of bifurcation, and presence of associated lesions. The external carotid artery is assessed mainly in terms of its branching pattern in order to identify a suitable branch for guidewire placement, evidence of abnormal vessel connections, embryonic bridges, or collateralization (note of warning: risk of distal and intracranial embolization), and evidence of previous embolic events. The internal carotid artery should be studied along its entire course to determine its course, branching pattern, the presence of main branches, collateral vessels (including its participation in the formation of the circle of Willis), and the presence of abnormal flow patterns (including competitive flow), and to identify associated anomalies such as embryonal vessels, the presence of associated lesions, the anatomic position of the take-off of the ophthalmic artery, and the form of the carotid T in order to estimate the risks of traumatization that are mainly due to guidewire or distal protection device (DPD) manipulation. Tortuosities, coilings, and kinkings may be associated with stenosis, and several projections could be required to define the anatomy. The proximity of the convoluted segments to the target lesion may affect the operator's ability to safely deploy the DPD. In addition, excessive meandering and elongation of the internal carotid artery may be increased if a stent is placed

with suboptimal longitudinal flexibility. To estimate the effect of stenting, imaging of the internal carotid artery in several different positions of the head may be helpful. Figure 7-2 shows the common collateral pathways of the cerebrovascular circulation as a potential source of intracranial embolization.[36]

The target lesion and the adjacent distal and proximal segments of the internal carotid artery are assessed for stent sizing, to measure the severity of the stenosis, and to define the morphology of the target lesion. The severity of the internal carotid artery stenosis is measured as a percentage reduction in the diameter of the patent lumen at the narrowest segment. Most frequently, automatic edge detection algorithms or densitometric quantitative techniques are employed; alternatively the measurements can be performed manually using calipers. Because of significant changes in size of the internal carotid artery at the bulbar level, precise definition of the employed

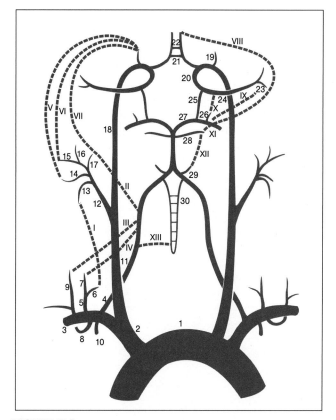

FIGURE 7-2. Collateral cerebrovascular circulation. *I,II,* collaterals between external carotid artery (ECA) and subclavian arteries and ECA and vertebral arteries (VA). *III,IV,* collaterals between subclavian arteries and vertebral arteries. *V–VII,* internal carotid arteries (ICA) and ECA. *VIII–X,* ICA and VA. *XI,XII,* VA and basilar arteries. *XIII,* VA and spinal arteries. *1,* Aortic arch; *2,* brachiocephalic trunk; *3,* subclavian artery; *4,* VA; *5,* thyrocervical trunk; *6,* inferior thyroid artery; *7,* ascending cervical artery; *8,* costothyroid artery; *9,* deep cervical artery; *10,* internal thoracic artery; *11,* common carotid artery; *12,* ECA; *13,* superior thyroid artery; *14,* facial artery; *15,* maxillary artery; *16,* superficial temporal artery; *17,* occipital artery; *18,* ICA; *19,* ophthalmic artery; *20,* anterior cerebral artery; *21,* anterior communicating artery; *22,* pericallosal artery; *23,* middle cerebral artery (parieto-occipital branches); *24,* anterior choroid artery; *25,* posterior communicating artery; *26,* posterior choroid artery; *27,* posterior cerebral artery; *28,* posterior cerebellar artery; *29,* posterior inferior cerebellar artery; *30,* spinal arteries. (Redrawn from Lusza G. *X-ray Anatomy of the Vascular System.* Philadelphia: JB Lippincott Co, 1963.)

methodology is required to allow reproducible measurements. According to the NASCET method, the shortest distance between the two opposing leading edges at the narrowest point and the lumen diameter of the adjacent healthy segment distal to the stenosis are compared. According to the European Carotid Surgery Trial (ECST) method, the luminal and the assumed nominal diameters at the site of maximum stenosis are compared. Finally, using the common carotid (CC) method, the minimum luminal diameter is compared with the luminal diameter in the proximal common carotid artery. Although the use of each of these three different techniques leads to the calculation of different absolute numbers for stenosis severity, the results are consistent, maintaining an almost linear relationship, and the equivalence of measurements has been determined: 50% NASCET stenosis is equivalent to a 65% ECST and CC stenosis, and 70% NASCET stenosis is equivalent to a 82% ECST and CC stenosis (for review, see references 24 and 37). Figure 7-3 shows a schematic comparison of quantitative methods to assess the severity of internal carotid artery stenoses. The principal morphologic aspects of the target lesion that are relevant to CAS include the presence of thrombi, surface morphology (ulcerations), calcifications, and the plaque burden.

On the basis of the anatomic information derived, the technical feasibility and strategy of CAS are formulated and potential interventional risks defined. The main issues include the estimated stability and backup of the support system required to overcome the anatomic adversities of the proximal vascular

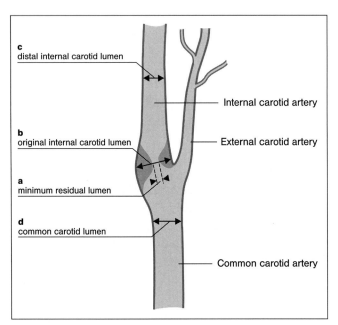

FIGURE 7-3. Quantitative measurements of the severity of internal carotid artery stenosis using three different methods. ESCT method: Stenosis = $[1 - (a/b)] \times 100$; NASCET method: Stenosis = $[1 - (a/c)] \times 100$; common carotid method: Stenosis = $[1 - (a/d)] \times 100$. Measurement *b*, the original internal carotid lumen, is made at the point of maximal stenosis (not necessarily the bulb) and is an estimate. In the original publication, a caliper was used for measurements. (Redrawn from Young GR, Humphrey PRD, Nixon TE, et al. Variability in measurements of extracranial internal carotid artery stenosis as displayed by both digital subtraction and magnetic resonance angiography. An assessment of three caliper techniques and visual impression of stenosis. *Stroke.* 1996;27:467–473.)

pathways, definition of the relevant external carotid artery branch for safe engagement of the support system, and evaluation of the interventional site, including the configuration, topography, and geometry of the flow divider (stent sizing and positioning), and features of the target lesion critical to guidewire use (position and diameter of the residual lumen with respect to the walls of the carotid bulb, and presence of ulcerations and tissue pockets), crossing of the DPD, and the need for predilatation (severity, calcification). Safe crossing ability of the DPD and adequate distal spacing between the target lesion and DPD are critical to overall procedural risk assessment.

To ensure quality, close adherence to established standards regarding procedural outcomes is required.[32] Although the achievement of perfect outcomes, that is, 100% success with 0% complications, is desirable, a certain level of complications may be considered acceptable on the basis of good clinical practice standards. The definition of thresholds of procedural indicators of outcome serves benchmarking. To allow consistent reporting of outcomes, unequivocal definition of procedural indicators such as complications is mandatory (Table 7-3). The suggested thresholds of neurologic and nonneurologic complications in performing quality, adult, diagnostic neuroangiography, as proposed by joint effort of the Society of Interventional Radiology, the American Society of Interventional and Therapeutic Neuroradiology, and the American Society of Neuroradiology, are summarized in Tables 7-4 and 7-5. To define the degree of severity of neurologic complications, modified Rankin disability score should be determined and reported (Table 7-6).

Diagnostic cerebrovascular angiograms should be evaluated by an interventionist, a vascular surgeon, and a neurologist; to select the optimum strategy of treatment, i.e., medical versus carotid artery endarterectomy (CAE) versus CAS, a consensus decision of the whole team is required. Provided that there exists a comparable level of interventional and surgical competence at a given institution, the indications for specific means of revascularization (CAE vs. CAS) depend primarily on estimates of the interventional and surgical risk (e.g., comorbidities, need

TABLE 7-3. Definition of Outcomes: Neurologic Complications, Minor and Major Complications

- Transient ischemic attack (TIA): neurologic deficits lasting less than 24 h
- Strokes: neurologic deficits lasting longer than 24 h
- Reversible strokes: neurologic deficits resolving within 7 days
- Permanent strokes: neurologic deficits lasting longer than 7 days
- Minor complications: either no therapy, no consequence or nominal therapy, no consequence; includes overnight admission for observation only
- Major complications: require therapy, minor hospitalization (<48 h); require major therapy, unplanned increase in level of care, prolonged hospitalization (>48 h); permanent adverse sequelae; death.

From Citron SJ, Wallace RC, Lewis CA, et al., for the Joint Standards of Practice Task Force of the Society of Interventional Radiology, the American Society of Interventional and Therapeutic Neuroradiology. Quality improvement guidelines for adult diagnostic neuroradiography. Cooperative study between ASITN, ASNR, and SIR. *J Vasc Intervent Radiol.* 2003;14:S257–S262.

TABLE 7-4.   Procedural Outcome Threshold of Neuroangiography in Adults: Neurologic Complications

	Reported Rate	*Suggested Complication-specific Threshold*
Reversible neurologic deficit (including transient ischemic attacks and reversible stroke)	0–2.3%	2.5%
Permanent neurologic deficit	0–5%	1%

From Citron SJ, Wallace RC, Lewis CA et al., for the Joint Standards of Practice Task Force of the Society of Interventional Radiology, the American Society of Interventional and Therapeutic Neuroradiology. Quality improvement guidelines for adult diagnostic neuroradiography. Cooperative study between ASITN, ASNR, and SIR. *J Vasc Intervent Radiol.* 2003;14:S257–S262.

TABLE 7-5.   Procedural Outcome Threshold of Neuroangiography in Adults: Nonneurologic Complications

	Reported Rate	*Suggested Complication-specific Threshold*
Renal failure	0–0.15%	0.2%
Arterial occlusion requiring surgical thrombectomy or thrombolysis	0–0.4%	0.2%
Arteriovenous fistula/pseudoaneurysm	0.01–0.22%	0.2%
Hematoma requiring transfusion or surgical evacuation	0.26–1.5%	0.5%

From Citron SJ, Wallace RC, Lewis CA et al., for the Joint Standards of Practice Task Force of the Society of Interventional Radiology, the American Society of Interventional and Therapeutic Neuroradiology. Quality improvement guidelines for adult diagnostic neuroradiography. Cooperative study between ASITN, ASNR, and SIR. *J Vasc Intervent Radiol.* 2003;14:S257–S262.

TABLE 7-6.   Modified Rankin Disability Score

0 = Grade	No signs or symptoms
1 = Grade	No significant disability; able to carry out all the usual activities of daily living (without assistance). Note: This does not preclude the presence of weakness, sensory loss, language disturbance, etc., but implies that these are mild and do not or have not caused patient to limit his/her activities (e.g., if employed before, is still employed at the same job).
2 = Grade	Slight disability; unable to carry out some previous activities, but able to look after own affairs without much assistance (e.g., unable to return to prior job; unable to do some household chores, but able to get along without daily supervision/help).
3 = Grade	Moderate disability, requiring some help but able to walk without assistance (e.g., needs daily supervision; needs assistance with small aspects of dressing, hygiene; unable to read or communicate clearly. Note: ankle-foot orthotic or cane does not imply needing assistance).
4 = Grade	Moderately severe disability; unable to walk without assistance and unable to attend bodily needs without assistance (e.g., needs 24-hr supervision and moderate-maximum assistance on several activities of daily living, but still able to do some activities by self, or with minimal assistance).
5 = Grade	Severe disability; bedridden, incontinent, and requiring constant nursing care and attention.
6 = Grade	Stroke, death
9 = Unknown (not obtainable from history or no follow-up)	

From Citron SJ, Wallace RC, Lewis CA, et al., for the Joint Standards of Practice Task Force of the Society of Interventional Radiology, the American Society of Interventional and Therapeutic Neuroradiology. Quality improvement guidelines for adult diagnostic neuroradiography. Cooperative study between ASITN, ASNR, and SIR. *J Vasc Intervent Radiol.* 2003;14:S257–S262.

for coronary artery bypass graft [CABG] surgery), presence of hostile neck conditions, and the angiographic substrate of the target lesion.

REVASCULARIZATION OPTIONS

It is customary in clinical practice to differentiate between symptomatic and asymptomatic carotid artery stenosis. The definition is based on the patient's history and physical examination; patients with documented carotid artery stenosis but no history of focal neurological signs and symptoms are considered asymptomatic, including those with detected "silent" infarcts on CT or MR imaging, regardless of the size and number of ischemic defects! In clinical practice, however, patients with radiographic evidence of ischemic defects in the distribution of a stenotic internal carotid artery are considered to have an active disease associated with a greater need for secondary prevention, including revascularization. The principal revascularization options are carotid artery surgery or CAS.

In 1954, Eastcott and colleagues published the first case report on revascularization of the carotid artery by resecting the 3–cm-long stenotic segment and repairing it using end-to-end anastomosis.[38] The first CAE was performed in 1956, as reported by DeBakey.[39] Evolution of carotid artery surgery for stroke prevention has been extensively reviewed and reported in the literature.[6,40]

It was not until 1991 that the benefits of CAE in symptomatic patients were reported in two large prospective and randomized trials, namely, ECST[41] and NASCET,[42] with final results and recommendations of both trials reported in 1998.[43,44] Recently, the evidence of data supporting the use of CAE for symptomatic carotid disease in relation to subgroups has been reviewed and presented.[45] Evidence of benefits of CAE in patients with asymptomatic carotid disease has been derived primarily from two large trials, namely, the Asymptomatic Carotid Atherosclerosis Study (ACAS)[46] and the Asymptomatic Carotid Surgery Trial (ACST)[47]; both trials have recently been commented on and reviewed.[48]

On the basis of current American Heart Association (AHA) guidelines, CAE appears beneficial for symptomatic patients with ipsilateral, 70% to 99% carotid artery stenosis, with a reported complication rate of $\leq$3%, whereas the indication for a 30% to 69% stenosis (measured by NASCET criteria) remained uncertain; it also appears beneficial for asymptomatic patients with carotid stenosis of $\geq$60%, a surgical risk of $\leq$3%, and a life expectancy of $\geq$5 years, irrespective of the status of the contralateral carotid artery (proven indication), as well as in patients with carotid stenosis of $\geq$60%, irrespective of the status of the contralateral carotid artery, who are scheduled for simultaneous CABG surgery (acceptable indication).[49] However, the latter strategy, which was introduced in 1972,[50] has remained a point of ongoing controversy.[51] On the basis of the recommendations of the American Academy of Neurology, the indications for CAE for severe (70% to 99%) symptomatic stenosis were endorsed. Moderate benefits were assigned to treatments of patients with a 50% to 69% symptomatic stenoses, and no indications were seen for patients with <50% stenosis, provided in all cases that the perioperative combined stroke and death rate was <3%. In patients with asymptomatic 60% to 99% stenosis the Academy saw fewer benefits than for symptomatic patients, and individual decisions were recommended.[52] CAE is presently the standard treatment for patients with symptomatic and asymptomatic extracranial carotid artery stenosis.

Percutaneous intervention for carotid artery stenosis in humans was first reported by Mathias in 1977.[53] Subsequently, sporadic studies on carotid balloon angioplasty were published, reporting technical success rates between 79% and 98%, and a risk of stroke between 4% and 6%.[54–57] In 1994, the first stent-supported carotid angioplasties using Palmaz medium biliary stents (Cordis, Miami, FL, USA), Flex-Stents (Cook, Bloomington, IN, USA), and Wallstents (Schneider, Zurich, Switzerland) were performed and reported.[58] Introduction of distal protection devices (DPDs) in 1996 [59] has increased procedural safety and has reduced the incidence of neurological complications.[60–62] Subsequently, in a number of single- and multicenter studies, improved endovascular techniques and technology have been used and CAS efficacy documented.[63] On the basis of early results and evolving evidence, an early advisory AHA statement[64] and more recent extensive guidelines for CAS performance have been formulated.[65]

Considering the indications for CAE in symptomatic and asymptomatic patients (Table 7-7) and on the basis of the evolving evidence available in 2003, the Collaborative Panel of the American Society of Interventional and Therapeutic Neuroradiology, the American Society of Neuroradiology, and the Society of the Interventional Radiology proposed indications and contraindications for CAS (Table 7-8).[65]

TABLE 7-7. Suggested Indications for Carotid Endarterectomy

Carotid Artery Status	Indication Level	
	Proven	Acceptable
Symptomatic	$\geq$70% stenosis and risk of death and major morbidity <6%	50%–69% and risk of death and major morbidity <6%
Asymptomatic	$\geq$60% stenosis and risk of death and major morbidity <3%	$\geq$60% stenosis and pending coronary artery bypass surgery

From Barr JD, Connors JJ, Sacks D, et al., for the ASITN, ASNR, and SIR Standards of Practice Committees. Quality improvement guidelines for the performance of cervical carotid angioplasty and stent placement. Developed by a Collaborative Panel of the American Society of Interventional and Therapeutic Neuroradiology, the American Society of Neuroradiology, and the Society of the Interventional Radiology. *J Vasc Intervent Radiol.* 2003;14:S321–S335.

CAROTID ARTERY STENTING: A CORONARYLIKE APPROACH

Within less than a decade, important advances have been made in dedicated CAS instrumentation, including the introduction of high-performance 0.035-in. and 0.014-in. guidewires, low-profile dilatation balloons, stents with improved design that provide greater radial force, better crossing, and scaffolding properties, and more efficacious and less traumatic distal protection devices. In addition, the coronarylike approach to CAS has been developed, which consists of telescopic coaxial techniques using low profile instrumentation to provide direct access to the target lesion and coronary equipment and rapid exchange techniques to accomplish the revascularization.[66,67]

With CAE representing the standard treatment of carotid artery disease, the rationale for CAS is to provide treatment options for patients with high surgical risk, patients with a "hostile neck" (i.e., high, above C2, and low, below the clavicle, internal carotid artery stenosis, prior neck radiation or neck surgery, medical conditions associated with cervical spinal immobility, extreme obesity with short neck, and requirements for tracheostomy), and patients with conditions associated with poor surgical outcomes (e.g., restenosis following an ipsilateral CAE). In addition patients with high surgical risk are considered. High surgical risk has been variously defined in the literature; those groups considered at such risk included patients with coronary artery disease requiring CABG surgery; patients with ongoing stable or unstable angina despite medication; patients with recent myocardial infarction, that is, within the past 30 days; patients with congestive heart failure, uncontrolled hypertension, contralateral carotid occlusion, renal insufficiency, or creatinine >1.5 mg/dL; and those with poorly controlled diabetes.[68–71]

To date, only one prospectively randomized trial study design has allowed direct comparison of the state-of-the-art coronary-approach CAS with CAE.[72,73] In this trial, 747 patients at 29 sites were evaluated between 1999 and 2002 for revascularization of internal carotid artery stenosis. A total of 334 patients were randomized, and 310 patients were treated; 406 patients were treated in the nonrandomized CAS, and seven patients in the nonrandomized CAE arm. Inclusion and exclusion criteria are

TABLE 7-8. Suggested Indications and Contraindications for Carotid Artery Stenting (CAS)

Acceptable Indications for CAS	*Relative Contraindications for CAS*	*Absolute Contraindications for CAS*
1. Symptomatic, severe stenosis that is surgically difficult to access (e.g., high bifurcation requiring mandibular dislocation)	1. Asymptomatic stenosis of any degree, except in particular circumstances, as described above	1. Carotid stenosis with angiographically visible intraluminal thrombus
2. Symptomatic, severe stenosis in a patient with significant medical disease that would make the patient high risk for surgery	2. Symptomatic stenosis associated with an intracranial vascular malformation	2. A stenosis that cannot be safely reached or crossed by an endovascular approach
3. Symptomatic severe stenosis *and* one of the following conditions:	3. Symptomatic stenosis in a patient with a subacute cerebral infarction	
a. Significant tandem lesion that may require endovascular therapy	4. Symptomatic stenosis in a patient with a significant contraindication to angiography	
b. Radiation-induced stenosis		
c. Restenosis after carotid endarterectomy		
d. Refusal to undergo carotid endarterectomy after proper informed consent		
e. Stenosis secondary to arterial dissection		
f. Stenosis secondary to fibromuscular dysplasia		
g. Stenosis secondary to Takayasu arteritis		
4. Severe stenosis associated with contralateral carotid artery occlusion requiring treatment before undergoing cardiac surgery		
5. Severe underlying carotid artery stenosis revealed after recanalization of carotid occlusion after thrombolysis for acute stroke (presumed to be the etiology of the treated occlusion) or to enable thrombolysis for acute stroke		
6. Pseudoaneurysm		
7. Asymptomatic preocclusive lesion in a patient otherwise meeting criteria 1–3		

Definitions: Severe stenosis is 70% or greater diameter stenosis by NASCET measurement criteria. Preocclusive stenosis is 90% or greater diameter stenosis by NASCET criteria or NASCET definition of "near occlusion."

From Barr JD, Connors JJ, Sacks D, et al., for the ASITN, ASNR, and SIR Standards of Practice Committees. Quality improvement guidelines for the performance of cervical carotid angioplasty and stent placement. Developed by a Collaborative Panel of the American Society of Interventional and Therapeutic Neuroradiology, the American Society of Neuroradiology, and the Society of the Interventional Radiology. *J Vasc Intervent Radiol.* 2003;14:S321–S335.

TABLE 7-9. SAPPHIRE Trial: Inclusion Criteria

Symptomatic patients with ≥50% stenosis

Asymptomatic patients with ≥80% stenosis of the native ipsilateral common or internal carotid artery measured by ultrasound or angiography

Consensus agreement by multidisciplinary team consisting of an interventionalist, consulting neurologist, and surgeon

Presence of ≥1 comorbid condition which increases the risk of endarterectomy

1. Anatomic (contralateral carotid occlusion; contralateral laryngeal nerve palsy; radiation therapy to neck; previous carotid endarterectomy with recurrent stenosis; difficult surgical access; severe tandem lesions)

2. Medical [congestive heart failure (class III/IV) and/or severe left ventricular dysfunction, i.e., left ventricular ejection fraction <30%; open heart surgery within 6 weeks; myocardial infarction 1 day to 4 weeks prior to treatment; angina at low workload or unstable angina (Canadian Cardiovascular Society class III/IV); severe pulmonary disease; age >80 years]

From Yadav JS, Wholey MH, Kuntz RE, et al. Protected carotid-artery stenting versus endarterectomy in high-risk patients. *N Engl J Med.* 2004;351:1493–1501, and Ouriel K. SAPPHIRE pivotal study. Available at: http://www.fda.gov/ohrms/dockets/ac/04/briefing/4033b1.htm. Accessed November 15, 2005.

summarized in Tables 7-9 and 7-10. The primary end points were death (all causes), any stroke, and myocardial infarction ≤30 days postprocedure, and death (all causes) and ipsilateral stroke between days 31 and 360 postprocedure.

The technical success for the stent delivery system (Precise, nitinol stent, Cordis Corp., Miami Lakes, FL, USA) was 99.4% (<50% residual stenosis) and 91.2% (<30% residual stenosis). The technical success rate for the ultimate placement rate of the protection system (Angioguard-XP, Cordis Corp., Miami Lakes, FL, USA) was 98.1%.

For the CAS and CAE groups, the cumulative incidence of death at 1 year was 7.4% versus 13.5%, and the cumulative incidence of stroke was 6.2% versus 7.9% at 1 year, respectively. The combined incidence of major adverse events (MAEs) between the two groups was 4.8% versus 9.8%, respectively. The incidence of MAE at 30 days and at 360 days is shown in Figures 7-4 and 7-5,

TABLE 7-10.   SAPPHIRE Trial: Exclusion Criteria

Ischemic stroke within previous 48 hr
Presence of intraluminal thrombus
Total occlusion of the target vessel
Vascular disease precluding use of catheter-based techniques
Intracranial aneurysm >9 mm in diameter
Need for more than two stents
History of bleeding disorder
Percutaneous or surgical intervention planned within next 30 days
Life expectancy <1 year
Ostial lesion of common carotid artery or brachiocephalic artery

From Yadav JS, Wholey MH, Kuntz RE, et al. Protected carotid-artery stenting versus endarterectomy in high-risk patients. *N Engl J Med.* 2004;351:1493–1501.

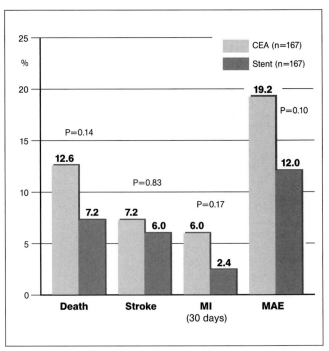

FIGURE 7-5.   Major adverse effects at 360 days, SAPPHIRE trial. (Redrawn from Ouriel K. SAPPHIRE pivotal study. Available at: http://www.fda.gov/ohrms/dockets/ac/04/briefing/4033b1.htm. Accessed November 15, 2005.)

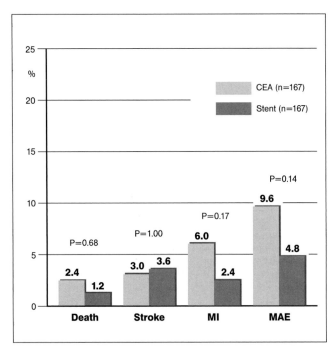

FIGURE 7-4.   Major adverse effects at 30 days, SAPPHIRE trial. (Redrawn from Ouriel K. SAPPHIRE pivotal study. Available at: http://www.fda.gov/ohrms/dockets/ac/04/briefing/4033b1.htm. Accessed November 15, 2005.)

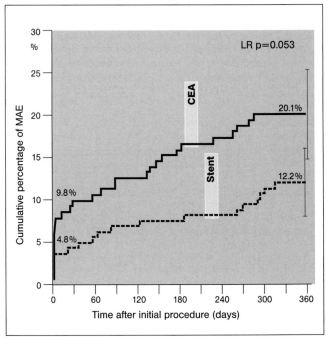

FIGURE 7-6.   Cumulative percentage of major adverse effects at 360 days, Kaplan-Meier analysis, SAPPHIRE trial. (Redrawn from Ouriel K. SAPPHIRE pivotal study. Available at: http://www.fda.gov/ohrms/dockets/ac/04/briefing/4033b1.htm. Accessed November 15, 2005.)

respectively. Figure 7-6 and Table 7-11 show the cumulative incidence of MAE at 1 year in patients treated with CAS and CAE. Cumulative incidence of MAE at 720 days is shown in Figure 7-7. The restenosis and target vessel revascularization rates at 360 days are shown in Table 7-12. At 2 years, the observed restenosis rate was higher with CAS than with CAE (38.7% vs. 26.6%).

In other early randomized trials in which CAS and CAE were compared, not all critical criteria required for evaluating the two techniques were met; in particular, no credentialing pretrial phase was required, thus allowing for important operator bias.[74–76]

Based on the current incomplete evidence, the recommendations for the use of coronarylike state-of-the-art CAS vary among professional societies, vendors, and health care providers. A representative example of current indication recommendations, definition of the high risk status, and the

institutional requirements to obtain reimbursement issued by a large health care provider is shown in Tables 7-13 to 7-15.[77] To answer the question of the long-term efficacy and safety of CAS, large prospective and randomized trials including Carotid

TABLE 7-11. Cumulative Incidence of Adverse Events within 1 Year Following Carotid Artery Stenting versus Carotid Endarterectomy, SAPPHIRE Trial

Event	Intention-to-Treat Analysis [Number (%)]			Actual-Treatment Analysis [Number (%)]		
	Stenting (n = 167)	*Endarterectomy (n = 167)*	*p value*	*Stenting (n = 159)*	*Endarterectomy (n = 151)*	*p value*
Death	12 (7.4)	21 (13.5)	0.08	11 (7.0)	19 (12.9)	0.08
Stroke	10 (6.2)	12 (7.9)	0.60	9 (5.8)	11 (7.7)	0.52
Major ipsilateral	1 (0.6)	5 (3.3)	0.09	0	5 (3.5)	0.02
Major nonipsilateral	1 (0.6)	2 (1.4)	0.53	1 (0.6)	1 (0.7)	0.97
Minor ipsilateral	6 (3.7)	3 (2.0)	0.34	6 (3.8)	3 (2.2)	0.37
Minor nonipsilateral	3 (1.9)	4 (2.7)	0.64	3 (2.0)	3 (2.1)	0.89
Myocardial infarction	5 (3.0)	12 (7.5)	0.07	4 (2.5)	12 (8.1)	0.03
Q-wave	0	2 (1.2)	0.15	0	2 (1.3)	0.15
Non-Q-wave	5 (3.0)	10 (6.2)	0.17	4 (2.5)	10 (6.7)	0.08
Cranial-nerve palsy	0	8 (4.9)	0.004	0	8 (5.3)	0.003
Target-vessel revascularization	1 (0.6)	6 (4.3)	0.04	1 (0.7)	6 (4.6)	0.04
Conventional end point (stroke or death at 30 days plus ipsilateral stroke or death from neurologic causes within 31 days to 1 yr)	9 (5.5)	13 (8.4)	0.36	8 (5.1)	11 (7.5)	0.40
Primary end point (death, stroke, myocardial infarction at 30 days plus ipsilateral stroke or death from neurologic causes within 31 days to 1 yr)	20 (12.2)	32 (20.1)	0.05	19 (12.0)	30 (20.1)	0.05

From Yadav JS, Wholey MH, Kuntz RE, et al. Protected carotid-artery stenting versus endarterectomy in high-risk patients. *N Engl J Med.* 2004;351:1493–1501.

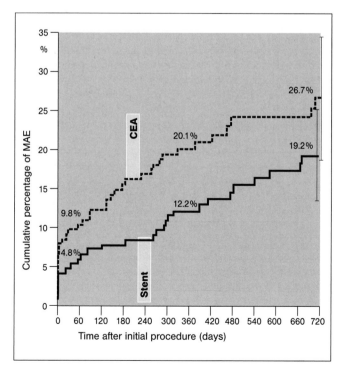

FIGURE 7-7. Cumulative percentage of major adverse effects at 720 days, Kaplan-Meier analysis, SAPPHIRE trial. (Redrawn from Ouriel K. SAPPHIRE pivotal study. Available at: http://www.fda.gov/ohrms/dockets/ac/04/briefing/4033b1.htm. Accessed November 15, 2005.)

Revascularization Endarterectomy versus Stent Trial (CREST), Carotid and Vertebral Artery Transluminal Angioplasty Study (CAVATAS II), Endarterectomy Versus Angioplasty in Patients with Severe Symptomatic Carotid Stenosis (EVA-3S), and Stent-protected Percutaneous Angioplasty of the Carotid versus Endarterectomy (SPACE) have been initiated, with results expected within the next 3 to 5 years. Until the base of evidence has been expanded, clinical practice for implementing CAS and CAE procedures will be based on the individual decisions of participating providers and institutions. The formation of teams with proven competence in CAS and CAE, and consensus indications for operating according to the established international standards, seems a safe interim strategy to provide optimum management in patients with carotid artery disease under the current circumstances.[78]

QUALITY ASSURANCE

Safe and efficacious performance of CAS requires appropriate patient selection, availability of at least one experienced operator. Physician qualifications and the means to obtain them by training and experience have been the subject of several guidelines and recommendations issued by the leading societies participating in neurovascular and vascular care.[65,79,80] In addition, standards of equipment quality, documentation, and outcome reporting for CAS have been proposed.[65] Tables 7-16 to 7-19 review examples of suggested standards for training in carotid stenting. Tables 7-20 and 7-21 show examples of proposed thresholds of outcomes in

TABLE 7-12. Restenosis Rates and Target Lesion Revascularization (TLR) at 360 days, SAPPHIRE Trial

In-Vessel Restenosis by U/S	Stent (n = 167)	CEA (n = 167)	p value
>50% diameter stenosis [a]	19.7% (24/122)	31.3% (30/96)	0.06
>70% diameter stenosis	0.8% (1/122)	5.2% (5/96)	0.09
>80% diameter stenosis	0.8% (1/122)	4.2% (4/96)	0.17
TLR—clinically driven (to 360 days)	0.6% (1/167)	3.6% (6/167)	0.12

CEA, carotid endarterectomy; U/S, ultrasound.

[a]Protocol definition.

From Ouriel K. SAPPHIRE pivotal study. Available at: http://www.fda.gov/ohrms/dockets/ac/04/briefing/4033b1.htm. Accessed November 15, 2005.

TABLE 7-13. Indications for Coronary Artery Stenting

Patients who are at high risk for carotid endarterectomy (CEA) and who also have symptomatic carotid artery stenosis ≥70%. Coverage is limited to procedures performed using FDA-approved carotid artery stenting systems and embolic protection devices

Patients who are at high risk for CEA and have symptomatic carotid artery stenosis between 50% and 70%, in accordance with the Category B IDE clinical trials regulation (42 CFR 405.201), as a routine cost under the clinical trials policy (Medicare NCD Manual 310.1), or in accordance with the National Coverage Determination on CAS post approval studies (Medicare NCD Manual 20.7)

Patients who are at high risk for CEA and have asymptomatic carotid artery stenosis ≥80%, in accordance with the Category B IDE clinical trials regulation (42 CFR 405.201), as a routine cost under the clinical trials policy (Medicare NCD Manual 310.1), or in accordance with the National Coverage Determination on CAS post approval studies (Medicare NCD Manual 20.7)

From Decision memo for carotid artery stenting (CAG-00085R); Decision summary. Available at: http://www.cms.hhs.gov/mcd/viewdecisionmemo.asp?id=157.

TABLE 7-14. Definition of High-risk Patients for Carotid Endarterectomy (CEA)

Patients at high risk for CEA are defined as having significant comorbidities and/or anatomic risk factors (i.e., recurrent stenosis and/or previous radical neck dissection), and would be poor candidates for CEA in the opinion of a surgeon. Significant comorbid conditions include but are not limited to:

- congestive heart failure (CHF) class III/IV
- left ventricular ejection fraction (LVEF) <30%
- unstable angina
- contralateral carotid occlusion
- recent myocardial infarction (MI)
- previous CEA with recurrent stenosis
- prior radiation treatment to the neck
- other conditions that were used to determine patients at high risk for CEA in the prior carotid artery stenting trials and studies, such as ARCHER, CABERNET, SAPPHIRE, BEACH, and MAVERIC II

From Decision memo for carotid artery stenting (CAG-00085R); Decision summary. Available at: http://www.cms.hhs.gov/mcd/viewdecision-memo.asp?id=157.

TABLE 7-15. List of Minimum Standards for Facilities to Meet in Order to Receive Coverage for Carotid Artery Stenting for High-risk Patients by CMS

Facilities must have necessary imaging equipment, device inventory, staffing, and infrastructure to support a dedicated carotid stent program. Specifically, high-quality x-ray imaging equipment is a critical component of any carotid interventional suite, such as high resolution digital imaging systems with the capability of subtraction, magnification, road mapping, and orthogonal angulation.

Advanced physiologic monitoring must be available in the interventional suite. This includes real time and archived physiologic, hemodynamic, and cardiac rhythm monitoring equipment, as well as support staff who are capable of interpreting the findings and responding appropriately.

Emergency management equipment and systems must be readily available in the interventional suite such as resuscitation equipment, a defibrillator, vasoactive and antiarrhythmic drugs, endotracheal intubation capability, and anesthesia support

Each institution should have a clearly delineated program for granting carotid stent privileges and for monitoring the quality of the individual interventionalists and the program as a whole. The committee overseeing this program should be empowered to identify the minimum case volume for an operator to maintain privileges, as well as the (risk-adjusted) threshold for complications that the institution will allow before suspending privileges or instituting measures for remediation. Committees are encouraged to apply published standards from national specialty societies recognized by the American Board of Medical Specialties to determine appropriate physician qualifications. Examples of standards and clinical competence guidelines include those published in the December 2004 edition of the American Journal of Neuroradiology and those published in the August 18, 2004 Journal of the American College of Cardiology.

To continue to receive Medicare payment for CAS under this decision, the facility or a contractor to the facility must collect data on all carotid artery stenting procedures done at that particular facility. This data must be analyzed routinely to ensure patient safety, and will also be used in the process of re-credentialing the facility. This data must be made available to CMS upon request. The interval for data analysis will be determined by the facility but should not be less frequent than every 6 months.

From Decision memo for carotid artery stenting (CAG-00085R); Decision summary. Available at: http://www.cms.hhs.gov/mcd/viewdecisionmemo.asp?id=157.

TABLE 7-16. Example of Suggested Cognitive Requirements for Performance of Carotid Stenting[a]

I. Pathophysiology of carotid artery disease and stroke
   a. Causes of stroke
      i. Embolization (cardiac, carotid, aortic, other)
      ii. Vasculitis
      iii. Arteriovenous malformation
      iv. Intracranial bleeding (subdural, epidural)
      v. Space-occupying lesion
   b. Causes of carotid artery narrowing
      i. Atherosclerosis
      ii. Fibromuscular dysplasia
      iii. Spontaneous dissection
      iv. Other
   c. Atherogenesis (pathogenesis and risk factors)
II. Clinical manifestations of stroke
   a. Knowledge of stroke syndromes (classic and atypical)
   b. Distinction between anterior and posterior circulation events
III. Natural history of carotid artery disease
IV. Associated pathology (e.g., coronary and peripheral artery disease)
V. Diagnosis of stroke and carotid artery disease
   a. History and physical examination
      i. Neurologic
      ii. Non-neurologic (cardiac, other)
   b. Noninvasive imaging and appropriate use thereof
      i. Duplex ultrasound
      ii. MRA
      iii. CTA
VI. Angiographic anatomy (arch, extracranial, intracranial, basic collateral circulation, common variants, and nonatherosclerotic pathologic processes)
VII. Knowledge of alternative treatment options for carotid stenosis and their results (immediate success, risks, and long-term outcome)
   a. Pharmacotherapy (e.g., antiplatelet agents, anticoagulation, lipid-lowering agents)
   b. Carotid endarterectomy
      i. Results from major trials (NASCET, ACAS, ECST, ACST)
      ii. Results in patients with increased surgical risk
   c. Stent revascularization
      i. Results with and without distal embolic protection
VIII. Case selection
   a. Indications and contraindications for revascularization to prevent stroke
   b. High risk criteria for carotid endarterectomy
   c. High risk criteria for percutaneous intervention
IX. Role of post-procedure follow up and surveillance

[a]Cognitive elements include the fund of knowledge regarding cerebrovascular disease, its natural history, pathophysiology, diagnostic methods, and treatment alternatives.

[b]In addition to baseline cognitive skills encompassed in the Competency document.

From Clinical competence statement on carotid stenting: training and credentialing for carotid stenting multispecialty consensus recommendations. A report of the SCAI/SVMB/SVS Writing Committee to develop a clinical competence statement on carotid interventions. *Cathet Cardiovasc Intervent.* 2005;64:1–11.

TABLE 7-17. Example of Suggested Technical Requirements for Performance of Carotid Stenting

Minimum numbers of procedures to achieve competence:
   I. Diagnostic cervicocerebral angiograms: 30 (≥half as primary operator)[b]
   II. Carotid stent procedures: 25 (≥half as primary operation)[b]
Technical elements for competence in both diagnostic angiography and interventional techniques:
   I. High level of expertise with antiplatelet therapy and procedural anticoagulation
   II. Angiographic skills
      a. Vascular access skills
      b. Selection of guidewires and angiographic catheters
      c. Appropriate manipulation of guidewires and catheters
      d. Use of "closed system" manifold
      e. Knowledge of normal angiographic anatomy and common variants
      f. Knowledge of Circle of Willis and typical/atypical collateral pathways
      g. Proper assessment of aortic arch configuration, as it affects carotid intervention
      h. Familiarity with use of angulated views and appropriate movement of the x-ray gantry
   III. Interventional skills
      a. Guide catheter/sheath placement
      b. Deployment and retrieval of embolic protection devices
      c. Pre- and postdilatation
      d. Stent positioning and deployment
   IV. Recognition and management of intraprocedural complications
      a. Cerebrovascular events
         i. Stroke or cerebrovascular ischemia
         ii. Embolization
         iii. Hemorrhage
         vi. Thrombosis
         v. Dissection
         vi. Seizure and loss of consciousness
      b. Cardiovascular events
         i. Arrhythmias
         ii. Hypotension
         iii. Hypertension
         iv. Myocardial ischemia/infarction
      c. Vascular access events
         i. Bleeding
         ii. Ischemia
         iii. Thrombosis
   IV. Management of vascular access
      a. Proper sheath removal and attainment of hemostasis
      b. Closure device utilization

[a]In addition to baseline cognitive skills encompassed in the Competency document.

[b]Angiograms and stenting procedures may be performed in the same sitting (e.g., in the same patients), provided that one performs 15 angiograms as primary operator before performing the first stent as primary operator.

From Clinical competence statement on carotid stenting: training and credentialing for carotid stenting multispecialty consensus recommendations. A report of the SCAI/SVMB/SVS Writing Committee to develop a clinical competence statement on carotid interventions. *Cathet Cardiovasc Intervent.* 2005;64:1–11.

TABLE 7-18. Example of Suggested Clinical Requirements for Performance of Carotid Stenting[a]

I. Determine the patient's risk/benefit for the procedure
II. Outpatient responsibilities
   a. Adjust medications preprocedure
   b. Counsel patient and family
III. Inpatient responsibilities
   a. Admit patients (privileges required) and write orders
   b. Obtain informed consent for procedures
   c. Provide pre- and postprocedure hospital care
      i. Neurological evaluation pre- and postprocedure
      ii. Postprocedure pharmacotherapy
      iii. Monitoring of hemodynamic and cardiac rhythm status
IV. Coordinate poststent surveillance and clinical outpatient follow-up

[a]Clinical elements include the ability to manage inpatients and outpatient care.

[b]In addition to baseline cognitive skills encompassed in the Competency document.

From Clinical competence statement on carotid stenting: training and credentialing for carotid stenting multispecialty consensus recommendations. A report of the SCAI/SVMB/SVS Writing Committee to develop a clinical competence statement on carotid interventions. *Cathet Cardiovasc Intervent.* 2005;64:1–11.

TABLE 7-19. Example of Suggested Training Requirements

Performance (under the supervision of a qualified physician and with at least 50% performed as the primary operator) of at least 200 diagnostic cervicocerebral angiograms with documented acceptable indications and outcomes for physicians with no prior catheter experience, or at least 100 diagnostic cervicocerebral angiograms with documented acceptable indications and outcomes for physicians with experience sufficient to meet the AHA requirements for peripheral vascular interventions.

Arterial stent experience as either:

1. Twenty-five noncarotid stent complete procedures, plus attendance at and completion of a "hands-on" course in performance of CAS, plus performance and completion of at least four successful and uncomplicated CAS procedures as principal operator under the supervision of an on-site qualified physician; this must be a comprehensive course in which the attendees earn at least 16 hours of AMA category I continuing medical education credit or

2. Ten consecutive CAS procedures as principal operator under the supervision of an on-site qualified physician on patients treated for appropriate indications documented by a log of cases performed and with acceptable success and complication rates according to the thresholds contained in this guideline and the ACR guideline for cervicocerebral angiography

Substantiation in writing by the director of the department, the chief of the medical staff, or the chair of the credentials committee of the institution in which the training procedures were performed and the institution in which privileges will be granted that the surgical team is familiar with all of the following: Indications and contraindications for CAS; preprocedural assessment and intraprocedural physiologic, cerebrovascular, and neurologic monitoring of the patient; appropriate use and operation of fluoroscopic and radiographic equipment and digital subtraction angiography systems; principles of radiation protection, hazards of radiation exposure to the patient and to the radiologic personnel, and radiation monitoring requirements; anatomy, physiology, and pathophysiology of the cerebrovascular system; pharmacology of contrast agents and cardiac antiarrhythmia drugs and recognition and treatment of adverse reactions to these substances; recognition and treatment of cardiac arrhythmias associated with CAS; technical aspects of performing CAS; recognition of any cerebrovascular abnormality or complication related to the CAS procedure;

postprocedural patient management, particularly the recognition and initial management of procedure complications

CAS, carotid artery stenting; AHA, American Heart Association; AMA, American Medical Association; ACR, American College of Radiology.

From Barr JD, Connors JJ, Sacks D, et al., for the ASITN, ASNR, and SIR Standards of Practice Committees. Quality improvement guidelines for the performance of cervical carotid angioplasty and stent placement. Developed by a Collaborative Panel of the American Society of Interventional and Therapeutic Neuroradiology, the American Society of Neuroradiology, and the Society of the Interventional Radiology. *J Vasc Intervent Radiol.* 2003;14:S321–S335.

TABLE 7-20. Suggested Definition of Neurologic Complications of Outcomes in Carotid Stenting

Neurologic complication: neurologic deterioration evidenced by an increase in the NIHSS score of one or more points

Transient deficit: a neurologic complication having complete resolution within 24 hr

Reversible stroke: a neurologic complication having a duration of >24 hr and up to 30 days

Permanent stroke: a neurologic complication having a duration of >30 days

Minor deficit: neurologic deterioration evidenced by an increase of the NIHSS score of less than four points without the presence of aphasia or hemianopsia

Major deficit: neurologic deterioration evidenced by an increase of the NIHSS score of four or more points or the presence of aphasia or hemianopsia

Technical success: inflation of angioplasty balloon/placement of stent in the carotid stenosis with improvement of the stenosis by 20% or more with a final residual stenosis of less than 50% using NASCET measurement criteria

NIHSS, National Institutes of Health Stroke Scale.

From Barr JD, Connors JJ, Sacks D, et al., for the ASITN, ASNR, and SIR Standards of Practice Committees. Quality improvement guidelines for the performance of cervical carotid angioplasty and stent placement. Developed by a Collaborative Panel of the American Society of Interventional and Therapeutic Neuroradiology, the American Society of Neuroradiology, and the Society of the Interventional Radiology. *J Vasc Intervent Radiol.* 2003;14:S321–S335.

carotid artery stenting. As much as interest in CAS for many physicians from various clinical backgrounds and specialties is understandable, ensuring patient safety and achieving the highest individual procedural benefits remain incontestably the highest priority. Because of the risk of permanent neurological deficits and death inextricably associated with the procedure, the aptitude of the candidate CAS interventionists requires an objective assessment and their learning curves must be optimized. Besides the creation of dedicated centers in endovascular therapy providing full clinical support, the availability of virtual-reality training facilities using dedicated simulators are a welcome adjunct in the efforts to assure care of excellence for patients with extracranial carotid artery disease.[80,81]

STANDARD PROCEDURE

INSTRUMENTATION

Selecting the optimum instrumentation for an each individual case is an important component of the planning and performance of the CAS procedure. To avoid intraprocedural complications,

TABLE 7-21. Suggested Thresholds for Outcome Measures of Carotid Stenting

Neurologic Complication	Complications Threshold	
	Asymptomatic Patient (%)	Symptomatic Patient (%)
Minor transient deficit	*	*
Major transient deficit	*	*
Minor reversible stroke	3.5	6
Major reversible stroke	2	3
Minor permanent stroke	3	4.5
Major permanent stroke	2	3
Death	0†	0†
Indications		
Meets the indications listed in Table 7-8		95%
Technical success		90%

From Barr JD, Connors JJ, Sacks D, et al., for the ASITN, ASNR, and SIR Standards of Practice Committees. Quality improvement guidelines for the performance of cervical carotid angioplasty and stent placement. Developed by a Collaborative Panel of the American Society of Interventional and Tutic Neuroradiology, the American Society of Neuroradiology, and the Society of the Interventional Radiology. *J Vasc Intervent Radiol.* 2003;14:S321–S335.

the operator must be thoroughly familiar with the technicalities of each device he plans to deploy. In some cases, certified training is required.

Introductory sheaths. Using the infrainguinal common femoral artery is used for access, 6 or 7F, 80- or 90-cm-long sheaths with stable backup are typically used (Arrow International, Corp. Reading, PA, USA, or Cook, Inc., Bloomington, IL, USA); 8F sheaths are required in technically demanding cases, particularly when guiding catheters are used to improve the ability to navigate the target vessel.

Guidewires. For stable support of the sheath 0.035-in. hydrophilic, floppy tip, and stiff or superstiff shaft guidewires are used (Roadrunner, Cook, Inc., Bloomington, IL, USA; Glidewire—regular or stiff, Terumo Cardiovascular Systems., Somerset, NJ, USA); 0.014-in. coronary guidewires with flexible and formable tips may be required in demanding cases to cross the target lesion.

Guiding catheters. Depending on the technique used to provide the access to the target lesions, conventional coronary guiding catheters (mostly Judkins right 3 or 4) may be used in conjunction with the introductory sheath to improve the stability of the system and thus to increase its tracking and pushing ability in patients with adverse vascular anatomy (see the co-axial telescopic technique below), or it may be used without a sheath support for direct access. In addition, guiding catheters may be useful in directing the guidewire of the distal protection device or the coronary guidewire in patients with complex or highly eccentric residual target lumen.

Balloon dilatation catheters. Dilatation catheters are used for pre- and postdilatations in conjunction with stent deployment. Typically, conventional rapid-exchange, low-profile, coronary balloon dilatation catheters with a nominal diameter of 1.5 to 3.5 mm and excellent refolding properties are selected for predilatations. Postdilatations are performed using rapid -exchange, peripheral balloon dilatation catheters,

also with excellent refolding properties. Postdilatations are usually performed using 5- or 6-mm-diameter balloons, or, exceptionally, 7 mm in postoperative cases or cases of internal carotid artery ectasia. If postdilatations of the common carotid artery are required, balloons matching the nominal size of the vessel (8 to 10 mm) are selected.

Stents. An expanding assortment of dedicated carotid artery stents, consisting of a variety of straight and tapered designs and using either the over-the-wire or rapid-exchange delivery systems, have been employed in clinical trials and become available for clinical practice after the device approval. Dedicated carotid stents approved for clinical use and deployed in clinical trials include the following:

- Carotid Wallstent Monorail Endoprosthesis (Boston Scientific, Natick, MA, USA) used in the BEACH trial
- OTW and RX Acculink (Guidant, Indianapolis, IN, USA) used in the ARCHeR 1-3, CREATE II, CREST, CAPTURE trials
- Precise, nitinol stent (Cordis Corp., Miami Lakes, FL, USA) used in the SAPPHIRE trial
- Xact Carotid Stent System (Abbott Vascular Devices, Redwood City, CA, USA) used in the SECuRITY trial

In the absence of comparative trials, individual carotid stent selection is based on the expected stent properties in terms of crossing ability, radial strength, longitudinal flexibility, vessel adaptability, and scaffolding properties as defined by the material and design of the stent. Stent size depends on the nominal diameter of the target vessel, the length of the lesion, and the operator's preference in remodeling the internal carotid artery (and common carotid artery) anatomy by deploying the stent. Typical stent sizes are 5 to 10 mm diameter and 20 to 50 mm length for vessel sizes ranging approximately between 4 and 9 mm. The compatibility of the diameter of the stent delivery system and the internal diameter of the sheath must be considered.

Distal protection devices. DPDs have become an obligatory component of CAS intervention and are typically employed to cross the target lesion; they are deployed first before any other manipulation takes place. Depending on the basic operating principle, distal balloon occlusion devices, distal filter devices, and proximal balloon occlusion devices can be distinguished. Dedicated carotid DPD approved for clinical use and deployed in clinical trials include the following:

- RX Accunet (Guidant, Indianapolis, IN, USA) used in the ARCHeR 3 trial
- FilterWire EX and EZ (EndoTex Interventional Systems, Inc., Cupertino, CA, USA) used in the BEACH and CABERNET trials
- Spider RX (ev3, Plymouth, MN, USA) used in the CREATE II trial
- Angioguard-XP (Cordis Corp., Miami Lakes, FL, USA) used in the SAPPHIRE and CASES trials
- EmboShield (Abbott Vascular Devices, Redwood City, CA, USA) used in the SECuRITY trial
- Rubicon Filter (Rubicon Medical Corp., Salt Lake City, UT, USA) used in the RULE Carotid trial
- MOMA (Invatec, Brescia, Italy) used in the MOMA and PRIAMUS trials

In selecting the DPD, important characteristics to consider include the nominal size of the vessel at the level of DPD deployment (warning note: mismatch between the size of the DPD and the target vessel may prevent optimum sealing or it may cause mechanical vessel wall irritation, spasm, and/or injury!), low crossing profile, atraumatic deployment, vessel wall adaptability, volume of the basket, size of the pores of the membrane (currently 100 to 150 mm), ease of retraction, and preparation and handling of the system.

BASIC STRUCTURE OF INTERNAL CAROTID ARTERY INTERVENTION

The basic structure of CAS is similar to that of any percutaneous intervention consisting of initialization, main interventional cycle and termination. CAS intervention is an iterative process designed to achieve optimum carotid artery revascularization at the lowest possible risk in smallest number of interventional steps. The number of interventional steps reflects primarily the complexity of the disease and skills of the operator. CAS consists of a number of individual steps linked by continuous risk/benefit considerations on the part of the operator (see Chapter 4).

Specifically, coronarylike CAS consists of two parts, namely, establishing direct access to the target lesion using a long sheath and/or coronary guiding catheter, and target carotid artery lesion revascularization; both of these steps are similar to coronary interventions. The distinctions between CAS and coronary interventions include the fact that access to the target lesion is typically more difficult, requiring greater expertise on the part of the operator, and the primary crossing of the target lesion by the guidewire of the DPD. In the following sections, coronarylike CAS using the co-axial telescopic approach is described.

Initialization

In context of this chapter initialization begins with establishing the vascular access and ends with providing direct access to the interventional site by placing the tip of the sheath or the guiding catheter proximal to the target lesion. All CAS procedures are performed using the transfemoral approach from the infrainguinal common femoral artery. The ability to reach the common carotid artery distal to the target lesion with the interventional system is the key to selecting the strategy for placing a safe and stable sheath or coronary guiding catheter. Depending on the vascular anatomy between the access site and the distal common carotid artery, particularly that of the aortic arch, the operator must anticipate the degree of technical difficulties and select the appropriate strategy and instrumentation. The co-axial telescopic approach provides a robust means to overcome anatomic adversities. The basic co-axial instrumentation set consists of a 0.035-in. stiff guidewire, diagnostic coronary catheter, usually with Judkins right configuration, and a long sheath with a dilator. The basic set can be upgraded by replacing the stiff guidewire with a superstiff guidewire and the coronary diagnostic catheter with a sheath dilator. In exceptionally difficult cases, a coronary guide with or without the additional support of the diagnostic coronary catheter may be employed instead of the sheath dilator. The first step is placement of a soft-tip diagnostic coronary catheter in conjunction with a hydrophilic, floppy, 0.035-in.

guidewire into the selected branch of the external carotid artery Stiff or superstiff, 0.035-in. guidewire is introduced to replace the diagnostic coronary catheter. Once securely positioned, this guidewire should not be moved throughout the entire placement of the sheath in the distal common carotid artery to avoid external carotid artery spasm or injury.

With the stiff or superstiff, 0.035-in. guidewire securely resting in the external carotid artery branch, the co-axial telescopic system is successively advanced to reach the target interventional site. Typically, the inside catheter is advanced first, then the outside catheter is slid over. In difficult cases, the forward push is combined with a slight retraction of the inside catheter. Despite the quite considerable forces sometimes required, the procedure must be conducted gently throughout to avoid uncontrolled bouncing and slipping of the deployed system. In particular, storage of energy within the system must be avoided and intermittent relaxation and position adjustments are required to avoid sudden and uncontrolled forward motion of the system. Once the adversities of the interposed vascular anatomy have been overcome, the tip of the sheath is positioned in the distal common carotid artery, typically about 2 cm proximal to the target lesion. With the sheath securely positioned, the 0.035-in. guidewire and the inner catheter are carefully withdrawn. After preinterventional angiograms of the extracranial interventional site and the intracranial internal carotid artery have been taken, the stage is set for the actual revascularization. Figure 7-8 demonstrates the co-axial telescopic technique of sheath placement in the distal common carotid artery.

Main Interventional Cycle: Assess, Intervene, Repeat

In context of this chapter main interventional cycle begins with the exploration and crossing of the target lesion and it ends with decision to terminate the intervention. On the basis of the preinterventional angiograms, a straight segment of the postbulbar internal carotid artery is selected for DPD placement. Adequate spacing between the DPD and the target lesion must be assured to allow free deployment. The tip of the DPD guidewire is then shaped in accordance with the morphology of the lesion and advanced to explore and cross the lesion. Extremely gentle exploration of the entry to the lesion is necessary to avoid dissections or embolization. Following guidewire engagement of the lesion, the DPD is advanced into its final position, where it projects distally to the base of the skull, and deployed. Full and symmetric deployment of the DPD should be clearly visualized on fluoroscopy. Passage of the DPD through the lesion is frequently the critical part of the procedure that determines the technical outcome. If DPD cannot cross the lesion, the procedure is usually terminated. Rarely, the operator might decide to cross the lesions with a coronary 0.014-in. soft-tip guidewire and predilate the lesion with a small, low-profile balloon catheter (≤2 mm diameter) to enable DPD crossing; this is done, however, at the expense of increasing the overall risk of the procedure. Figure 7-9 provides an example of an aborted CAS because the DPD was unable to cross the lesion.

Following the deployment of the DPD, the operator must decide whether to predilate or to directly stent the lesion. Most lesions and nearly all complex high-grade lesions require

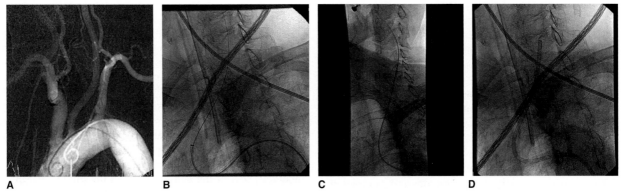

A   **B**   **C**   **D**

FIGURE 7-8. Co-axial telescopic technique of sheath placement in the distal common carotid artery in a patient with a left internal carotid artery (ICA) stenosis. **A:** Aortic arch angiogram in left anterior oblique (LAO) projection. Distal elongation and elevation with dorsocranial take-off of the brachiocephalic trunk and technically more demanding access to the interventional site. **B:** A hydrophilic 0.035-in. guidewire has been placed in the left external carotid artery (ECA). The tip of the long introductory sheath has been positioned at the ostium of the common carotid artery (CCA). **C:** A hydrophilic 0.035-in. guidewire was exchanged via diagnostic Judkins right 4 catheter, positioned with the tip at the take-off of the left ECA for a superstiff 0.035-in. guidewire placed in the thyroid superior branch of the ECA. The tip of the long introductory sheath appears just distal to its final position in the CCA. **D:** The superstiff 0.035-in. guidewire and the diagnostic catheter have been carefully retracted; the tip of the long introductory sheath has reached its final position in the distal CCA ready for preinterventional angiogram before resuming the ICA intervention.

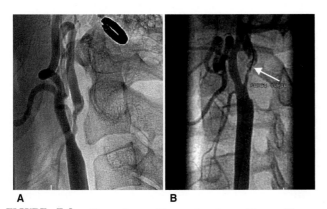

A   **B**

FIGURE 7-9. Aborted carotid stenting in a 45-year-old man. **A:** High-grade, long complex, internal carotid (ICA) lesion at the level of the bulb. **B:** Distal protection device (PercuSurge, Medtronic, Inc, Santa Rosa, CA, USA) is shown "frozen" across the lesion (*arrow*).

predilatation, whereas only selected lesions that carry a high likelihood of safe crossing and adequate stent expansion appear to be amenable to direct stenting. Predilatation is performed using low-profile coronary balloon dilatation catheters that allow high-pressure inflation as well as rapid and complete refolding. Successful predilatation demonstrates distensibility at the neck of the lesion, which is important to know prior to stent deployment. In addition, it allows assessment of the sensitivity of the carotid sinus to mechanical irritation and the consecutive hemodynamic response. The severity and extent of the blood pressure and heart rate response determine the need for atropine administration or temporary transvenous pacing during stenting. Routine prophylactic placement of a right ventricular pacing electrode is not recommended. In a few cases, predilatation even with very high inflation pressures (up to 20 bar and more) may fail, and the intervention must be aborted.

Certain lesions may be stented directly because they do not usually require predilatation; these include ulcerated lesions of moderate severity, intimal flaps, and suture dehiscence lesions and dissections.

As the next step, a rapid-exchange self-expanding stent delivery system is brought carefully up and across the target lesion. Radiopaque markers allow precise positioning so that the entire lesion is fully covered. In nitinol stents, the longitudinal shortening of the stent following deployment is very small, such that the proximal marker approximately corresponds to the stent end after deployment. By contrast, if a Carotid Wallstent is used, there is considerable shortening after deployment, depending on the lumen and the taper of the target vessel. Therefore, when this stent design is used, approximately two-thirds of the entire stent length indicated by the proximal and distal markers is placed proximally with respect to the lesion. This placement strategy allows for asymmetrical longitudinal shortening due to the greater width of the common carotid artery. It should be noted that at present the Carotid Wallstent is the only design that allows positioning to be corrected during deployment; nitinol stents do not allow repositioning once the deployment has been initiated. To allow optimum vessel adaptation, the proximal stent segment should appose the distal common carotid artery, whereas the distal segment should end distal to the bulb in a healthy, and if possible straight internal carotid artery segment. Shorter stents may be used for revascularization of focal postbulbar stenoses or postoperative scar-related stenoses. In these cases, the proximal end of the stent is deployed at the level of the distal to middle bulb, leaving the carotid bifurcation stent-free. Where there are large differences between the lumen of the common and internal carotid arteries, tapered stents may improve vessel wall adaptation. Stents that are inadequately expanded and deployed cannot be safely removed by endovascular means. Because of the elevated risk of distal embolization despite aggressive antiplatelet management, operative stent extraction should be discussed with the vascular surgeon.

To allow optimum strut-to-wall apposition and optimum scaffolding following stent deployment, postdilatations are frequently required. Postdilatations are particularly important where there is locally irregular stent strut architecture, indicating incomplete stent apposition and the formation of "tissue pockets" and residual stenoses. Although 0% residual stenosis is the goal, up to 30% diameter residual stenosis is usually considered acceptable. Postdilatations are performed using brief (5 to 20 seconds) dilatations of short (≤20 mm), high-pressure balloons that can be rapidly and completely refolded. To avoid traumatization, postdilatations are usually not required in covering dissections when optimum results were achieved according to angiographic visualization, that is, regular strut geometry, normal flow pattern, and adequate scaffolding of flaps and floating tissue debris were documented in calcified plaques and in cases of 0% residual stenosis. In patients who require stent-in-stent implantations ("sandwich technique") because of long lesions or the presence of protruding plaque tissue components, postdilatations or any other mechanical manipulations are contraindicated as a rule.

The adaptability of stents to the anatomy of the internal carotid artery appears to be variable. Particularly in elongated vessels and convoluted segments, any interventional device, DPD, or stent will attempt to stretch any mobile vascular segment. Because the total length of the vessel remains the same, new tortuosities may be created or existing tortuosities may be increased. In these segments, secondary kinking and spasms are particularly prevalent. These anatomic corrections are usually temporary and resolve, at least partially, following retraction of the devices. Newly created convolutions distal to the implanted stents do not seem to be of any pathophysiological relevance in most cases. However, optimum vessel adaptability of the stents without anatomic corrections is desirable. Depending on the angiographic result, and always with the patient status in mind, the operator decides whether to proceed with postdilatation or to terminate the procedure. According to the recommendations of the Collaborative Panel of the American Society of Interventional and Therapeutic Neuroradiology, the American Society of Neuroradiology, and the Society of the Interventional Radiology, technical success is achieved when inflation using stent angioplasty has resulted in stenosis improvement of at least 20%, with a final residual stenosis of <50% using NASCET measurement criteria.[65] Before terminating the intervention, the operator confirms the integrity of the stent, complete stent deployment, symmetric strut pattern, and overall geometry.

Several examples of different material behavior during the CAS are shown in Figures 7-10 to 7-14. Figure 7-10 shows an example of excellent stent adaptation in a case with marked internal carotid artery elongation. Figure 7-11 shows an example of excellent stent adaptation to a massive plaque with a highly irregular surface. Figure 7-12 shows excellent adaptation of the stent to variable calibers in the course of the vessels. Figure 7-13 shows anatomic correction of an elongated vessel. Figure 7-14 shows suboptimal stent adaptation to difficult plaque anatomy.

Termination

In context with this chapter termination begins with angiographic documentation of final results and ends with sheath removal. When a final result has been achieved, the instrumentation is withdrawn carefully in the reverse order to initial deployment. To avoid late procedural embolizations, aspiration of the blood from the sheath and from the proximal internal carotid artery should be performed before retracting the DPD. To avoid stent damage during the DPD retraction maneuver, care must be taken to avoid friction between the device and the deployed stent. Following DPD retraction, the final results are documented via the sheath, including DSA of the extracranial and the intracranial internal carotid artery in two projections. Following documentation of the final results the sheath is removed and hemostasis performed. To avoid proximal dissections, the long introductory sheath is withdrawn over the reintroduced 0.035-in. guidewire and diagnostic coronary catheter or sheath dilator. "Bouncing" the sheath must be avoided during retraction. Figures 7-15 to 7-18 show typical examples of carotid artery stenting using the coronarylike approach in four different settings.

Peri-interventional Patient Care

Peri-interventional patient care can be divided into pre-, intra-, and postprocedural management and care. Preprocedural patient evaluation includes the same components used in evaluating patients undergoing noncarotid interventions (see Chapter 8) as well as carotid artery-specific components. The latter include documentation of the preprocedural neurological status of the patient, preferably performed by a neurologist, recent angiographic documentation of the target site, and intracranial vasculature and recent CT or MR brain imaging. DSA documentation includes selective angiography of both carotid arteries; in complex cerebrovascular anatomy, selective angiography of both vertebral arteries is also performed.

Informed consent is an important part of the medicolegal preinterventional documentation. The consent format must comply with the existing laws, and regulatory and institutional policies. The risks cited should include the typical complications of interventional procedures (see Chapter 8). In addition, the risk of transient and permanent neurological deficits and the risk of death should be explicitly stated. Rather than referring to the data reported in the literature, the local institutional incidence of major complications should be stated. Separate informed consents are required for each separate invasive procedure or intervention. The completed and signed informed consent becomes an important part of the patient chart.

The patient should be well hydrated on entering the procedure, and in some patients, preventive placement of a urinary bladder catheter may improve the patient's comfort during the intervention. An example of suggested preprocedural management is shown in Table 7-22.[65,82,83]

During the procedure, standard cardiovascular and respiratory monitoring according to the applicable standards and recommendations is required (see Chapter 8). Throughout the entire procedure, a close rapport with the patient is required so that any changes in the neurological status can be recognized immediately. The presence of a neurologist is not required

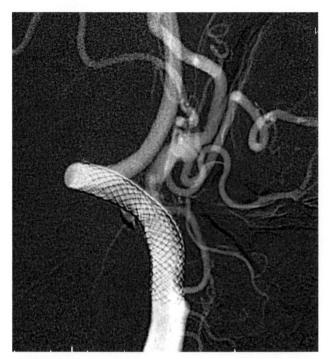

FIGURE 7-10. Stent follows anatomy. Elongation of the internal carotid artery. Excellent stent adaptation to vessel anatomy.

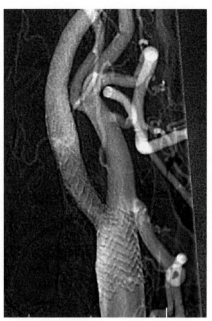

FIGURE 7-12. Stent follows anatomy. An excellent stent adaptation to marked differences in caliber along the course of the common and internal carotid arteries.

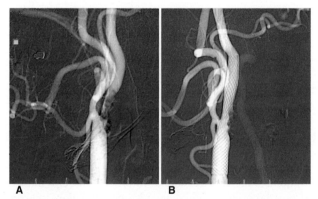

FIGURE 7-11. Stent follows anatomy. **A:** Highly complex, high-grade proximal internal carotid artery stenosis. **B:** Excellent stent adaptation to the highly irregular surface of the lesion. Regular strut pattern is maintained; the huge mass of the plaque is completely excluded. Radial stent force appears sufficient to withstand the recoil force, maintain lumen patency, and preserve laminar flow. The stent scaffold perfectly fits the irregular plaque surface thanks to the mesh stent principle represented by the Carotid Wallstent (see Chapter 5).

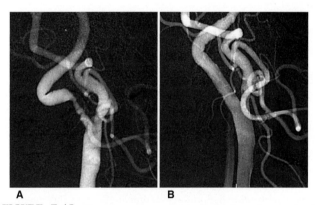

FIGURE 7-13. Stent corrects anatomy. **A:** High-grade, proximal, internal carotid artery stenosis. **B:** Stent stretches the entire proximal segment and displaces the elongation distally.

during the procedure. Transcranial Doppler (TCD) monitoring may be implemented, but does not add any immediate procedural advantage. Experience, atraumatic working style and undivided concentration are far more important than any technical monitoring accessory. However, TCD plays an important role in evaluating new CAS techniques and technologies and should be a consistent part of clinical research protocols. An example of suggested procedural management is provided in Table 7-23.

Following the procedure, in most cases a closure device may be applied for hemostasis, and the patient is then transferred to a monitored bed and observed for up to 24 hours. In uncomplicated cases, rapid ambulation is recommended to improve the patient's comfort, and to reduce the symptoms and duration of the postprocedural hypotension that is frequently encountered. Although blood pressure and ECG monitoring should be maintained for 12 to 24 hours, ambulation at the bedside and around the room within 2 to 4 hours is encouraged in all uncomplicated cases where a plug or suture closure device has been applied successfully. Table 7-24 shows an example of recommendations for postprocedural care after carotid artery stenting.

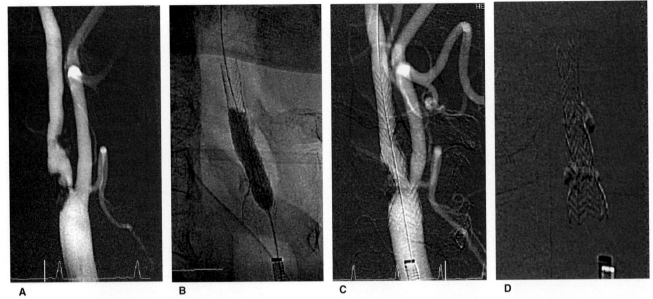

FIGURE 7-14. Suboptimal stent adaptation on difficult plaque anatomy. **A:** Complex, high-grade proximal, internal carotid artery stenosis with high plaque burden, irregular mass distribution, and moderate angiographic calcification. **B:** Postdilatation with nearly complete dilatation balloon expansion at high pressure. **C:** Following postdilatation, regular stent position and luminal expansion. Local recoil corresponding to the sites of the maximum plaque burden with distortion of the segmental stent geometry resulting from interactions between the radial forces of the stent and segmental recoil of the vessel wall. **D:** Subtracted digital subtraction angiography (DSA) image without contrast agent injection. Regular stent position and luminal expansion. Local recoil corresponding to the sites of the maximum plaque burden with distortion of the segmental stent geometry.

ADJUVANT MEDICATION

Patients with documented internal carotid artery stenosis scheduled for CAS receive 100 (70 to 300) mg per day acetyl-salicylic acid (ASA), and 75 mg per day clopidogrel (minimum 3 days prior to the intervention to prevent appositional thrombi at the site of the intervention; alternatively, on the morning of the intervention 300 to 600 mg loading dose). Other recommended medication with proven efficacy for secondary prevention includes statins and angiotensin II–converting enzyme inhibitors.

On the day of the intervention, the patient's medication is continued, except blood pressure medication, which is withheld for the day of the intervention.

Prior to the intervention, the patient receives a single bolus of 5000 U unfractionated heparin (UFH) to a target activated clotting time (ACT) of 200 to 250 seconds; direct thrombin antagonists may provide a useful alternative. In patients with a history of hypotensive responses, prophylactic administration of an intravenous bolus of 0.5 mg atropine should be considered. Target baseline heart rate ranging between 80 and 90 beats per minute and blood pressure in a normal range appear desirable. In patients unresponsive to atropine and patients with critical comorbidities such as left main coronary artery disease prior to surgery, a temporary transvenous pacing lead should be placed prior to the procedure. Adequate hydration is accomplished using a slow intravenous infusion of a crystalline solution; typically 500 to 1000 mL is administered during the procedure.

Sedatives may disguise neurological symptoms, and their use is discouraged.

CAROTID ARTERY STENTING: RISK REDUCTION AND COMPLICATION MANAGEMENT

Prevention is the best treatment. All procedural steps must be performed thoroughly and diligently, and meticulous interventional technique is required. Optimum strategic decisions and accomplished fluency of all mechanical manipulations during brachiocephalic interventions are the most important means of prevention. Any distractions to the operator during the intervention must be avoided. The operator must focus fully his attention on all details of the carotid intervention throughout the entire procedure.

It is important to realize that in all brachiocephalic interventions, as opposed to most other vascular interventions, embolizations may be life threatening. Therefore, avoidance of distal injury has the highest priority. TCD monitoring has clearly identified interventional steps associated with the peak microembolic signal (MES) transits. Although MES may remain asymptomatic, their outbursts clearly coincide with the critical mechanical steps of the intervention such as sheath placement, guidewire manipulation, and DPD retraction.[84] It is, therefore, particularly during these stages of the intervention that utmost gentleness and care are required. Thus, careful use of the mechanical advantages

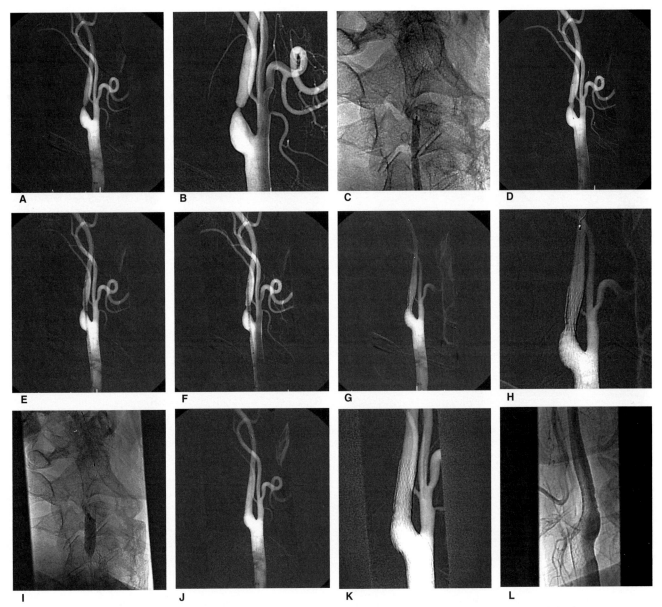

FIGURE 7-15. Standard carotid stenting. High-grade, proximal stenosis of the carotid bulb. **A:** Digital subtraction angiogram (DSA) of a high-grade, proximal, internal carotid artery stenosis and deployed distal protection device. **B:** Close-up DSA, confirmation of the findings. **C:** Predilatation. **D:** Result of predilatation. **E:** Stent positioning. **F:** Stent repositioning before deployment. **G:** Result following stent deployment. **H:** Close-up DSA of the result following stent deployment. **I:** Postdilatation. **J:** Final result. **K:** Close-up, final result shows excellent anatomic result. **L:** Second projection of the final result.

of the coaxial telescopic technique reduces the degree of trauma during sheath placement. Gentle handling of a bent guidewire tip adapted to the morphology of the stenosis and the width and elongation of the target vessel facilitates exploration of the neck of the target lesion and allows safe and atraumatic crossing. This gentle, explorative, manual manipulation of the guidewire may be compared to the smooth stereotactic guidance of the guidewire when external magnetic coils are used. Full deployment of the DPD with a full vessel-wall adaptation and avoidance of inadvertent repositioning during the procedure, frequent aspirations of the entire sheath/catheter system contents, prior

injections of contrast agents, and complete blood withdrawal from the system before retraction of the DPD all reduce the risk of distal embolizations. In addition, the operator must be aware of any angiographic deformations of the deployed stents and the completeness of plaque scaffolding as potential sources of late embolizations. In patients with a large plaque burden, optimum anatomic stent adaptation to the surface plaque morphology might be preferable to removing the residual stenosis "at any cost" (Fig. 7-11). It should be remembered that, in contrast to most coronary interventions, removal of the sheath or guiding catheter also represent a critical part of the intervention. Gentle

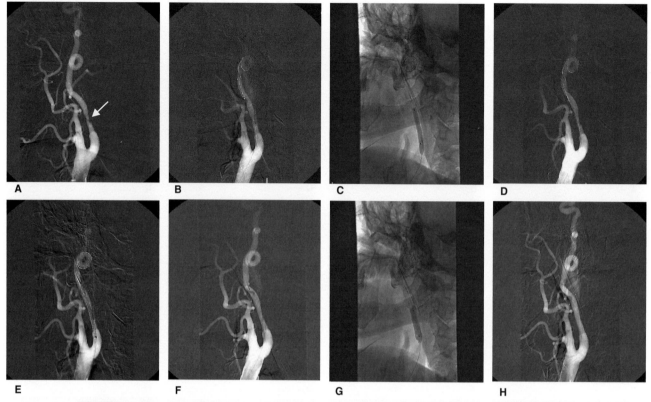

FIGURE 7-16.   Carotid stenting. Internal carotid artery stenosis with thrombus. **A:** Digital subtraction angiogram (DSA) with a high-grade, proximal, internal carotid artery stenosis and central thrombus (*arrow*). Note the downstream coiling. **B:** Distal protection device deployed. **C:** Predilatation. **D:** Residual stenosis after predilatation; in an asymptomatic patient, thrombus no longer seen. **E:** Stent positioning across the lesion. **F:** Residual stenosis after the stent deployment. **G:** Postdilatation. **H:** Final result.

removal using the reversed coaxial telescopic technique avoids injury and "surprise" late embolizations following what appeared to be a successful intervention.

It is important to remember that during and after CAS, a number of fully reversible changes, sensations, and alterations may occur that have no prognostic significance. In these cases, it is important to avoid overtreatment that might in itself become injurious. These events are in their sum a result of complex circulatory reflectory and neurohumoral adaptations related to the intermittent impairments of cerebral perfusion, local mechanical vascular irritations, and systemic traumatization caused by the procedure itself. These reversible events include "foreign body" sensations ipsilateral to the side of the intervention in the neck or in the submandibular region. These sensations usually disappear within several hours of intervention without any specific treatment. Furthermore, during the balloon inflations, particularly in the vicinity of the base of the skull, quite severe headache-like pains may occur. The pain subsides with balloon deflation. Postinterventional hypotension frequently accompanies CAS and is well tolerated in most patients, with volume supplementation the only treatment necessary. In any case, mild hypotension is preferable to postinterventional hypertension or to large blood-pressure swings. Similarly, postinterventional bradycardia is usually well tolerated and requires intravenous atropine treatment in only a minority of patients.

Peri-interventional fatigue represents a symptom of cerebral malperfusion and subsides following hemodynamic stabilization of the patient. Similarly, a transient, prognostically benign, sudden loss of consciousness with retrograde amnesia may result from prolonged episodes of interrupted cerebral perfusion during prolonged (usually >10 to 15 seconds) and repetitive balloon inflations The symptoms are fully reversible following balloon deflation or with shortening of the inflation time. In addition, repetitive transient cerebral ischemia associated with prolonged inflation times may cause ischemic pseudoseizures and contralateral extremity weakness. These symptoms are usually fully reversible on restoration of the antegrade blood flow. However, in all patients with transient focal and nonfocal neurological symptoms, close observation is mandatory until the symptoms have fully resolved.

Persistent symptoms or any complications before, during, or after the intervention are medical emergencies and must be managed as such. In the following sections, possible scenarios relevant specifically to CAS are discussed.

HEMODYNAMIC INSTABILITY

Hemodynamic and electrical instability associated with CAE has been well recognized for years and attributed to transient dysfunction of adventitial baroreceptors on direct mechanical

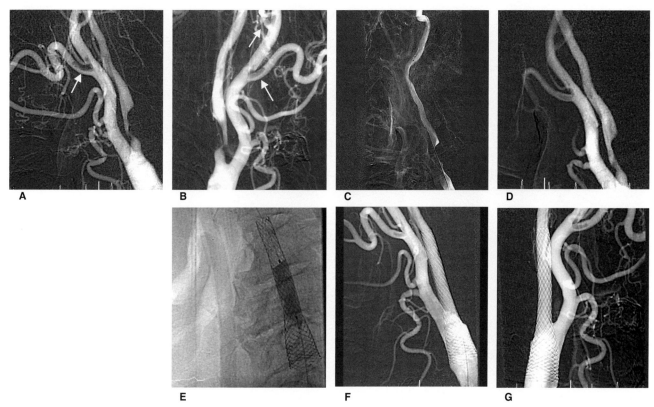

FIGURE 7-17. Carotid stenting. Internal carotid artery stenosis with evidence of earlier thrombotic events in the distribution of the external carotid artery. **A:** High-grade, eccentric, proximal, internal carotid artery stenosis. Thrombus overriding the bifurcation of the external carotid artery (*arrow*). **B:** Second projection. Thrombi are seen on two different bifurcations (*arrows*). **C:** Distal protection device placement. **D:** Result following predilatation. **E:** Postdilatation following stent deployment. **F:** Final result. Unchanged appearance of the distal external carotid artery thrombus. **G:** Final result, second projection. Unchanged appearance of the distal external carotid artery thrombus.

stimulation associated with tissue removal.[85,86] Bradycardia and hypotension during the early postoperative period were related to increased activity of the carotid sinus nerve or carotid baroreceptors secondary to the postoperative stretch with consecutive reflectory responses.[87] In CAS, transient hemodynamic instability is also frequent; the reported frequency of periprocedural hypotension (systolic blood pressure <90 mm Hg), hypertension (systolic blood pressure >160 mm Hg), and bradycardia (heart rate <60/min) is 22.4%, 38.8%, and 27.5%, respectively.[88] In this study, all events were transient and had resolved within a mean of 25.7 hours (range 18 to 43 hours). Hemodynamic instability associated with CAS appears to be related to the mechanical irritation (stretch) of the baroreceptors situated within the carotid sinus, and reflex inhibition of nucleus tractus solitarius located in the caudal medulla, with consecutive inhibition of the afferent sympathetic fibers during the CAS intervention. Active treatment is not required in the majority of cases; early ambulation in uncomplicated cases might reduce symptoms and shorten the phase of hemodynamic instability.[89]

General prevention of hemodynamic instability consists of withholding blood pressure medication on the day of the intervention, adequate hydration using intravenous access, and administration of 0.5 to 1.0 mg atropine intravenously, if needed. In patients with symptomatic and persistent hypotension (systolic blood pressure <80 mm Hg), active hemodynamic support using the infusion of volume expanders may be implemented. Only in the most severe cases should low-dose intravenous dobutamine, if necessary in combination with dopamine, be administered. Because of the risk of severe hypertension, norepinephrine and adrenalin should be avoided, unless for vital indications. Oxygen supplementation via nasal prongs stabilizes the patient and improves oxygenation. In patients with severe coronary artery disease (left main disease, multivessel disease) awaiting coronary surgery, and in patients with unstable cardiac bradyarrhythmias, prophylactic pacing may be required. Unchecked bradyarrhythmias or episodes of asystole with ensuing myocardial ischemia might be particularly deleterious in these patients.

In patients with persistent hypertension (systolic blood pressure >160 mm Hg), gentle blood-pressure reduction using intravenous nitroglycerin is suggested. However, blood-pressure depression and blood-pressure swings must be avoided.

CEREBRAL HYPERPERFUSION SYNDROME

CAE may be associated with ipsilateral intracerebral hemorrhage in <1% (0.4% to 2.7%) of patients.[90–92] Breakdown of the autoregulation of the cerebral blood flow on reperfusion (hypothesis of "normal perfusion pressure breakthrough")[93]

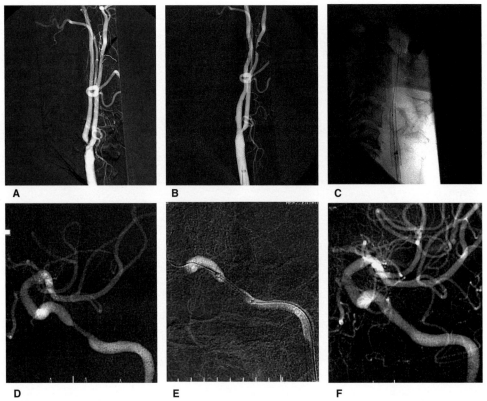

FIGURE 7-18.   Tandem lesions of the internal carotid artery. **A:** Filiform short proximal internal carotid artery stenosis involving the common carotid artery. **B:** Post dilatation following stent placement. **C:** Final result. **D:** Concentric tandem stenosis of the intracranial internal carotid artery (pars petrosa). **E:** Direct stenting. **F:** Final result.

TABLE 7-23.   Example of Procedural Care Recommendations

Vital signs should be obtained and recorded at regular intervals during the course of the procedure

Cardiac rhythm should be monitored continuously

Intravenous access must be available for administration of fluids and drugs

If the patient is to receive conscious sedation, pulse oximetry must be used; administration of sedation should be in accordance with the ACR Standard for Conscious Sedation; anesthesia personnel, a registered nurse, or other appropriately trained personnel should be present and have primary responsibility for monitoring the patient; all medication doses and times should be recorded

Neurologic deterioration should be documented and quantified by the NIHSS[a]

ACR, American College of Radiology.
[a]NIHSS, National Institutes of Health Stroke Scale; for reference see Brott T, Adams HP Jr, Olinger CP, et al. Measurements of acute cerebral infarction: a clinical examination scale. *Stroke.* 1989; 20: 864–870, and NIH Stroke Scale. Available at: http://www.ninds.nih.gov/doctors/NIH_Stroke_Scale.pdf. Accessed November 18, 2005.

From Barr JD, Connors JJ, Sacks D, et al., for the ASITN, ASNR, and SIR Standards of Practice Committees. Quality improvement guidelines for the performance of cervical carotid angioplasty and stent placement. Developed by a Collaborative Panel of the American Society of Interventional and Therapeutic Neuroradiology, the American Society of Neuroradiology, and the Society of the Interventional Radiology. *J Vasc Intervent Radiol.* 2003;14:S321–S335.

TABLE 7-22.   Example of Preprocedural Care Requirements

The history and indications for the procedure must be recorded in the patient's medical record; relevant medications, allergies, and bleeding disorders should be noted

The vital signs and physical (general and neurologic) examination must be documented

Neurologic assessment must include documentation of the National Institutes of Health Stroke Scale (NIHSS[a])

[a]NIHSS, National Institutes of Health Stroke Scale; for reference see Brott T, Adams HP Jr, Olinger CP, et al. Measurements of acute cerebral infarction: a clinical examination scale. *Stroke.* 1989; 20: 864–870, and NIH Stroke Scale. Available at: http://www.ninds.nih.gov/doctors/NIH_Stroke_Scale.pdf. Accessed November 18, 2005.

From Barr JD, Connors JJ, Sacks D, et al., for the ASITN, ASNR, and SIR Standards of Practice Committees. Quality improvement guidelines for the performance of cervical carotid angioplasty and stent placement. Developed by a Collaborative Panel of the American Society of Interventional and Therapeutic Neuroradiology, the American Society of Neuroradiology, and the Society of the Interventional Radiology. *J Vasc Intervent Radiol.* 2003;14:S321–S335.

TABLE 7-24. Example of Postprocedural Care Recommendations

A procedure note must be written in the patient's medical record summarizing the procedure, any immediate complications, and the patient's status at the end of the procedure; this information should be communicated to the referring physician as soon as possible; the note may be brief if the formal report will be dictated and available the same day

All patients should be carefully observed during the postprocedure period; the patient's vital signs and neurologic examination, along with the status of the puncture site and the peripheral pulses should be monitored at regular intervals by a nurse or other qualified personnel

The physician performing the procedure or a qualified designee (physician or nurse) should evaluate the patient after the initial postprocedure period; these findings should be recorded in a progress note in the patient's medical record; the physician and/or designee should be available for continuing care before and after the patient's discharge from the hospital

Neurologic assessment must include documentation of the NIHSS
NIHSS, National Institutes of Health Stroke Scale.
From Barr JD, Connors JJ, Sacks D, et al., for the ASITN, ASNR, and SIR Standards of Practice Committees. Quality improvement guidelines for the performance of cervical carotid angioplasty and stent placement. Developed by a Collaborative Panel of the American Society of Interventional and Therapeutic Neuroradiology, the American Society of Neuroradiology, and the Society of the Interventional Radiology. *J Vasc Intervent Radiol.* 2003;14:S321–S335.

has been thought to trigger the intracerebral bleeding. Indeed, severe hypertension or chronic hemispheric hypoperfusion with impaired autoregulation are major risk factors for perioperative intracerebral bleeding.[94]

Hyperperfusion syndrome was reported in 5.0% of patients with CAS, occurring within 2 to 18 hours of the procedure and associated with moderate to severe headaches, sensory disturbances, and focal neurological deficits; although no death was reported, permanent disability occurred in 30% of patients.[95] In a later report, a lower incidence of the hyperperfusion syndrome (1.1%) was reported, but here the outcome was worse (mortality rate 0.44%). In this series, the symptoms developed within a median of 10 hours (range 6 hours to 4 days) following CAS.[96]

Stable blood-pressure control represents the only recognized means of prevention of the CSA-related hyperperfusion syndrome. Vigorous treatment of blood pressure in either direction should be avoided in all cases; however, in patients with hypertension or pre-existing impaired cerebral perfusion, for example, high-grade stenosis in the presence of incompetent intracerebral collateralization, abrupt iatrogenic blood pressure changes may be particularly deleterious. Intravenous nitroglycerin and calcium channel blockers are the preferred medication to control sustained hypertension. Before starting blood pressure medication, other causes of elevated blood pressure such as urinary bladder urgencies, pain, and anxiety must be excluded. Patients with hypertensive syndrome complicated by intracerebral hemorrhage require immediate termination of the procedure, reversal of anticoagulation using protamine, and an emergency brain CT. Sudden loss of consciousness preceded by a headache, in the absence of intracranial vessel occlusion and the presence of moderate mass effect on angiography, should alert the operator to this devastating event. Conditions associated with intracerebral hemorrhage in conjunction with CAS are reviewed in Table 7-25.[97]

TABLE 7-25. Conditions Associated with Intracerebral Hemorrhage in Conjunction with Carotid Artery Stenting (CAS)

CAS on preocclusive or occluded artery

Excessive anticoagulation

Poorly controlled hypertension

Stenting in the presence of a recent ischemic stroke (<3 weeks)

Presence of a vulnerable aneurysm

From Vitek JJ, Roubin GS, New G, et al. Carotid stenting. Available at: http://www.fac.org.ar/scvc/llave/stroke/vitek/viteki.htm. Accessed January 6, 2006.

SPASM

Spasms of the internal carotid artery are frequently provoked by mechanical irritation of the vessel walls. Therefore, all endovascular instruments should be handled gently in the target artery, and guidewires and DPD should not be moved or repositioned after initial placement, unless it is absolutely necessary (warning note: because of the coaxial telescopic principle, any motion from the outside catheters is translated to the inside device, unless their motion is restricted; when repositioning guides or sheath, hold the wire!). In addition, the nominal size of the internal carotid artery should be matched; refrain from oversizing stents and the DPD! If distal internal carotid artery spasms occur, no treatment is needed in the majority of patients because the spasm resolves spontaneously following withdrawal of the instrumentation. In cases of persistent distal spasm, angiographic exclusion of a dissection is required in multiple projections. In patients with pre-existing intimal folds in elongated and kinked segments, it may be difficult to distinguish among spasm, infolding, and dissection.

If spasm is confirmed, nitroglycerin might be considered (100 to 300 μg internal carotid artery bolus). To avoid injury and escalating the problem, mechanical attempts to "dilatate" spasms are not recommended. Figure 7-19 shows a spasm due to the deployment of a DPD, with spontaneous resolution following retraction of the device.

SLOW-FLOW, NO-FLOW

Compromised antegrade flow in the target artery that is not related to balloon inflation must be addressed immediately. The timing of its occurrence narrows down the possible causes: Before DPD deployment, severe spasm, massive distal embolization, or extensive dissection may be responsible. Following DPD deployment, acute stent thrombosis or filter plugging appears more likely.

In cases of impaired flow secondary to a documented or suspected dissection, retaining the initial intraluminal position of the primary guidewire with the tip at the base of the skull is most critical for safe passage of the subsequent instrumentation. Retraction of the primary guidewire or exploration of the interventional site with a secondary guidewire must be avoided! Puff injection of a contrast agent followed by angiography, if needed, should provide anatomic orientation. Careful low-inflation-pressure dilatation with an undersized balloon at the site of the occlusion, followed by deployment of a flexible stent, might quickly resolve the situation.

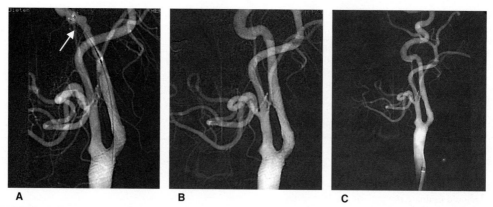

FIGURE 7-19.   Internal carotid artery spasm due to distal protection device. **A:** Distal spasm at the level of the deployed distal protection filter (*arrow*). **B:** Spontaneous spasm resolution following retraction of the distal protection device. **C:** Overview angiogram, normal morphology.

Plugging of the distal protection filter was the suspected cause of impaired flow in a retrospective, monocenter registry observed in 10.1% (42 of 414) of patients, corresponding to 9.3% (42 of 453) of procedures.[98] Impaired flow was associated with stent deployment and poststent dilatation, and it was fully reversible following retrieval of the DPD. However, patients with impaired flow had an increased incidence of stroke or death (9.5% vs. 2.9%) at 30 days follow-up; the difference was mainly influenced by the higher rates of stroke (9.5% vs. 1.7%). Although it has been documented that 50% of the microemboli released during CAS are <100 μm,[99] the small pore size of the filter membrane might increase the incidence of filter thrombosis in addition to the containment capacity of the device being overwhelmed when large emboli are released.[100] Frequent aspiration of blood from the sheath and the internal carotid artery segment below the DPD may reduce the risk of filter plugging. In addition, optimum scaffolding of lesions with a large plaque burden along with complete exclusion of the remaining plaque tissue is important. Once plugging has occurred, the DPD filter must be retracted, sometimes in a half-open condition.

Stent thrombosis is a rare cause of no flow. An example of recommendations for the prevention of acute stent thrombosis is provided in Table 7-26.[97]

In cases of persistent flow impairment due to massive embolization, revascularization efforts using mechanical embolectomy or fibrinolysis—possibly combined with administration of GPIIb/IIIA receptor inhibitors—represent difficult options.

NEUROLOGICAL COMPLICATIONS

Spontaneous MES detected by TCD[101] may accompany asymptomatic, that is, clinically silent, and symptomatic, that is, manifest by history or physical examination, carotid artery stenosis.[102] In fact, detection of MES has been proposed as a marker of stroke risk in symptomatic[103] as well as asymptomatic[104] patients. It has been shown that unprotected carotid angioplasty is associated with significantly more MES than CAE (fourfold increase in mean numbers) with no significant differences in neurological outcomes[105] and that the use of DPDs markedly reduces the frequency of MES.[84] Furthermore, it has been shown that unprotected CAS,

TABLE 7-26.   Example of Recommendations for Prevention of Acute Stent Thrombosis Associated with Carotid Stenting

Compulsive and appropriate use of adjunctive antiplatelet therapy

Meticulous stenting technique including (1) stenting only in the presence of brisk flow without significant inflow or outflow obstruction; (2) stenting from normal segment to normal segment, if possible; and (3) ensuring proper stent sizing (oversizing in the case of self-expanding stents) and careful opposition to the vessel wall

From Vitek JJ, Roubin GS, New G, et al. Carotid stenting. Available at: http://www.fac.org.ar/scvc/llave/stroke/vitek/viteki.htm. Accessed January 6, 2006.

even if performed by highly experienced operators (several hundred CAS procedures each) may result in cerebral ischemia detectable with diffusion-weighted brain MR imaging.[106] However, the clinical relevance of MES remains unclear: There has been reported evidence of impairment[107] as well as of improvement[108] in postprocedural neuropsychological functions, as measured by a battery of neuropsychological tests. With incoming data, the issue of the clinical relevance of MES will soon be clarified. Because of the inability of TCD to discriminate between thrombus and atheroma, the source of MES during CAS remains open to debate; for clinical practice, consistent antithrombotic management and meticulous CAS technique must once again be emphasized for prevention.

Whereas microemboli (~100-μm diameter) might remain clinically silent, distal macroembolization into the intracerebral vascular territory probably produces neurological symptoms in all cases. Procedural actions that increase the incidence of distal embolization are summarized in Table 7-27. Other causes of macroembolizations may include inefficient capture, with particles or debris bypassing the DPD because of incomplete vessel wall apposition; squeezing out debris into the bloodstream from the basket during the DPD retraction maneuver; or shaving off plaque remnants or thrombi during the withdrawal of the introductory sheath. Paying attention to all technical details throughout the entire course of the intervention minimizes the risk of embolization, yet it appears highly unlikely that the <1% of neurological complications demanded for CAS indications in

TABLE 7-27. Procedural Actions Increasing the Incidence of Distal Embolization

Very Important	Less Important
Predilatation with oversized peripheral balloon	Initial angiographic access
Forcing stent across a lesion (particularly if heavily calcified)	Crossing the lesion with guidewire
Aggressive postdilatation and/or oversizing	
Persistent, aggressive attempts to access a tortuous, highly atherosclerotic common carotid artery with the sheath	

Modified from Vitek JJ, Roubin GS, New G, et al. Carotid stenting. Available at: http://www.fac.org.ar/scvc/llave/stroke/vitek/viteki.htm. Accessed January 6, 2006.

low-risk asymptomatic patients[104] will be achieved. Definitions of neurological complications in patients with CAS are stated in Table 7-20; an example of their incidence in high-risk patients is shown in Table 7-11. Full and thorough, preferably independent, documentation of all neurological complications must be ensured in all institutions that provide CAS treatments.

In patients with intracerebral macroembolizations, angiographic documentation of the embolic site is required. Interventionalists familiar with intracerebral interventional techniques will attempt embolectomy or local fibrinolytic pharmacotherapy, frequently with a rather uncertain outcome. Emergency CT or MRI[109] and neurological intensive care management are required in all patients.

RESTENOSIS

As with catheter-based interventions in other vascular beds, CAS is limited by in-stent restenosis, technically defined as >50% diameter recurrent luminal obstruction.

Reported data on CAE suggest restenosis rates for ≥70% stenosis ranging from 0.1% at a median follow-up of 7.1 years[110] to 7.7% at a median follow-up of 5.9 years.[111] In centers performing >500 CAE annually, the reported incidence of restenosis for stenoses >30% to >70% ranged between 0.1% and 7.9% (for review, see reference 110). Systematic review of restenosis rates following carotid angioplasty with and without stenting for ≥50% and ≤70% stenoses at 1 and 2 years were at the 6% and 7.5% level, respectively. The restenosis rate at 2 years for ≥70% stenosis was 4%.[112] However, in-stent restenosis rates reported in studies that directly compared CAS and CAE suggest higher restenosis rates for CAS. Thus, in CAVATAS the reported in-stent restenosis rate for ≥70% stenosis was 18.5% for CAS and 5.2% for CAE.[113] The incidence of in-stent restenosis determined in SAPPHIRE is shown in Table 7-12.[72,73]

The presence of a mild to moderate (up to 70%) angiographic in-stent restenosis alone is not an indication for reintervention; in asymptomatic patients, close ultrasound follow-up (every 3 to 6 months) is currently recommended, yet better means of risk stratification (such as, perhaps, TCD) should provide more objective case selection in the future. Asymptomatic patients with severe in-stent restenosis and symptomatic patients with moderate to severe in-stent restenosis, particularly those with significant concomitant lesions of the contralateral internal carotid artery, should be considered for reintervention. Figures 7-20 and 7-21 show examples of diffuse and focal in-stent carotid artery restenosis.

Reinterventions are performed according to the same rules applicable to de novo lesion interventions. Although the smooth appearance of in-stent restenosis on ultrasound and angiography makes it tempting to forego distal embolization protection, small thrombi can never be excluded, and DPD is obligatory in all patients.

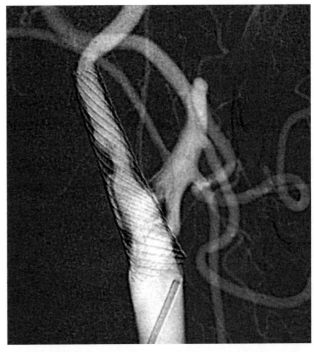

FIGURE 7-20. Carotid artery in-stent restenosis, 6 months follow-up. Moderate diffuse and moderate to severe focal in-stent restenosis at the level of the carotid bulb is shown.

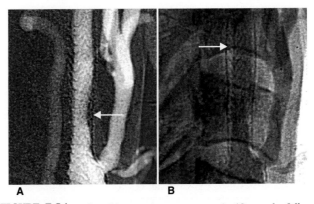

FIGURE 7-21. Carotid artery in-stent restenosis, 12 months follow-up. Smooth diffuse layer of neointima associated with a mild restenosis shown on digital subtraction angiography (DSA) (*arrow*) **(A)** and DSA without a mask (*arrow*) **(B)**.

REFERENCES

1. Mohr JP, Albers GW, Amarenco P, et al. Etiology of stroke. *Stroke.* 1997;28:1501–1506.
2. Barnett HJM, Mohr JP, Stein BM, et al. (eds.). *Stroke. Pathophysiology, Diagnosis and Management.* 3rd ed. New York: Churchill Livingstone, 1998:355–480.
3. Alberts MJ, Tournier-Lasserve E. Update on the genetics of stroke and cerebrovascular disease 2004. *Stroke.* 2005;36:179–181.
4. American Stroke Association and American Heart Association. Heart disease and stroke statistics—2005 update. Available at www.americanheart.org, Publications&Resources; Statistics. Accessed January 1, 2006.
5. Sacco RL, Benjamin EJ, Broderick JP, et al. Risk factors. *Stroke.* 1997;28:1507–1517.
6. Thompson JE. The evolution of surgery for the treatment and prevention of stroke. The Willis lecture. *Stroke.* 1996;27:1427–1434.
7. Hunt JR. The role of the carotid arteries in the causation of vascular lesions of the brain, with remarks on certain special features of the symptomatology. *Am J Med Sci.* 1914; 147:704–713.
8. Estol CJ. Dr C. Miller Fisher and the history of carotid artery disease. *Stroke.* 1996;27:559–566.
9. Giddens DP, Zarins CK, Glagov S, et al. Flow and atherogenesis in the human carotid bifurcation. In: Schettler C, Nerem RM, Schmid-Schönbein H, et al., eds. *Fluid Dynamics as a Localizing Factor for Atherosclerosis.* Berlin: Springer Verlag, 1983:38–45.
10. Caro CG, Fitz-Gerald JM, Schroter RC. Atheroma and arterial wall shear: observation, correlation and proposal of a shear dependent mass transfer mechanism of atherogenesis. *Proc R Soc Lond B Biol Sci.* 1971;177:109–159.
11. Wells DR, Archie JP Jr, Kleinstreuer C. Effect of carotid artery geometry on the magnitude and distribution of wall shear stress gradients. *J Vasc Surg.* 1996;23:667–678.
12. Younis HF, Kaazempur-Mofrad MR, Chan RC, et al. Hemodynamics and wall mechanics in human carotid bifurcation and its consequences for atherogenesis: investigation of interindividual variation. *Biomechan Model Mechanobiol.* 2004;3:17–32.
13. Takiuchi S, Rakugi H, Honda K, et al. Quantitative ultrasonic tissue characterization can identify high-risk atherosclerotic alteration in human carotid arteries. *Circulation.* 2000; 102:766–770.
14. Gronholdt ML, Nordestgaard BG, Bentzon J, et al. Macrophages are associated with lipid-rich carotid artery plaques, echolucency on B-mode imaging, and elevated plasma lipid levels. *J Vasc Surg.* 2002;35:137–145.
15. Imbesi SG, Kerber CW. Why do ulcerated atherosclerotic carotid artery plaques embolize? A flow dynamic study. *AJNR Am J Neuroradiol.* 1998;19:761–766.
16. Rothwell PM, Gibson R, Warlow CP on behalf of the European Carotid Surgery Trialists's Collaborative Study. Interrelation between plaque surface morphology and degree of stenosis on carotid angiograms and the risk of ischemic stroke in patients with symptomatic carotid stenosis. *Stroke.* 2000;31:615–621.
17. European Carotid Surgery Trialists' Collaborative Group. MRC European Carotid Surgery Trial: Interim results for symptomatic patients with severe (70–99%) or with mild (0–29%) stenosis. *Lancet.* 1991;337:1235–1243.
18. North American Symptomatic Carotid Endarterectomy Trial Collaborators. Beneficial effect of carotid endarterectomy in symptomatic patients with high-grade carotid stenosis. *N Engl J Med.* 1991;325:445–453.
19. Streifler JY, Eliasziw M, Fox AJ, et al. Angiographic detection of carotid plaque ulceration. Comparison with surgical observations in multicenter study. *Stroke.* 1994;25:1130–1132.
20. Lovett JK, Gallagher PJ, Hands LJ, et al. Histological correlates of carotid plaque surface morphology on lumen contrast imaging. *Circulation.* 2004;110:2190–2197.
21. Huston J 3rd, James, EM, Brown, RD Jr, et al. Redefined duplex ultrasonographic criteria for diagnosis of carotid artery stenosis. *Mayo Clin Proc.* 2000; 75:1133–1141.
22. Mathiesen EB, Bonaa KH, Joakimsen O. Echolucent plaques are associated with high risk of ischemic cerebrovascular events in carotid stenosis: the tromso study. *Circulation.* 2001; 103:2171–2175.
23. Moneta GL, Edwards JM, Chitwood RW, et al. Correlation of North American Symptomatic Carotid Endarterectomy Trial (NASCET) angiographic definition of 70 percent to 99 percent internal carotid artery stenosis with duplex scanning. *J Vasc Surg.* 1993;17:152–158.
24. Wilterdink JL, Furie KL, Kistler JP. Evaluation of carotid artery stenosis. Available at: http://patients.uptodate.com/topic.asp?file=cva_dise/4600&title=Carotid+artery+stenosis. Accessed January 2, 2006.
25. Wilterdink JL, Feldmann E, Furie KL, et al. Transcranial Doppler ultrasound battery reliably identifies severe internal carotid artery stenosis. *Stroke.* 1997; 28:133–136.
26. Sloan MA, Alexandrov AV, Tegeler CH, et al. Assessment: Transcranial doppler ultrasonography. Report of the Therapeutics and Technology Assessment Subcommittee of the American Academy of Neurology. *Neurology.* 2004;62:1468–1491.
27. Oliviera-Filho J, Koroshetz WJ. Neuroimaging of acute ischemic stroke. Available at: http://patients.uptodate.com/topic.asp?file=cva_dise/12684&title=Neuroimaging. Accessed January 2, 2006.
28. Moniz E. L'encephalographic arterielle: son importance dans la localization des tumeurs cerebrales. *Rev Neurol (Paris).* 1927;2:72–90.
29. Seldinger SI. Catheter replacement of the needle in percutaneous arteriography. *Acta Radiol [Diagn] (Stockholm).* 1953;39:368–376.
30. Geddes LA, Geddes LE. *The Catheter Introducers.* Chicago: Mobius Press, 1993.
31. Brody R. Digital subtraction angiography. *IEEE Trans Nucl Sci.* 1982;29:1176–1180.
32. Citron SJ, Wallace RC, Lewis CA et al. for the Joint Standards of Practice Task Force of the Society of Interventional Radiology, the American Society of Interventional and Therapeutic Neuroradiology. Quality improvement guidelines for adult diagnostic neuroradiography. Cooperative study between ASITN, ASNR, and SIR. *J Vasc Intervent Radiol.* 2003;14:S257–S262.
33. Teitelbaum GP, Higashida RT. Cerebrovascular angiography. In: Lanzer P, Rösch J, eds. *Vascular Diagnostics: Periinterventional Evaluations.* Berlin: Springer Verlag, 1994:207–242.
34. Moran CJ, Kido DK, Cross DT III. Cerebral vascular angiography: indications, technique, and normal anatomy of head. In: Baum S, ed. *Abram's Angiography.* 4th ed. Boston: Little, Brown and Company,1997:241–283.
35. Morris P. *Practical Neuroangiography.* Philadelphia: Lippincott Williams & Wilkins, 1997.
36. Lusza G. *X-ray Anatomy of the Vascular System.* Philadelphia: JB Lippincott Co, 1963.
37. Young GR, Humphrey PRD, Nixon TE, et al. Variability in measurements of extracranial internal carotid artery stenosis as displayed by both digital subtraction and magnetic resonance angiography. An assessment of three caliper techniques and visual impression of stenosis. *Stroke.* 1996;27:467–473.
38. Eastcott HHG, Pickering GW, Rob CG. Reconstruction of internal carotid artery. *Lancet.* 1954;i:994–996.
39. DeBakey ME. Successful carotid endarterectomy for cerebrovascular insufficiency. Nineteen-year follow-up. *JAMA.* 1975;233:1083–1085.
40. Moore WS. Extracranial cerebrovascular disease: The carotid artery. In: Moore WE, ed. *Vascular Surgery: A Comprehensive Review.* 6th ed. Philadelphia: WB Saunders, 2002:585–626.
41. European Carotid Surgery Trialists' Collaborative Group. MRC European Carotid Surgery Trial: Interim results for symptomatic patients with severe (70–99%) or with mild (0–29%) stenosis. *Lancet.* 1991;337:1235–1243.
42. North American Symptomatic Carotid Endarterectomy Trial Collaborators. Beneficial effect of carotid endarterectomy in symptomatic patients with high-grade carotid stenosis. *N Engl J Med.* 1991;325:445–453.
43. European Carotid Surgery Trialists' Collaborative Group. Randomised trail of endarterectomy for recently symptomatic carotid stenosis: final results of the MRC European Carotid Surgery Trial (ECST). *Lancet.* 1998;351:1379–1387.
44. Barnett HJM, Taylor DW, Eliasziw M, et al. For the North American Symptomatic Carotid Endarterectomy Trial Collaborators. Benefit of carotid endarterectomy in patients with symptomatic moderate or severe stenosis. *N Engl J Med.* 1998;339:1415–1425.
45. Rothwell PM, Eliasziw M, Gutnikov SA, et al. Endarterectomy for symptomatic carotid stenosis in relation to clinical subgroups and timing of surgery. *Lancet.* 2004;363:915–924.
46. Executive Committee for the Asymptomatic Carotid Atherosclerosis Study. Endarterectomy for asymptomatic carotid artery stenosis. *JAMA.* 1995; 273:1421–1428.
47. MRC Asymptomatic Carotid Surgery Trial (ACST) Collaborative Group. Prevention of disabling and fatal strokes by successful carotid endarterectomy in patients without recent neurological symptoms: randomised controlled trial. *Lancet.* 2004;363:1491–1502.
48. Rothwell PM, Goldstein LB. Carotid endarterectomy for asymptomatic carotid stenosis. Asymptomatic carotid surgery trial. *Stroke.* 2004;35:2425–2427.
49. Biller J, Feinberg WM, Castaldo JE, et al. Guidelines for carotid endarterectomy. A statement for healthcare professionals from a special writing group of the Stroke Council, American Heart Association. *Circulation.* 1998;97:501–509.
50. Bernhard VM, Johnson WD, Peterson JJ. Carotid artery stenosis: association with surgery for coronary artery disease. *Arch Surg.* 1972;105:837–840.
51. Huh J, Wall J Jr., Soltero ER. Treatment of combined coronary and carotid artery disease. *Curr Opin Cardiol.* 2003;18:447–453.
52. Chaturvedi S, Bruno A, Feasby T, et al. Carotid endarterectomy—an evidence based review. Report on the therapeutics and technology assessment subcommittee of the American Academy of Neurology. *Neurology.* 2005;65:794–801.
53. Mathias K. Ein neuartiges Katheter-System zur perkutanen transluminalen Angioplastie von Karotisstenosen. *Fortschr Med.* 1977;95:1007–1011.
54. Tsai FY, Matovich V, Hieshima G, et al. Percutaneous transluminal angioplasty of the carotid artery. *AJNR Am J Neuroradiol.* 1986;7:349–358.
55. Kachel R, Basche S, Heerklotz I, et al. Percutaneous transluminal angioplasty (PTA) of supra-aortic arteries especially the internal carotid artery. *Neuroradiology.* 1991;33:191–194.
56. Higashida RT, Tsai FY, Halbach W, et al. Cerebral percutaneous transluminal angioplasty. *Heart Dis Stroke.* 1993;2:497–502.
57. Kachel R. Results of balloon angioplasty in the carotid arteries. *J Endovasc Surg.* 1996;3:22–30.
58. Yadav JS, Roubin GS, Iyer S, et al. Electives tenting of the extracranial carotid arteries. *Circulation.* 1997;95:376–381.
59. Theron JG, Paylelle GG, Coskun O, et al. Carotid artery stenosis: treatment with protected balloon angioplasty and stent placement. *Radiology.* 1996;201:627–636.
60. Al-Mubarak N, Colombo A, Gaines PA, et al. Multicenter evaluation of carotid artery stenting with a filter protection system. *J Am Coll Cardiol.* 2002;39:841–846.
61. Kastrup A, Gröschel K, Krapf H, et al. Early outcome of carotid angioplasty and stenting with and without cerebral protection devices. A systematic review of the literature. *Stroke.* 2003;34:813–819.
62. Zahn R, Mark B, Niedermaier N, et al. for the Arbeitsgemeinschaft Leitende Kardiologische Krankenhausärzte (ALLK). Embolic protection devices for carotid artery stenting: better results than stenting without protection? *Eur Heart J.* 2004;25:1550–1558.
63. Coward LJ, Featherstone RL, Brown MM. Percutaneous transluminal angioplasty and stenting for carotid artery stenosis (Cochrane Review). Available at: www. Cochrane.org/ Cochrane/revabstr/AB000515.htm. Accessed November 14, 2005.
64. Bettmann MA, Katzen BT, Whisnant J, et al. Carotid stenting and angioplasty. A statement for healthcare professionals from the councils on Cardiovascular Radiology, Stroke, Cardio-Thoracic and Vascular Surgery, Epidemiology and Prevention, and Clinical Cardiology, AHA. *Circulation.* 1998;97:121–123.
65. Barr JD, Connors JJ, Sacks D, et al. for the ASITN, ASNR, and SIR Standards of Practice Committees. Quality improvement guidelines for the performance of cervical carotid angioplasty and stent placement. Developed by a Collaborative Panel of the American Society of Interventional and Therapeutic Neuroradiology, the American Society of Neuroradiology, and the Society of the Interventional Radiology. *J Vasc Intervent Radiol.* 2003;14:S321–S335.
66. Roubin GS, New G, Iyer SS, et al. Immediate and late clinical outcomes of carotid artery stenting in patients with symptomatic and asymptomatic carotid artery stenosis; a 5-year prospective analysis. *Circulation.* 2001;103:532–537.

67. New G, Roubin GS, Iyer SS, et al. Carotid artery stenting: rationale, indications, and results. *Compr Ther.* 1999;25:438–445.

68. Rothwell PM, Slattery J, Warlow CP. Clinical and angiographic predictors of stroke and death from carotid endarterectomy: systematic review. *BMJ.* 1997;317:1571–1577.

69. Sundt TM Jr, Sandok BA, Whisnant JP. Carotid endarterectomy. Complications and preoperative assessment of risk. *Mayo Clin Proc.* 1975;50:301–306.

70. McCrory DC, Goldstein LB, Samsa GP, et al. Predicting complications of carotid endarterectomy. *Stroke.* 1993;24:1285–1291.

71. Goldstein LG; Samsa GP, Matchar DB, et al. Multicenter review of preoperative risk factors for endarterectomy for asymptomatic carotid artery stenosis. *Stroke.* 1998;29:750–753.

72. Yadav JS, Wholey MH, Kuntz RE, et al. Protected carotid-artery stenting versus endarterectomy in high-risk patients. *N Engl J Med.* 2004;351:1493–1501.

73. Ouriel K. SAPPHIRE pivotal study. Available at: http://www.fda.gov/ohrms/dockets/ac/04/briefing/4033b1.htm. Accessed November 15, 2005.

74. Carotid and Vertebral Artery Transluminal Angioplasty Study (CAVATAS) Investigators. Endovascular versus surgical treatment in patients with carotid stenosis in the Carotid and Vertebral Artery Transluminal Angioplasty Study (CAVATAS): a randomized trial. *Lancet.* 357:1729–1737.

75. Naylor AR, Bolia A, Abbott RJ, et al. Randomized study of carotid angioplasty and stenting versus carotid endarterectomy: a stopped trial. *J Vasc Surg.* 1998;28:326–334.

76. Brooks WH, McClure RR, Jones MR, et al. Carotid angioplasty and stenting versus carotid endarterectomy: randomized trial in a community hospital. *J Am Coll Cardiol.* 2001; 38:1589–1595.

77. Decision Memo for carotid artery stenting (CAG-00085R); Decision summary. Available at: http://www.cms.hhs.gov/mcd/viewdecisionmemo.asp?id=157.

78. Lanzer P, Weser R, Prettin C. Carotid-artery stenting in high risk patient population; single-center, single-operator results. *Clin Res Cardiol.* 2006;95:4–12.

79. Higashida RT, Hopkins LN, Berenstein A, et al. Program requirements for residency fellowship education in neuroendovascular surgery/interventional neuroradiology: a special report on graduate medical education. *AJNR Am J Neuroradiol.* 2000;21:1153–1159.

80. Clinical competence statement on carotid stenting: training and credentialing for carotid stenting multispecialty consensus recommendations. A report of the SCAI/SVMB/SVS Writing Committee to develop a clinical competence statement on carotid interventions. *Cathet Cardiovasc Intervent.* 2005;64:1–11.

81. Gallagher AG, Cates CU. Approval of virtual reality training for carotid stenting. *JAMA.* 2004;292:3024–3026.

82. Brott T, Adams HP Jr, Olinger CP, et al. Measurements of acute cerebral infarction: a clinical examination scale. *Stroke.* 1989; 20: 864–870.

83. NIH Stroke Scale. Available at: http://www.ninds.nih.gov/doctors/NIH_Stroke_Scale.pdf. Accessed November 18, 2005.

84. Al-Mubarak N, Roubin GS, Vitek JJ, et al. Effect of the distal-balloon protection system on microembolization during carotid stenting. *Circulation.* 2001;104:1999–2002.

85. Bove EL, Fry WJ, Gross WS, et al. Hypotension and hypertension as consequences of baroreceptor dysfunction following carotid endarterectomy. *Surgery.* 1979;85:633–637.

86. Satiani B, Vasko JS, Evans WE. Hypertension following carotid endarterectomy. *Surg Neurol.* 1979;11:357–359.

87. Tarlov E, Schmidek H, Scott RM, et al. Reflex hypotension following carotid endarterectomy: mechanism and management. *J Neurosurg.* 1973;39:323–327.

88. Qureshi AI, Luft AR, Sharma M, et al. Frequency and determinants of postprocedural hemodynamic instability after carotid angioplasty and stenting. *Stroke.* 1999;30:2086–2093.

89. Roubin GS. Rapid ambulation after CAS. *Endovasc Today.* April 2005; 45–46.

90. Ouriel K, Shortell CK, Illig KA, et al. Intracerebral hemorrhage after carotid endarterectomy: Incidence, contribution to neurologic morbidity, and predictive factors. *J Vasc Surg.* 1999;29:82–89.

91. Piepgras DG, Morgan MK, Sundt TF, et al. Intracerebral hemorrhage after carotid endarterectomy. *J Neurosurg.* 1988;68:532–536.

92. Solomon RA, Loftus CM, Quest DO, et al. Incidence and etiology of intracerebral hemorrhage following carotid endarterectomy. *J Neurosurg.* 1986;64:29–34.

93. Spetzler RF, Wilson CB, Weinstein P, et al. Normal perfusion pressure breakthrough theory. *Clin Neurosurg.* 1978;25:651–672.

94. Breen JC, Caplan LR, DeWitt LD, et al. Brain edema after carotid surgery. *Neurology.* 1996;46:175–181.

95. Meyers PM, Higashida RT, Phatouros CC, et al. Cerebral hyperperfusion syndrome after percutaneous transluminal stenting of the craniocervical arteries. *Neurosurgery.* 2000;47:335–345.

96. Abou-Chebl A, Yadav JS, Reginelli JP, et al. Intracranial hemorrhage and hyperperfusion syndrome following carotid artery stenting. *J Am Coll Cardiol.* 2004;43:1596–1601.

97. Vitek JJ, Roubin GS, New G, et al. Carotid stenting. Available at: http://www.fac.org.ar/scvc/llave/stroke/vitek/viteki.htm . Accessed January 6, 2006.

98. Casserly IP, Abou-Chebl A, Fathi RB, et al. Slow-flow phenomenon during carotid artery intervention with embolic protection device. *J Am Coll Cardiol.* 2005;46:1466–1472.

99. Whitlow PL, Lylyk P, Londero H, et al. Carotid artery stenting protected with an emboli containment system. *Stroke.* 2003;33:1308–1314.

100. Kindel M, Spiller P. Transient occlusion of an Angioguard protection system by massive embolization during angioplasty of a degenerated aortocoronary saphenous vein graft. *Cathet Cardiovasc Intervent.* 2002;55:501–504.

101. Ringelstein EB, Droste DW, Babikian VL, et al. Consensus on microembolus detection by TCD. *Stroke.* 1998;29:725–729.

102. Markus HS. Microembolic signal detection in cerebrovascular disease. In: Babikian VL, Wechsler L, eds. *Transcranial Doppler Ultrasonography.* 2nd ed. Boston: Butterworth-Heinemann; 1999.

103. Markus HS, MacKinnon A. Asymptomatic embolization detected by Doppler ultrasound predicts stroke risk in symptomatic carotid artery stenosis. *Stroke.* 2005;36:971–975.

104. Spence JD, Tamayo A, Lownie SP, et al. Absence of microemboli on transcranial Doppler identifies low-risk patients with asymptomatic carotid stenosis. *Stroke.* 2005;36:2373–2378.

105. Crawley F, Clifton A, Buckenham T. Comparison of hemodynamic cerebral ischemia and microembolic signals detected during carotid endarterectomy and carotid angioplasty. *Stroke.* 1997;28:2460–2464.

106. Jaeger HJ, Mathias KD, Hauth E, et al. Cerebral ischemia detected with Diffusion-Weighted MR Imaging after stent implantation in the carotid artery. *AJNR Am J Neuroradiol.* 2002;23:200–207.

107. Crawley F, Stygall J, Lunn S, et al. Comparison of microembolism detected by transcranial Doppler and neuropsychological sequelae of carotid surgery and percutaneous transluminal angioplasty. *Stroke.* 2000;31:1329–1334.

108. Moftakhar R, Turk AS, Niemann DB, et al. Effects of carotid or vertebrobasilar stent placement on cerebral perfusion and cognition. *AJNR Am J Neuroradiol.* 2005;26: 1772–1780.

109. Oliviera-Filho J, Koroshetz WJ. Neuroimaging of acute ischemic stroke. Available at: http://patients.uptodate.com.

110. Ecker RD, Pichelmann MA, Meissner I, et al. Durability of carotid endarterectomy. *Stroke.* 2003;34:2941–2944.

111. LaMuraglia GM, Brewster DC, Moncure AC, et al. Carotid endarterectomy at the millennium: what interventional therapy must match. *Ann Surg.* 2004;240:535–544.

112. Gröschel K, Riecker A, Schulz JB, et al. Systematic review of early recurrent stenosis after carotid angioplasty and stenting. *Stroke.* 2005;36:367–373.

113. McCabe DJH, Pereira AC, Clifton A, et al. Restenosis after carotid angioplasty, stenting, or endarterectomy in the Carotid and Vertebral Artery Transluminal Angioplasty Study (CAVATAS). *Stroke.* 2005;36:281–286.

Peter Lanzer

L.D. Timmie Topoleski*

CHAPTER **8**

Coronary Arteries

Since their introduction in the late 1970s, coronary interventions have gradually become technically less demanding and safer. This is primarily due to the introduction of low-profile high-technology products, stents, and microcatheter-based techniques. In fact, the greater facility of endocoronary instrumentation combined with the systematic use of guiding catheters for better steering and device manipulation in a highly vulnerable microenvironment has become a model approach for an increasing number of noncoronary endovascular interventions as well. Although the facility and quality of the instrumentation are important, the individual professional competence of the operator remains the most critical factor in the success of coronary interventions. Integral parts of professional competence are a thorough understanding of the principles of coronary image acquisition and interpretation, reliable risk and benefit definition for individual patients, and accomplished operational skills. To review the essentials of coronary interventions as they apply to real-life clinical practice, the traditional textbook approach of reciting the established medical facts and pronouncing treatment recommendations based solely on customary statistical evidence has been abandoned in this chapter. Instead, following a brief historical retrospective, practice-relevant principles of the coronary interventions have been reviewed. This review is systematic, starting with the description of the mechanical effects of coronary interventions, and includes the current requirements for interventional coronary competence, patient- and lesion-related risk factors, instrumentation, the basic structure of coronary interventions, complication management, and treatment strategies in standard clinical situations. Although a linear approach to reading the individual chapter may be preferable, each section is self-contained, and a study of selected topics of interest is fully acceptable for an advanced reader.

RETROSPECTIVE

Following experimental and postmortem studies,[1,2] the first intraoperative catheter-based coronary artery dilatation in a human was performed by Andreas Grüntzig, native of Dresden, Germany, in St. Mary's Hospital in San Francisco in 1976.[3] Subsequently, the first coronary intervention in a catheterization laboratory was performed by Grüntzig at the University Hospital Zürich, Switzerland, on September 16, 1977. The second procedure was also performed by Grüntzig, assisted by Martin Kaltenbach, at the University Hospital in Frankfurt am Main, Germany, on October 18, 1977, with the third and fourth procedures performed in Zürich and Frankfurt, respectively.[4] Surgical stand-by on these procedures was provided by Ake Senning in Zürich and Peter Satter in Frankfurt am Main.

These first European experiences using the new technique of percutaneous transluminal coronary angioplasty (PTCA) were soon followed by procedures performed in the United States by Richard Myler at St. Mary's Hospital, San Francisco, and Simon Stertzer at Lenox Hill Hospital, New York City. Between September 1977 and March 1980, a total of 377 PTCA interventions were reported (131 in Zürich, 67 in Frankfurt, 94 in San Francisco, and 85 in New York).[5] By 1982 four institutions reported >300 cases (Zürich-Atlanta, Frankfurt am Main, San Francisco, and New York City).[6]

The first PTCA procedures were performed using 8F or 9F sheath and guiding catheter systems. Balloon catheters had a shaft diameter ranging from 0.5 to 1.25 mm (2F to 4F) and had

---

*Coauthor: Principles of percutaneous coronary interventions

two lumina, one for contrast media injections and one for balloon inflation. Inflatable polyvinyl chloride (PVC) balloons ranged in size from 3.0 × 10 mm to 3.8 × 10 mm and were attached to the distal end of the catheter shaft. At the distal end of the shaft a short wire was attached for steering. The coronary artery was typically dilated at 5-bar pressures for 15 to 20 seconds. Because steering was difficult, stenoses of the left main and proximal coronary segments were dilated.[7,8] These "fixed balloon" systems were manufactured by Schneider Meditang AG in Zürich at a rate of five sterile balloon catheters per week in 1977.[9]

PTCA got off to a slow start and met mistrust and skepticism. However, following Grüntzig's transfer to the University of Atlanta, in September 1980, and important improvements in technology, PTCA entered mainstream cardiology and has proceeded to achieve the unprecedented success that we witness today.[10] Several important milestones and technical improvements shall be reviewed in this context.

In 1980 a movable 175-cm-long guidewire was introduced by John Simpson and Edward Robert at Stanford University that allowed better steering of the dilatation system, a technique later called balloon over the wire (OTW).[11] Thus, the next generation of dilatation balloon catheters was manufactured using the coaxial double-lumen (Advanced Cardiovascular Systems, ACS) or eccentric guidewire lumen design (Schneider Meditang and United States Catheter and Instrument, Inc., USCI). The extra-long (300 cm) guidewire technique ("long wire") introduced by Martin Kaltenbach in 1984 allowed exchange of dilatation balloon catheters without recrossing the target lesion.[12] In 1986, extension ("docking") wires that could be attached to the distal end of regular-length guidewires became available. Greater safety and the possibility of multiple balloon exchanges during the procedure markedly improved the use of PTCA, allowing more complete treatments of a greater number of lesions. A major extension of PTCA techniques followed the introduction of dilatation balloon catheters with a short guidewire lumen limited to the distal tip. Use of this monorail or rapid-exchange system (designed by Tasilo Bonzel, University Freiburg/Breisgau[13]) made possible multiple rapid balloon exchanges using regular-length guidewires, which markedly accelerated the time required to perform coronary interventions.

Perhaps the most significant event in the short but eventful history of PTCA was the introduction of coronary stents by the groups led by Ulrich Sigwart[14] and Joel Puel[15] in 1987. Coronary stent implantation primarily employed as a "bailout" in selected patients after unsuccessful PTCA has drastically changed the basic approach to catheter-based coronary therapy in the course of less than two decades. Stenting has led to a reduction in restenosis rates; an improved clinical outcome, and the greater safety of endocoronary interventions, which in turn have recently opened up a new era in pharmacotherapy[16] and stent technology; the use of bioabsorbable materials[17] promises to rapidly transform mechanical endovascular "plumbing" into biological vessel repair. However, it is important to remember that the wide clinical acceptance of intracoronary stenting only became possible after the thrombotic and bleeding complications have been brought under control through the use of powerful ADP receptor and GPIIb/IIIa receptor inhibitors (for review, see references 18 and 19).

In addition to conventional "plain old balloon angioplasty" (POBA) and stent-supported PTCA, several other techniques of coronary artery revascularization have been introduced into clinical practice. In 1985 John Simpson, of Stanford University, introduced directional coronary atherectomy (DCA) to permit debulking of protruding components of atherosclerotic plaques.[20] In 1987 another debulking technique, high-speed rotational atherectomy, was introduced by Kenneth Kensey and John Nash, from the Michael Reese Hospital in Chicago.[21] Excimer laser coronary atherectomy (ELCA), which allows partial plaque removal and modification by evaporation of soft tissue components, was introduced in 1989 by Frank Litvack, from Cedars-Sinai Medical Center, Los Angeles.[22] Finally, the introduction of intracoronary radiation therapy (brachytherapy) represented an important step toward efficacious treatment of coronary restenotic lesions.[23]

This brief review of memorable developments in endocoronary therapy would remain incomplete without several important milestones in acute coronary revascularization therapy being mentioned. The use of selective intracoronary fibrinolysis was introduced into broad clinical practice by the group led by Peter Rentrop, University of Göttingen.[24] The subsequent systemic application was introduced by Rolf Schröder and his group at the Free University of Berlin in the early 1980s.[25]

PRINCIPLES OF PERCUTANEOUS CORONARY INTERVENTIONS

Atherosclerosis is considered a complex biological response, primarily inflammatory in nature, of the vessel wall and blood constituents to vessel wall injury ("response-to-injury" hypothesis).[26] Following decades of study, proposals have been made for the temporal evolution, classification, and nomenclature of atherosclerotic lesions.[27–29] Similarly, many of the biological events leading to the progression and rupture of atherosclerotic plaque have been elucidated (for review, see Chapter 1). In itself remarkable and noteworthy is the long and arduous path necessary to turn an initial observation of the cause-and-effect relationships between thrombus and myocardial infarction[30] and between thrombus and plaque rupture taking multiple stages[31–35] into clinically accepted facts[36] and design of causal therapy.[24,25] Whereas pharmacotherapy primarily aims at removing the last link in a long chain of events, that is, thrombosis and thrombus formation and more recently plaque pacification, the goal of angioplasty and other catheter-based techniques is the removal or modification of hemodynamically relevant and unstable atherosclerotic lesions. The principle behind angioplasty is the acute mechanical stretch and subsequent biological remodeling of the vessel wall.

MECHANICAL RESPONSE OF CORONARY ARTERY LESIONS: GEOMETRY, BOUNDARY CONDITIONS, AND MATERIAL PROPERTIES

Predicting the mechanical response of any material subject to external forces requires a full understanding of three fundamental elements: (i) the *geometry* of the material, (ii) the *boundary conditions*, which include not only the forces applied, but also the other constraints on the material, and (iii) the *mechanical properties* of the material. This is also true for predicting or understanding the response of an atherosclerotic lesion subject to balloon inflation during angioplasty. A discussion of how each of these elements influences the deformations of a body will be useful before specific topics regarding lesion deformation are examined.

Although the geometry of lesions may be the most accessible of the three elements required to predict mechanical behavior, it is by no means easy to determine. Histological reconstruction of an atherosclerotic lesion is useful for continued research on the mechanical effects of angioplasty, but is of little immediate use to the patient. Although a technique such as intravascular ultrasound (IVUS) provides potentially useful images of an atherosclerotic lesion, the use of ultrasound to determine an exact geometry and tissue composition (for example, the thickness of a calcified lesion) requires knowledge of the material properties related to ultrasound backscatter, the speed of sound in the different materials, and the boundary-wave reflection and transmission characteristics (which depend on the acoustic impedance of the different materials). If the plaque contains two or more distinct tissues (i.e., if it is partly fibrotic and partly calcified), then the reconstructed ultrasonic image may not show the exact geometry (and thus not lead to a correct judgment) if the ultrasound properties of the materials are not known.

To illustrate the role that geometry plays in a material's response to externally applied loads, consider the simple analogy of a soft substance sandwiched between two harder plates, such as jam or jelly between two crackers. If the jam layer is thin and the crackers practically touch, then the sandwich responds almost like two crackers alone. If the jam layer is thick, then the sandwich initially responds almost as jam alone and the jam is extruded as the crackers are pushed together. Thus, without knowing the exact geometry and tissue composition of the lesion, the prediction of the material's (i.e., the lesion's) response to loading will likely be invalid.

Because plaque is generally irregularly shaped and it is irregularly embedded within the underlying vessel wall, the forces applied by a smooth dilatation balloon will be irregularly distributed and highly complex. In some engineering systems, simplified models of applied forces and geometry can lead to usable designs or solutions, often "averaging out" the effects of material inconsistencies and irregular geometries and forces. In such cases, however, local effects of the irregularities do not greatly influence the overall behavior of the material. In the case of atherosclerotic lesions, however, it is likely that local geometric effects play an important role in determining how and when a lesion will rupture.[37,38] Because understanding the detailed (local) response of the plaque is essential for determining how the plaque will respond, researchers such as Holzapfel et al.[39–41] use intricate numerical simulations, such as the finite-element method, to investigate plaque responses at the local level.

The finite-element method (FEM, also known as finite-element analysis or FEA) is a powerful numerical technique for predicting stress and strains in a body under a system of loads (in fact, FEM can also be used for many applications, including fluid flow and magnetic fields). The method is based on representing an irregularly shaped body (such as an atherosclerotic plaque) by a network (called a "mesh" or "grid") of regularly shaped "elements," usually rectangles or triangles (Fig. 8-1).

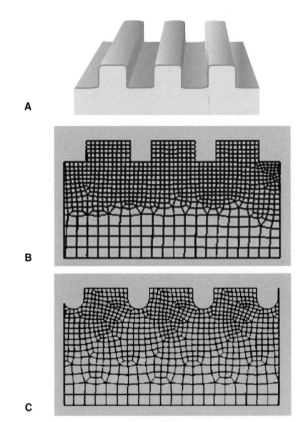

FIGURE 8-1.   Examples of finite elements. **A:** 3D rendering of simple square channels in a material. **B:** Head-on view of the same material, broken into many discrete elements (the finite element "mesh" or "grid"). **C:** Channels with a different cross section, showing a different finite element.

Both two-dimensional and three-dimensional analyses are applied to many problems. For an FEM analysis, the geometry of a lesion may be obtained from histological sections. The full three-dimensional geometry can be reconstructed from sequential histological slices. Equations for stress and strain are solved on an element-by-element basis, and then the stress and strain fields, which provide the prediction of the material's response to loading, are reconstructed for the entire body. Although FEM is invaluable for analysis, it remains only a *model* of the physical system. Its usefulness as a predictive tool depends on its accuracy in reproducing the geometry, boundary conditions, and material properties of the object being analyzed. To properly interpret FEM results, and thus obtain useful information, it is essential that FEM users, especially when studying complex systems such as biological tissues, understand the limitations of the method and interpret the results accordingly. For any model to be treated as a "black box," where the results are taken as absolute fact without users having an understanding of the limitations of the model, can lead to erroneous and even dangerous conclusions.

In the case of balloon angioplasty, forces are imparted to the lesion by the balloon catheter. Balloon catheters are designed to open up or to dilate occluded or stenotic vascular segments. Inflating small longitudinal balloons filled with fluid—a mixture of normal saline and contrast media—under high pressure generates radial forces that are exerted onto the vessel walls, causing expansion of the dilated segment associated with loosening of the vessel wall architecture, limited tears of the subintimal layers, and mainly longitudinal plaque redistribution.

Boundary conditions include all of the forces applied to a material or structure, and all constraints on the material's deformation. Consider, for example, a heavy box placed in the center of a round table. The table is subject to a force—a distributed load—at each point where the box contacts the table and the center of the table sags toward the ground. The legs of the table are presumably in contact with the floor, which prevents the table legs from moving further toward the ground. In engineering terms we may say that the vertical displacement of the table legs is zero. In this illustration, there are examples of both load and displacement boundary conditions (the effect of the contact of the mass of the box, and the effect of the contact of the table legs with the floor, respectively). It becomes much more difficult to predict how much the table would sag if there were different springs or flooring types under each table leg, or if the loads on the table top were uneven and not centered on the table.

A balloon catheter is fairly symmetric and cylindrical when inflated. The radial force applied to the vessel (lesion) wall, at a first approximation, is similar to an internal pressure acting on the vessel wall. An internal pressure, however, is uniform at every point and acts perpendicular to the surface; the forces imparted by the balloon to the vessel wall are, in contrast, probably not uniform because of the irregular contact surface and heterogeneous composition of the lesions.

The lesion sits on or is embedded in the underlying vessel wall. The vessel wall thus constrains the movement or deformation of the lesion, but since it itself is *not* rigid, it will deform under loads. In this case, the mechanical properties of the underlying vessel will define a boundary condition on the lesion. If the vessel is included explicitly in an analysis, then the geometry and material properties of the vessel must be known. The tissue surrounding the vessel is then the source of the boundary condition(s). If the vessel is in contact with or embedded in muscle tissue, for example, then the boundary conditions, and hence the vessel response to loads, will change depending on whether the muscle is relaxed or contracted.

A further complexity of enormous import that may be included in the discussion of boundary conditions is the way that different tissue types in a diseased vessel—plaque cap, underlying lesion, modified media, vessel, for example—are connected. The *interfaces* between the materials and the manner in which those interfaces behave will have a pivotal influence on plaque response. The influence is especially obvious when plaque dissection, or "lift-off" from the vessel wall, is considered. Little is known of the behavior of lesion material interfaces, and this knowledge is essential for understanding critical responses of lesions as well as a lesion's vulnerability to rupture or dissection.

Even sophisticated state-of-the-art computer analyses of the responses of atherosclerotic lesions to the forces of balloon angioplasty are limited by the extent to which the material properties of the lesions and underlying vessel walls are known. Without knowledge of the material properties, accurately predicting lesion response is impossible even if the geometry is known precisely. We gain little if we know the exact thickness of the jam in the previous example, but assume or believe that it behaves like hard cheese. Few investigators have accepted the challenges of studying the mechanical properties of atherosclerotic lesions.[42,43] Experimental studies to date show that most lesions share some general characteristics: for example, the mechanical responses are nonlinear and exhibit hysteresis (Fig. 8-2), that is, they behave differently when loading and unloading. It is also clear that detailed responses are lesion specific. The studies also concluded that relatively little is known about the mechanical properties and that much additional work is necessary to develop an understanding of lesions' responses.

There are, of course, many limitations inherent in determining the material properties of biological tissue. Since material properties must be determined by mechanical testing, the mechanical testing of lesion response to forces is performed primarily on dissected vessels and lesions. The ex vivo specimens are usually removed from their natural loading environment (the pulsatile blood flow) for several hours to perhaps nearly 2 days before testing. It is well documented that healthy blood vessels undergo a "relaxation" when they are removed from their loading environment. Researchers usually perform a series of loading-unloading cycles, called "preconditioning," to return the specimens, in theory, to their physiological state. The specimens are subject to a number of loading-unloading cycles sufficient to demonstrate that the mechanical response repeats from one cycle to the next, and are then considered preconditioned. A critical assumption, however, is that the vessels have been returned to their physiological state since that state is unknown.

An example of an investigation of plaque's mechanical properties is found in a series of studies by Topoleski, Salunke, Humphrey, and Mergner.[44,45] Isolated plaques from diseased arteries were dissected and tested in tension and unconfined compression. The specimens were subjected to 15 loading-unloading cycles (preconditioned), allowed to rest for 15 minutes, and then subjected to another 15 loading-unloading cycles. The relationship between the responses to the first loading protocol and those to the second proved to be a function of the type of lesion (atheromatous, fibrous, or calcified) (Fig. 8-2). More recently, Holzapfel et al.[43] performed tensile tests on isolated components of diseased vessels (plaque cap, intima, media, adventitia) to investigate their mechanical properties. Their results further underscore the highly complex character of the mechanical response of a diseased artery. It remains imperative to develop an understanding of the mechanical properties and responses of atherosclerotic tissue.

Isolating lesions for mechanical testing may provide insights into the local behavior of the lesions, but in vivo the lesions are usually intimately entwined with the underlying vessel tissue. Today there is no way to accurately predict or understand the interaction between the lesion and underlying tissue, and therefore no way to predict the response of the lesion-tissue system to the forces imparted by balloon angioplasty. Nonetheless, it is essential to understand the behavior of isolated lesions and tissue segments as a first step toward understanding the response of lesions in the context of diseased vessels with different pathologies.

The geometry, boundary conditions, and material properties interact to produce a unique stress state in a lesion. Only by understanding the detailed contributions of each can we truly understand how a specific lesion will respond to forces applied during angioplasty. A generalized model of lesion

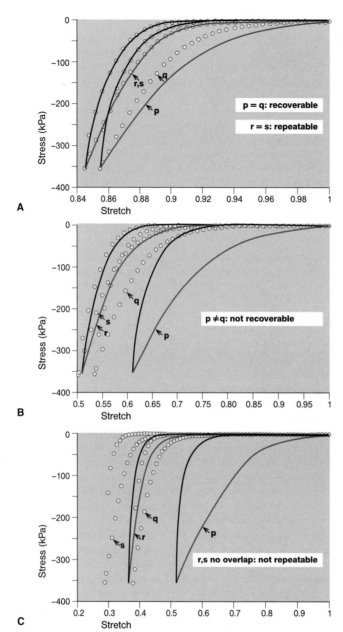

FIGURE 8-2. Ex vivo studies of mechanical properties of atherosclerotic plaques with different tissue composition. In this series of experiments, dissected plaques were subjected to 15 cycles of radial compressive loading (phase I), and then allowed to "rest" for 10 min. The specimen was subjected to a second set of 15 cycles (phase II). In each figure, only the first and 15th cycle for each phase are presented for clarity. In each case, the specimens were classified by mechanical behavior before histological analysis. Curve **p** is the first loading cycle of the first phase, and **r** is the 15th loading cycle of the first phase; curve **q** is the first loading cycle of the second phase, and **s** is the 15th loading cycle of the second phase. **A:** Curves **p** and **q** are very close on loading and overlap during unloading. This behavior was termed "recoverable," indicating the specimen's apparent recovery to its initial state (i.e., from curve **r** to curve **q**) during the rest period. Also, curves **r** and **s** overlap (the 15th cycles for each phase), which was termed "repeatable," indicating that the stress-stretch behavior was consistent (or had reached a state of equilibrium) for each phase by the time the 15th cycle was reached. **B:** **p** and **q** do not overlap, hence the specimen did not recover during the rest period; however, curves **r** and **s** overlap, indicating that although the specimen did not recover, the behavior apparently reached the same state of equilibrium by the 15th cycle for both phases. **C:** Neither **p** and **q**, nor **r** and **s** showed any relationship, indicating that the specimen neither recovered nor reached a state of equilibrium after 15 cycles. Histological analysis showed that the behavior represented in **A** was associated with calcified plaques. The calcification may have contributed an elastic component to the material that allowed the recovery. The behavior in **B** was associated with fibrous plaques. The first loading phase apparently compressed the plaque beyond its ability to recover in the experimental time frame, but the plaque reached a state of equilibrium. The behavior in **C** was associated with atheromatous plaques. It is possible that material from the viscous or liquid core was forced out of the fibrous tissue network during the entire test, and thus the plaques neither recovered nor reached a state of equilibrium.

behavior, however, can be described in a relatively straightforward manner.

As a result of the forces applied by the balloon catheter, the lesion and vessel wall undergo radial compression, which generally acts to compress the lesion and wall thickness. In addition to compressing the vessel wall, the forces exerted by the dilatation balloon tend to expand the vessel diameter, creating circumferential tension (or "hoop stresses") in the vessel wall. By expanding a relatively small length of a vessel, defined by the length of the balloon, longitudinal tension is also generated, especially near the shoulders of the balloon catheter. Movement of the balloon during inflation may also result in shear forces being applied to the lesion (vessel) wall surface. Even this simple analysis describes a complex, multifaceted loading of the vessel wall from a balloon catheter, resulting in complex stresses and deformations, or strains, in the expanded vessel (for example, see reference 46).

The goal of angioplasty is to create a permanent deformation (leading to an expanded lumen) of either the vessel wall or the atherosclerotic lesion, or both, without producing collapse of the wall.

Regardless of the complexity of the deformations, they are reversed if the deformations are "elastic." Permanent (or "nonelastic") deformations, such as fracture or rupture of the lesion, or permanent deformations from other mechanisms, are necessary for the shape of the lumen to change. Mechanisms that are responsible for permanent deformations, and hence the open lumen, are not well understood. For example, microcracking of a calcified lesion is a possible mechanism for permanent deformation (this may be analogous to bending a "green" twig from a tree: the twig will develop cracks and remain bent, but will not snap apart like a dried twig). "Overstretching" of the plaque or the vessel wall is another way of saying "nonelastic" or permanent deformations. The local mechanisms by which overstretching keeps the lumen of a vessel open are not known: This is in contrast to the mechanisms for plastic deformation of a metal, for example. Knowledge of the plastic deformation mechanisms in metals has allowed materials scientists and engineers to use those mechanisms advantageously to design better materials for specific applications. A better understanding of the mechanisms by which an occluded blood vessel retains an expanded lumen following dilation would probably lead to techniques for improving the outcomes of angioplasty.

If the lumen stays open by creating nonelastic deformations, *residual stresses* are developed within the material. Neither the extent nor the location of the residual stresses is known, nor how they may affect the subsequent (long-term) response and any possible reocclusion of the vessel.

Furthermore, even though the forces applied to the lesion or vessel wall through the balloon catheter are ostensibly radially compressive, the response of the lesion may not be compressive. For example, a theory of mechanics known as "beam on elastic foundation" predicts the behavior of one material (the "beam") as it undergoes externally applied loading while it sits on another material (the "elastic foundation") (see for example the treatment by Haslach and Armstrong[47]) Although beam on elastic foundation may not be a completely accurate model of the lesion-vessel wall system, the theory illustrates an important result that we may not overlook. Under certain combinations of geometry, boundary conditions, and compressive loading, parts

of the beam (the lesion) will, in fact, tend to lift away from the underlying vessel wall (Fig. 8-3). Consider again the analogy of a green twig: If someone steps on a green twig lying, for example, on concrete, then the concrete fully supports the twig and nothing much happens. The twig may not even respond or deform. In contrast, if the twig is lying on compliant soil, then stepping on the center of the twig can cause the ends of the twig to lift off the ground. Similarly, if the ends of a lesion are pulled away from the underlying vessel wall, then the result might be further rupture or perhaps thrombosis in the resulting fissure. Thus, if we apply the beam on elastic foundation theory, it is vital for us to understand how the relationship between the size of the lesion and the size of the balloon (the balloon "coverage") can affect the response of specific lesions in specific vessels.

In current clinical practice, a stent is generally deployed at the site of the occlusion after balloon expansion. A stent acts as a permanent mechanical barrier to the potential elastic "recoil" of the open lumen, regardless of whether the recoil originates in the plaque or the underlying vessel. The stent is essentially a "retaining wall" to keep the lumen in place. It in fact creates new boundary conditions on the lesion. The mechanics following stent placement are also not well understood, although it is clear that residual stresses are present, probably in both the plaque and the underlying vessel. The stents are subject to the same cyclic loading as the lumen (pulsatile loads) and may be subject to fatigue failure in the long term.

Through mechanical intervention, it is possible to change the geometry of the lesion, reopening the lumen for improved blood flow. Given our current knowledge base, however, the complex geometry, boundary conditions, and material properties of a diseased vessel make it practically impossible to make detailed predictions of vessel responses. Once these elements

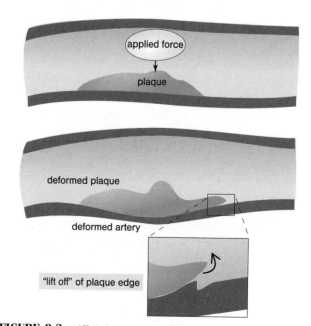

FIGURE 8-3. (*Top*) A concentrated force applied to an irregularly shaped plaque. The deformations would be analogous for a more distributed load, for example, from the surface of a balloon. (*Bottom*) The loaded configuration (deformation). (*Inset*) How the ends of the dissimilar materials—plaque and vessel wall—may tend to separate.

are known, however, we must still create clinical protocols to specifically target and activate mechanisms that will keep the lumen open, and not activate those that are potentially harmful, such as changes in lesion geometry that could lead to renarrowing and thrombus formation.

MECHANICAL EFFECTS OF ANGIOPLASTY

The local changes in tissue response that lead to permanent deformations, and hence successful angioplasty, are a specific subset of the lesion's material properties. In engineering materials, for example, the yield stress of a material marks the onset of permanent deformation; it is a property specific to each material that must be determined experimentally.

Grüntzig assumed plaque compression to be the principle mechanism of coronary angioplasty ("footprints in the snow"). Although initial studies performed by Kaltenbach at the Mayo Clinic in 1978 seemed to confirm this hypothesis,[48] later studies showed that the stretching of the vessel wall associated with plaque rupture and plaque redistribution are the main mechanisms of stenosis dilatation.[49,50] The combination of focal plaque rupture, wall dissection, and radial and longitudinal wall stretch has been documented as being an important sequelae of angioplasty in both native coronary arteries and venous coronary bypass vessels.[51-53] Plaque compression and distal embolization of plaque components were considered less important components of dilatation. Unwanted results of coronary artery dilatation associated with angioplasty include complete destruction of the vessel wall architecture, extensive dissections, thrombus formation, vessel closure, and perforation. Successful angioplasty activates those mechanisms that retain the open lumen while avoiding the detrimental results.

It is poorly understood how the expansion of the balloon is translated into stresses and strains in the tissue, how much a specific tissue deforms, and whether the deformation is permanent or transient. Despite the need for more extensive and detailed research, some basic and general concepts can be developed from simple analyses. As a starting point, the principal stresses developed in the vessel wall may be calculated using a simplification of Laplace's equation for circumferential (hoop) σ_θ, radial σ_r, and longitudinal (axial) σ_l stresses:

$$\sigma_\theta = pd/2t \tag{1a}$$

$$\sigma_l = pd/4t \tag{1b}$$

$$\sigma_r = p \tag{1c}$$

where p is the internal pressure acting on the vessel wall, d is the mean diameter of the vessel, and t is the mean thickness of the vessel wall. According to the equations, both the radial and the hoop stresses are greater than the longitudinal stress. If the balloon is just at its full extension and is pressing uniformly against the vessel wall (i.e., applying uniform pressure to the vessel wall), then we can estimate the stresses in the vessel by

$$\sigma_\theta^* = p_b d_b/2t \tag{2a}$$

$$\sigma_l^* = p_b d_b/4t \tag{2b}$$

$$\sigma_r^* = p_b \tag{2c}$$

where p_b and d_b are the balloon inflation pressure (N/cm^2) and the balloon diameter at the balloon inflation pressure

p_b (cm), respectively. However, these relationships will hold only if the internal pressure in the balloon and the balloon diameter are good approximations of the pressure on the vessel wall and the diameter of the vessel. Since the balloon is opening an obstructed or occluded vessel and its size is adjusted to the nominal size of the adjacent nonstenotic coronary artery segment, allowing reasonably accurate matching between balloon and vessel diameters, the pressure-diameter relationship is likely to remain approximately linear. However, the pressure-diameter relationship within the balloon may become nonlinear because of significant deformations of the inflated, not fully noncompliant balloons, such as in rigid, highly irregular stenoses. When the pressure-diameter relationship is nonlinear, the pressure in the balloon p_b may not be a good approximation of the pressure on the vessel wall.

Several important conditions must be met for Equations 1 and 2 to apply to angioplasty. First, the material under pressure (i.e., the blood vessel wall with or without plaque) must be linear, homogeneous, elastic, and isotropic. Note that here, in engineering terms, the meaning of *elastic* is not that commonly understood in the medical literature. *Elastic* means that material will return to its original state once the load that causes a deformity—for example, an artery stretched by internal pressure—is removed; it does not necessarily mean that the material is "stretchy" (extensible) or rubbery. *Homogeneous* means that the mechanical properties and the mechanical response to applied forces are the same everywhere in the material. If the nature of the material changes, for example, the composition changes from area to area, then the material is likely not to be homogeneous (described as "inhomogeneous"). *Isotropic* means that the material properties as well as the mechanical response to applied forces are the same regardless of the direction in which the forces are applied. Materials with preferred fiber orientations, for example, have different material properties in different directions (e.g., along the fiber direction vs. perpendicular to the fiber direction), and are therefore not isotropic (described as "anisotropic"). In fact, blood vessels are not linear, homogeneous, or isotropic; consequently, Equations 1 and 2 give only a very rough, first-order estimate of the stresses in the blood vessel.

Another complication is that Equations 1 and 2 hold only for what is termed a "thin-walled" cylinder, where the thickness is at most 10% of the vessel radius. The equations assume that the stresses are uniform throughout the vessel wall, which is only true when the wall is thin and homogeneous (in fact, the stresses may begin to vary when the wall is as little as 3% to 5% of the radius).

If the vessel wall is "thick," that is, >10% of the luminal radius, as is the case in many blood vessels, then a different theory is used to predict the stresses:

$$\sigma_r^t = \frac{a^2 p_i}{b^2 - a^2}\left(1 - \frac{b^2}{r^2}\right) \tag{3a}$$

$$\sigma_\theta^t = \frac{a^2 p_i}{b^2 - a^2}\left(1 + \frac{b^2}{r^2}\right) \tag{3b}$$

where a and b are the inner radius and outer radius of the vessel, respectively, p_i is the internal pressure (assuming there is only internal pressure acting on the vessel), and r is the radius of interest within the vessel wall (e.g., at the center of the vessel wall, $r = a + (b - a)/2$).

Both sets of equations were originally derived for a cylinder made of an engineering material, such as a metal, under internal pressure. The strains, or deformations, of such pressurized cylinders are very small. For the equations to be accurate, the strains must be small, for which "small" means less than a 10% change. Because the deformations of a blood vessel, either under blood pressure or during balloon angioplasty, may not be small, the equations have limited predictive power.

The system of a vessel wall and an atherosclerotic lesion is certainly nonelastic, inhomogeneous, and anisotropic. In addition, the irregular geometry of the occluded vessel results in complex loading over the lesion surface. Given the irregular geometry, the complicated system of applied loads, and the complex nature of the material properties, understanding the lesion's response to the balloon angioplasty procedure, and the mechanisms of permanent deformation that are activated during it, is a formidable problem. This prompted modern biomechanical studies of stresses in blood vessels. One of the first and widely applicable theories was developed by Fung et al. in 1979.[54] The complex treatment of stresses in nondiseased vessels is well summarized by Humphrey.[55] More recent, and more involved, theories of stresses in nondiseased vessels are found, for example, in Gleason et al.[56] and Haslach.[57]

The limitations of the pressure vessel theory can be illustrated by a relevant example. Based on the thick-walled model, overstretching the vessel by 10% of its diameter is associated with an increase in circumferential stress of approximately 10%. Based on the more advanced and physiologically reasonable model by Fung et al.,[54] the same increase of 10% in diameter can result in a 23% increase in stress.[1] Further overextension, to 30% of vessel diameter, for example, results in a 30% stress increase based on the thick-walled model but in 116% increase according to the model of Fung et al. Neither model takes into account the irregularities of an atherosclerotic lesion; the models both assume that the vessel is not diseased. The presence of disease complicates calculations of the stress and strains in the lesion and the vessel. It must be emphasized that increasing the balloon pressure, regardless of the model used, increases the associated stresses, markedly increasing the risk of rupture. It is important that investigations of balloon induced stresses be continued in order to reduce the potential for plaque rupture. Furthermore, and perhaps more pertinent to angioplasty, none of the models discussed is able to predict the stress at which a permanent deformation mechanism is activated.

Following balloon deflation, the plastic and elastic forces within the coronary artery wall—antagonistic by their very nature—become operative. Lesion or vessel material that has plastically deformed remains in the deformed shape. In contrast, adjacent material that has only been elastically deformed, and which would return to its original shape in the absence of any constraint, is prevented from doing so. Thus, new *residual stresses* are created within the lesion and the vessel.

---

[1]Even a summary treatment of more advanced and realistic models of arterial behavior is beyond the scope of this chapter. It is important to note that the calculations of Fung's model, or any of the other models, must be based on physically measured parameters, which are difficult to obtain in their own right.

The consequences of such induced residual stresses in the diseased vessel are not known. They may include initiating or mediating biological responses, such as remodeling of the vessel wall or endothelial cell proliferation, and long-term mechanical responses, such as rendering the lesion susceptible to future rupture caused by lesion fatigue under applied pulsatile loads.

MECHANICAL EFFECTS OF STENT IMPLANTATION

The inflation of balloons with crimped stents—in contrast to conventional balloons—causes the vessel walls to become permanently distended at the stented segments. Neglecting a certain amount of elastic recoil allowed by the stent, the forces exerted against the walls remain operative until termination of the vessel's remodeling process. At the edges of the stent, there is a sharp change in the stresses affecting the vessel, causing a major redistribution of stresses between the stented and nonstented adjacent segments. In many engineering systems, areas of high stress gradients (where the stress changes quickly over small distances) sometimes result in *stress concentrations* and are vulnerable to failure or unwanted deformations. Such stress concentrations may cause the proliferation of endothelial cells observed in some stented vessels at the transition points. However, the relationships between the stresses on the vessel and the biological responses are not known.

BIOLOGICAL EFFECTS OF ANGIOPLASTY AND STENT IMPLANTATION

Arterial vessel wall remodeling is a result of biological adaptation at atherosclerotic plaque sites.[58] Based on morphometric measurements, three basic responses to an increasing plaque burden can be distinguished: expansion, lack of change, and shrinkage, corresponding to positive, absent, and negative remodeling, respectively. Using IVUS, the remodeling ratio (RR) is defined as the ratio of the external elastic membrane (EEM) area at the lesion site to the EEM area at a defined proximal reference site.[59] Positive remodeling of the culprit lesions' sites is associated with unstable coronary presentation[60] and has been observed more frequently in fibrofatty lesions.[61] Following angioplasty, serial IVUS data show a healing defect associated with positive, intermediate, or negative remodeling. Dilatation sites with the largest initial gain showed a greater propensity for restenosis on follow-up at 1 to 6 months.[62] Implantation of a bare metal stent (BMS) effectively prevents remodeling at the implantation sites but it does not fully prevent an in-stent restenosis due to myointimal hyperplasia. Positive peri-BMS remodeling appears to be associated with a lower incidence of in-stent restenosis (see reference 63; for review, see Chapter 1).

PERCUTANEOUS CORONARY INTERVENTIONS

Percutaneous coronary intervention (PCI) represents first-line emergency treatment in patients with ST segment-elevation myocardial infarction who present early (up to 12 to 24 hours) following the onset of symptoms and in the majority of patients with non-ST segment-elevation myocardial infarction. Furthermore, elective PCI represents an important therapy option in patients with chronic coronary artery syndromes. In the subsequent sections, selected principal issues relevant to the clinical practice of PCI will be reviewed. However, a fully comprehensive review of the available literature neither has been intended nor will be provided.

RELEVANCE

Since their introduction in 1977 and 1987, respectively, percutaneous transluminal coronary angioplasty (PTCA), also termed in colloquial usage *plain old balloon angioplasty* (POBA),[3,4] and stent-supported angioplasty, also termed in a broader sense *percutaneous coronary intervention* (PCI),[14,15] have become increasingly important strategies in routine management of patients with acute and chronic syndromes of coronary artery disease (CAD). Although representative figures of the number of procedures performed are difficult to obtain, a few selected examples easily illustrate the astounding proliferation of catheter-based CAD treatments in Western countries (Tables 8-1 and 8-2, Figures 8-4 to 8-6).[64,65] However, the absolute number of procedures performed in the West is likely to appear modest when compared with future data from the new rapidly growing economies of China and India.

EVIDENCE

The efficacy of coronary artery bypass graft surgery (CABG)[66] and its superiority over medical treatment in patients with CAD have been documented (for review, see references 67 and 68). Figures 8-7 and 8-8 show the overall benefits of CABG surgery and those derived by selected subgroups of patients.

Similarly, the efficacy and superiority of PTCA[3,4] over medical treatment in patients with CAD has been demonstrated in terms of relieving angina and improved quality of life (for review, see reference 69). Comparisons of PTCA and CABG during the present era showed no statistical difference in mortality and combined cardiac outcomes (cardiac death and nonfatal myocardial infarction). However, patients randomized to CABG were less likely to experience postprocedural symptoms and were less likely to require subsequent revascularization (Table 8-3).[67] Among subgroups, PTCA was superior to CABG in patients with single-vessel and two-vessel disease without high-grade ($\geq$95%) left anterior descending (LAD) disease. In patients with three-vessel and patients with two-vessel disease and $\geq$95% LAD disease, CABG was superior as shown in Figure 8-9 (for review, see reference 67).

Comparisons between bare metal stent, BMS-supported angioplasty and CABG disclosed trends similar to those observed in PTCA and CABG studies; however the gap in prevention of reinterventions on follow-up and total event rates has narrowed (Table 8-4).[67] Results of the more recent Arterial Revascularization Therapies Study (ARTS) randomized trials

TABLE 8-1. Estimated Number of Percutaneous Transluminal Coronary Angioplasty (PTCA) Procedures Performed in the United States 1995–2000

Year	1995	1996	1997	1998	1999	2000
Numbers	434,000	666,000	686,363	925,500	1,069,302	1,024,875

Source: http://www.tdrdata.com/IPD/IPD_Samples_Procedure.asp.

TABLE 8-2. German Registry of Percutaneous Coronary Interventions (PCI) 1984–2002

Year	Number of PCIs Reported	Annual Relative Increase (%)
GERMANY, WEST		
1984	2,809	
1985	4,491	+ 59.9
1986	7,999	+ 78.1
1987	12,083	+ 51.1
1988	16,923	+ 40.0
1989	23,360	+ 38.0
1990	32,459	+ 39.0
GERMANY, UNIFIED		
1991	44,528	
1992	56,267	+ 26.4
1993	69,804	+ 24.0
1994	88,380	+ 26.6
1995	109,669	+ 11.5
1996	125,840	+ 8.0
1997	135,925	+ 12.7
1998	153,257	+ 8.4
1999	166,132	+ 8.5
2000	180,336	+ 8.3
2001	195,280	+ 6.6
2002	208,178	+ 6.6
2003	221,867	+ 6.6
2004	248,909	+ 11.2

Modified from van Buuren F, Horstkotte D. Ergebnisse der gemeinsamen Umfrage der Kommission für Klinische Kardiologie und Arbeitsgruppen Interventionelle Kardiologie (für die ESC) und Angiologie der Deutschen Gesellschaft für Kardiologie – Herz- und Kreislaufforschung über das Jahr 2004;21. Bericht über die Leistungszahlen der Herzkatheterlabore in der Bundesrepublik Deutschland. Source: http://leitlinien.dgk.org/files/Leistungszahlen2004.pdf. Accessed May 21, 2006.

showed comparable results for BMS-supported angioplasty and CABG in terms of mortality and incidence of stroke and myocardial infarction, but superiority of CABG in terms of the need of repeat revascularization and recurrence of angina on a 5-year follow-up in patients with multivessel disease (Fig. 8-10).[70] These results have been confirmed by the Argentine Randomized Study: Coronary Angioplasty with Stenting Versus Coronary Bypass Surgery (ERACI II) trial.[71]

Comparison of PTCA and BMS-supported angioplasty has shown the superiority of stenting in terms of reducing the number of major adverse cardiac events (MACE), which was higher in high-risk patients, and restenosis rates. These studies were not powerful enough, however, to determine the impact on mortality and the subgroup effects (Fig. 8-11) (for review, see reference 72).

Following the introduction drug-eluting stents (DESs), their superiority over BMS has been demonstrated in a number of trials primarily in terms of the in-stent restenosis rates (Figs. 8-12, 8-13). The superiority was not shown convincingly for mortality and nonfatal myocardial infarction (for review, see reference 72). A more recent review of the data confirms the evidence (for review, see reference 73) and suggests differences in outcome with different drug-eluting agents.[74,75]

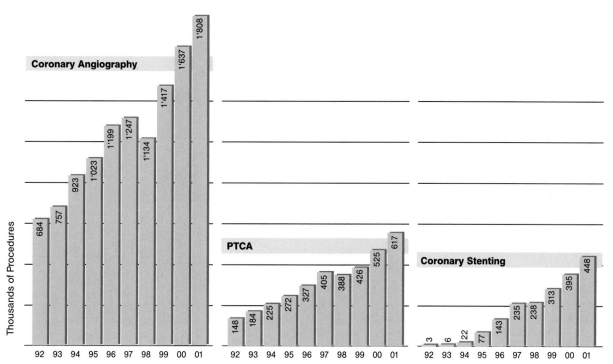

FIGURE 8-4. Coronary angiograms, percutaneous transluminal coronary angioplasty (PTCA), and coronary stenting from 1992 to 2001 in Europe in thousands of procedures. (Modified from Togni M, Balmer F, Pfiffner D, et al. Percutaneous coronary interventions in Europe 1992–2001. *Eur Heart J.* 2004;25:1208–1213.)

Trials comparing DES-supported angioplasty and CABG, such as SYNergy, SYNTAX, and ARTS II, are underway and will provide more definite evidence regarding the current state of the art interventional and surgery strategies for elective coronary artery revascularization in different patient populations.

TRAINING

Initially, the process of learning angioplasty was an informal matter of learning by doing. This corresponded to the grass-roots style of the courses organized by Grüntzig in Zürich and Atlanta in the late 1970s and early 1980s, rather than being based

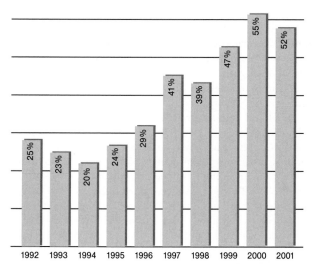

FIGURE 8-5. Ad hoc percutaneous transluminal coronary angioplasty (PTCA) from 1992 to 2001 in Europe (percent of total). (Modified from Togni M, Balmer F, Pfiffner D, et al. Percutaneous coronary interventions in Europe 1992–2001. *Eur Heart J.* 2004;25:1208–1213.)

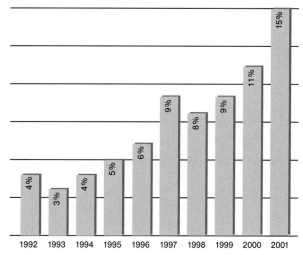

FIGURE 8-6. Percutaneous transluminal coronary angioplasty (PTCA) for acute myocardial infarction from 1992 to 2001 in Europe (percent of total). (Modified from Togni M, Balmer F, Pfiffner D, et al. Percutaneous coronary interventions in Europe 1992–2001. *Eur Heart J.* 2004;25:1208–1213.)

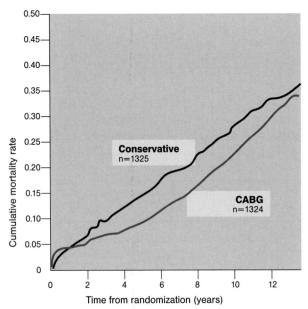

FIGURE 8-7. Cumulative mortality derived from trials comparing coronary artery bypass surgery (CABG), and medical therapy. (Modified from Yusuf S, Zucker D, Peduzzi P, et al. Effects of coronary artery bypass graft surgery on survival: overview of 10-year results from randomized trials by the Coronary Artery Bypass Graft Surgery Trialists Collaboration. *Lancet.* 1994;344:563–570.)

on theory and structured teaching. Since the mid-1980s curricula and formal training requirements have been successively introduced in angioplasty and interventional cardiology. Current fellowships in interventional cardiology typically require a minimum of 1 year of training following a formal training in cardiology. For example, in the United States the current guidelines for training in interventional cardiology stated by the American Board of Internal Medicine (ABIM)[76] include "a minimum of 250 therapeutic interventional cardiac procedures during 12 months of accredited interventional cardiology fellowship training." Trainees are required (selected excerpts) to:

- Be currently certified in cardiovascular disease by the ABIM
- Have satisfactorily completed the requisite training
- Demonstrated clinical competence in the care of patients
- Met the licensure requirements
- Passed the secure exam for that discipline
- Follow the training and practice pathways prescribed

To receive credit for performance of a therapeutic interventional cardiac procedure in the training pathway, a fellow must meet the following criteria:

- Participate in procedural planning including indications for the procedure and the selection of appropriate procedure or instruments.
- Perform critical technical manipulations of the case. (Regardless of how many manipulations are performed in any one "case," each case may count as only one procedure.)
- Be substantially involved in postprocedural management of the case.
- Be supervised by the faculty member responsible for the procedure. (Only one fellow can receive credit for each case even if others were present.)

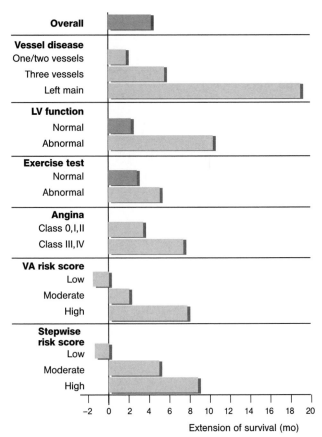

FIGURE 8-8. Survival after 10 years of follow-up after coronary artery bypass graft surgery in various subgroups of patients, from a meta-analysis of seven randomized studies. LV, left ventricular; VA, Veterans Administration. Angina class according the Canadian Cardiology Society Classification. (Modified from Yusuf S, Zucker D, Peduzzi P, et al. Effects of coronary artery bypass graft surgery on survival: overview of 10-year results from randomized trials by the Coronary Artery Bypass Graft Surgery Trialists Collaboration. *Lancet.* 1994;344:563–570.)

To attest clinical competence, "The Board requires documentation that candidates for certification are competent in (1) patient care (which includes medical interviewing, physical examination, and procedural skills), (2) medical knowledge, (3) practice-based learning and improvement, (4) interpersonal and communication skills, (5) professionalism, and (6) systems-based practice."

Recognizing the critical importance of competence and qualification, the majority of U.S. hospitals now grant privileges to interventional cardiologists on an individual basis following a detailed and extensive review and documentation of clinical skills and track record in addition to ABIM certification.

In Europe there are diverse national curricula for the interventional cardiology subspecialty, and European guidelines for interventional training have been formulated but not yet inaugurated. The European curriculum foresees 2 years of structured formal training in institutions performing a minimum of 800 procedures annually with the availability of at least two supervisors who have performed at least 1000 percutaneous coronary interventions (PCIs) and/or have a minimum of 5 years of experience dedicated to interventional cardiology. Advanced optional training includes formal training in peripheral interventional techniques.[77] Some of these concepts have been proposed in earlier communications.[78]

TABLE 8-3. Comparison of Trials: Percutaneous Transluminal Coronary Angioplasty (PTCA) versus Coronary Artery Bypass Graft (CABG)

Trial	Age/ (% ♀)	CAD	No Pat.	Death CABG/ PCI	Q-MI CABG/ PCI	AP CABG/ PCI	RR (%) CABG/ PCI	Primary End Points	Primary End Points (Total %) CABG/PCI	Follow-up (Years)
BARI	61/26	MV	1829	15.6/19.1	19.6/21.3	—	7/1	D	15.6/19.1	8
EAST	61/26	MV	392	17/21	19.6/16.6	12/20	13/54	D+MI+T	27.3/28.8	8
GABI	—/20	MV	359	6.5/2.6	9.4/4.5	26/29	6/44	A	26/29	1
Toulouse	67/23	MV	152	10.5/13.2	1.3/5.3	5.3/21.1	9/29	A	5.2/21.1	5
RITA	57/19	SV+MV	1011	3.6/3.1	5.2/6.7	21.5/31.3	4/31	D+MI	8.6/9.8	2.5
ERACI	58/13	MV	127	4.7/9.5	7.8/7.8	3.2/4.8	6/37	D+MI+A+RR	23/53	3
MASS	56/42	SV(LAD)	142	—	—	2/18	0/22	D+MI+RR	3/24	3
Lausanne	56/20	SV(LAD)	134	1.5/0	1.5/2.9	5/6	3/25	D+MI+RR	7.6/36.8	2
CABRI	60/22	MV	1054	2.7/3.9	3.5/4.9	10.1/13.9	9/36	D	2.7/3.9	1

PCI, percutaneous coronary intervention; CAD, coronary artery disease; QW, Q wave; MI, myocardial infarction; Hosp CABG, required CABG after PCI and before hospital discharge; RR, repeated revascularization; F/U, follow-up; BARI, Bypass Angioplasty Revascularization Investigation; EAST, Emory Angioplasty Surgery Trial; GABI, German Angioplasty Bypass-surgery Investigation; RITA, Randomized Intervention Treatment of Angina; ERACI, Estudio Randomizado Argentino de Angioplastia vs Cirugia; MASS, Medicine, Angioplasty, or Surgery Study; CABRI, Coronary Angioplasty versus Bypass Revascularization Investigation; SoS, the Stent or Surgery Trial; ERACI II, Coronary Angioplasty with Stenting vs Coronary Artery Bypass in patients with MV disease; ARTS, Arterial Revascularization Therapies Study; AWESOME, Angina with Extremely Serious Operative Mortality Evaluation; SIMA, Stenting vs Internal Mammary Artery; LEIPZIG, Stenting vs Minimally Invasive Bypass Surgery; MV, multivessel; D, death; T, thallium defect; A, angina; SV, single vessel; and LAD, left anterior descending coronary artery. Modified from Eagle KA, Guyton RA, Davidoff R, et al. ACC/AHA 2004 guideline update for coronary artery bypass graft surgery. *Circulation.* 2004;110:e340-e437. Only late results are shown.

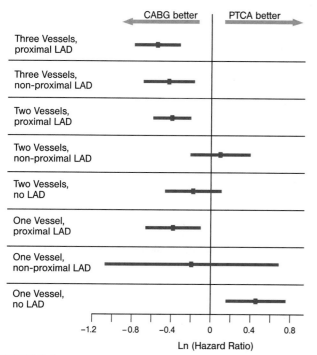

FIGURE 8-9.   Adjusted hazard ratio (ln) with 95% confidence interval, for mortality, between percutaneous transluminal coronary angioplasty (PTCA) and coronary artery bypass graft surgery (CABG). (Modified from Eagle KA, Guyton RA, Davidoff R, et al. ACC/AHA 2004 guideline update for coronary artery bypass graft surgery. *Circulation.* 2004;110:e340–e437.)

QUALITY

The principles of quality management based on international standards (International Organization for Standardization, ISO), have been introduced and are now well established in most interventional cardiology programs. These quality assurance guidelines regulate, standardize, and monitor all major areas of interventional activity. Important examples of national and international quality assurance guidelines that have broad international recognition and impact include:

- Cardiac catheterization laboratory equipment and personnel[80]
- Radiation protection in catheterization laboratory[81]
- PCI indications and performance[82,83]
- Terminology and documentation[84]
- PCI documentation forms[85]

Institutional participation in standardized registries such as ACC-NCD[84] allows consistent benchmarking and process control. Increasing awareness of the importance of adherence to evolving standards along with peer and market pressures continually reinforce the importance of stringent quality management, particularly in interventional therapy.

At least two conditions must be satisfied to allow external and internal comparisons of data between institutions, namely the precise definition of all the assessed outcome variables and consistent and honest reporting. Some of the variables frequently used in interventional cardiology to measure outcome are reviewed next.

Outcome

Unequivocally defined targets are required to enable a reliable assessment of the results of coronary interventions. Target variables include success, failure, and complications.

DEFINITION OF SUCCESS. Success of the procedure can be defined by angiographic, procedural, and clinical criteria applicable to a specific time or time period following the intervention.

TABLE 8-4.   Comparison of Trials: Stent-percutaneous Transluminal Coronary Angioplasty (PTCA) versus Coronary Artery Bypass Graft (CABG)

Trial	Age/ (% ♀)	CAD	No Pat.	Death CABG/ PCI	Q-MI CABG/ PCI	AP CABG/ PCI	RR (%) CABG/ PCI	Primary End Points	Primary End Points (Total %) CABG/PCI	Follow-up (Years)
SOS	61/21	MV	988	2/5	19.6/21.3	21/34	6/21	RR	6/21	1
ERACI II	62/21	MV	450	8/3	19.6/16.6	8/15	5/17	D+MI+CVA+RR	19/23	1.6
ARTS	61/24	MV	1205	3/3	9.4/4.5	10/21	4/21	D+MI+CVA+RR	12/26	1
AWESOME	67/—	MV	454	2/5	—	—	—	D	21/20	3
SIMA	59/21	SV	121	3.6/3.1	4/2	5/9	0/24	D+MI+RR	7/31	2.4
LEIPZIG	62/25	SV	220	4.7/9.5	2/0	21/38	8/29	D+MI+RR	15/31	0.5

For abbreviations, see Table 8-3.

Modified from Eagle KA, Guyton RA, Davidoff R, et al. ACC/AHA 2004 guideline update for coronary artery bypass graft surgery. *Circulation.* 2004;110:e340–e437.

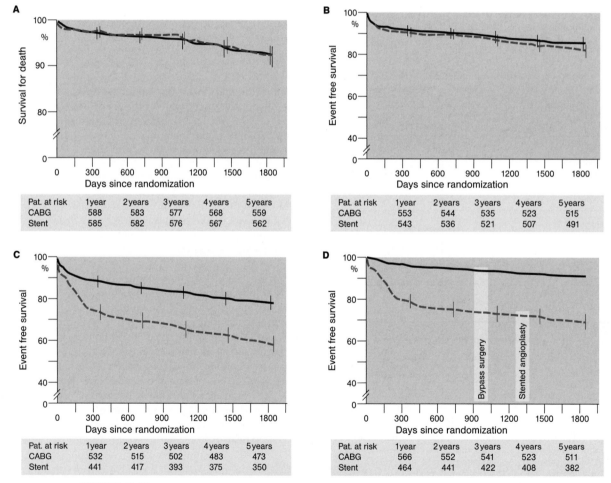

FIGURE 8-10.   Comparison between coronary artery bypass grafting (CABG) and percutaneous coronary intervention (PCI) using bare-metal stents at 5-year follow-up; results from the Arterial Revascularization Therapies Study (ARTS) randomized trial. **A:** Kaplan-Meier curves showing freedom from death. **B:** Kaplan-Meier curves showing freedom from death, cerebrovascular accident, or myocardial infarction or revascularization. **C:** Kaplan-Meier curves showing freedom from death, cerebrovascular accident, or myocardial infarction or revascularization. **D:** Kaplan-Meier curves showing freedom from revascularization. (Adapted from Serruys PW, Ong ATL, van Herwerden LA, et al. Five-year outcomes after coronary stenting versus bypass surgery for the treatment of multivessel disease. The final analysis of the Arterial Revascularization Therapies Study (ARTS) randomized trial. *J Am Coll Cardiol.* 2005;46:575–581.)

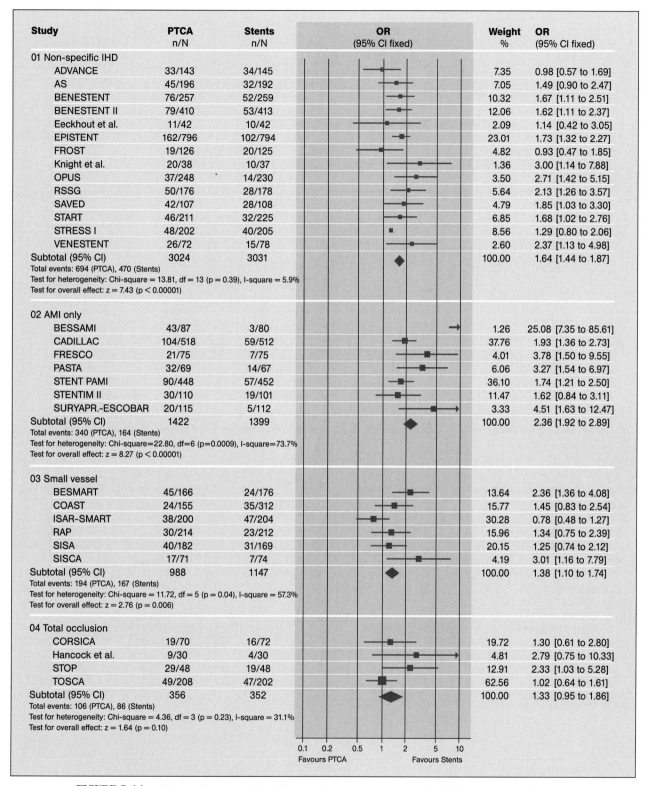

Study	PTCA n/N	Stents n/N	OR (95% CI fixed)	Weight %	OR (95% CI fixed)
01 Non-specific IHD					
ADVANCE	33/143	34/145		7.35	0.98 [0.57 to 1.69]
AS	45/196	32/192		7.05	1.49 [0.90 to 2.47]
BENESTENT	76/257	52/259		10.32	1.67 [1.11 to 2.51]
BENESTENT II	79/410	53/413		12.06	1.62 [1.11 to 2.37]
Eeckhout et al.	11/42	10/42		2.09	1.14 [0.42 to 3.05]
EPISTENT	162/796	102/794		23.01	1.73 [1.32 to 2.27]
FROST	19/126	20/125		4.82	0.93 [0.47 to 1.85]
Knight et al.	20/38	10/37		1.36	3.00 [1.14 to 7.88]
OPUS	37/248	14/230		3.50	2.71 [1.42 to 5.15]
RSSG	50/176	28/178		5.64	2.13 [1.26 to 3.57]
SAVED	42/107	28/108		4.79	1.85 [1.03 to 3.30]
START	46/211	32/225		6.85	1.68 [1.02 to 2.76]
STRESS I	48/202	40/205		8.56	1.29 [0.80 to 2.06]
VENESTENT	26/72	15/78		2.60	2.37 [1.13 to 4.98]
Subtotal (95% CI)	3024	3031		100.00	1.64 [1.44 to 1.87]

Total events: 694 (PTCA), 470 (Stents)
Test for heterogeneity: Chi-square = 13.81, df = 13 (p = 0.39), I-square = 5.9%
Test for overall effect: z = 7.43 (p < 0.00001)

Study	PTCA n/N	Stents n/N	OR (95% CI fixed)	Weight %	OR (95% CI fixed)
02 AMI only					
BESSAMI	43/87	3/80		1.26	25.08 [7.35 to 85.61]
CADILLAC	104/518	59/512		37.76	1.93 [1.36 to 2.73]
FRESCO	21/75	7/75		4.01	3.78 [1.50 to 9.55]
PASTA	32/69	14/67		6.06	3.27 [1.54 to 6.97]
STENT PAMI	90/448	57/452		36.10	1.74 [1.21 to 2.50]
STENTIM II	30/110	19/101		11.47	1.62 [0.84 to 3.11]
SURYAPR.-ESCOBAR	20/115	5/112		3.33	4.51 [1.63 to 12.47]
Subtotal (95% CI)	1422	1399		100.00	2.36 [1.92 to 2.89]

Total events: 340 (PTCA), 164 (Stents)
Test for heterogeneity: Chi-square=22.80, df=6 (p=0.0009), I-square=73.7%
Test for overall effect: z = 8.27 (p < 0.00001)

Study	PTCA n/N	Stents n/N	OR (95% CI fixed)	Weight %	OR (95% CI fixed)
03 Small vessel					
BESMART	45/166	24/176		13.64	2.36 [1.36 to 4.08]
COAST	24/155	35/312		15.77	1.45 [0.83 to 2.54]
ISAR-SMART	38/200	47/204		30.28	0.78 [0.48 to 1.27]
RAP	30/214	23/212		15.96	1.34 [0.75 to 2.39]
SISA	40/182	31/169		20.15	1.25 [0.74 to 2.12]
SISCA	17/71	7/74		4.19	3.01 [1.16 to 7.79]
Subtotal (95% CI)	988	1147		100.00	1.38 [1.10 to 1.74]

Total events: 194 (PTCA), 167 (Stents)
Test for heterogeneity: Chi-square = 11.72, df = 5 (p = 0.04), I-square = 57.3%
Test for overall effect: z = 2.76 (p = 0.006)

Study	PTCA n/N	Stents n/N	OR (95% CI fixed)	Weight %	OR (95% CI fixed)
04 Total occlusion					
CORSICA	19/70	16/72		19.72	1.30 [0.61 to 2.80]
Hancock et al.	9/30	4/30		4.81	2.79 [0.75 to 10.33]
STOP	29/48	19/48		12.91	2.33 [1.03 to 5.28]
TOSCA	49/208	47/202		62.56	1.02 [0.64 to 1.61]
Subtotal (95% CI)	356	352		100.00	1.33 [0.95 to 1.86]

Total events: 106 (PTCA), 86 (Stents)
Test for heterogeneity: Chi-square = 4.36, df = 3 (p = 0.23), I-square = 31.1%
Test for overall effect: z = 1.64 (p = 0.10)

0.1   0.2   0.5   1   2   5   10
Favours PTCA   Favours Stents

FIGURE 8-11. Six-month event rate in trials comparing percutaneous transluminal coronary angioplasty with and without stent. (Modified from Hill R, Bagust A, Bakhai A, et al. Coronary artery stents: a rapid systematic review and economic evaluation. *Health Technol Assessment.* 2004;35. Available at: www.ncchta.org/execsumm/ summ835.htm. Accessed September 20, 2005.)

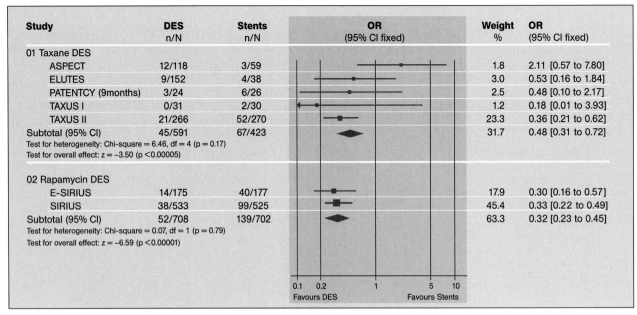

FIGURE 8-12.   Results of trials comparing drug-eluting stents (DES) and bare-metal stents (BMS) in terms of 6-month adverse event rates (n, number of events, N, number of cases). (Modified from Hill R, Bagust A, Bakhai A, et al. Coronary artery stents: a rapid systematic review and economic evaluation. *Health Technol Assessment.* 2004;35. Available at: www.ncchta.org/execsumm/summ835.htm. Accessed September 20, 2005.)

Angiographic success, that is, the removal of a coronary obstruction, has been defined by several criteria. In the present era, angiographic success was mostly defined as reduction of stenosis diameter to <50%, the %DS (binary definition).[85] Later a minimum luminal diameter (MLD), a continuous variable, was employed to better characterize the gradual nature of the degree

of severity of residual stenoses (for review, see reference 86). Today zero degree residual stenosis is considered the optimal result of stent-supported angioplasty, and a residual stenosis <30% is considered an acceptable "stentlike" result of balloon angioplasty (for review, see reference 87). Angiographic calculation of the cross-sectional luminal area, although probably a

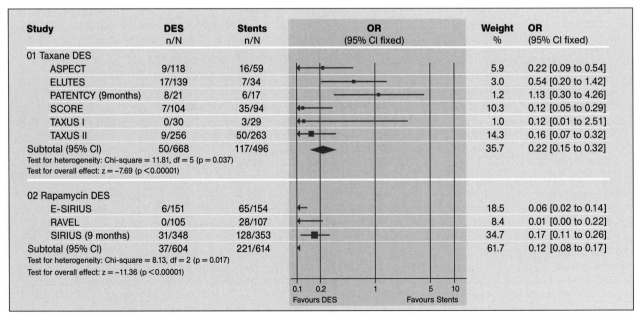

FIGURE 8-13.   Results of trials comparing drug-eluting stents (DES) and bare-metal stents (BMS) in terms of binary (>50%) restenosis rate at 6 months (n - number of events, N - number of cases). (Modified from Hill R, Bagust A, Bakhai A, et al. Coronary artery stents: a rapid systematic review and economic evaluation. *Health Technol Assessment.* 2004;35. Available at: www.ncchta.org/execsumm/summ835.htm. Accessed September 20, 2005.)

more accurate indicator than linear measurements, has not been widely applied in clinical practice.[88] Normal antegrade coronary artery flow in the target vessel (thrombolysis in myocardial infarction, TIMI, III) should also be present. Angiographic success is determined following the intervention. In patients undergoing plain angioplasty, the immediate gain representing the maximum luminal expansion following dilatation is usually slightly reduced because of recoil ("early loss") when measurement has been deferred.

On follow-up (typically 6 months), restenosis and in-stent restenosis of the target lesion and coronary flow of the target vessel are described using the same parameters stated earlier (%DS, MLD, and TIMI). Restenosis usually refers to a reoccurrence of any stenosis >50% DS. This >50% or <50% status has been termed *binary restenosis*, and its frequency in a defined population of lesions and/or patients has accordingly been termed the *binary restenosis rate* (BRR). Alternatively, the actual degree of loss immediately after dilatation ("early loss") and on follow-up ("late loss") is indicated in percent or in absolute numbers (usually millimeters) at a specific point in time during follow-up. Currently, MLD measured at the narrowest point of the target lesion is the most frequently used parameter in clinical settings.

At present, angiographic definitions of success do not include any intermediate results or associated coronary damage such as side-branch closure, extensive stenting for an initially short lesion, or compromise of a nontarget vessel. It appears likely that additional angiographic criteria of success are required to enable us to discriminate results better in order for us to achieve better prognostication and to better assess new and emerging technologies. Examples of large differences in outcomes of interventions hidden within the current definition of angiographic success are provided in Figures 8-14 and 15.

Procedural success denotes angiographic success in absence of any clinically relevant complications. Procedural complications are most frequently summarized in quality assurance and clinical research protocols as major adverse cardiac (and cerebral) events (MAC[C]E) and include cardiac and noncardiac death, nonfatal myocardial (and cerebral) infarction, and target vessel revascularization (TVR) at predefined times during follow-up (up to 24 hours after the intervention, during the hospital stay, within 30 days, 6 months, and others). Complications concerning the access site include bleeding and vascular injuries. The former are standardized based on TIMI trial definitions for major (overt clinical bleeding with a drop in hemoglobin >5g/dL or in hematocrit >15%), minor (drop in hemoglobin >3g/dL and ≤5g/dL or hematocrit >9% and ≤15%), and none (bleeding event that does not meet the major or minor criteria).[83] The last include iatrogenic dissections, fistulas, and pseudoaneurysms.

Peri-interventional myocardial injury (PMI) denotes any postprocedural rise in cardiac enzymes (cardiac troponins with peak values at 24 to 48 hours, CKMB with peak values at 24 hours) above the upper limit of normal (ULN[89]). Typical sampling intervals are at baseline, 6 to 9 hours, 12 to 24 hours, and as needed after the intervention. Cardiac troponins I and T are the preferred cardiac marker proteins because of their high sensitivity and specificity. The MB (muscle-brain) fraction of creatine kinase (CK) is preferred in patients with elevated cardiac markers at baseline because the serum kinetics are more favorable (Fig. 8-16).[90] The incidence, prognostic significance, causes, prevention, and treatment of PMI have recently been reviewed.[91]

Clinical success denotes procedural success associated with relief of symptoms and freedom from adverse events over time. Restenosis and bypass attrition are the major limiting factors affecting long-term clinical success in coronary interventions and coronary surgery, respectively.

DEFINITION OF PROCEDURAL FAILURE AND COMPLICATIONS. Procedural failure is present when the target lesion was not successfully revascularized for technical reasons such as an inability to cross or to dilate the lesion (target vessel failure, TVF). Nontechnical causes of failed revascularization such as a suspension of intervention because of systemic adverse effects such as contrast agent allergy are not considered TVF. Procedural failure may be accompanied by complications as outlined in the previous section. Definitions of some of the frequent procedural complications contained in the current ACC/AHA guidelines are summarized in Table 8-5.[81] The patient-, lesion- and procedure-related factors of PMI have been reviewed and discussed elsewhere.[91]

DEFINITION OF THE QUALITY OF INTERVENTIONS. The technical quality of interventions is hardly documented by the current quality assurance protocols. Surrogate indicators of quality include an elevated periprocedural serum concentration of cardiac markers of injury, procedural and fluoroscopy time, radiation exposure, and the use of contrast agents. Tables 8-6 and 8-7 provide examples of such surrogate measures. Documentation of more specific indicators of the technical quality of coronary interventions, such as suboptimal stent apposition, stent damage, underdilatation, incomplete lesion coverage, side-branch closure, or an impaired microcirculation, would probably improve analyses of outcomes and data interpretations. Extensive efforts to document results are, however, unrealistic in current clinical practice, and a broad implementation of expert interventional techniques might be a preferable course of action.

PERCUTANEOUS CORONARY INTERVENTIONS: COMPONENTS

Percutaneous coronary intervention (PCI) is a complex process of an initialization followed by a number of iterative cycles, each consisting of image acquisition, intervention, and reassessment and concluded by a termination. The dynamics of each intervention depend on operator's decisions to proceed or to terminate the procedure based on a continuous series of instant benefit and risk assessments. The ultimate criterion of a successful outcome is the sum of benefits to the patient. The outcome of the intervention is affected by factors related to the lesion, the patient, and the operator. Since these factors are incompletely defined and difficult to measure, direct measures of PCI process quality are not available. Surrogate criteria such as cost effectiveness must be interpreted with care and within the context of individual interventions.

An ideal PCI consists of an initialization, a single iterative cycle, and a termination. Ideal "real-world" PCI consists of an initialization, a minimum number of cycles converging in an optimum revascularization of the target lesion, and a termination.

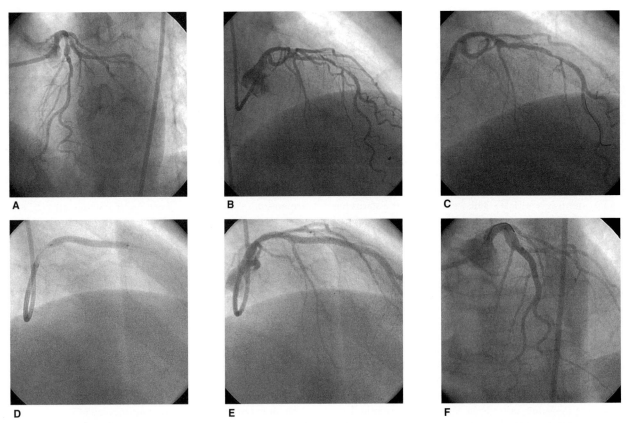

FIGURE 8-14. Long, proximal left anterior descending (LAD) artery stenosis, drug-eluting stenting (DES). 66-year-old male with Canadian Cardiology Society (CCS) III° angina on exertion and anterior wall ischemia documented by stress echocardiography. Angiogram revealed high proximal long LAD up to 90% stenosis **(A,B)**. Following guidewire placement **(C)** 3.5/32 mm Taxus (Boston Scientific, Natick, MA, USA) was deployed at 14 bar and after dilated to improve the strut apposition and to optimize the proximal transition between native vessel wall and stent **(D)**. Final angiograms revealed complete LAD revascularization **(E,F)**.

In contrast to operator-independent mathematical automated iterative processes, PCI is highly operator dependent and its outcome is affected by a large number of frequently initially "hidden" variables. In simple terms, the PCI operator sets the stage by calling certain findings on coronary angiography an indication for catheter-based treatment and by defining the strategy of the intervention. Following the initialization, which ends with the last angiogram taken before guidewire placement, the main cycle of the intervention begins. During the main cycle the operator performs an interventional action, monitors the result, and, based on his interpretation, terminates the procedure or proceeds with the next cycle of the intervention. The operator's decisions are based on his estimates of expected benefits and potential risks of his actions. The ability to avoid and to predict impending risks and to resolve materialized risky situations are hallmarks of experienced operators. In addition, secondary factors including incurred procedural costs, potential legal implications, patients' wishes, psychological disposition of the operator, and other variables also affect the decision process. Besides avoiding unnecessary risks and staying in control in difficult situations, the master operator also typically uses a minimum number of required iterative cycles to achieve technically and clinically excellent results, while keeping the complication rates and material costs low compared to less accomplished operators. These attributes produce the impression of seeming simplicity, straightforwardness, and elegance. The strategic considerations

concerning PCI have been outlined in Chapter 4. In the subsequent section, general considerations and patient- and lesion-related factors concerning PCI are discussed.

GENERAL CONSIDERATIONS

Initial steps in setting the stage for performing PCI include stating the indication, obtaining informed consent, and examining the patient.

Indications

PCI is principally considered in patients with documented coronary artery lesions causing myocardial ischemia or adversely affecting the prognosis of the patient. PCI is indicated when based on evidence it appears more beneficial to the patient compared to other forms of treatment. The indications change in time as a consequence of progress in understanding the pathophysiology of CAD and as a result of evolving technologies. Although the appropriateness of PCI is usually not contested in patients with acute coronary syndromes, PCI indications in patients with chronic coronary syndromes appear less straightforward. Although the guidelines provide a useful framework for PCI indications (Tables 8-8 to 8-10),[67,81,82] they by no means replace the decision process needed to address the specific needs of individual patients. Frequently, to decide

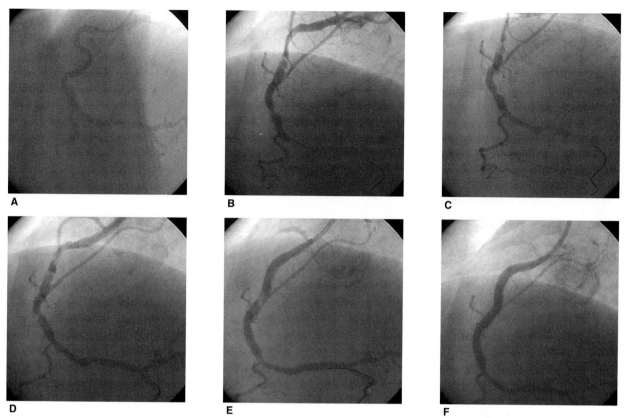

FIGURE 8-15. Full metal jacket coronary artery reconstruction: 51-year-old man with inferior wall ST elevation myocardial infarction (STEMI). Angiogram showed single-vessel coronary disease, AHA segment 3 right coronary artery (RCA) "culprit" lesion in a moderately tortuous, diffusely diseased infarct-related RCA (**A**). Following guidewire placement, diffuse atherosclerosis with multiple plaques, spasms, and proximal (AHA segment 1) dissection were seen (**B**). Dilatation of the "culprit" lesion was performed using a 3.0/20-mm balloon and resulted in RCA closure (**C**). Following stent placement (3.0/18 mm Lekton motion, Biotronik at 10 bar) antegrade coronary blood flow was restored (**D**). Subsequently, because of multiple proximal segment plaques and plaque shifts occurring after each subsequent stent implantation, four successive distal to proximal overlapping stent placements were required (3.5/8 mm, 4.0/13 mm 2×, 4.0/20 mm, all Lekton motion, Biotronik at 14 bar) (**E**). Final angiogram documented "full metal jacket" RCA AHA segment 1 and 2 revascularization and spot "culprit" lesion revascularization (**F**).

on the most appropriate treatment for individual patients, a thorough discussion of findings followed by consensus decisions between interventionist and surgeon involving the patient is required.

Informed Consent

Performance of PCI is contingent on consent of the patient. Thus, in all cases an informed consent must be signed by the patient well ahead of the intended intervention; typically, in elective cases 24 hours is considered adequate. In severely compromised or unconscious patients, as is often the case in emergency procedures, informed consent may be difficult to obtain. In these cases it is customary to assume that the physician acts in the best interest of his patient; a brief written statement describing the circumstances leading to the decision to perform PCI is usually considered sufficient. However, because any interventions without patient's explicit prior consent are open to different legal interpretations, the operator should clearly understand the customary legal practices in his environment.

An interview with the patient and a core physical examination including chest auscultation, auscultation and palpation of peripheral pulses, and the Allen test for radial procedures must be conducted before an informed consent is obtained. Usually a printed standard consent form is used and modified as necessary for individual patients. The main purpose of the interview is to convey full information to the patient regarding the expected benefits and risks of the planned treatment. The interview should be conducted unhurriedly in a quiet environment. All the information should be communicated honestly, clearly, and understandably. The explanation of expectations and risks must be complete and realistic. Although risk statistics are available in the literature (Tables 8-11 and 8-12,[81,92] it is preferable to use the actual data from the operator's institution (Table 8-13). Other individual risks should be explicitly stated. In patients undergoing multiple interventions during a single hospital stay, separate informed consent is needed for each intervention. In high-risk procedures it is advisable to conduct the interview in the presence of a third person cosigning the document. Signed and dated consent becomes a part of the patient's medical chart confirming to the legal requirements.

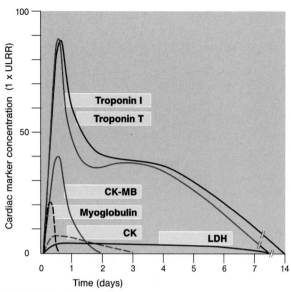

FIGURE 8-16. Kinetic profiles of cardiac marker proteins associated with ST elevation myocardial infarction. (Modified from French JK, White HD. Clinical implications of the new definition of myocardial infarction. *Heart.* 2004;90:99–106.)

Peri-PCI Orders and Evaluations

Before PCI, standard evaluations performed in all patients, include resting 12-lead ECG and laboratory examinations (potassium, creatinine, prothrombin time, platelets count, TSH, glucose (<24 hours before PCI), and chest x-ray (optional).

Suggested written pre-PCI orders are stated as follows:

- Shave and prep both groins or prepare other access site as specified
- Keep NPO (nothing by mouth) after midnight except for clear liquids; for patients scheduled for the second half of the day, a light breakfast is allowed; avoid dehydration!
- Maintain medication except long-acting diuretics and biguanides (metformin; see later discussion)
- Establish the intravenous line prior to transport to the catheterization laboratory
- Have patient void on call and put on hospital gown
- Administer sedatives, such as diazepam 5 mg PO, if necessary

Following an uncomplicated PCI, the patient is transferred for up to 24-hours monitoring. Post-PCI orders typically include:

- Timing of sheath removal (if patient remains asymptomatic)
- Method of hemostasis
- Duration of compression required in hours (if no closure device was used)
- Protocol to check puncture site for bleeding
- Protocol to check blood pressure and peripheral pulse, e.g., q15min ×2, q30min ×4, q60min ×3h
- Requirements for ECG monitoring (in hours)
- Fluid intake requirements, orally and/or intravenously; if inadequate, loop diuretic requirements
- Timing of intake of patient's usual medication

Patients with complex or complicated procedures are transferred to a fully monitored bed, usually an intensive care unit. Post-PCI orders state the planned management. Unstable patients do not leave catheterization laboratory until stable.

RISK ASSESSMENT; PATIENT-RELATED FACTORS

Comprehensive evaluation of all risk factors is critical to estimate the risk of the intervention. The overall latent risk of PCI (see Chapter 4) comprises primarily patient- and lesion-related risk factors. Knowledge of patient-related risk factors prior to the intervention allows risk reduction by targeting their prevention, their stabilization, and in some cases even their elimination. Principal patient-related risk factors are reviewed.

Low-Risk Patients

Low-risk patients are considered those with no record of any of the established patient- and/or lesion-related risk factors such as exemplified by a healthy young man with single-vessel CAD and type A target lesion in a side branch. However, even in low-risk patients the complications are not zero, and it is precisely in this group where any major complication seems to weigh double. The best prevention of avoidable unexpected complications is by adopting the same thorough fully concentrated approach to the intervention as if a technically demanding case were being treated.

Patients with Poor Left Ventricular Function

Left ventricular function (LVF) is usually assessed by quantitative echocardiography or angiography. Global systolic LV dysfunction may be graded as light (left ventricular ejection fraction, LVEF >45%), moderate (LVEF ~30% to 45%), or severe (LVEF <30%). The segmental systolic LVF is also assessed[93] and related to distribution of coronary artery lesions. Diastolic LVF is not routinely evaluated prior to PCI.

The latent PCI risk increases with decreasing systolic LVF. Segmental LVF is important to differentiate between healthy and dysfunctional myocardium and myocardial scar. In some cases, the viability of the myocardium may be assessed. Matching the segmental LVF with coronary lesions allows better risk assessment and prognostication, and it is useful in decisions on PCI targets. The jeopardy score[94] shown in Table 8-14 provides a means to assess the risk from PCI based on the severity of CAD and segmental LVF.

Patients with moderate to severe systolic LV dysfunction require optimal management of heart failure including adequate hydration and stable medication (ACE inhibitors, beta-blockers, diuretics, antialdosterone agents) prior to elective PCI. Patients with persistent heart failure despite optimal medical management with LVEF <20% to 30% and a jeopardy score >3 are candidates for prophylactic mechanical support during PCI. Patients who should receive mechanical support routinely as soon as possible prior to PCI are those with marked hemodynamic compromise in the settings of an acute coronary syndrome or with cardiogenic shock defined by systolic blood pressure <90 mm Hg or a value 30 mm Hg below basal levels for at least 30 minutes, an elevated arteriovenous oxygen difference (>5.5 mL/dL), and a depressed cardiac index

TABLE 8-5. Definitions of Procedural Complications

Procedural Complications	Definitions
Primary cause of death	Patient died during this period of hospitalization
Periprocedural myocardial infarction (MI)	The new presence of a myocardial infarction as documented by at least 1 of the following criteria: 1. Evolutionary ST-segment elevations, development of new Q-waves in 2 or more contiguous ECG leads, or new or presumably new left bundle branch block pattern on the ECG 2. Biochemical evidence of myocardial necrosis; this can be manifested as (1) CK-MB ≥3× the upper limit of normal or if CK-MB not available (2) total CK ≥3× upper limit of normal. Because normal limits of certain blood tests may vary, please check with your lab for normal limits for CK-MB and total CK

Coronary artery bypass graft (CABG) during this admission	If the patient had a CABG during this admission indicate the CABG status using the following categories:
	 I. Elective: The procedure could be deferred without increased risk of compromised cardiac outcome
	 II. Urgent: All of the following conditions are met:
	   A. Not elective
	   B. Not emergency
	   C. Procedure required during same hospitalization in order to minimize chance of further clinical deterioration
	 III. Emergency: The patient's clinical status includes any of the following:
	   A. Ischemic dysfunction (any of the following):
	     1. Ongoing ischemia including rest angina despite maximal medical therapy (medical and/or intra-aortic balloon pump)
	     2. Acute evolving MI within 24 h before intervention
	     3. Pulmonary edema requiring intubation
	   B. Mechanical dysfunction (either of the following):
	     1. Shock with circulatory support
	     2. Shock without circulatory support
	 IV. Salvage: The patient is undergoing CPR en route to the Operating Room

Cerebrovacular accident (CVA/stroke)	Patient experienced a CVA as documented by a loss of neurological function caused by an ischemic event with residual symptoms at least 24 h after onset
Vascular complications Bleeding	Blood loss at the site of arterial or venous access or due to perforation of a traversed artery or vein requiring transfusion and/or prolonging the hospital stay, and/or causing a drop in hemoglobin >3.0 gm/dL. Bleeding attributable to the vascular site could be retroperitoneal, a local hematoma >10 cm diameter or external
Occlusion	A total obstruction of the artery usually at the site of access requiring surgical repair. Occlusion is defined as total obstruction of the artery by thrombus, dissection or other mechanism, usually at the site of access, requiring surgical repair. Occlusion may be accompanied by absence of palpable pulse or Doppler signal and associated with signs and symptoms of an ischemic limb requiring surgical intervention
Dissection	A dissection occurred at the site of percutaneous entry. Dissection is defined as disruption of an arterial wall resulting in splitting and separation of the intimal (or subintimal) layers
Pseudoaneurysm	Pseudoaneurysm is defined as the occurrence of an aneurysmal dilatation of the artery at the site of catheter entry demonstrated by arteriography or ultrasound
AV fistula	AV fistula is defined as a connection between the access artery (e.g., femoral) and access vein (e.g., femoral) that is demonstrated by an imaging study (arteriography or ultrasound) and most often characterized by a continuous bruit
Renal failure	After the lab visit—but before any subsequent lab visits only: Indicate if the patient experienced acute renal insufficiency resulting in an increase in serum creatinine to more than 2.0 mg/dL (or a 50% or greater increase over an abnormal baseline) measured prior to procedure, or requiring dialysis

Reproduced with permission from Smith SC, Dove JT, Jacobs AK, et al. ACC/AHA guidelines for percutaneous coronary intervention (Revision of the 1993 PTCA guidelines) *J Am Coll Cardiol.* 2001;37:2239–2300.

TABLE 8-6. Selected Surrogate Indicators of Quality of Interventions (Heart Centre Coswig, 2004)

Procedure	Procedure Time[a]— Averages (min)	Mean Fluoroscopy and Cine Time ±SD (min)	Mean Fluoroscopy and Cine Exposure ± SD (cGy/cm²)	Mean Iodine Contrast (mL) ± SD
Ad hoc PCI	49.3 ± 28.9	11.3 ± 8.1	3.690 ± 300	70 ± 40

Ad hoc percutaneous coronary intervention (PCI) includes approximately 2/3 emergency and 1/3 elective cases
[a]Procedure time is the time from placing on and removing the patient from the table.
SD, standard deviation.

TABLE 8-7. Mean Fluoroscopy and Cine Times of Coronary Interventions and Diagnostics (Mean ± SD) (Heart Centre Coswig, 2004)

Intervention	Number of Interventions	Mean Fluoroscopy and Cine Time ± SD (min)
PCI only	124	10.7 ± 7.9
PCI and angiography	742	11.3 ± 8.1
Coronary angiography only	1436	2.9 ± 2.8

($<$2.2 L/min/m^2 body-surface area) in the presence of elevated pulmonary-capillary wedge pressure ($>$15 mm Hg).[95] Indications for mechanical support other than severe reversible systolic LV dysfunction include:

- Multivessel coronary artery disease and ongoing ischemia scheduled for delayed revascularization
- Multivessel coronary artery disease and ongoing ischemia not amenable to revascularization (selected cases)

- High-risk PCI such as that of unprotected left main or complex multivessel lesions in patients with moderate to severe LV dysfunction

In patients considered for mechanically supported PCI, significant aortic and peripheral artery occlusive disease must be excluded before device implantation. The intra-aortic balloon pump (IABP)[96] is the mechanical support device most frequently used in the catheterization laboratory (for review, see reference 97). Although percutaneous implantation from the contralateral femoral artery site is usually straightforward, several limitations should be kept in mind:

- Limited intravascular residence time ($<$3 maximally 7 to 10 days)
- Reduced efficacy in patients with arrhythmias
- Limited efficacy in the presence of mild aortic insufficiency
- Need for residual authentic LV function
- Requirements for therapeutic anticoagulation
- Presence of any of the exclusion criteria

In patients with severe intractable LV dysfunction and/or cardiogenic shock due to reversible causes such as acute

TABLE 8-8. Indications for Percutaneous Coronary Intervention (PCI), European Society of Cardiology Recommendations

Indication	Class of Recommendation	Level of Evidence
CHRONIC CORONARY SYNDROMES		
Objective large myocardial ischemia (in presence of any lesion subsets, except chronic total occlusions which cannot be crossed)	I	A
Chronic total occlusion	IIa	C
High surgical risk	IIa	B
Multivessel disease	IIb	C
Unprotected left main in the absence of other revascularization options	IIb	C
Routine stenting of de novo stenosis; native artery, venous grafts	I	A
ACUTE CORONARY SYNDROMES		
NSTEMI and instable angina pectoris (early PCI, high risk group)	I	A
STEMI (primary PCI; unselected patients)	I	A
STEMI (primary PCI, contra-indication to fibrinolysis)	I	A
STEMI (primary PCI, presentation 3–12 h after onset of symptoms)	I	A
STEMI (primary PCI, routine stenting)	I	A
STEMI (facilitated PCI following fibrinolysis)	No recommendation	—
STEMI (facilitated PCI following GP IIb/IIIa inhibitors)	No recommendation	—
STEMI (rescue PCI after failed fibrinolysis)	I	B
STEMI (primary PCI, cardiogenic shock)	I	C
STEMI (routine angiography after successful fibrinolysis)	I	A
STEMI (PCI for ischemia following successful fibrinolyis)	I	B

NSTEMI, non-ST elevation myocardial infarction; STEMI, ST elevation myocardial infarction.

Modified from Silber S, Albertsson P, Aviles FF, et al. Guidelines for percutaneous coronary interventions. The Task Force for Percutaneous Coronary Interventions of the European Society of Cardiology. 2005;26:804–847.

TABLE 8-9. ACC/AHA Recommendations for Percutaneous Coronary Interventions Based on Clinical Symptoms: Asymptomatic/CCS Class I Angina patients

Indications	Level of Recommendation	Level of Evidence
Patients who do not have treated diabetes with asymptomatic ischemia or mild angina with 1 or more significant lesions in 1 or 2 coronary arteries suitable for PCI with a high likelihood of success and a low risk of morbidity and mortality. The vessels to be dilated must subtend a large area of viable myocardium.	I	B
The same clinical and anatomic requirements for Class I, except the myocardial area at risk is of moderate size or the patient has treated diabetes.	IIa	B
Patients with asymptomatic ischemia or mild angina with ≥3 coronary arteries suitable for PCI with a high likelihood of success and a low risk of morbidity and mortality. The vessels to be dilated must subtend at least a moderate area of viable myocardium. In the physician's judgment, there should be evidence of myocardial ischemia by ECG exercise testing, stress nuclear imaging, stress echocardiography, or ambulatory ECG monitoring or intracoronary physiologic measurements.	IIb	B
Patients with asymptomatic ischemia or mild angina who do not meet the criteria as listed under Class I or Class II and who have: a. Only a small area of viable myocardium at risk b. No objective evidence of ischemia c. Lesions that have a low likelihood of successful dilatation d. Mild symptoms that are unlikely to be due to myocardial ischemia e. Factors associated with increased risk of morbidity or mortality f. Left main disease g. Insignificant disease <50%	III	C

Modified from Smith SC, Dove JT, Jacobs AK, et al. ACC/AHA guidelines for percutaneous coronary intervention (Revision of the 1993 PTCA guidelines). *J Am Coll Cardiol.* 2001;37:2239–2300.

TABLE 8-10. ACC/AHA Recommendations for Percutaneous Coronary Intervention (PCI) Based on Clinical Symptoms: CCS Class II–IV Angina Patients with Single- or Multivessel Coronary Disease on Medical Therapy

Indications	Level of Recommendation	Level of Evidence
Patients with 1 or more significant lesions in 1 or more coronary arteries suitable for PCI with a high likelihood of success and low risk of morbidity or mortality. The vessel(s) to be dilated must subtend a moderate or large area of viable myocardium and have high risk.	I	B
Patients with focal saphenous vein graft lesions or multiple stenoses who are poor candidates for reoperative surgery.	IIa	C
Patient has 1 or more lesions to be dilated with reduced likelihood of success or the vessel(s) subtend a less than moderate area of viable myocardium. Patients with 2- or 3-vessel disease, with significant proximal LAD CAD and treated diabetes or abnormal LV function.	IIb	B
1. Patient has no evidence of myocardial injury or ischemia on objective testing and has not had a trial of medical therapy, or has a. Only a small area of myocardium at risk b. All lesions or the culprit lesion to be dilated with morphology with a low likelihood of success c. A high risk of procedure-related morbidity or mortality. 2. Patients with insignificant coronary stenosis (e.g., <50% diameter). 3. Patients with significant left main CAD who are candidates for CABG.	III	C

Modified from Smith SC, Dove JT, Jacobs AK, et al. ACC/AHA guidelines for percutaneous coronary intervention (Revision of the 1993 PTCA guidelines). *J Am Coll Cardiol.* 2001;37:2239–2300.

myocardial ischemia, cardiopulmonary support (CPS) and extracorporeal membrane oxygenation (ECMO) assist devices provide excellent short-term support.[98] Depending on the size of the CPS cannula and volume status, a patient's circulation can be maintained for a short period of time (<3 days) regardless of cardiac rhythm and residual output. However, in contrast to IABP, CPS does not unload LV and does not improve coronary perfusion. Supported PCI is a technically demanding

TABLE 8-11. In-hospital Rates of Major Complications

Study	Year	Complication Rates (%)				
		Death	STEMI	Emergency CABG	Major Neurological	Major Vascular
NHLBI-DR	2000	1.9	2.8	0.4	0.3	3.8
SCA&I	2000	0.5	N/A	0.5	0.1	0.2
BARI	1996	0.7	2.8	4.1	0.2	0.2
NY State (Balloon)	1997	0.85	N/A	2.7	N/A	N/A
NY State (Stent)	1997	0.71	N/A	1.66	N/A	N/A
North, New England	1996	1.2	2.0	1.3	N/A	N/A
Medicare	1997	2.5	N/A	3.3	N/A	N/A
EPILOG (Abciximab)	1997	0.3	0.4	0.4	0.2	1.1
EPILOG (Placebo)	1997	0.8	0.8	1.7	0.0	1.1
EPISTENT (Abciximab)	1998	0.3	0.9	0.8	0.4	2.9
EPISTENT (Placebo)	1996	0.6	1.4	1.1	0.1	1.7

STEMI, ST elevation myocardial infarction; CABG, coronary artery bypass grafting.

Modified from Smith SC, Dove JT, Jacobs AK, et al. ACC/AHA guidelines for percutaneous coronary intervention (Revision of the 1993 PTCA guidelines). *J Am Coll Cardiol.* 2001;37:2239–2300.

TABLE 8-12. In-hospital Rates of Major Complications Related to Underlined Coronary Artery Disease and Procedure

Indication	Myocardial Infarction (%)		TIA/ Stroke (%)		In-hospital Death (%)		Access Site (%)		Pulmonary Embolism (%)		CPR (%)	
	Cath	PCI	Cath	PCI	Cath	PCI	Cath	PCI	Cath	PCI	Cath	PCI
Stable AP	0.08	0.69	0.1	0.1	0.21	0.26	0.58	1.14	0.06	0.01	0.1	0.28
Unstable angina	0.26	0.59	0.17	0.13	0.48	0.55	0.39	1.43	0.1	0.1	0.3	0.26
NSTEMI	0.25	0.75	0.25	0.18	1.74	1.44	1.06	1.44	0.0	0.0	0.43	0.66
STEMI	0.34	1.68	0.05	0.22	2.84	4.27	0.77	1.4	0.0	0.4	0.87	2.07
Cardiogenic shock		4.08		0.68		33.11		0.68		0.0		18.82

NSTEMI, non-ST elevation myocardial infarction; STEMI, ST elevation myocardial infarction; TIA, transient ischemic attacks; CPR, cardiopulmonary resuscitation; PCI, percutaneous coronary intervention.

Modified from Zeymer U, Weber M, Zahn R, et al. Indications and complications of invasive diagnostic procedures and percutaneous interventions in the year 2003. *Z Kardiol.* 2005;94:392–398.

TABLE 8-13. In-hospital Rates of Major Complications of Percutaneous Coronary Intervention (PCI)

Procedural Complication	Complications of Total Procedures (%)
Access site[a]	0.4
Myocardial infarction	0.3
Emergency coronary surgery	0.4
Major stroke	0.0
Death	0.1

(Data Heart Centre Coswig 2003; all cases included, 1/3 elective and 2/3 emergency PCI).

[a]Represents the sum of major and minor bleedings based on TIMI classification pseudoaneurysms and fistulas (ACC clinical data standards—reference guide. American College of Cardiology key data elements and definitions for measuring the clinical management and outcome of patients with acute coronary syndromes. Available at www.acc.org/clinical/data_standards/ACS/acs_index.htm. Accessed May 28, 2005).

TABLE 8-14. Calculation of Baseline Left-ventricular (LV) Dysfunction in Patients with Coronary Artery Disease—Jeopardy Score

Coronary Artery Segment	LV Region Supplied by Target Vessel	LV Region Supplied by Vessel with Stenosis >70%	LV Region with Hypokinesia Supplied by Vessel without Stenosis
RIVA (LAD)	1	1	0.5
Rd	1	1	0.5
Rs	1	1	0.5
RCx (LCx)—marginal	1	1	0.5
RCx (LCx)—distal	1	1	0.5
RIVP (PDA)	1	1	0.5

RIVA, ramus interventricularis anterior; LAD, left anterior descending; Rd, ramus diagonalis; Rs, ramus septalis; RCx, ramus circumflexus; LCx, left circumflex; RIVP, ramus interventricularis posterior; PDA, posterior desceding artery.

Modified from Almany SL. Interventional strategies in patients with left ventricular dysfunction. In: Freed M, Grines C, Safan RD, eds. *The New Manual of Interventional Cardiology.* Birmingham: Physician's Press, 1997:157.

procedure demanding complete revascularization in one stage and the lowest possible complication rates, and should therefore be performed only by experienced operators. In patients with protracted or irreversible LV dysfunction, weaning from the mechanical support device might be difficult and in some cases even impossible. Other mechanical LV support devices, such as the left atrial-femoral artery bypass and surgically implanted left ventricular assist devices, have not been primarily designed for mechanical support in the catheterization laboratory and do not play a significant role in PCI[99]

Diabetic Patients

Type II diabetes is a critical risk factor for vascular multimorbidity[100] and a strong independent predictor for cardiovascular events.[101] In context with PCI, high rate of left main lesions, multivessel and diffuse CAD, large plaque burden, and poor collateralization are of particular relevance.[102–104] Correspondingly, the complication rates, long-term mortality, and restenosis rates of diabetics undergoing PCI are greater compared with nondiabetics.[105,106] Clinical outcomes of PCI using balloon dilatation alone[107,108] and BMS with GPIIb/IIIa inhibitors were worse compared to patients treated with surgery.[109–111] Although DESs have been shown to be superior to BMSs in diabetic patients as well,[112] their efficacy compared to bypass surgery still remains unclear; important trials such as FREEDOM and BARI 2D may clarify the questions of the most appropriate treatment for diabetics with multivessel (MVD) CAD and are underway. Based on the available evidence, surgery is the better option for elective treatment of diabetics with MVD, particularly when internal mammary artery (IMA) grafts to the LAD can be used.[113] In patients with single nonproximal LAD vessel disease, percutaneous treatment using DES and GPIIb/IIIa receptor inhibitors should be considered, whereas in those with single proximal LAD disease, either one of the two revascularization strategies may be considered.[114] Patients with acute coronary syndromes, particularly those with ST elevation myocardial infarction (STEMI), are treated by PCI.[115]

Adverse morphology of diabetic CAD associated with multiple associated functional abnormalities[116,117] and worse PCI outcomes of diabetics versus nondiabetics in all subgroups[113,114] mandate a number of specific considerations in planning PCI in diabetics versus nondiabetics:

- Greater likelihood of underestimation of the severity and extent of the coronary disease
- Greater likelihood of vascular and organ multimorbidity
- Metabolic instability
- Greater likelihood of contrast agent–induced nephropathy
- Greater potential of side effects from medications, especially biguanides
- Greater likelihood of immune incompetence and healing defects

Optimal management of diabetics undergoing PCI requires optimal management of all identified risk factors, meticulous PCI technique, and thorough aftercare. The risk of contrast-induced nephropathy (CIN), particularly in patients with preexisting renal insufficiency, mandates a close surveillance of renal function during the peri-interventional period (Table 8-15)[118] and adequate hydration. To avoid metabolic complications, tight metabolic control and adjustments in medication are also important. Table 8-16 provides a check list for diabetics undergoing PCI.

Patients with Renal Disease

The presence of pre-existing renal disease is a marker of poor outcome in patients undergoing PCI[119,120] and CABG.[121,122] Although patients with renal insufficiency have benefited from the introduction of coronary stenting[123] and off-pump coronary surgery,[124] the negative prognostic implications of renal disease persist.[125] For patients with end-stage renal disease in the present era, CABG was favored over angioplasty[122]; however, no conclusive data comparing PCI and CABG utilizing recent revascularization strategies are available. Therefore, at present both strategies of coronary revascularization should

TABLE 8-15. Stages of Renal Insufficiency in Patients with Type II Diabetes

Stage	Albumin (mg/L)	Creatinine Clearance (mL/min/1.73 m^2)
1. Renal damage with preserved excretory function		
1a. with microalbuminuria	20–200	>90
1b. with macroalbuminuria	>200	>90
2. Renal damage with excretory insufficiency		
2a. light	>200	60–89
2b. moderate	>200	30–59
2c. severe	Falling	15–29
2d. terminal	Falling	<15

Reproduced with permission from National Kidney Foundation—K/DOQL. Clinical practice guidelines for chronic kidney disease evaluation, classification and stratification. *Am J Kidney Dis.* 2002;39:S1–266.

be considered, yet the least aggressive technique allowing complete revascularization should be selected. Guidelines applicable to coronary revascularization of patients on chronic hemodialysis are provided by the National Kidney Foundation.[126]

In clinical practice the detection of renal disease and exact definition of the degree of renal dysfunction prior to PCI are of key importance in avoiding the risk of contrast-induced nephropathy (CIN), defined as ≥25% increase in serum creatinine from baseline or absolute increase by 44.2 μmol/L (0.5 mg/dL) within 48 hours after application of a contrast agent lasting for a minimum of 2 days.[127,128] Patients at risk for developing CIN include:

- Patients with pre-existing renal disease
- Patients with type II diabetes regardless of age
- Elderly, aged, and dehydrated patients
- Patients on nephrotoxic medication
- Patients following prolonged hypotension
- Patient following high contrast media exposure (>200 mL), repeated contrast media exposures, or the application of high-osmolarity agents

Measures to prevent CIN are summarized in Table 8-17.

Admission and procedural rules for high-risk CIN patients undergoing PCI include:

- Hospitalization 2 days prior to PCI
- Adequate hydration and judicious use of diuretics!
- Staging diagnostic coronary angiography and PCI by >10 days
- Avoiding other procedures requiring contrast agents
- Using biplane angiography, if available
- Consideration of preventive hemodialysis in high-risk patients with high contrast exposure[129]

In patients developing CIN despite preventive measures, the severity of renal dysfunction can be determined using the glomerular filtration rate (GFR) or using measurements of

creatinine clearance calculated with the Cockcroft and Gault equation[130]: Creatinine clearance (mL/min) = (140 − age in years) × (body weight in kg)/72 × creatinine concentration in serum (mg/100 mL). When creatinine serum concentrations are measured in SI units (μmol/L), it is necessary to multiply the results by 0.82 in males and 0.85 in females.[131] Table 8-18 is a summary of stages of chronic renal insufficiency based on GFR measurements.

Management of patients with established CIN includes:

- Transfer to intensive care unit where acute hemodialysis is available
- Close monitoring of input and output
- Daily determination of creatinine, urea, electrolytes for 5 days as needed
- Consultations with nephrologists as needed

Table 8-19 summarizes recommended measures for treating CIN.

In addition to the negative prognostic significance of renal insufficiency, the high incidence of extensive coronary artery calcifications in these patients should be taken into consideration when determining the revascularization strategy.[132,133]

Patients with Thyroid Disease

Application of iodinated contrast agents during PCI is associated with massive iodine exposure. However, although ~15 to 100 g of iodine, corresponding to 1500 to 10,000 times the total iodine content of the human body, is applied, only a fraction of this amount, approximately 0.1 to 0.001%(0.5 to 36 μg/mL) is biologically active free inorganic iodine. In addition, some free iodine is generated by deiodination of the organically bound iodine (~0.1 to 0.2% of the total administered dose within 1 hour of exposure).[134] The free iodine may, however, induce thyrotoxicosis in susceptible patients such as those with hyperthyroid disease, immunologically based thyroid disease, or autonomic thyroid tissue, and multinodular goiter in individuals living in endemic iodide-deficient regions and in patients receiving certain medications (e.g., amiodarone, expectorants) and having particular nutritional habits (e.g., kelp ingestion).

Iodide-induced thyrotoxicosis (IIT) may be associated with sustained adverse cardiovascular effects including atrial and ventricular arrhythmias, conduction abnormalities, and heart failure. Life-threatening symptoms of persistent heart failure and dysrhythmias may occur in compromised patients.[135,136]

To reduce the risk of IIT, systematic screening is required prior to PCI. A standard checklist includes:

- Assessment of the history of thyroid disease
- Exclusion of offensive medication
- Palpation of the thyroid gland
- Laboratory examinations (thyroid-stimulating hormone [TSH] assay is performed; if below normal, free triiodothyronine [T3] and, less frequently, free tetraiodothyronine [fT4] are measured).

Preventive measures prior to PCI are recommended in patients at risk for IIT. Extended drug treatment is mandatory in patients at risk and in those with thyrotoxicosis and vital indications for PCI (Table 8-20). In stable patients with overt hyperthyroidosis, PCI is deferred until the thyroid function has been normalized.

TABLE 8-16. Check list and Recommendations for Percutaneous Coronary Intervention (PCI) Admission of Patients with Type II Diabetes

Time	Recommendation	Comment
DAY 1 BEFORE INTERVENTION	Admission	Check and stabilize
	Laboratory studies	
	Blood glucose	Normal fasting range 80–120 mg% (4.4–6.7 mmol/L); Glucose >140 mg% (6.7 mmol/L) correct and recheck in 2 h as needed
	Hemoglobin HbA_{1c}	$HbA_{1c} \geq 6.5\%$ suboptimal long-term control of glycemia indicates greater metabolic instability
	Albumin in urine	Normal range 20–200 µg/min; albumin >200 µg/min or >300 mg/24 h or >200 mg/L indicates renal nephropathy
	Creatinine cleareance	Normal range >90mL/min, creatinine clearance <15 mL/min corresponds to terminal renal failure
	Medication	
	Continue all standard medication	
	Stop long-acting diuretics in dehydrated patients	Encourage fluid intake and/or start intravenous infusion in severely dehydrated patients intravenous infusion
	Stop biguanides (metformin!) from at least 24 h before to 24 h after PCI	Small but defined danger of lactic acidosis with potentially intractable circulatory shock secondary to biguanides!
	Prescribe 600 mg acetylcystein qd for 3 weeks	
	Scheduling	
	Schedule PCI for early morning	
DAY OF PCI	Perform PCI in early morning	
	Laboratory studies	
	Blood glucose q 2–4 h	Correct with short-acting intravenous or subcutaneous insulin or 5% glucose IV as needed
	Creatine, creatinine clearance, urea, potassium, natrium	Correct with fluids and/or electrolytes
	Urine output (mL/h) as needed	Place urinary catheter as needed
	Strict input-output records in advanced renal insufficiency	Arrange for post-PCI hemodialysis as needed
	Medication	
	Continue all medication except biguanides	
	Give half regular insulin dose while patient NPO (nulla per os; nil by mouth)	
	Encourage fluid intake, hydrate as needed	
DAY 1 AFTER PCI	*Laboratory studies*	
	Blood glucose q 6 h as needed	
	Creatine, creatinine clearance, urea, potassium, natrium daily post PCI to reach baseline function	
	Medication	
	Continue all medication except biguanides	

Patients with Allergy

Adverse responses to iodine contrast agents (ICA) occur in ~5% to 10% of patients, although they are very mild in the majority of cases. Moderate to severe adverse responses have been estimated at 1% to 2% and fatalities at ~0.001% (0.0003% to 0.0026%) of ICA applications. Use of nonionic low-osmolality contrast agents is associated with less patient discomfort and may be safer.[137] The differences between contrast agents have been rarely statistically meaningful in the conducted trials because of the low frequency of target events.[138]

Allergylike and true allergy responses are more common in patients with a history of:

- Asthma
- Food allergies to iodine containing seafood and shellfish (e.g., scallops and shrimp)
- Metal allergies such as nickel, cobalt, manganese
- Allergies to medications

In predisposed patients, the symptoms are not only more frequent but also frequently more severe.

TABLE 8-17. Prevention of Contrast-induced Nephropathy (CIN)

Issue	Measure
Nephrotoxic medication, long acting diuretics	Discontinue all nonessential offenders such as nonsteroidal anti-inflammatory drugs (NSAID)
	Stop long-acting diuretics 48–72 h prior to PCI; warning: Patients with heart failure
Contrast agent	Use iso-osmolar, dimeric, nonionic iodinated contrast agents (e.g., iodixanol)
	Avoid high-osmolar contrast media
	Limit dose to a minimum
Hydration	Encourage fluid intake
	Provide IV fluids, e.g., 0.9% NaCl 1 mL/kg/h for 6–12 h before and 12–24 h after PCI; warning: Patients with heart failure
N-acetylcysteine	600 bid p.o. or 150 mg/kg IV 30 min infusion
Laboratory examinations	Check creatinine and electrolytes daily for 2–3 days after PCI
Diuresis	Check daily input and output for 2–3 days after PCI

Modified from Gleeson TG, O'Dwyer J, Bulugahapitiya S, et al. Contrast-induced nephropathy. *Br J Cardiol.* 2004;11:53–61.

Although the exact mechanism of adverse responses to ICA has not been established, usually nonanaphylactoid (chemotoxic, vasovagal, and idiopathic) and anaphylactoid (idiosyncratic "allergylike" and true allergic) responses are distinguished. Nonanaphylactoid chemotoxic responses may be dose dependent and include primarily nephrotoxic and neurotoxic as well as some cardiovascular effects (e.g., arrhythmogenicity). Anaphylactoid responses may be nonspecific reactions due to as yet unknown mediators or they may be mediated by antibodies (IgE) or T lymphocytes. Nearly all severe responses occur within minutes (≤20 minutes) following ICA exposure. In some cases late responses (up to 7 and more days), consisting usually of mild urticaria, bronchospasm, or renal dysfunction, may occur.

Based on the symptoms, several grades of severity may be distinguished. The majority of responses are very mild, consisting of urticaria, pruritus, and diaphoresis without systemic symptoms (grade 1). Grade 2 is associated with mild to moderate dyspnea due to laryngeal edema and bronchospasm, hypotension due to vasodilatation, and abdominal symptoms (nausea, vomiting, abdominal pain). In grade 3 moderate to severe dyspnea and

TABLE 8-18. Stages of Chronic Renal Insufficiency (CRI)

Stage	Description	GFR (mL/min/1.73 m²)
1	Renal damage with normal or elevated GFR	≥90
2	Renal damage with mildly decreased GFR	60–89
3	Renal damage with moderately decreased GFR	30–59
4	Renal damage with severely decreased GFR	15–29
5	Kidney failure	<15

GRF, glomerular filtration rate.

Modified from National Kidney Foundation. K/DOQI clinical practice guidelines for chronic kidney disease: evaluation, classification and stratification. 2002;39(2suppl1):S1–S266.

TABLE 8-19. Suggested Management of Patients with Contrast-Induced Nephropathy (CIN)

Issue	Measure
Hyperkalemia	
<5.0 mmol/L	Restrict dietary intake (<40 mmol/day)
	Stop potassium-sparing diuretics
5.0–6.5 mmol/L	Give potassium binding ion-exchange resin (e.g., 15 g resonium tid or qid)
	Give loop diuretics (warning: oliguria)
>6.5 mmol/L	Give insulin-dextrose IV infusion (10 U short-acting insulin in 50 mL 50% dextrose)
	Give 50–100 mmol sodium bicarbonate IV infusion
	Give 10 mL 10% calcium gluconate IV short infusion over 5 min
	Consider hemodialysis if treatment resistant and/or with arrhythmias
Volume overload	Restrict fluid intake (<1 L/day)
	Restrict NaCl (2–4 g/day)
	Give loop diuretics and thiazides as needed
	Consider hemodialysis if resistant and/or heart failure
Metabolic acidosis	Restrict protein intake (0.6–0.8 g/kg/day)
	Give sodium bicarbonate IV infusion as needed for pH art. >7.2
Hyperphosphatemia	Restrict phosphate intake (<800 mg/day)
	Give phosphate binders (e.g., calcium carbonate or aluminum hydroxide)
Acute renal failure	Rapidly rising urea and creatinine, falling urine output (oliguria 100–400 mL/day, anuria <100 mL/day; if urine output <0.5 mL/kg/hr for >2 hours investigate!; if creatinine >500–1000 μmol/L, urea >20 mmol/L, hyperkalaemia >7.5 mmol/L, metabolic acidosis pH <7.2 get nephrologist involved early, plan for hemodialysis

Modified from Kolonko A, Wiecek A. Contrast-associated nephropathy—old clinical problem, and new therapeutic perspectives. *Nephrol Dial Trasplant.* 1998;13:803-806.

profound hypotension occur. Grade 4 refers to severe cardiocirculatory and pulmonary compromise and/or arrest.

Prophylactic medication is recommended for all predisposed patients and for those with previous adverse responses to ICA. The suggested oral regimen among accepted protocols consists of:

- Prednisone 50 mg PO 12, 6, and 1 hour prior to exposure
- Diphenhydramine, H1-antihistamine, 50 mg PO 12 and 1 hour prior to exposure
- Ranitidine, H2-histamine receptor blocker, 50 mg PO 1 hour prior to exposure.

TABLE 8-20. Prevention of Iodine-induced Hyperthyroidism in Patients Undergoing Percutaneous Coronary Interventions

Prevention in susceptible patients	900 mg (20 drops t.i.d.) perchlorate/day (300 mg = 1 mL = 20 drops)
	Give at least 2 to 4 h prior to contrast exposure
	Continue for 14 days
Prophylaxis in patients with overt hyperthyroidosis	900 mg (20 drops t.i.d.) perchlorate/day 20-80 mg thiamizole/day
	Give at least 2 to 4 h prior to contrast exposure
	Continue as needed

An intravenous regimen can alternatively be given in patients unable to take oral medication.

Immediate treatment is necessary when symptoms suggestive of adverse responses to ICA occur during PCI. In patients with moderate to severe symptoms, immediate supplementary oxygen, intravenous administration of fluids, and intramuscular administration of adrenalin (0.5 mL of 1:1000 solution) are required. Because of the potential, albeit small, risk of cardiopulmonary arrest, the PCI operator must be thoroughly familiar with manifestations and management of anaphylactic shock and full-scale resuscitation (for review, see references 139–141). Table 8-21 provides a summary of the recommended adverse reaction ICA management.

In patients with pronounced vasovagal responses during PCI, typical treatment consists of:

- Fluid intravenous (IV) supplementation using crystalline solution (e.g., Ringer lactate) or plasma expander (e.g., starch derivatives such as HAES 6%)
- Atropine 0.5 to 1.0 mg IV
- Catecholamines (dopamine, dobutamine) IV, if needed.

PCI should not be resumed before stable blood pressure (systolic BP ≥100 mm Hg) and heart rate have been restored in a fully asymptomatic patient.

Elderly and Aged Patients

At present the majority of patients undergoing PCI are 60 to 75 years old with the proportion of patients >75 years of age (including those older than 85) growing. Advancing age has been associated with worse outcome following plain balloon angioplasty[142,143] and stent-supported angioplasty.[144,145] In fact, the outcome progressively worsens with an increase in age indicated as a continuous and discrete variable.[146] Typical examples of the effects of advancing age on outcome following coronary intervention are shown in Tables 8-22 and 23 and Figure 8-17.

Although not necessarily a risk factor by itself, age serves as a pathophysiological marker for a more advanced coronary artery disease (greater complexity of CAD, greater proportion of multivessel disease) and increasing incidence of comorbidities as shown in Table 8-24.[147]

Although the current ACC/AHA PCI guidelines abstained from special recommendations regarding PCI in the elderly[81] (except for recommendations regarding primary PCI in cardiogenic shock), it is obvious that elderly and aged patients considered for coronary interventions constitute a special group requiring special considerations and strategic planning, including those concerning complete versus palliative revascularization, procedural staging, and early mobilization to reduce procedural risk.

TABLE 8-21. Recommended Prevention and Treatments for Adverse Responses to Iodinated Contrast Agents

PREVENTION (HIGH RISK PATIENT)	*50 mg diphenhydramine or equivalent antihistamine iv* *300 mg cimetidine or equivalent H2-receptor antagonist iv* *50 mg prednisolone or equivalent corticosteroid*		

TREATMENT

	Severity		
Symptom	Mild	Moderate	Severe
Urticaria	50 mg diphenhydramine or equivalent antihistamine IV	50 mg diphenhydramine or equivalent antihistamine IV 300 mg cimetidine or equivalent H2-receptor antagonist IV 50 mg prednisolone or equivalent corticosteroid	50 mg diphenhydramine or equivalent antihistamine IV 300 mg cimetidine or euuivalent H2-receptor antagonist IV 125 mg prednisolone or equivalent corticosteroid
Bronchospasm	Oxygen 2–4 L/min via nasal prongs Bronchodilator, e.g., 2 puffs β-2 agonist fenoterol	Oxygen via face mask Epinephrine 1:1000 (1 mg = 1 mL) 0.1–0.3 mL sc q 10–15 min up to 1 mL (= 1 mg epinephrine)	Oxygen via face mask Epinephrine 1:1000 (1 mg = 1mL dilute with 0.9% NaCl up to 10 mL with resulting 1:10,000) 10 mL IV bolus over 5 min, repeat q 10 min as needed Prepare for intubation and mechanical ventilation
Laryngeal edema	Oxygen via face mask Epinephrine 1:1000 (1 mg = 1 mL) 0.1–0.3 mL sc q 10–15 min up to 1 mL (= 1 mg epinephrine)	Oxygen via face mask Epinephrine 1:1000 (1 mg =1 ml) 0.1–0.3 mL sc q 10–15 min up to 1 mL (=1 mg epinephrine) Prepare for intubation and mechanical ventilation	Epinephrine 1:1000 (1 mg = 1 mL dilute with 0.9% NaCl up to 10 mL with resulting 1:10,000) 10 mL IV bolus over 5 min, repeat q 10 min as needed Intubate
Massive dyspnoe, hypotension, clouding of consciousness. incontinence	Shock management including high volume supplementation and catecholamines		
Cardiopulmonary arrest	Full scale cardiopulmonary resuscitation		

Adapted from Siddiqui NH. Contrast medium reactions, recognition and treatment. Available at: www.emedicine.com/ radio/topic864.htm. Accessed June 12, 2005.

TABLE 8-22. Outcomes of Percutaneous Coronary Intervention at 30 Day and 1 Year Stratified by Age

| | Age, Years | | | | |
	<55	55–65	65–75	>75	*p*
PATIENTS, *N*	749	590	470	273	
30-D OUTCOMES, %					
Death	0.8	1.2	3.6	4.8	<0.0001
Reinfarction	0.8	1.0	1.1	0.0	0.41
Disabling stroke	0.0	0.2	0.2	0.4	0.52
Ischemic target vessel revascularization	3.5	3.2	3.2	4.1	0.91
Composite major adverse events	4.6	4.8	7.3	8.8[a]	0.02
Subacute thrombosis	1.1	0.7	1.3	0.4	0.55
Moderate/severe bleeding	1.7	3.6	4.1	6.3	0.002
Any stroke	0.4	0.5	1.9	1.1	0.027
Intracranial hemorrhage	0.0	0.0	0.2	0.0	0.32
1-Y OUTCOMES, %					
Death	1.6	2.1	7.1	11.1	<0.0001
Cardiac	1.1	1.2	5.1	7.2	<0.0001
Noncardiac	0.5	0.9	2.0	3.9	0.0005
Reinfarction	1.9	2.6	3.4	1.6	0.35
Disabling stroke	0.3	0.3	0.9	1.2[b]	0.23
Ischemic target vessel revascularization	15.4	11.8	11.7	13.3	0.15
Composite major adverse events	17.5	14.1	18.9	23.6	0.004
Subacute or late thrombosis	1.1	0.7	1.5	0.4	0.40
Moderate/severe bleeding	2.2	3.6	5.1	8.0	0.003
Any stroke	0.7	1.0	3.3	3.1	0.001
Intracranial hemorrhage, %	0.0	0.5	0.6	0.8	0.14

[a]*p*<0.01 vs. age <55 years.
[b]*p* = 0.08 vs. age <55 years.
Reproduced with permission from Guagliumi G, Stone GW, Cox DA, et al. Outcome in elderly patients undergoing primary coronary intervention for acute myocardial infarction: results from the controlled abciximab and device investigation to lower late angioplasty complications (CADILLAC) trial. *Circulation.* 2004;110:1598–1604.

TABLE 8-23. Outcomes of Percutaneous Coronary Intervention at 1 Year Stratified by Age

| | Incidence (%) by Age | | |
Adverse Event	<65 Years (*n* = 2377)	65–79 Years (*n* = 1690)	≥80 years (*n* = 286)
Death	2.1	4.9	11.0
MI	5.8	7.0	9.4
CABG	6.5	7.1	6.4
Death/MI	6.8	10.1	16.7
Death/MI/CABG	12.2	16.3	22.6

MI, myocardial infarction; CABG, coronary artery bypass grafting.
Modified from Cohen HA, Williams DO, Holmes DR Jr., et al. Impact of age on procedural and 1-year outcome in percutaneous transluminal coronary angioplasty: a report from the NHLBI dynamic registry. *Am Heart J.* 2003;146:513–519.

Panvascular Patients

Patients with clinically significant disease in at least two major vascular territories (panvascular patients) are mostly diabetics at any age and the elderly (>65 and <75 years) individuals carrying a higher risk of interventions.[100,148] Knowledge of the panvascular status based on a more extensive pre-PCI vascular workup is important for implementing risk reduction strategies. In addition, comprehensive panendovascular or hybrid strategies of global revascularizations might reduce the overall procedural risk and should be considered in all relevant cases.[149]

Severely Ill Patients

Severely and terminally ill patients (assumed life expectancy ≤6 months) include patients with a chronic terminal disease complicated by CAD and patients with life-threatening CAD

A Age <70

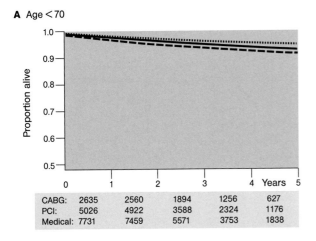

CABG:	2635	2560	1894	1256	627
PCI:	5026	4922	3588	2324	1176
Medical:	7731	7459	5571	3753	1838

B Age 70–79

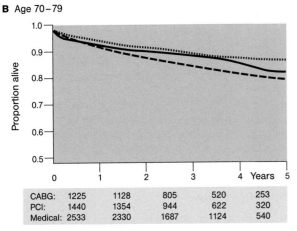

CABG:	1225	1128	805	520	253
PCI:	1440	1354	944	622	320
Medical:	2533	2330	1687	1124	540

C Age 80+

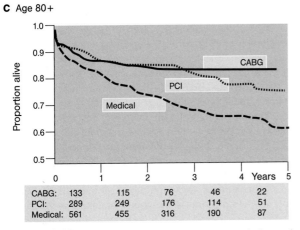

CABG:	133	115	76	46	22
PCI:	289	249	176	114	51
Medical:	561	455	316	190	87

FIGURE 8-17. Kaplan-Meier curves of patient survival over time for three age groups A–C as outlined, following percutaneous coronary intervention. (Adapted from Graham MM, Ghali WA, Faris PD, et al. Survival after coronary revascularization in the elderly. *Circulation.* 2002;105:2378.)

associated with major neurological deficits, and/or multiorgan failure without prior terminal disease.

Patients with terminal disease complicated by CAD are usually not considered candidates for surgical revascularization, and definitive or palliative PCI represents an option in principle in most cases. In patients with life-threatening CAD, percutaneous treatment is offered in most cases as a primary mode of treatment. In contrast to conventional emergency PCI, in this cohort of severely ill patients not only the target lesions but all critical coronary lesions should be revascularized in one stage. To avoid futile treatments, however, an interdisciplinary consensus and the patient's declared will are required. Decision making should consider:

- Degree of severity and expected reversibility of the hemodynamic and electrical compromise
- Severity, complexity, and technical accessibility of the CAD
- Severity and expected reversibility of the LV dysfunction
- Status of the terminal disease
- Presence and expected reversibility of major neurological deficits
- Presence and severity of other comorbid conditions
- Critical risk and benefit assessment

In patients with terminal disease presenting with a critical CAD, all medical and relevant social aspects of the disease and intended treatment should be broached and discussed.

RISK ASSESSMENT; TARGET LESION-RELATED FACTORS

Assessment of diagnostic coronary angiograms in patients considered for PCI includes determining the status of the target interventional site (target lesion, target vessel, target ostium) and that of nontarget vessels (see Chapter 3B for details). In addition, LVF, the ascending aorta and aortic arch, and the vascular path from the access to the target ostium are evaluated. Based on these factors the strategy of the intervention and instrumentation is selected. Selection of the strategy depends on a clear understanding of the risks and benefits. Selection of the instrumentation depends on the understanding of the performance characteristics of the endovascular instrumentation to meet the anatomical requirements. Lack of direct visual inspection of the interventional site in interventional techniques (as opposed to surgery) explains some of the intricacies facing the interventionist. Thus, for an optimal PCI correct reading and interpretation of the angiograms are the most critical issues in design and execution of the individual interventions. Whereas during the planning stage the operator makes theoretical assumptions based on his previous experience, during the intervention he must integrate visualization (imaging equipment), vision (eye), interpretation (brain), and tactile feedback of manipulation (hand) into a real-time and frequently instantaneous action. To become eventually an informed intuition common to master operators, each step of this process must be understood, studied, and trained.

The prognostic relevance of target lesion and target vessel morphology for the outcome of coronary interventions was pointed out by the 1988 American College of Cardiology/American Heart Association (ACC/AHA) angiographic classification of coronary artery lesions into A–C types.[150] At that time the expected success rates were >85% for type A lesions, 60% to 85% for moderately complex type B lesions, and <60% for complex type C lesions. Successful angioplasty was defined as a ≥20% increase in luminal diameter with the final diameter stenosis <50% in the absence of major complications including death, acute myocardial infarction, or the need for emergency bypass.[150] The clinical relevance of the ACC/AHA lesion classification has been proven by several

TABLE 8-24. Increase in Multimorbidity with Age

Variables and Comorbidities	Age		
	<65 Years (n = 2537)	65–79 Years (n = 1776)	≥80 Years (n = 307)
Female (%)[a]	27.7	43.6	59.0
Prior PCI (%)	27.4	31.8	26.4
Prior CABG (%)[a]	12.3	22.3	19.9
Prior MI (%)	35.4	37.1	35.8
History of diabetes	27.3	29.8	26.6
History of CHF (%)[a]	5.4	13.5	25.2
CHF during hospitalization (%)[a]	5.1	10.5	15.8
History of hypertension (%)[a]	55.6	68.9	70.7
History of hypercholesterolemia (%)[a]	65.3	60.5	44.8
Noncardiac disease (%)[a]	24.0	40.0	47.0
Cerebrovascular (%)[a]	3.8	8.5	12.8
Renal (%)[a]	3.0	5.4	6.6
Peripheral vascular disease (%)[a]	5.2	9.5	11.2
Pulmonary (%)[a]	5.9	9.6	13.2
Cancer (%)[a]	2.9	9.5	14.8

[a]$p < 0.001$.

Selected demographic and clinical characteristics are shown (4620 patients treated with percutaneous coronary intervention, PCI, between 1997–1999 and stratified by age <65 years, 65–79 years and ≥80 years). CABG, coronary artery bypass grafting; MI, myocardial infarction; CHF, congestive heart failure. Modified from Cohen HA, Williams DO, Holmes DR Jr., et al. Impact of age on procedural and 1-year outcome in percutaneous transluminal coronary angioplasty: a report from the NHLBI dynamic registry. *Am Heart J.* 2003;146:513–519.

investigators.[151–153] Ellis et al. proposed further subclassification of type B lesions into B1 (i.e., lesions with one B criterion) and B2 (i.e., lesions with >1 B criterion).[151] In the same study, high-grade, bend, and bifurcation stenoses, chronic total occlusions, and male gender were highlighted as negative prognostic factors. An analogous subclassification of type C lesions was introduced by Myler et al.[152] In this study, the presence of a thrombus, increasing lesion length, diffuse disease, calcification, and angulated, high-grade (>95%) and bifurcation lesions were identified as negative prognostic factors.

In an attempt to improve the prognostic significance of angiographic coronary lesions, the Society of Coronary Angiography and Interventions (SCAI) introduced a group I–IV classification.[154] However, with the broad availability of stents, evolving instrumentation, and better technical skills, the prognostic implications of lesion morphology has begun to change, reducing the overall need for complex classifications. Thus, although different lesions are still associated with different prognoses with regard to technical success and long-term outcome, the use of stents and antiplatelet medication has clearly attenuated the prognostic significance of their morphology. At present the majority of coronary lesions (>90%) can be revascularized with results comparable to those of type A lesions on the ACC/AHA classification. The remaining ~10% of lesions are technically more difficult to treat and have a higher risk of complications. Whereas in the former group the operator's experience and mastery may not be as critical, in the latter group they are the most critical determinant of outcome. At present, as in 1980s, the lowest technical success rates are achieved in revascularizations of chronic total occlusions (CTOs); defined as occlusions older than 3 months.

Uncomplicated Lesions

ACC/AHA type A[150] or SCAI type I lesions[154] are considered uncomplicated, and technical and procedural success is >90%. The majority of direct stenting PCI is performed on this subset of lesions. However, the availability of stents and particularly of DES has considerably expanded the scope of angiographic lesions which now may be considered prognostically equivalent to uncomplicated lesions. Figure 8-14 provides an example of a formal type C (lesion >20 mm) ACC/AHA classification lesion now considered amenable to direct stenting. Thus, lesions without a thrombus, heavy calcification, and/or highly complex morphology may be considered prognostically equivalent to uncomplicated lesions. It should be kept in mind that an uncomplicated lesion can become complicated if the proximal access is difficult. Moreover, angiographic visualization might not tell the whole story: "surprise" complexity of a presumably uncomplicated lesion (and vice versa!) might become evident only in the course of the intervention. It is the dynamics of changes of lesions undergoing interventions that ultimately decides on their dignity. Careful attention to the findings of the intermediary angiograms throughout the intervention is important to recognize a lesion initially classified as benign that is turning critical during the course of the intervention.

Thrombotic Lesions

Thrombotic lesions have been considered high-risk type B or type C on the ACC/AHA classification.[150,152,155] Although the advent of stents and antiplatelet agents has mitigated some of the adversities associated with the mechanically and biologically unstable thrombotic lesions,[156,157] their treatment still carries a higher risk of complications. In fact, full prognostic significance of thrombotic lesions as the source of proximal (target site) and distal (microcirculatory) complications has only recently been fully recognized (for review, see reference 158). Thrombus formation accompanies unstable lesions; in patients with acute coronary syndromes it is almost obligatory. However, compared to coronary angioscopy, the ability of coronary angiography to detect a thrombus is limited (Figs. 8-18 to 8-20).[159] Using angioscopy as a point of reference, angiography detects only ~20% of thrombi.[160,161] Although the presence of thrombi is associated with increased interventional risk of, for example, reocclusion, reinfarction, and death, the actual degree of risk may vary considerably.[155–157] In addition to *primary* thrombi detected on the initial angiograms, *secondary* thrombus formation may occasionally be visualized in the course of an intervention in patients with multiple critical lesions, poor coronary flow, poor LVF, procoagulatory syndromes, or inadequate anticoagulation, and patients undergoing long and complex procedures.

Acute totally occlusive coronary thrombi are depicted as occluded vessels lacking collaterals, and subtotally occlusive thrombi are shown as intraluminal fixed or floating filling defects in stenotic segments. In emergency interventions in patients with multiple coronary artery occlusions it is critical for the operator to identify the "culprit" acute occlusion. Attempts to revascularize chronic total occlusions while leaving the infarct lesion untouched may be fatal in high-risk patients. In the absence of collateral vessels the distinction between acute closure and CTO might be difficult. Careful review of angiograms before beginning the intervention is critical. In difficult crossing, another careful review of angiograms may give the operator cues to revise PCI strategy.

Particularly in high-risk patients and in patients presenting with a protracted prehospital course, multiple thrombi may be found. Some thrombi may be sharply demarcated while others are displayed as intraluminal haziness. In some cases even large thrombi are angiographically visible only by indirect signs such as "no flow" or "slow flow." The distinction between a thrombus and an embolus on angiography is unreliable. The absence of

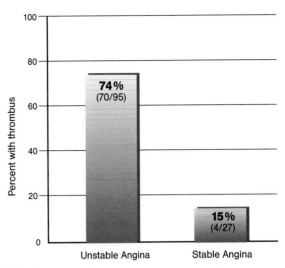

FIGURE 8-19. Incidence of angioscopic thrombi in patients with unstable and stable angina pectoris. (Modified from White CJ, Ramee SR, Collins TJ, et al. Coronary thrombi increase PTCA risk: angioscopy as a clinical tool. *Circulation.* 1996;93:253–258.)

angiographic evidence for atherosclerosis (smooth endothelial interfaces) and the presence of arrhythmias or intracardiac masses suggest embolus.

The principle treatment options include mechanical extraction, dilatation/stenting with the administration of GIIb/IIIa platelet aggregation inhibitors, fibrinolysis, or any combination of these with or without thromboembolic protection devices.

Mechanical extraction shows promise in proximal fresh totally occlusive thrombi, provided it can be performed by an experienced operator. Before deploying the thrombectomy device, the feasibility and the risks of mechanical injury and downstream embolization should be assessed. In most devices, ≥7F systems are required, and a concomitant administration of GIIb/IIIa platelet inhibitors is obligatory in the absence of contraindications. In patients with distal thrombi, diffuse disease, difficult proximal segment, or high plaque burden, mechanical thrombectomy

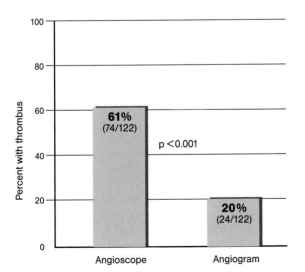

FIGURE 8-18. Incidence of angiographic versus angioscopic thrombi. (Modified from White CJ, Ramee SR, Collins TJ, et al. Coronary thrombi increase PTCA risk: angioscopy as a clinical tool. *Circulation.* 1996;93: 253–258.)

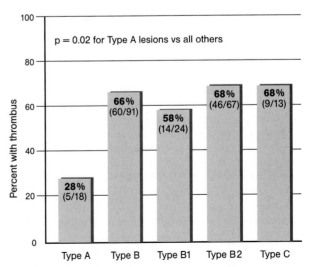

FIGURE 8-20. Incidence of angioscopic thrombi among ACC/AHA lesion categories. (Modified from White CJ, Ramee SR, Collins TJ, et al. Coronary thrombi increase PTCA risk: angioscopy as a clinical tool. *Circulation.* 1996;93:253–258.)

cannot be recommended. Figure 8-21 provides an example of failed mechanical thrombectomy in a distal location.

The majority of thrombotic lesions are presently treated by administering GP IIb/IIIa platelet receptor inhibitors early and using a guidewire and balloon to recanalize occlusions and stenting the culprit lesion. Distal protection devices (DPDs) should be considered in all interventions involving saphenous vein grafts (SVGs) (exception: diffusely degenerated SVG), in large thrombus masses, and whenever possible in "the last remaining" vessel, in cases with reduced LVF or a large amount of jeopardized rest myocardium. To successfully deploy the DPD the target vessel should be large (≥3.5 mm diameter) and allow for deployment distal to the target lesion.

Fibrinolytic agents are rarely used to treat thrombotic lesions in the catheterization laboratory because of their low efficacy compared to PCI. Possible exceptions are patients with highly diffuse coronary artery disease and multiple thrombotic lesions, and patients in whom PCI access to the target lesion failed. In the absence of contraindications, superselective or locoregional intracoronary fibrinolysis should be considered in these patients. In these cases one of the second- or third-generation selective thrombolytic agents should be administered via OTW catheters. The efficacy of fibrinolytic agents as a measure of last resort in resilient cases associated with distal embolizations, subtotal distal occlusions, and slow antegrade coronary artery flow is, however, doubtful. In contrast, in all cases, the definite risk of bleeding complications must be taken into account.

The formation of *secondary de novo* thrombi during PCI prompts an immediate review of angiograms to exclude mechanical causes (intimal flaps, dissections, deformed struts). In addition, activated clotting time (ACT) is assessed. Mechanical causes of thrombus formation must be addressed and eliminated immediately. ACT <250 seconds is corrected by an additional dose of unfractionated heparin (up to 5000 U UFH). In addition, in the absence of contraindications, GP IIb/IIIa platelet receptor inhibitors are administered, preferably using the intracoronary route. Fibrinolytic agents are usually not indicated. In rare cases, persistent thrombosis associated with clinical instability may require prompt consultation with a cardiac surgeon to review surgical options.

Calcified Lesions

Vascular calcifications are hydroxyapatite crystal deposits within the intima and, less frequently, the media[162] resulting from passive physicochemical and active cellular processes.[163]

Coronary artery lesions are frequently calcified, yet the low sensitivity of angiography often leaves them undetected. Thus, compared to IVUS, coronary angiography detects only 25% of one-quadrant calcium, 50% of two-quadrant calcium, 60% of three-quadrant calcium, and 85% of four-quadrant calcium lesions (Table 8-25 and Fig. 8-22). In addition, better angiographic visibility of superficial and extensively circumferential calcifications has been described (Figs. 8-23, 8-24).[164]

Because the mass attenuation coefficient of calcium is greater than that of soft tissues,[165] calcium deposits are seen as dark and usually irregularly shaped spots or "railroad tracks" in the course of the coronary artery on native films. They are typically located in the proximal to middle coronary segments. With increasing energy (kilo–electron volts, keV) of x-ray radiation, the difference between the mass attenuation coefficients for

calcium and soft tissues decreases, making detection of calcifications more difficult, as seen for example in obese patients.

Calcified lesions may be "bad" or "good" news.[166,167]: they may destabilize the lesion by increasing the heterogeneity of stress distribution across the arterial wall (primarily probable in plaques with superficial calcification), but they may also increase the mechanical stability via a "natural stenting" effect (most likely in deeper calcifications). In addition, the prevention of positive remodeling might actually contribute to plaque stabilization (see Chapter 1 for review).

Heavily calcified lesions are rigid and therefore more difficult to dilate; dilatations require higher inflation pressures associated with lower technical success[168] and a higher risk of complications,[169] particularly of dissections.[170]

In patients with proximal high-grade extensively calcified lesions, IVUS should be considered to assess the feasibility and risk of the intervention. Yet, the accessibility of these lesions to IVUS probes is frequently limited, leaving the operator no other option but to rely on angiography. To reduce risk, heavily calcified high-grade proximal LAD lesions that are difficult to assess should be operated in most cases. In patients with less heavily calcified lesions, standard DES-supported angioplasty can usually be performed safely. Stents with greater radial force may be required to counteract the low mechanical instability of dilated calcified lesions. Primary debulking using rotational atherectomy may be considered in some cases.[171,172]

Low-grade (<50%) proximal calcified lesions may complicate access to more distal high-grade (calcified or noncalcified) target lesions. "Unplanned" interventions on these proximal sites should be avoided by selecting the lowest profile instrumentation available, a gentle and meticulous technique associated with, and the least possible number of passages. Optimal selection of the guidewire is important to conduct PCI atraumatically. Medium stiffness of the tip, high shape retention, and high slipperiness are preferable in most cases. Increasing complexity of the target lesions increases the need for improved crossing ability, and thus for greater stiffness and better force transmission of the shaft. However, if shafts are too stiff they may stretch the artery by directing the advancing equipment into the walls. In doing so, the operator increases not only the friction (and force needed to overcome the resistance) but also the risk of dissection. In these cases, the potentials of different strategies, such as using two guidewires, should be explored. Once the guidewire has crossed the target lesion and has been securely placed, low-profile high-track balloon dilatation catheters and low-profile firm crimp stent delivery systems are critical to success. Direct stenting of calcified lesions requires a prior assessment of the dilatability of the lesion. Undersized balloon predilatations appear preferable in most cases.

Patients with extensive diffuse calcifications are poor candidates for PCI and coronary surgery, and consensus decisions of interventionists and surgeons usually determine the optimal approach. In patients selected for PCI, the principal options are focal and palliative coronary repair, plaque modification using excimer laser angioplasty, and extensive stenting using DES.

High Plaque Burden Lesions

Arterial enlargement may let an advanced atherosclerosis remain "hidden" without luminal encroachment[173] and keep it from being visualized by angiography. In addition, compared to

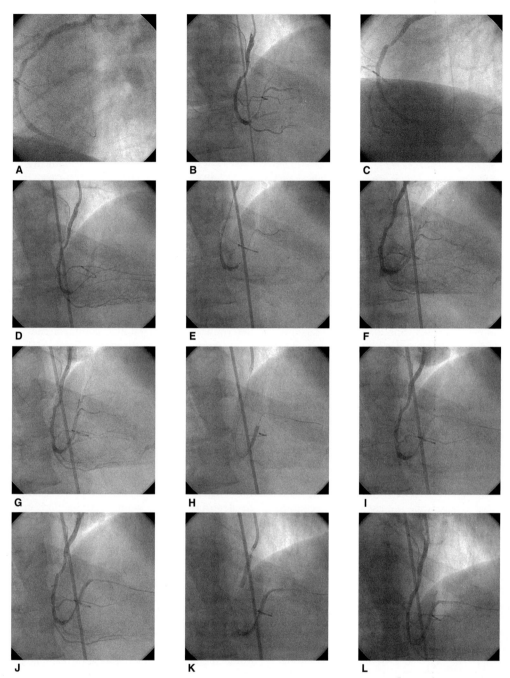

FIGURE 8-21. Failed thrombectomy percutaneous coronary intervention (PCI), right coronary artery (RCA). A 49-year-old man with an acute inferior ST elevation myocardial infarction (STEMI) involving the right ventricle, complete atrioventricular block requiring transvenous pacing, rhythm instability, and severe hemodynamic compromise requiring high catecholamine support and fibrinolysis prior to admission. Following intra-aortic balloon pump (IABP) placement, coronary angiography revealed two-vessel disease (RCA and left anterior descending artery, LAD) with marked right dominance. The infarct-related artery (IRA) RCA was a diffusely diseased vessel with a distal subtotal thrombotic occlusion (**A–C**). Guidewires were placed into the inferior interventricular and posterolateral ramus of the RCA (**D**). As outpatient thrombolytic treatment had failed, the decision was made to extract the thrombus using a thrombectomy device (Pronto, Vascular Solutions). Following device placement (**E**), the thrombus was removed, and the device retracted. Subsequent angiography revealed an extensive dissection distal to the crux, associated with a dissecting occlusion of the posterolateral ramus and subtotal occlusion of the inferior interventricular ramus (**F**). To allow stenting, a guidewire placed in the inferior interventricular ramus had to be removed, then two stents were placed in the posterolateral ramus (Lekton motion 3.0/25 mm and 3.5/25 mm at 10 bar, Biotronik) with "no-reflow" (**G–I**). Subsequently, the proximal dissection (**J**) was stented (3.5/25 mm Coroflex, Braun at 12 bar) (**K**) and TIMI II° into the posterolateral ramus, with persistent occlusion of the inferior interventricular ramus was achieved. Despite multiple redilatations and extensive pharmacotherapy including two additional intracoronary boluses of eptifibatide, "slow-flow" into the posterolateral ramus and "no-flow" of the inferior interventricular ramus persisted (**L**). Following consultation with cardiac surgeons the patient was referred for immediate coronary artery bypass surgery.

TABLE 8-25. Relation of Angiographic versus Intravascular Ultrasound Definition
of Coronary Lesions Calcification Patterns

	Coronary Angiography			
	None/Mild	Moderate	Severe	*p*
Number of lesions	715	306	134	
Intravascular ultrasound				
Target lesion calcium, n (%)	436 (61)	274 (90)	141 (98)	<.0001
Arc of calcium, degrees	71 ± 83	165 ± 106	238 ± 104	<.0001
Length of calcium, mm	2.5 ± 3.2	4.5 ± 3.5	6.2 ± 4.7	<.0001
Superficial calcium, n (%)	261 (37)	219 (72)	123 (92)	<.0001
Arc of superficial calcium, degrees	44 ± 74	124 ± 110	215 ± 119	<.0001
Length of superficial calcium, mm	1.5 ± 2.6	3.2 ± 3.1	5.7 ± 5.0	<.0001
Reference arc of calcium, degrees	25 ± 63	61 ± 93	87 ± 98	<.0001
Length of reference calcium, mm	1.0 ± 2.6	2.6 ± 4.8	3.3 ± 4.1	<.0001
Total length of calcium, mm	3.6 ± 4.4	7.2 ± 6.4	9.7 ± 6.4	<.0001

Modified from Mintz GS, Popma JJ, Pichard AD, et al. Patterns of clarification in coronary artery disease:
a statistical analysis of intravascular ultrasound and coronary angiography in 1155 lesions. *Circulation.*
1995;91:1959–1965.

IVUS, the ability of angiography to detect the geometry and morphology of lesions appears limited. Specifically, cross-sectional geometry (Tables 8-26 and 8-27; Fig. 8-25),[174] the longitudinal extent of atherosclerosis,[175] and atherosclerotic remodeling (Fig. 8-26) are imperfectly visualized by angiography (for review, see reference 176). Thus, in interpreting coronary angiograms the operator must be keenly aware of the fact that the true intramural extent and severity of coronary atherosclerosis may be underestimated and the true lesion morphology may be distorted.

Atherosclerotic lesions with a large plaque burden are either focal or diffuse. The amenability of focal high-grade lesions to dilatation depends on their tissue composition and circumferential distribution. Dilatability decreases with increasing rigidity and circumferential extent, while the risk of complications, dissection, and rupture increases at the same time. Because of

the limited ability of angiography to detect either of the two determinants of dilatability, complementary IVUS guidance is recommended in proximal focal high plaque burden lesions. When such lesions span the entire circumference, bypass revascularization should be considered. Alternatively, primary debulking using DCA, with or without IVUS guidance, may be reasonable.[177–179]

Coronary angiography may not detect lesions with a diffusely distributed large plaque burden (Fig. 8-27). In some cases diffuse discrete endoluminal irregularities, particularly when associated with distal stenoses or diffusely narrowed arteries supplying large territories, indicate a severe diffuse disease. In these patients flow-pressure wire measurements may be helpful in determining the optimal revascularization strategy. The hemodynamic relevance of both focal and diffuse disease can

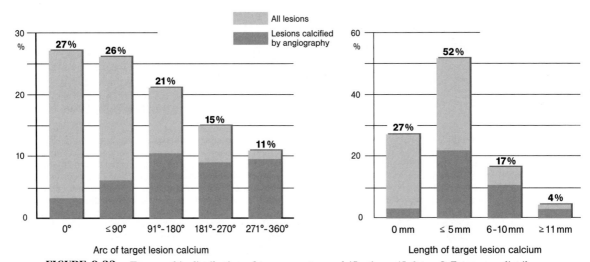

FIGURE 8-22. Topographic distribution of coronary artery calcifications. (*Left panel*) Frequency distribution of the maximum arc of intravascular ultrasound target lesion calcium. Coronary angiography detected 25% of one-quadrant calcium, 50% of two-quadrant calcium, 60% of three-quadrant calcium, and 85% of four-quadrant calcium. (*Right panel*) Frequency distribution of the lengths of intravascular ultrasound target lesion calcium. Coronary angiography detected 42% of calcium ≤5 mm in length, 63% of calcium 6 to 10 mm in length, and 61% of calcium >11 mm in length. (Modified from Mintz GS, Popma JJ, Pichard AD, et al. Patterns of calcification in coronary artery disease: a statistical analysis of intravascular ultrasound and coronary angiography in 1155 lesions. *Circulation.* 1995;91:1959–1965.)

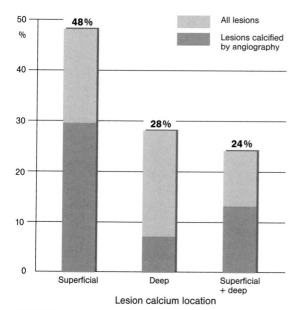

FIGURE 8-23. Distribution of lesion calcium locations according to depth. Coronary angiography detected superficial target lesion calcium, either alone (sensitivity, 60%) or in combination with deep calcium (sensitivity, 54%), more often than it detected isolated deep target lesion calcium (sensitivity, 24%, *P* <.0001). (Modified from Mintz GS, Popma JJ, Pichard AD, et al. Patterns of calcification in coronary artery disease: a statistical analysis of intravascular ultrasound and coronary angiography in 1155 lesions. *Circulation.* 1995;91:1959–1965.)

be determined using the pullback technique. Vigorous medical management is indicated in patients with distally decreased fractional flow reserve (FFR) and gradual normalization on pullback, whereas conventional PCI appears justified in patients with a focal significant decrease documented by FFR. In patients with both a diffuse and a focal reduction in FFR, additional factors such as limiting symptoms, risk profile, and

previous response to medical treatment are helpful to determine the most desirable approach to further management. In patients selected for PCI, focal atraumatic repair and maximum prevention are required.

INSTRUMENTATION

Angiographic findings determine the operator's selection of instrumentation, and optimal instrumentation is critical to technical success, procedural time, material costs, and minimizing the risk of the procedure. In this section, selected instrumentation for coronary interventions is reviewed; a more extensive discussion is provided in Chapter 5.

Puncture Needle, Introductory Guidewire, and Vascular Sheath

PUNCTURE NEEDLES

Purpose. Puncture needles are designed to allow smooth penetration of the skin and underlined tissue, atraumatic puncture of the vessel's front wall, and stable positioning of the tip within the lumen.

Requirements. Ideally, puncture needles are sharp and relatively stiff, allowing smooth penetration and good steering even in highly fibrotic or calcified tissues. A large bore is required to allow optimal blood jet return, which is indicative of complete vessel wall penetration and unobstructed endoluminal seating.

Materials and Design. Puncture needles are metallic tubes with a sharp distal tip and proximal plastic hub for firm grip and contain a Luer-Lok connector. Most needles are manufactured from thin-walled, large-bore tubes of stainless steel. Two-piece (outer needle and stylet) and three-piece (outer needle, stylet, and obturator) needles are now rarely used in current interventional practice.

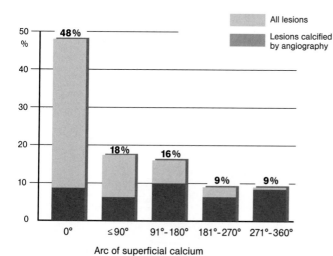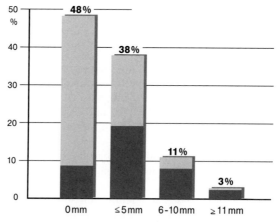

FIGURE 8-24. Topographic distribution of coronary artery calcifications. (*Left*) Frequency distribution of the arc of superficial target lesion calcium. Coronary angiography detected 34% of one-quadrant superficial calcium, 59% of two-quadrant superficial calcium, 69% of three-quadrant superficial calcium, and 86% of four-quadrant superficial calcium. (*Right*) Frequency distribution of the lengths of superficial target lesion calcium. Coronary angiography detected 50% of superficial calcium ≤5 mm in length, 67% of superficial calcium 6 to 10 mm in length, and 65% of superficial calcium >11 mm in length. Thus, the sensitivity of coronary angiography increased with an increasing arc or length of lesion-associated superficial calcium (both *P* <.0001). (Modified from Mintz GS, Popma JJ, Pichard AD, et al. Patterns of calcification in coronary artery disease: a statistical analysis of intravascular ultrasound and coronary angiography in 1155 lesions. *Circulation.* 1995;91:1959–1965.)

TABLE 8-26. Comparison of Lesions Measured by Intravascular Ultrasound (IVUS) and Quantitative Coronary Angiography According to Severity of IVUS Eccentricity of ≥3.0 and <3.0

	Normal Arc of Arterial Wall within Lesion (Group 1, n = 219)	IVUS Eccentricity Index ≥3.0 (Group 2, n = 441)	IVUS Eccentricity Index <3.0 (Group 3, n = 786)	ANOVA p
EEM CSA, mm²	16.1 ± 6.8	19.2 ± 6.7	18.8 ± 6.3	<.0001
Lumen CSA, mm²	4.1 ± 4.7	2.5 ± 2.3	2.1 ± 1.8	<.0001
CSN, %	75.0 ± 18.5	86.9 ± 9.2	88.1 ± 8.1	<.0001
Arc of calcium, degrees	62 ± 68	95 ± 93	121 ± 108	<.0001
QCA reference lumen diameter	3.11 ± 0.66	3.15 ± 0.57	3.10 ± 0.59	NS
QCA MLD	1.44 ± 0.75	1.22 ± 0.70	1.11 ± 0.66	<.0001
QCA percent diameter stenosis	54 ± 21	61 ± 20	64 ± 19	<.0001

EEM, external elastic membrane; CSA, cross-sectional area; CSN, cross-sectional narrowing; QCA, quantitative coronary angiography; MLD, minimum lumen diameter; ANOVA, analysis of variance.

Reproduced with permission from Mintz GS, Popma JJ, Pichard AD, et al. Limitations of angiography in the assessment of plaque distribution in coronary artery disease a systematic study of target lesion eccentricity in 1446 lesions. *Circulation* 1996;93:924–931.

TABLE 8-27. Comparisons of Angiographic Eccentric and Concentric Lesions with Quantitative Intravascular Ultrasound (IVUS) Parameters

	Eccentric by Angiography (n = 795)	Concentric by Angiography (n = 651)	p
EEM CSA, mm²	19.1 ± 6.3	19.4 ± 6.9	NS
Lumen CSA, mm²	2.3 ± 1.9	3.0 ± 3.6	.0002
CSN, %	87.4 ± 10.0	84.7 ± 13.0	.0003
IVUS eccentricity index	3.8 ± 2.7	3.2 ± 2.3	.0010
Eccentric by IVUS, n (%)	393 (49)	267 (41)	.0048
Arc of normal arterial wall, n (%)	126 (15)	93 (14)	NS

EEM, external elastic membrane; CSA, cross-sectional area; CSN, cross-sectional narrowing; QCA, quantitative coronary angiography; MLD, minimum lumen diameter.

Reproduced with permission from Mintz GS, Popma JJ, Pichard AD, et al. Limitations of angiography in the assessment of plaque distribution in coronary artery disease a systematic study of target lesion eccentricity in 1446 lesions. *Circulation* 1996;93:924–931.

Occasionally, a soft two-piece Teflon catheter-over-needle is employed, permitting the safe use of hydrophilic guiding catheters.

Standard puncture needles for femoral, brachial, and axillary artery access are 9 to 10 cm, and for the radial access approximately 5 cm long. The outer and inner diameters of the puncture needles are usually indicated in gauges (which originally—in 19th-century England—was an industrial measure for the diameter of wire). Gauge sizes (G) are indicated in fractions of an inch (1 in. = 2.54 cm) (Table 8-28).

Standard puncture needles and Teflon catheter-over-needle for access via the transfemoral, transbrachial, and transaxillar arteries are 18G (0.049 in. outer/0.042 in. inner diameter), and for transradial access 21G (0.032 in. outer/0.022 in. inner diameter) to allow smooth passage of 0.035-in. and 0.021-in. introductory guidewires, respectively.

INTRODUCTORY GUIDEWIRES

Purpose. Following successful vascular puncture, an introductory J-curve guidewire is used for needle replacement to secure

vascular access, a maneuver termed the Seldinger procedure after its inventor.[180]

Requirements. The most important requirements for introductory guidewires are atraumatic design, and the adequate length and support for the introduction of the sheath.

Material and Design. Introductory guidewires are typically 30 cm long with an 0.018-in. (radial) and a 0.021-in. or 0.035-in. (other sites) diameter. They are usually J-tipped and manufactured out of stainless steel or polymers.

INTRODUCTORY SHEATH

Purpose. Following stable endoluminal introductory guidewire placement, a sheath is used to establish stable percutaneous vessel access, which allows safe introduction and exchange of the catheter.

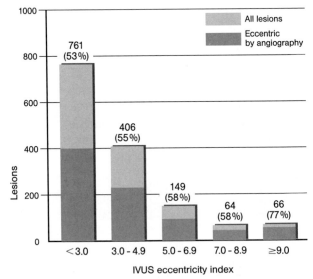

FIGURE 8-25. Frequency distribution of the intravascular ultrasound (IVUS) eccentricity index. The total number of lesions in each IVUS group is shown with the percentage of lesions with eccentricity by angiography shown in parentheses. (Modified from Mintz GS, Popma JJ, Pichard AD, et al. Limitations of angiography in the assessment of plaque distribution in coronary artery disease a systematic study of target lesion eccentricity in 1446 lesions. *Circulation.* 1996;93:924–931.)

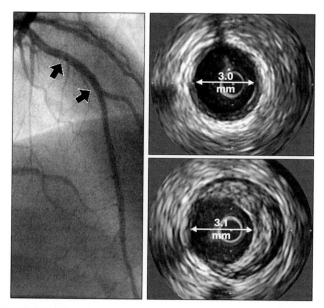

FIGURE 8-26. Example of coronary remodeling. (*Left*) Normal left anterior descending (LAD) artery on angiography displays mild concentric (*upper right*) and moderate eccentric (*lower right*) degree of atherosclerosis on IVUS, as shown at two selected sites. Positive remodeling at the more distal site (*lower right*) prevents detection of atherosclerosis by angiography. (Reproduced with permission from Nissen SE, Yock P. Intravascular ultrasound novel pathophysiological insights and current clinical applications. *Circulation.* 2001;103:604–616.)

Requirements. The vascular sheath should allow atraumatic passage through tissue, including the vessel wall. Requirements are high flexibility, high kink resistance, a soft atraumatic tip, and biological compatibility (including low thrombogenicity).

Material and Design. A vascular sheath typically consists of a shaft with a pneumatic seal, side arm, and inside dilator.

A fixation or lock mechanism between the two parts is needed to prevent separation of the sheath and the dilator during advancement. A standard introductory sheath is 15 cm long. The version whose internal diameter ranges from 4F to 5F (French size F, named in commemoration of the 19th-century French manufacturer of surgical instruments Joseph-Frederic-Benoit Charriere; 1F corresponds to 0.33 mm) is used for diagnostic catheterization, and the 5F to 7F version typically for percutaneous interventions. Longer (30, 45, 65, 80, and 90 cm) and bigger (up to 26F) introductory sheaths are available to facilitate access to the target vessel through elongated or tortuous vascular paths or to permit the use of larger devices during endovascular interventions.

Guiding Catheter

Mechanical Properties. The flexural stiffness (flexibility) is one of the most important properties of endovascular instruments. A wide range of bending properties are required for successful treatments. Typically, the proximal part of instruments requires greater flexural stiffness to achieve precise transmission of the movement of the operator's hands up to the tip of the instrument, whereas the distal end of instruments has to be softer, with low bending stiffness and high ductility to avoid injuries. The degree of congruency between the mechanical properties of the instrumentation needed to successfully navigate the vascular system and the manual dexterity of the operator will determine the procedural success.

The main factors governing flexural stiffness of guiding catheters include the outer and inner diameters, the thickness of the wall, the mechanical properties of the materials, and their mutual arrangement. A simple means to measure flexural stiffness of endovascular instruments is shown in Figure 8-28. The bending force F_{bend} is applied perpendicular to the free end of the specimen and causes the bending deflection δ. A

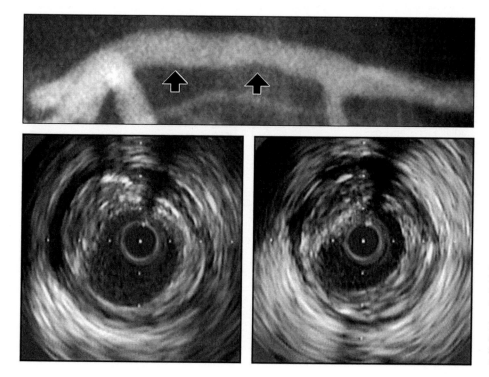

FIGURE 8-27. Angiographic underestimation of coronary artery atherosclerosis. Minor angiographic luminal irregularities (*top*) appeared on intravascular ultrasound (IVUS) as a diffuse atherosclerosis, shown at two sites (*arrows*). (Reproduced with permission from Nissen SE, Yock P. Intravascular ultrasound novel pathophysiological insights and current clinical applications. *Circulation.* 2001;103:604–616.)

TABLE 8-28.   Gauge, Inch, and Millimeter Sizes of Puncture Needles

	Outer Diameter		Inner Diameter	
Gauge	In.	Millimeter	In.	Millimeter
12	0.104	2.6	0.091	2.3
13	0.092	2.3	0.077	1.9
14	0.080	2.0	0.071	1.8
15	0.072	1.8	0.059	1.5
16	0.064	1.6	0.052	1.3
17	0.056	1.4	0.046	1.1
18	0.048	1.2	0.042	1.0
19	0.040	1.0	0.031	0.8
20	0.036	0.9	0.025	0.6
21	0.032	0.8	0.022	0.6

thin wire can be used to transmit the bending force onto the tested object. To allow objective definition of the bending process and to avoid sagging the bending length a has to be small ($a \approx 50$ mm or smaller). At small δ, F_{bend} exhibits a linear dependence on bending deflection δ. Thus, for $\delta \leq 0.1a$, the flexural stiffness S_{bend} can be calculated as

$$S_{bend} = \frac{a^3 \Delta F_{bend}}{3 \Delta \delta},$$

where $\frac{\Delta F_{bend}}{\Delta \delta}$ is the slope of the measured bending force as a function of the bending deflection within its linear range as determined by linear fitting (Fig. 8-29). By determining the slope, the bending of the specimen due to gravitational force is also eliminated. The unit for S_{bend} is N mm². Note that the bending stiffness depends on the cube of the bending length. Hence, the bending length a has to be determined very precisely. The propensity of a guiding catheter to kink can be measured as the bending deflection δ at which kinking occurs. Other relevant mechanical properties of the guiding catheters include crush resistance of the shaft, defined as a force needed to squash the catheter, and curve retention, measured as angle deviation from the original form following a defined amount of use. Examples of measured flexural stiffness of different guiding catheters are shown in Table 8-29 and Figure 8-30.

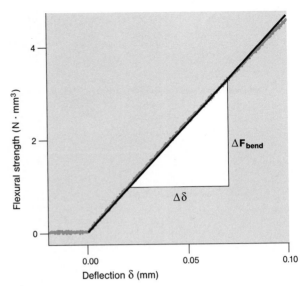

FIGURE 8-29.   Measurements from a two-point bending test of a thin guiding wire. The noisy curve represents the measuring points. The straight line is a linear fit according to the equation $S_{bend} = \frac{a^3}{3} \frac{\Delta F_{bend}}{\Delta \delta}$, the horizontal part at the outset coming from connecting the end of the instrument to the force transducer. In this example, a value $S_{bend} = 123$ N mm² is obtained for flexural stiffness. (Courtesy Dr. Wünsche, Kunstoff-Zentrum, Leipzig.)

Purpose. Guiding catheters (guides) provide a transport corridor for the delivery of endovascular devices to the ostium of the target vessel, improve the steering of the endovascular devices, and ensure their backup during interventions. To perform well, guiding catheters are expected to provide:

- Optimal shape to accommodate the topography of the aortic arch and target vessel ostia of individual patients
- Atraumatic ostial seating and, if needed, endoluminal insertion
- Stable backup and shape retention even in difficult and lengthy procedures
- Resistance to kinking and compression
- Large internal diameter for delivery of large instruments and small outer diameter to minimize injury to the access site
- Low friction of the luminal interface
- Low thrombogenicity and high biological compatibility.

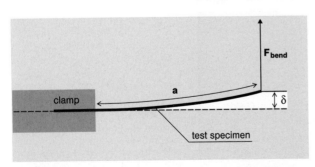

FIGURE 8-28.   Diagram for measuring flexural stiffness in a two-point arrangement. The value a is the bending length, δ the bending deflection, and F_{bend} the bending force. The left end of the specimen has to be horizontally clamped in a careful manner, e.g., without changing the sectional shape in case of catheters. (Courtesy Dr. Wünsche, Kunstoff-Zentrum, Leipzig.)

TABLE 8-29.   Flexural Stiffness of Four Dilatation Catheters

		Flexural Stiffness (N · mm²)	
Catheter	Diameter (French)	Distal	Proximal
1	6	420	410
2	6	340	520
3	8	1490	2270
4	8	580	640

Courtesy Dr. Wünsche, Kunstoff-Zentrum, Leipzig.

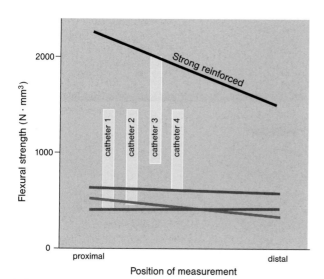

FIGURE 8-30. Flexural stiffness of 8F guiding catheters (*upper line*) compared with 6F catheters. (Courtesy Dr. Wünsche, Kunstoff-Zentrum, Leipzig.)

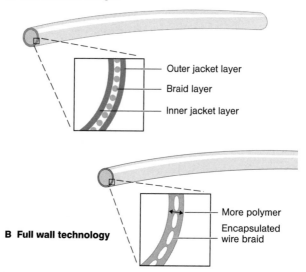

FIGURE 8-31. Guiding catheter walls in conventional and full-wall design.

Material, Design, and Form. Two basic designs of guiding catheter tubes are available: conventional and full wall. In the conventional design, the tube of the guiding catheter consists of three layers:

- An outer jacket manufactured from a soft and smooth material, such as nylon, polyester elastomer, silicone
- A braid of round or flattened stainless steel wire
- An inner jacket made of the same material as outer jacket and coated with a low-friction material such as Teflon (polytetrafluoroethylene, PTFE) or silicone.

To increase flexibility and torque transmission while maximizing resistance to kinking and compression in full-wall technology, the inner and the outer layers are molded together with a flat wire braid encapsulation. To reduce friction, the internal surface of the polymer is typically covered with silicon. To improve visibility, barium sulfate, barium carbonate, or bismuth is added. To accommodate the different needs for optimal backup (see the later discussion of secondary curve), for which greater stiffness is required, and atraumatic ostial insertion (primary curve), for which a soft tip is required, several transitional zones of gradually changing stiffness are implemented. Figure 8-31 shows the walls of a guiding catheter in conventional and full-wall design. Figure 8-32 shows an example of the transitional zones at the catheter's distal end.

Standard guides are 100-cm (90- to 115-cm) long tubes whose outer diameter ranges from 5F to 10F. They consist of a proximal hub, a long straight segment, and a shaped coaxial segment. The straight shaft is primarily responsible for torque transmission and resistance to kinking and compression during positioning. The configuration and shape of the coaxial segment of the transitional zones and the coaxial segment with the tip are, in contrast, decisive determinants of the backup and ostial seating. A number of catheter forms and shapes have been designed and implemented to ensure optimal seating and backup while accommodating the specific anatomy of the aortic arch and topography of the coronary ostia. The basic catheter forms employed in coronary interventions have been designed by Mason Sones,[181] Melvin Judkins,[182] and Kurt Amplatz.[183] The classical Judkins left and right coronary catheter configurations are shown in

Figure 8-33. These classical designs have been redesigned and modified by numerous engineers and operators. Still, new designs continue to surface, improving intubations of difficult ostia, coaxial seating, or catheter backup. To allow residual perfusion of the target vessel during interventions, the coaxial segment of the guide may carry side holes. Drawbacks of side holes are the greater use of contrast agents (50% to 80%), lower image quality, and potential of damaging guidewire tips. Guides with particularly soft or short tips are available to allow atraumatic ostial positioning in patients with severe proximal disease.

The French size of the guiding is the primary determinant of flexural stiffness, torque transmission, and kinking and crushing propensity. The internal diameter, in contrast, is the factor determining the maximum diameter of the deliverable endovascular instrumentation. Although the majority of PCIs are performed using 6F guides, 5F guides are fully adequate for straightforward interventions. Technically more demanding procedures usually require 7F size systems. Table 8-30 shows comparisons of the internal diameters of selected guiding catheters. For "double balloon" techniques, guiding catheters with a minimum internal diameter of 0.071 in. are needed; however, guides with bigger internal diameters are usually selected for greater comfort and better imaging.

The suitability of a specific guiding catheter for a given patient depends on the degree of concordance between the mechanical properties that are required and provided. Criteria for selection include:

- Access site (majority of guides are designed for the transfemoral approach and accommodate the anatomy of the vascular access path and transmission of forces from this access site best)
- Expected complexity of the case (a bigger French size provides greater freedom in executing the PCI process and usually works better in difficult cases)
- Anatomy of the aortic arch and of the target ostium (consider using special guiding catheter forms and shapes for special cases, but try the simplest shape first)

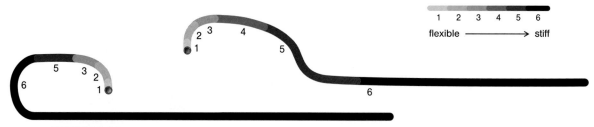

FIGURE 8-32.   Transitional zones of two different guiding catheters.

- Expected necessary backup (consider extra-support shaped catheters with optimal shape retention and catheters allowing deep seating for difficult cases in which a greater use of force may be required)

Standard catheter shapes are usually adequate for the majority of patients. In patients in whom the anatomy of the vascular access pathway is difficult or aberrant, however, special catheter forms and shapes as well as longer sheaths, which provide additional support, may be required. In selecting the catheter shape, standard recommendations should be followed (Table 8-31); in difficult cases, the trial-and-error approach represents the strategy of last resort. In difficult anatomy or high-crossing-resistance stenoses or occlusions, guiding catheters with extra support can be useful. These catheters provide stronger backup because they exert more pressure horizontally on the aortic wall opposite the ostium. Examples of extra-support guiding catheter shapes are the EBU configuration for the left coronary ostium and ECR configuration for the right coronary ostium (both Medtronic, Santa Rosa, CA, USA). However, the operator must take extra caution in seating these catheters because of the higher risk of ostial dissection.

Optimal seating of the guide is characterized by a perfect coaxial alignment with the ostium and the proximal segment of the target vessel and flexible, yet firm ostial intubation. Seating that is too firm bears the danger of dissections with their inevitable consequences, whereas seating that is too loose or misalignments may cause poor backup, dislocations, and instability during the procedure. In patients with ostial stenoses or spasms and in unstable patients, guiding catheters with side holes may be required, which allow continuous coronary perfusion at the expense of poorer coronary artery visualization, greater contrast medium consumption, and potential guidewire damage. The robustness of the system is primarily determined by the French size; backup is also the result of the overall stiffness of the primary and secondary curves (greater stiffness provides greater backup). Interplay between degrees of stiffness and flexibility of the primary and secondary curves determines the propensity of the catheter for passive (peripheral ostial) or active (deep ostial) seating. A softer primary curve and stiffer secondary curve allow for deep intubation while retaining reasonable backup. With active seating, the risk of traumatization increases with the stiffness and French size of the guide. For example, selecting a 6F instead of a 5F Z2 and Launcher guiding catheter increases the stiffness of the coaxial segment by 33% and 64%, respectively. Objective ranking of the relevant mechanical properties of guiding catheters by noncommercial certified institutions would be helpful in improving our understanding of their handling and selection. Table 8-32 provides an example of ranking of three commercially available guiding catheters. Furthermore, operators would welcome industry support for a standardized set of indicators of the clinical performance of guiding catheters, which could be contained in marketing

Normal left takeoffs

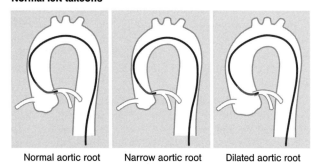

Normal aortic root   Narrow aortic root   Dilated aortic root

Normal right takeoffs

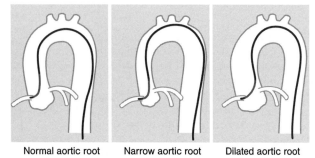

Normal aortic root   Narrow aortic root   Dilated aortic root

FIGURE 8-33.   Left and right Judkins catheters.

TABLE 8-30.   Comparisons of Internal Diameters of Selected Guiding Catheters

Guiding Catheter	5F (in.)	6F (in.)	7F (in.)	8F (in.)
Zuma (Medtronic)	0.058	0.068	0.081	0.091
Z2 (Medtronic)	0.058	0.070	0.081	0.091
Launcher (Medtronic)	0.058	0.071	0.081	0.090
Viking (Guidant)		0.068	0.078	0.091
Heartrail (Terumo)	0.059	0.071	0.081	0.091

French size corresponds to the outer diameter.

TABLE 8-31. Selection of Guiding Catheter Shapes Recommended for Typical Anatomic Variants Relevant to Percutaneous Coronary Interventions (PCI)

Anatomic Location of the Ostium	Left Coronary Ostium	Right Coronary Ostium
Anterior take-off	Amplatz left 1 or 2	Amplatz left 1, Amplatz right 2
Posterior take-off	EBU type	Amplatz left 1, Amplatz right 2
High take-off	Judkins left 3.0 or 3.5, Amplatz left 3, Multiple purpose	Amplatz right 2, Judkins right 3.0 or 3.5, Multiple purpose
Upward take-off (superior)	Amplatz left 2 short tip EBU type 3.5 or larger	Amplatz left 1, Amplatz right 2, Hockey stick-type, 3 D right coronary type
Downward take-off (inferior)	Judkins left 4—modified	Judkins right 4—modified
Bypass—aortic anastomosis	Left coronary bypass type Multiple purpose Judkins right 4.0 Amplatz right 1	Multiple-purpose Judkins right 4.0 Amplatz right 1
Bypass—internal mammary	Internal mammary	Internal mammary, Judkins right 3.5 or 4.0

information improving selection. The notion of "one size fits all" may work for standard PCI cases, but not for difficult ones. A set of performance indicators could include measures of length (cm), shape, internal and external diameters (in inches and millimeters), measures of stiffness and the rate of change of stiffness of the shaft, coaxial segment, and the tip, thermostability, resistance to kinking, and shape retention. Until more objective data on individual products become available, careful assessment of the clinical performance of individual products remains the only option. Table 8-33 summarizes some of the advantages and limitations of 5F, 6F, and 7F guiding catheters.

Guidewire

Purpose. Guidewires are wires designed for safe placement of endovascular instrumentation. Although they are relatively simple-looking devices, guidewires display an extraordinary variety of properties and characteristics that may allow a safe navigation of virtually any vascular territory within the human body. The safe tracking of endovascular pathways and overcoming of obstacles require a unique combination of flexibility and stiffness present in different proportions along the entire length of the guidewire depending on product specifications. Since reinforcing one of the desired properties usually requires compromises on other properties, guidewire design and manufacturing belong to the most difficult technological enterprises. The ultimate criteria for guidewire assessment include tracking ability, support, and safety. The simplest way to differentiate guidewires is based on their thickness, usually indicated in fractions of an inch. The most frequently used guidewires are 0.035 in. (0.89 mm) and 0.014 in. (0.36 mm) thick (for comparison, the diameter of a human hair is approximately 0.001 in. or 0.0254 mm).

Material and Design. The thickness of commercially available guidewires ranges from 0.007 in. (0.178 mm) to 0.078 in. (1.98 mm), and their length varies from 140 cm to 450 cm. However, typically guidewires for rapid exchange instrumentation are typically about 170 cm long (range 140 to 190 cm) and those for over-the-wire (OTW) instrumentation are 260 to 300 cm long. To allow the conversion of a rapid-exchange intervention into an OTW procedure, extension wires allowing docking onto the distal end of the guidewire are available. Standard guidewires are manufactured either with a straight or preshaped

TABLE 8-32. Comparison of Some Relevant Performance Parameters of Selected Guiding Catheters

Product	Inner Sliding Resistance (Low-to-high)	Distal Tip Flexibility (Low-to-high)	Shaft Stiffness (High-to-low)	Compression Resistance (High-to-low)	Kink Resistance (High-to-low)
Z/M	3	2	3	3	3
V/G	2	3	1	1	1
H/T	1	1	2	2	2

Ranking in arbitrary units 1–3; same French size catheters compared (undisclosed source).

TABLE 8-33.   Advantages and Limitations of 5F, 6F, and 7F Guiding Catheters

	Advantages	*Drawbacks*
5F	Active engagement of the ostium Deep and very deep seating for greater backup Avoidance of using guiding catheters with side holes in presence of moderately severe ostial lesions in some cases Lower rate of peripheral complications	Suboptimal backup on passive engagement of the ostium Poor visualization while instrumentation in place due to low flow of the contrast agent Marked limitations in complex procedures and complications Prevention of more complex techniques (e.g., double-wire, "kissing" dilatations)
6F	Reasonable compromise for standard interventions Availability of side holes	Limitations in using complex techniques (e.g., "kissing" dilatation) Limitations in using larger diameter devices with need of matching inner lumen to the diameter of interventional devices (e.g., >3.25-mm "cutting balloons," thrombectomy catheters)
7F	Optimum backup primarily on passive engagement of the ostium Optimum freedom of selecting required instrumentation and performing complex procedures virtually in any intervention Adequate contrast visualization while instrumentation in place Availability of side holes	Limited active engagement of the ostium Limited deep seating of the guiding catheter Higher rate of peripheral complications

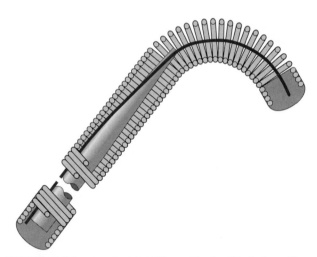

FIGURE 8-34.   Standard 0.035-in. guidewire (Cook, Inc., Bloomington, IN, USA). The guidewire consists of a core 0.21-in. diameter mandrel, with a progressive diameter reduction over the final 15 cm to 0.12-in. diameter, with attached 0.005- to 0.002-in. filament. Mandrel material and thickness are primarily responsible for guidewire stiffness and support; the filament provides the shaping characteristics of the tip. Up to the tip, the mandrel is surrounded by a 0.024- to 0.052-in. wire coil. Mandrel and coil are soldered together at the distal end with a hemisphere. Over the distal end, the spiral is slightly movable with respect to the filament, thus allowing stretching of the J-curve by a backward pull. The soft distal end is 15 cm in length. All components are manufactured from stainless steel. The coils are covered with silicone coating.

tip. However, for steering, the straight tip must be shaped. The shape given the tip depends on the anatomy of target vessel and morphology of the target lesion.

0.035-IN. GUIDEWIRES. Guidewires with a thickness of 0.035 in. and with a J-curve or straight tip are primarily designed to guide the diagnostic and guiding catheters to the proximity of the ostia of target vessels. In addition, interventional 0.035-in. guidewires are designed to navigate target vessels, to cross the target lesions, and to support the positioning of the interventional instrumentation.

A standard 0.035-in. guidewire (Cook Inc., Bloomington, IN) is shown in Figure 8-34. The 0.035-in. stiff or superstiff guidewires provide better support for introducing larger and bulkier devices and include the Amplatz super stiff (Boston Scientific, Natick, MA) and Lunderquist (Cook Inc., Bloomington, IN).

Examples of interventional 0.035-in. guidewires designed to provide support, steering and crossing ability, and greater slipperiness include Roadrunner (Cook Inc., Bloomington, IN) and Terumo guidewires (Terumo, Shibuya-ku, Tokyo).

0.014-IN. GUIDEWIRES. Guidewires with a thickness of 0.014 in. are nearly exclusively used in coronary interventions, although their use in other vascular territories has been rising. Only highly specialized interventions employ 0.007, 0.009, 0.010, 0.011, 0.012, and 0.018 in. guidewires. The shaft and tip should be distinguished because each exhibits markedly different design and mechanical properties.

Shaft. The shaft consists of a core mandrel surrounded by a coil spring or polymer jacket covered by a hydrophilic or hydrophobic coating. The basic physical properties of the shaft—stiffness, longitudinal flexibility, and torque transmission—are determined by the material of the core mandrel (e.g., 304v stainless steel, nitinol, and its alloys), its thickness, and its taper. The stiffness of the shaft, that is, the resistance to bending or kinking, can be measured as a force (grams per millimeter) needed to bend the wire. The stiffness of the shaft of the wire is primarily responsible for the support the guidewire provides for the tracking of endovascular devices. To classify wires by shaft stiffness, four categories of guidewires are usually distinguished: low, standard, stiff, and extra stiff (Table 8-34). The jacket covering the core consists either of metallic (e.g., 304v stainless steel, platinum, or platinum-nickel) coils or polymeric (e.g., polyurethane, silicone, Teflon). The outer layer of the wire consists of a hydrophilic or hydrophobic coating, responsible for slipperiness, smoothness, and biological compatibility.

Tip. The distal tip of the guidewire is mainly responsible for its tracking and crossing abilities. There are two basic designs of the tip, core to tip and shaping ribbon. The core-to-tip design is characterized by a bottom-to-tip core mandrel. This design is associated with better torque transmission and finer steering ability. The shaping-ribbon design is characterized by a tapered shaft with a fine wire plate or filament firmly attached distally. This design provides greater flexibility and pliability of the tip. To improve the flexibility of the tip, the core is gradually tapered toward the distal end. In the conventional design the taper is graded in a staircase fashion, whereas in the parabolic design the transitions are smooth. The parabolic design improves torque transmission. The length of the tapered segment also affects wire behavior. Longer taper usually allows better tracking and lower propensity for the wire prolapse frequently observed in stenotic sharp bends or kinks. Similar to the shaft, the stiffness of the tip can be measured as the force required deflecting the tip by a given distance. The core mandrel of the tip is covered by either a tightly wound coil or a polymer covered by coating. To improve radiographic visibility, x-ray radiation absorbing materials such as tungsten are admixed to the polymer of the tip. To steer the guidewire, the tip must be shaped. The shaping is performed either using a shaping tool, usually a guidewire introducer, or by pressing the tip against the tip of the thumb. Gentle shaping is required to preserve the mechanical properties of the tip. Optimal

steering is usually achieved with simple short (approximately 2 mm long) bends and rounded 45- to 60-degree angles. In more complex target anatomy, the person shaping the tip should take into consideration anatomical features such as the angulation of the take-off of the target vessel and, if different, of the vessel of destination, the morphology of the proximal segment of the target vessel, and the complexity of the target lesion. Larger bends are necessary in large-diameter vessels (>3.5 mm) and sharp take-off angles, where the vertical length of the bend should be approximately 15% to 20% less than the diameter of the target vessel to allow the tip some play while advancing toward the target lesion. Some basic rules for shaping the tip include:

- Treat the tip gently
- Keep the shape simple; more than one bend is rarely really helpful
- Avoid reshaping; the shape should be based on the most critical feature if the anatomy is complex
- Keep the bend rounded; avoid kinking
- Before exchanging the wire, check whether the shape of the tip has changed

Figure 8-35 shows the core-to-tip and shaping ribbon design of a 0.014-in. guidewire. Figure 8-36 shows conventional and parabolic tip designs.

Ideal guidewire provides excellent:

- Tracking
- Crossing
- Steering
- Support
- Atraumatic navigation and passage
- High biocompatibility

These performance parameters require:

- Balanced stiffness and flexibility of shaft and tip
- Torque and push stability
- Atraumatic design
- Low friction of shaft and tip
- Form retention of the tip
- Kinking-resistant tip

Modeling, integration, and translation of these parameters into high-performance products remain a daunting task for the industry. On the part of the operator, two main tasks need to be accomplished:

- Selection ("best bet")
- Handling ("best go")

The guidewire (tip and shaft) should match the requirements of the target site. Thus, it should permit safe navigation and crossing while providing optimal support to shuttle the endovascular instruments back and forth. In some cases, more than one guidewire might be needed to meet the anatomic requirements. Typically, the operator's initial choice of guidewire is based on his assessment of the target vessel and target lesion with regard to tracking, steering, crossing, pushing, support, and vulnerability. In most anatomically uncomplicated

TABLE 8-34. Grading of Stiffness of 0.014-in. Guidewire Shaft and Tip on Arbitrary Scale 1–4

Product Name	Shaft Stiffness/ Support (Grades 1–4)	Tip Stiffness (Grades 1–4)
Standard wires		
Balance	2	1
Middleweight		
Universal Balance	1	1
High support wires		
Balance Heavyweight	3	2
Extra S'Port	4	2
High finesse wires		
Whisper LS	1	1
Whisper MS	1	2
Recanalization wires		
Cross-It 100XT	2	3
Cross-It 200XT	2	4
HT Pilot 150	2	3

Modified from Guidant, Indianapolis, IN, USA.

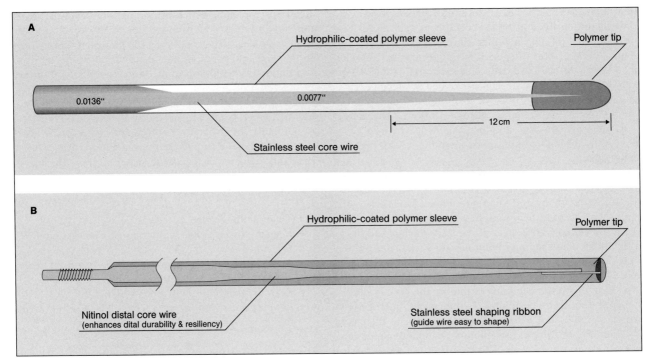

FIGURE 8-35.   A 0.014-in. guidewire with a core-to-tip and shaping ribbon design.

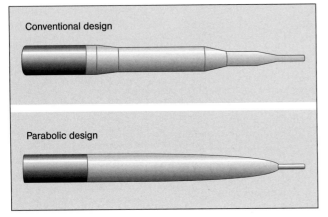

FIGURE 8-36.   A 0.014-in. guidewire tip with conventional and parabolic designs.

cases, "universal" guidewires are efficacious and safe, and should be selected. In other cases specialized guidewires are preferable:

- Tortuous proximal segments: Guidewires with excellent tracking ability are required
- Diffuse disease: An atraumatic soft tip is necessary
- High-grade target stenosis: Places high demands on steering ability and shape retention of the tip
- Long and tight lesions: Make an efficient force and torque transmission down to the tip necessary
- Extremely angulated take-off: A very gradual decrease in stiffness toward the tip is necessary to avoid prolapse

- Chronically occluded target artery: More than one guidewire is frequently required, preferably combined with an OTW system.

Although in most cases the systematic approach makes it possible to select the most appropriate guidewire, an operator must occasionally resort to a trial-and-error approach.

The guidewire tip is then carefully shaped for optimal steering. Simple bends help the tip retain its finesse. The angle and length of the bend depend on the diameter of the target vessel and branching angles to be overcome before reaching the target lesion. Examples of the required guidewire properties for typical clinical situations are given in Table 8-35.

It should be remembered that a selection based on one particular property may result in others being compromised. Guidewire selection should therefore be primarily be based on the parameter considered most important for crossing the target lesion, along with safety considerations. A dissection or perforation due to a stiff tip or an untoward motion during intervention may mar even the best repair of a proximal target vessel. A stiffer shaft may provide better support by stretching the vessel, but it also may decrease the stability of the system if it exceeds the backup provided by the guiding catheter. Excessive stiffness may also press the guidewire against the wall, directing the device into plaques and cause dissection. A guidewire with a stiffer tip may transmit push and torque better but at the expense of tracking ability. On the other hand, a guidewire with a softer tip may enter the lesion easily but may "freeze" and buckle within it. Furthermore, with excessive force the exceedingly soft or slippery tip may burrow under the plaque and cause a dissection. A stiff shaft and a stiffer tip tend not to give at obstacles, easily causing a perforation. Selection

TABLE 8-35.   Examples of Required 0.014-in. Guidewire Properties for Typical Clinical Situations

| Clinical Situation | Main Required Property | | Comments |
	Shaft	Tip	
Tight, complex target lesion	High torque transmission	Flexible, reinforced	Good steering and push required
Tight complex target lesion in distal segment	High torque transmission, stiffness	Torque transmission to tip; high shape retention	Excellent steering and push required; consider second guidewire in tortuous target vessels
Highly calcified target lesion	High flexural stiffness	Flexible, reinforced; shape retention; low friction	Good push and shape retention are required for crossing
Total occlusion, acute	Medium flexural stiffness	Soft; good steering ability	Careful probing exploration to avoid trauma
Total occlusion, subacute	Medium flexural stiffness	Medium flexibility; medium steering ability	More push and more extensive punctual probing required
Total occlusion, chronic	Medium to high flexural stiffness	Medium to high flexural stiffness	Push transmission to tip required; slow decisive and consistent probing
Vulnerable target vessel/ diffuse disease	High flexibility	High flexibility	Work with light hand required, guidewire passes obstacles by combination of gentle push and rotation of the tip
Sharp take-off of target vessel	Medium flexural stiffness	High push transmission to tip; highest shape retention	Smooth transition of decreasing flexural stiffness to tip required to avoid prolapse and digression to nontarget vessels
Tortuous target vessel	Medium flexural stiffness	High flexibility	Second wire to gently straighten up target vessel might be required

of the appropriate guidewire for a given PCI situation necessitates compromises among various needs, yet is rewarding because it is often the key to a successful intervention.

Dilatation Balloon Catheter

Purpose. Balloon catheters are devices designed to restore normal blood flow in occluded or stenotic arteries by inflating small longitudinal balloons filled with a mixture of saline and contrast media. Inflation under high pressure exerts hoop (radial) and longitudinal (axial) forces onto the wall, producing stretch, redistribution, and compression of stenotic tissue, and, ideally, restoration of the lumen.

Dilatation pressures between 2 and 14 bar are usually employed, but pressure up to 24 bar can be required to dilate highly fibrotic or calcified lesions. Naturally, with increasing inflation pressure the danger of balloon rupture and resulting vessel wall dissection or rupture increases. A ruptured balloon discharges pressure primarily in the longitudinal direction tearing mostly at the balloons' ends rather than in the middle, thus reducing the danger of vessel wall damage. For dilatation to be efficient, the balloon (including the balloon shoulders) must be expanded symmetrically in the radial and longitudinal directions with the balloon in close contact with the wall surfaces. During balloon deflation and withdrawal, the balloon must be refolded optimally and the balloon catheter retracted very carefully under fluoroscopy in order to avoid damage to the wall or to the deployed stents.

Ideal balloon catheters are characterized by the following qualities (where H means high and L low):

- Pushing ability (H): complete transmission to the tip of the force exerted at the distal end
- Tracking ability (H): ability to navigate through a tortuous path
- Crossing ability (H): the ability to overcome tight stenoses
- Balloon compliance (L): minimum change in size and shape at high pressures and with hard lesions
- Pressure resistance (H): resistance to rupture at high inflation pressures
- Refolding properties (H): complete and fast refolding following repeated inflations
- Atraumatic behavior (H): ability to track the guidewire in to-and-fro movements without causing vessel wall damage

Material and Design. Balloon catheters are available in two basic designs. These are the "over-the-wire" (OTW) and rapid exchange (Rx), or monorail, systems. OTW is the older system, which has been available since the early 1980s. It utilizes a continuous proximal-to-distal wire lumen and a separate lumen for balloon inflation. The Rx system, available since the mid-1980s, provides an alternative with a short distal wire lumen with the wire entering the shaft at the tip and exiting usually 30 cm distal, and a single lumen for balloon inflation. The original fixed-balloon, single-lumen catheters with or without a short guidewire attached to the tip have become obsolete in standard interventions.

Advantages of the OTW balloon catheters include (a) greater support since the guidewire reinforces the shaft, permitting better push and torque transmission, (b) stable endoluminal placement of the balloon, permitting multiple exchanges of guidewires with protected advancements and without the need to recross the lesion, and (c) the ability to administer superselective contrast media or a pharmacologic agent via the guidewire lumen. The major drawback of the OTW system compared to the Rx system is that balloon exchange is more cumbersome, requiring the use of wire extensions or long exchange wires. The Rx system is used more frequently in standard endovascular interventions because of the rapidity of balloon exchange and the ease of handling.

The principal parts of balloon catheters are:

- Proximal plastic hub
- Proximal long double-lumen (OTW) or single-lumen (Rx) straight shaft consisting of a PTFE-coated hypo tube, which is usually reinforced by stainless steel or manufactured from a polymer
- Transition zone
- Distal, coaxial (OTW and Rx systems) polymer, frequently nylon reinforced by stainless steel wire, shaft with dilatation balloon tightly wrapped around the shaft, and tapered tip

In the OTW system, the proximal shaft contains two lumina for the guidewire and balloon inflation-deflation, versus a single lumen for balloon inflation-deflation in the Rx system. The more flexible distal coaxial shaft typically spans 30 cm and in both systems contains two lumina. The full length of a balloon catheter is typically 140 cm. The proximal shaft has an outer diameter between 2.0F and 2.5F; the distal part of the shaft containing the balloon usually has an outer diameter from 2.5F to 3.2F. To reduce outer friction, the shaft is coated with silicone or hydrophilic polymers. The guidewire exit port in the Rx system is usually located 25 to 30 cm from the crossing tip of the catheter and carries radiopaque marker.

The standard balloon is a cylindrical body with distal and proximal cones and necks. The shoulders of drug-delivery balloons may be shaped differently in order to exhibit various important properties, such as low crossing friction and low balloon slipping. The rounded, conical, and offset necks result in different balloon shapes (conical/square, conical/spherical, tapered, square, long spherical, offset, and others). Coronary dilatation balloons are typically 10 to 30 mm long and carry either one central or two peripheral radiopaque markers to facilitate positioning. Balloons are manufactured from a large number of noncompliant, semicompliant, and compliant polymers that support inflation pressures that range from 2 to 24 bar. Different abrasion and puncture resistant coatings usually cover the coaxial segment of the balloon catheter to increase or decrease slipperiness and to allow drug delivery and drug release.

Dilatation balloon catheters can be characterized by the following properties:

- *Diameter* of a balloon inflated to nominal pressure
- *Length* of a balloon, indicating the full working length or the length of the straight segment
- *Balloon (crossing) profile*, the maximum diameter of the balloon when mounted, wrapped, and deflated on the catheter
- *Balloon (entry) profile*, the minimum diameter of the balloon, usually at or close to the tip of the balloon
- *Nominal pressure*, the inflation pressure required for a balloon to expand to its nominal size
- *Rated burst pressure*, the maximum pressure to which a balloon can be inflated without rupturing, defined as a 95% degree of confidence and a 99.9% guarantee level for 40 inflations in vitro at normal body temperature (37.0°C)
- *Mean burst pressure*, the average pressure required for a balloon to rupture
- *Balloon compliance*, the rate of change in diameter with increasing inflation

The ability of balloon catheters to accomplish set tasks of reaching, crossing, and successfully dilating the lesion without causing damage to the target vessel or its tributaries depends on the design, the materials, and manufacturing quality. An example of a successful dilatation balloon technology is shown in Figure 8-37 (Ryujin catheter, Terumo, Shibuya-ku, Tokyo). For a more extensive review, see Chapter 5.

Balloons for coronary artery dilatations are typically 10 to 30 mm long. The length of balloon selected should match the length of the stenosis so that the flat portion of the balloon spans the full length of the lesion and the balloon shoulders go beyond its edges. Noncompliant balloons and balloons with

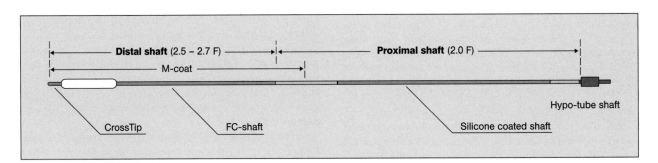

FIGURE 8-37. Ryujin dilatation balloon catheter (Terumo, Shibuya-ku, Tokyo). The Ryujin catheter consists of a hypotube shaft coated with silicone and a different, undisclosed, coating on the transition zone and distal coaxial shaft to minimize friction. To maximize the rate of force transmission to the tip (pushing ability) while retaining high flexibility (tracking ability), a novel flexible-corrugated, 2.5F to 2.7F coaxial shaft design has been introduced, providing a gradual increase in flexibility toward the tip while retaining the required strength. The balloon has a double conical shape with the proximal neck longer and more gradual (2.5 to 5 mm for 1.25- to 3.25-mm diameter balloons) than the shorter and steeper distal neck (2.5 to 4.0 mm for 1.25- to 3.25-mm diameter balloons). The smooth transit section of the balloon-holding shaft to the cross tip measures 3 mm. The balloon entry profile measures 0.43 mm, and the maximum balloon profile measures from 0.66 mm (0.026 in.) up to 0.94 mm (0.037 in.) for 1.5- to 4.0-mm diameter balloons. The standardized deflation time ranges from 0.7 seconds for 1.25 × 15 mm diameter balloons to 6.0 seconds for 4.0 × 10 mm diameter balloons.

short shoulders are preferred in order to reduce the risk of edge traumatization. A rational basis is still lacking for the use of larger diameter balloons inflated at lower pressures versus smaller diameter balloons inflated to higher pressures to achieve the desired target diameter, that is, nominal diameter of the target vessel at the target segment, and for the optimal duration and speed of step-up of application of distending pressures. Intuitively, the use of larger balloons is preferred in lesions with less diffuse noncalcified lesions, whereas smaller balloons seem to perform better in patients with diffuse heavily calcified plaques. However, the use of oversized balloons at high pressures bears the risk of dissections and ruptures and must be avoided. Selection of the diameter of the dilation balloon is commonly termed *sizing*. Balloons are sized using visual estimates, quantitative coronary angiography (QCA), or IVUS. In routine clinical practice, visual estimates are most frequently performed. Individual balloon inflations typically last between 20 and 120 seconds. Longer inflation times may be required in attempts to tack on dissecting flaps in lesions not amenable to stenting. In these cases balloon catheters permitting antegrade coronary perfusion are preferable.

Stents

Purpose. Stents are cylindrical, generally metallic implants designed to remove stenoses by scaffolding the vessel and preventing recoil, to prevent restenoses, and to smooth out the intimal interface following dilatation.

Material and Design. Stents are cylindrical structures consisting of cells formed by struts with repetitive patterns to ensure optimal scaffolding. Stents are delivered to the target lesion by delivery systems, that is, they are usually crimped onto conventional balloon catheters. Set free, they self-expand or are dilated to two to four times their crimped diameter. Permanently implanted stents are exposed to high mechanical stresses in a biologically complex environment requiring the following properties:

- *Radial strength*: the infinite elastic modulus to prevent recoil by the opposing and withstanding repetitive compressive loading forces of pulsatile and nonpulsatile vessel wall motion resulting in tension, torsion, and bending of the implanted stent
- *Tensile strength*: achievement of the highest radial strength using a minimum of material (thin struts, optimal cell size)
- *Steep work-hardening rate* for optimal increase in stiffness during expansion
- *Flexibility* to allow delivery of intact stents along any vascular path to any desired vascular location against frontal and lateral loading forces
- *Conformability* to allow complete circumferential stent-vessel wall contact (apposition) in corrugated surfaces
- *Ductility* to resist deformation during expansion
- *Optimal yield strength* to allow stent expansion at acceptable balloon inflation pressures while allowing firm crimping onto the delivery system (high stent retraction forces required)
- *Longevity* to provide long-term scaffold avoiding corrosion and material fatigue (except bioabsorbable stents)
- *Radiopacity* to permit precise positioning and stent identification
- *Biological compatibility* to minimize thrombogenicity, inflammatory responses, and restenosis
- *Preservation* of side-branch access

- *Adaptability* to serve as platform for drug delivery, coverage of perforation sites, and other functions
- *Large strains* with optimal stress-strain relationships (superelastic behavior)
- *Optimal hysteresis* between loading and unloading conditions, balancing minimum compression against maximum shape recoverability

In an attempt to satisfy this multitude of partially contradictory and mutually exclusive requirements, a stream of constantly improving stent designs and stent materials have been proposed and marketed. Some of the common stent materials are discussed next.

METALS
- Stainless steels[*] (e.g., 316L with 18% chromium, 14% nickel, 2.9% molybdenum, 2.0% manganese, 0.75% silicon, 0.03% carbon)
- Cobalt alloys (e.g., cobalt with 20% chromium, 35% nickel, 10% molybdenum, 1.0% titanium, 1.0% iron, 0.15% manganese, 0.15% silicon, 0.025% carbon)
- Titanium alloys
- Nitinol (martensitic, cold worked 40%, superelastic)[**]
- Magnesium

POLYMERS
- Silicones
- Gore-Tex (ePTFE)
- Polyethylenes
- Polyurethanes

BIODEGRADABLE POLYMERS
- Poly(glycolic acid)
- Poly(lactic acid)
- Metallic

The majority of today's balloon-expandable stents are manufactured from stainless steel alloys, and most self-expandable stents are made of nitinol. Typically, the area directly supported by the stent strut for 17% to 19% of the total stented area. The thickness of the individual struts varies between 80 μm and 140 μm, and the deflation time of the stent delivery system (SDS) balloons varies between 2 seconds and 7 seconds according to manufacturers' information. The force required to withdraw or dislodge the stent from the SDS varies between individual products from 1.4 N to 4.3 N. Specific designs include reinforced stents for ostial implantations, stents designed to improve access to side branches, bifurcation stents, stents covered with membranes to seal off severely dissected or ruptured vessels, stents for drug delivery (DESs), and biodegradable stents. Stent surfaces interacting with the body environment may be coated to increase smoothness or hydrophilicity, to alter charge, and to prevent leachables from entering the body.

---

[*]Stainless steels with manganese, chromium substituted for nickel are available.

[**]Martensitic—balloon expandable, contracts on heating, exceptionally flexible because of long and low initial stress–strain plateau followed by a steep increase in stiffness. Cold worked: 40% high elasticity with large recoverable strains and ductility; superelastic: high recoverable strain, modifiable by processing and altering the nickel–titanium relationship.

From the perspective of PCI, ideal stents are:

- Technically easy and safe to deliver
- Easy to deploy
- Highly durable and resistant to fatigue, fracture, cracking, wear, creep, and corrosion
- Optimally visible
- Highly biologically compatible
- Consistent with long-term healing without restenosis
- Compatible with magnetic resonance imaging (MRI) and computed tomography (CT) environments

For SDS to permit a technically easy and atraumatic delivery of an intact stent to a tight calcified target bifurcation lesion located in a distal segment of a tortuous, diffusely atherosclerotic coronary artery (the equivalent of an operator's nightmare), the stent itself must be highly flexible, accept a firm crimp, and exhibit a low profile, and the carrier balloon catheter must exhibit excellent tracking and pushing ability. Further requirements are that there be smooth and longitudinal geometry on bends to avoid "fish-scale" effects (abstaining struts on bends), optimal apposition along with avoidance of "trumpet" effects (asymmetric stent expansion at the ends), and satisfactory access to the side branches. In other clinical situations other specific requirements might become important. Thus:

- Greater radial strength is needed in heavily fibrotic and/or calcified ostial lesions and lesions located in the intramural segment
- High recoverable strain is required in vascular segments spanning joints and other exponent body locations
- High visibility becomes critical in stenting critical lesions in obese patients
- Small cell size is favored in lesions with large plaque burden associated with prolapsing tissue debris
- Optimal interplay between the hardening (stiffening) of the stent on expansion and the homogenous expansion characteristics of the stent delivery system is critical for symmetrical strut apposition in complex fibrotic and calcified lesions, particularly in vein grafts
- Avoidance of "dog boning" (overexpansion of delivery balloons beyond the edges of the stent in balloons with long shoulders and/or high compliance) is particularly important in diffusely diseased vessels
- Rapid and geometrically optimal refolding of the balloon is critical to prevent damage to stents with thin struts or to vulnerable vessels

For the operator to be able to select the optimal stent in any given clinical situation, he must have knowledge and understanding of stents' performance characteristics. Defining clinically relevant performance parameters for which manufacturers would be required to provide information would be helpful in achieving this goal. Some of the clinically relevant performance parameters are:

- Diameter of a fully expanded stent [mm] by nominal pressure [bar]
- Length of the stent [mm], usually corresponding to the inside balloon markers
- Radial (recoil) and longitudinal shortening following full expansion by nominal pressure [% diameter, % length]

- Maximum diameter of the stent when crimped on the deflated balloon of the catheter [French size, inches, millimeters] (crossing profile)
- Minimum diameter of the stent, usually at or close to the tip of the SDS [French size, inches, millimeters] (entry profile)
- Strut thickness [inches, millimeters]
- Scaffolded area [mm^2]
- Unsupported surface area (USA) [mm^2]
- Metal-to-artery ratio [%]
- Radial strength of fully expanded stent at nominal pressure
- Kinetics of stent (hardening) with expansion (stress-strain curve)
- Longitudinal flexibility [N]
- Firmness of crimp (dislodgement force) [N]
- Recrossing ability
- Accessibility of side branches (cell size of symmetrically, at nominal pressure fully expanded stent)
- Material, with complete chemical definition of the alloy
- Material surface properties (corrosion, leachability, charge, biocompatibility)
- Radiopacity
- Stent apposition geometry: imprint of cells in straight and bended vascular segments
- Nominal pressure, rated burst pressure, mean burst pressure [bar] of the delivery balloon
- Compliance of the delivery balloon
- Refolding characteristics of the delivery balloon (refolding mechanism, time to completely refold) [seconds]
- Documented restenosis rate
- Expected documented longevity (number of loaded cycles before material fatigue)

With the emergence of DESs, BMSs now serve primarily as a delivery platform for drugs and backup systems in difficult stent deployments. Nevertheless, the mechanical properties outlined hold for DESs with permanent or bioabsorbable platforms regardless of future designs.

Few topics in coronary angioplasty have been discussed as fervently as the question of the appropriate balloon or stent "sizing." To prevent injuries, dilatation balloons were initially sized up to the nominal diameter of the target vessel determined by angiography.[184] Difficult lesions were dilated with slightly oversized balloons and/or repeated high-pressure or prolonged dilatations. However, oversized dilatations precipitated the risk of dissections and other procedural complications and were discouraged.[185–187] However, based on data indicating that the minimal luminal diameter (MLD) achieved by PTCA is a powerful predictor of restenosis, the notion that the maximum diameter should be achieved has been suggested as a new target to prevent restenosis during the early stent era ("bigger is better" hypothesis).[188–192] To reduce the risks while maximizing the benefits of up-sized dilatations, IVUS guidance has been shown to improve the angiographic results,[193–197] but not necessarily the clinical outcome.[198] At present balloons and stents in angiography-guided interventions are sized to the nominal diameter of the target vessel adjacent to the target lesion ±10%. For IVUS guidance, MUSIC or CLOUT trial criteria represent acceptable standards.[194,195] Advent of temporary stenting using bioabsorbable stents holds a great promise for a truly biological vessel wall repair.[17]

BASIC STRUCTURE OF CORONARY ARTERY INTERVENTION

Although the performance of PCI appears highly individual, a repetitive pattern can be recognized that is common to all interventions. In this section three basic components of this general pattern are described in some detail: *initialization*; the *main procedural cycle*, consisting of an assessment, intervention, and reassessment linked together and driven by the decisions of the operator into series of repetitive iterations designed to achieve the optimum result by using the fewest procedural cycles; and finally *termination*. The number of procedural cycles required reflects commonly the complexity of the disease and skills of the operator (see Chapter 4).

INITIALIZATION

In context of this chapter, intialization begins with establishing the vascular access and ends with providing direct access to the interventional site by placing the tip of the guiding catheter proximal to the target coronary or bypass vessel followed by acquisition of the preinterventional coronary angiograms. Although the actual intervention has not yet been resumed, the procedural risks associated with the placement of the sheath and seating of the guiding catheter at the coronary artery ostium may already materialize at this stage. Therefore, great care is needed to avoid complications. High quality of the baseline coronary angiograms is critical to the appropriate selection of strategy and instrumentation.

Vascular Access

PCI can be performed using both common femoral, brachial, and radial arteries[199–202] (for review, see also Chapter 12). The vast majority of coronary interventions is performed from the right common femoral artery (CFA). Although comparable complication rates for the different access sites have been reported,[203] there are important differences. CFA provides the most versatile and robust access, allowing upsizing (up to 22F) and optimal backup for coronary interventions (most coronary guiding catheters are preshaped to accommodate coronary ostia and the aortic arch from the CFA access!). Typical complications of the CFA access include large hematoma (1.3%), retroperitoneal bleeding (0.4%), false aneurysm (0.4%), vessel closure (0.1%), infection (0.1%), and embolization (0.1%).[204] Transfemoral access should be avoided in patients with severe abdominal aortic or iliofemoral disease and in patients with iliofemoral bypass grafts.

Compared with the CFA access transbrachial route provides a shorter intravascular path, better control of the puncture site, and early mobilization. Limitations include a propensity to spasms, limits to the system size (≤6F), frequently suboptimal backup (except in LIMA PCI), and the need for prompt sheath removal following intervention. For coronary interventions both brachial arteries are acceptable; for coronary procedures the right brachial access is usually preferred because of a shorter intravascular path, an advantage opposed by a small but definite added risk of cerebrovascular thromboembolic complications.

The transradial access has been propagated by some interventionists. Clinically relevant limitations include marked propensity to spasms, particularly with multiple catheter exchanges, suboptimal ostial seating and backup, limited upsizing (5F, maximally 6F), and small but not negligible risk of hand injury in case of radial artery closure. In addition, greater use of radial arteries for coronary conduits also limits the clinical utility of this access. Contraindications include patients with severe generalized vascular calcinosis, patients on hemodialysis, and those with vascular multimorbidity. Allen test and preferably duplex examination are required to document functional collaterization.[205,206]

The size of the sheath and the system depends on the size of the interventional instrumentation and also the expected technical complexity of the case. At present the majority of PCIs are performed using 6F systems, whereas in PCI requiring kissing techniques, multiple guidewires, or adjuvant revascularization techniques the use of 7F systems and greater may be required. In straightforward cases 5F systems are sufficient. Choice of the sheath depends on tortuosity of the ipsilateral pelvic arteries and the aorta. In most cases, sheaths with a standard length are selected. However, longer sheaths (up to 90 cm) may be required to recover steerability of the guiding catheter in patients with adverse peripheral vascular anatomy.

Placement of the Guiding Catheter

Guiding catheters are selected in order to allow safe delivery of the interventional instruments into the target sites, and seating of the guide at the ostium can be thought of as an extension of the peripheral arterial access to the proximity of a distant interventional situs. Atraumatic seating of the tip and optimal backup during the entire intervention are the two factors critical to the success of the procedure. Optimal seating is achieved when the tip of the guide becomes coaxially aligned with the target ostium; optimal backup is achieved when the guide is stably yet gently ostially seated and a stable contact with the opposite aortic wall, providing the right flexibility and "play" required for passive and/or active seating of the guide. Angiographic criteria for optimum seating include:

- Tip just touches and exerts a gentle forward pressure onto the target ostium (passive seating)
- Tip is seated intraluminally without traumatizing or obstructing the target artery (active seating)
- Primary and secondary curves of the guiding catheter and the proximal segment of the target artery form a single, preferably vertically oriented plane
- Primary curve of the guiding catheter and the proximal segment of the target artery are coaxial
- Secondary curve is fully developed and "leans" against the aortic wall opposite the ostium, permitting stability, flexibility, and "play"

Suboptimal seating prompts repositioning, selection of a different guide, or in extreme cases a different access site. Difficult seating is frequently associated with the following conditions:

- Abnormalities of the aortic root (e.g., wide root, horizontal root) and ascending aorta (e.g., aneurysm)

- Abnormalities (e.g., elongation, flat or steep arch) and anomalies (any abnormal development of the embryological fourth arterial arch) of the aortic arch
- Excessive elongation or tortuosity of the aorta and iliac arteries
- Anomalous origins of the coronary artery ostia
- Aortic plaque obstructing the target ostium
- Ostial lesions
- Jets due to aortic valve disease
- Any combination of the above

Suboptimal seating of the guide may perpetuate technical difficulties, and an early correction during the initialization phase is strongly encouraged. Unstable seating, uncontrolled movements ("jumping") of the tip, and undue pressure against the ostium invite complications and must be corrected at once. In rare cases anatomical or functional adversities cannot be overcome and suboptimal seating must be accepted.

Ventricularization and overt damping of the pressure curve or myocardial ischemia following placement of the guide may indicate serious complications and must be clarified at once. Leaning of the tip against the wall is usually harmless and can be easily corrected; potentially more serious causes, particularly in deep seating, include ostial lesions, ostial or proximal injuries, and thrombus formation, each of which requires immediate clarification. Repositioning or replacing of the guiding catheter resolves the problem in most cases. Confirmed injury usually requires an immediate repair. Guides with side holes should be used in patients with ostial lesions and ischemic response upon seating.

Baseline Angiograms

Following the seating of the guiding catheter, a series of baseline coronary angiograms are taken to document the baseline status and to provide the best projections of the interventional site to guide the intervention. Representative images of the interventional site are stored on the monitor for immediate reference.

MAIN INTERVENTIONAL CYCLE: ASSESS, INTERVENE, AND REPEAT

Assess

Baseline angiograms are reviewed to confirm the indication and strategy.

Intervene (Four Movements to a Symphony)

Coronary interventions require rhythm and a steady flow of action combining decision making and acting out the decisions in narrowly spaced repetitive cycles. The sum of these cycles could be thought of as a symphony consisting of four movements. In the first movement the guidewire is introduced through the Tuohy-Borst port, advanced close to the tip of the guiding catheter, and then positioned. Care must be taken not to damage the preshaped tip during this simple movement. To avoid damage to the tip and to the

coronary ostium, the final advancement of the guidewire for approximately the last 20 cm before reaching the tip of the guide should be fluoroscopy guided. This is particularly important when guides with side holes have been used. Following the gentle entry of the guidewire into the coronary ostium, it is navigated downstream of the vessels using gentle probing and a slow rotating forward push. Guidewires with a floppy tip may be advanced faster, yet always in a controlled and careful manner. Once the tip reaches the target lesion, it is aligned with the presumed entry point of the lesion and then carefully advanced. If crossing is barred, the entry to the lesion is explored using a gentle to-and-fro motion in different directions. In difficult cases, use of an OTW system may improve steering and crossing ability. After crossing the lesion, the guidewire is advanced and the guidewire tip parked in the distal segment of the target artery for maximum support. In technically difficult cases, however, it may be preferable to park the tip more proximally or in a side branch to avoid target vessel perforations resulting from possible forceful inadvertent forward guidewire motion. Correct placement of the guidewire must be documented by angiography; at least two different projections are required to confirm correct placement and absence of injury.

In the second movement, the selected dilatation balloon catheter or stent delivery device is advanced to the tip of the guide, directed to and positioned across the target lesion. Fluoroscopy is required to monitor the entry of the device into the coronary artery and any motion of the device thereafter. It should be remembered that during the forward push onto the device the generated force is transmitted not only to the tip but also via friction onto the guidewire, which transmits the force along its length forward to its tip and back to the guiding catheter; thus from the mechanical standpoint the system functions as a unity. Precise tactile feedback is required to control the forces employed to overcome obstacles during the advancement of the device to avoid injury. Depending on the anatomy and morphology of the proximal access and the target site flexibility, tracking, pushing, or crossing ability of the device will determine successful delivery. However, keeping the principle of mechanical unity of the entire system in mind, successful placement of the device across the target lesion can be achieved in almost all cases. The final position of the device should be documented on a cine film.

In the third movement, the actual intervention is performed, typically consisting of inflating a dilatation balloon with high pressure sustained for a short period of time, usually 20 to 120 seconds, and deflating it.

In the fourth movement the device is retracted, the results documented on cine films, and, based on the interpretation of the results, either the intervention is terminated or the next step of the intervention is planned. Before retracting the device, the negative pressure is released to permit refolding, softening of the folds, and smoothing of the edges. To avoid damage to the vessel walls and, if applicable, to the already-deployed stents, the retracting maneuver is performed with care and circumspection under fluoroscopy. Full withdrawal of the device is usually required when a 5F system is used; in bigger systems partial withdrawal is sufficient to allow adequate flow of the contrast agent. To allow comprehensive evaluation, at least two projections of the site are usually required.

Repeat

Proceeding with the intervention and repeating the main interventional cycle may imply a number of actions ranging from minor repositioning of the guidewire to replacing the entire system. Usually, however, balloon dilatation, using a larger balloon or higher inflation pressure, or stent deployment is performed. In rare cases, a complete reinitialization of the procedure, including establishment of a new arterial access, may be required.

TERMINATION

The decision to terminate is the key step of the intervention. Whereas it may be straightforward in cases with an optimal outcome, it becomes more involved in difficult cases requiring multiple main cycles and possibly involving multiple target lesions. The intervention is usually terminated when the criteria for optimal angiographic success (i.e., 0° residual stenosis, TIMI III° coronary flow) in an asymptomatic and stable patient are achieved. The termination criteria may, however, be modified to accommodate less than optimal and palliative results also.

As with anything in life, it is also always important in coronary interventions to learn when it is time to stop. Timely termination after accepting a "good" result might avoid unnecessary escalations associated with multiple stenting, and in worst cases drifting into driven cascades of multiple interventional steps and uncertain outcomes. Although the main cycle usually ends with the complete removal of the instrumentation from the coronary artery to document the results, in some cases only a partial retraction of the devices and the guidewire might be preferable to allow unobstructed view of the interventional site while avoiding recrossing of stents or unstable lesions. However, the final angiograms should be acquired without any hardware left in place in at least two projections, preferably using a standard imaging protocol (see Chapter 3B). Occasionally, the final angiograms reveal complications requiring return to the main interventional cycle. Following final angiograms, usually the patient is undraped, the sheath is removed, hemostasis performed, and the patient transferred to the unit for 12 to 24 hours of monitoring. Termination finishes with the completion of the hemostasis.

STENTING, ADJUNCT MEDICATION, HEMOSTASIS

Since the introduction of PTCA (or POBA) in the 1970s, BMSs and intracoronary DESs have become essential components of catheter-based coronary interventions, as has the use of multiple adjuvant medications. In the following sections a few key points of stenting and adjunct medication are outlined; for more complete coverage, the reader is referred to the literature.[207,208]

INTRACORONARY STENTING

Intracoronary stenting, which was initially introduced as a bailout in cases where angioplasty failed,[14,15] has now become a routine coronary procedure. Following a series of setbacks including a high incidence of acute stent thrombosis[209,210] and later of bleeding complications due to aggressive anticoagulation protocols,[191,192] the introduction of efficacious antiplatelet agents[7] paved the way for a broad clinical acceptance of intracoronary stenting.[211] The advent of stents armed with antiproliferative agents,[16] the development of biodegradable stents,[17] and the potential of both concepts being combined have opened a new era of endocoronary therapy.

Based on the available evidence, BMS-supported PCI performs better than POBA based on the criteria of either stentlike results (<30% residual stenosis) or conventional angioplasty results (<50% residual stenosis) (for review, see reference 212). Similarly, angiographic and presumably also clinical results favor DES over BMS.[72,73] Furthermore, emerging evidence appears to support unconditional (i.e., routine) DES stenting in increasing numbers of subgroups of patients and indications. Yet, the wisdom of unrestricted unconditional stenting should be questioned for the following reasons:

1. The current DESs are relatively high profile and do not allow successful deployment in all clinical settings.
2. DESs prevent positive remodeling permanently.
3. Unconditional stenting increases the incidence of vessel wall injuries potentially associated with multiple stent deployments, in extreme cases in a "full metal jacket" repair.
4. Even innocuous stent-related edge injuries get frequently stented.
5. Deployed stents might interfere with surgical revascularization, if later needed.
6. Deployed stents might interfere with reinterventions in patients with disease progression.
7. Deployed stents might prevent the use of future technologies such as bioabsorbable stents.

Because of these limitations unconditional stenting based only on evidence must be rejected in clinical practice and a more differentiated approach is required. For example, it clearly makes a difference whether a main vessel or a side branch ought to be stented, or whether the first or the 10th stent ought to be placed. Unfortunately, physiological guidance by IVUS or pressure/flow wire data in patients with stentlike results following angioplasty did not improve stent indications.[213–215] Thus, until still better stents and more objective decision criteria become available, individual decisions taking into account expected risks and benefits prior to each stent deployment are recommended. Although DES appears to be an obvious choice in most if not all cases, secondary considerations such as tracking ability in difficult anatomy and high radial force requirements may tilt the decision toward BMS.

Selection of the best stent for a given lesion includes the decision on sizing. Stent sizing up to ±10% of the nominal target vessel diameter appears to be acceptable in angiography-guided interventions. In the IVUS-guided stenting MUSIC trial[195] or CLOUT trial[194] criteria targeting 0% residual stenosis (average 5% residual stenosis has been typical in large trials) are acceptable. The length of the expanded stent should fully cover the target lesion.

In dissections, stenting of the proximal entry point might suffice in some cases; however, complete lesion coverage is usually preferred because of uncertainties in identifying entry points exactly and potentials of creating secondary entry sites in the dissection membranes due to spot stenting.

In long and/or discontinuous lesions, placement of a single stent is preferred. If a single long stent cannot be delivered or discontinuities of lesions >5 mm are present, multiple stents with or without overlap might be required. In overlapping stents one ring overlap usually suffices. In multilocular lesions frequently the most distal stent is placed first to avoid recrossing. However, in numerous cases distal stenoses become less significant or even disappear when proximal stenosis is removed and a full antegrade flow has been restored. Thus, a reverse order of stent placement (from most proximal to most distal) might be also justified, particularly in emergency cases with a pronounced coronary vasomotion.

In all cases, however, it is critical to deliver an intact stent to fully cover the lesion. Stent damage, stent loss or incomplete lesion coverage due to "freezing" of the stent might trigger serious complications. With stents optimally positioned complete stent deployment and optimum strut-wall apposition while preserving the three-dimensional stent geometry are required. To learn more about the issues of optimal inflation pressures and IVUS guidance the reader is referred to the literature.[216–221] In this context it should be emphasized that particular care must be paid to avoid strut damage threatened to occur throughout the procedure. Particularly, stents with a low strut thickness are prone to damage mostly resulting from excessive manipulation. Key factors include meticulous technique of stent delivery avoiding a buildup of friction, and a careful withdrawal of a completely evacuated delivery balloon (in some cases balloons exposed to a negative pressure might incompletely refold causing stent damage by the stiff folds of the balloon, particularly when abruptly retracted). Furthermore, to avoid damage of the deployed stent, recrossing maneuvers and afterdilatations should be kept to a minimum. Figures 8-38 and 8-39 provide examples of single stent intervention and escalating stent procedures resulting in extensive metal coverage.

Better stents allowed primary stenting using a direct approach.[222–227] Currently, in large-volume centers approximately 30% of the stent-supported coronary angioplasties are performed directly, trends rising. Although direct stenting might appear to be the technique of choice in a significant number of patients, it is necessary to carefully assess the entire intracoronary access pathway as well as the severity and rigidity of the target lesion prior to stenting. In cases with highly complex and rigid lesions, direct stenting is not recommended. In these cases in which direct stenting has been already initiated, timely retraction of the stent delivery system and predilatation represent the best prevention of avoidable complications. Some of the potential advantages and drawbacks of direct stenting are summarized in Table 8-36.

ADJUVANT MEDICATION

Peri-interventional medical management focuses on anticoagulants and antiplatelet agents.

During the early present era, 10,000 U intravenous unfractionated heparin (UFH) was typically administered to prevent thromboembolism. During the late present era, activated clotting time (ACT) was introduced to better steer the anticoagulation. Based on the early experience of surgeons[228] and interventionists,[229–231] target ACT values for coronary angioplasty (e.g., 250 to 300 seconds for the HemoTec device and 300 to 350 seconds for the Hemochron device) were established.

With the introduction of stents, the incidence of stent thrombosis and the excessive bleeding that was subsequent to more aggressive anticoagulation regimen have stimulated new work on peri-interventional management of thromboses. Peri-interventional antithrombotic regimens have grown more complex since the introduction of new anticoagulants such as low-molecular-weight heparins (LMWH) and hirudins (for review, see references 232 and 233), and the use of increasingly potent antiplatelet agents. Based on evidence[81,82] and assuming similar outcomes and incidence of bleeding complications with UFH and low-molecular-weight heparins, LMWH,[234] a number of periinterventional antithrombotic regimens have been proposed. Typically, a single intravenous bolus of 5000 U or 60 U/kg (ranging from 30 to 100 U/kg) UFH is given prior to PCI. In patients receiving GPIIb/IIIa receptor inhibitors, lower dose ranges are preferable (target ACT >200 seconds). In patients not receiving GPIIb/IIIa receptor inhibitors, a target ACT of 250 to 350 seconds is recommended. In uncomplicated elective cases, postinterventional anticoagulation following PCI is not indicated; for details in different clinical settings, see references 81, 82, and 235.

The pivotal role that platelets play in initiating acute atherothrombotic syndromes[236] and peri-interventional complications during coronary interventions[237] (for review, see reference 238) has been increasingly appreciated over the past two decades. Since the recognition of the importance of aspirin in coronary prevention[239] and the importance of platelets in pathophysiology of atherosclerosis (for review, see reference 240) and acute coronary syndromes (for review, see references 241–243), efficacious antiplatelet strategies (for a review, see reference 244) have been implemented in peri-interventional settings (for a review, see reference 245). The use of acetylsalicylic acid (for review, see reference 244), thienopyridines (for review, see reference 246), and glycoprotein IIb/IIIa receptor inhibitors (see reference 208 for a review and references 247 and 248 on their limitations due to resistance) during PCI is the subject of numerous guidelines and recommendations.[81,82,235] A representative example of the current recommendations is provided in Table 8-37[235] and Tables 8-38 and 8-39.[81,82] Table 8-40 provides an example of comparisons of GP IIb/IIIa receptor inhibitors based on pharmacokinetics, adverse effects, and costs. Potentials of an intracoronary application of GP IIb/IIIa receptor inhibitors[249] and a triple oral

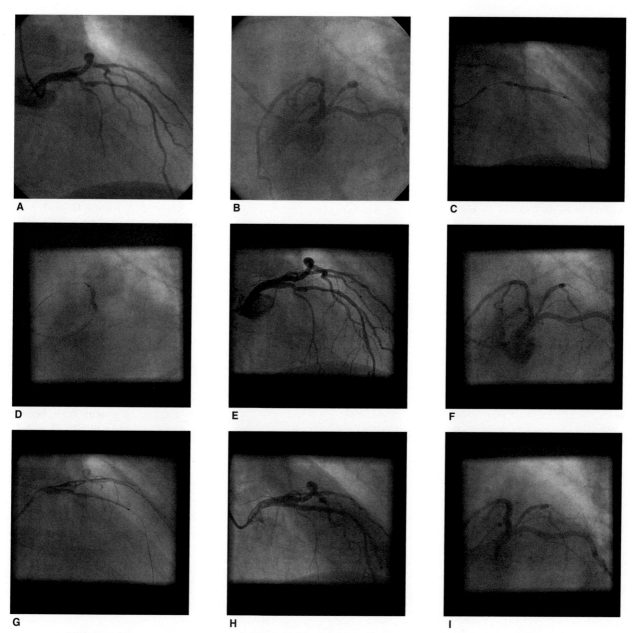

FIGURE 8-38. Primary stenting, uncomplicated emergency percutaneous coronary intervention (PCI). A 62-year-old woman with non-ST elevation myocardial infarction (NSTEMI). Emergency angiography shows single-vessel disease with a long proximal (AHA segment 6) 70% left anterior descending artery (LAD) stenosis as the "culprit" lesion **(A,B)**. Predilation with 10 bar was performed using a 2.0/30-mm balloon catheter **(C,D)**. Subsequently, 50% restenosis **(E,F)** was primarily stented using a 3.0/30-mm Driver (Medtronic) at 12 bar **(G)**, resulting in 0% residual stenosis **(H,I)**. Note the semipermeable filters in **C–I** to reduce the radiation exposure during the intervention.

antiplatelet treatment (acetylsalicylic acid, clopidogrel, cilostazol, a selective phosphodiestrase III inhibitor)[250] are under clinical investigation.

To reduce the incidence of peri-interventional bleeding complications in patients receiving potent antithrombotic medication, we recommend a meticulous atraumatic technique of arterial puncture, the use of smaller French size systems, early sheath removal (<2 hours in uncomplicated cases), and optimal hemostasis. Protamine can be used to reverse UFH (1.0–1.3 mg for each 1000 IU UFH); slow intravenous injection is recommended[251] because of the potential of anaphylactic reaction (<2%). Coronary bypass surgery in patients

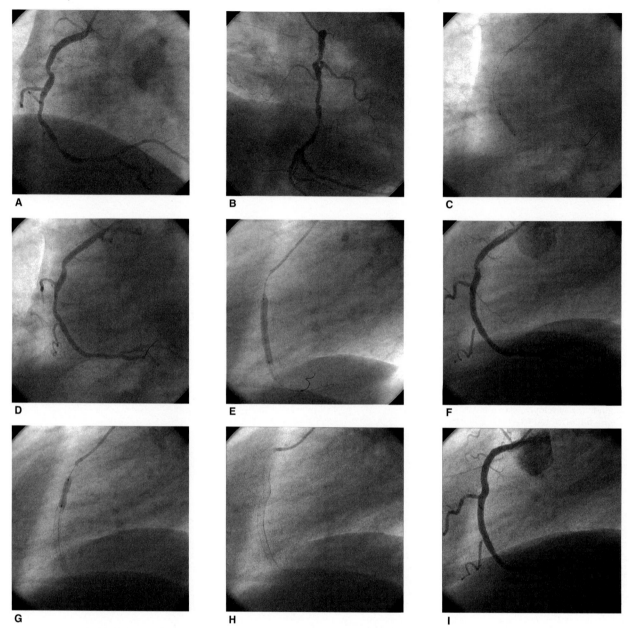

FIGURE 8-39. A 51-year-old man with crescendo angina, Canadian Cardiology Society (CCS) III°. Percutaneous coronary intervention on right coronary artery (RCA). **A:** Diagnostic cine angiogram, right coronary artery (RCA), right anterior oblique (RAO) 45 degrees. Target 80% lesion distal RCA, diffuse disease mid-RCA segment. **B:** Diagnostic cine angiogram, RCA, left anterior oblique (LAO) 30 degrees. Target lesion with projectional shortening, diffuse disease mid-RCA. **C:** Direct stenting distal RCA target lesion. **D:** Successful revascularization of the target lesion. Diffuse disease of mid-RCA appears borderline on angiography. **E:** Long-segment direct stenting of the entire mid-RCA with distal stent overlap with the first stent by one ring. **F:** Successful revascularization of the mid-RCA with proximal axial plaque shift and accentuation of the pre-existing stenosis. **G:** Direct stenting. Deployment of a second stent with distal overlap with the second stent by one ring is shown. On nominal inflation pressure, incomplete stent deployment is visualized. **H:** Full-metal jacket. The entire mid-RCA segment has been stented by successive, overlapping stent implantations (from distal to proximal, conventional approach). **I:** Final angiogram. Satisfactory angiographic result. No residual stenoses. TIMI III°.

TABLE 8-36. Potential Advantages and Drawbacks of Direct Stenting

Potential Advantages	Potential Drawbacks
Avoidance of multiple exchanges	Failure to track
Less trauma	Failure of precise positioning, incomplete deployment
Lower rate of "no-reflow"	Stent damage or loss
Shorter procedural time	Incomplete apposition
Lower procedural costs	Traumatization of the target vessel
	Unconditional stenting

receiving GP IIb/IIIa receptor inhibitors may be associated with higher bleeding complications;[252] yet it can be performed safely if these agents have been stopped prior to or at the time of the operation and fresh platelet concentrates are available if needed.[253]

HEMOSTASIS

Although the sheath may be removed and hemostasis performed in the catheterization laboratory at the end of the procedure, it is

TABLE 8-37. Summary Recommendation for Antithrombotic Therapy in Peri-interventional Settings

PATIENTS UNDERGOING PERCUTANEOUS CORONARY INTERVENTION (PCI): ORAL ANTIPLATELET THERAPY

Aspirin
1. For patients undergoing PCI, the guideline developers recommend pretreatment with aspirin, 75 to 325 mg (**Grade 1A**).
2. For long-term treatment after PCI, the guideline developers recommend aspirin, 75 to 162 mg/d (**Grade 1A**).
3. For long-term treatment after PCI in patients who receive antithrombotic agents such as clopidogrel or warfarin, the guideline developers recommend lower-dose aspirin, 75 to 100 mg/d (**Grade 1C+**).

Thienopyridine Derivatives
Pretreatment with Thienopyridines prior to PCI
1. The guideline developers recommend a loading dose of 300 mg of clopidogrel at least 6 h prior to planned PCI (**Grade 1B**). If clopidogrel is started <6 h prior to PCI, the guideline developers suggest a 600-mg loading dose of clopidogrel (**Grade 2C**).
2. If ticlopidine is administered, the guideline developers recommend a loading dose of 500 mg at least 6 h before planned PCI (**Grade 2C**).

Aspirin-Intolerant Patients
1. For PCI patients who cannot tolerate aspirin, the guideline developers recommend that the loading dose of clopidogrel (300 mg) or ticlopidine (500 mg) be administered at least 24 h prior to the planned PCI (**Grade 2C**).

Duration of Thienopyridine Therapy after Stent Placement
1. After PCI, the guideline developers recommend, in addition to aspirin, clopidogrel (75 mg/d) for at least 9 to 12 months (**Grade 1A**).
2. If ticlopidine is used in place of clopidogrel after PCI, the guideline developers recommend ticlopidine for 2 weeks after placement of a bare metal stent in addition to aspirin (**Grade 1B**).
3. In patients with low atherosclerotic risk, such as those with isolated coronary lesions, the guideline developers recommend clopidogrel for at least 2 weeks after placement of a bare metal stent (**Grade 1A**), for 2 to 3 months after placement of a sirolimus-eluting stent (**Grade 1C+**), and 6 months after placement of a paclitaxel-eluting stent (**Grade 1C**).

PATIENTS UNDERGOING PCI: GLYCOPROTEIN (GP) IIb-IIIa INHIBITORS

1. For all patients undergoing PCI, particularly those undergoing primary PCI, or those with refractory unstable angina (UA) or other high-risk features, the guideline developers recommend use of a GP IIb-IIIa antagonist (abciximab or eptifibatide) (**Grade 1A**).
2. In patients undergoing PCI for ST-segment elevation myocardial infarction (STEMI), the guideline developers recommend abciximab over eptifibatide (**Grade 1B**).
Remark: Whenever possible, abciximab should be started prior to balloon inflation.
3. The guideline developers recommend administration of abciximab as a 0.25 mg/kg bolus followed by a 12-h infusion at a rate of 10 μg/min (**Grade 1A**) and eptifibatide as a double bolus (each 180 μg/kg administered 10 min apart), followed by an 18-h infusion of 2.0 μg/kg/min^{-1} (**Grade 1A**).
4. In patients undergoing PCI, the guideline developers recommend **against** the use of tirofiban as an alternative to abciximab (**Grade 1A**).
5. For patients with non-ST-segment elevation myocardial infarction (NSTEMI)/UA who are designated as moderate-to-high risk based on thrombolysis in myocardial infarction (TIMI) score, the guideline developers recommend that upstream use of GP IIb-IIIa antagonist (either eptifibatide or tirofiban) be started as soon as possible prior to PCI (**Grade 1A**).
6. In NSTEMI/UA patients who receive upstream treatment with tirofiban, the guideline developers recommend that PCI be deferred for at least 4 h after initiating the tirofiban infusion (**Grade 2C**).
7. With planned PCI in NSTEMI/UA patients with an elevated troponin level, the guideline developers recommend that abciximab be started within 24 h prior to the intervention (**Grade 1A**).
Underlying values and preferences: These recommendations for the use of GP IIb-IIIa inhibitors place a relatively high value on preventing cardiovascular events and a relatively low value on cost and bleeding complications.

(Continued)

TABLE 8-37. (*Continued*)

PATIENTS UNDERGOING PCI: UNFRACTIONATED HEPARIN (UFH)

1. In patients receiving a GP IIb-IIIa inhibitor, the guideline developers recommend a heparin bolus of 50 to 70 IU/kg to achieve a target activated clotting time (ACT) >200 seconds (**Grade 1C**).

2. In patients not receiving a GP IIb-IIIa inhibitor, the guideline developers recommend that heparin be administered in doses sufficient to produce an ACT of 250 to 350 s (**Grade 1C+**). The guideline developers suggest a weight-adjusted heparin bolus of 60 to 100 IU/kg (**Grade 2C**).

3. In patients after uncomplicated PCI, the guideline developers recommend **against** routine postprocedural infusion of heparin (**Grade 1A**).

Patients Undergoing PCI: Low-Molecular-Weight Heparin (LMWH)

1. In patients who have received LMWH prior to PCI, the guideline developers recommend that administration of additional anticoagulant therapy is dependent on the timing of the last dose of LMWH (**Grade 1C**). If the last dose of enoxaparin was administered ≤8 h prior to PCI, the guideline developers suggest no additional anticoagulant therapy (**Grade 2C**). If the last dose of enoxaparin was administered between 8 h and 12 h before PCI, the guideline developers suggest a 0.3 mg/kg bolus of intravenous (IV) enoxaparin at the time of PCI (**Grade 2C**). If the last enoxaparin dose was administered >12 h before PCI, the guideline developers suggest conventional anticoagulation therapy during PCI (**Grade 2C**).

Patients Undergoing PCI: Direct Thrombin Inhibitors

1. For patients undergoing PCI who are not treated with a GP IIb-IIIa antagonist, the guideline developers recommend bivalirudin (0.75 mg/kg bolus followed by an infusion of 1.75 mg/kg/h^{-1} for the duration of PCI) over heparin during PCI (**Grade 1A**).

2. In PCI patients who are at low risk for complications, the guideline developers recommend bivalirudin as an alternative to heparin as an adjunct to GP IIb-IIIa antagonists (**Grade 1B**).

3. In PCI patients who are at high risk for bleeding, the guideline developers recommend bivalirudin over heparin as an adjunct to GP IIb-IIIa antagonists (**Grade 1B**).

Patients Undergoing PCI: Vitamin K Antagonists

1. In patients who undergo PCI with no other indication for systemic anticoagulation therapy, the guideline developers recommend **against** routine use of warfarin (or other vitamin K antagonists) after PCI (**Grade 1A**).

Dose adjustments of eptifibatide and tirofiban in patients with renal insufficiency should be implemented according to the specifications of the manufacturers.

Reproduced with permission from Popma JJ, Berger P, Ohman EM, et al. Antithrombotic therapy during percutaneous coronary intervention. The Seventh ACCP Conference on Antithrombotic and Thrombolytic Therapy. *Chest* 2004;126:576S–599S.

TABLE 8-38. Suggested Dual Antithrombotic Peri-interventional Regimen with Special Consideration of Bare Metal Stents (BMSs) and Drug-eluting Stents (DESs)

Timing	Drug	
	ASA	Clopidogrel
Pre-treatment PCI	≥2 h before PCI 100 mg (75–325 mg) po or 500 mg IV. (empirical dosage)	≥6 h 300 mg <6h 6600 mg (loading dose)
During PCI	—	—
Long-term after PCI	100 mg/d (75–162 mg/d; 75–100 mg in patients receiving thienopyridines) for life	75 mg/d for 6–12 months, alternatively 3–4 weeks after BMS, 6–12 months after DES, 12 months after brachytherapy

PCI, percutaneous coronary intervention; ASA, acetylsalicylic acid.

Based on Smith SC, Dove JT, Jacobs AK, et al. ACC/AHA guidelines for percutaneous coronary intervention (Revision of the 1993 PTCA guidelines). *J Am Coll Cardiol.* 2001;37:2239-2300; and Silber S., Albertson P, Aviles FF, et al. Guidelines for percutaneous coronary interventions. The Task Force for Percutaneous Coronary Interventions of the European Society of Cardiology. 2005;26:804-847.

safer to monitor the patient for 2 to 4 hours before the sheath removal. Criteria for sheath removal include the absence of symptoms, negative cardiac markers, systolic blood pressure <140 mm Hg, and ACT <180 seconds. The principal options to achieve hemostasis are:

- Mechanical compression; manual or using mechanical devices, e.g., FemoStop (Radi Medical Systems, Inc.)
- Sealing the puncture site using chemicals designed to enhance the body's natural hemostasis, e.g., collagen type I (VasoSeal, Datascope Corp.)
- Sandwiching the puncture site between a bioabsorbable anchor and collagen sponge
- Suturing (e.g., Perclose device, Abbott Vascular)

Selection of the method of hemostasis depends on a number of factors including the patient's constitution and mobility, status of the arterial puncture site, vessel wall calcification, systemic blood pressure, and patient's comfort. An early closure of the arterial access and timely mobilization are probate means to prevent complications. Although closure devices might not lower the incidence of local complications,[254] they

TABLE 8-39. Suggested Antithrombotic Peri-interventional Regimen Using Glycoprotein IIb/IIIa Receptor Inhibitors

Indication	Medication	Recommendation/ Evidence Level
Stable CAD with complex lesions, threatening and actual vessel closure, visible thrombus, no/ slow flow	Abciximab, eptifibatide, tirofiban	IIa/C
NSTEMI in high-risk patients immediately before PCI	Abciximab, eptifibatide	I/C
NSTEMI in high-risk patients before diagnostic angiography and possible PCI <48 h	Eptifibatide, tirofiban	I/C
NSTEMI in high-risk patients with known coronary anatomy <24 h before planned PCI	Abciximab	IC
STEMI in all patients with primary PCI	Abciximab	IIa/A

CAD, coronary artery disease; NSTEMI, non-ST elevation myocardial infarction; PCI, percutaneous coronary intervention; STEMI, ST elevation myocardial infarction.

Based on Smith SC, Dove JT, Jacobs AK, et al. ACC/AHA guidelines for percutaneous coronary intervention (Revision of the 1993 PTCA guidelines). *J Am Coll Cardiol.* 2001;37:2239-2300; and Silber S. Albertsson P, Aviles FF, et al. Guidelines for percutaneous coronary interventions. The Task Force for Percutaneous Coronary Interventions of the European Society of Cardiology. 2005;26:804–847.

greatly improve the aftercare. Closure devices should not be used in morbidly obese patients and in patients with severely calcified arteries. In patients with synthetic grafts their use is contraindicated.

FOLLOW-UP

Following uncomplicated PCI, patients are typically discharged 24 hours after sheath removal. To ensure patients' safety, contrary to some opinions,[255] outpatient PCI is not recommended for routine clinical practice. Table 8-41 provides an example of post-PCI orders in uncomplicated procedures.

Following complex or complicated PCI and in patients scheduled for staged procedures, the sheath is left in place and the patient is transferred for monitoring. Because of the risk of peripheral complications, the sheath should be removed within 24 hours. Low-dose heparin, e.g., 800 U/h UFH until 4 hours before sheath removal (ACT <180 seconds) is recommended to prevent thromboembolism.

MANAGING COMPLICATIONS

Complications are unexpected, adverse events directly related to the procedure that usually occur shortly after the intervention (<24 to 48 hours). Less frequently, late complications occur due to aneurysm or fistula formation (days) or material fatigue (months to years). In a broader sense, even minor technical adversities such as unintended guidewire withdrawal or the necessity to change the guiding catheter may also be regarded as complications potentially leading to clinical events, particularly when they occur in critical situations such as emergency procedures. Thus, optimal strategy and meticulous technique are the best means to prevent complications.

In the absence of standardized reporting of intermediate complications, the elevation of cardiac markers following PCI represents the best means of monitoring procedural complications (for review, see reference 91). Predictors of postprocedural cardiac marker elevation include transient vessel closure, side branch closure, prolonged spasms, distal embolizations, multivessel disease, procedures on saphenous vein grafts, high-grade stenoses, slow flow/no reflow, coronary dissections worse than NHLBI type C classification, prolonged nonperfusion balloon inflation, prolonged ischemia, thrombosis, hemodynamic instability and intervention in patients with acute coronary

TABLE 8-40. Comparisons of Glycoprotein (GP) IIb/IIIa Receptor Inhibitors Based on Pharmacokinetics, Adverse Effects and Costs

Agent	Recommended Indications	Time to 80% Inhibition	Half-Time, Plasma	Half-Time, Platelet-bound	Adverse Effects				Costs
Abciximab	Stable CAD, NSTEMI, STEMI	<10 min	30 min	12–16 h	B	T	A	H	+++
Eptifibatide	Stable CAD, NSTEMI	<15 min (180 μg)	48–168 min	Seconds	B	T	—	H	++
Tirofiban	Stable CAD, NSTEMI	30 min	72–120 min	Seconds	B	T	—	—	++

B, bleeding; T, thrombocytopenia; A, anaphylaxis; H, hypotension; NSTEMI, non-ST elevation myocardial infarction; STEMI, ST elevation myocardial infarction; CAD, coronary artery disease.

Adapted from Brouse S, Roberts K. Medical advisory panel; Drug class review: Glycoprotein (GP) IIb/IIIa receptor inhibitors for use in Acute Coronary Syndromes (ACS) & Percutaneous Coronary Intervention (PCI). Available at: www.vapbm.org/reviews/glycoproteinreview.pdf. Accessed August 20, 2005.

TABLE 8-41. An Example of Post Percutaneous Coronary Intervention Orders (PCI) Following Uncomplicated PCI Using a 5F system

ECG monitoring/telemetry	≤24 h
12-lead ECG	Immediately and 6 h post-PCI or as needed
Laboratory controls	CKMB and creatinine 3 (6 h) and 12 h after PCI, alternatively cardiac troponins T/I if normal range at baseline
Femoral sheath removal	ACT ≤180 s (2–4 h after PCI)
Hemostasis	Manual compression, check for pulses and bleeding q 30 min for 2 h, relax compression after 4 h, dressing for 5 h total, check for complete hemostasis before removal
Mobilization	Gradual, e.g., sit up and walk ~2 h, after dressing removal
Medication	100 mg ASA q day, 75 mg clopidogrel q day + other as prescribed

CKMB, creatine kinase MB isoenzyme; ACT, active clotting time; ASA, acetylsalicylic acid.

syndromes. In addition, the experience of the interventionist might also be important.[256–259] Patients with postprocedural elevated levels of cardiac markers have a worse prognosis than those undergoing uncomplicated PCI (for review, see reference 260). Furthermore, the prognosis correlates with the magnitude of the elevation.[261–263] In PCI settings cardiac markers are measured at baseline and usually at 3 to 6 hours and 12 hours. The results are entered into the PCI quality protocols. Complications arising at the site of the intervention are addressed immediately to prevent escalation. Systemic complications resulting from acute heart failure, cardiac arrhythmias, pericardial tamponade, and peripheral thromboembolism are subject to standard critical care management.[264] Tables 8-42 and 8-43 provide representative examples of major and minor complications associated with PCI complications reported.

PLAQUE SHIFT

Circumferential and longitudinal plaque distribution varies greatly among lesions. Using the pathological definition of eccentricity (presence of an arc of disease-free wall within the plaque), the majority of coronary artery lesions are eccentric[265,266] Angiographic eccentricity, defined as luminal asymmetry of the lesion (type B lesion, ACC/AHA nomenclature), has been identified as a negative prognostic factor,[150] but the ability of angiography to identify eccentricity is limited. Compared to intracoronary ultrasound, the concordance was low depending on the definition and criteria (Table 8-44).[267] The IVUS eccentricity index has been defined as the ratio of maximum to minimum plaque plus media thickness. Using index values ≥3.0 as a cutoff, the concordance between IVUS and angiographic eccentricity was 53.8%. Thus, the ability of angiography to depict plaque distribution is low.[268–271]

Angioplasty-associated "controlled" injury denoted also as acute plaque remodeling results from plaque shifts, fissuring, rupture, dissection, embolization, compression, thrombus formation, and hemorrhage.[272] Depending on the direction of induced stresses within the walls, plaque redistribution (plaque shift or "snowplow effect") occurs mainly in the axial direction with the circumferential and radial shifts being less prominent. Axial plaque shifts redistribute the plaque toward the lesion's periphery and into adjacent segments.[273,274] Angiography may depict some plaque shifts by visualizing the changes in the endoluminal silhouette. Unable to see the site directly, the operator fully depends on correct reading and interpretation of images.

Because the angiographic definition of lesions' morphology is suboptimal (see Chapter 3B), a great deal of experience is required for appropriate treatment decisions. For example, minor plaque shifts might not require repair at all, a decision based on a thorough evaluation of multiple target site projections. Whereas antegrade axial shifts in nonproximal segments are generally benign and usually require no further intervention, retrograde axial shifts might be more significant, eventually requiring a stent coverage. Figure 8-40 shows a typical example of a distal axial plaque shift requiring stent coverage.

TABLE 8-42. Representative Example of the Incidence of Major Percutaneous Coronary Intervention (PCI) Complications in a Large-volume, Experienced Center

Years	1980–1987	1988–1991	1992–1995	1996–1998	Total
Number of patients	7254	6591	6367	6417	26,629
Number of lesions	8885	9068	8321	8342	34,616
Complication-free success (%)	88	90	90	94	91
Emergency bypass surgery (%)	3.4	2.1	1.3	1.5	2.1
STEMI (%)	1.6	1.0	0.8	0.3	1.0
In-hospital death (%)	11.2	0.5	0.6	0.7	0.5

Of treated patients, 48% had single-vessel disease and 52% multivessel disease; multivessel PCI was performed in 9% of patients.

Emory University Hospital. Available at: www.rjmatthewsmd.com/Definitions.angiogramm.htm. Accessed August 24, 2005.

TABLE 8-43. Representative Example of the Incidence of Minor PCI complications

Complication	Frequency (%)
Dissection	29
Side branch occlusion	1.7
DC shock for ventricular arrhythmia	1.5
Emergency recatheterization	0.8
Femoral access repair	0.6
Blood transfusion	0.3
Coronary embolization	0.1
Cardiac tamponade	0.1
Stroke	0.03

Emory University Hospital. Available at: www.rjmatthewsmd.com/Definitions/angiogramm.htm. Accessed August 24, 2005.

TABLE 8-44. Comparison of Pathological Equivalent, Angiographic, and Ultrasound Eccentricity

Parameter	Eccentric by Angiography (n = 795)	Concentric by Angiography (n = 651)	Significance (p value)
EEM CSA, mm²	19.1 ± 6.3	19.4 ± 6.9	NS
Lumen CSA, mm²	2.3 ± 1.9	3.0 ± 3.6	0.0002
CSN, %	87.4 ± 10.0	84.7 ± 13.0	0.0003
IVUS eccentricity index	3.8 ± 2.7	3.2 ± 2.3	0.0010
Eccentric by IVUS, n (%)	393 (49)	267 (41)	0.0048
Arc of normal arterial wall, n (%)	126 (15)	93 (14)	NS

IVUS, intravascular ultrasound; EEM, external elastic membrane; CSA, cross-sectional area; CSN, cross-sectional narrowing; IVUS eccentricity index, ratio of maximum to minimum plaque plus media thickness (i.e., eccentricity index of 1 ~ concentric lesion).

Modified from Mintz GS, Popma JJ, Pichard AD, et al. Limitations of angiography in the assessment of plaque distribution in coronary artery disease. *Circulation.* 1996;93:924–931.

VESSEL WALL DISSECTION

Limited dissections are a common pathological finding following angioplasty[275] and can be visualized in about 30% of angiograms, in many instances without any apparent negative prognostic significance (such as restenosis or clinical adverse events) if no other complicating factors have been present.[276,277] Even the depth or extent of dissection as documented by IVUS may not be related to adverse outcomes.[278] Small stenting-related edge dissections, documented in 10.7% of all stent implantations, remained clinically silent and healed at 6-month IVUS follow-up.[279] Common predictors of iatrogenic dissections seen on angiography included complex lesions, calcified lesions, long lesions, eccentric lesions, and vessel tortuosity.[280–284]

The angiographic classification of dissections according to the NHLBI PTCA registry is based on the presence of intraluminal filling defects, extravasation of contrast agents, and abnormal peri- or extraluminal staining (see Chapter 3B). The classification of coronary dissections based on IVUS differentiates between the following types:

- *Intimal:* limited to the atheroma and/or intima
- *Medial:* extending into the media
- *Adventitial:* extending through the external elastic membrane (EEM)
- *Intramural hematoma:* "an accumulation of blood within the medial space, displacing the internal elastic membrane inward and EEM outward. Entry and/or exit points may or may not be observed"
- *Intrastent:* "separation of neointimal hyperplasia from stent struts, usually seen only after treatment of in-stent restenosis"

The IVUS severity of a dissection is based on the following criteria:

1) depth (into plaque—useful only in describing intimal dissections that do not reach the media); 2) circumferential extent (in degrees of arc) using a protractor centered on the lumen; 3) length using motorized transducer pullback; 4) size of residual lumen (CSA, cross-sectional area); and 5) CSA of the luminal dissection. Additional descriptors of a dissection may include the presence of a false lumen, the identification of mobile flap(s), the presence of calcium at the dissection border, and dissections in close proximity to stent edges.[285]

Coronary dissections are either spontaneous or iatrogenic. Spontaneous dissections may be associated with coronary artery disease or, less frequently, they may be caused by spasms, collagen and immune system disorders, chest trauma, strenuous exercise, cocaine abuse, and other conditions.[286] Unlike atherosclerotic dissections originating from the intima, spontaneous non-atherosclerotic dissections frequently occur in the outer layers, media, and adventitia, where they are associated with degeneration and inflammation.[287] The preponderance of cases reported in women in the peripartal period is striking.[288]

Spontaneous atherosclerotic dissections are usually associated with acute coronary syndromes. They may cause vessel closure or a partial obstruction. Complete stent coverage with precise stent placement spanning the entire length of the lesion is usually required. In patients with culprit lesions associated with extensive distal dissections, the operator must decide whether to stent only the entry site (usually the most proximal part of the lesion) or the entire dissection. Because of the attending risks (oversight of multiple entry points, incomplete coverage of the lesion), stenting limited to the entry site should probably be considered only in IVUS-guided interventions. If more than one stent is needed to cover the lesion, in most cases the more distal stent should be implanted first to close off the re-entry and to avoid bulging of the dissection sac, with the possibility of secondary injury. The stent overlap usually spans one ring; intussusceptions of intimal flaps or secondary dissections must be avoided. To prevent self-perpetuating traumatization, conservative sizing and lower inflation pressures are recommended. When longer stents are used (>20 mm), postdeployment dilatations with shorter balloons are usually required to ensure optimum strut apposition of the struts.

Iatrogenic dissections are caused by guidewires, guiding catheters, or any of the endovascular instruments. Figure 8-41 provides an example of iatrogenic dissections due to guidewire and guiding catheter injuries. Guidewire-related dissections are the most frequent iatrogenic dissections. The risk of guidewire-related dissection increases with the stiffness of the tip, stiffness of the shaft, slipperiness of the tip, and difficulty of the anatomic substrate such as with total and subtotal occlusions, complex lesions, and advanced diffuse disease. Other dissection-prone substrates include highly vulnerable tortuous vessels (indicative of long-standing hypertension) and vasospastic and small arteries. Gender-based differences in coronary artery vulnerability are possible, yet largely speculative.

Because of the forward motion involved in advancing the guidewire, the majority of guidewire-related dissections in coronary interventions are antegrade. Antegrade dissections are prone to expansion and in extreme cases to vessel closure and may be prone to distal propagations. Retrograde propagations are less common. To reduce the risk of dissections, the stiffness of the tip and shaft, the speed and force of push, and the extent of the rotating forward motion should be adjusted to the anatomic substrate. To prevent damage, the tip should be shaped and introduced into the guide carefully (note: avoid reshaping and

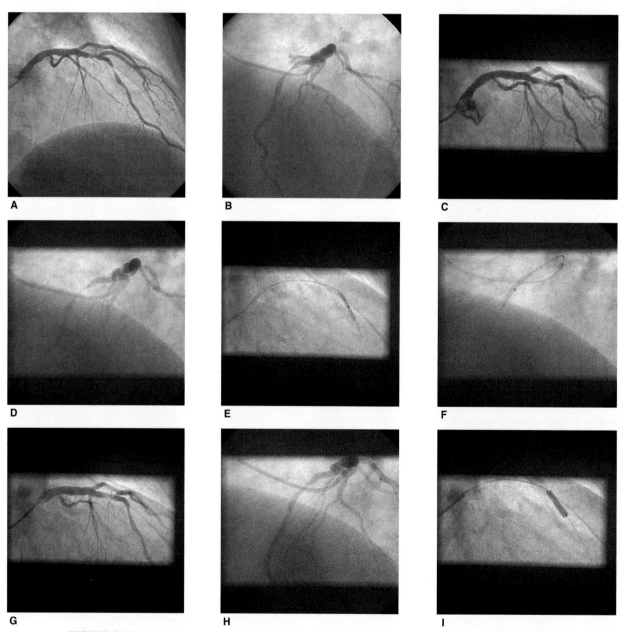

FIGURE 8-40.   Plaque shift. A 51-year-old man with anterior wall ST elevation myocardial infarction (STEMI). Diagnostic angiograms (23-cm image magnification) revealed 95% "culprit" lesion left anterior descending artery (LAD) stenosis in AHA segment 7 **(A,B)**. Reference percutaneous coronary intervention (PCI) images were taken using 14-cm image magnification **(C,D)**, and PCI was initiated. Following predilatation using 2.5/20-mm balloon at 7 bar **(E,F)**, residual 60% residual stenosis was demonstrated **(G,H)** and a 3.5/18-mm Vision stent (Guidant) at 12 bar was implanted **(I)**. Subsequent angiography revealed moderate distal plaque shift requiring deployment of a second stent (3.0/15-mm Vision, Guidant, 10 bar, one crown distal overlap) **(L,M)**. **J,K:** A satisfactory revascularization result was documented in the final angiograms **(N,O)**. (*Continued*)

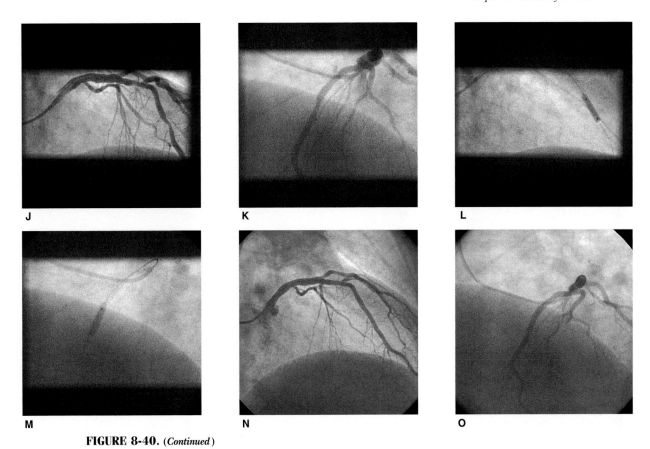

FIGURE 8-40. (*Continued*)

complex shapes). Using fluoroscopy for guidance, the guidewire enters the ostium, avoiding side holes of the guide if present. Brisk entry into the vessel may cause high proximal dissections and should be avoided. Thus, before advancing the guidewire into the ostium, unobstructed flow and coaxial alignment between the tip of the guide and the proximal segment of the vessel at the entry point should be confirmed. To avoid trapping the tip under plaque (recognized by deformation or buckling of the tip), continuous fluoroscopic guidance is mandatory. If the guidewire has been trapped, it is retracted just enough to straighten up and free the tip, and then slowly readvanced. Once the tip has reached the proximal end of the target lesion, slow and gentle, probing, rotational advancement is recommended for safe crossing. If guidewire dissections occur, the guidewire is retracted and angiography performed. Spontaneously sealed guidewire dissections do not require any additional treatment, except when the left main, last remaining vessel, or other critical vessel has been involved. In these cases IVUS monitoring is recommended to exclude angiographically silent dissections. Persistent, stable uncomplicated dissections (NHLBI types A and B) should be initially treated by plain dilatation (1:1 balloon sizing, low inflation pressure). In large vessels or if a large portion of the myocardium is at risk, direct stenting is recommended. Persistent, unstable, or expanding type A and B dissections and any dissections graded at least NHLBI type C require immediate stent repair. To ensure placement in the true lumen, the guidewire should move, rotate, and enter the side branches freely. Subsequent distal explorative passage of a small, low-profile dilatation balloon is recommended before dilatation or stenting.

Dissections caused by guiding catheters are usually ostial or high proximal. With active seating of the guide, more distal dissections are also possible. As the vessel wall damage may be extensive, careful angiographic evaluation followed by an immediate stent repair is required.

Dissections due to "Dottering" may propagate in any direction and may be extensive. Careful evaluation of angiograms in multiple projections is necessary to plan repair.

VESSEL WALL PERFORATION AND RUPTURE

Coronary artery wall perforations and ruptures represent a rare complication in coronary interventions.[289] Predisposing factors include oversizing, balloon ruptures, use of debulking devices, stiff or slippery hydrophilic guidewires, total occlusions, and complex lesions.[290–294] Although the use of GP IIb/IIIa receptor inhibitors and anticoagulants may not increase the incidence of coronary perforations, it certainly may unmask small and otherwise unapparent fissures and may also aggravate the severity of extravasation.[295] The severity of extravasation (see Chapter 3B)[290] and the efficacy of treatment are the primary determinants of outcome. Table 8-45 summarizes the clinical outcome of coronary artery perforations in four studies.

In clinical practice the majority of perforations are distal guidewire perforations, and the majority of ruptures are assssociated with oversized dilatations in vulnerable vessels. Coronary perforations may be self-limiting or persisting. Small guidewire perforations are usually self-limiting and seal off spontaneously

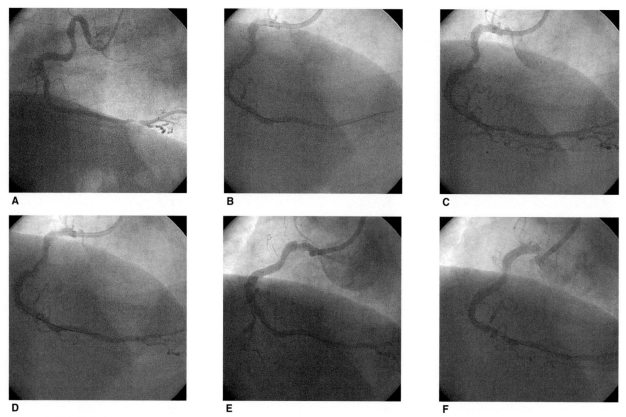

FIGURE 8-41. Single-vessel disease, tortuous vessel, distal lesion, guide and guidewire dissections. A 76-year-old male presenting with non-ST elevation myocardial infarction (NSTEMI) and persistent angina. Angiography revealed single vessel right coronary artery (RCA) disease with a distal stenosis (AHA segment 3) in a tortuous vessel **(A).** A Choice PT^2 (Boston Scientific) guidewire was placed distally, while a second guidewire (Heavy weight, Guidant) was placed into the third segment for better support and straightening of the target vessel **(B).** With some difficulty, Lekton motion 3.0/9-mm was advanced via the Choice PT^2 and deployed at 10 bar **(C).** Angiography showed guide dissection following deep seating in the proximal segment and a guidewire dissection in the middle segment **(D,E).** Both dissections required stenting (3.5/15-mm Lekton motion, Biotronik at 14 bar and 4.0/18-mm Driver, Medtronic at 14 bar). Final angiograms revealed complete revascularization and intact ostium **(F).**

TABLE 8-45. The Effect of Severity of Extravasation Based on Ellis et al.'s Classification of Coronary Perforations[a] on Clinical Outcome in Four Studies

Study by Author	Perforation Ellis I-III (Number of Cases)	Pericardial Tamponade %	Myocardial Infarction %	Emergency CABG %	Death %
Ellis et al.	I (13)	8	0	15	0
	II (31)	13	13	10	0
	III (16)	63	51	63	19
	III—cavity spilling (2)	0	0	0	0
Ajluni et al.	I/II (17)	6	29	24	6
	II (10)	20	30	60	20
Gruberg et al.	I/II/III	31	35	39	10
Dippel et al.	I (0)	—	—	—	—
	II (19)	5	—	0	0
	III (14)	43	—	50	21
	III—cavity spilling (2)	0	—	0	0

CABG, coronary artery bypass grafting

[a]Ellis SG, Ajluni S, Arnold SZ, et al. Increased coronary perforation in the new device era. Incidence, classification, management, and outcome. *Circulation.* 1994;90:2725–2302.

Modified from Rogers JH, Lasala JM. Coronary artery dissection and perforation complicating percutaneous coronary intervention. *J Invasive Cardiol.* 2004;16:493–499.

within minutes. On control angiograms no extravasation is detected and echocardiograms reveal no hemorrhage or a small pericardial one. Repeat echocardiograms and overnight monitoring are customary, and discontinuation of antithrombotic agents is usually not required. Ellis type III closed perforations (spilling of the contrast agent into contained structures such as cardiac chambers) are usually clinically benign: Although they may persist for years, they do not produce any clinical symptoms (coronary steal has not been reported) and therefore do not justify closure in most cases. Persisting coronary artery perforations require immediate attention. Treatment depends on the severity of the hemodynamic compromise, the magnitude of extravasation and pericardial hemorrhage, and technical accessibility. In hemodynamically stable patients with Ellis I perforations and accessible lesions, prolonged balloon inflation and stenting, if needed, are employed. In hemodynamically stable patients with moderate perforations (Ellis II) and accessible lesions, rapid angiographic definition of the perforation site followed by immediate stent repair is required. In patients with signs of pericardial tamponade, emergency pericardiocentesis is followed by stenting. In technically accessible lesions, PTFE-covered stents should be tried first. In severe free perforations (Ellis III), tamponade followed by cardiogenic shock is imminent and requires immediate pericardial decompression followed by perforation site closure, preferably using a PTFE-covered stent. If unsuccessful (e.g., the bulky PTFE-covered stent does not track), stent-in-stent stenting with conventional BMSs may resolve the situation. If pericardiocentesis or stenting fails, the target vessel is blocked by balloon inflation and the patient is transferred for immediate emergency surgery. In patients with coronary artery wall rupture and cardiogenic shock, immediate resuscitation followed by an immediate surgical repair may be life-saving. Antithrombotic agents should be discontinued for 12 to 24 hours or as needed in all cases of successfully treated free perforations to prevent recurrence. Useful algorithms of coronary artery perforation management have been provided in the literature.[296]

VESSEL CLOSURE AND NO-REFLOW

Acute coronary artery closure may occur spontaneously or be associated with interventions. It may be permanent, temporary, or intermittent. The most frequent causes of closure include thrombosis, dissection (NHLBI classification type F), elastic recoil, or vasoconstriction. Mechanical or functional closure produces ischemia of the subtended myocardium, the result such as myocardial stunning, myocardial hibernation, or myocardial cell death depends on the duration, the presence of pre-existent collaterals, and other factors.[297–299]

Procedure-related coronary artery closure occurs in <2% of coronary procedures. Predictive factors are the length of the stenosis, stenosis located at a bend point >45 degrees or at a branch point, the presence of thrombus, the presence of other stenoses in the same vessel, multivessel disease, female gender, and other factors.[300] Threatened and actual acute coronary artery closure was the first[14,15] and remains the most persuasive indication for stent implantation.[301]

In clinical practice nearly all spontaneous acute actual or threatened coronary artery closures are seen in patients presenting with ST-segment elevation, and less frequently with non-ST-segment elevated myocardial infarction. Interventional treatment consists of guidewire placement and careful crossing (note: use the least offensive guidewire first), explorative passage of a 1.25- to 2.0-mm-diameter low-profile balloon down to the distal segment of the target artery, and, if it is unobstructed, predilatation to unmask the lesion and to allow antegrade blood flow into the occluded vessel. In patients with sluggish antegrade flow, the intracoronary administration of GPIIb/IIIa receptor inhibitors[302] may improve visualization of the target artery and facilitate the intervention.

The "no-reflow" phenomenon is distinguished from acute vessel closure by the absence of mechanical epicardial coronary artery obstruction.[303] Following demonstration of no-reflow during experimental myocardial infarction,[304] no-reflow and slow flow were documented in patients with myocardial infarction treated by fibrinolytics[305] and PCI.[306] The angiographic definition contains two components: TIMI flow grade 0 or <III and lack of mechanical obstructions. No-reflow occurs in up to 2.0% of PCI; it most frequently involves emergency, SVG, and ablative interventions and represents a negative prognostic indicator.[307,308] The pathogenesis of no-reflow remains uncertain, at least as far as the precise role of coronary microcirculation is concerned.[309,310]

Because we do not clearly understand the underlying pathogenesis, the clinical management of no-reflow remains largely an empirical matter. In patients with angiographic coronary artery occlusion, the possibility of mechanical obstruction must first be excluded by probing the target vessel with a small-diameter (≤2 mm) dilatation balloon following guidewire placement. If passage of the dilatation balloon is free and extraluminal guidewire placement is excluded or appears unlikely, multiple, sequential, overlapping low-pressure (4 to 6 bar) dilatations are performed, followed by inflations of larger balloons (≤3 mm) if needed. In cases with proximal occlusive intimal flaps or massive recoil, stent implantation might be required to ensure patency and to confirm no-reflow. However, because of the possibility of inducing no-reflow in some cases by implanting the stent, restrictive use of stents, if justified, is recommended in these situations. Vasodilatatory agents and platelet inhibitors are usually administered after confirmation of proximal patency and include 100-μg boluses of verapamil,[311] 10-mg boluses of papaverine,[312] 30- to 50-μg boluses of adenosine,[313,314] or 0.3- to 0.9-μg/kg boluses of sodium nitroprusside,[315] all of which are administered intracoronarily. In addition, intracoronary boluses of a GP IIb/IIIa inhibitor abciximab or eptifibatide may be given.[316] Thrombolytics and nitroglycerin are not recommended. In patients with no-reflow complicating PCI and in patients with acute coronary syndrome who do not respond to any of the foregoing measures, prolonged (<12 hours) empirical treatment using intravenous infusion of abciximab may be considered. However, the definite increase in the risk of bleeding complications must be weighed against unclear benefits.

SIDE BRANCH COMPROMISE AND CLOSURE

Side branch compromise and closure may occur in bifurcation lesions when parent vessel dilatation leads to involvement of a side branch either directly by radial plaque shift, dissection, spasm, or "edema" because a balloon dilatation or stenting was performed across the side branch ostium, or indirectly by axial plaque shift, dissection, or spasm. Occasionally side branches that are innocent bystanders may become compromised or closed during interventions for nonbifurcation lesions. In these cases the collateral damage is usually due to shearing off plaques during the intravasal passage of the instrumentation or intentional or inadvertent placement of guidewires into the side branch and consecutive side-branch injury. Side-branch injury results in regional myocardial ischemia or in regional myocardial infarction. Attending electrical or hemodynamic instability is possible but relatively rare. Clinical management depends on a number of factors including the size of the side branch and the size of the myocardium in jeopardy,[317–319] but also on the coronary status of the patients, emergency or elective settings, technical accessibility, possible reversibility, and other factors.

In assessing the size of the side branch, either the luminal diameter in millimeters or a qualitative assessment (bypassable, not bypassable) is used. In general, vessels <1.5 (2) mm are usually not considered for interventions and vessels ≥2.0 to 2.5 mm are the principal candidates for intervention. Bypassable side branches are always candidates for rescue revascularization. The size of the myocardium in jeopardy can be estimated on the basis of the segmental approach[93] and the corresponding coronary distribution. The functional impact of the compromise is assessed using the TIMI scale where TIMI I–II° flow grades are considered a functional and TIMI III° a total occlusion. The need to revascularize an iatrogenic side branch compromise or closure is greater in patients with multivessel disease and compromised left ventricular function and in young individuals. In contrast, a lengthy attempt to revascularize a spontaneously or iatrogenically occluded side branch in an emergency setting may expose the patient to undue risks and should be carefully considered before embarking on potentially difficult and unrewarding interventions. It becomes futile, particularly in stable patients, if performed at the expense of compromising the already successfully revascularized parent vessel. In patients with compromised but not totally occluded side branches in an emergency setting, a

staged procedure should be considered; attempts to intervene on total occlusions are better justified and more frequent.

Before resuming a side-branch intervention, 100 to 300 μg intracoronary nitroglycerin should be given to exclude ostial spasm. Then the baseline angiogram should be reviewed to assess the side branch at the outset of the procedure as to the presence of an ostial lesion and associated distal lesions. In compromised side branches with pre-existent ostial lesions and diffuse distal disease, attempts at intervention may endanger the parent vessel and are rarely justified in small nonbypassable vessels. A de novo lesion in a side branch >2 mm should be approached in most cases, but not at the expense of the parent vessel, particularly when the parent vessel is an artery related to an infarct. The intervention strategy is similar to a standard PCI in bifurcation lesions.

STENT THROMBOSIS

In the early period of coronary stenting, stent thrombosis represented a frequent early complication.[191,192] The incidence of stent thrombosis was considerably reduced following the introduction of more potent antithrombotic regimen (for review, see references 245 and 320), improved implantation techniques,[321,322] and possibly improved stent design.[323]

The pathogenesis of stent thrombosis is likely multifactorial, including a number of stent-, patient-, and lesion-related causes such as those shown in Figure 8-42.[324] Recently, platelet activation related to stent deployment was also documented to be a potential thrombogenic factor.[325] In addition, incomplete strut apposition, underdilatation, residual high-grade stenosis, proximal or distal uncovered dissection not covered by stent, vessel diameter <3 mm, TIMI flow <3 at the final angiogram, inflow or outflow obstruction, stent length and the number of deployed stents,[326–328] gene polymorphisms,[329] and resistance to aspirin[247] and thienopyridines[330] were all associated with an increased risk

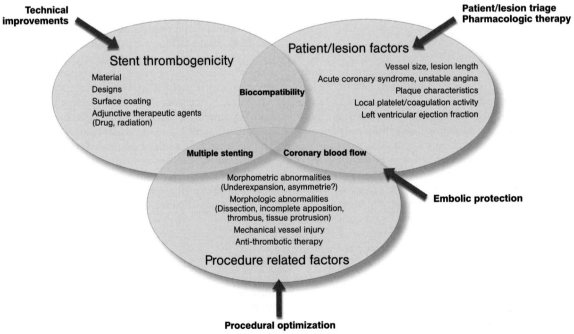

FIGURE 8-42. Risk factors associated with stent thrombosis and targets of risk reduction (arrows). (Modified from Honda Y, Fitzgerald PJ. Stent thrombosis; an issue revisited in a changing world. *Circulation.* 2003;108:2–5.)

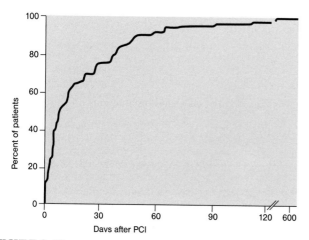

FIGURE 8-43. Cumulative incidence of stent thrombosis following bare-metal stent (BMS) implantation. (Adapted from Wenaweser P, Rey C, Eberli FR, et al. Stent thrombosis following bare-metal stent implantation: success of emergency percutaneous coronary intervention and predictors of adverse outcome. *Eur Heart J.* 2005;26:1180–1187.)

of stent thrombosis. In addition, specific risk factors for late stent thrombosis are stenting across ostia of major branches, radiation therapy, nonstented plaque disruptions, stenting of a markedly necrotic lesion, and diffuse in-stent restenosis.[331]

Based on the temporal occurrence, acute (≤24 hours following the stent implantation), subacute (>24 hours within 30 days), and late (>30 days) stent thromboses can be distinguished. In a large series using BMSs and including 6058 patients enrolled between 1995 and 2003, the overall incidence of stent thrombosis was 1.6% with a median onset of 8 days ranging between 0 and 639 days after PCI; 11% were acute, 64% subacute, and 25% late stent thromboses.[332] Figure 8-43 shows the cumulative incidence of stent thrombosis following BMS implantation. In a pooled analysis of 10 randomized studies, the overall incidence of stent thrombosis was 0.58%.[333] Table 8-46 shows the incidence of stent thrombosis in 10 randomized studies using DES implantations. Figure 8-44 shows a comparison between the incidence of overall and late stent thrombosis in patients receiving DES and BMS. Figure 8-45 documents the impact of stent length (DES) on acute thrombosis. Using data from a routine clinical practice, the incidence of stent thrombosis (DES) was higher (1.3%) than that reported in randomized trials (0.58%), and differences were noted between sirolimus- (0.8%) and paclitaxel- (1.7%) eluting stents. Importantly, renal failure, diabetes, and poor left ventricular function have been also identified as important risk factors for stent thrombosis, heightening their importance in real-life scenarios as opposed to a clinical study setting.[334] Tables 8-47 and 8-48 document the factors associated with stent thrombosis following DES implantation at 9 months follow-up.

In patients with acute stent thrombosis following BMS implantation, the majority of events seem to occur within the first few hours after the implantation,[335,336] whereas intraprocedural stent thrombosis appears rare (<0.01%) and primarily associated with acute coronary syndromes and thrombotic lesions.[337] Although the issue of late stent thrombosis associated with DES implantations[338] deserves further long-term evaluation, significant differences between DES and BMS have thus far not been documented according to the available

evidence. The increased occurrence of late stent thrombosis observed in procedures involving brachytherapy has been reduced to a level comparable to that of conventional stenting by implementing long-term antiplatelet therapy.[339]

Preventive strategies include a meticulous stent implantation technique combined with an optimal pharmacologic management.[235] Despite the overall low incidence of stent thrombosis, its prevalence continues to rise as a result of the increasing number of stent-supported angioplasties.[324] Both the poor prognosis[326,327] and the high costs[340] associated with stent thrombosis mandate the development of improved strategies for preventing stent thrombosis.[250]

Stent thrombosis presents typically as unstable angina, myocardial infarction, and in some cases as sudden coronary death.[334] Although the reported primary technical success rates are high (>90%), a significant number of patients (16%) may suffer an early recurrence within a median of 5.0 ± 8.5 days of the emergency PCI. Emergency angiograms show total thrombotic occlusion in the majority of cases (83%); less frequently subocclusive thrombi (17%) are visualized.[332] Following balloon angioplasty or thrombectomy[341] re-establishing the antegrade coronary flow, angiograms should be evaluated to exclude mechanical causes of thrombus formation such as incomplete coverage of the lesion, edge dissections, protruding tissue flaps due to incomplete scaffolding, and tissue intussusceptions in overlapping stent placements and to allow repair. A second stent is deployed in the presence of proximal or distal edge dissections. In the presence of suspected underdilatation, incomplete strut apposition, or stent damage, careful high-pressure dilatation may suffice to resolve the situation. In patients with suspected incomplete scaffolding and protruding tissues, IVUS imaging is preferably performed to assess the site, usually requiring a high-pressure redilatation followed by stent-in-stent placement. In patients with suspected tissue intussusceptions, IVUS-guided placement of a bridging stent or surgical revascularization, especially with large tissue flaps, may be required. In all patients with documented stent thrombosis, the early administration of GPIIb/IIIa receptor inhibitors and extended administration of the dual antiplatelet therapy (minimum 6 months) is recommended.

DISTAL EMBOLIZATION

White, platelet-rich and red, fibrin-rich thrombus formation regularly accompanies physiological wound closure.[342] Thrombi represent a frequent finding during coronary interventions at coronary sites with spontaneous or iatrogenic plaque ruptures.[159–161] Furthermore, peripheral spontaneous embolization possibly secondary to weaker adhesion of platelets during appositional growth[343] or iatrogenic embolizations due to mechanical manipulations are frequent.[344,345] Coronary embolizations initially thought to be primarily associated with interventions in specific settings, such as for thrombotic lesions, emergencies, degenerated SVG, and atherectomy devices,[346–348] have been more recently recognized to accompany a number of coronary interventional settings, including PCI in native coronary arteries (for review, see reference 158).

Distal embolization protection strategies include optimal pharmacologic peri-interventional management, meticulous atraumatic technique, particularly in fragile lesions, diffuse disease or preexistent thrombi, and in some cases deployment of

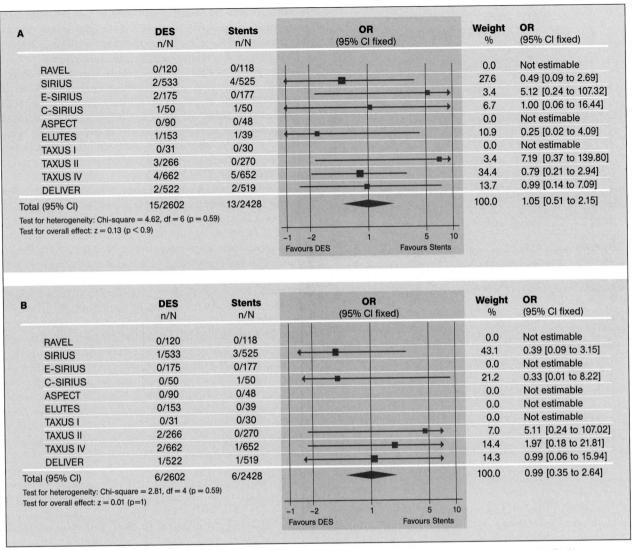

FIGURE 8-44. Comparison between the incidence of the overall (**A**) and late stent thrombosis (**B**) in patients receiving drug-eluting (DES) and bare-metal stents in 10 randomized studies in the pooled population. (Adapted from Moreno R, Fernandez C, Hernandez R, et al. Drug-eluting stent thrombosis. Results from a pooled analysis including 10 randomized studies. *J Am Coll Cardiol.* 2005;45:954–959.)

DPDs. Whereas the value of the former two strategies remains undisputed, the role of DPDs in thromboembolic protection and prevention of distal myocardial injury has not yet been fully ascertained. Filter, distal, and proximal occlusive devices of various designs and thrombus extraction devices have been employed in SVG and acute coronary interventions in several trials (for review, see reference 349). Thus, whereas improved clinical outcome seems to support the use of DPD in SVG interventions,[350,351] their use in patients with acute coronary syndromes appears more doubtful.[352,353] Results of ongoing trials using new-generation devices such as RULE-SVG (Rubicon Filterwire) and AMEthyst (Interceptor Filterdevice) may provide answers needed to clarify the indications for use of DPD in coronary interventions. Clearly, an individual's benefit from DPD will depend on the risk of embolization associated with unprotected intervention versus the risk of injury associated with DPD deployment. Therefore, particularly in patients with complex multilocular target-vessel lesions, atraumatic and

user-friendly design of the DPD and skills of the operator will ultimately determine the outcome and clinical acceptance.

The low sensitivity of coronary angiography to detect a thrombus is well known and has been already discussed. De novo thrombi that occasionally form during interventions in cases with impaired coronary flow or suboptimal anticoagulation usually respond quickly to improved flow or pharmacologic interventions such as the intracoronary injection of abciximab, if indicated in the presence of adjusted ACT. In severe cases, the withdrawal of endovascular instrumentation including the guidewire might be required to gain control of the excessive thrombogenicity. In patients with large pre-existing proximal thrombi in large vessels or last remaining vessels, extraction under distal protection should be considered prior to stenting. In nonproximal lesion sites and nonvital vessels the thrombus is "tacked on" by primary stenting. Using the currently available generation of DPDs, thromboembolic protection still appears problematic in patients with a difficult anatomy or a thrombus located distally.

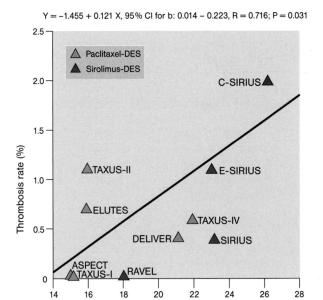

Y = −1.455 + 0.121 X, 95% CI for b: 0.014 – 0.223, R = 0.716; P = 0.031

FIGURE 8-45. The impact of stent length on stent thrombosis in 10 randomized studies. (Adapted from Moreno R, Fernandez C, Hernandez R, et al. Drug-eluting stent thrombosis. Results from a pooled analysis including 10 randomized studies. *J Am Coll Cardiol.* 2005;45:954–959.)

RARE COMPLICATIONS

Less frequent complications of coronary interventions include loss or entrapment of endovascular instruments, persistent spasms, and air embolization.

Stent loss was primarily associated with the use of manually crimped stents. In complete stent delivery systems, it is rare.[354] Other materials lost in the coronary arteries include broken-off guidewire tips, ruptured balloon catheters, and delivery devices.

Stents may slip backward from the balloon during the forward motion of the delivery system or, more frequently, are lost on withdrawal. In either case, an attempt can be made to gently reintroduce the balloon into the stent, inflate the balloon up to 2–4 bar, and carefully withdraw the partially loaded stent into the guiding catheter. When this maneuver fails or when the guidewire is disengaged, a retrieval device, a "goose-neck" loop snare or retrieval basket is guided distally to the stent and deployed to trap and to retrieve the stent. In some cases of partial slippage of the stents and difficult retrieval, stent deployment in a nontarget location might be considered. Snare loop retrieval is indicated in all patients in whom there is intracoronary embolization of defective equipment such as uncoiled or broken guidewires (see Chapter 15).

Transient focal coronary spasms are common and frequently associated with mechanical endocoronary manipulations in susceptible vessels.[355] The initial measure to relieve spasms is pharmacologic intervention, usually in the form of intracoronary nitroglycerin administered as a repeated 100- to 300-μg bolus. The efficacy of other coronary vasodilators such as magnesium sulfate, papaverine, or calcium blockers remains unproven.[356] In resilient cases, guidewire withdrawal beyond the narrowed segment should be weighed against the risk of possible difficulties re-entering a possible dissection. Alternatively, low-pressure dilatation with an undersized balloon may be attempted to resolve the spasm. The angiographic distinction between spasm and damaged wall might not be possible if the narrowing persists despite intracoronary vasodilation and guidewire withdrawal. In this case, de novo stenosis is assumed and treated. The introduction of endovascular instrumentation, in particular stiff guidewires, in fragile, usually tortuous, and elongated arteries lacking extramural support may cause intense corrugations, foldings, and invaginations of the target coronary artery (concertina or accordion effect).[357–359] Although inappropriate stenting should be avoided, it may prove challenging in difficult anatomy and technically demanding cases to distinguish between multiple intima lesions and invaginations. In addition to plaques and microdissections, adventitial hematoma has been reported to trigger peri-interventional coronary spasms.[360] Occlusive, persistent peri-interventional spasms manifested by

TABLE 8-46. Incidence of Stent Thrombosis in 10 Randomized Studies Using Drug-eluting Stents (DESs) and Relevant Stent- and Lesion-related Factors

Study	DES Thrombosis	Mean Lesion Length (mm)	Mean Stented Length (mm)	Stented/ Lesion Length Ratio	No. of Stents per Patient	Mean RVD (mm)	Mean MLD Postprocedure (mm)	Mean Stenosis Postprocedure
RAVEL (1)	0.0%	9.60	18.0	1.88	1.00	2.60	2.43	11.90%
SIRIUS (2)	0.4%	14.40	21.5	1.49	1.40	2.80	2.67	5.40%
E-SIRIUS (3)	1.1%	14.90	23.0	1.70	1.50	2.55	2.43	7.70%
C-SIRIUS (4)	2.0%	14.50	26.2	1.80	1.60	2.65	2.53	6.10%
ASPECT (5)	0.0%	11.10	15.0	1.35	1.00	2.94	2.84	3.00%
ELUTES (6)	0.7%	10.80	16.0	1.48	1.07	2.90	2.70	9.60%
TAXUS–I (7)	0.0%	10.70	15.0	1.40	1.00	2.99	2.95	13.56%
TAXUS–II (8)	1.1%	10.40	15.9	1.52	1.06	2.75	2.53	10.90%
TAXUS–IV (9)	0.6%	13.40	21.7	1.58	1.08	2.75	2.26	19.10%
TAXUS–IV (10)	0.4%	11.70	19.8	1.69	1.11	2.85	2.86	2.7%

MLD, minimum lumen diameter; RVD, reference vessel diameter.
Reproduced with permission from Moreno R, Fernandez C, Hernandez R, et al. Drug-eluting stent thrombosis. Results from a pooled analysis including 10 randomized studies. *J Am Coll Cardiol.* 2005;45:954–959.

TABLE 8-47. Univariate Predictors of Cumulative Stent Thrombosis

Variables	Incidence of Stent Thrombosis, No./Total (%)	Hazard Ratio (95% Confidence Interval)	p value
CATEGORICAL VARIABLES			
Premature antiplatelet therapy discontinuation	5/17 (29)	152 (152–442)	<.001
Prior brachytherapy	2/23 (8.7)	7.49 (1.78–31.49)	.006
Renal failure	8/127 (6.2)	11.67 (5.17–26.35)	<.001
Bifurcation with two stents	13/336 (3.9)	4.62 (2.22–9.62)	<.001
Bifurcation lesion	18/507 (3.6)	6.50 (3.02–13.98)	<.001
Unprotected left main artery	3/92 (3.3)	0.95 (0.67–1.36)	.81
Diabetes	15/591 (2.5)	3.45 (1.66–7.18)	<.001
Thrombus	1/50 (2)	1.58 (0.21–11.65)	.65
Unstable angina	8/590 (1.4)	1.24 (0.56–2.73)	.58
Male sex	22/1907 (1.2)	0.80 (0.30–2.11)	.66
B2 or C type	21/1698 (1.2)	1.19 (0.48–2.94)	.69
Calcification	4/392 (1)	0.74 (0.26–2.14)	.58
Sirolimus-eluting stent	9/1062 (0.8)	0.50 (0.22–1.10)	0.09
CONTINUOUS VARIBALES[a]			
Age, y	68 (10)	1.05 (1.01–1.09)	.004
Balloon diameter, mm	3.0 (0.3)	1.22 (0.54–2.72)	.62
Balloon-to-artery ration	1.2 (0.2)	2.71 (0.82–8.97)	.10
Left ventricular ejection fraction per 10% decrease	45 (9)	1.07 (1.04–1.11)	<.001
Lesion length, mm	19.46 (13.43)	1.01 (0.98–1.03)	.39
Preintervention reference vessel diameter, mm	2.55 (0.44)	1.22 (0.54–2.72)	.22
Postintervention minimal lumen diameter, mm	2.30 (0.71)	0.58 (0.33–1.00)	.06
Stent length, mm	33.67 (23.24)	1.01 (0.98–1.03)	.32
Stent per-lesion ration	1.37 (0.6)	1.49 (0.85–2.63)	.16

[a]Continuous variables are presented as mean (SD) in patients who developed stent thrombosis.

Reproduced with permission from Iakovou I, Schmidt T, Bonizzoni E, et al. Incidence, predictors, and outcome of thrombosis after successful implantation of drug-eluting stents. *JAMA.* 2005;293:2126–2130.

diffuse vessel constriction and major hemodynamic compromise appear to be rare.[361] Subselective locoregional or local administration of vasodilating agents using OTW-type catheters has been recommended in these difficult cases.[362]

Air embolism has been known and feared since the early days of coronary interventions.[363] The most severe incidents of air embolism result from incompletely aspirated guiding catheters, from incompletely secured vents, or from damaged parts connected with the dilatation or guiding catheter lumen located outside the patient's body. Less threatening air embolism usually results from balloon rupture or incompletely removed air bubbles in syringes used for coronary injections. Hemodynamic responses range from clinically silent passage of air bubbles to cardiogenic shock. The severity of responses depends on the amount of air injected, the size of the acutely ischemic myocardium, and the patient's baseline conditions. Air embolism may be far more threatening in patients treated for acute coronary syndromes than in those treated electively. In patients with light to moderate myocardial ischemic response, general supportive measures such as oxygen, volume, and administration

of an antianginal agent usually appear to be sufficient. With moderate to severe responses, deep seating of the guiding catheter with immediate suction, massive catecholamine support, and full-scale resuscitation, if needed, may be life-saving. As with any peri-interventional complications, the best treatment is always prevention. Constant awareness of possible equipment failure and repeated aspiration before injections or introduction of any new equipment represent the best prevention.

ELECTIVE CORONARY ARTERY INTERVENTION IN SELECTED SETTINGS

The strategy followed in coronary endovascular interventions is determined by the angiographic appearance of the target lesion, the target vessel, the patient's status, and the operator's decision on all these factors. The primary determinants, however, are lesion morphology and the site of the intervention. Selected examples of typical interventional settings are reviewed in the following sections.

TABLE 8-48. Independent Predictors of Stent Thrombosis

Variables	*Hazard Ratio (95% Confidence Interval)*	*p value*
SUBACUTE STENT THROMBOSIS		
Premature antiplatelet therapy discontinuation	161.17 (26.03–997.94)	<.001
Renal failure	10.06 (3.13–32.35)	<.001
Bifurcation lesion	5.96 (1.90–18.68)	.002
Diabetes	5.84 (1.74–19.55)	.004
Left ventricular ejection fraction per 10% decrease	1.12 (1.06–1.19)	<.001
Stent length, per 1-mm increase	1.03 (1.00–1.05)	.01
LATE STENT THROMBOSIS		
Premature antiplatelet therapy discontinuation	57.13 (14.84–219.96)	<.001
Bifurcation lesion	8.11 (2.50–26.26)	.001
Left ventricular ejection fraction per 10% decrease	1.06 (1.01–1.12)	.03
CUMULATIVE STENT THROMBOSIS		
Premature antiplatelet therapy discontinuation	89.78 (29.90–269.60)	<.001
Renal failure	6.49 (2.60–16.15)	<.001
Bifurcation lesion	6.42 (2.93–14.07)	<.001
Diabetes	3.71 (1.74–7.89)	.001
Left ventricular ejection fraction per 10% decrease	1.09 (1.05–1.13)	<.001

Reproduced with permission from Iakovou I, Schmidt T, Bonizzoni E, et al. Incidence, predictors, and outcome of thrombosis after successful implantation of drug-eluting stents. *JAMA.* 2005;293:2126–2130.

LEFT MAIN LESION

In view of the poor prognosis of medical therapy,[364,365] coronary artery bypass graft (CABG) surgery has become a standard form of treatment of patients with left main coronary artery disease (LMCAD).[366–369]

Grüntzig et al.[8] were the first to report the successful performance of PTCA in patients with left main disease. Because of the high risk associated with the procedure at that time, however, LMCAD was subsequently considered a contraindication for PTCA.[370] Nevertheless, with improving technology and led on by data from several experienced centers, percutaneous treatment of left main disease has continued to evolve. Yet despite some early encouraging results,[371,372] the outcome of left main coronary artery interventions was considered suboptimal throughout the entire prestent era, and CABG was recommended for all eligible patients.[373] The introduction of BMS renewed the scientific debates and clinical interest in percutaneous treatment of unprotected left main disease in various subgroups of patients.[374–378] Based on a pooled registry of data on patients treated for LMCAD in 25 experienced centers between 1994 and 1996, results similar to those for CABG were observed in a selected group of low-risk patients defined as age <65 years, LVEF >30%, and the absence of cardiogenic shock and myocardial infarction.[375] Other candidate groups for unprotected LMCAD included inoperable patients and patients at a high surgical risk.[379] Table 8-49 shows an example of the baseline angiographic characteristics of patients with unprotected left main coronary artery interventions; note the high jeopardy score and high percentage of distal lesions. Table 8-50 shows the 9-month results for the same group of patients. Figure 8-46 highlights the independent negative prognostic significance of emergency presentation with acute myocardial infarction and poor left

TABLE 8-49. Baseline Angiographic Characteristics of 107 Patients with Unprotected Left Main Coronary Artery Interventions Treated in 25 Centers

Jeopardy score (0–6), mean	4.7 ± 1.0
Lesion length, mm	4.7 ± 3.0
Lesion location,[a] %	
Ostial	43.7
Midshaft	31.1
Distal	61.2
LVEF, %	49 ± 17
No. of diseased vessels, %	
Two	50.5
Three	49.5
Reference dimension, mm	3.9 ± .9
Percent stenosis, median/interquartile range	58/69/81

LVEF, left ventricular ejection fraction.

[a] >30% narrowing (numbers sum to >100%).

Reproduced with permission from Ellis SG, Tamai H, Nobuyoshi M, et al. Contemporary percutaneous treatment of unprotected left main coronary stenoses. Intital results from a multicenter registry analysis 1994–1994. *Circulation.* 1997;96:3867–3872.

ventricular function. The initial experience with sirolimus-eluting stents for unprotected LMCAD showed improved 12-month clinical outcome (freedom from death, myocardial infarction, and target lesion revascularization) with DES compared to BMS.[380] In another early study implementing sirolimus- and paclitaxel-eluting stents for LMCAD, the rate of MACE was lower in patients with DES at 6 months compared to historical BMS controls.[381] The results of prospective randomized trials comparing state of the art DES and CABG for treating LMCAD (SYNTAX, Phase III; Study of the German Heart Center Munich,

TABLE 8-50.   Nine-month Results of 107 Patients with Unprotected Left Main Coronary Artery Interventions Treated in 25 Centers

	Restenosis, %	9-mo Survival, %	9-mo EFS, %
AMI	a	31.3 ± 12.1	12.5 ± 7.8
Not AMI			
CABG candidate (*n* = 68)	17.4	84.3 ± 4.6	81.2 ± 4.9
Stable angina (*n* = 43)	9.8	90.6 ± 4.4	87.9 ± 4.6
New onset angina (*n* = 8)	28.6	85.7 ± 12.8	85.7 ± 12.8
Progressive/rest angina (*n* = 17)	37.5	69.3 ± 10.4	50.0 ± 11.9
High risk (*n* = 25)	31.2	70.1 ± 8.5	52.8 ± 8.8
Not high risk (*n* = 43)	10.0	84.5 ± 4.9	85.8 ± 4.9
LVEF ≥40 (*n* = 51)	13.5	87.3 ± 4.5	86.0 ± 4.6
LVEF <40 (*n* = 9)	a	26.5 ± 10.0	22.3 ± 12.0
Not CABG candidate (*n* = 23)	a	29.5 ± 9.6	26.5 ± 9.7
Rx with stent (*n* = 51)	14.3	70.5 ± 6.6	62.8 ± 6.1
Rx with DCA (*n* = 25)	16.7	88.0 ± 6.5	88.0 ± 6.5
Rx with PTCA (*n* = 9)	50.0	44.4 ± 16.6	44.4 ± 16.6
Ostial (*n* = 43)	30.8	66.6 ± 7.2	65.6 ± 7.3
Distal (*n* = 51)	14.8	69.7 ± 6.5	66.3 ± 6.8
Stent (*n* = 26)	12.5	68.0 ± 8.3	60.0 ± 8.5
DCA (*n* = 17)	12.5	82.4 ± 7.4	82.4 ± 7.4
Total (*n* = 107)	20.8	66.0 ± 4.7	60.7 ± 4.8

EFS, event-free survival; AMI, acute myocardial infarction; CABG, coronary artery bypass graft surgery; LVEF, left ventricular ejection fraction; Rx, treatment; DCA, directional coronary atherectomy; PTCA, percutaneous transluminal coronary angioplasty.

a *n*<5 with data.

Modified from Ellis SG, Tamai H, Nobuyoshi M, et al. Contemporary percutaneous treatment of unprotected left main coronary stenoses. Intital results from a multicenter registry analysis 1994–1994. *Circulation.* 1997;96:3867–3872.

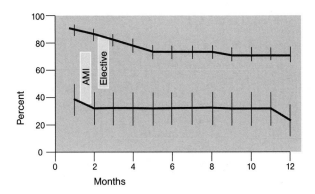

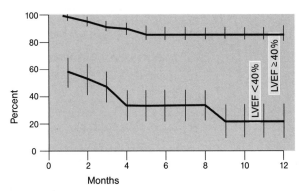

FIGURE 8-46.   Kaplan-Meier survival curves for patients with acute myocardial infarction and elective patients and in patients with left ventricular ejection fraction (LVEF) greater and less than 40%. (Reproduced with permission from Ellis SG, Tamai H, Nobuyoshi M, et al. Contemporary percutaneous treatment of unprotected left main coronary stenoses. Initial results from a multicenter registry analysis 1994–1996. *Circulation.* 1997;96:3867–3872.)

Phase IV) may help to identify the optimal concepts and strategies. Until a sufficient database on DES LMCAD revascularization has been established, Dr. Samuel Johnson's (1709–1784) dictum "Sir, a man is not obliged to do all that he can" may be of some assistance in determining indications and treatment.

In patients considered for unprotected (no bypass present) LMCAD interventions, several important issues need to be clarified prior to any definitive decision. Because the goal is to assess objectively the risks and benefits of two treatment options individually in each patient, all three parties involved—interventionist, surgeon, and patient—should concur in the decision. A risk-benefit assessment includes consideration of emergency or elective settings, left ventricular function, comorbidities, age, and life expectancy, as well as the angiographic findings and the experience and expertise of the interventionist operators directly involved. Optimal angiographic definition of the LMCAD and of the interventional site including the branching main coronary vessels is necessary to plan the strategy of revascularization. The primary determinants relevant to catheter-based treatments include the severity (moderate to severe, subtotal), complexity (thrombus, calcification, eccentricity), and location (ostium, shaft, distal, number of branches involved) of the target lesion. In addition, the presence, number, and location of an associated secondary target and nontarget lesions are important. Based on the concept of actional risk (see Chapter 4) it is evident that the justification increases with the urgency of the situation, in particular if alternative options are lacking. It must be firmly kept in mind

that the level of actional risk increases with the technical complexity and inexperience of the operator. Thus, for example, the actional risk might become exceedingly high in patients with acute coronary syndromes, hemodynamic compromise, and presence of angiographic complex bifurcation LMCAD in the setting of a complex multivessel disease. This high level of risk can hardly be compensated regardless of the expertise of the operator. In contrast, the procedural risk associated with revascularization of type A left main coronary artery lesions performed by experienced operators in most cases appears to be acceptable in both elective and, in particular, emergency settings. Surgical standby is recommended in all LMCAD interventions, with the possible exception of emergency interventions in hospitals without direct access to coronary surgery.

Given the suboptimal angiographic definition of LMCAD,[382,383] the use of IVUS has been proposed to improve the anatomic resolution,[384] which, however, does not unequivocally improve the outcome.[385] Furthermore, its use is limited in patients with unsuitable coronary anatomy including tortuous vessels, sharp bends and take-offs, or high-grade and particularly calcified lesions because of lack of passage of the stiff ultrasound transducer. Although debulking does effectively reduce the plaque burden prior to stenting and may reduce restenosis,[386] its relevance to the clinical outcome remains uncertain. Therefore, it is not routinely performed in standard procedures.

Although LMDCA interventions are governed by the same principles as non-LMCDA procedures, strategic flexibility, straightforward planning that is always a step ahead of the action, meticulous, quick, and atraumatic execution of each interventional step without any "messing around," and short inflation and deflation times to avoid prolonged myocardial ischemia and coronary blood-flow stasis appear even more critical to ensure success of the intervention. In addition, maintenance of optimal anticoagulation levels with ACT adjusted to 250 to 300 seconds throughout the entire procedure appears also critical. To maximize the operator's flexibility, the choice of larger systems is always preferable; therefore, although a 6F system may be technically sufficient, a 7F sheath and guiding catheters are recommended, particularly in complex procedures. Stable seating of the guide must be achieved to avoid dislocation and repositioning in the middle of the procedure. Guides with side holes are usually required in ostial left main lesions. Direct stenting, if technically feasible, may shorten the intervention and actually increase the safety of the procedure in recoil- or dissection-prone lesions. DES is highly recommended and if technically possible should be utilized in all

LMCAD interventions. Prophylactic use of mechanical left ventricular support devices in uncomplicated LMCAD interventions does not improve the outcome and is not recommended. Unintended LM interventions in patients with subcritical LM stenoses and distal CAD should be avoided by meticulous technique and atraumatic traffic of instrumentation across the LM lesion. In these cases, however, the operator should be keenly aware of the possible need for unplanned LM interventions and should select the size of the system accordingly. Figure 8-47 shows an example of escalating intervention in a patient with primarily subcritical LMCAD.

OSTIAL LESION

Ostial lesions are usually defined as lesions within 3 mm of the take-off of a major coronary artery. Native aorto-ostial, aorto-graft-ostial, and branch-ostial lesions can be distinguished. Aorto-ostial and aorto-graft-ostial lesions result from

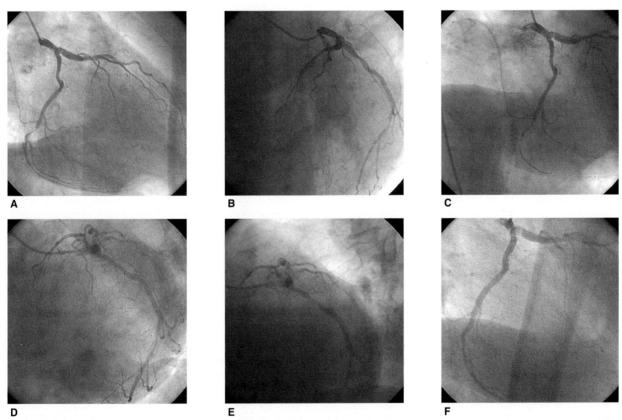

FIGURE 8-47. Left main disease, escalating intervention, (left circumflex artery, LCx, left main artery, LM). A 61-year-old man admitted with non-ST elevation myocardial infarction (NSTEMI) with nonspecific ST-T lateral ECG changes following an elective LCx intervention in the referring hospital. Angiogram revealed severe coronary disease with 50% distal LM stenosis, subtotal stenosis within the proximal third of the posterolateral ramus (culprit lesion) of the diffusely diseased LCx, 80% proximal diagonal ramus (Rd) stenosis, and diffuse left anterior descending (LAD) and right coronary artery (RCA) vessel wall irregularities **(A,B).** Because of angiographically borderline LM stenosis, intravascular ultrasound (IVUS) was performed, revealing an eccentric, moderately calcified, 56% cross-sectional area with 30% diameter stenosis. Because of acute myocardial infarction and LM stenosis that was not hemodynamically significant, the decision was made to perform an LCx percutaneous coronary intervention (PCI), using a 5F system, and staged Rd PCI. A guidewire was placed, and the LCx lesion dilated (2.5/20 mm at 8 bar) resulting in vessel closure **(C).** Following redilatations antegrade blood flow was restored, and after multiple predilatations, a 2.75/15-mm Lekton motion (Biotronik) at 12 bar was successfully placed. On the subsequent angiogram, 70% LCx stenosis in AHA segment 11 was revealed, dilated **(D),** and stented **(E).** In the following angiographic sequence, the LM stenosis appeared more severe **(F)** and caudal right anterior oblique (RAO) projection revealed a now hemodynamically significant ostial LCx stenosis **(G)** requiring revascularization. Following predilatation of the LM/LCx ostium with 3.0/15 mm, a 4.0/15-mm Driver (Medtronic) stent was placed at 14 bar, resulting in removal of the LCx ostial stenosis and major plaque shift into the LAD **(H,I).** A second guidewire was placed in the LAD **(J)** and, following predilatation with 3.0/15 mm at 10 bar, the LAD ostial lesion was stented (4.0/15-mm Driver, Medtronic at 16 bar) using the "culotte" technique **(K).** Because of the limitations of the 5F system, final "kissing" balloon dilatation could not be implemented and both ostial LM stents were sequentially dilated at 14 bar, resulting in angiographically reconstructed LM bifurcation **(L).** *(Continued)*

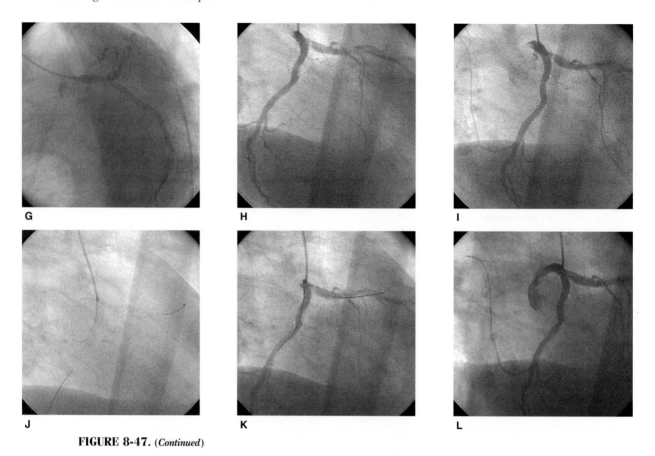

FIGURE 8-47. (*Continued*)

atherosclerosis of the aorta or the most proximal arterial segment. Probably because of the different tissue composition of the transitional zones between the elastic aorta and muscular arteries at branching points,[387] ostial plaques appear more densely fibrotic and calcified, and therefore more rigid and prone to postdilatation recoil, dissections, and restenosis than nonostial lesions.[388] Use of debulking devices[389] and stents[390,391] has improved the acute and long-term outcome. The clinical use of DES has further decreased in-stent restenosis rates.[392] The advantages of DES compared to BMS with regard to reduction in MACE, including lower rates of revascularization and reduced in-stent restenosis rates, strongly favor the use of DES in ostial interventions. The rate of debulking atherectomy procedures in the presented study (3.1% DES and 6% BMS) reflects the current infrequent use of these techniques in clinical practice. Table 8-51 shows an example of the characteristics of patients and treated lesions in a recent study, and Table 8-52 and Figure 8-48 document the clinical outcome and angiographic results from the same study.

Treatments of native and bypass-related aorto-ostial lesions appear to be technically more demanding for a number of reasons. Aortic plaques frequently prevent stable and coaxial seating of the guiding catheters. Occasionally multiple attempts are required to seat the guide, thus increasing the risk of a dissection. Once seating is achieved, later repositioning or even guide exchange (different shape, side holes, short tip) may become required because of ostial obstructions, blood-flow stasis, thrombus formation, or severe ischemia developing in the

course of the procedure. Selection of the guide with the "best fit" regarding the shape, allowing the minimum number of seating attempts, and a smooth transition between the primary curve of the guide and the ostium while avoiding deep insertions and active engagement, as well as the size for stable yet flexible "backup" are critical to reduce the risk of guide-related complications and to facilitate the conduct of the intervention. Undue pressure of the tip of the guide onto the ostium must be avoided. Gentle handling of the guide without storage of energy by torque, twist, or flexion usually prevents the guide from uncontrolled jumps and associated risk of ostial injury. In cases with ostial RCA lesions prophylactic placement of a 5F femoral vein sheath is recommended to allow for rapid placement of a transvenous pacing lead if need arises. In patients with unstable cardiac rhythm, prophylactic pacing lead placement is useful. Surgical standby is usually not required for treatments of ostial lesions in experienced centers, yet availability of coronary surgery on short call is required.

Once optimal ostial seating of the guide is achieved, close attention must be paid to the navigation and crossing of the lesion by the guidewire. Because of the frequently suboptimal angiographic definition of the residual patent channel and limited space for navigation, guidewire manipulation must be executed with the outmost care to avoid proximal dissection or closure. Atraumatic, soft-tip steerable guidewires with optimal shape retention are used for gentle steering and navigation across the lesion. However, even with the soft-tip guidewires, robust and vigorous guidewire manipulations can result in a

TABLE 8-51. Selected Patient- and Lesion-related Characteristics in 82 Patients with Bare-metal and Drug-eluting Stenting of Ostial lesions

	SES	BMS	p value
PATIENT CHARACTERISTICS			
Patients (*n*)	32	50	
Male gender, *n* (%)	27 (84)	41 (82)	0.7
Age (y)	62 ± 10	63 ± 11	0.9
Unstable angina, *n* (%)	8 (25)	22 (44)	0.06
Diabetes, *n* (%)	3 (9.4)	6 (12)	0.7
Multivessel disease, *n* (%)	22 (69)	39 (77)	0.7
Left ventricular ejection fraction, *n* (%)	51 ± 8	55 ± 9	0.04
LESION CHARACTERISTICS			
Lesions (*n*)	32	50	
Vessels treated			0.4
Left main artery, *n* (%)	10 (31)	10 (20)	
Right coronary artery, *n* (%)	17 (53)	28 (56)	
Saphenous vein graft, *n* (%)	5 (16)	12 (24)	
Lesion characteristics			
Calcium, *n* (%)	4 (13)	6 (12)	0.9
Eccentric, *n* (%)	16 (67)	32 (64)	0.8
In-stent restenosis, *n* (%)	12 (38)	11 (22)	0.2
Preintervention TIMI flow grade 0 to 2, *n* (%)	8 (25)	6 (12)	0.2
Total occlusion, *n* (%)	2 (6)	1 (2)	0.3
Thrombus, *n* (%)	0	3 (6)	0.1

Values are presented as numbers (relative percentages), or mean ± SD.

BMS, bare metal stent; MI, myocardial infarction; PCI, percutaneous coronary intervention; SES, sirolimus-eluting stent; TIMI, Thrombolysis In Myocardial Infarction.

Modified from Iakovou I, Ge L, Michev I, et al. Clinical and angiographic outcome after sirolimus-eluting stent implantation in aorto-ostial lesions. *J Am Coll Cardiol.* 2004;44:967-971.

TABLE 8-52. Quantitative Coronary Angiography at Baseline, After Intervention, and at 10-Month Follow-up in 82 Patients with Bare-metal and Drug-eluting Stenting of Ostial Lesions

Quantitative Coronary Angiography	SES	BMS	p value
Lesions (*n*)	32	50	
PREINTERVENTION			
RVD (mm)	3.17 ± 0.59	3.47 ± 0.74	0.1
MLD (mm)	1.09 ± 0.69	1.48 ± 0.74	0.07
DS (%)	66 ± 19	58 ± 17	0.1
Lesion length (mm)	10.20 ± 7.27	8.47 ± 4.01	0.1
POSTINTERVENTION			
RVD (mm)	3.59 ± 0.52	3.97 ± 0.51	0.01
MLD (mm)	3.18 ± 0.55	3.66 ± 0.53	0.005
DS (%)	11 ± 7	9 ± 7	0.2
FOLLOW-UP			
Angiography done, *n* (%)	28 (88%)	35 (70%)	0.1
RVD (mm)	3.61 ± 0.43	3.50 ± 0.83	0.6
MLD (mm)	3.13 ± 0.59	1.60 ± 1.36	<0.0001
DS (%)	15 ± 13	55 ± 34	<0.0001
Late loss (mm)	0.21 ± 0.31	2.06 ± 1.37	<0.0001
Restenosis, *n* (%)	3 (11)	18 (51)	0.001

Values are presented as numbers (relative percentages), or mean ± standard deviation.

DS, diameter stenosis; MLD, minimal lumen diameter; RVD, reference vessel diameter; SES, sirolimus-eluting stents; BMS, bare-metal stents.

Modified from Iakovou I, Ge L, Michev I, et al. Clinical and angiographic outcome after sirolimus-eluting stent implantation in aorto-ostial lesions. *J Am Coll Cardiol.* 2004;44:967–971.

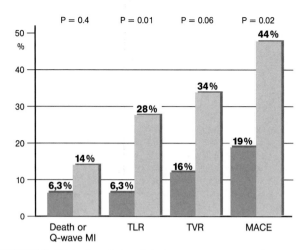

FIGURE 8-48. Cumulative clinical outcome at 10-month follow-up in 82 patients with bare-metal and drug-eluting stenting of ostial lesions. (*Dark bars*) Bare-metal stent; (*light bars*) sirolimus-eluting stent. MACE, major adverse cardiac events; MI, myocardial infarction; TLR, target lesion revascularization; TVR, target vessel revascularization. (Modified from Iakovou I, Ge L, Michev I, et al. Clinical and angiographic outcome after sirolimus-eluting stent implantation in aorto-ostial lesions. *J Am Coll Cardiol.* 2004;44:967-971.)

recoil and dislocation of the guide from the ostium, increasing the risk of a dissection and requiring frequently cumbersome reseating. Once the guidewire securely passes the ostial lesions and is placed in the distal segment of the target vessel, angiographic definition of the ostium should be updated to determine the need for cutting, ablation, or predilatation of the lesion. Predilatation, typically using undersized balloons at high pressures, may be useful to inform the operator about the dilatability of the lesion while improving the visualization of the distal target vessel and stent delivery. However, the downside of ostial predilatation is the risk of massive recoil or dissection with threatened or actual vessel occlusion potentially associated with immediate hemodynamic instability. Thus, in cases with suitable anatomy allowing stent crossing and precise ostial positioning, direct stenting is preferable; in all other cases predilatation or plaque ablation may be required. Use of a "cutting balloon" employing three or four longitudinally attached atherotomes 0.18 mm in height, and 0.70 to 0.76 mm thick[393–396] for ostial predilatation, sometimes after conventional predilatation, might be helpful to redistribute the atheroma and to reduce the risk of major dissections. Once the lesion has been prepared, it should be stented using stents with a large radial strength, virtually without any exception. To deliver an intact stent and to avoid strut damage, in well-prepared lesions a careful deeper engagement of the guide might prove helpful. In these cases the deeply inserted guide is gently withdrawn along with the stent in the inside position. Close to the ostium, the stent is deployed and the guide gently disengaged, still in close touch with the ostium. The final position of the proximal stent end is controlled in a strictly perpendicular ostial projection, with the proximal ring of the stent matching the plane of the ostium. Strict perpendicular projections of the ostium are required to perform this maneuver and stent placement with precision. Extensive disengagement or "popping

out" of the guide may cause not only a complete recoil and disengagement of the guide, but also ejection of the stent delivery system along with the guidewire. In these cases, the instrumentation should be withdrawn and the guide carefully re-engaged for immediate angiographic control to assess the status and to prepare for rewiring of the target vessel and continuation of the procedure. In patients with ostial ectasia or aneurysm, more complete ostial coverage and stent adaptation using slightly oversized balloons and higher inflation pressures with the gently disengaged guide and balloon catheter moved radially along the ostial circumference with individual stent-modifying inflations may be required.

In graft-ostial anastomotic lesions, chronic and acute postoperative lesions should be distinguished. In chronic lesions, successive predilatations with increasingly large balloons are usually required to overcome the resistance of the "stricture-like" fibrotic lesions that are frequently present; this is followed by stenting. In acute postoperative ostial lesions, interventions should be avoided, if possible, because of the high risk of vessel wall rupture and because of the uncertain and usually angiographically undetermined cause of the obstruction. Dilatation attempts on an acute postoperative anastomotic edema or thrombus formation might have disastrous consequences. If emergency intervention is mandatory to relieve major ischemia, angioplasty using conservatively sized balloons and low inflation pressures should be employed. Because of the risk of mechanical damage within the highly vulnerable site, stenting should be, if possible, deferred in the acute setting. Ostial-branch lesions represent a subgroup of bifurcation lesions (see the next section).

BIFURCATION LESIONS

Bifurcations and branching points have been recognized as predilection sites for atherosclerosis, and the importance of the disturbed flow for atherosclerotic plaque formation has been acknowledged.[397] Contrary to the initial assumption,[398] low shear stress (i.e., frictional contact force transmitted to the vessel walls by flow) has been recognized as the major atherogenic force.[399] More recently, the importance of flow dynamics on the topographic distribution of coronary[400] and carotid[401,402] lesions has been recognized and extensively studied.

Bifurcation lesions are a subset of type B AHA/ACC lesions[150] and are usually considered significant if >50% stenosis in the main branch and/or in the side branch has been documented by angiography. A side branch >2 mm in diameter or those that can be bypassed are considered candidate vessels for revascularization. On the basis of the angulation between the main branch and side branch, bifurcations are classified as Y-shaped (angulation <70 degrees, side branch usually with easier access, plaque shift more likely) and T-shaped (angulation >70 degrees). Following guidewire engagement in both vessels, the bifurcation angle frequently changes. According to the topographic distribution of the atheroma at the flow divider, different classifications have been introduced (Fig. 8-49A–D)[403–406] that serve as templates in the strategic planning of revascularization.

Complete main-branch and side-branch repair represents the guiding clinical principle of bifurcation lesion revascularization. However, despite the existence of numerous stenting concepts, bifurcation interventions continue to have lower

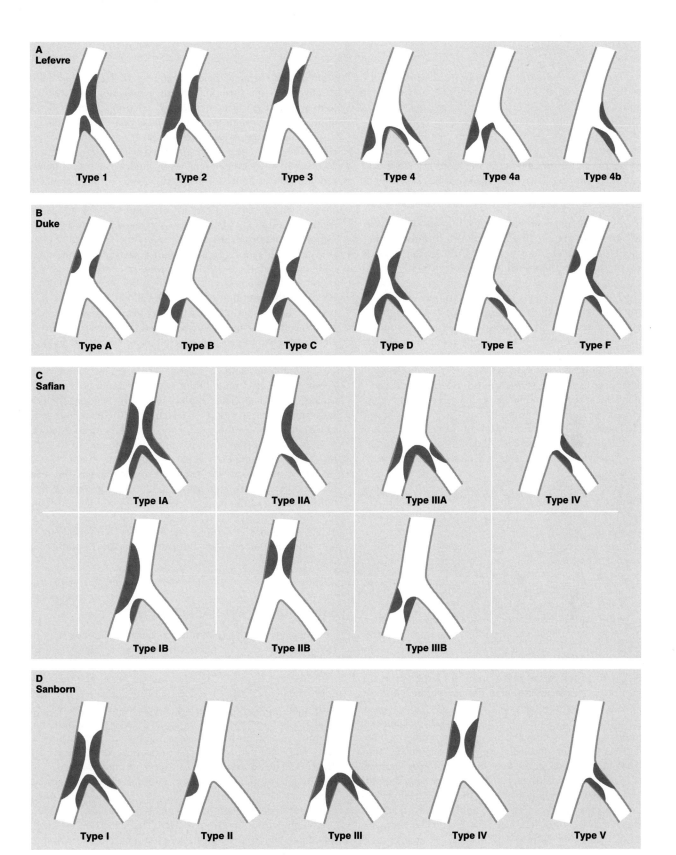

FIGURE 8-49. A–D: Classification of bifurcation lesions based on topographic distribution of lesions reported in the literature. (Modified from Lefevre T, Louvard Y, Morice M-C, et al. Stenting of bifurcation lesions: a rational approach. *J Interv Cardiol.* 2001;14:573–586; Pompa J, Bashore T. Qualitative and quantitative angiography—Bifurcation lesions. In: Topol E, ed. *Textbook of Interventional Cardiology.* Philadelphia: WB Saunders, 1994:1055–1058; Koller P, Safian RD. Bifurcation stenosis. In: Freed M, Grinces C, Safian RD, eds. *The New Manual of Interventional Cardiology.* Birmingham, MI: Physicians Press, 1996:229–243; Spokojny AM, Sanborn TM. The bifurcation lesion. In: Ellis SG, Holmes DR, Jr., eds. *Strategic Approaches in Coronary Intervention.* Baltimore: Williams & Wilkins, 1996:288.)

primary success rates, higher restenosis rates, and worse clinical outcome than do nonbifurcation interventions, and the optimum approach remains elusive.[407–413] Although the causes of the suboptimal outcome of bifurcation intervention have not been clearly elucidated, crosstalk between main-branch and side-branch interventions, associated with unfavorable hemodynamics and negative remodeling in the main branch following side-branch stenting, have been observed in experimental studies,[414] and the wisdom of complete revascularization strategies has been questioned.[415]

At present, one-stent (main branch) techniques with or without side-branch dilatation and two-stent techniques (main branch and side branch) can be distinguished. Surprisingly, although two-stent techniques initially achieve better angiographic results, their clinical outcome may actually be worse.[416] The principal two-stent (bare-metal) techniques by design (intention to treat) include the following: V-technique,[417] simultaneous kissing stent technique,[418] crush techniques (standard, step, reverse),[419] T-technique (standard, modified, provisional),[420] Y-technique,[421] skirt,[422] and culotte[423] techniques. The one-stent technique by design is the simplest and potentially most promising technique when DESs are used.[424] A modified one-stent technique using dedicated stent systems might also represent a promising alternative in suitable and accessible lesions.[425] Preparation of lesions using predilatation may be critical in complex high-grade lesions or when higher profile stent delivery systems are used. Debulking strategies are rarely used at present.[426,427]

The technical aspects of the present stent techniques have been eloquently reviewed in the literature[428,429] and will not be repeated in this context. Instead, several practical aspects of percutaneous bifurcation interventions will be addressed.

As with any intervention, the initial angiographic findings regarding the actual morphology and topographic distribution of the lesion, in this case a bifurcation lesion, determine the interventional strategy. Besides the conventional criteria, proximal accessibility, angulation of the flow divider, topographic distribution of the plaque, diameter of the side branch, and clinical setting (i.e., elective, emergency, availability of surgical standby) are critically reviewed. In all cases that can be bypassed or where a side branch is ≥2 to 2.5 mm in diameter, two guidewires should be used. On the basis of the interventionist's experience, the options for secure revascularization of the main branch and the advantages and disadvantages of leaving the side branch untouched should be considered first. This initial consideration is supported by emerging evidence that in a fair number of bifurcation lesions the least traumatic approach—employing one-stent (DES) implantation in the least number of interventional steps—might actually yield the best clinical if not angiographic results, raising serious questions about the current dogma of complete revascularization of all bifurcation lesions. If indeed main-branch and side-branch intervention has proven necessary, a nonstent angioplasty (provisional stenting) strategy should probably be considered first. The necessity to implant a second stent (actual or threatened side-branch closure) might be based on the intermediate angiographic result and requires the use of one of the established two-stent techniques. Here again, the least traumatic approach in the given setting should be selected. With increasing complexity of the intervention, the need for final balloon-kissing dilatation becomes more pressing. In summary, it appears that experienced operators, instead of assuming a rigid

approach to revascularization strategy of bifurcation lesions strictly based on their angiographic morphology ("intention-to-treat" strategy), are increasingly adopting a more flexible approach based on the response of individual bifurcation lesions to the initial steps of the intervention ("go-with-the-flow" strategy). The use of the latter approach is conditional on initial securing of all relevant branches by guidewires and, if needed, modification of the lesion by predilatations or plaque ablation. The initial broad spectrum of possible next-step interventions successively narrows down as the intervention progresses. At each step the next best option is selected based on the experience of the interventionist. Because of the tendency of plaque shifts in the direction of least resistance, usually the ostia, kissing-balloon techniques should be used not only in escalating bifurcation interventions but also already at the plaque modification stages. Early careful use of kissing-balloon techniques might produce acceptable results actually reducing the need for side-branch stenting. Final kissing-balloon dilatations are required in all two-stent techniques to assure full strut deployment and apposition. Dilatation balloons with optimal deflation characteristics should be used, and a careful successive retraction of the deployed balloons under fluoroscopy guidance is required to avoid stent damage. The length of the kissing balloons should be sufficient to span the entire axial length of the main-branch and side-branch lesions; the sum of the diameters of both balloons should closely approximate the nominal diameter of the proximal adjacent segment of the parent vessel.

Clearly, to improve the strategies and ultimately the results of endocoronary treatments of bifurcation lesions, a better understanding of the biology biomechanics and hemodynamics of coronary flow dividers is required, not just better stent designs. Tables 8-53 and 8-54 demonstrate examples of the angiographic and clinical outcome of bifurcation versus nonbifurcation interventions.

SAPHENOUS VEIN GRAFT LESION

The long-term outcome of aortocoronary saphenous vein graft (SVG) surgery[430,431] is limited by early graft failure (approximately 10% prior to hospital discharge, 5% to 10% within 1 to 12 months) and late graft failure (annual attrition rate initially approximately 2%, after 6 years, 4% to 5% annually).[432] Whereas early graft failure is mostly due to technical factors including small size and degeneration of the target artery, late graft failure is due to restenosis secondary to myointimal hyperplasia followed by graft atherosclerosis (for review, see reference 433). Figure 8-50 demonstrates SVG attrition over time compared with the long-term patency of the internal mammary grafts.[434] Predictors of late-progression of SVG atherosclerosis include graft age, current cigarette smoking, hypertension, dyslipidemia (low high-density lipoprotein, HDL, high low-density lipoprotein, LDL, high triglycerides), poor left ventricular function, and prior myocardial infarction,[435,436] whereas the importance of diabetes remains uncertain. Antiplatelet agents, aspirin[437] and probably clopidogrel,[438] lipid-lowering agents,[439] and probably angiotensin-converting enzyme (ACE) inhibitors[440] are beneficial for long-term SVG patency.

In patients presenting with postbypass recurrence of angina or acute coronary syndromes, SVG disease is the more likely cause than is the progression of native coronary artery disease,

TABLE 8-53. Quantitative Angiographic Characteristics and Results of Bifurcation or Nonbifurcation Interventions

	Nonbifurcation Lesion (n = 2474)	One or more Bifurcation Lesion (n = 349)	p value
BEFORE PCI			
Percentage diameter stenosis	73.8 ± 16.2	74.1 ± 14.3	0.68
Reference diameter	2.9 ± 0.6	2.8 ± 0.6	0.020
Minimal luminal diameter	0.8 ± 0.5	0.7 ± 0.4	0.14
AFTER PCI			
Percent diameter stenosis	9.9 ± 13.4	13.0 ± 16.4	<0.001
Reference diameter	3.0 ± 0.5	2.9 ± 0.6	0.029
Minimal luminal diameter	2.7 ± 0.6	2.6 ± 0.7	<0.001
Acute gain	1.9 ± 0.7	1.8 ± 0.7	0.008
FOLLOW-UP (9-MONTH)			
≥50% loss of gain	798 (32)	122 (35)	0.31
Late loss	1.0 ± 0.8	1.0 ± 0.8	0.96
Late loss index	0.5 ± 0.5	0.5 ± 0.6	0.44
≥50% narrowing	551 (22)	97 (28)	0.022

Diameters in mm; numbers in parentheses are percentages of the total.

PCI, percutaneous coronary intervention.

Reproduced with permission from Garot P, Lefevre T, Savage M, et al. Nine-month outcome of patients treated by percutaneous coronary interventions for bifurcation lesions in the recent era. A report from the Prevention of Restenosis with Translat and Its Outcomes (PRESTO) Trial. *J Am Coll Cardiol.* 2005;46:606–612.

TABLE 8-54. Major Adverse Cardiac Events at 9 Months Follow-up in Bifurcation or Nonbifurcation Interventions

Variable/Event	Nonbifurcation Lesions (n = 10,068)	One or More Bifurcation Lesions (n = 1412)	p value
Death, MI, or TVR	1499(15)	256(18)	0.002
Death or MI	247(2)	29(2)	0.36
Death	119(1)	13(1)	0.39
MI	141(1)	17(1)	0.55
TVR	1367(14)	241(17)	<0.001
PTCA	1427(14)	229(16)	0.041
CABG	373(4)	81(6)	<0.001
PTCA or CABG	1711(17)	290(21)	0.001

Numbers in parentheses are percentages of the total.

MI, myocardial infarction; TVR, target vessel revascularization; PTCA, percutaneous transluminal coronary angioplasty; CABG, coronary artery bypass grafting.

Reproduced with permission from Garot P, Lefevre T, Savage M, et al. Nine-month outcome of patients treated by percutaneous coronary interventions for bifurcation lesions in the recent era. A report from the Prevention of Restenosis With Translat and its Outcomes (PRESTO) Trial. *J Am Coll Cardiol* 2005;46:606–612.

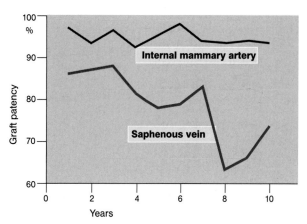

FIGURE 8-50. Attrition of saphenous vein graft bypasses compared with internal mammary grafts over time. (Adapted from Loop FD, Lytle BW, Cosgrove DM, et al. Influence of the internal-mammary-artery graft on 10-year survival and other cardiac event. *N Engl J Med.* 1986;314:1–6.)

as the time progresses (Fig. 8-51).[441] The principal treatment options in patients with unstable angina include reoperation or coronary intervention. Because of the higher risk of reoperation,[442] SVG intervention is preferred, if technically feasible, in the majority of patients. However, SVG angioplasty is associated with a worse outcome and higher complication rates than native coronary artery interventions.[443] Whereas stenting has improved the outcome of SVG interventions (Table 8-55; Figure 8-52),[444] no added benefit of GPIIb/IIIa receptor antagonists was detected in a pooled analysis of five randomized trials.[445]

In high-volume centers, up to 10% of coronary interventions are performed on SVG, of which approximately two-thirds are performed electively. Angiographic findings in patients with SVG disease include high-grade stenosis, and subtotal or total occlusions associated with a diffuse or focal, ostial, body, or distal anastomosis graft atherosclerosis.[446,447] Although procedural complications of SVG interventions are qualitatively similar to those observed in native coronary interventions, "slow-flow" and "no-reflow",[448,449] distal embolization,[450] and significant (more than three times the upper limit of normal) periprocedural creatine kinase isoenzyme MB (CK-MB) elevation[451] appear more frequent, possibly because of the greater vulnerability and friability of graft lesions.[452] Identified risk factors for complications include emergency procedures, thrombotic and ulcerated lesions, large vessel diameter, slow flow, large plaque volume, poor status of the runoff vessel, earlier endovascular treatment, nonostial location of the lesion, large subtended myocardial territory, last remaining vessel, graft in place for >3 years, and diffuse graft degeneration. Additional risk factors include the use of an atherectomy device, patient age, and the presence of comorbidities. Although, a number of techniques have been proposed and implemented to reduce the risk and to improve the outcome,[453–456] thus far and only on the basis of limited experience, the use of DPDs[457,458] and DESs[459] has proved beneficial. Figure 8-53 shows the improvement in clinical outcome with the use of DES compared to BMS for SVG disease.

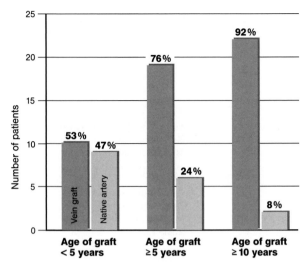

FIGURE 8-51. Etiology of unstable angina following coronary artery bypass graft (CABG) over time. Progression of native vessel disease and that of saphenous vein graft disease are compared. (Modified from Chen L, Theroux P, Lesperance J, et al. Angiographic features of vein grafts versus ungrafted coronary arteries in patients with unstable angina and previous bypass surgery. *J Am Coll Cardiol.* 1996;28:1493–1499.)

TABLE 8-55. Procedural Outcome and Early Clinical Adverse Events after Following Plain Balloon and Stent-supported Angioplasty in Patients with Saphenous Vein Graft Interventions

Variable	Stent Group (n = 108)	Angioplasty Group (n = 107)	p value
PROCEDURAL OUTCOME[a]			
Angiographic success (%)	97	86	<0.01
Procedural efficacy (%)	92	69	<0.001
Crossover to stenting (%)	—	7	—
Hospital stay (days)	7 ± 6	4 ± 7	<0.001
IN-HOPITAL EVENTS (%)			
Death	2	2	0.79
Q-wave myocardial infarction	2	1	0.99
Non-Q-wave myocardial infarction	2	7	0.10
CABG	2	4	0.45
Abrupt vessel closure	1	1	0.99
Repeated PTCA	1	1	0.99
Any event	6	11	0.13
BLEEDING AND VASCULAR COMPLICATIONS AT 0–30 DAYS (%)			
Stroke	0	0	0.99
Vascular surgery	5	3	0.72
Transfusion	15	3	<0.01
Any event	17	5	<0.01

Plus–minus values are means ±SD. CABG denotes coronary-artery bypass graft surgery, and PTCA percutaneous transluminal coronary angioplasty. Five of the 220 patients originally enrolled were excluded because of protocol violations.

[a]Angiographic success was defined as residual stenosis of <50% of the vessel diameter immediately after the procedure. Efficacy was defined as angiographic success achieved with the signed therapy and the absence of a major in-hospital complication.

Reproduced with permission from Savage MP, Douglas JS, Fischman DL, et al. for the Saphenous Vein De Novo Trial Investigators, Stent placement compared with balloon angioplasty for obstructed coronary by pass grafts. *N Engl J Med.* 1997;337:740–747.

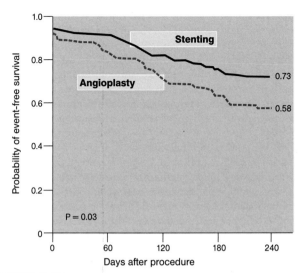

FIGURE 8-52. Cardiac adverse effect free survival of patient with saphenous vein graft (SVG), angioplasty, and stenting. Kaplan-Meier survival curves for freedom from major cardiac events at 240-day follow-up. (Modified from Savage MP, Douglas JS, Fischman DL, et al. for the Saphenous Vein De Novo Trial Investigators. Stent placement compared with balloon angioplasty for obstructed coronary bypass grafts. *N Engl J Med.* 1997;337:740–747.)

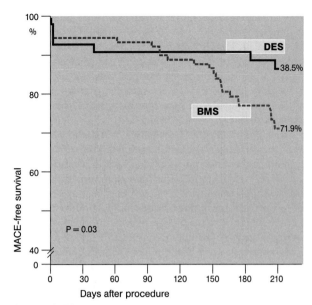

FIGURE 8-53. Kaplan-Meier survival curves for freedom from major adverse cardiac events (MACE) at 6-month follow-up. BMS, bare-metal stents; DES, drug-eluting stents. (Modified from Ge L, Iakovou I, Sangiorgi GM, et al. Treatment of saphenous vein graft lesions with drug- eluting stents. Immediate and midterm outcome. *J Am Coll Cardiol.* 2005;45:989–994.)

The principal points to consider in evaluating preinterventional SVG angiograms are the status of the target graft (focal vs. diffuse degeneration), degree of stenosis/occlusion, topographic location and complexity of the target lesion (ostium, body, distal anastomosis, runoff artery, and thrombus), and the presence of competitive flow. In addition, the anatomic course of the graft (upsloping, twisted, tortuous), presence of venous valves, and degree of step-down between the graft and native vessel are assessed. Furthermore, the status of the bypassed native coronary artery needs to be evaluated and the risks and benefits of native vessels versus bypass revascularization should be considered. The intervention strategy is tailored to the individual case. For example, diffusely narrowed and chronically degenerated SVGs are highly resilient to dilatation attempts and have a high tendency to recoil. Because of their high rigidity, these grafts are highly sensitive to oversized dilatations and may produce extensive tears and ruptures when challenged. In contrast, large and diffusely degenerated grafts may be expected to be filled with a large, highly friable plaque burden that is likely to be associated with thrombi. Distal protection and a most careful atraumatic approach are required to lower the risk of embolization and "no-reflow." Large SVGs with moderate degeneration and slow flow are prone to thrombotic complications, and meticulous anticoagulation, little instrumentation, and a short interventional time are required. In addition, empirical administration of GPIIb/IIIa receptor inhibitors may be considered in these cases.

In distal graft anastomotic lesions, significant differences in the diameter of the graft and native vessel may need to be addressed. Introduction of a second guidewire usually prevents balloon slipping ("watermelon-seed" phenomenon). Successful stenting might require overlapping placement of two stents with different diameters, because the radial strength of the presently available self-expanding stents usually does not suffice to prevent recoil and stent deformation. Cases of early graft failure require optimum anatomic definition of the interventional site

and interpretation of the findings with the assistance of the surgeon. Because of high vulnerability, the most conservative approach to the intervention (undersizing, low inflation pressures) is required. In some cases, a staged approach with initial palliative stabilization might be preferable. In some cases, a staged approach with initial palliative stabilization might be preferable. In cases with a high competitive flow, concomitant visualization of the native bypassed artery from a different access site might be needed to visualize the target lesion.

ARTERIAL GRAFT LESION

The internal mammary artery (IMA) was introduced into coronary bypass surgery initially for direct intramyocardial revascularization (Vineberg procedure)[460] and later for coronary revascularization.[461] Initial acceptance was restricted because of the perceived dominance of coronary surgery using the SVG.[462–464] However, following documentation of excellent long-term patency, the IMA has become a favored and widely used graft in coronary surgery.[465,466] In a recent trial, a 10-year IMA graft patency of 85% was documented,[467] and similar results using the right IMA for coronary grafting were reported.[468] The radial artery was used as a free graft (excised segment of the radial artery anastomosed with the aorta and the coronary artery) in coronary surgery in the early 1970s[469] and was reintroduced later following better preparation techniques as a free, composite (proximal anastomosis at the SVG site) and direct (coronary-to-coronary) graft in the 1990s.[470–472] Although conflicting findings regarding long-term patency have been reported,[473–476] the advantage of radial versus SVG coronary grafting has been documented in a randomized trial.[477] When it occurs, radial graft failure is usually due to a diffuse graft narrowing on angiography ("string sign") that is not amenable to PCI. The cause of this radial graft failure remains uncertain; undue sensitivity to a number of vasoconstrictors such as endothelin-1, angiotensin, and 5-hydroxytryptamine[478] and strong competitive flow[477] have been discussed. The right gastroepiploic artery, a branch of the gastroduodenal artery, was introduced as a pedicled conduit (if ≥2mm diameter) for single or sequential coronary artery grafting in the early 1990s.[479] Despite impressive long-term results,[480] in situ gastroepiploic grafting has not become widely popular, mainly because of the need for concomitant abdominal surgery and limited availability.[481] Because of the long anatomic course leading from the ostium of the celiac trunk via the common hepatic and gastroduodenal arteries to the gastroepiploic artery, percutaneous interventions of this vessel are not technically feasible.

IMA graft disease is most frequently related to stenosis of anastomoses, graft damage (e.g., clipping), suboptimal graft length (redundant with kink stenosis; short on lung inflation), or competitive flow. In addition, incomplete removal of side branches such as the large pectoral branch may participate in the pathophysiology of IMA graft dysfunction. In contrast, IMA graft atherosclerosis appears exceedingly rare. Although the incidence of IMA graft failures is low, it might have become more frequent with the introduction of minimally invasive direct coronary artery bypass (MIDCAB) grafting, mainly left IMA-to-LAD.[482]

In patients with IMA graft dysfunction, angiography may demonstrate focal stenoses with or without diffuse graft narrowings with normal or reduced antegrade flow, diffusely narrowed grafts without identifiable focal stenoses, or graft occlusions. Ostial, body, and anastomotic IMA lesions can be all corrected by endovascular means. The majority of lesions are anastomotic and mostly related to insertions into plaque or technical problems. The lesions involving the body of the graft are usually located in kinked or clipped segments. Proximal ostial lesions are rare, and their cause remains uncertain; catheter-induced injury should be kept in mind as a potential offender. Diffusely narrowed IMA grafts with preserved antegrade flow may represent morphologic adaptation onto low-flow states related to the presence of a pronounced competitive flow via the native vessel. In some patients the diminished flow through the graft appears to be associated with the distal location of the distal graft anastomosis, with upstream occlusion of the native vessel and consequently a small amount of the subtended myocardium. Diffusely narrowed IMA grafts with poor antegrade flow usually represent late stages of IMA graft degeneration secondary to mechanical obstructions, graft damage, or disuse in the presence of a vigorous competitive flow.

IMA graft angioplasty has been associated with a high technical success and acceptable clinical outcomes.[483–486] Introduction of stent-supported angioplasty has improved the clinical outcomes.[487]

In preparing for IMA graft interventions, native vessel and bypass graft coronary angiograms are evaluated to determine whether the IMA graft or the native artery should be revascularized. Taking into account the technical accessibility and severity of the target vessel disease, the functionally more important vessel should be revascularized. In patients considered for IMA graft intervention, the ipsilateral subclavian artery and the brachiocephalic trunk in presence of right IMA graft lesions must be assessed[488]; stenoses with a translesional gradient ≥20 mm Hg should be revascularized prior to coronary interventions. In cases of flow-limiting lesions following the placement of the guide, stenosis should be revascularized regardless of the magnitude of the gradient. Alternatively, the ipsilateral brachial artery might be considered for access.

In approaching IMA graft interventions the operator should take into account the greater vulnerability, propensity to vasospasm, and focal thrombus formations of IMA grafts.[489] In addition, the operator should be familiar with the angiographic appearance of the mechanical refolding of the vessel associated with vessel shortening following the guidewire or dilatation balloon placement, sometimes described as the "concertina" or "accordion effect,"[357–359] and "pseudo-transection."[490] Distinguishing between functional responses to mechanical irritations and vessel wall injuries is critical to avoid unnecessary escalations of interventions. For spasm prevention, an intracoronary bolus of verapamil (e.g., 100 µg) and nitroglycerin (e.g., 100 µg) is usually administered empirically before resuming the procedure. In addition, in extremely tense and anxious patients, early sedation (e.g., diazepam 5 mg intravenously) is recommended. To avoid thrombotic complications ACT should be adjusted to the upper range of 250 to 300 seconds prior to the intervention and maintained at that level throughout the entire procedure.

The use of highly flexible low-profile instrumentation, in combination with a gentle and meticulous interventional technique, usually prevents spasms induced by mechanical irritation. Vessel traumatization can usually be avoided by gentle passive seating of the guide, the use of a hydrophilic soft tip and soft-to-medium-shaft guidewires, and by minimizing the number of interventional steps and instrumentation exchanges. If spasm has been induced, it may become difficult to exclude dissection on angiographic grounds alone. Because of the low efficacy of vasospasmolytic pharmacotherapy, removal of the guidewire and sometimes even disengagement of the guide may be required to resolve the spasm. However, instead of retracting the guidewire with attending difficulties and risks associated with rewiring the IMA in cases of dissection, replacement of the guidewire with a highly tracking microcatheter that removes the mechanical stretch on the vessel and allows distal injection of contrast agent to assess distal patency appears preferable.[491] Following this maneuver and in the absence of dissections, the spasm usually resolves. In cases with angiographically proven or suggested dissections, full mechanical reconstruction of the integrity of the vessel wall is usually required to restore antegrade blood flow and to resolve the spasm. In presence of the usually severe ongoing ischemia and hemodynamic instability, revascularization becomes urgent. In total IMA occlusion and complete lack of the antegrade blood flow, a second access might be required to visualize the interventional situs via the native vessel, if possible. Following the angiographic definition of the target site, direct stenting of the target lesion is preferred, if feasible. In rare intractable cases a switch to a native-vessel, usually RIVA, intervention might become necessary. Surgical bailout always represents the last-resort option. Figure 8-54 provides an example of a persistent vasospasm complicating an emergency IMA graft anastomosis stenosis revascularization.

Ostial IMA graft lesions and dissections are rare. Endovascular treatment is technically feasible, with excellent short-term and poor long-term outcome.[492] The optimal approach to this type of lesion has not yet been identified. In these cases surgical revascularization options should be always considered.

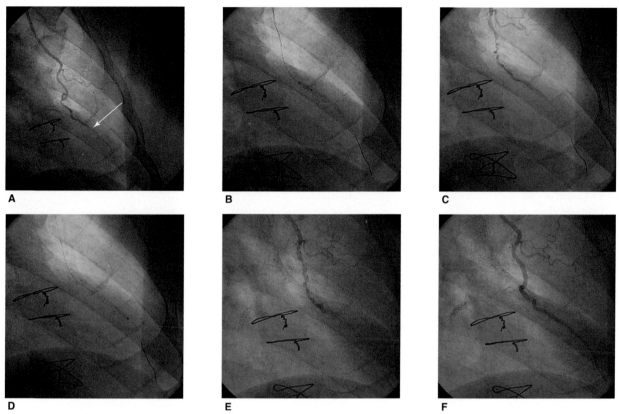

FIGURE 8-54. Left internal mammary artery (LIMA) percutaneous coronary intervention (PCI). A 54-year-old man with non-ST elevation myocardial infarction (NSTEMI) and single LIMA-to-left anterior descending (LAD) artery bypass. Emergency angiography showed 70% stenosis of the distal LIMA anastomosis as the "culprit" lesion (*arrow*) **(A).** Following guidewire placement, the distal anastomosis was dilated with a 2.5/30-mm balloon at 8 bar **(B).** Following dilatation, a subtotal LAD occlusion and massive LIMA spasm occurred **(C);** 200 μg nitroglycerin was injected into the graft, and a 3.0/18-mm Driver stent (Medtronic) was positioned across the culprit lesion and deployed at 12 bar **(D).** Following stenting, the LIMA spasm resolved only partially **(E).** Complete resolution of the spasm followed after intracoronary administration of 300 μg nitroglycerin and guidewire withdrawal **(F).**

CHRONIC TOTAL OCCLUSION

Chronic total occlusion (CTO) (no flow for >3 months) is present in up to 50% of patients with significant coronary artery disease on angiography.[493] Successful CTO recanalization appears to improve outcome and to confer long-term clinical benefits at 10-year follow-up.[494] These results have been confirmed in a recent study.[495] Table 8-56 shows the relationship between selected demographic and lesion-dependent factors on the technical success or failure of CTO revascularization. Figure 8-55 documents the improvement in 5-year clinical outcome in patients with a successful CTO revascularization.

In contrast, studies designed to prove the validity of the "open artery hypothesis" [496] by subacute recanalizations of occluded coronary arteries following acute coronary syndromes have produced ambivalent results.[497–499] The ongoing NHLBI-sponsored prospective and randomized trial (Occluded Artery Trial, OAT) is "designed to test the hypothesis that opening an occluded infarct related artery 3–28 days following a myocardial infarction will reduce the composite endpoint of mortality, recurrent myocardial infarction, and New York Heart Association class IV heart failure over a 3-year follow-up"; the results of this trial will provide answers to questions regarding the clinical benefits of a postacute total occlusion revascularization.

Since the early reports, angioplasties on CTO classified as type C ACC/AHA lesions[150] have been associated with lower technical success rates and a worse clinical outcome than non-CTO interventions.[500] Although the introduction of BMS[501] has improved these outcomes, mainly by preventing restenosis, reocclusion, and target vessel revascularization, the overall results remained below those achieved in the treatment of stenotic lesions.[502–510] An example of differences in immediate angiographic outcomes and at 9.1 $\pm$ 3.3 months follow-up in patients with CTO revascularization using plain balloon angioplasty and BMS is shown in Table 8-57. A summary of the outcomes of CTO-PTCA and BMS interventions of four studies is shown in Table 8-58. Initial data suggest that the angiographic and clinical outcomes may be further improved when DES rather than BMS are used.[511,512] Figure 8-56 demonstrates the 6-month clinical benefits of DES over BMS stenting in CTO interventions.

The decision to perform CTO revascularization and the technical approach to it are determined by patient-, angiography-, and interventionist-related factors. Although successful CTO

TABLE 8-56. Demographics and Target Vessel–related Factors: Effect on Success and Failure of Chronic Total Occlusion (CTO) Revascularization Procedure

	CTO Success (n = 567)	CTO Failure (n = 304)	p value
Age (years)	59.6 ± 10.8	60.5 ± 10.4	0.2
Male sex (%)	73.6	72.2	1.0
Diabetes mellitus (%)	12.0	9.1	0.2
Hypertension (%)	20.3	21.0	0.7
Hypercholesterolaemia (%)	48.6	43.3	0.2
Family history of coronary disease (%)	21.9	18.8	0.3
Impaired LV function (%)	32.5	38.1	0.5
Previous myocardial infarction (%)	55.7	49.2	0.2
Previous PCI (%)	24.3	23.0	0.9
Previous CABG (%)	8.7	10.4	0.4
VESSEL DISEASE			0.03
Single-vessel (%)	46.0	32.6	
Two-vessel (%)	36.2	40.5	
Three-vessel (%)	17.8	27.0	
Number of lesions	573	306	
TARGET VESSEL OF THE LESION			0.8
RCA (%)	42.2	52.6	
LAD (%)	33.2	26.5	
LCX (%)	24.4	20.6	
LMS (%)	0.2	0.3	

PCI, percutaneous coronary intervention; CABG, coronary artery bypass grafting; LAD, left anterior descending artery; RCA, right coronary artery; LCX, left circumflex artery; LMS, left main stem artery.

Reproduced with Permission from Hoye A, van Domburg RT, Sonnenschein K, et al. Percutaneous coronary intervention for chronic total occlusions: The Thoraxcenter experience 1992–2002. *Eur Heart J* 2005;26:2630–2636).

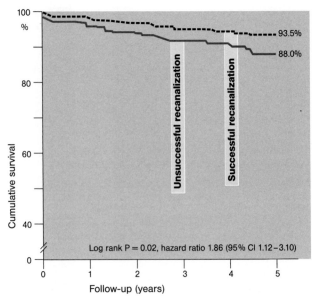

FIGURE 8-55. Cumulative survival at 5 years with regard to the outcome of attempted recanalization of a chronic total occlusion (CTO). Improved outcome in patients with successful CTO revascularization is documented. (Modified from Hoye A, van Domburg RT, Sonnenschein K, et al. Percutaneous coronary intervention for chronic total occlusions: the Thoraxcenter experience 1992–2002. *Eur Heart J.* 2005;26:2630–2636.)

revascularization appears beneficial according to statistical evidence, it might not be so in individual patients if it has not been successful or if it was associated with clinically relevant complications.[494,495] Furthermore, in patients with reocclusion of CTO following an initially successful revascularization the transient anatomic success might be in fact detrimental because of the potentially ensuing loss of the established collaterals.[513] Thus, the decision to attempt CTO recanalization requires a careful consideration of prospective individual risks and benefits in each patient. Angiographic signs predicting the technical success and outcome include the morphology of the target vessel stump (blunt vs. tapered), length of the occlusion, residual antegrade flow, retrograde definition of the occluded artery, and the presence of collaterals, particularly of collateral bridging with a direct take-off from the target vessel stump. Other critical factors affecting the technical success and outcome include the age of the CTO and the skill and perseverance of the interventionist.[514–518] Older occlusions are more resistant to crossing because of progressive fibrocalcific tissue transformation and intraluminal remodeling.[519] Functional occlusions (TIMI >0 degrees) are associated with higher rates of technical success than complete occlusions (TIMI 0 degrees). In CTO with a favorable anatomy (tapered stump, no bridging collaterals, short length of the occlusion, occlusion duration <3 months), technical success rates of >80% can be expected. In contrast, CTO with an adverse anatomy (blunt stump, bridging collaterals, long segmental occlusion, occlusion duration >3 months) may have technical success rates as low as 20%. Overall, CTO of >35 mm are associated with a higher incidence of restenosis.[520] Procedural complications of CTO interventions are similar to those of a standard PCI for non-CTO lesions, except for the higher incidence of guidewire dissections and perforations. However, if dilatations of the perforating sites have been avoided, these perforations are usually self-limiting and require no treatment.

In conventional CTO recanalizations, the operator attempts to find and to reopen the true coronary lumen. Although a great number of endovascular devices have been designed and marketed specifically for CTO interventions, the conventional principle remains the same: engagement, penetration and crossing of the cap of the occlusive plaque, and distal intraluminal passage of the guidewire, frequently requiring negotiation of the more distal former culprit lesion and successively upsizing dilatations. The operator may either try to identify the weakest spot of the occluding cap using a soft or medium-stiffness tip and hydrophilic guidewire, or attempt to penetrate the cap by force at any spot using a stiff or superstiff guidewire. Using the hydrophilic guidewires, the entire cap is carefully and gently explored to avoid dissections or perforations. If dissection occurs, the guidewire is retracted and the probing maneuver repeated. Stiff guidewires may allow penetration of the cap at any suitable location at the expense of poor steering and higher risk of distal vessel wall injury and dissection. Although a staged approach with increasingly aggressive instrumentation (rapid

TABLE 8-57. Example of Quantitative Coronary Angiographic Outcomes of Plain Balloon Angioplasty and Bare-metal Stenting at 9.1 ± 3.3 Months Follow-up in 97 Patients (88% of Initially Studied Patients)

	Stent *(n = 56)*	*PTCA* *(n = 54)*	*p value*
BEFORE PROCEDURE			
Proximal vessel diameter (mm)	3.02 ± 0.69	2.92 ± 0.48	0.37
AFTER PROCEDURE			
RD (mm)	3.01 ± 0.48	2.92 ± 0.55	0.34
MLD (mm)	2.46 ± 0.50	1.91 ± 0.49	<0.0001
DS (%)	18.2 ± 11.2	34.5 ± 10.3	<0.0001
AT FOLLOW-UP			
RD (mm)	2.99 ± 0.51	2.85 ± 0.48	0.15
MLD (mm)	1.74 ± 0.88	0.85 ± 0.75	<0.0001
DS (%)	42.3 ± 26.6	69.2 ± 26.8	<0.0001
Restenosis rate (% of pts)	32.0	68.1	0.0008
Reocclusion rate (% of pts)	8.0	34.0	0.0035
CHANGE IN MLD			
All lesions			
Late loss (mm)	0.76 ± 0.71	1.06 ± 0.80	0.06
Loss index	0.32 ± 0.31	0.55 ± 0.38	0.002
Only nonoccluded vessels at follow-up			
Late loss (mm)	0.61 ± 0.52	0.55 ± 0.36	0.54
Loss index	0.26 ± 0.24	0.30 ± 0.21	0.03

Mean value ± SD or percentage of patients (pts).

DS, diameter stenosis; MLD, minimal lumen diameter; PTCA, percutaneous transluminal coronary angioplasty; RD, reference diameter.

Reproduced with permission from Rubartelli P, Niccoli L, Verna E, et al. Stent implantation versus balloon angioplasty in chronic coronary occlusions: results from GISSOC trial. *J Am Coll Cardiol.* 1998;32:90–6).

exchange followed by OTW in combination with increasingly stiff guidewires) may reduce the risk, frequently in clinical practice the best available CTO guidewire in OTW approach is tried first. With successful engagement and proximal penetration of the cup, the guidewire may "freeze" or it may follow an extra-anatomic path on exerted pressure. Careful probing maneuvers, redirecting the tip, and advancing the tip of the OTW balloon catheter closer to the tip of the guidewire might improve crossing ability without increasing the risk of penetration. Following successful crossing, the guidewire is advanced to the distal segment of the target vessel while exploring the side branches along the path to ensure intraluminal placement. Subsequently, a low-profile OTW balloon is passed down to the vessel to confirm the intraluminal guidewire position. If a low-profile, small-size (1.25- to 2.0-mm diameter) OTW balloon will not pass or severe resistance has been met, in some cases an 0.8-mm diameter excimer laser probe may be helpful in opening up and remodeling the reopened channel. Where there is an extra-anatomic course of the guidewire, it is important to ensure that the guidewire tip has re-entered the true lumen at some distal point confirmed by the unhampered intraluminal motion of the tip freely entering side branches. After intraluminal placement of the guidewire has been confirmed, successive, overlapping, undersized (≤2-mm diameter) balloon dilatations are performed, advancing in the caudocranial direction. If no blood flow returns, dilatations with a larger balloon should be considered. In all cases, a proximal focal occlusive lesion or intimal flap preventing the inflow must be excluded before proceeding with the intervention. Before focal stenting, the true size of the occluded artery should be assessed using intracoronary administration of nitroglycerin. Because of excessively high reocclusion rates, extensive stenting of CLO should be avoided whenever possible. In cases with sufficient reflow in the absence of flow-limiting or unstable lesions, a staged approach with definite revascularization in 8 to 12 weeks might be preferable to allow reflow-directed positive remodeling of the target vessel.

The intentional subintimal tracking and reentry (STAR) technique is similar to techniques employed in recanalization of chronic occlusions of the superficial femoral artery (see Chapter 12). It was recently introduced to improve the technical success of coronary CTO interventions. STAR employs partial extra-anatomical recanalization, with re-entry at some distal point, and confirmation of the distal re-entry by a super-selective injection of a contrast agent administered via a high-tracking microcatheter.[521] This technique requires a great deal of experience and technical dexterity, yet based on a limited data the technical success rates are higher than for the conventional approach. Understanding the clinical importance of CTO revascularization, a number of novel approaches have been proposed and reviewed in the literature.[522]

RESTENOSIS AND IN-STENT RESTENOSIS

Plain balloon coronary angioplasty causes immediate luminal expansion (acute or early gain) followed by a partial early loss due to recoil, and in approximately 30% to 70% of cases late loss due to renarrowing associated with late mechanical (mainly plastic) and biological (mainly myointimal hyperplasia) remodeling. In stent-supported coronary angioplasty, early loss and negative remodeling are prevented (assuming perfect scaffolding), leaving the myointimal hyperplasia as the single cause of renarrowing. Biological cascades triggered by mechanical stretch and vessel wall injury are complex, and their details are still incompletely understood.[523–525] Postangioplasty coronary wall changes may result in positive or negative remodeling.[526] The healing and/or restenotic process is usually completed within 3 to 6 months of the angioplasty injury, although minor additional luminal losses up to 3 years following angioplasty have been reported.[527]

Table 8-59 shows the results of quantitative angiographic and IVUS measurements before and after plain balloon angioplasty and on follow-up. Figure 8-57 reviews the temporal sequence of major biological responses following angioplasty injury leading to repair and restenosis. The risk factors associated with restenosis and in-stent restenosis are similar (Table 8-60).

Angiographic restenosis has been arbitrarily defined as recurrence >50% luminal diameter (binary definition)[85] or any change in the minimal luminal diameter (MLD) on a continuous basis (for review, see reference 86). Quantitative coronary angiography measurements, albeit highly reproducible, appear to systematically underestimate the MLD measured by IVUS.[528,529] The issue of the ability to distinguish between different techniques of

TABLE 8-58. Clinical Trials Comparing Percutaneous Transluminal Coronary Angioplasty (PTCA) versus Stenting in Patients with Nonacute Coronary Artery Occlusions

Trial	No Patients	Reocclusion PTCA	Reocclusion Stent	Reocclusion p value	Restenosis PTCA	Restenosis Stent	Restenosis p value	Target vessel revascularization PTCA	Target vessel revascularization Stent	Target vessel revascularization p value
Stenting in Chronic Coronary Occlusion[a]	114	26%	16%	0.058	74%	32%	<0.001	42%	22%	0.025
Gruppo Italiano di Studio sulla Stent nelle Occlusioni coronariche[b]	110	34%	8%	0.004	68%	32%	0.0008	22%	5%	0.04
Mori et al.[c]	96	11%	7%	0.04	57%	28%	0.005	49%	28%	<0.05
Stent versus Percutaneous Angioplasty in Chronic Total Occlusion[d]	85	24%	3%	0.01	64%	32%	0.01	40%	25%	NS
Total Occlusion Study of Canada[e]	410	20%	11%	0.02	70%	55%	<0.01	15%	8%	0.03

[a]Simes PA, Golf S, Myreng Y, et al. Stenting in Chronic Coronary Occlusion (SICCO): a randomized, controlled trial of adding stent implantation after successful angioplasty. *J Am Coll Cardiol.* 1996;28:1444–1451.

[b]Rubartelli P, Niccoli L, Verna E, et al. Stent implantation versus balloon angioplasty in chronic coronary occlusions: results from GIS-SOC trial. *J. Am Coll Cardiol.* 1998;32:90–96.

[c]Mori M, Kurogane H, Hayashi T, et al. Comparison of results of intracoronary implantation of Palmaz-Schatz stent with conventional balloon angioplasty in chronic total coronary artery occlusion. *Am J Cardiol.* 1996;78:958–959.

[d]Hoher M, Wohrle J, Grebe OC, et al. A randomized trial of elective stenting after balloon recanalization of chronic total occlusions. *J Am Coll Cardiol.* 1999;34:722–729.

[e]Buller CE, Dzavik V, Carere RG, et al. Primary stenting versus balloon angioplasty in occluded coronary arteries; the total occlusion study of canada (TOSCA). *Circulation.* 1999;100:236–242.

Modified from Sadanandan S, Buller C, Menon V, et al. The late open artery hypothesis—a decade later. *Am Heart J.* 2001;142:411–421.

coronary revascularization on the basis of angiographic surrogate end points has been recently reviewed.[530]

Recurrent stenosis represents a major drawback of endocoronary interventions, with reported restenosis rates ranging on average between 25% and 50%, and reaching up to >70% in high-risk populations for plain balloon angioplasty.[531,532] The incidence of restenosis has been reduced by the introduction of BMS support of coronary angioplasty.[191,192] Depending on study and stent design, the incidence of in-stent restenosis ranged between 15% and 35% in most studies reported in the literature.[533–535] Low strut thickness was associated with a lower incidence of restenosis.[536] Figure 8-58 provides an example of comparisons between BMS-supported and plain balloon angioplasty on restenosis rates at 6 months.

In the 1990s brachytherapy using γ (iridium-192) and β (yttrium-90, strontium-90, phosporus-32, and rhenium-188 or -186) radiation implemented on intracoronary radioactive seeds, trains, and wires was successfully introduced for the prevention and treatment of restenosis. A significant reduction in 6-month angiographic restenosis rates, ranging between 41% and 66%,

TABLE 8-59. Quantitative Angiographic and Intravascular Ultrasound (IVUS) Measurements at Baseline, after the Intervention, and on Follow-up after Plain Balloon Angioplasty

	Baseline	Postintervention	Follow-up	Δ(Post vs. Follow-up)	P (Post vs. Follow-up)
ANGIOGRAPHIC RESULTS					
MLD, mm	0.90 ± 0.48	2.42 ± 0.59	1.44 ± 0.88	−0.94 ± 0.79	<.0001
DS, %	68 ± 16	17 ± 13	49 ± 28	32 ± 27	<.0001
IVUS RESULTS					
EEM CSA, mm²	18.5 ± 6.3	20.1 ± 6.4	18.2 ± 6.4	−1.9 ± 3.6	<.0001
Lumen CSA, mm²	1.7 ± 0.9	6.6 ± 2.5	4.0 ± 3.7	−2.6 ± 3.3	<.0001
P+M CSA, mm²	16.8 ± 6.2	13.5 ± 5.5	14.2 ± 5.4	0.7 ± 2.3	<.0001

DS, diameter stenosis; MLD, minimal lumen diameter; EEM, external elastic membrane; CSA, cross-sectional area.

Adapted from Mintz GS, Popma JJ, Pichard AD, et al. Arterial remodeling after coronary angioplasty. *Circulation.* 1996;94:35–43.

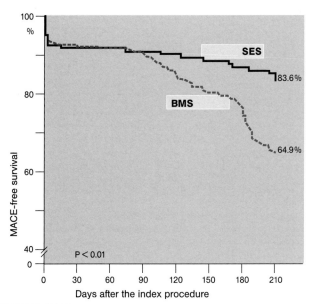

FIGURE 8-56. Comparison of clinical outcomes in patients with chronic total occlusion (CTO) revascularization. Kaplan-Meier survival curves for freedom from MACE at 6-month follow-up in patients with DES compared with BMS stenting in CTO interventions. (Modified from Ge L, Iakovou I, Cosgrave J, et al. Immediate and long-term outcomes of sirolimus-eluting stent implantation for chronic total occlusions. *Eur Heart J.* 2005;26:1056–1062.)

and a significant decrease in MACE, due to reduction of target-vessel revascularization ranging between 36% and 75% compared with nonradiation controls, were reported in several prospective randomized trials. Recurrent stenosis at the proximal and distal edges of the irradiated coronary segments ("candy-wrapper" effects), and late thrombosis observed following both γ and β radiation represented limitations of this approach and prompted changes in strategy, including extended length of the irradiated segment and longer duration of the postprocedural antiplatelet therapy.[527,537–540] Figure 8-59 shows an example of the rate of angiographic restenosis (>50% diameter) using ^{192}Ir versus

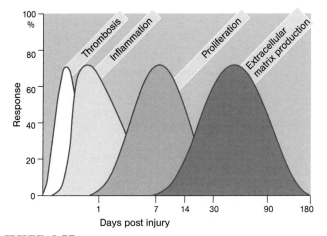

FIGURE 8-57. Temporal sequence of major biological responses associated with restenosis. (Modified from Nikol S, Huehns TY, Hofling B. Molecular biology and post-angioplasty restenosis. *Atherosclerosis.* 1996;123:17–31.)

TABLE 8-60. Risk Factors for Restenosis after Percutaneous Coronary Interventions

Risk Factor Family	*Specific Factors*
Clinical characteristics	Male gender Old age Unstable coronary syndromes Diabetes Hypertension
Target lesion-/target vessel–related characteristics	Thrombus Restenosis Multiple irregularities Length Number of stenoses LAD location Graft lesion Severity Residual stenosis Acute gain Relative gain Absence of intima tear Plaque burden (IVUS)
Procedural characteristics	Stent design, number of stents, total stent length, stent overlap, mean inflation time, type of the device
Biology-related (markers)	C-reactive protein, serum amyloid A, plasminogen activator inhibitor type-I, plasmin-plasmin inhibitory complex, P-selectin, endothelin, insulin, Lp(a), CMV seropositivity
Genetic factors	Gene polymorphisms of angiotensin-converting enzyme, platelet glycoprotein IIIa/IIb and Ia, matrix metalloproteinase-3, apolipoprotein-E, interleukin-1 receptor antagonist

LAD, left anterior descending; IVUS, intravascular ultrasound; CMV, cytomegalovirus.

Modified from Agema WRP, Jukema JW, Pimstone WN, et al. Genetic aspects of restenosis after percutaneous coronary interventions: towards more tailored therapy. *Eur Heart J.* 2001;22:2058–2074.

placebo at 6-month and 3-year follow-up. Figure 8-60 provides an example of MACE-free survival benefit with the use of brachytherapy versus placebo.

The introduction of DES into clinical practice was associated with a significant reduction in angiographic in-stent restenosis rates, a significant reduction in TVR, and a correspondingly reduced MACE rate compared with BMS without a reduction in mortality from all causes.[541] Inhibition of in-stent myointimal hyperplasia by drug elution[542] was associated with a lesser late lumen loss at 6 to 9 months (0.2 to 0.4 mm in DES vs. 0.9 to 1.0 mm in BMS),[543–545] with reported overall restenosis rates ranging between 5% and 10%.[546,547] A long-term benefit of DES implantation at 4 years (sirolimus) and up to 2 years (paclitaxel) was also documented.[548,549] In-stent and persistent restenosis associated with sirolimus-eluting stent implantation appears to be related to gaps in stent coverage, inadequate stent expansion, or procedure-related vessel wall injury.[550–552]

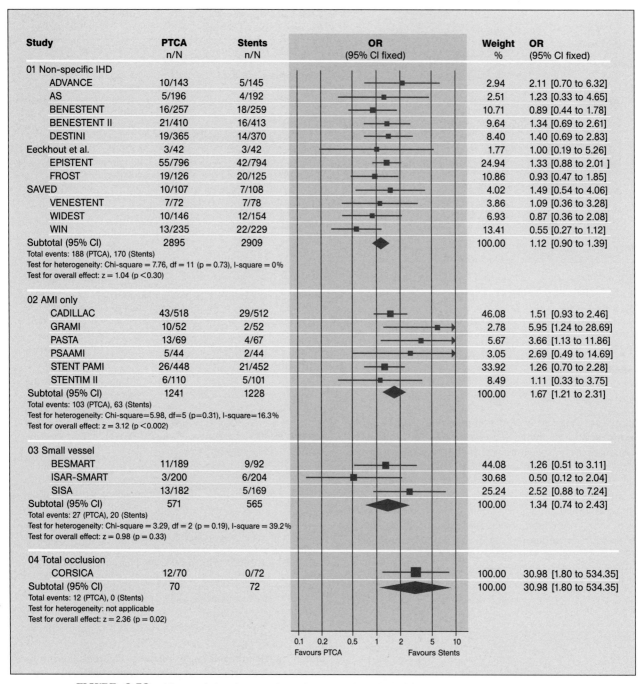

FIGURE 8-58. Meta-analysis of comparisons between plain balloon angioplasty and stent-supported angioplasty for coronary artery disease. Six-month restenosis rates. (Adapted from Hill R, Bagust A, Bakhai A, et al. Coronary artery stents: a rapid systematic review and economic evaluation. Available at: www.ncctha.org/execsumm/summ835.htm. Accessed November 11, 2005.)

stressing the importance of a meticulous implantation technique (i.e., smooth delivery to the target, full and symmetrical stent expansion, complete strut-to-wall apposition, full length lesion coverage). Other predictors of in-stent restenosis with sirolimus-eluting stents included in-stent restenosis target lesion, ostial location of lesion, long lesion (>36 mm), small vessel (<2.2 mm), presence of type II diabetes,[553] and possibly regions with stent overlaps. Direct comparisons between sirolimus- and paclitaxel-eluting stents suggested sirolimus

stents to be more advantageous with regard to angiographic restenosis rates and TVR rates at higher costs.[554–557] Comparison between sirolimus-eluting and thin-strut stents evealed an advantage of sirolimus-eluting stents, with possibly only a marginal benefit in large vessels (≥2.8 mm).[558] Figure 8-61 provides a summary of results comparing DES and BMS with regard to composite event rates defined as MACE, target vessel failure, or event-free survival as primary reported end points in different studies.

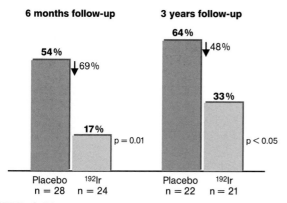

6 months follow-up

3 years follow-up

54%

↓69%

17%

p = 0.01

Placebo
n = 28

192Ir
n = 24

64%

↓48%

33%

p < 0.05

Placebo
n = 22

192Ir
n = 21

FIGURE 8-59. Rate of angiographic restenosis (>50% diameter stenosis of stent and/or stent margin) in ^{192}Ir versus placebo patients at 6-month and 3-year follow-up. (Modified from Tierstein PS, Massullo V, Jani S, et al. Three-year clinical and angiographic follow-up after intracoronary radiation: results of a randomized clinical trial. *Circulation.* 2000;101:360–365.)

The current generation of DESs incorporates primarily two antiproliferative drugs, sirolimus and paclitaxel. Sirolimus (rapamycin), a macrolide antibiotic with potent antifungal, immunosuppressive, and antimitotic properties, is produced by *Streptomyces hygroscopicus*, an actinomycete found in soil. Sirolimus inhibits T lymphocyte activation and proliferation that occurs in response to antigenic and cytokine (interleukin [IL]-2, IL-4, and IL-15) stimulation. Inside the cell, sirolimus effects require binding to immunophilin FK binding-protein-12

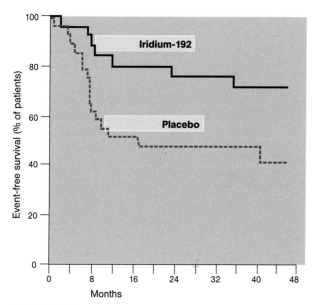

FIGURE 8-60. Kaplan-Meier curves of major adverse cardiac event free survival following intracoronary irradiation with iridium-192 compared to placebo; a 3-year follow-up. (Redrawn from Tierstein PS, Massullo V, Jani S, et al. Three-year clinical and angiographic follow-up after intracoronary radiation: results of a randomized clinical trial. *Circulation.* 2000;101:360–365.)

(FKBP12), which is present only on smooth muscle cells and T lymphocytes, to generate an immunosuppressive complex. Antimitotic activity of the rapamycin-FKBP12 complex is based on inhibition of the cytokine-dependent kinase mTOR (mammalian target of rapamycin), a key regulatory kinase, and consecutive suppression of cytokine-driven T-cell proliferation, inhibiting the progression from the G1 phase (cell growth) to the S phase (DNA replication).[559] Stent design and the pharmacokinetics of the drug release have been reported.[560] In the first published randomized trial using the sirolimus-eluting Cypher BxVelocity balloon expandable stent (Cordis Inc., Miami, FL, USA) in the treatment of patients with de novo native coronary artery lesions (RAVEL), no restenosis was observed in the sirolimus stent group compared with 27% restenosis in the BMS group at 6-month follow-up, along with a reduced rate of major cardiovascular events (5.8% vs. 28.8%).[561]

Paclitaxel, an antimicrotubule agent, originally isolated from the bark of the Pacific yew, is an antineoplastic agent, clinically used primarily in the treatment of ovarian and breast cancer. Paclitaxel promotes the assembly of microtubules from tubulin dimers and stabilizes microtubules by preventing their depolymerization, resulting in inhibition of the normal dynamic reorganization of the microtubule network that is essential for normal cellular functions during mitosis. Paclitaxel-induced abnormal arrays or "bundles" of microtubules interfere with cell proliferation, migration, and intracellular signal transduction.[562] Paclitaxel has been incorporated into a carrier system of the NIRx-Express stent (Boston Scientific, Natick, MA, USA); the stent design and pharmacokinetics of the drug release has been reviewed in the product description.[563] In the first published randomized trial using the paclitaxel-eluting TAXUS NIRx balloon expandable stent (Boston Scientific Corp., Natick, MA, USA) in the treatment of patients with de novo native coronary artery lesions (TAXUS I), no restenosis was observed in the paclitaxel stent group compared with 10% restenosis in the BMS group at 6-month follow-up, along with a reduced rate of major cardiovascular events (3% vs. 10%) at 12 months in a highly selected group of patients.[564]

Although a variety of pharmacological approaches have been proposed and evaluated to reduce restenosis, including systematic treatment with GPIIb/IIIa receptor inhibitors,[565] unfractionated[566–568] and low-molecular[569,570] heparin, oral anticoagulants,[571] corticosteroids,[572,573] sirolimus,[574,575] statins,[576] homocysteine-lowering agents,[577] ACE inhibitors,[578,579] carvedilol,[580] trapidil,[581] and tranilast,[582] with the possible exception of the antioxidant probucol[583] clinical trials have provided disappointing results. Recently, encouraging results have been reported using oral cilostazol, a potent phosphodiesterase-3 inhibitor and antithrombotic agent.[584] Gene therapy holds a great potential for reducing restenosis by a number of mechanisms, yet the available clinical evidence is extremely limited.[585]

Although compared with BMS, DES has proved more beneficial in a number of patient subsets and specific settings, including left main disease,[380,381,386,586] LAD disease[587,588] including ostial location,[589] small vessels,[590,591] long[591,592] and ostial[392,589] lesions, and importantly in diabetic patients,[593–595] the potential limitations may include suboptimal outcome in complex lesions[596] and bifurcation lesions.[424] In addition, the issues of the use of multiple DESs, overlapping stents, optimum stent

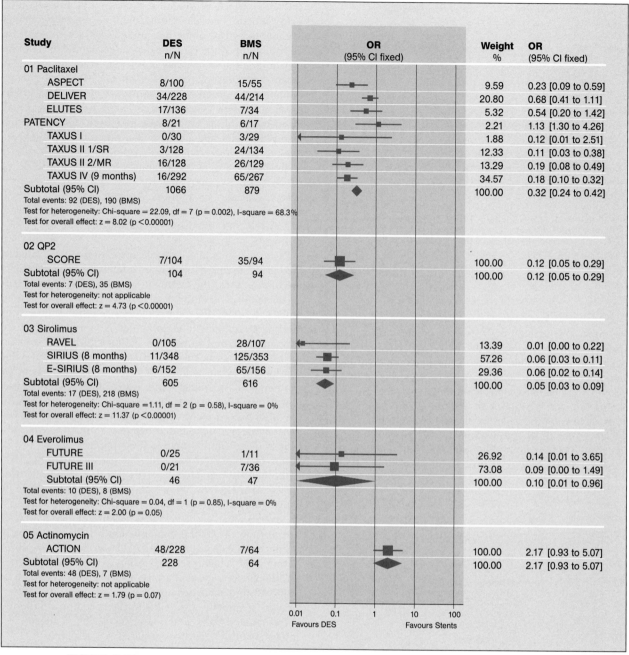

FIGURE 8-61. Summary of results comparing the drug-eluting (DES) and bare-metal stents (BMS) with regard to composite event rates, defined as major adverse cardiac events (MACE), target vessel failure, or event-free survival, as reported primary reported end points in different studies. (Redrawn from Hill RA, Dŭndar Y, Bakhai A, et al. Drug-eluting stents: an early systematic review to inform policy. *Eur Heart J.* 2004;25:902–919.)

length, late restenosis, and late thrombosis require further attention and evaluation.[597-601]

At present on the basis of the available evidence, the first-line approach to restenosis prevention, restenosis, and in-stent restenosis treatment is DES-supported coronary angioplasty.[602] Current evidence suggests that sirolimus-eluting stents have some advantages in terms of angiographic and clinical endpoints over paclitaxel-eluting stents; however, the selection of a particular DES will depend on additional factors including

deliverability and costs.[603] In selected institutions, brachytherapy will probably retain a limited role in the treatment of restenoses in particularly resilient cases.[540] The clinical utility of other proposed experimental strategies such as intravascular sonography, photodynamic therapy, endoluminal low-energy laser, and photophoresis remains to be determined.

The technical approach to treating restenosis is similar to that used for de novo lesions. Although the angiographic appearance of in-stent restenosis appears smooth and patterned compared with postangioplasty restenosis,[604] and therefore may suggest a more straightforward crossing, careful guidewire exploration of the in-stent restenosis entry site and circumscript intrastent passage are mandatory to avoid subsent guidewire passage. Unrecognized substent guidewire placement with subsequent attempts on dilatation will destroy the stent and might induce technically demanding or even irreparable vessel closure. Following guidewire placement and depending on the severity of restenosis, DES stenting with or without predilatation is implemented. If DES is not available, conventional or "cutting" balloon angioplasty with or without stenting for edge restenoses is implemented. Debulking techniques are rarely used in restenosis treatment and prevention in the present scenarios. The development of bioabsorbable stents allowing antiproliferative drug elution represents a promising new target in restenosis treatment and prevention.

MULTIPLE LESIONS IN ONE VESSEL

Coronary atherosclerosis is a diffuse process typically associated with multiple simple and complex lesions[605,606] in a single vessel. The distribution of lesions along the coronary artery is uneven; the majority of clinically relevant plaques are located in the proximal segments of the coronary arteries, with the largest fall-off over distance in the LAD.[607,608] The major predilection sites include the flow dividers opposite the major branches and the inner sides of curvatures.[609–612] Furthermore, multiple plaques and plaque ruptures at sites other than the culprit lesion were demonstrated by IVUS in patients with acute coronary syndromes.[613] Annual progression of plaques from silent to a clinical state occurs in approximately 6% of patients undergoing PCI.[614]

In a clinical setting, the finding of multiple lesions in a single coronary artery is relatively frequent, particularly in patients with advanced disease. To determine the strategy of the intervention, the hemodynamic relevance of individual lesions is assessed or estimated. Usually, only stenotic lesions >70% diameter are considered candidates for intervention. In the presence of more than one hemodynamically relevant lesion in a single coronary artery, usually all lesions are revascularized in one stage starting with the most distal one and proceeding from distal to proximal. This approach bears the advantage of avoiding the necessity of recrossing of already revascularized lesions. However, the dynamic character of lesions with incomplete circumferential plaque extension and angiographically apparent crosstalk between serial lesions may call for a different order of the sequence. For example, the intervention may be started with the most proximal lesion addressed first. Re-establishing the antegrade coronary blood flow may change the angiographic appearance of distal lesions, leading to rearrangement of the order of interventions. In some cases, the lesion initially considered significant might virtually "disappear." Taking the dynamic behavior of lesions into account,[615] intracoronary nitroglycerin should always be administered prior to each intervention. Because, in patients with single or multiple intermediate ("borderline") lesions in a single vessel, angiography is unlikely to identify the flow-limiting lesions and guide the intervention, the flow/pressure wire is usually employed for guidance. In this scenario only the relevant focal lesions are addressed. Catheter-based interventions are not indicated in patients in whom a continuous fall off in translesional pressure is detected, and vigorous medical treatment is prescribed instead. In patients with multiple <50% stenoses, the stenoses are left untouched and secondary prevention is reinforced.

In patients with very distal significant lesions, conservative therapy without any catheter-based intervention is usually preferred, mainly because of the risk of compromising the upstream segment of the vessel in case of complications and distal closure. In addition, distal stenting associated with low distal coronary blood flow and typically a vessel diameter <2 mm carries a high risk of restenosis when BMS have been used. In patients with closely spaced tandem superimposed lesions (separation <5 mm), the lesions are usually treated as a single lesion. In patients with a diffuse disease and multiple superimposed lesions, surgical options should be considered and discussed with the surgeon. Figure 8-62 provides an example of emergency PCI in a patient with single-vessel RCA disease and multiple lesions requiring multiple sequential stent implantations.

MULTIPLE LESIONS IN DIFFERENT VESSELS: MULTIVESSEL DISEASE

Based on a classic definition, multivessel disease (MVD) is a coronary disease in which there is

a greater than 50% diameter stenosis in two of the three major epicardial coronary vessels or surgically bypassable branches thereof. When the right coronary artery was nondominant and failed to supply any of the left ventricular myocardium, the first two moderately sized or large obtuse marginal branches of the circumflex were considered to supply one vascular territory, and the distal obtuse marginal branches and the posterior descending coronary artery were said to supply a different vascular territory.[616]

Other MVD definitions include coronary artery disease with presence of >70% stenoses in at least two coronary arteries or ≥70% stenosis in one coronary artery and ≥50% stenosis in a second coronary artery.[617,618]

Without any objective data on the hemodynamic severity of coronary lesions and corresponding myocardial viability, in most early studies interventionists and surgeons divided coronary artery lesions into three categories:

- *Clinically important:* responsible for ischemic symptoms and signs in a vessel sufficiently large to justify revascularization
- *Borderline:* revascularization judged to be not required
- *Irrelevant:* distal territory small or nonviable as outlined in the Bypass Angioplasty Revascularization Investigators (BARI) trial criteria.[619]

The strategic targets of myocardial revascularization in patients with MVD may be:

- Complete anatomic revascularization, that is, revascularization of all coronary segments >1.5 mm in diameter with ≥50% diameter stenosis
- Incomplete anatomic/adequate functional revascularization, that is, revascularization of all coronary segments with ≥50% diameter stenosis supplying viable myocardium

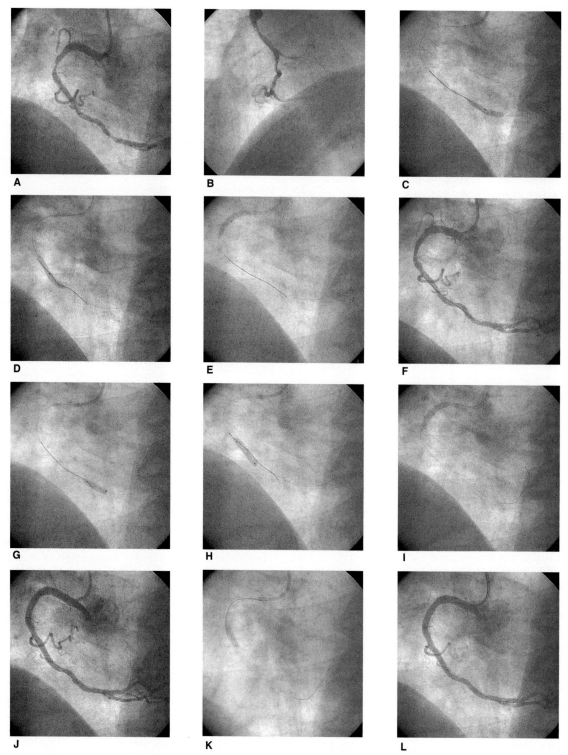

FIGURE 8-62. Multiple lesions, single-vessel disease. A 68-year-old man admitted with uncomplicated non-ST elevation myocardial infarction (NSTEMI). Angiography revealed single-vessel right coronary artery (RCA) disease with three stenoses in the proximal (80%), middle (80%), and distal (70%) segments (AHA segments 1, 2 and 3) **(A,B).** A Whisper M (Guidant) guidewire was placed distally, and a second guidewire (Heavy-weight, Guidant) was placed in the middle RCA segment for support. Consecutive predilatations of all three lesions from distal to proximal using 2.5/20-mm and 3.0 × 20-mm balloons at 8 bar were performed **(C–E).** Angiography revealed the diffuse character of the disease, with residual 40% and 50% stenoses **(F).** Following stenting of all three lesions (one with 3.5/12 mm, two with 4.0/15 mm; all Driver, Medtronic, at 14 bar) over the Whisper M guidewire **(G–I),** dissection and plaque shift between the two proximal stents was detected **(J),** requiring placement of a fourth stent (4.0/10-mm Lekton motion, Biotronik) **(K).** This resulted in complete revascularization at the expense of extensive stenting **(L).**

- Incomplete functional revascularization, that is, failure to revascularize all coronary segments with ≥50% diameter stenosis supplying viable myocardium (for review, see reference 620)

Traditionally, the principal target of surgical revascularization in patients with MVD was complete anatomic revascularization associated with an improved clinical outcome, including lower mortality, lesser anginal symptoms, and reduced need for repeat revascularizations.[621,622] However, over the past two decades the justification for this approach has been questioned, and eventually a far more differentiated approach was adopted in most institutions. Thus, in the attempt to minimize the risk associated with extensive revascularization procedures, a number of factors including the presence of diabetes, renal disease, and left ventricular dysfunction, entry indication, emergency versus elective settings, age and life expectancy of the patient, and a host of other factors are usually considered, resulting in individually customized strategic considerations.[620]

Angioplasty has been offered to patients with MVD as an alternative to coronary bypass surgery for >20 years.[616,623–625] Initially, the surgical approach was adopted and complete anatomical revascularization was targeted in angioplasty interventions.[624] Thus, in the late 1980s and early 1990s, interventions on >10 lesions were common in many laboratories. However, despite the fact that at times all angiographic lesions were addressed in one stage, complete anatomic revascularization was less frequently achieved using catheter-based interventions compared with surgery, particularly in patients with CTO. With better understanding of the restenotic process, the principal importance of the viability of the dependent myocardium, left ventricular function, and long-term clinical outcomes, the targets of MVD revascularization have become gradually modified.[626–628] At present, functionally adequate revascularization represents a reasonable target in the majority of patients undergoing PCI for MVD.

In a number of studies comparing plain balloon- and BMS-supported angioplasty with CABG for treating patients with MVD, the superiority of the surgical approach in terms of the lower incidence of recurrent angina and lower need for target vessel revascularization was repeatedly documented.[67,73,630] Even the results of the two recent trials comparing BMS-supported coronary angioplasty and CABG at 5-year follow-up (the ARTS and the ERACI II trials[70,71]) confirmed these results. In the ARTS trial the incidence of repeat revascularization and the composite event-free survival rate were significantly different between two groups: stent group (30.3%), CABG group (8.8%; p <0.001; relative risk, 3.46; 95% confidence interval, 2.61 to 4.60), and 58.3% in the stent group and 78.2% in the CABG group (p <0.0001; relative risk, 1.91; 95% confidence interval, 1.60 to 2.28), respectively. Overall freedom from death, stroke, or myocardial infarction did not differ significantly between the groups (18.2% in the stent group vs. 14.9% in the surgical group; p = 0.14; relative risk, 1.22; 95% confidence interval, 0.95 to 1.58).[70] In the ERACI II trial, survival and freedom from nonfatal acute myocardial infarction did not differ statistically between patients treated with PCI and those who underwent CABG (92.8% vs. 88.4% and 97.3% vs. 94% respectively, p = 0.16). However, freedom from repeat revascularization procedures

(PCI/CABG) and freedom from MACE were significantly lower with PCI than with CABG (71.5% vs. 92.4%, p = 0.0002 and 65.3% vs. 76.4%; p = 0.013, respectively[71]; Fig. 8-10). However, the use of drug-eluting stents to treat patients with MVD might change this perspective. In a preliminary report, the 1-year results of the follow-up Arterial Revascularization Therapies Study (ARTS-II trial) comparing the outcome of the sirolimus-eluting stent PCI (3.7 stents per patient) with the outcome of the previous ARTS-I trial showed favorable results, that is, lower 1-year adjusted MACE of sirolimus-eluting stent PCI compared to both the CABG and the BMS-PCI historical arms.[631] The data from this study and the results of subsequent trials might redefine the evolving role PCI in revascularization strategies for patients with MVD. Given the presently incomplete evidence, decisions about revascularization strategies in individual patients include consensus by an interventionist and surgeon that is based on the diffuse or focal character of the disease, the functional state and vitality of the myocardium, left ventricular function, and relevant patient-related factors as stated earlier. In some patients, hybrid revascularization might represent the therapy of choice.[632] In patients selected for angioplasty, DES should preferably be used in all cases.

Functionally adequate percutaneous revascularization requires definition of all the target lesions and their approximate ranking. In addition, their relevance to staging is considered. In approaching the MVD intervention, typically the hemodynamically most critical lesion is revascularized first, followed by other lesions in descending order of importance. However, experienced interventionists maintain a considerable flexibility as far as the order of addressed target lesions is concerned. For example, in high-risk interventions, arguably the least risky lesion or the lesion with the highest functional yield may be revascularized first to improve the myocardial perfusion, setting the stage for the intervention on higher risk lesions. In patients with MVD including CTO, initial CTO revascularization may also reduce the procedural risk of the intervention. In patients with limiting coexistent morbidities, other considerations such as length of the intervention, radiation exposure, amount of contrast agent used, and patient comfort may also become important. In summary, in patients with MVD various patient-related factors must be considered in addition to the angiographic status of the CAD in order to select the individually optimal strategy of revascularization. The most important noncoronary factors affecting the choice of strategy include the presence of type II diabetes, renal dysfunction, cardiac function, and myocardial viability.

ACUTE CORONARY ARTERY INTERVENTION

Acute coronary artery interventions were initially performed for bailout following failed thrombolysis. Since the early 1980s, however, the potential of PTCA as the primary treatment of patients with acute coronary syndromes has been recognized and explored.[633,634] Subsequent to the first randomized trials comparing acute coronary interventions with systemic thrombolysis,[635,636] acute coronary catheter-based interventions have grown to become a standard of care in patients presenting with acute coronary syndromes.[81,82]

In clinical practice, emergency PCI differs considerably from elective coronary interventions. They are characterized by the immediate urgency of the procedure and greater procedural risk associated with the evolving myocardial ischemia or infarction, associated with instability of the patient and potential threat to the patient's life. Depending on the severity of the presenting symptoms, management (the scope and the speed) of the emergency intervention must be scaled up to include interventions under the conditions of a full-scope resuscitation, hemodynamic support, and mechanical ventilation, or scaled down to a lower emergency level.

The hallmarks of emergency interventions are time constraints and dealing with an unstable lesion and ongoing myocardial ischemia. To save time and to assure the best available treatment to all patients requires a functioning rescue chain consisting of an early alert, sophisticated prehospital management, quick transportation, and professional hospital staff supported by established hospital critical pathways operating on the basis of 24/7/365 availability.

In patients with confirmed ST-elevation myocardial infarction, direct admission to the catheterization laboratory saves time and reduces complications. In patients requiring resuscitation or advanced hemodynamic or respiratory support, in addition to the operator an anesthesiologist or other qualified physician is required to attend to the patient, allowing the interventionist to focus without restriction on the intervention. In stable patients with non-ST-segment elevation acute coronary syndromes, admission to the coronary care unit may be preferable to complete diagnostics and to prepare the patient for early angiography.

Once arterial access is established, diagnostic coronary angiography is performed. A limited number of views is required to identify the culprit lesion, to assess the coronary status, and to determine the left ventricular function. Unequivocal identification of the culprit lesion is critical to avoid futile revascularization attempts on CTOs or addressing secondary lesions in patients with MVD or previous coronary bypass surgery. In patients with multiple concurrent potential "culprit" lesions on angiography, the patient's history, ECG, and echocardiography might be needed to assist identification. Following unequivocal identification of the culprit lesion, the strategy of the intervention is determined and the lesion is addressed immediately. In the vast majority of patients, only the "culprit" lesion of the infarct-related artery (IRA) should be addressed! All attempts at revascularization of nonculprit lesions in an acute setting in patients with MVD should be resisted and deferred, unless absolutely necessary! Exemptions to this rule include hemodynamically unstable patients despite successful culprit lesion revascularization, and patients with severe LV dysfunction, including those in cardiogenic shock. In addition, in unstable patients with failed culprit lesion revascularization, nonculprit lesions may be considered for emergency revascularization in an attempt to optimize myocardial perfusion. Alternative strategies in unstable patients presenting with MVD and LV dysfunction include emergency culprit lesion revascularization, mechanical LV support with short-term "cooling off" and stabilization, and staged completion of revascularization by PCI or bypass surgery. However, this strategy bears the risk of successive and protracted multiorgan dysfunction, particularly in patients with incomplete revascularization, ongoing myocardial ischemia, and marked pre-existent LV dysfunction. Therefore, in these patients a particularly close monitoring is mandatory to avoid the point of no return. Figure 8-63 shows an example of a "bridging-to-surgery" emergency intervention in a patient with multivessel disease and severe LV dysfunction. Patients presenting for emergency angiography shortly after coronary bypass surgery should be reviewed in close rapport with the operating surgeon. Because of the high risk of either surgical revision or coronary intervention, a consensus decision is required to determine the optimal course of action. If percutaneous intervention appears the most appropriate approach, it is most important to proceed with the least offensive interventional strategy by avoiding oversizing and high-pressure inflations. However, in many cases reoperation might be required for unstable patients.

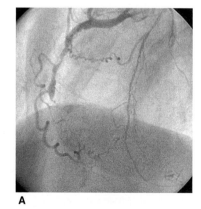
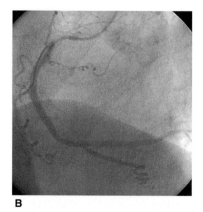

A   **B**

FIGURE 8-63.   Emergency "bridging-to-surgery" percutaneous coronary intervention (PCI): right coronary artery (RCA) and severe myocardial dysfunction. An 80-year-old woman with subacute inferior wall ST elevation myocardial infarction (STEMI) and severe hemodynamic compromise. Angiography revealed thrombotic RCA occlusion (infarct-related artery), occluded left anterior descending (LAD) artery, and partial retrograde LAD filling via collaterals **(A).** Following guidewire placement and predilatation using a 2.5/30-mm balloon at 8 bar, a 3.5/38-mm Driver stent (Medtronic) at 18 bar was deployed, resulting in an acceptable angiographic result **(B)** and rapid hemodynamic stabilization of the patient.

The conduct of emergency PCI does not allow lesion-based stratification common in elective procedures; all lesions qualify to the same degree and must be addressed for an immediate repair and revascularization. To bring the patient out of the risk zone associated with ongoing myocardial ischemia or evolving myocardial infarction as quickly as possible, the strategy of the intervention should be as straightforward and atraumatic as possible. The necessity to deal effectively with virtually any type of unstable coronary artery lesions in unstable and potentially threatened patients under considerable time constraints provides the obvious evidence for the need of an experienced operator supported by an experienced catheterization laboratory team. It is these experienced operators and their teams who will most likely do "the right thing in the right order at the right time," thus maximizing the chances of patients with acute coronary syndromes for the best possible outcome.

REFERENCES

1. Grüntzig A, Riedhammer HH, Turina M, et al. Eine neue Methode zur perkutanen Dilatation von Koronarstenosen. Tierexperimentelle Prüfung. *Verh Dtsch Ges Kreislforsch.* 1976;42:282–385.
2. Grüntzig A, Schneider J. Die perkutane Dilatation chronischer Koronarstenosen—Experiment und Morphologie. *Schweiz Med Wschr.* 1977;107:1588.
3. Grüntzig A, Myler R, Hanna ES, et al. Coronary transluminal angioplasty. *Circulation.* 1977;56(Abstract):84.
4. Grüntzig A. Transluminal dilatation of coronary artery stenosis [letter]. *Lancet.* 1978;i:263.
5. Kaltenbach M, Kober G, Satter P, et al. Koronare Eingefäberkrankung. *Verh Dtsch Ges Herz Kreislforsch.* 1980;46:130–137.
6. Kaltenbach M. Evolution of interventional cardiology in Germany. *J Intervent Cardiol.* 2002;15:33–39.
7. Grüntzig A, Hirzel H, Goebel N, et al. Die perkutane transluminale Dilatation chronischer Koronarstenosen: erste Erfahrungen. *Schweiz Med Wschr.* 1978;108:1721–1723.
8. Grüntzig A, Senning A, Siegenthaler WE. Nonoperative dilation of coronary-artery stenoses. *N Engl J Med.* 1979;301:61–68.
9. Beck A, Grüntzig A. *Eine Idee verändert die Medizin.* Konstanz: Clio-Verlag, 1999:2373.
10. King SB III, Meier B. Interventional treatment of coronary heart disease and peripheral vascular disease. *Circulation.* 2000;102:IV-81-IV-86.
11. Simpson JB, Baim DS, Robert E, et al. A new catheter system for coronary angioplasty. *Am J Cardiol.* 1982;29:1216–1221.
12. Kaltenbach M. Neue Technik zur steuerbaren Ballondilatation von Kranzgefäßverengungen. *Z Kardiol.* 1984;73:699–673.
13. Bonzel T, Wollschläger H, Just H. Ein neues Kathersystem zu mechanischen Dilatation von Koronarstenosen mit austauschbaren intrakoronaren Kathetern, höherem Kontrastmitteluß und verbesserter Steuerbarkeit. *Biomed Technik.* 1986;21:195–201.
14. Sigwart U, Puel J, Mirkovitch V, et al. Intravascular stents to prevent occlusion and restenosis after transluminal angioplasty. *N Engl J Med.* 1987;316:701–706.
15. Puel J, Joffre F, Rousseau F, et al. Endo-protheses coronariennes auto-expansives dans le prevention des restenoses apres angioplastie transluminale. *Arch Mal Coeur.* 1987;8:1311–1312.
16. Sousa JE, Costa MA, Abizaid A, et al. Lack of neointimal proliferation after implantation of sirolimus-coated stents in human coronary arteries: a quantitative coronary angiography and three-dimensional intravascular ultrasound study. *Circulation.* 2001;103:192–195.
17. Heublein B, Rohde R, Kaese V, et al. Biocorrosion of magnesium alloys: a new principle in cardiovascular implant technology? *Heart.* 2003;89:651–656.
18. Quinn MJ, Fitzgerald DJ. Ticlopidine and clopidogrel. *Circulation.* 1999;100:1667–1672.
19. Brophy JM, Joseph L. Medical decision making with incomplete evidence—choosing a platelet glycoprotein IIbIIIa receptor inhibitor for percutaneous coronary interventions. *Med Decis Making.* 2005;25:222–228.
20. Simpson JB, Johnson DE, Thapliyal HV, et al. Transluminal atherectomy: a new approach to the treatment of atherosclerotic vascular disease [abstract]. *Circulation.* 72(suppl II):111–146.
21. Kensey KR, Nash JE, Abrahams L, et al. Recanalization of obstructed arteries with a flexible, rotating tip catheter. *Radiology.* 1987;165:387–389.
22. Litvack F, Grundfest W, Hickey A, et al. Percutaneous coronary excimer laser angioplasty in animals and humans. *J Am Coll Cardiol.* 1989;13:61A.
23. Teierstein PC, Massullo V, Jani S, et al. Catheter-based radiotherapy to inhibit restenosis after coronary stenting. *N Engl J Med.* 1997;336:1697–1703.
24. Rentrop P, Blanke H, Karsch KR, et al. Selective intracoronary thrombolysis in acute myocardial infarction and unstable angina pectoris. *Circulation.* 1981;63:307–317.
25. Schröder R, Biamino G, Enz-Rudiger L. Intravenous short-term infusion of streptokinase in acute myocardial infarction. *Circulation.* 1983;63:536–548.
26. Ross R. Atherosclerosis: an inflammatory disease. *N Engl J Med.* 1999;340:115–126.
27. Stary HC, Chandler AB, Glagov S, et al. A definition of initial, fatty streak, and intermediate lesions of atherosclerosis: a report from the Committee on Vascular Lesions of the Council on Arteriosclerosis, American Heart Association. *Arterioscler Thromb.* 1994;14:840–856.
28. Stary HC, Chandler AB, Dinsmore RE, et al. A definition of advanced types of atherosclerotic lesions and a histological classification of atherosclerosis: a report from the Committee on Vascular Lesions of the Council on Arteriosclerosis, American Heart Association. *Arterioscler Thromb.* 1995;15:1512–1531.
29. Stary HC. *Atlas of Atherosclerosis Progression and Regression.* New York: Parthenon, 1999.
30. Herrick JB. Clinical features of sudden obstruction of the coronary arteries. *JAMA.* 1912;23:2015–2020.
31. Benson RL. The present status of coronary arterial disease. *Arch Pathol.* 1926;2:876–916.
32. Duguid JB. Thrombosis as a factor in the pathogenesis of coronary atherosclerosis. *J Pathol.* 1946;58:207–212.
33. Chapman I. Morphogenesis of occluding coronary artery thrombosis. *Arch Pathol.* 1965;80:256–261.
34. Constantinides P. Plaque fissuring in human coronary thrombosis. *J Atheroscler Res.* 1966;6:1–17.
35. Chandler AB, Chapman I, Erhardt LR, et al. Coronary thrombosis in myocardial infarction. Report of a workshop on the role of coronary thrombosis in the pathogenesis of acute myocardial infarction. *Am J Cardiol.* 1974:34:823–833.
36. DeWood MA, Spores J, Notske R, et al. Prevalence of total coronary occlusion during the early hours of transmural myocardial infarction. *N Engl J Med.* 1980;303:897–902.
37. Richardson PD, Davies MJ, Born GVR. Influence of plaque configuration and stress distribution on fissuring of coronary atherosclerotic plaques. *Lancet.* 1989;i:941–944.
38. Richardson PD. Biomechanics of plaque rupture: progress, problems, and new frontiers. *Ann Biomech Eng.* 2002;3:524–536.
39. Holzapfel GA, Stadler M, Gasser TC. Towards a computational methodology for optimizing angioplasty treatments with stenting. In: Holzapfel GA, Ogden RW, eds. *Mechanics of Biological Tissue.* Heidelberg: Springer-Verlag, 2005:207–220.
40. Holzapfel GA, Stadler M, Gasser TC. Changes in the mechanical environment of stenotic arteries during interaction with stents: computational assessment of parametric stent designs. *ASME J Biomech Eng.* 2005;127:166–180.
41. Gasser TC, Holzapfel GA. A rate-independent elastoplastic constitutive model for (biological) fiber-reinforced composites at finite strains: continuum basis, algorithmic formulation and finite element implementation. *Comput Mech.* 2002;29:4–5, 340–360.
42. Salunke NV, Topoleski LDT. Biomechanics of atherosclerotic plaque. *Crit Rev Bioeng.* 1997;25(3):243–285.
43. Holzapfel GA, Sommer G, Regitnig P. Anisotropic mechanical properties of tissue components in human atherosclerotic plaques. *J Biomech Eng.* 2004;126:657–665.
44. Topoleski LDT, Salunke NV, Humphrey JD, et al. Composition- and history-dependent radial compressive behavior of human atherosclerotic plaque. *J Biomed Mat Res.* 1997;35(1):117–127.
45. Salunke NV, Topoleski LDT, Humphrey JD, et al. Compressive stress-relaxation of human atherosclerotic plaque. *J Biomed Mat Res.* 2001;55(2):236–241.
46. Topoleski LDT. Biomechanics: mechanical properties and behavior of atherosclerotic plaque. In: Lanzer P, Topol EJ, eds. *PanVascular Medicine: Integrated Clinical Management.* Heidelberg: Springer Verlag, 2002:340–352.
47. Haslach HW Jr., Armstrong RW. *Deformable Bodies and Their Material Behavior.* New York: Wiley, 2004:193–199.
48. Kaltenbach M. The first angioplasties in Germany (personal communication).
49. Castaneda-Zuniga WR, Formanek A, Tadavarthy M, et al. The mechanism of balloon angioplasty. *Radiology.* 1980;135:565–571.
50. Block PC, Myler RK, Sterzer S, et al. Morphology after transluminal angioplasty in human beings. *N Engl J Med.* 1981;305:382–385.
51. Waller BF, Garfinkel HJ, Rogers FJ, et al. Early and late morphologic changes in major epicardial coronary arteries after percutaneous transluminal coronary angioplasty. *Am J Cardiol.* 1984;53:42C–47C.
52. Waller BF. Coronary luminal shape and the arc of disease-free wall: morphologic observations and clinical relevance. *J Am Coll Cardiol.* 1986;6:1100–1101.
53. Waller BF, Rothbaum DA, Garfinkel HJ, et al. Morphologic observations following percutaneous transluminal balloon angioplasty of early and late aortocoronary saphenous vein bypass grafts. *J Am Coll Cardiol.* 1984;4:784–792.
54. Fung YC, Fronek K, Patitucci P. Pseudoelasticity of arteries and the choice of its mathematical expression. *Am J Physiol.* 1979;237(5):H620-H631.
55. Humphrey JD. Mechanics of the arterial wall: review and directions. *Crit Rev Biomed Eng.* 1995;23(1–2):1–162.
56. Gleason RL, Hu JJ, Humphrey JD. Building a functional artery: issues from the perspective of mechanics. *Front Biosci.* 2004;9:2045–2055.
57. Haslach H. Nonlinear viscoelastic, thermodynamically consistent, models for biological soft tissue. *Biomech Model Mechanobiol.* 2005;3(3):172–189.
58. Glagov S, Weisenberg E, Zarins CK, et al. Compensatory enlargement of human atherosclerotic coronary arteries. *N Engl J Med.* 1987;316:1371–1375.
59. Pasterkamp G, Borst C, Gussenhoven EJ, et al. Remodeling of de novo atherosclerotic lesions in femoral arteries: impact on mechanism of balloon angioplasty. *J Am Coll Cardiol.* 1995;26:422–428.
60. Schoenhagen P, Ziada KM, Kapadia SR, et al. Extent and direction of arterial remodeling in stable versus unstable coronary syndromes. *Circulation.* 2000;101:598–603.
61. Fujii K, Carlier SG, Mintz GS, et al. Association of plaque characterization by intravascular ultrasound virtual histology and arterial remodeling. *Am J Cardiol.* 2005;96:1476–1483.
62. Mintz GS, Kimura T, Nobuyoshi M, et al. Relation between preintervention remodeling and late arterial responses to coronary angioplasty or atherectomy. *Am J Cardiol.* 2001;87:392–396.
63. Nakamura M, Yock PG, Bonneau HN, et al. Impact of peri-stent remodeling on restenosis. A volumetric intravascular ultrasound study. *Circulation.* 2001;103:2130–2132.

64. Togni M, Balmer F, Pfiffner D, et al. Percutaneous coronary interventions in Europe 1992–2001. *Eur Heart J.* 2004;25:1208–1213.

65. Buuren F, Horstkotte D. Ergebnisse der gemeinsamen Umfrage der Kommission für Klinische Kardiologie und Arbeitsgruppen Interventionelle Kardiologie (für die ESC) und Angiologie der Deutschen Gesellschaft für Kardiologie—Herz- und Kreislaufforschung über das Jahr 2004; 21. Bericht über die Leistungszahlen der Herzkatheterlabore in der Bundesrepublik Deutschland. Source: http://leitlinien.dgk.org/files/Leistungszahlen2004.pdf. Accessed May 21, 2006.

66. Garrett HE, Dennis EW, DeBakey ME. Aortocoronary bypass with saphenous vein graft. Seven-year follow up. *JAMA.* 1973;223:792–794.

67. Eagle KA, Guyton RA, Davidoff R, et al. ACC/AHA 2004 guideline update for coronary artery bypass graft surgery. *Circulation.* 2004;110:e340-e437.

68. Yusuf S, Zucker D, Peduzzi P, et al. Effects of coronary artery bypass graft surgery on survival: overview of 10-year results from randomized trials by the Coronary Artery Bypass Graft Surgery Trialists Collaboration. *Lancet.* 1994;344:563–570.

69. Sculpher MJ, Petticrew M, Kelland JL, et al. Resource allocation for chronic stable angina: a systematic review of effectiveness, costs and cost-effectiveness of alternative interventions. *Health Technol Assessment* 1998;2. Available at: www.ncchta.org/fullmono/mon210.pdf. Accessed September 20, 2005.

70. Serruys PW, Ong ATL, van Herwerden LA, et al. Five-year outcomes after coronary stenting versus bypass surgery for the treatment of multivessel disease. The final analysis of the Arterial Revascularization Therapies Study (ARTS) randomized trial. *J Am Coll Cardiol.* 2005;46:575–581.

71. Rodriquez AE, Baldi J, Pereira CF, et al. Five-year follow-up of the Argentine Randomized Study: Coronary Angioplasty with Stenting Versus Coronary Bypass Surgery in patients with multiple vessel disease (ERACI II) trial. *J Am Coll Cardiol.* 2005;46:582–588.

72. Hill R, Bagust A, Bakhai A, et al. Coronary artery stents: a rapid systematic review and economic evaluation. *Health Technol Assessment.* 2004;35. Available at: www.ncchta.org/execsumm/summ835.htm. Accessed September 20, 2005.

73. Hill RA, Dündar Y, Bakhai A, et al. Drug-eluting stents: an early systematic review to inform policy. *Eur Heart J.* 2004;25:902–919.

74. Dibra A, Kastrati A, Mehilli J, et al. Paclitaxel-eluting or sirolimus-eluting stents to prevent restenosis in diabetic patients. *N Engl J Med.* 2005;353:653–662.

75. Windecker S, Remondino A, Eberli FR, et al. Sirolimus-eluting and paclitaxel-eluting stents for coronary revascularization. *N Engl J Med.* 2005;353:663–670.

76. American Board of Internal Medicine. Policies for Added Qualifications in Interventional Cardiology: Eligibility for Certification and Board Policies. Available at: www.abim.org/cert/policiesaqic.shtm. Accessed August 27, 2005.

77. Kearney P. European Society of Cardiology (personal communication).

78. Rodevand O. The European cardiologist. *Circulation.* 1996;94:594–595.

79. Bashore TM, Bates ER, Berger PB, et al. American College of Cardiology/Society for Cardiac Angiography and Interventions clinical expert consensus document on cardiac catheterization laboratory standards: a report of the American College of Cardiology Task Force on Clinical Expert Consensus Document. *J Am Coll Cardiol.* 2001;37:2170–2214.

80. Hirschfeld JW Jr., Balter S, Brinker JA, et al. ADDF/AHA/HRS/SCAI clinical competence statement on physician knowledge to optimize patient safety and image quality in fluoroscopically guided invasive cardiovascular procedures. *J Am Coll Cardiol.* 2004;44:2259.

81. Smith SC, Dove JT, Jacobs AK, et al. ACC/AHA guidelines for percutaneous coronary intervention (Revision of the 1993 PTCA guidelines). *J Am Coll Cardiol.* 2001;37:2239–2300.

82. Silber S, Albertsson P, Aviles FF, et al. Guidelines for percutaneous coronary interventions. The Task Force for Percutaneous Coronary Interventions of the European Society of Cardiology. *Eur Heart J.* 2005;26:804–847.

83. ACC Clinical data standards—reference guide. American College of Cardiology key data elements and definitions for measuring the clinical management and outcome of patients with acute coronary syndromes. Available at: www.acc.org/clinical/data_standards/ACS/acs_index.htm. Accessed May 28, 2005.

84. ACC-National Cardiovascular Data Registry Cath Lab Module v3.04 Data Collection Form available at: www.accncdr.com/WebNCDR/NCDRDocuments/DataCollectionFormv30.pdf. Accessed May 28, 2005.

85. Roubin GS, King SB III, Douglas JS Jr. Restenosis after percutaneous transluminal coronary angioplasty: the Emory University Hospital experience. *Am J Cardiol.* 1987;60:39B-43B.

86. Umans VAWM, Strauss BH, Keane D, et al. Quantitative coronary angiography in interventional cardiology. In: Lanzer P, Rösch J, eds. *Vascular Diagnostics: Periinterventional Evaluations.* Berlin: Springer, 1994:277–293.

87. Anderson HV, Carabello BA. Provisional versus routine stenting. Routine stenting is there to stay. *Circulation.* 2000;102:2910–2914.

88. Wiesel J, Grunwald AM, Tobiasz C, et al. Quantitation of absolute area of a coronary arterial stenosis: experimental validation with a preparation in vivo. *Circulation.* 1986;74:1099–1106.

89. Alpert JS, Thygessen K, Antman E, et al. Myocardial infarction redefined—a consensus document of the Joint European Society of Cardiology/American College of Cardiology Committee for the redefinition of myocardial infarction. *J Am Coll Cardiol.* 2000;36:959–969.

90. French JK, White HD. Clinical implications of the new definition of myocardial infarction. *Heart.* 2004;90:99–106.

91. Herrmann J. Peri-procedural myocardial injury: 2005 update. *Eur Heart J.* 2005;26:2493–2519.

92. Zeymer U, Weber M, Zahn R, et al. Indications and complications of invasive diagnostic procedures and percutaneous interventions in the year 2003. *Z Kardiol.* 2005;94:392–398.

93. Cerqueira MD, Weismann NJ, Dilsizian V, et al. A statement for healthcare professionals from the Cardiac Imaging Committee of the Council on Clinical Cardiology of the American Heart Association, American Heart Association Writing Group on Myocardial Segmentation and Registration for Cardiac Imaging: Standardized myocardial segmentation and nomenclature for tomographic imaging of the heart. *Circulation.* 2002;105: 539–542.

94. Almany SL. Interventional strategies in patients with left ventricular dysfunction. In: Freed M, Grines C, Safian RD, eds. The New Manual of Interventional Cardiology. Birmingham: Physician's Press, 1997:157.

95. Califf RM, Bengtson JR. Cardiogenic shock. *N Engl J Med.* 1994;330:1724–1730.

96. Kantrowitz A, Tjouneland S, Freed PS, et al. Initial clinical experience with intraaortic balloon pumping. *JAMA.* 1968;203:113–118.

97. Peterson JC, Cook DJ. Systematic review: intra-aortic balloon counterpulsation pump therapy: a critical appraisal of the evidence for patients with acute myocardial infarction. *Crit Care.* 1998;2:3–8.

98. Ludwig K, von Segesser LK. Cardiopulmonary support and extracorporeal membrane oxygenation for cardiac assist. *Ann Thorac Surg.* 1999;68:672–677.

99. Jessup M. Mechanical cardiac-support devices—dreams and devilish details. *N Engl J Med.* 2001;345:1490–1493.

100. Lanzer P. Vascular multimorbidity in patients with a documented coronary artery disease. *Z Kardiol.* 2003;92:650–659.

101. Resnick HE, Howard BV. Diabetes and cardiovascular risk. *Ann Rev Med.* 2002;53:245–267.

102. Waller BF, Palumbo PJ, Lie JT, et al. Status of the coronary arteries at necropsy in diabetes mellitus with onset of age 30 years: analysis of 229 diabetic patients with and without clinical evidence of coronary heart disease and comparison to 183 control subjects. *Am J Med.* 1980;69:498–506.

103. Ledru F, Ducimetiere P, Battaglia S, et al. New diagnostic criteria for diabetes and coronary artery disease: insights from an angiographic study. *J Am Coll Cardiol.* 2001;37:1543–1550.

104. Goraya TY, Leibson CL, Palumbo PJ, et al. Coronary atherosclerosis in diabetes mellitus: a population based autopsy study. *J Am Coll Cardiol.* 2002;40:946–953.

105. Kip KE, Faxon DP, Detre KM, et al. Coronary angioplasty in diabetic patients: the National Heart, Lung and Blood Institute Percutaneous Transluminal Angioplasty Registry. *Circulation.* 1996;94:1818–1825.

106. Cutlip DE, Chauban MS, Baim DS, et al. Clinical restenosis after coronary stenting: perspectives from multicenter clinical trials. *J Am Coll Cardiol.* 2002;40:2082–2089.

107. Bypass Angioplasty Revascularization Investigation (BARI) Investigators. Comparison of coronary bypass surgery with angioplasty in patients with multivessel disease. *N Engl J Med.* 1996;335:217–225.

108. King SB, Kosinski AS, Guyton RA, et al., EAST Investigators. Eight-year mortality in the Emory Angioplasty versus Surgery Trial (EAST). *J Am Coll Cardiol.* 2000;35:1116–1121.

109. Sedlis SP, Morrison DA, Lorin JD, et al. Percutaneous coronary intervention versus coronary bypass graft surgery for diabetic patients with unstable angina and risk factors for adverse outcomes with bypass: outcome of diabetic patients in the AWESOME randomized trial and registry. *J Am Coll Cardiol.* 2002;40:1555–1566.

110. Abizaid A, Costa MA, Centemero M, et al. Clinical and economic impact of diabetes mellitus on percutaneous and surgical treatment of multivessel coronary disease patients: insights from the Arterial Revascularization Therapy Study (ARTS) trial. *Circulation.* 200;104:533–538.

111. Legrand VM, Serruys PW, Unger F, et al. Three-year outcome after coronary stenting versus bypass surgery for the treatment of multivessel disease. *Circulation.* 2004;109: 1114–1120.

112. Dibra A, Kastrati A, Mehili J, et al. Paclitaxel-eluting or sirolimus-eluting stents to prevent restenosis in diabetic patients. *N Engl J Med.* 2005;353:663–670.

113. King SB 3rd. Is surgery preferred for the diabetic with multivessel disease? Surgery is preferred for the diabetic with multivessel disease. *Circulation.* 2005;112:1500–1507.

114. Flaherty JD, Davidson CL. Diabetes and coronary revascularization. *JAMA.* 2005;293: 1501–1508.

115. Nesto RW. Correlation between cardiovascular disease and diabetes mellitus: current concepts. *Am J Med.* 2004;116(suppl 5A):11S-22S.

116. Creager MA, Lüscher TF, Cosentino F, et al. Diabetes and vascular disease: pathophysiology, clinical consequences, and medical therapy: part I. *Circulation.* 2003;108:1527–1532.

117. Lüscher TF, Creager MA. Diabetes and vascular disease: pathophysiology, clinical consequences, and medical therapy: part II. *Circulation.* 2003;108:1655–1661.

118. National Kidney Foundation—K/DOQL. Clinical practice guidelines for chronic kidney disease evaluation, classification and stratification. *Am J Kidney Dis.* 2002;39:S1–266.

119. Reusser L, Osborn L, White H, et al. Increased morbidity after coronary angioplasty in patients on chronic hemodialysis. *Am J Cardiol.* 1994;73:965–967.

120. Naidu SS, Selzer F, Jacobs A, et al. Renal insufficiency is an independent predictor of mortality after percutaneous coronary interventions. *Am J Cardiol.* 2003;92:1160–1164.

121. Anderson R, O'Brien M, Ma Whinney S, et al. Renal failure predisposes patients to adverse outcome after coronary artery bypass surgery. *Kidney Int.* 1999;55:1057–1062.

122. Rinehart AL, Herzog CA, Collins AJ, et al. A comparison of coronary angioplasty and coronary artery bypass grafting outcomes in chronic dialysis patients. *Am J Kidney Dis.* 1995;25:281–290.

123. Rubenstein MH, Harrell LC, Sheynberg BV, et al. Are patients with renal failure good candidates for percutaneous coronary revascularization in the new device era? *Circulation.* 2000;102:2966–2972.

124. Erentug V, Akinci E, Kirali K, et al. Complete off-pump coronary revascularization in patients with dialysis-dependent renal disease. *Tex Heart Inst J.* 2004;31:153–156.

125. Rihal CS, Textor SC, Grill DE, et al. Incidence and prognostic importance of acute renal failure after percutaneous coronary intervention. *Circulation.* 2002;105:2259–2264.

126. National Kidney Foundation. Clinical Practice Guidelines for Cardiovascular Disease in Dialysis Patients available at: http://www.kidney.org/professionals/KDOQI/guidelines_cvd/index.htm. Accessed June 7, 2006.

127. Gleeson TG, O'Dwyer J, Bulugahapitiya S, et al. Contrast-induced nephropathy. *Br J Cardiol.* 2004;11:53–61.

128. Kolonko A, Wiecek A. Contrast-associated nephropathy—old clinical problem, and new therapeutic perspectives. *Nephrol Dial Transplant.* 1998;13:803–806.

129. Marenzi G, Marana I, Lauri G, et al. The prevention of radiocontrast agent-induced nephropathy by hemofiltration. *N Engl J Med.* 2003;349:1333–1340.

130. Cockcroft DW, Gault MH. Prediction of creatinine clearance from serum creatinine. *Nephron.* 1976;16:31–41.
131. National Kidney Foundation. Clinical Practice Guidelines for Chronic Kidney Disease: Evaluation, Classification, and Stratification available at: http://www.kidney.org/professionals/KDOQI/guidelines_ckd/toc.htm. Accessed June 7, 2006.
132. Mintz GS, Pichard AD, Popma JJ, et al. Determinants and correlates of target lesion calcium in coronary artery disease: a clinical, angiographic and intravascular ultrasound study. *J Am Coll Cardiol.* 1997;29:268–274.
133. Schwarz U, Buzello M, Ritz E, et al. Morphology of coronary atherosclerotic lesions in patients with end-stage renal failure. *Nephrol Dial Transplant.* 2000;15:218–223.
134. Acland JD. The interpretation of the serum protein-bound iodine: a review. *J Clin Pathol.* 1971;24:187–218.
135. Polikar R, Burger AG, Scherrer U, et al. The thyroid and the heart. *Circulation.* 1993;87: 1435–1441.
136. Klein I, Ojamaa K Thyroid hormone and the cardiovascular system. *N Engl J Med.* 2001;344:501–509.
137. Siddiqui NH Contrast medium reactions, recognition and treatment. Available at: www.emedicine.com/radio/topic864.htm. Accessed June12, 2005.
138. Bettmann MA, Heeren T, Greenfield A, et al. Adverse events with radiographic contrast agents: results of the SCVIR Contrast Agent Registry. *Radiology.* 1997;203:611–620.
139. Bush WH, Swanson DP. Acute reactions to intravascular contrast media: types, risk factors, recognition, and specific treatment. *Am J Radiol.* 1991;157:1153–1161.
140. Morcos SK, Thomsen HS. Adverse reactions to iodinated contrast media. *Eur Radiol.* 2001;11:1267–1275.
141. Morcos WH. Acute serious and fatal reactions to contrast media: our current understanding. *Br J Radiol.* 2005;78:686–693.
142. Mock MB, Holmes DR Jr., Vliestra RE, et al. Percutaneous transluminal coronary angioplasty (PTCA) in the elderly patient: experience in the National Heart, Lung and Blood Institute PTCA Registry. *Am J Cardiol.* 1984;53:89C-91C.
143. Kelsey SF, Miller DP, Holubkov R, et al. Results of percutaneous transluminal coronary angioplasty in patients greater or equal to 65 years of age (from the 1985 to 1986 National Heart, Lung and Blood Institute's Coronary Angioplasty Registry). *Am J Cardiol.* 1990;66:1033–1038.
144. Graham MM, Ghali WA, Faris PD, et al. Survival after coronary revascularization in the elderly. *Circulation.* 2002;105:2378.
145. Guagliumi G. Stone GW, Cox DA, et al. Outcome in elderly patients undergoing primary coronary intervention for acute myocardial infarction: results from the controlled abciximab and device investigation to lower late angioplasty complications (CADILLAC) trial. *Circulation.* 2004;110:1598–1604.
146. Holmes DR Jr., White HD, Pieper KS, et al. Effect of age on outcome with primary angioplasty versus thrombolysis. *J Am Coll Cardiol.* 1999;33:412–419.
147. Cohen HA, Williams DO, Holmes DR Jr., et al. Impact of age on procedural and 1-year outcome in percutaneous transluminal coronary angioplasty: A report from the NHLBI dynamic registry. *Am Heart J.* 2003;146:513–519.
148. Lanzer P, Zuehlke H, Jehle P, et al. Cardiovascular multimorbidity, emerging coalescence of the integrated panvascular approach. *Z Kardiol.* 2004;93:259–265.
149. Lanzer P, Weser R, Prettin C. Carotid-artery stenting in a high-risk patient population: single centre, single operator results. *Clin Res Cardiol.* 2006;95:4–12.
150. Ryan TJ, Faxon DP, Gunnar RM, et al. Guidelines for percutaneous transluminal angioplasty. A report of the American College of Cardiology/American Heart Association Task Force on Assessment of Diagnostic and Therapeutic Cardiovascular Procedures (Subcommittee on Percutaneous Transluminal Coronary Angioplasty). *Circulation.* 1988;78:486–502.
151. Ellis SG, Vandormael MG, Cowley MJ, et al. Coronary morphologic and clinical determinants of procedural outcome with angioplasty for multivessel coronary disease. Implications for patient selection. *Circulation.* 1990;82:1193–1202.
152. Myler RK, Shaw C, Stertzer SH, et al. Lesion morphology and coronary angioplasty: current experience and analysis. *J Am Coll Cardiol.* 1992;19:1641–1652.
153. Tan K, Sulke N, Taub N, et al. Clinical and lesion morphological determinants of coronary angioplasty success and complications: current experience. *J Am Coll Cardiol.* 1995;25:855–865.
154. Krone RJ, Laskey WK, Johnson C, et al. for the Registry Committee of the Society for Cardiac Angiography and Interventions. A simplified lesion classification for predicting success and complications of coronary angioplasty. *Am J Cardiol.* 2000;85:1179–1184.
155. Mabin TA, Holmes DR Jr., Smith HC, et al. Intracoronary thrombus: role in coronary occlusion complicating percutaneous transluminal coronary angioplasty. *J Am Coll Cardiol.* 1985;5:198–202.
156. Reeder GC, Bryant SC, Suman VJ, et al. Intracoronary thrombus: still a risk factor for PTCA failure? *Cathet Cardiovasc Diagn.* 1995;34:191–195.
157. Khan MM, Ellis SG, Aguirre FV, et al. Does intracoronary thrombus influence the outcome of high risk percutaneous transluminal coronary angioplasty? Clinical and angiographic outcomes in a large multicenter trial. *J Am Coll Cardiol.* 1998;31:31–36.
158. Topol EJ, Yadav JS. Recognition of the importance of embolization in atherosclerotic vascular disease. *Circulation.* 2000;101:570–580.
159. White CJ, Ramee SR, Collins TJ, et al. Coronary thrombi increase PTCA risk: angioscopy as a clinical tool. *Circulation.* 1996;93:253–258.
160. den Heijer P, Foley DP, Escaned J, et al. Angioscopic versus angiographic detection of intimal dissection and intracoronary thrombus. *J Am Coll Cardiol.* 1994;24:649–654.
161. Tierstein PC, Schatz RA, DeNardo SJ, et al. Angioscopic versus angiographic detection of thrombus during coronary interventional procedures. *Am J Cardiol.* 1995;75: 1083–1087.
162. Stary HC. Natural history of calcium deposits in atherosclerosis progression and regression. *Z Kardiol.* 2000;89(suppl 2):II28-II35.
163. Epple M, Lanzer P. How much interdisciplinarity is required to understand vascular calcifications? Formulation of four basic principles of vascular calcification. *Z Kardiol.* 2001;90 (Suppl 3):III2-III5.
164. Mintz GS, Popma JJ, Pichard AD, et al. Patterns of calcification in coronary artery disease: a statistical analysis of intravascular ultrasound and coronary angiography in 1155 lesions. *Circulation.* 1995,91:1959–1965.
165. Kamm K-F, Onnasch DGW. X-ray angiography. In: Lanzer P, Lipton M, eds. *Diagnostics of Vascular Diseases: Principles of Technology.* Berlin: Springer Verlag, 1997:63–98.
166. Burke AP, Taylor A, Farb A, et al. Coronary calcification: insights from sudden coronary death victims. *Z Kardiol.* 2000;89(suppl 2):II49-II53.
167. Huang H, Virmani R, Younis H, et al. The impact of calcification on the biomechanical stability of atherosclerotic plaques. *Circulation.* 2001;103:1051–1056.
168. Ellis SG, Gallison L, Grines CL, et al. Incidence and predictors of early recurrent ischemia after successful percutaneous transluminal coronary angioplasty for acute myocardial infarction. *Am J Cardiol.* 1989;63:263–268.
169. Myler RK, Schaw RE, Stertzer SH, et al. Lesion morphology and coronary angioplasty: current experience and analysis. *J Am Coll Cardiol.* 1992;19:1641–1652.
170. Fitzgerald PJ, Ports TA, Yock PG. Contribution of localized calcium deposits to dissection after angioplasty. An observational study using intravascular ultrasound. *Circulation.* 1992;86:64–70.
171. Fourrier JL, Stankowiak C, Lablanche JM, et al. Histopathology after rotational angioplasty of peripheral arteries in human beings. *J Am Coll Cardiol.* 1988;11:109A.
172. Mintz GS, Potkin BN, Keren G, et al. Intravascular ultrasound evaluation of the effect of rotational atherectomy in obstructive atherosclerotic coronary artery disease. *Circulation.* 1992;86:1383–1393.
173. Lafont A, Topol EJ, eds. *Arterial Remodelling: A Critical Factor in Restenosis.* New York: Springer, 1997.
174. Mintz GS, Popma JJ, Pichard AD, et al. Limitations of angiography in the assessment of plaque distribution in coronary artery disease a systematic study of target lesion eccentricity in 1446 lesions. *Circulation.* 1996;93:924–931.
175. Tuzcu EM, DeFranco AC, Goormastic M, et al. Dichotomous pattern of coronary atherosclerosis 1 to 9 years after transplantation: insights from systematic intravascular ultrasound imaging. *J Am Coll Cardiol.* 1996;27:839–846.
176. Nissen SE, Yock P. Intravascular ultrasound novel pathophysiological insights and current clinical applications. *Circulation.* 2001;103:604–616.
177. Topol EJ, Leya F, Pinkerton CA, et al. A comparison of atherectomy with coronary angioplasty in patients with coronary artery disease. *N Engl J Med.* 1993;329:221–227.
178. Adelman AG, Cohen EA, Kimball BP, et al. A comparison of directional atherectomy with balloon angioplasty for lesions of the left anterior descending artery. *N Engl J Med.* 1993;329:228–233.
179. Simonton CA, Leon MB, Baim DS, et al. 'Optimal' directional coronary atherectomy: final results of the Optimal Atherectomy Restenosis Study (OARS). *Circulation.* 1998;97:332–339.
180. Seldinger SI. Catheter replacement of the needle in percutaneous arteriography. *Acta Radiol [Diagn] (Stockh).* 1953;39:368–376.
181. Sones FM. Cine coronary arteriography. *Mod Conc Cardiovasc Dis.* 1962;31:735–738.
182. Judkins MP. Selective coronary arteriography. Part I: A percutaneous transfemoral technic. *Radiology.* 1967;89:815–824.
183. Amplatz K, Formanek G, Stanger P, et al. Mechanics of selective coronary artery catheterization via femoral approach. *Radiology.* 1967;89:1040–1047.
184. Grüntzig A, Senning A, Siegenthaler WE. Nonoperative dilatation of coronary-artery stenosis. *N Engl J Med.* 1979;301:61–68.
185. Saffitz JE, Rose TE, Oaks JB, et al. Coronary artery rupture during angioplasty. *Am J Cardiol.* 1983;51:902–906.
186. Roubin GS, Douglas JS Jr., King SB, et al. Influence of balloon size on initial success, acute complications, and restenosis after percutaneous transluminal angioplasty: a prospective randomized study. *Circulation.* 1988;78:557–565.
187. Nichols AB, Smith R, Berke AD, et al. Importance of balloon size in coronary angioplasty. *J Am Coll Cardiol.* 1989;13:1094–1100.
188. Rensing BJ, Hermans WRM, Deckers JP, et al. Lumen narrowing after percutaneous transluminal coronary balloon angioplasty follows a near Gaussian distribution: a quantitative angiographic study of 1,445 successfully dilated lesions. *J Am Coll Cardiol.* 1992;19:939–945.
189. Beatt KV, Serruys PW, Luijten HE, et al. Restenosis after coronary angioplasty: the paradox of increased lumen diameter and restenosis. *J Am Coll Cardiol.* 1992;19:258–266.
190. Kuntz RE, Gibson CM, Nobuyoshi M, et al. Generalized model of restenosis after conventional balloon angioplasty, stenting and directional atherectomy. *J Am Coll Cardiol.* 1993;21:15–25.
191. Fischman DL, Leon MB, Baim DS, et al. for the Stent Restenosis Study Investigators. A randomized comparison of coronary-stent placement and balloon angioplasty in the treatment of coronary artery disease. *N Engl J Med.* 1994;331:496–501.
192. Serruys PW de Jaegere P, Kiemeneij F, et al. for the BENETEST Study Group. A comparison of balloon-expandable-stent implantation with balloon angioplasty in patients with coronary artery disease. *N Engl J Med.* 1994;331:489–495.
193. Haase KK, Athanasiadis A, Marholdt H, et al. Acute and 1-year follow-up results after vessel size adopted PTCA using intracoronary ultrasound. *Eur Heart J.* 1998;19:263–272.
194. Stone GW, Hodgson JM, St Goar FG, et al. Improved procedural results of coronary angioplasty with intravascular ultrasound-guided balloon sizing: the CLOUT pilot trial. *Circulation.* 1997;95:2044–2052.
195. de Jaegere P, Mudra H, Figulla H, et al. Intravascular ultrasound-guided optimized stent deployment. Immediate and six months clinical and angiographic results form the Multicentric Ultrasound Stenting in Coronaries Study (MUSIC Study). *Eur Heart J.* 1998;19:1214–1223.
196. Frey AW, Hodgson JM, Müller C, et al. Ultrasound-guided strategy for provisional stenting with focal balloon combination catheter: results from the randomized strategy for intracoronary ultrasound-guided PTCA and stenting (SIPS) trial. *Circulation.* 2000;102:2497–2502.
197. Fitzgerald PJ, Oshima A, Hayase M, et al. Final results of the Can Routine Ultrasound Influence Stent Expansion (CRUISE). *Circulation.* 2000;102:523–530.
198. Mudra H, di Mario C, de Jaegere P, et al. Randomized comparison of coronary stent implantation under ultrasound or angiographic guidance to reduce stent restenosis (OPTICUS Study). *Circulation.* 2001;104:1343–1352.

199. Sones FM. Cine coronary arteriography. *Mod Conc Cardiovasc Dis.* 1962;31:735–738.

200. Judkins MP. Selective coronary arteriography. Part I: A percutaneous transfemoral technic. *Radiology.* 1967;89:815–824.

201. Campeau L. Percutaneous radial artery approach for coronary angiography. *Cathet Cardiovasc Diagn.* 1989;16:3–7.

202. Kiemeneij F, Laarman GJ. Percutaneous transradial artery approach for coronary stent implantation. *Cathet Cardiovasc Diagn.* 1993;30:173–178.

203. Kiemeneij F, Laarman GJ, Odekerken D, et al. A randomized comparison of percutaneous transluminal angioplasty by radial, brachial and femoral approaches: the access study. *J Am Coll Cardiol.* 1997;29:1269–1275.

204. Johnson LW, Esenta P, Giambartolomei A, et al. Peripheral vascular complications of coronary angioplasty by the femoral and brachial techniques. *Cathet Cardiovasc Diagn.* 1994;31:165–172.

205. Safian RD, Freed M. Coronary intervention: preparation, equipment and technique. In: Freed M, Grines C, Safian RD, eds. *The New Manual of Interventional Cardiology.* Birmingham: Physician's Press, 1997:1–63.

206. Yakubov SJ, George BS. Brachial and radial approach to coronary intervention. In: Freed M, Grines C, Safian RD, eds. *The New Manual of Interventional Cardiology.* Birmingham: Physician's Press, 1997:65–73.

207. Serruys PW, Colombo A, Leon MB, et al., eds. *Coronary Lesions: A Pragmatic Approach.* London: Marin Dunitz, 2002.

208. Lincoff AM, ed. *Platelet Glycoprotein IIb/IIIa Inhibitors in Cardiovascular Disease.* Totowa, NJ: Humana Press, 2003.

209. Serruys PW, Strauss BH, Beatt KJ, et al. Angiographic follow-up after placement of a self-expanding coronary artery stent. *N Engl J Med.* 1991;324:13–17.

210. Roubin GS, Cannon AD, Agrawal SK, et al. Intracoronary stenting for acute and threatened closure complicating PTCA. *Circulation.* 1992;85:916–927.

211. Eeckhout W, Wijns W, Meier B, et al. Indications for intracoronary stent placement: the European view. *Eur Heart J.* 1999;20:1014–1019.

212. Anderson HV, Carabello BA. Provisional versus routine stenting. Routine stenting is here to stay. *Eur Heart J.* 2000;102:2910–2914.

213. Rodriquez A, Ayala F, Bernardi V, et al. Optimal coronary balloon angioplasty with provisional stenting versus primary stent (OCBAS): immediate and long term results. *J Am Coll Cardiol.* 1998:82.1351–1357.

214. Bech GJ, Pijls NH, de Bruyne B, et al. Usefulness of fractional flow reserve to predict clinical outcome after balloon angioplasty. *Circulation.* 1999;99:883–888.

215. Serruys PW, de Bruyne B, Carlier S, et al. Randomized comparison of primary stenting and provisional balloon angioplasty guided by flow velocity measurement. *Circulation.* 2000;102:2930–2937.

216. Colombo A, Hall P, Nakamura S, et al. Intracoronary stenting without anticoagulation accomplished with intravascular ultrasound guidance. *Circulation.* 1995;91:1676–1688.

217. Nakamura S, Hall P, Gaglione A el al. High pressure assisted coronary stent implantation accomplished without intravascular ultrasound guidance and subsequent anticoagulation. *J Am Coll Cardiol.* 1997;29:21–27.

218. de Jaegere P, Mudra H, Figulla H, et al. Intravascular ultrasound-guided optimized stent deployment. Immediate and six months clinical and angiographic results form the Multicentric Ultrasound Stenting in Coronaries Study (MUSIC Study). *Eur Heart J.* 1998;19:1214–1223.

219. Dirschinger J, Kastrati A, Neumann F-J, et al. Influence of balloon pressure during stent placement in native coronary arteries on early and late angiographic and clinical outcome: a randomized evaluation of high-pressure inflation. *Circulation.* 1999;100:918–923.

220. Mudra H, di Mario C, de Jaegere P, et al. Randomized comparison of coronary stent implantation under ultrasound or angiographic guidance to reduce stent restenosis (OPTICUS Study). *Circulation.* 2001;104:1343–1352.

221. Berry E, Kelly S, Hutton J, et al. Intravascular ultrasound-guided interventions in coronary artery disease: a systematic literature review, with decision-analytic modelling, of outcomes and cost-effectiveness. Health Technology Assessment NHS R&D HTA Programme. Available at: www.hta.nhsweb.nhs.uk/fullmono/mon435.pdf. Accessed December 15, 2005.

222. Figulla HR, Mudra H, Reifart N, et al. Direct coronary stenting without predilatation: a new therapeutic approach with a special balloon catheter design. *Cathet Cardiovasc Diagn.* 1998;43:245–252.

223. Herz I, Assali A, Solodoky A, et al. Coronary stenting without predilatation (SWOP): applicable technique in everyday practice. *Cathet Cardiovasc Intervent.* 2000;49:384–388.

224. Martinez-Elbal L, Ruiz-Nodar JM, Zueco J, et al. for the DISCO investigators. Direct coronary stenting versus stenting with balloon pre-dilatation: immediate and follow-up results of a multicentre, prospective, randomized study. The DISCO trial. *Eur Heart J.* 2002;23:633–640.

225. Brito FS Jr., Caixeta AM, Perin MA, et al. on behalf of the DIRECT Study Investigators. Comparison of direct stenting versus stenting with predilatation for the treatment of selected coronary narrowings. *Am J Cardiol.* 2002;89:115–120.

226. Antoniucci D, Valenti R, Migliorini A, et al. Direct infarct artery stenting without predilation and no-reflow in patients with acute myocardial infarction. *Am Heart J.* 2001;142:684–690.

227. Vecchia LL, Vincenzi P, Favero L, et al. Frequency and determinants of direct stenting in routine percutaneous coronary interventions: data on 835 consecutive procedures in a single center. *Ital Heart J.* 2004;5.749–754.

228. Bull BS, Huse WM, Bauer FS, et al. Heparin therapy during extracorporeal circulation. The use of dose-response curve to individualize heparin and protamin dosage. *J Thorac Cardiovasc Surg.* 1975;69:685–689.

229. Rath B, Bennett DH. Monitoring the effect of heparin by measurement of activated clotting time during and after percutaneous transluminal coronary angioplasty. *Br Heart J.* 1990;63:18–21.

230. Dougherty KG, Gaos CM, Bush HS, et al. Activated clotting times and activated partial thromboplastin times in patients undergoing coronary angioplasty who receive bolus doses of heparin. *Cathet Cardiovasc Diagn.* 1992;26:260–263.

231. Fergusson JJ, Dougherty KG, Gaos CM, et al. Relation between procedural ACT and outcome after PTCA. *J Am Coll Cardiol.* 1994;23:1061–1065.

232. O'Donnell M, Turpie AGG. Low-molecular-weight heparin in acute coronary syndromes. *Heart Drug.* 2004;4:111–118.

233. de Areneza DP, Flather MD, Shibata MC, et al. Systematic review of hirudin in acute coronary syndromes and percutaneous coronary interventions. *Curr Intervent Cardiol Rep.* 2001;3:156–162.

234. Mahaffey KW, Cohen M, Garg J, et al. High-risk patients with acute coronary syndromes treated with low-molecular-weight of unfractionated heparin. *JAMA.* 2005;294:2594–2600.

235. Popma JJ, Berger P, Ohman EM, et al. Antithrombotic therapy during percutaneous coronary intervention. The Seventh ACCP Conference on Antithrombotic and Thrombolytic Therapy. *Chest.* 2004;126:576S-599S.

236. Willerson JT, Campbell WB, Winniford MD, et al. Conversion from chronic to acute coronary artery disease: speculation regarding mechanisms. *J Allergy Clin Immunol.* 1984;54:1349–1354.

237. Harker LA. Role of platelets and thrombosis in mechanisms of acute occlusion and restenosis after angioplasty. *Am J Cardiol.* 1987;60(suppl):20B-28B.

238. Topol EJ. Toward a new frontier in myocardial reperfusion therapy: emerging platelet prominence. *Circulation.* 1998;97:211–218.

239. Craven LL. Experiences with aspirin (acetylsalicylic acid) in the non-specific prophylaxis of coronary thrombosis. *Miss Val Med J.* 1953;75:38–44.

240. Ross R, Glomset JA. The pathogenesis of atherosclerosis, part I and II. *N Engl J Med.* 1976;295:369–377, 420–425.

241. Davies MK, Thomas AC. Plaque fissuring: the cause of acute myocardial infarction, sudden ischemic death, and crescendo angina. *Br Heart J.* 1985;53:363–373.

242. Falk E Why do plaques rupture? *Circulation.* 1992;86(suppl III):III30-III42.

243. Virmani R, Kolodgie RD, Burke AP, et al. Lessons from sudden coronary death: a comprehensive morphological classification scheme for atherosclerotic lesions. *Arterioscler Thromb Vasc Biol.* 2000;20:1262–1275.

244. Awtry EH, Loscalzo J. Aspirin. *Circulation.* 2000;101:1206–1218.

245. Gawaz M, Neumann F-J, Ott I, et al. Platelet activation and coronary stent implantation. *Circulation.* 1996;94:279–285.

246. Quinn MJ, Fitzgerald DJ. Ticlopidine and clopidogrel. *Circulation.* 1999;100:1667–1672.

247. Mason PJ, Jacobs AK, Freedman JE. Aspirin, resistance and antithrombotic disease. *J Am Coll Cardiol.* 2005;46:986–993.

248. Wiviott SD, Antman EM. Clopidogrel resistance. A new chapter in a fast-moving story. *Circulation.* 2004;109:3064–3067.

249. Burzotta F, Romagnoli E, Trani C, et al. Intracoronary administration of abciximab acutely increases flow through culprit vessels of patients with acute coronary syndromes undergoing percutaneous coronary intervention. *Circulation.* 2003;108:e138.

250. Lee S-W, Park S-W, Hong M-K, et al. Triple versus dual antiplatelet therapy after coronary stenting. *J Am Coll Cardiol.* 2005;46:1833–1837.

251. Levy JH. *Anaphylactic Reactions in Anaesthesia and Intensive Care.* New York: Butterworth-Heinemann, 1992.

252. Gammie JS, Zenati M, Kormos RL, et al. Abciximab and excessive bleeding in patients undergoing emergency cardiac operations. *Ann Thorac Surg.* 1998;65.465–469

253. Lemmer JH, Metzdorff MT, Krause AH, et al. Emergency coronary artery bypass surgery in abciximab treated patients. Ann Thorac Surg. 2000;69:90–95.

254. Koreny M, Riedmüller E, Nikfardjam M, et al. Arterial puncture closing devices compared with standard manual compression after cardiac catheterization systematic review and meta-analysis. *JAMA.* 2004;291:350–357.

255. Slaboom T, Kiemeneij F, Laarman GJ, et al. Outpatient coronary angioplasty: feasible and safe. *Cathet Cardiovasc Intervent.* 2005;64:421–427.

256. Black AJR, Anderson HV, Ellis SG. *Complications of Coronary Angioplasty.* New York: Marcel Dekker, 1991.

257. Shook TL, Sun GW, Burstein S, et al. Comparison of percutaneous transluminal coronary angioplasty outcome and hospital costs for low-volume and high-volume operators. *Am J Cardiol.* 1996;77(5):331–336.

258. Ellis SG, Weintraub W, Holmes D, et al. Relation of operator volume and experience to procedural outcome of percutaneous coronary revascularization at hospitals with high interventional volumes. *Circulation.* 1997;95:2479–2484.

259. Harjai KJ, Berman AD, Grines CL, et al. Impact of interventionalist volume, experience, and board certification on coronary angioplasty outcomes in the era of stenting. *Am J Cardiol.* 2004;94:421–426.

260. Abdelmeguid AE, Topol EJ. The myth of the myocardial "infarctlet" during percutaneous coronary revascularization procedures. *Circulation.* 1996;94:3369–3375.

261. Abdelmeguid AE, Topol EJ, Whitlow PL, et al. Significance of mild transient release of creatine kinase-MB fraction after percutaneous coronary interventions. *Circulation.* 1996;94:1528–1536.

262. Ellis SG, Chew D, Chan A, et al. Death following creatine kinase-MB elevation after coronary intervention: identification of an early risk period: importance of creatine kinase-MB level, completeness of revascularization, ventricular function, and probable benefit of statin therapy. *Circulation.* 2002;106:1205–1211.

263. Kini A, Marmur JD, Kini S. Creatine kinase-MB elevation after coronary intervention correlates with diffuse atherosclerosis, and low-to-medium elevation has a benign clinical course: implications for the early discharge after coronary intervention. *J Am Coll Cardiol.* 1999;34:663–671.

264. Fink MP, Abraham E, Vincent J-L, et al., eds. *Textbook of Critical Care.* 5th ed. Philadelphia: WB Saunders, 2005.

265. Vlodaver Z, Edwards JE. Pathology of coronary atherosclerosis. *Prog Cardiovasc Dis.* 1971;14:256–274.
266. Waller BF. The eccentric coronary atherosclerotic plaque: morphologic observations and clinical relevance. *Clin Cardiol.* 1989;12:14–20.
267. Mintz GS, Popma JJ, Pichard AD, et al. Limitations of angiography in the assessment of plaque distribution in coronary artery disease. *Circulation.* 1996;93:924–931.
268. Myler RK, Shaw RE, Stertzer SH, et al. Lesion morphology and coronary angioplasty: current experience and analysis. *J Am Coll Cardiol.* 1992;19:1641–1652.
269. Ellis SG, Vandormael MG, Cowley MJ, et al. Coronary morphologic and clinical determinants of procedural outcome with angioplasty for multivessel coronary disease: implications for patient selection. *Circulation.* 1990;82:1193–1202.
270. Uretsky BF, Denys BG, Counihan PC, et al Angioscopic evaluation of incompletely obstructing coronary intraluminal filling defects: comparison to angiography. *Cathet Cardiovasc Diagn.* 1994;33(4):323–329.
271. Waxman S, Sassower MA, Mittelman MA, et al. Angioscopic predictors of early adverse outcome after coronary angioplasty in patients with unstable angina and non-q-wave myocardial infarction. *Circulation.* 1996;93:2106–2113.
272. Waller BF. "Crackers, breakers, stretchers, drillers, scrapers, shavers, burners, welders, and melters": the future treatment of atherosclerotic coronary artery disease. A clinical-morphological assessment. *J Am Coll Cardiol.* 1989;13:969–987.
273. Mintz GS, Pichard AD, Kent KM, et al. Axial plaque redistribution as a mechanism of percutaneous transluminal coronary angioplasty. *Am J Cardiol.* 1996;77:427–430.
274. Ahmed JM, Mintz GS, Weissman NJ, et al. Mechanism of lumen enlargement during intracoronary stent implantation: an intravascular ultrasound study. *Circulation.* 2000;102:7–10.
275. Buja LM, Willerson JT, Murphree SS. Pathobiology of arterial wall injury, atherosclerosis, and coronary angioplasty. In: Black AJR, Anderson HV, Ellis SG, eds. *Complications of Coronary Angioplasty.* New York: Marcel Dekker, 1991:11–34.
276. Leimgruber PP, Roubin GS, Anderson HV, et al. Influence of intimal dissection on restenosis after successful angioplasty. *Circulation.* 1985;72:530–535.
277. TAUSA Investigators, Ambrose JA, Almeida OD, Sharma SK, et al. Angiographic evolution of intracoronary thrombus and dissection following percutaneous transluminal coronary angioplasty (The Thrombolysis and Angioplasty in Unstable Angina [TAUSA] trial). *Am J Cardiol.* 1997;79:559–563.
278. Peters JRG, Kok WEM, Di Carlo C, et al. Prediction of restenosis after coronary balloon angioplasty: results of PICTURE (Post-IntraCoronary Treatment Ultrasound Result Evaluation), a prospective multicenter Intracoronary ultrasound imaging study. *Circulation.* 1997;95:2254–2261.
279. Sheris SJ, Canos MR, Weissman NJ. Natural history of intravascular ultrasound-detected edge dissections from coronary stent deployment. *Am Heart J.* 2000;139:59–63.
280. Sharma SK, Israel DH, Kamean JL, et al. Clinical, angiographic, and procedural determinants of major and minor coronary dissection during angioplasty. *Am Heart J.* 1993;126:39–47.
281. Hermans WR, Rensing BJ, Foley DP, et al. Therapeutic dissection after successful coronary balloon angioplasty: no influence on restenosis or on clinical outcome in 693 patients. The MERCATOR Study Group. *J Am Coll Cardiol.* 1992;20:767–780.
282. Lincoff AM, Popma JJ, Ellis SG, et al. Abrupt vessel closure complicating coronary angioplasty: clinical, angiographic and therapeutic profile. *J Am Coll Cardiol.* 1992;19:926–935.
283. Koul AK, Hollander G, Moskovits N, et al. Coronary artery dissections during pregnancy and the postpartum period: two case report and review. *Cathet Cardiovasc Intervent.* 2001;52:88–94.
284. Cowley MJ, Dorros G, Kelseay SF, et al. Acute coronary events associated with percutaneous transluminal coronary angioplasty. *Am J Cardiol.* 1984;53:12C.
285. Mintz GS, Nissen SE, Anderson WD, et al. American College of Cardiology Clinical Expert Consensus Document on standards for acquisition, measurement and reporting on intravascular ultrasound studies (IVUS). *J Am Coll Cardiol.* 2001;37:1480–1492.
286. Almeda FQ, Barkatullah S, Kavinsky CJ. Spontaneous coronary artery dissection. *Clin Cardiol.* 2004;27:377–380.
287. Bulkey BH, Roberts WE. Dissecting aneurysm (hematoma) limited to coronary artery. A clinicopathologic study of six patients. *Am J Med.* 1973;55:747–756.
288. Sage MD, Koelmeyer TD, Smeeton WM. Fatal postpartum coronary artery dissection. A light—and electron—microscope study. *Am J Forens Med Pathol.* 1986;7:107–111.
289. Gunning MG, Williams IL, Jewitt DE, et al. Coronary artery perforation during percutaneous intervention: incidence and outcome. *Heart.* 2002;88:495–498.
290. Ellis SG, Ajluni S, Arnold SZ, et al. Increased coronary perforation in the new device era. Incidence, classification, management, and outcome. *Circulation.* 1994;90:2725–2302.
291. Ajluni SC, Glazier S, Blankenship L, et al. Perforations after percutaneous coronary interventions: clinical, angiographic, and therapeutic observations. *Cathet Cardiovasc Diagn.* 1994;32:206–223.
292. Gruberg L, Pinnow E, Flood R, et al. Incidence, management, and outcome of coronary artery perforation during percutaneous coronary intervention. *Am J Cardiol.* 2000;86: 680–682.
293. Stankovic G, Orlic D, Corvaja N, et al. Incidence, predictors, in-hospital, and late outcomes of coronary artery perforations. *Am J Cardiol.* 2004;93(2):213–216.
294. Witzke CF, Martin-Herrero F, Clarke SC, et al. The Changing Pattern of Coronary Perforation During Percutaneous Coronary Intervention in the New Device Era. *J Invasive Cardiol.* 2004;16:297–301.
295. Dippel EJ, Kereiakes DJ, Tramuta DA, et al. Coronary perforation during percutaneous coronary intervention in the era of abciximab platelet glycoprotein IIb/IIIa blockade: an algorithm for percutaneous management. *Cathet Cardiovasc Intervent.* 2001;52: 279–286.
296. Rogers JH, Lasala JM. Coronary artery dissection and perforation complicating percutaneous coronary intervention. *J Invasive Cardiol.* 2004;16:493–499.
297. Kloner RA, Jennings RB. Consequences of brief ischemia: stunning, preconditioning, and their clinical implications. Part 1. *Circulation.* 2001;104:2981–2989.
298. Kloner RA, Jennings RB. Consequences of brief ischemia: stunning, preconditioning, and their clinical implications. Part 2. *Circulation.* 2001;104.3158–167.
299. Kloner RA, Bolli R, Marban E, et al. Medical and cellular implications of stunning, hibernation and preconditioning. *Circulation.* 1998;97:1848–1867.
300. Ellis SG, Roubin GS, King SB III, et al. Angiographic and clinical predictors of acute closure after native vessel coronary angioplasty. *Circulation.* 1988;77:372–379.
301. Balcon R, Beyar R, Chierchia S, et al. Recommendations on stent manufacture, implantation and utilization. *Eur Heart J.* 1997;18:1536–1547.
302. Wöhrle J, Grebe OC, Nusser T, et al. Reduction of major adverse cardiac events with intracoronary compared with intravenous bolus application of abciximab in patients with acute myocardial infarction or unstable angina undergoing coronary angioplasty. *Circulation.* 2001;107: 1840–1843.
303. Kloner RA, Ganote CE, Jennings RB. The "no-reflow" phenomenon after temporary coronary occlusion in the dog. *J Clin Invest.* 1974;54:1496–1508.
304. Krug A, de Rochemont WM, Korb G. Blood supply of the myocardium after temporary coronary occlusion. *Circ Res.* 1966;19:57–62.
305. Schofer J, Montz R, Matthey D. Scintigraphic evidence of the "no-reflow" phenomenon in human beings after coronary thrombolysis. *J Am Coll Cardiol.* 1985;5:593–598.
306. Wilson RF, Laxson DD, Lesser JR, White CW. Intense microvascular constriction after angioplasty of acute thrombotic coronary artery lesions. *Lancet.* 1989;i:807–811.
307. Piana RN, Paik GY, Moscucci M, et al. Incidence and treatment of "no-reflow" after percutaneous coronary intervention. *Circulation.* 1994,89:2514–518.
308. Williams MS, Coller BS, Vaananen HJ, et al. Activation of platelets in platelet-rich plasma by rotablation is speed-dependent and can be inhibited by abciximab (c7E3 Fab; ReoPro). *Circulation.* 1998;98:742–748.
309. Rezkalla SH, Kloner RA. No-reflow phenomenon. *Circulation.* 2002;105:656–662.
310. Eeckhout E, Kern MJ. The coronary no-reflow phenomenon: a review of mechanisms and therapies. *Eur Heart J. 2001*;22:729–739.
311. Pomerantz RM, Kuntz RE, Diver DJ, et al. Intracoronary verapamil for the treatment of distal microvascular coronary artery spasm following PTCA. *Cathet Cardiovasc Diagn.* 1991;24:283–285.
312. Ishihara M, Sato H, Tateishi H, et al. Attenuation of the no-reflow phenomenon after coronary angioplasty for acute myocardial infarction with intracoronary papaverine. *Am Heart J.* 1996;132:959–963.
313. Fischell TA, Carter AJ, Foster MT, et al. Reversal of no-reflow during vein graft stenting using high velocity boluses of intracoronary adenosine. *Cathet Cardiovasc Diagn.* 1998;45.360–365.
314. Assali AR, Sdringola S, Ghani M, et al. Intracoronary adenosine administered during percutaneous intervention in acute myocardial infarction and reduction in the incidence of no-reflow phenomenon. *Cathet Cardiovasc Intervent.* 2000;51:27–31.
315. Parham WA, Bouhasin A, Ciaramita JP, et al. Coronary hyperaemic dose responses of intracoronary sodium nitroprusside. *Circulation.* 2004;109:1236–1243.
316. Rawitscher D, Levin DN, Cohen I, et al. Rapid reversal of no-reflow using abciximab after coronary device intervention. *Cathet Cardiovasc Diagn.* 1997,42:187–190.
317. Meier B, Grüntzig AR, King SB III, et al. Risk of side branch occlusion during coronary angioplasty. *Am J Cardiol.* 1984;53:10–14.
318. Boxt LM, Meyerovitz MF, Taus RH, et al. Side branch occlusion complicating percutaneous transluminal angioplasty. *Radiology.* 1986,161:681–683.
319. Arora RR, Raymond RE, Dimas AP, et al. Side branch occlusion during coronary angioplasty: incidence, angiographic characteristics, and outcome. *Cathet Cardiovasc Diagn.* 1989;18:210–212.
320. Urban P, Macaya C, Rupprecht HJ, et al. Randomized evaluation of anticoagulation versus antiplatelet therapy after coronary stent implantation in high-risk patients: multicenter aspirin and ticlodipine trial after intracoronary stenting (MATTIS). *Circulation.* 1998;98:2126–2132.
321. Colombo A, Hall P, Nakamura S, et al. Intracoronary stenting without anticoagulation accomplished with intravascular ultrasound guidance. *Circulation.* 1995;91:1676–1688.
322. Nakamura S, Hall P, Gaglione A el al. High pressure assisted coronary stent implantation accomplished without intravascular ultrasound guidance and subsequent anticoagulation. *J Am Coll Cardiol.* 1997;29:21–27.
323. Campbell R, Edelman ER. Endovascular stent design dictates experimental restenosis and thrombosis. *Circulation.* 1995;91:2995–3001.
324. Honda Y, Fitzgerald PJ. Stent thrombosis: an issue revisited in a changing world. *Circulation.* 2003;108:2–5.
325. Gurbel PA, Bliden KP, Guyer K, et al. Platelet reactivity in patients with recurrent events pos-stenting: Results of the PREPARE POST-STENTING study. *J Am Coll Cardiol.* 2005;46:1820–1826.
326. Cheneau E. Leborgne L, Mintz GS, et al. Predictors of subacute stent thrombosis: results of a systemic intravascular ultrasound study. *Circulation.* 2003;108:43–47.
327. Cutlip DE, Baim DS, Ho KK, et al. Stent thrombosis in the modern era: a pooled analysis of multicenter coronary stent clinical trials. *Circulation.* 2001;103:1967–1971.
328. Orford JL, Lennon R, Melby S, et al. Frequency and correlation of coronary stent thrombosis in the modern era: analysis of a single center registry. *J Am Coll Cardiol.* 2002;40:1567–1572.
329. Kastrati A, Koch W, Gawaz M, et al. PIA polymorphism of glycoprotein IIIa and risk of adverse events after coronary stent placement. *J Am Coll Cardiol.* 2000;36:84–89.
330. Gurbel PA, Bliden KP, Hiatt BL, et al. Clopidogrel for coronary stenting: response variability, drug resistance, and the effect of pretreatment platelet reactivity. *Circulation.* 2003;107:2908–2913.
331. Farb A, Burke AP, Kolodgie FD, et al. Pathological mechanisms of fatal late coronary thrombosis in humans. *Circulation.* 2003;108:1701–1706.

332. Wenaweser P, Rey C, Eberli FR, et al. Stent thrombosis following bare-metal stent implantation: success of emergency percutaneous coronary intervention and predictors of adverse outcome. *Eur Heart J.* 2005;26:1180–1187.
333. Moreno R, Fernandez C, Hernandez R, et al. Drug-eluting stent thrombosis. Results from a pooled analysis including 10 randomized studies. *J Am Coll Cardiol.* 2005;45:954–959.
334. Iakovou I, Schmidt T, Bonizzoni E, et al. Incidence, predictors, and outcome of thrombosis after successful implantation of drug-eluting stents. *JAMA.* 2005;293:2126–2130.
335. Kandzari DE,Mark DB. Intracoronary brachytherapy: time to sell short? *Circulation.* 2002;106(6):646–648.
336. Assali AR, Sdringola S, Ghani M, et al. Timing of coronary stent thrombosis in patients treated with prophylactic tirofiban. *J Invasive Cardiol.* 2000;12(9):460–463.
337. Chieffo A, Bonizzoni E, Orlic D, et al. Intraprocedural stent thrombosis during implantation of sirolimus-eluting stents. *Circulation.* 2004;109:2732–2736.
338. Vimani R, Guagliumi G, Farb A, et al. Localized hypersensitivity and late coronary thrombosis secondary to a sirolimus-eluting stent. Should we be cautious? *Circulation.* 2004;109:701–705.
339. Teierstein P, Reilly JP. Late stent thrombosis in brachytherapy: the role of long-term antiplatelet therapy. *J Invasive Cardiol.* 2002;14:109–114.
340. Reynolds MR, Rinaldi DE, Pinto DS, et al. Current clinical characteristics and economic impact of subacute stent thrombosis. *J Invasive Cardiol.* 2002;14:363–368.
341. Silva JA, White CJ, Ramee SR, et al. Treatment of coronary stent thrombosis with rheolytic thrombectomy: results from a multicenter experience. *Cathet Cardiovasc Intervent.* 2003;58:11–17.
342. Brummel KE, Jenny NS, Mann KG. Molecular and cellular hemostasis and fibrinolysis. In Lanzer P, Topol EJ, eds. *PanVascular Medicine: Integrated Clinical Approach.* New York: Springer-Verlag, 2002:287–318.
343. van Gestel MA, Heemskerk JWM, Slaaf DW, et al. Real-time detection of activation patterns in individual platelets during thromboembolism in vivo: differences between thrombus growth and embolus formation. *J Vasc Res.* 2002;39:534–543.
344. Keeley EC, Velez CA, O'Neill WW, et al. Long-term clinical outcome and predictors of major adverse cardiac events after percutaneous interventions on saphenous vein grafts. *J Am Coll Cardiol.* 2001;38:659–665.
345. Henrique JP, Zjilstra F, Ottervanger JP, et al. Incidence and clinical significance of distal embolization during primary angioplasty for acute myocardial infarction. *Eur Heart J.* 2002;23:1112–1117.
346. MacDonald RG, Feldman RL, Conti CR, et al. Thromboembolic complications of coronary angioplasty. *Am J Cardiol.* 1984;54:916–917.
347. Weyne AE, Heyndricks GR, Vanderckhove YR, et al. Embolization complicating coronary angioplasty in the presence of an intracoronary thrombus. *Clin Cardiol.* 1986;9:463–465.
348. Topol EJ, Leya F, Pinkerton CA, et al. for the CAVEAT-study group. A comparison of coronary angioplasty with directional atherectomy in patients with coronary artery disease. *N Engl J Med.* 1993;329:221–227.
349. Gorog DA, Foale RA, Malik I. Distal myocardial protection during percutaneous coronary intervention. *J Am Coll Cardiol.* 2005;46:1434–1445.
350. Grube E, Schofer JJ, Webb J, et al. Evaluation of a balloon occlusion and aspiration system for protection from distal embolization during stenting saphenous grafts. *Am J Cardiol.* 2002;89:941–945.
351. Baim DS, Wahr D, George B, et al. Randomized trial of a distal embolic protection device during percutaneous intervention of saphenous vein aorto-coronary bypass grafts. *Circulation.* 2002;105:1285–1290.
352. Yip HK, Wu CJ, Chang HW, et al. Effect of PercuSurge GuardWire device on the integrity of microvasculature and clinical outcomes during primary transradial coronary intervention in acute myocardial infarction. *Am J Cardiol.* 2003;92:1331–1335.
353. Stone GW, Webb J, Cox DA, et al. Distal microcirculatory protection during percutaneous coronary intervention in acute ST-segment elevation myocardial infarction. *JAMA.* 2005;293:1063–1072.
354. Garratt KN. Coronary stent retrieval: devices and techniques. In: Ellis SG, Holmes DR Jr., eds. *Strategic Approaches in Coronary Interventions.* Philadelphia: Lippincott Williams & Wilkins, 2000;441–451.
355. Fischell T. Coronary artery spasm after percutaneous transluminal coronary angioplasty: pathophysiology and clinical consequences. *Cathet Cardiovasc Diagn.* 1990;19:1–3.
356. Mohri M, Shimokawa H, Takeshita A. Coronary artery spasm: clinical aspects. In Lanzer P, Topol EJ, eds. *PanVascular Medicine: Integrated Clinical Approach.* New York: Springer-Verlag, 2002:921–929.
357. Grewe K, Presti CF, Perez JA. Torsion of an internal mammary graft during percutaneous transluminal coronary angioplasty: a case report. *Cathet Cardiovasc Diagn.* 1990;19: 195–197.
358. Deligonul U, Tatineni S, Johnson R, et al. Accordion right coronary artery: an unusual complication of PTCA guidewire entrapment. *Cathet Cardiovasc Diagn.* 1991;23:111–113.
359. Rauh RA, Ninneman RW, Joseph D, et al. Accordion effect in tortuous right coronary arteries during percutaneous transluminal coronary angioplasty. *Cathet Cardiovasc Diagn.* 1991;23:107–110.
360. Ziada KM, Roffi M, Crowe TD, et al. Adventitial hematoma triggering coronary spasm during percutaneous coronary intervention. *J Invasive Cardiol.* 2001;13:464–466.
361. Wong A, Cheng A, Chan C, et al. Cardiogenic shock caused by severe coronary artery spasm immediately after coronary stenting. *Tex Heart J.* 2005;32.78–80.
362. Rashid H, Marshall RJ, Diver DJ, et al. Spontaneous and diffuse coronary artery spasm unresponsive to conventional intracoronary pharmacological therapy: a case report. *Cathet Cardiovasc Intervent.* 2000;49:188–191.
363. Kahn JK, Hartzler GO. The spectrum of symptomatic coronary air embolism during balloon angioplasty: causes, consequences, and management. *Am Heart J.* 1990;119: 1374–1377.
364. Bruschke AVG, Proudfit WI, Sones FM. Progress study of 590 consecutive nonsurgical cases of coronary artery disease followed 5–9 years. *Circulation.* 1973;47:147–153.
365. Lim JS, Proudfit WI, Sones FM. Left main coronary arterial obstruction: Long term follow up of 141 nonsurgical cases. *Am J Cardiol.* 1975;36: 131–135.
366. Conley MJ, Ely RL, Kisslo J, et al. The prognostic spectrum of left main stenosis. *Circulation.* 1978;57:947–952.
367. Takaro T, Peduzzi P, Detre KM, et al. Survival in subgroups of patients with left main coronary artery disease. Veterans Administration Cooperative Study of Surgery for Coronary Arterial Occlusive Disease. *Circulation.* 1982;66:14–22.
368. Yusuf S, Zucker D, Peduzzi P, et al. Effect of coronary artery bypass graft surgery on survival: overview of 10-year results from randomised trials by the Coronary Artery Bypass Graft Surgery Trialists Collaboration. *Lancet.* 1994;344:563–570.
369. Eagle KA, Guyton RA, Davidoff R, et al. ACC/AHA 2004 guideline update for coronary artery bypass graft surgery: summary article: a report of the American College of Cardiology/American Heart Association Task Force on Practice Guidelines (Committee to update the 1999 guidelines for coronary artery bypass graft surgery). *Circulation.* 2004;110:1168–1176.
370. Bentivoglio LG, VanRaden MJ, Kelsey SF, et al. Percutaneous transluminal coronary angioplasty (PTCA) in patients with relative contraindications: Results of the National Heart, Lung and Blood Institute PTCA registry. *Am J Cardiol.* 1984;53: 82C-88C.
371. Stertzer SH, Myler RK, Insel H, et al. Percutaneous transluminal coronary angioplasty in left main stem coronary stenosis: a five-year appraisal. *Int J Cardiol.* 1985;9:149–159.
372. Hartzler GO, Rutherford BD, McConahay DR, et al. 'High-risk' percutaneous transluminal coronary angioplasty. *Am J Cardiol.* 1988;62(suppl):33G-37G.
373. O'Keefe JH Jr., Hartzler GO, Rutherford BD, et al. Left main coronary angioplasty: early and late results of 127 acute and elective procedures. *Am J Cardiol.* 1989;64:144–147.
374. Marso SP, Steg G, Plokker T, Holmes D, et al. Catheter-based reperfusion of unprotected left main stenosis during an acute myocardial infarction: the ULTIMA experience. *Am J Cardiol.* 1999;83:1513–1517.
375. Tan WA, Tamai H, Park S-J, et al. for the ULTIMA investigators. Long-Term Clinical Outcomes after unprotected left main trunk percutaneous revascularization in 279 patients *Circulation.* 2001;104:1609–1614.
376. Sperker W, Gyongyosi M, Kiss K, et al. Short and long term results of emergency and elective percutaneous interventions on left main coronary artery stenoses. *Cathet Cadiovasc Intervent.* 2002;56:22–29.
377. Neri R, Migliorini A, Moschi G, et al. Percutaneous reperfusion of left main coronary disease complicated by acute myocardial infarction. *Cathet Cadiovasc Intervent.* 2002;56:31–34.
378. Park S-J, Lee CW, Kim Y-H, et al. Technical feasibility, safety, and clinical outcome of stenting of unprotected left main coronary artery bifurcation narrowing. *Am J Cardiol.* 2002;90:374–378.
379. Ellis SG, Tamai H, Nobuyoshi M, et al. Contemporary percutaneous treatment of unprotected left main coronary stenoses. Initial results from a multicenter registry analysis 1994–1996. *Circulation.* 1997;96:3867–3872.
380. Park S-J, Kom Y-H, Lee B-K, et al. Sirolimus-eluting stent implantation for unprotected left main coronary artery stenosis. *J Am Coll Cardiol.* 2005;45:351–356.
381. Chieffo A, Stankovic G, Bonizzoni E, et al. Early and mit-term results of drug- eluting stent implantation in unprotected left main. *Circulation.* 2005;111:791–795.
382. Isner JM, Kishel J, Kent KM, et al. Accuracy of angiographic determination of left main coronary arterial narrowing. Angiographic-histologic correlative analysis in 28 patients. *Circulation.* 1981;63:1056–1064.
383. Cameron A, Kemp HG Jr., Fisher LD, et al. Left main coronary artery stenosis: angiographic determination. *Circulation.* 1983;68:484–489.
384. Fassa A-A, Wagatsuma K, Higano ST, et al. Intravascular ultrasound-guided treatment for angiographically indeterminate left main coronary artery disease: a long term follow-up study. *J Am Coll Cardiol.* 2005,45.204–211.
385. Valgimigli AP, Van Mieghem CA, Rodriquez-Granillo GA, et al. Comparison of early outcome of percutaneous coronary intervention for unprotected left main coronary artery disease in the drug-eluting stent era with versus without intravascular ultrasonic guidance. *Am J Cardiol.* 2005;95:644–647.
386. Park SJ, Hong M, Lee CW, et al. Elective stenting of unprotected left main coronary artery stenosis. Effect of debulking before stenting and intravascular ultrasound guidance. *J Am Coll Cardiol.* 2001;38:1054–1060.
387. Janzen J, Lanzer P, Rothenberger-Janzen K, et al. Variable extension of the transitional zone in the medial structure of the carotid artery tripod. *VASA.* 2001;30:101–107.
388. Topol EJ, Ellis SG, Fishman J, et al. Multicenter study of percutaneous transluminal angioplasty for right coronary artery ostial stenosis. *J Am Coll Cardiol.* 1987;9:1214–1218.
389. Tank KH, Sulke N, Taub N, et al. Percutaneous coronary angioplasty of aorto ostial, non-aorta ostial, and branch ostial stenoses: acute and long-term outcome. *Eur Heart J.* 1995;16:631–639.
390. Sabri MN, Cowley MJ, DiSciascio G, et al. Immediate results of interventional devices for coronary ostial narrowing with angina pectoris. *Am J Cardiol.* 1994;73:122–125.
391. Rocha-Singh K, Morris N, Wong SC, et al. Coronary stenting for treatment of ostial stenoses of native coronary arteries or aortocoronary saphenous venous grafts. Am J Cardiol 1995;75:26–9.
392. Iakovou I, Ge L, Michev I, et al. Clinical and angiographic outcome after sirolimus-eluting stent implantation in aorto-ostial lesions. *J Am Coll Cardiol.* 2004;44:967–971.
393. Umeda H, Iwase M, Kanda H, et al. Promising efficacy of primary gradual and prolonged balloon angioplasty in small coronary arteries: a randomized comparison with cutting balloon angioplasty and conventional balloon angioplasty. *Am Heart J.* 2004;147:E4.
394. Mauri L, Bonan R, Weiner BH, et al. Cutting balloon angioplasty for the prevention of restenosis: results of Cutting Balloon Global Randomized Trial. *Am J Cardiol.* 2002;90:1079–1083.
395. Mauri L, Bonan R, Weiner BH, et al. Cutting balloon angioplasty for the prevention of restenosis: results of Cutting Balloon Global Randomized Trial. *Am J Cardiol.* 2002;90:1079–1083.

396. Albiero R, Silber S, De Mario C, et al. Cutting balloon versus conventional balloon angioplasty for the treatment of in-stent restenosis: results of restenosis cutting balloon evaluation trial (RESCUT). *J Am Coll Cardiol.* 2004;43:943–949.
397. Schettler G, Nerem RM, Schmid-Schönbein H, et al., eds. *Fluid Dynamics as a Localizing Factor for Atherosclerosis.* Berlin: Springer Verlag, 1983.
398. Fry DL. Acute vascular endothelial changes associated with increased blood velocity gradients. *Circ Res.* 1968;22:165–197.
399. Caro CG, Fitz-Gerald JM, Schroter RC. Atheroma and arterial wall shear: servation, correlation and proposal of a shear dependent mass transfer mechanism for atherogenesis. *Proc R Soc Lond B Biol Sci.* 1971;177:109–159.
400. Asakura T, Karino T. Flow patterns and spatial distribution of atherosclerotic lesions in human coronary arteries. *Circ Res.* 1990;66:1045–1066.
401. Younis HF, Kaazempur-Mofrad MR, Chan RC, et al. Hemodynamics and wall mechanics in human carotid bifurcation and its consequences for atherogenesis: investigation of inter-individual variation. *Biomech Model Mechanobiol.* 2004;3:17–32.
402. Irace C, Cortese C, Fiaschi E, et al. Wall shear stress is associated with intima-media thickness and carotid atherosclerosis in subjects at low coronary heart disease risk. *Stroke.* 2004;35:464–468.
403. Lefevre T, Louvard Y, Morice M-C, et al. Stenting of bifurcation lesions: a rational approach. *J Intervent Cardiol.* 2001;14:573–586.
404. Pompa J, Bashore T. Qualitative and quantitative angiography—bifurcation lesions. In: Topol E, ed. *Textbook of Interventional Cardiology.* Philadelphia: WB Sounders, 1994: 1055–1058.
405. Koller P, Safian RD. Bifurcation stenosis. In: Freed M, Grinces C, Safian RD, eds. *The New Manual of Interventional Cardiology.* Birmingham, MI: Physicians Press, 1996:229–243.
406. Spokojny AM, Sanborn TM. The bifurcation lesion. In Ellis SG, Holmes DR Jr., eds. *Strategic Approaches in Coronary Intervention.* Baltimore: Williams & Wilkins, 1996:288.
407. George BS, Myler RK, Stertzer SH, et al. Balloon angioplasty of coronary bifurcation lesions: the kissing balloon technique. *Cathet Cardiovasc Diagn.* 1986;12:124–138.
408. Renkin J, Wijns W, Hanet C, et al. Angioplasty of bifurcation stenoses. *Cathet Cardiovasc Diagn.*;22:167–173.
409. Weinstein JS, Baim DS, Sipperly ME, et al. Salvage of branch vessels during bifurcation lesion angioplasty: acute and long-term follow-up. *Cathet Cardiovasc Diagn.* 1991;22:1–6.
410. Aliabadi D, Tilli FV, Bowers TR, et al. Incidence and angiographic predictors of side-branch occlusion following high-pressure intracoronary stenting. *Am J Cardiol.* 1997;80:994–997.
411. Al Suwaidi J, Berger PB, Rihal CS, et al. Immediate and long-term outcome of intracoronary stent implantation for true bifurcation lesions. *J Am Coll Cardiol.* 2000;35:929–936.
412. Brueck M, Scheinert D, Flachskampf FA, et al. Sequential vs. kissing balloon angioplasty for stenting of bifurcation coronary lesions. *Cathet Cardiovasc Intervent.* 2002;55:61–66.
413. Garot P, Lefevre T, Savage M, et al. Nine-month outcome of patients treated by percutaneous coronary interventions for bifurcation lesions in the recent era. A report from the Prevention of Restenosis with Tranislat and Its Outcomes (PRESTO) Trial. *J Am Coll Cardiol.* 2005;46:606–612.
414. Richter Y, Groothuis A, Seifert P, et al. Dynamic flow alterations dictate leucocyte adhesion and response to endovascular interventions. *J Clin Invest.* 2004;113:1607–1614.
415. Alexander RW. Getting stents to go with the flow. *J Clin Invest.* 2004;113:1532–1534.
416. Yamashita T, Nishida T, Adamian MG, et al. Bifurcation lesions†: two stents versus one stent—immediate and follow-up results. *J Am Coll Cardiol.* 2000;35:1145–1151.
417. Schampaert E, Fort S, Adelman AG, et al. The V-stent: a novel technique for bifurcation stenting. *Cathet Cardiovasc Diagn.* 1993;39:320–326.
418. Sharma SK, Choudhury A, Lee J, et al. Simultaneous kissing stents (SKS) technique for treating bifurcation lesions in medium-to-large size coronary arteries. *Am J Cardiol.* 2004;94:913–917.
419. Colombo A, Stankovic G, Orlic D, et al. Modified T-stenting technique with crushing for bifurcation lesions: immediate results and 30-day outcome. *Cathet Cardiovasc Intervent.* 2003;60:145–151.
420. Teierstein PS. Kissing Palmaz-Schatz stents for coronary bifurcation stenosis. *Cathet Cardiovasc Diagn.* 1996;37:307–310.
421. Fort S, Lazzam C, Schwartz L. Coronary "Y" stenting: a technique for angioplasty of bifurcation stenoses. *Can J Cardiol.* 1996;12:678–682.
422. Baim DS. Is bifurcation stenting the answer? *Cathet Cardiovasc Diagn.* 1996;37:314–316.
423. Chevalier B, Glatt B, Royer T, et al. Placement of coronary stents in bifurcation lesions by the "culotte" technique. *Am J Cardiol.* 1998;82:943–949.
424. Colombo A, Moses JW, Morice MC, et al. Randomized study to evacuate sirolimus-eluting stents implanted at coronary bifurcation lesions. *Circulation.* 2004;109:1244–1249.
425. Lefevre T, Ormiston J, Guagliumi G, et al. The Frontier stent registry: safety and feasibility of a novel dedicated stent for the treatment of bifurcation coronary artery lesions. *J Am Coll Cardiol.* 2005;46:592–598.
426. Simonton CA III. The bifurcation lesion. B. The role of coronary atherectomy. In Ellis SG, Holmes DR Jr., eds. Philadelphia: Lippincott Williams & Wilkins, Strategic Approaches in Coronary Intervention, 2ed. 2000:229–232.
427. Stankovic G, Colombo A, Bersin R, et al. Comparison of directional coronary atherectomy an stenting versus stenting alone for the treatment of de novo and restenotic coronary artery narrowing. *Am J Cardiol* .2004;93.953–958.
428. Reimers B, Colombo A. The bifurcation lesion. A. The role of stents. In Ellis SG, Holmes DR Jr., eds. Philadelphia: Lippincott Williams & Wilkins, Strategic Approaches in Coronary Intervention, 2ed.2000:211–229.
429. Iakovou I, Ge L, Colombo A. Contemporary stent treatment of coronary bifurcations. *J Am Coll Cardiol.* 2005;46:1446–1455.
430. Favaloro RG. Saphenous vein graft in the surgical treatment of coronary artery disease: operative technique. *J Thorac Cardiovasc Surg.* 1969;58:178–185.
431. Garrett HE, Dennis EW, DeBakey ME. Aortocoronary bypass with saphenous vein graft: seven-year follow-up. *JAMA.* 1973;223:792–794.
432. Aranki S, Aroesty JM. Long-term outcome after coronary artery bypass graft surgery. Available at: www.patients.uptodate.com. Accessed December 22, 2005)
433. Motwani JG, Topol EJ. Aortocoronary saphenous vein graft disease: pathogenesis, predisposition, and prevention. *Circulation.* 1998;97:916–931.
434. Loop FD, Lytle BW, Cosgrove DM, et al. Influence of the internal-mammary-artery graft on 10-year survival and other cardiac event. *N Engl J Med.* 1986;314:1–6.
435. Goldman S, Zadina K, Moritz T, et al. Long-term patency of saphenous vein and left internal mammary artery grafts after coronary artery bypass surgery: results from a Department of Veterans Affairs Cooperative Study. *J Am Coll Cardiol.* 2004;44:2149.
436. Domanski MJ, Borkowf CB, Campeau L, et al. Prognostic factors for atherosclerosis progression in saphenous vein grafts: the Postcoronary Artery Bypass Graft (Post-CABG) trial. Post-CABG Trial Investigators. *J Am Coll Cardiol.* 2000;36:1877–1883.
437. Sanz G, Pajaron A, Alegria E, et al. Prevention of early aortocoronary bypass occlusion by low dose aspirin and dipyridamole. Grupo Espanol para el Seguimiento del Injerto Coronario (GESIC) *Circulation.* 1990;82:769–773.
438. Bhatt DL, Chew DP, Hirsch AT, et al. Superiority of clopidogrel versus aspirin in patients with prior cardiac surgery. *Circulation.* 2001;103:363–368.
439. MRC/BHF Heart Protection Study of cholesterol lowering with simvastatin in 20,536 high-risk individuals: a randomised placebo-controlled trial. *Lancet.* 2002;360:7–12.
440. Kjoller-Hansen L, Steffensen R, Grande P. The Angiotensin-converting Enzyme Inhibition Post Revascularization Study (APRES). *J Am Coll Cardiol.* 2000;35:881–888.
441. Chen L, Theroux P, Lesperance J, et al. Angiographic features of vein grafts versus ungrafted coronary arteries in patients with unstable angina and previous bypass surgery *J Am Coll Cardiol.* 1996 28: 1493–1499.
442. Loop FD, Lytle BW, Cosgrove DM, et al. Reoperation for coronary atherosclerosis: changing practice in 2509 consecutive patients. *Ann Surg.* 1990;212:378–386.
443. de Feyeter PJ, van Suylen RJ, de Jaegere PP, et al. Balloon angioplasty for the treatment of lesions in saphenous vein grafts. *J Am Coll Cardiol.* 1993;21:1539–1549.
444. Savage MP, Douglas JS, Fischman DL, et al. for the Saphenous Vein De Novo Trial Investigators. Stent placement compared with balloon angioplasty for obstructed coronary bypass grafts. *N Engl J Med.* 1997;337:740–747.
445. Roffi M, Mukherjee D, Chew DP, et al. Lack of benefit from intravenous platelet glycoprotein IIb/IIIa receptor inhibition as adjunctive treatment for percutaneous interventions of aortocoronary bypass grafts. A pooled analysis of five randomized clinical trials. *Circulation.* 2002;106:3063–3067.
446. ChoussatR, BlackAJ, Bossi I, et al. Long-term clinical outcome after endoluminal reconstruction of diffusely degenerated saphenous vein grafts with less-shortening Wallstents. *J Am Coll Cardiol.* 2000;36:387–394.
447. Gruberg L, Hong MK, Mehran R, et al. In-hospital and long-term results of stent deployment compared with balloon angioplasty for treatment of narrowing at the saphenous vein graft distal anastomosis site. *Am J Cardiol.* 1999;84:1381–1386.
448. Sdringola S, Assali AR, Ghani M, et al. Risk assessment of slow- and no-reflow phenomenon in aorto coronary vein graft percutaneous intervention. *Cathet Cardiovasc Intervent.* 2001;54:318–324.
449. Popma JJ, Holper EE, Kuntz RE. Distal protection devices during percutaneous saphenous vein graft intervention: has a new standard of care been established? *Curr Intervent Cardiol Rep.* 2001;3:275–278.
450. Lefkovits J, Holmes DR, Califf R, et al. Predictors and sequelae of distal embolization during saphenous vein graft intervention from the CAVEAT-II trial. *Circulation.* 1995;92:734–740.
451. Hong M, Mehran R, Dangas G. Creatine-kinase-MB enzyme elevation following successful saphenous vein graft intervention is associated with late mortality. *Circulation.* 1999;100:2400–2405.
452. MautnerSL, Mautner GC, Hunsbarger SA, et al. Comparison of composition of atherosclerotic plaques in saphenous veins used as aortocoronary bypass conduits with plaques in native coronary artery in the same men. *Am J Cardiol.* 1992;70:1380–1385.
453. Holmes DR Jr., Topol EJ, Califf RM, et al. A multicenter, randomized trial of coronary angioplasty versus directional atherectomy for patients with saphenous vein bypass graft lesions. *Circulation.* 1995;91:1966–1974.
454. Bittl JA, Sanborn TA, Yardley DE, et al. Predictors of outcome of percutaneous excimer laser coronary angioplasty of saphenous vein bypass graft lesions. *Am J Cardiol.* 1994;74:144–148.
455. Singh M, Rosenschein U, Kalon KL, et al. Treatment of saphenous vein grafts with ultrasound thrombolysis: a randomized study. *Circulation.* 2003;107:2331–2336.
456. Stone GW, Cox DA, Low R, et al. for the X-tract Investigators. Safety and efficacy of a novel device for treatment of thrombotic and atherosclerotic lesions in native coronary arteries and saphenous vein grafts: results from the multicenter X-sizer for treatment of thrombus and atherosclerosis in coronary applications trial (X-TRACT) study. *Cathet Cardiovasc Intervent.* 2003;58:419–427.
457. Baim DS, Wahr D, George B, et al. Saphenous vein graft Angioplasty Free of Emboli Randomized (SAFER) Trial Investigators. Randomized trial of a distal embolic protection device during percutaneous intervention of saphenous vein aorto-coronary bypass grafts. *Circulation.* 2002;105:1285–1290.
458. Stone GW, Rogers C, Hermiller J, et al. Randomized comparison of distal protection with a filter-based catheter and a balloon occlusion and aspiration system during percutaneous intervention of diseased saphenous vein aorto-coronary bypass grafts. *Circulation.* 2003;108:548–553.
459. Ge L, Iakovou I, Sangiorgi GM, et al. Treatment of saphenous vein graft lesions with drug-eluting stents. Immediate and midterm outcome. *J Am Coll Cardiol.* 2005;45:989–994.
460. Vineberg AM. Development of an anastomosis between the coronary vessels and a transplanted internal mammary artery. *Can Med Assoc J.* 1946;55:117–119.
461. Kolesov VI. Mammary artery-coronary artery anastomosis as method of treatment for angina pectoris. *J Thorac Cardiovasc Surg.* 1967;54:535–544.
462. Garrett HE, Dennis EW, DeBakey ME. Aortocoronary bypass with saphenous vein graft. Seven-year follow-up. *JAMA.* 1973;223:792–794.

463. Favaloro RG. Saphenous vein autograft replacement of severe segmental coronary artery occlusion: operative technique. *Ann Thorac Surg.* 1968;5:334–339.
464. Favaloro RG. Landmarks in the development of coronary artery bypass surgery. *Circulation.* 1998;98:466–478.
465. Loop FD. Internal-thoracic-artery grafts: biologically better coronary arteries. *N Engl J Med.* 1996;334:263–265.
466. Cameron A, Davis KB, Green G, et al. Coronary bypass surgery with internal thoracic artery grafts: effects on survival over a 15-year period. *N Engl J Med.* 1996;334:216–219.
467. Goldman S, Zadina K, Moritz T, et al. Long-term patency of saphenous vein and left internal mammary artery grafts after coronary artery bypass surgery: results from a Department of Veterans Affairs Cooperative Study. J Am Coll Cardiol. 2004;44:2149.
468. Ura M, Sakata R, Nakayama Y, et al. Long-term patency rate of right internal thoracic artery bypass via the transverse sinus. *Circulation.* 1998;98:2043–2048.
469. Carpentier A, Guermonprez JL, Deloche A, et al. The aorta-to-coronary radial artery bypass graft. A technique avoiding pathological changes in grafts. *Ann Thorac Surg.* 1973;16:111–121.
470. Conklin LD, Ferguson ER, Reardon MJ. The technical aspects of radial artery harvesting. *Tex Heart Inst J.* 2001;28(2):129–131.
471. Acar C, Jebara VA, Porthogese M, et al. Revival of the radial artery for coronary artery bypass grafting. *Ann Thorac Surg.* 1992;54:652–660.
472. Manasse E, Sperti G, Suma H, et al. Use of the radial artery for myocardial revascularization. *Ann Thorac Surg.* 1996;62:1076–1083.
473. Zacharias A, Habib RH, Schwann TA, et al. Improved survival with radial artery versus vein conduits in coronary bypass surgery with left internal thoracic artery to left anterior descending artery grafting. *Circulation.* 2004;109:1489–1496.
474. Weinschelbaum EE, Macchia A, Caramutti VM, et al. Myocardial revascularization with radial and mammary arteries: initial and mid-term results. *Ann Thorac Surg.* 2000;70:1378–1383.
475. Iaco AL, Teodori G, Di Giammarco G, et al. Radial artery for myocardial revascularization: long-term clinical and angiographic results. *Ann Thorac Surg.* 2001;72:464–469.
476. Khot UN, Friedman DT, Pettersson G, et al. Radial artery bypass grafts have an increased occurrence of angiographically severe stenosis and occlusion compared with left internal mammary arteries and saphenous vein grafts. *Circulation.* 2004;109:2086–2091.
477. Desai ND, Cohen EA, Naylor CD, et al. A randomized comparison of radial-artery and saphenous-vein coronary bypass grafts. *N Engl J Med.* 2004;351:2302–2309.
478. Nottin R, Grinda JM, Anidjar S, et al. Coronary-coronary bypass graft: an arterial conduit-sparing procedure. *J Thorac Cardiovasc Surg.* 1996;112:1223–1230.
479. Barner HB. New arterial conduits for coronary bypass surgery. *Semin Thorac Cardiovasc Surg.* 1994;6:78–80.
480. Grandjean GJ, Boonstra PW, den Heyer P, et al. Arterial revascularization with the right gastroepiploic artery and internal mammary arteries in 300 patients. *J Thorac Cardiovasc Surg.* 1994;107:1309–1315.
481. Dietl CA, Benoit CH, Gilbert CL, et al. Which is the graft of choice for the right coronary and posterior descending arteries? Comparison of the right internal mammary and the right gastroepiploic artery. *Circulation.* 1995;92(suppl II):II-92-II-97.
482. Bonchek LI, Ullyot DJ. Minimally invasive coronary bypass: a dissenting opinion. *Circulation.* 1998;98:495–497.
483. Kereiakes DJ, George B, Sterzter SH, et al. Percutaneous angioplasty of left internal mammary artery grafts. *Am J Cardiol.* 1985;55:1215–1216.
484. Pinkerton CA, Slack JD, Orr CM, et al. Percutaneous transluminal angioplasty involving the internal mammary artery bypass grafts: a femoral approach. *Cathet Cardiovasc Diagn.* 1987;13:414–418.
485. Shimshack TM, Giorgi LV, Johnson WL, et al. Applications of PTCA to the internal mammary artery graft. *J Am Coll Cardiol.* 1988;12:1205–1214.
486. Hearne SE, Davidson CJ, Zidar JP, et al. Internal mammary artery graft angioplasty: acute and long-term outcome. *Cathet Cardiovasc Diagn.* 1998;44:153–156.
487. Sharma AK, McGlynn S, Apple S, et al. Clinical outcome following stent implantation in internal mammary artery grafts. *Cathet Cardiovasc Intervent.* 2003;59:436–441.
488. Osborn L, Vernon S, Reynolds B, et al. Screening for subclavian artery stenosis in patients who are candidates for coronary bypass surgery. *Cathet Cardiovasc Intervent.* 2002;66: 162–165.
489. Boston DR, Malouf A, Barry WH. Management of intracoronary thrombosis complicating percutaneous transluminal coronary angioplasty. *Clin Cardiol.* 1996;19:536–542.
490. Blankenship JC. Right coronary artery pseudo-transection due to mechanical straightening during coronary angioplasty. *Cathet Cardiovasc Diagn.* 1995;36:43–45.
491. Sharma S, Makkar RM. Percutaneous intervention on the LIMA: tackling the tortuosity. *J Invasive Cardiol.* 2003;15:359–362.
492. Jacq L, Lancelin B, Brenot P, et al. Percutaneous transluminal angioplasty of ostial lesions of internal mammary artery grafts. *Cathet Cardiovasc Intervent.* 2001;52:368–372.
493. Christofferson RD, Lehmann KG, Martin GV, et al. Effect of chronic total coronary occlusion on treatment strategy. *Am J Cardiol.* 2005;95:1088–1091
494. Suero JA, Marso SP, Jones PG, et al. Procedural outcomes and long-term survival among patients undergoing percutaneous coronary intervention of a chronic total occlusion in native coronary arteries: a 20-year experience. *J Am Coll Cardiol.* 2001;38:409–414.
495. Hoye A, van Domburg RT, Sonnenschein K, et al. Percutaneous coronary intervention for chronic total occlusions: the Thoraxcenter experience 1992–2002. *Eur Heart J.* 2005;26:2630–2636.
496. Kim CB, Braunwald E. Potential benefits of late reperfusion of infarcted myocardium. The open artery hypothesis. *Circulation.* 1993;88:2426–2436.
497. Topol EJ, Califf RM, Vandormael M, et al. A randomized trial of late reperfusion therapy for acute myocardial infarction. *Circulation.* 1992;85:2090–2099.
498. Dzavik V, Beanlands DS, Davies RF, et al. Effects of late percutaneous transluminal coronary angioplasty of an occluded infarct-related coronary artery on left ventricular function in patients with a recent (<6 weeks) Q-wave myocardial infarction (Total Occlusion post-Myocardial Infarction Intervention Study [TOMIIS])—a pilot study. *Am J Cardiol.* 1994;73:856–861.
499. Sadanandan S, Buller C, Menon V, et al. The late open artery hypothesis—a decade later. *Am Heart J.* 2001;142:411–421.
500. Heyndrickx GR, Serruys PW, van de Brand M, et al. Transluminal angioplasty after mechanical recanalization in patients with chronic occlusion of coronary artery. *Circulation.* 1982;66:II-5A.
501. Maiello L, Colombo A, Almagor Y, et al. Coronary stenting with balloon-expandable stent after the recanalization of chronic total occlusions. *Cathet Cardiovasc Diagn.* 1993;28: 293–296.
502. Simes PA, Golf S, Myreng Y, et al. Stenting in Chronic Coronary Occlusion (SICCO): a randomized, controlled trial of adding stent implantation after successful angioplasty. *J Am Coll Cardiol.* 1996;28:1444–1451.
503. Mori M, Kurogane H, Hayashi T, et al. Comparison of results of intracoronary implantation of Palmaz-Schatz stent with conventional balloon angioplasty in chronic total coronary artery occlusion. *Am J Cardiol.* 1996;78:958–959.
504. Rubartelli P, Niccoli L, Verna E, et al. Stent implantation versus balloon angioplasty in chronic coronary occlusions: results from GISSOC trial. *J Am Coll Cardiol.* 1998;32:90–96.
505. Lotan C, Rozenman Y, Hendler A, et al. Stents in total occlusion for restenosis prevention: the multicentre randomized STOP study. *Eur Heart J.* 2000;21:1960–1966.
506. Hoher M, Wohrle M, Grebe OC, et al. A randomized trial of elective stenting after balloon recanalization of chronic total occlusions. *J Am Coll Cardiol.* 1999,34:722–729.
507. Sievert H, Rohde S, Utech A, et al. Stent or angioplasty after recanalization of chronic coronary occlusions? (The SARECCO trial). *Am J Cardiol.* 1999;84:386–390.
508. Buller CE, Dzavik V, Carere RG, et al. Primary stenting versus balloon angioplasty in occluded coronary arteries: the Total Occlusion Study of Canada (TOSCA). *Circulation.* 1999;100:236–242.
509. Hoher M, Wohrle J, Grebe OC, et al. A randomized trial of elective stenting after balloon recanalization of chronic total occlusions. *J Am Coll Cardiol.* 1999;34:722–729.
510. Werner GS, Bahrmann P, Mutschke O, et al. Determinants of target vessel failure in chronic total coronary occlusions after stent implantation: the influence of collateral function and coronary hemodynamics. *J Am Coll Cardiol.* 2003;42:219–225.
511. Werner GS, Krack A, Schwarz G, et al. Prevention of lesion recurrence in chronic total coronary occlusions by paclitaxel-eluting stents. *J Am Coll Cardiol.* 2004;44:2301–2306.
512. Ge L, Iakovou I, Cosgrave J, et al. Immediate and long-term outcomes of sirolimus-eluting stent implantation for chronic total occlusions. *Eur Heart J.* 2005;26:1056–1062.
513. Werner GS, Emig U, Mutschke O. Regression of collateral function after recanalization of chronic total coronary occlusions: a serial assessment by intracoronary pressure and Doppler recordings. *Circulation.* 2003;108:2877–2827.
514. Serruys PW, Umans V, Heyndrickx GR, et al. Elective PTCA of totally occluded coronary arteries not associated with acute myocardial infarction: short-term und long-term results. *Eur Heart J.* 1985;6:2–12.
515. Maiello L, Colombo A, Gianrossi R, et al. Coronary angioplasty of chronic occlusions: factors predictive of procedural success. *Am Heart J.* 1992;124:581–584.
516. Meier B. "Occlusion angioplasty". light at the end of the tunnel or dead end? *Circulation.* 1992;85:1214–1216.
517. Stewart JT, Denne L, Bowker TJ, et al. Percutaneous transluminal coronary angioplasty in chronic coronary artery occlusion. *J Am Coll Cardiol.* 1993;21:1371–1376.
518. Dzavik V. Restenosis and reocclusion after recanalization of an occluded coronary artery: is there a light at the end of the tunnel? *Curr Intervent Cardiol Rep.* 2001;3:311–317.
519. Suzuki T, Hosokawa H, Yokoya K, et al. Time-dependent morphological characteristics in angiographic chronic total coronary occlusions. *Am J Cardiol.* 2001;88:167–169.
520. Kobayashi Y, De Gregorio J, Kobayashi N, et al. Stented segment length as an independent predictor of restenosis. *J Am Coll Cardiol.* 1999;34:651.
521. Colombo A, Mikhail GW, Michev I, et al. Treating chronic total occlusions using subintimal tracking and reentry: The STAR technique. *Cathet Cardiovasc Intervent.* 2005;407–411.
522. Segev A, Strauss BH. Novel approaches for the treatment of chronic total coronary occlusions. *J Intervent Cardiol.* 2004;17:411–416.
523. Schwartz SM, deBlois D, O'Brien ER. The intima. Soil for atherosclerosis and restenosis. *Circ Res.* 1995;77:445–465.
524. Nikol S, Huehns TY, Hofling B. Molecular biology and post-angioplasty restenosis. *Atherosclerosis.* 1996;123:17–31.
525. Agema WRP, Jukema JW, Pimstone WN, et al. Genetic aspects of restenosis after percutaneous coronary interventions: towards more tailored therapy. *Eur Heart J.* 2001;22:2058–2074.
526. Mintz GS, Popma JJ, Pichard AD, et al. Arterial remodelling after coronary angioplasty. *Circulation.* 1996,94:35–43.
527. Tierstein PS, Massullo V, Jani S, et al. Three-year clinical and angiographic follow-up after intracoronary radiation: results of a randomized clinical trial. *Circulation.* 2000;101:360–365.
528. Nissen SE, Gurley JC, Grines CL, et al. Intravascular ultrasound assessment of lumen size and wall morphology in normal subjects and patients with coronary artery disease. *Circulation.* 1991;84:1087–1099.
529. Bruining N, Sabate N, de Feyter PJ, et al. Quantitative measurements of in-stent restenosis: a comparison between quantitative coronary ultrasound and quantitative coronary angiography. *Cathet Cardiovasc Intervent.* 1999;48:133–142.
530. Kereiakes DJ, Kuntz RE, Mauri L, et al. Surrogates, substudies, and real clinical end-points in trials of drug-eluting stents. *J Am Coll Cardiol.* 2005;45:1206–1212.
531. Casterella PJ, Teirstein PS. Prevention of coronary restenosis. *Cardiol Rev.* 1999;7:219–231.
532. Gilbert J, Raboud J, Zinman B. Meta-analysis of the effect of diabetes on restenosis rates among patients receiving coronary angioplasty stenting. *Diabetes Care.* 2004;27:990–1012.

533. Kastrati A, Dirschinger J, Boekstegers P, et al. Influence of stent design on 1-year outcome after coronary stent placement: a randomized comparison of five stent types in 1, 147 unselected patients. *Cathet Cardiovasc Intervent.* 2000;50:290–297.

534. Radke PW, Kaiser A, Frost C, et al. Outcome after treatment of coronary in-stent restenosis: results from a systematic review using meta-analysis techniques. *Eur Heart J.* 2003;24:266–273.

535. Levin T, Cutlip D, Baim DS. Intracoronary stent restenosis. Available at: http://patients.uptodate.com/topic.asp?file=chd/55508. Accessed November 8, 2005.

536. Kastrati A. Mehili J, Dirschinger J, et al. Intracoronary stenting and angiographic results: strut thickness effect on restenosis outcome. *Circulation.* 2001;103:2816–2821.

537. Leon MB, Tierstein PS, Moses JW, et al. Localized intracoronary gamma-radiation therapy to inhibit the recurrence restenosis after stenting. *N Engl J Med.* 2001;344:250–256.

538. Popma JF, Suntharalingam M, Lansky A, et al. Randomized trial of 90Sr/90Y γ-radiation versus placebo control for treatment of in-stent restenosis. *Circulation.* 2002;106: 1090–1096.

539. Waksman R, Raizner AE, Yeung AC, et al. Use of localised intracoronary beta radiation in treatment of in-stent restenosis: the INHIBIT randomised controlled trial. *Lancet.* 2002;359: 551–557.

540. Waksman R, Weinberger J. Coronary brachytherapy in the drug-eluting stent era. Don't bury it alive. *Circulation.* 2003;108:386–388.

541. Babapulle MN, Joseph L, Belisle P, et al. A hierarchical Bayesian meta-analysis of randomised clinical trials of drug-eluting stents. *Lancet.* 2004;364:583–589.

542. Costa MA, Simon DI. Molecular basis of restenosis and drug-eluting stents. *Circulation.* 2005;111:2257–2263.

543. Moses JW, Leon MB, Popma JJ, et al. Sirolimus-eluting stents versus standard stents in patients with stenosis in a native coronary artery. *N Engl J Med.* 2003;349:1315–1319.

544. Schofer J, Schluter M, Gershlick AH, et al. Sirolimus-eluting stents for treatment of patients with long atherosclerotic lesions in small coronary arteries: double-blind, randomised controlled trial (E-SIRIUS). *Lancet.* 2003;362:1093–1097.

545. Stone GW, Ellis SG, Cox DA, et al. A polymer-based, paclitaxel-eluting stent in patients with coronary artery disease. *N Engl J Med.* 2004;350:221–226.

546. Mauri L, Orav EJ, O'Malley AJ, et al. Relationship of late loss in lumen diameter to coronary restenosis in sirolimus-eluting stents. *Circulation.* 2005;111:321–328.

547. Mauri L, Orav EJ, Kuntz RE. Late loss in lumen diameter and binary restenosis for drug-eluting stent comparison. *Circulation.* 2005;111:3435–3442.

548. Sousa JE, Costa MA, Abizaid A, et al. Four-year angiographic and intravascular ultrasound follow-up of patients treated with sirolimus-eluting stents. *Circulation.* 2005;111: 2326–2332.

549. Grube E, Silber S, Hauptmann KE, et al. Two-year-plus follow-up of a paclitaxel-eluting stent in de novo coronary narrowings (TAXUS I). *Am J Cardiol.* 2005;96:79.

550. Carrozza JP Jr. Sirolimus-eluting stents: does a great stent still need a good interventionalist? *J Am Coll Cardiol.* 2004;43:1116–1121.

551. Lemos PA, Saia F, Ligthart JM, et al. Coronary restenosis after sirolimus-eluting stent implantation: morphological description and mechanistic analysis from a consecutive series of cases. *Circulation.* 2003;108:257–262.

552. Fujii K, Mintz GS, Kobayashi Y, et al. Contribution of stent underexpansion to recurrence after sirolimus-eluting stent implantation for in-stent restenosis. *Circulation.* 2004;109:1085–1090.

553. Lemos PA, Hoye A, Goedhart D, et al. Clinical, angiographic, and procedural predictors of angiographic restenosis after sirolimus-eluting stent implantation in complex patients: an evaluation from the Rapamycin-Eluting Stent Evaluated At Rotterdam Cardiology Hospital (RESEARCH) study. *Circulation.* 2004;109:1366–1371.

554. Ong AT, Serruys PW, Aoki J, et al. The unrestricted use of paclitaxel- versus sirolimus-eluting stents for coronary artery disease in an unselected population: one-year results of the Taxus-Stent Evaluated at Rotterdam Cardiology Hospital (T-SEARCH) registry. *J Am Coll Cardiol.* 2005;45:1135–1141.

555. Windecker S, Remondino A, Eberli FR, et al. Sirolimus-eluting and paclitaxel-eluting stents for coronary revascularization. *N Engl J Med.* 2005;353:653–659.

556. Dibra A, Kastrati A, Mehilli J, et al. Paclitaxel-eluting or sirolimus-eluting stents to prevent restenosis in diabetic patients. *N Engl J Med.* 2005;353:663–671.

557. Kastrati A, Dibra A, Eberle S, et al. Sirolimus-eluting stents vs paclitaxel-eluting stents in patients with coronary artery disease: meta-analysis of randomized trials. *JAMA.* 2005;294:819–826.

558. Pache J, Dibra A, Mehili J, et al. Drug-eluting stents compared with thin-strut bare stents for the reduction of restenosis: a prospective, randomized trial. *Eur Heart J.* 2005;26:1262–1268.

559. Sirolimus: mechanism of action. Available at: www.rxlist.com/cgi/generic2/sirolimus_cp.htm. Accessed December 26, 2005.

560. Cordis, Johnson and Johnson. Instruction for Use Cypher TM Sirolimus-eluting coronary stent on raptor over-the-wire delivery system and Cypher TM Sirolimus-eluting coronary stent on raptorrail rapid exchange delivery system available at: http://www.fda.gov/cdrh/PDF2/p020026c.pdf. Accessed June 7, 2006.

561. Morice MC, Serruys PW, Sousa JE, et al. A randomized comparison of a sirolimus-eluting stent with a standard stent for coronary revascularization. *N Engl J Med.* 2002;346:1773–1780.

562. Albumin bound paclitaxel: mechanism of action. Available at: www.rxlist.com/cgi/generic3/abraxane_cp.htm. Accessed December 26, 2005.

563. Taxus Express Coronary Stent System. Summary of safety and effectiveness data. Available at: www.fda.gov/cdrh/pdf3/P030025b.pdf. Accessed December 26, 2005.

564. Grube E, Silber S, Hauptmann KE, et al. Six- and twelve-month results from a randomized, double-blind trial on a slow-release paclitaxel-eluting stent for de novo coronary lesions. *Circulation.* 2003;107:38–42.

565. The ERASER Investigators Acute platelet inhibition with abciximab does not reduce In-stent restenosis (ERASER study). *Circulation.* 1999;100:799–806.

566. Wilensky RL, Tanguay JF, Ito S, et al. Heparin infusion prior to stenting (HIPS) trial: final results of a prospective, randomized, controlled trial evaluating the effects of local vascular delivery on intimal hyperplasia. *Am Heart J.* 2000;139:1061–1067.

567. Ellis SG, Roubin GS, Wilentz J, et al. Effect of 18- to 24-hour heparin administration for prevention of restenosis after complicated coronary angioplasty. *Am Heart J.* 1989;117:777–783.

568. Serruys PW, Herrman JP, Simon R, et al. A comparison of hirudin with heparin in the prevention of restenosis after coronary angioplasty. Helvetica Investigators. *N Engl J Med.* 1995;333:757–762.

569. Faxon DP, Spiro TE, Minor S, et al. Low molecular weight heparin in prevention of restenosis after angioplasty. Results of Enoxaparin Restenosis (ERA) Trial. *Circulation.* 1994;90:908–913.

570. Gimple LW, Herrmann HC, Winniford M, et al. Usefulness of subcutaneous low molecular weight heparin (ardeparin) for reduction of restenosis after percutaneous transluminal coronary angioplasty. *Am J Cardiol.* 1999;83:1524–1560.

571. Ten Berg JM, KelderJC, Suttorp MJ, et al. A randomized trial assessing the effect of coumarins started before coronary angioplasty on restenosis: Results of the 6-month angiographic substudy of the Balloon Angioplasty and Anticoagulation Study (BAAS). *Am Heart J.* 2003;145:58–63.

572. Pepine CJ, Hirshfeld JW, Macdonald RG, et al. A controlled trial of corticosteroids to prevent restenosis after coronary angioplasty. M-HEART Group. *Circulation.* 1990;81:1753–1758.

573. Lee CW, Chae JK, Lim HY, et al. Prospective randomized trial of corticosteroids for the prevention of restenosis after intracoronary stent implantation. *Am Heart J.* 1999;138:60–66.

574. Hausleiter J, Kastrati A, Mehilli J, et al. Randomized, double-blind, placebo-controlled trial of oral sirolimus for restenosis prevention in patients with in-stent restenosis: the Oral Sirolimus to Inhibit Recurrent In-stent Stenosis (OSIRIS) trial. *Circulation.* 2004;110:790–795.

575. Waksman R, Ajani AE, Pichard AD, et al. Oral rapamycin to inhibit restenosis after stenting of de novo coronary lesions: the Oral Rapamune to Inhibit Restenosis (ORBIT) study. *J Am Coll Cardiol.* 2004;44:1386–1392.

576. Serruys PW, de Feyter P, Macaya C, et al. Fluvastatin for prevention of cardiac events following successful first percutaneous coronary intervention: a randomized controlled trial. *JAMA.* 2002;287:3215–3220.

577. Lange H, Suryapranata H, De Luca G, et al. Folate therapy and in-stent restenosis after coronary stenting. *N Engl J Med.* 2004;350:2673–2677.

578. Does the new angiotensin converting enzyme inhibitor cilazapril prevent restenosis after percutaneous transluminal coronary angioplasty? Results of the MERCATOR study: a multicenter, randomized, double-blind placebo-controlled trial. Multicenter European Research Trial with Cilazapril after Angioplasty to Prevent Transluminal Coronary Obstruction and Restenosis (MERCATOR) Study Group. *Circulation.* 1992;86:100–110.

579. Desmet W, Vrolix M, De Scheerder I, et al. Angiotensin-converting enzyme inhibition with fosinopril sodium in the prevention of restenosis after coronary angioplasty. *Circulation.* 1994;89:385–392.

580. Serruys PW, Foley DP, Hofling B, et al. Carvedilol for prevention of restenosis after directional coronary atherectomy: final results of the European Carvedilol Atherectomy Restenosis (EUROCARE) trial. *Circulation.* 2000;101:1512–1518.

581. Serruys PW, Foley DP, Pieper M, et al. The TRAPIST Study. A multicentre randomized placebo controlled clinical trial of trapidil for prevention of restenosis after coronary stenting, measured by 3-D intravascular ultrasound. *Eur Heart J.* 2001;22:1938–1947.

582. Holmes DR Jr., Savage M, LaBlanche JM, et al. Results of Prevention of REStenosis with Tranilast and its Outcomes (PRESTO) trial. *Circulation.* 2002;106:1243–1250.

583. Daida H, Kuwabara Y, Yokoi H, et al. Effect of probucol on repeat revascularization rate after percutaneous transluminal coronary angioplasty (from the Probucol Angioplasty Restenosis Trial [PART]). *Am J Cardiol.* 2000;86:550–558.

584. Douglas JS, Holmes DR Jr., Kereiakes DJ, et al. Coronary stent restenosis in patients treated with cilostazol. *Circulation.* 2005;112:2826–2832.

585. Kutryk MJ, Foley DP, van den Brand M, et al. Local intracoronary administration of antisense oligonucleotide against c-myc for the prevention of in-stent restenosis. Results of the randomized Investigation by the Thoraxcenter of Antisense DNA using Local delivery and IVUS after Coronary Stenting (ITALICS) trial. *J Am Coll Cardiol.* 2002;39:281–287.

586. Arampatzis CA, Lemos PA, Tanabe K, et al. Effectiveness of sirolimus-eluting stent for treatment of left main coronary artery disease. *Am J Cardiol.* 2003;92:327–342.

587. Sawhney N, Moses JW, Leon MB, et al. Treatment of left anterior descending coronary artery disease with sirolimus-eluting stents. *Circulation.* 2004;110:374–380.

588. Dangas G, Ellis SG, Shlofmitz R, et al. Outcomes of paclitaxel-eluting stent implantation in patients with stenosis of the left anterior descending coronary artery. *J Am Coll Cardiol.* 2005;45:1186–1191.

589. Seung KB, Kim YH, Park DW, et al. Effectiveness of sirolimus-eluting stent implantation for the treatment of ostial left anterior descending artery stenosis with intravascular ultrasound guidance. *J Am Coll Cardiol.* 2005;46:787–792.

590. Ardissino D, Cavallini C, Bramucci E, et al. Sirolimus-eluting vs uncoated stents for prevention of restenosis in small coronary arteries: a randomized trial. *JAMA.* 2004;292:2727–2734.

591. Schofer J, Schluter M, Gershlick AH, et al. Sirolimus-eluting stents for treatment of patients with long atherosclerotic lesions in small coronary arteries: double-blind, randomised controlled trial (E-SIRIUS). *Lancet.* 2003;362:1093–1098.

592. Lemos PA, Hoye A, Goedhart D, et al. Clinical, angiographic, and procedural predictors of angiographic restenosis after sirolimus-eluting stent implantation in complex patients: an evaluation from the Rapamycin-Eluting Stent Evaluated At Rotterdam Cardiology Hospital (RESEARCH) study. *Circulation.* 2004;109:1366–1370.

593. Moussa I, Leon MB, Baim DS, et al. Impact of sirolimus-eluting stents on outcome in diabetic patients: a SIRIUS (SIRolImUS-coated) Bx Velocity balloon-expandable stent in the treatment of patients with de novo coronary artery lesions) substudy. *Circulation.* 2004;109:2273–2278.

594. Hermiller JB, Raizner A, Cannon L, et al. Outcomes with the polymer-based paclitaxel-eluting TAXUS stent in patients with diabetes mellitus: the TAXUS-IV trial. J Am Coll Cardiol. 2005;45:1172–1179.

595. Dibra A, Kastrati A, Mehili J, et al. Paclitaxel- eluting or sirolimus eluting stents to prevent restenosis in diabetic patients. *N Engl J Med*. 2005;353:663–670.

596. Stone GW, Ellis SG, Cox DA, et al. A polymer-based paclitaxel-eluting stent in patients with complex coronary artery disease: a randomized trial. *JAMA*. 2005;294:1215–1223.

597. Wessely R, Kastrati A, Schömig A. Development of late restenosis in patients receiving a polymer coated sirolimus-eluting stent subsequently to appropriate 6-month angiographic follow-up. *Ann Intern Med*. 2005;143:392–394.

598. Virmani R, Guagliumi G, Farb A, et al. Localized hypersensitivity and late coronary thrombosis secondary to a sirolimus-eluting stent: should we be cautious? *Circulation*. 2004;109:701–705.

599. Stabile EP, Stabile E, Regar E, et al. Late thrombosis in drug-eluting coronary stents after discontinuation of antiplatelet therapy. *Lancet*. 2004;364:1519–1521.

600. Wong SC, Hong MK, Ellis SG, et al. Influence of stent length to lesion length ratio on angiographic and clinical outcomes after implantation of bare metal and drug-eluting stents (the TAXUS-IV study). *Am J Cardiol*. 2005;95:1043–1048.

601. Mauri L, O'Malley AJ, Popma JJ, et al. Comparison of thrombosis and restenosis risk from stent length of sirolimus-eluting stents versus bare metal stents. *Am J Cardiol*. 2005;95:1140–1147.

602. Neumann F-J, Desmet W, Grube E, et al. Effectiveness and safety of sirolimus-eluting stents in the treatment of restenosis after coronary stent placement. *Circulation*. 2005;111:2107–2111.

603. Moliterno DJ. Healing Achilles—sirolimus versus paclitaxel. *N Engl J Med*. 2005;353:724–727.

604. Mehran R, Dangas G, Abizaid AS, et al. Angiographic patterns of in-stent restenosis: classification and implications for long-term outcome. *Circulation*. 1999, 100: 1872–1879.

605. Daoud AS, Florentin RA, Goodale F. Diffuse coronary arteriosclerosis versus isolated plaque in the etiology of myocardial infarction. *Am J Cardiol*. 1964;14:69–74.

606. Fuster V, Moreno PR, Fayad ZA, et al. Atherothrombosis and high-risk plaque: Part I: evolving concepts. *J Am Coll Cardiol*. 2005;46:937–954.

607. Gibson CM, Kirtane AJ, Murphy SA, et al. Distance from the coronary ostium to the culprit lesion in acute ST-elevation myocardial infarction and its implications regarding the potential prevention of proximal plaque rupture. *J Thromb Thrombol*. 2003;15:189–193.

608. Wang JC, Normand S-L T, Mauri L, et al. Coronary artery spatial distribution of acute myocardial infarction occlusions. *Circulation*. 2004;110:278–284.

609. Grottum P, Swindland A, Walloe L. Localization of atherosclerotic lesions in the bifurcation of the left main coronary artery. *Atherosclerosis*. 1983;47:55–62.

610. Sabbah HN, Khaja F, Brymer JF, et al. Blood velocity in the right coronary artery in relation to the distribution of atherosclerotic lesions. *Am J Cardiol*. 1984;53:1008–1012.

611. Asakura T, Karino T. Flow pattern and spatial distribution of atherosclerotic lesions in human coronary arteries. *Circ Res*. 1990;66:1045–1066.

612. Tsutsui H, Yamagashi M, Uematsu M, et al. Intravascular ultrasound evaluation of plaque distribution at curved coronary segments. *Am J Cardiol*. 1998;81:977–981.

613. Rioufol G, Finet G, Ginon I, et al. Multiple atherosclerotic plaque rupture in acute coronary syndrome. A three vessel intravascular ultrasound study. *Circulation*. 2002;106:804–808.

614. Glaser R, Selzer F, Faxon DP, et al. Clinical progression of incidental, asymptomatic lesions discovered during culprit vessel coronary intervention. *Circulation*. 2005;111:143–149.

615. Gould KL. Methods for pressure-flow analysis and arteriography. In: Gould KL, ed. *Coronary Artery Stenosis and Reversing Atherosclerosis*. London: Arnold, 1999:31–53.

616. Ellis SG, Vandormael MG, Cowley MJ, et al. Coronary morphologic and clinical determinants of procedural outcome with angioplasty for multivessel coronary disease. *Circulation*. 1990;82:1193–1202.

617. Stevens T, Kahn JK, McCallister BD, et al. Safety and efficacy of percutaneous transluminal coronary angioplasty in patients with left ventricular dysfunction. *Am J Cardiol*. 1991;68:313–318.

618. Bell MR, Bailey KR, Reeder GS, et al. Percutaneous transluminal angioplasty in patients with multivessel coronary disease: how important is complete revascularization for cardiac event-free survival? *J Am Coll Cardiol*. 1990;16:553–539.

619. Botas J, Stadius ML, Bourassa MG, et al. Angiographic correlates of lesion relevance and suitability for percutaneous coronary angioplasty and coronary artery bypass grafting in the Bypass Angioplasty Revascularization Investigation study (BARI). *Am J Cardiol*. 1996;77:805–814.

620. Zimarino M, Calafiore AM, De Caterina R. Complete myocardial revascularization: between myth and reality. *Eur Heart J*. 2005;26:1824–1830.

621. Jones EL, Craver J, Guyton RA, et al. Importance of complete revascularisation in performance of the coronary bypass operation. *Am J Cardiol*. 1983;51:7–13.

622. Lawrie GM, Morris GC Jr., Silvers A, et al. The influence of residual disease after coronary bypass on the 5-year survival rate of 1274 men with coronary artery disease. *Circulation*. 1982;66:717–724.

623. Holmes DR Jr., Reeder GS, Vliestra RE. Role of percutaneous transluminal coronary angioplasty in patients with multivessel disease. *Am J Cardiol*. 1988;61:94–101.

624. Vandormael MG, Chaitman BR, Ischinger T, et al. Immediate and short-term benefit of multilesion coronary angioplasty: influence of degree of revascularization. *J Am Coll Cardiol*. 1985;6:983–988.

625. Mabin TA, Holmes DR Jr., Smith HC, et al. Follow-up clinical results in patients undergoing percutaneous transluminal coronary angioplasty. *Circulation*. 1985;71:94–98.

626. Bourassa MG, Holubkov R, Yeh W, et al. Strategy of complete revascularisation in patients with multivessel coronary artery disease (a report from the 1985–1986 NHLBI PTCA Registry). *Am J Cardiol*. 1992;70:174–185.

627. Hasdai D, Berger PB, Bell MR, et al. The changing face of coronary interventional practice: The Mayo Clinic Experience. *Arch Intern Med*. 1997;157:677–684.

628. Faxon DP, Ghalili K, Jacob AK. The degree of revascularisation and outcome after multivessel coronary angioplasty. *Am Heart J*. 1997;123:854–860.

629. Hill R, Bagust A, Bakhai A, et al. Coronary artery stents: a rapid systematic review and economic evaluation. Available at: www.nccthA.org/execsumm/summ835.htm. Accessed November 11, 2005.

630. Patil CV, Nikolsky E, Boulos M, et al. Multivessel coronary artery disease†: current revascularization strategies. *Eur Heart J*. 2000;22:1183–1197.

631. Serruys PW for the ARTS-II Investigators. ARTS-II: Arterial Revascularization Therapies Study Part II of the sirolimus-eluting stent in the treatment of patients with multivessel de novo coronary lesions. Late Breaking Trial. Presented at the American College of Cardiology, 54th Annual Meeting, Orlando, Florida, March 2005.

632. Riess FC, Schofer J, Kremer P, et al. Beating heart operations including hybrid revascularization: initial experiences. *Ann Thorac Surg*. 1998;66:1076–1081.

633. Hartzler GO, Rutherford BD, McConnahay DR, et al. Percutaneous transluminal coronary angioplasty with and without thrombolytic therapy for treatment of acute myocardial infarction. *Am Heart J*. 1983;106:965–973.

634. Hartzler GO, Rutherford BD, McConnahay DR, et al. Percutaneous transluminal coronary angioplasty: application for acute myocardial infarction. *Am J Cardiol*. 1984;53:117C–121C.

635. Grines CL, Browne KF, Marco J, et al. A comparison of immediate angioplasty with thrombolytic therapy for acute myocardial infarction. *N Engl J Med*. 1993;328:673–679.

636. Stone W, Grines CL, Browne KF, et al. Predictors of in-hospital and 6-month outcome after acute myocardial infarction in the reperfusion-era: the Primary Angioplasty in Myocardial Infarction (PAMI) trial. *J Am Coll Cardiol*. 1995;25:370–377.

Tim C. Rehders
Hüseyin Ince
Stephan Kische
Christoph A. Nienaber

CHAPTER **9**

Thoracic Aorta

ENDOVASCULAR TREATMENT OF AORTIC DISSECTION

Acute aortic dissection is an uncommon but potentially catastrophic illness that occurs with an incidence of approximately 2.9 per 100,000 per year with at least 7000 cases per year in the United States. Early mortality is as high as 1% per hour if untreated, but survival may be significantly improved by the timely institution of appropriate therapy. Prompt clinical recognition and definitive diagnostic testing are therefore essential in the management of patients with aortic dissection. Conventional treatment of *Stanford type A* (De Bakey type I and II; see Fig. 9-1) dissection consists of surgical reconstruction of the ascending aorta with complete or partial resection of the dissected aortic segment; thus in type A dissections interventional endovascular strategies have no clinical application except to relieve critical malperfusion prior to surgery of the ascending aorta by distal fenestration in cases of thoracoabdominal extension (De Bakey type I) and peripheral ischemic complications. Conversely, stent-graft placement aims at remodeling of the thoracic descending aorta typically in type B dissection by sealing one (or multiple) proximal entry tears with a Dacron-covered stent, thus initiating thrombosis of the false lumen.[1–4] In addition reconstruction of a collapsed true lumen might result in re-establishment of side-branch flow (Fig. 9-2). Various scenarios of malperfusion syndrome are amenable to endovascular management. These include static or dynamic (by intima invagination) collapse of the aortic true lumen (so called "pseudocoarctation"; Fig. 9-3), static or dynamic occlusion of one or more vital side branches (Fig. 9-4), or enlarging false aneurysm due to patent proximal entry tear.

Although peripheral pulse deficits can be acutely reversed with surgical repair of the dissected thoracic aorta in approximately 90%, patients with mesenteric or renal ischemia do not fare well. Mortality of patients with renal ischemia is 50% to 70% and as high as 87% with mesenteric ischemia.[5–7] Surgical mortality rates in patients with acute peripheral vascular ischemic complications are similar to those with mesenteric ischemia, reaching an 89% in-hospital mortality rate.[8–11] Operative mortality of surgical fenestration varies from 21% to 61%, which encouraged percutaneous interventional management by endovascular balloon fenestration of a dissecting aortic membrane to treat mesenteric ischemia, a concept discussed as a niche indication in such complicated cases of malperfusion.[10–12]

The interventional management of *Stanford type B* (De Bakey type III) dissection and the use of stent grafts evolved slowly in anticipation of the risk of paraplegia from spinal artery occlusion as seen in up to 18% after open surgery.[11,12] With further technical improvement a large series of cases has now been successfully treated in various specialized centers by endovascular stent-graft placement covering entry tears in the descending aorta and even in the aortic arch. Recent studies have demonstrated that closure of proximal entry tears is essential to reconstruct the aortic wall and reduce total aortic diameter. Entry tear closure promotes depressurization of false lumen, thrombus formation in the false lumen (Fig. 9-5), and remodeling of the entire aorta.[2,3,12] In the near future combined surgical and interventional procedures even for proximal dissection are likely to evolve.[13–15]

CURRENT INDICATIONS FOR FENESTRATION AND ENDOVASCULAR AORTIC REPAIR

The exact role of percutaneous fenestration and stent grafting in the treatment of *aortic dissection* is not fully established yet. There appears to be a role for interventional concepts in the treatment

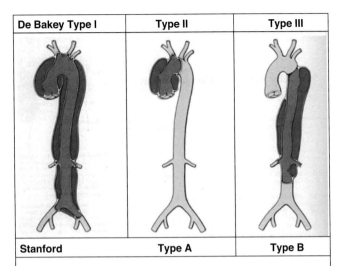

De Bakey Type I	Type II	Type III

Stanford	Type A	Type B

De Bakey

Type I   Originates in the ascending aorta, propagates at least to the
         aortic arch and often beyond it distally

Type II   Originates in and is confined to the ascending aorta

Type III Originates in the descending aorta and extends distally down the
         aorta or, rarely, retrograde into the aortic arch and ascending
         aorta

Stanford

Type A   All dissections involving the ascending aorta,
         regardless of the site of origin

Type B   All dissections not involving the ascending aorta

FIGURE 9-1. The most common classifications of thoracic aortic dissection: Stanford and De Bakey.

of static or dynamic obstruction of aortic branch arteries; static obstruction of a branch can be overcome by placing endovascular stents in the ostium of the compromised side branch, and dynamic obstruction may benefit from stents in the aortic true lumen with or without additional balloon fenestration or side-branch stenting. In classic aortic dissection, successful fenestration leaves true lumen pressure unchanged.[16] Sometimes bare stents deployed from the true lumen into side branches are useful to buttress the flap in a stable position.[17] In chronic dissection where fenestration of a fibrosed dissecting membrane may result in collapse of the connection between true and false lumen, a stent may be necessary to keep the fenestration open. A rare use of fenestration is to create a re-entry tear for the dead-end false lumen back into the true lumen with the aim to prevent thrombosis of the false lumen and compromise of branches fed exclusively from the false lumen or jointly from the false and true lumen, a concept, however, that lacks clinical proof of benefit. Conversely, fenestration may increase the long-term risk of aortic rupture because a large re-entry tear promotes flow in the false lumen and provides the basis for aneurysmal expansion of the false lumen. There is also a risk of peripheral embolism from a patent but partly thrombosed false lumen.[17,18]

The most effective method to exclude an enlarging and aneurysmal dilated false lumen is the sealing of proximal entry tears with a customized stent graft; the absence of a distal re-entry tear is desirable for optimal results but not a prerequisite. Adjunctive treatment by fenestration and/or ostial bare stents may help establish flow to compromised aortic branches. Compression of the true aortic lumen cranial to the main abdominal branches with distal malperfusion (so called pseudocoarctation) may also

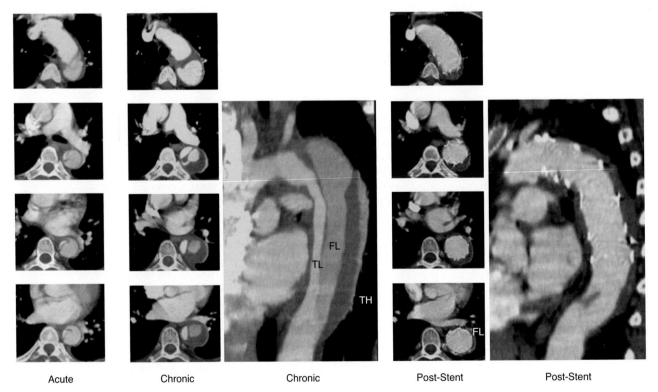

| Acute | Chronic | Chronic | Post-Stent | Post-Stent |

FIGURE 9-2. Type B aortic dissection in a 48-year-old man; note the dynamic obstruction of the true lumen (*TL*) in the acute phase. After stent-graft placement across the proximal thoracic entry, the entire true lumen of the thoracic aorta is reconstructed with time, with complete "healing" of the dissected aortic wall and shrinking of the completely thrombosed false lumen (*FL*). Other abbreviations: Th Thrombus.

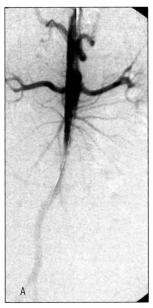
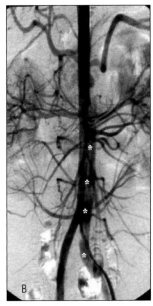

FIGURE 9-3. Digital subraction angiography in thoraco-abdominal type B dissection. **A:** Dynamic obstruction of the true lumen distally to the renal arteries causing malperfusion of the mesentery and both lower extremities. **B:** At follow-up (3 months after stent-graft placement in the proximal descending aorta) the true lumen has widened as a consequence of aortic remodeling and the patient is asymptomatic. However, the false lumen (white stars) in the abdominal aorta is not completely thrombosed.

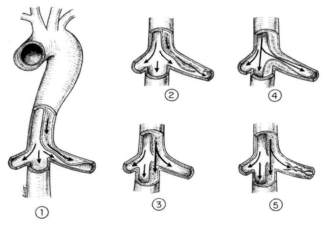

FIGURE 9-4. Possible variants of static or dynamic occlusion of aortic side branches in aortic dissection.

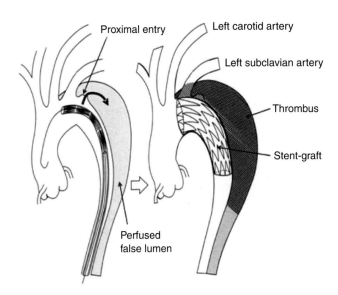

FIGURE 9-5. Concept of interventional reconstruction of the dissected aorta with sealing of the proximal entries, depressurization of the false lumen and initiation of false lumen thrombosis.

TABLE 9-1. Considerations for Surgical, Medical, and Interventional Therapy in Aortic Pathologies

- Surgery
  - Treatment of choice in acute type A dissection
  - Acute type B dissection complicated by the following:
    - Retrograde extension into the ascending aorta
    - Dissection in Marfan syndrome
    - Rupture or impending rupture (historically classic indication)
    - Progression with compromise of vital organs
- Medical therapy
  - Treatment of choice in *un*complicated type B dissection
  - Stable, isolated arch dissection
  - Stable type B dissection (chronic, ≥2 weeks of onset)
- Interventional therapy
  - Stent grafts to seal entry to false lumen of aortic dissection and to enlarge compressed true lumen
    - Complicated (unstable) type B dissection
    - Malperfusion syndrome (proximal aortic stent graft and/or distal fenestration/stenting of branch arteries)
    - Stable type B dissection (under study)
  - Stent grafts to exclude thoracic aortic aneurysm (≥5.5 cm)
  - Stent grafts to cover perforating aortic ulcers (especially deep, progressive ulcers)
  - Stent grafts to reconstruct the thoracic aorta after traumatic injury
  - Stent grafts as an emergency treatment of evolving or imminent aortic rupture

be corrected by stent grafts that enlarge the compressed true lumen and improve distal aortic blood flow.[2,3,10,12] Depressurization and shrinking of the false lumen is the most beneficial result to be gained, ideally followed by complete thrombosis of the false lumen and remodeling of the entire dissected aorta (Fig. 9-2), and in rare occasions even in retrograde type A dissection.[14] Similar to previously accepted indications for surgical intervention in complicated type B dissection, scenarios such as intractable pain with descending dissection, rapidly expanding false lumen diameter, extra-aortic blood collection as a sign of imminent rupture, or distal malperfusion syndrome are accepted indications for emergent stent-graft placement.[15,17–19] Moreover, late onset of complications such as malperfusion of vital aortic side branches may justify endovascular stent grafting of an occlusive lamella (or fenestration) to improve distal true lumen flow as a first option. Only after an unsuccessful attempt may surgery still be employed, considering that surgical repair failed to prove superior to interventional treatment even in uncomplicated cases; in complicated cases the concept of endoluminal treatment is currently replacing open surgery in advanced aortic centers.[1–3,17–20] A summary of treatment options is listed in Table 9-1.

TECHNIQUE OF AORTIC STENT-GRAFT PLACEMENT

Aortic stent grafts are primarily used to correct compression of the supplying true lumen cranial to major aortic branches and to increase distal flow. Moreover, proximal communications should be sealed to depressurize the false lumen, direct flow to the true lumen, and induce thrombosis in the false lumen with fibrotic transformation and subsequent remodeling of the aortic wall. Stent-graft placement across the origin of the celiac, superior mesenteric, and renal arteries is strongly discouraged for empiric reasons.

Based on the measurements obtained during angiography, transesophageal echocardiography (mandatory for detection of small entries), contrast-enhanced spiral CT scanning (best technique for unstable patients in an emergency situation), magnetic resonance angiogram (contraindicated for patients with pacemakers or implantable defibrillators), or intravascular ultrasound, customized stent grafts should be used in covering up to 20 cm (and sometimes even more) of dissected aorta and the major tear(s). The procedure is best performed in the catheterization and imaging laboratory using digital angiography and under general anesthesia. The femoral artery is the most popular access site and can usually accommodate a 24F stent-graft system. Using the Seldinger technique a 260-cm stiff wire is placed over a pigtail catheter navigated with a soft wire in the true lumen under both fluoroscopic and transesophageal ultrasound guidance. In complex cases with multiple re-entries in the abdominal aorta, the "embracement technique" with the use of two pigtail catheters is useful (Fig. 9-6). A pigtail catheter that has been installed in the true aortic lumen via the left brachial artery picks up the femoral pigtail catheter in the true lumen of the abdominal aorta and pulls it up into the aortic arch. This procedure ensures definite positioning of the stiff guide wire in the true lumen, which is essential for correct deployment of the stent graft. Carefully advanced over the stiff wire, the launching of the

stent-graft is performed with systolic blood pressure briefly lowered to 50 to 60 mm Hg by infusing sodium nitroprusside to prevent dislodgement.[21] After deployment, short inflation of a latex balloon may be used to improve apposition of the stent struts to the aortic wall, but only if proximal sealing of thoracic communications is incomplete. Both Doppler ultrasound and contrast fluoroscopy are instrumental for documenting the immediate result or initiating adjunctive maneuvers. For thoracic aortic aneurysm or ulcers, the navigation of wires and instruments is markedly easier, but meticulous imaging using ultrasound and fluoroscopy simultaneously is equally important. A frequent anatomical consideration is the close vicinity between the origin of the left subclavian artery (LSA) and the primary tear in type B dissections. For this reason complete coverage of the ostium to the LSA has to be accepted at times to perform endovascular aortic repair in this aortic pathology adjacent to the LSA. According to observational evidence, prophylactic surgical maneuvers are not imperatively required for safety reasons, but may be relegated to an elective measure after an endovascular aortic intervention when intolerable signs or symptoms of ischemia occur.[22] However, prior to intentional LSA occlusion, careful attention has to be paid to potential supra-aortic variants (e.g., presence of a lusorian artery, a nonintact vertebral-basilar system, or vertebral arteries, which originate directly from the aortic arch) and pathologies detected in the course of preinterventional imaging.

INTERVENTIONAL THERAPY IN AN ELECTIVE SETTING

With the use of bare stents in aortic side branches and sometimes performance of fenestrating maneuvers, compromised flow can be restored in >90% (range 92% to 100%) of vessels obstructed from aortic dissection. The average 30 day mortality rate is 10% (range 0% to 25%) and additional surgical revascularization is rarely needed.[23] Most patients remain asymptomatic over a mean follow-up time of about 1 year. Fatalities related to the interventional procedure may occur as a result of nonreversible ischemic complications, progression of the dissection, or complications of additional reconstructive surgical procedures on the thoracic aorta.[1–3,17,20] Potential problems may arise from unpredictable hemodynamic alterations in the true and false lumen after fenestration and side-branch stenting. These alterations can result in loss of previously well-perfused arteries, or in loss of initially salvaged side branches.

Recent reports suggest that percutaneous stent-graft placement in the dissected aorta is safer and produces better results than surgery for type B dissection. Paraplegia may occur after use of multiple stent grafts but still appears to be a rare phenomenon, especially when the stented segment does not exceed 16 cm. Results of short-term follow-up are excellent with a 1-year survival rate of >90%; tears can be readapted and aortic diameters generally decrease with complete thrombosis of the false lumen. This suggests that stent placement may facilitate healing of the dissection, sometimes of the entire aorta, including abdominal segments (Fig. 9-2). However, late reperfusion of the false lumen has been observed occasionally, underlining the need for stringent MR or CT follow-up imaging. Therefore postinterventional imaging should be done 3 months and 12 months after the procedure, followed by further examinations in yearly intervals. In some patients, follow-up imaging has revealed tears that had initially been overlooked, but required additional stents.

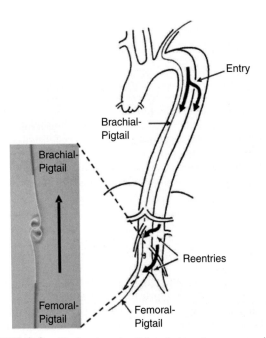

FIGURE 9-6. "Embracing pigtails" technique to ensure navigation of the guidewire in the true lumen before stent-graft placement.

INTERVENTIONAL THERAPY IN AN EMERGENT SETTING

Recently, inclusion criteria for endovascular treatment of acute type B aortic dissection have been reported by Shimono et al.[24]; in our opinion the following criteria should apply when an emergent stent-graft placement is considered:

1. Identification of a least one patent primary entry tear in the descending thoracic aorta
2. Major tear located in the descending aorta proximal to the 10th thoracic vertebra
3. Absence of severe dilatation (>38 mm in diameter) and/or severe atherosclerotic alterations in the landing zone for stent grafting
4. Exclusion of severe aortic regurgitation
5. Exclusion of coronary artery or aortic arch branch ischemia
6. Femoral and iliac arteries of sufficient size and quality (absence of kinking or significant stenosis) to permit passage of at least a 22F catheter (vessel diameter ≥7.5 mm).

Few cases of emergent stent-graft placement have been so far described. We have recently reported a series of 11 patients treated by emergent endovascular aortic repair of dissection and compared with historic-matched control patients subjected to conventional therapy. All the patients had acute type B aortic dissection complicated by loss of blood into the periaortic space. All procedures were performed successfully with no evidence of periprocedural morbidity, aborted leakage, and ensured reconstruction of the dissected aorta; at a mean follow up of 15 ± 6 months, no deaths were seen in the stent-graft group, whereas four patients had died with conventional treatment. Also, as previously seen in elective endovascular procedures, emergent aortic dissection stent grafting was not associated with excessive peripheral or neurological complications.[18]

Nevertheless, whereas patients who suffer from postsurgery aortic dissection and receive stent grafting seem to show better outcome than those in whom a second surgical intervention is attempted,[25] endovascular repair in impending rupture or para-aortic leakage has not yet proved to be always effective.

ENDOVASCULAR TREATMENT OF TRUE ANEURYSMS IN THE THORACIC AORTA

INTRODUCTION

Thoracic aortic aneurysms (TAAs) are uncommon compared to infrarenal abdominal aortic aneurysms, composing no more than 2% to 5% of the total spectrum of degenerative aortic aneurysms. We must recognize the inherent bias of data from university referral-center populations, and only a few reports exist from population-based studies or investigations based on autopsy. The reported incidence of TAAs in population-based studies is between 5.9% and 10.4% per 100,000 person-years. TAAs may involve one or more aortic segments (aortic root, ascending aorta, arch, or descending aorta) and are classified accordingly. Sixty percent of thoracic aortic aneurysms involve the aortic root and/or ascending aorta, 40% the descending aorta, 10% the arch, and 10% show a thoracoabdominal extension (involving >1 segment). Etiology, natural history, and treatment of thoracic aneurysms differ for each of these segments.[26]

The natural history of thoracic aortic aneurysms is not yet well defined. One reason for this is that both etiology and location of an aneurysm may have an impact on its growth rate and propensity for dissection or rupture. A second reason is that it is rare, in the era of modern imaging, to actually allow a known aneurysm to grow until rupture, because surgery is usually performed when aneurysms are just large enough to be considered at significant risk for rupture. When patients with large aneurysms do not undergo surgery, they are usually elderly or have important comorbidities, thus increasing their mortality, irrespective of the aneurysm.

From longitudinal observation, Davies et al.[27] found that the average rate of growth for thoracic aneurysms is 0.1 centimeter per year. The rate of growth, however, was greater in aneurysms of the descending than ascending aorta, greater for dissected than nondissected aneurysms, and higher in patients with Marfan syndrome than in non-Marfan patients. Initial size is an important predictor of the growth rate in thoracic aneurysms. However, even controlling for initial aneurysm size, there is still substantial variation,[28] thus making it difficult to prospectively predict growth for a given aneurysm. With regard to aneurysm size and the risk of rupture or dissection, Davies et al.[27] found an annual rate of 2% at a diameter of <5 cm, 3% for aneurysms between 5 and 5.9 cm, and 7% for aneurysms ≥6 cm in diameter. Therefore, the risk appears to rise exponentially as thoracic aneurysms reach a size of 6 cm.

An alternative approach for the repair of descending thoracic aneurysms is the use of transluminally placed endovascular stent grafts (Fig. 9-7). This technique has the advantage of a nonsurgical procedure, with potentially fewer postoperative complications and lower morbidity. Ellozy et al.[29] recently reported a series of 84 patients receiving endovascular stent grafts to treat descending thoracic aortic aneurysms. Primary technical success was achieved in 90%, and successful exclusion of the aneurysm was achieved in 82%. However, major procedure-related or device-related complications occurred in 38%, including proximal attachment failure (8%), distal attachment failure (6%), mechanical device failure (3%), periprocedural death (6%), and late aneurysm rupture (6%). More encouraging was the fact that only 3% suffered persistent neurological complications. In addition, a preliminary series from our institution demonstrated a promising potential of endovascular stent-graft treatment for patients with late aneurysm formation after complex surgical repair of coarctation.[30] Compared with open surgical repair, endovascular stent grafting does appear to have low perioperative morbidity and mortality; nevertheless but clearly, technical refinements and miniaturization of the housing are awaited for before use as a routine treatment for any aneurysm. At present, it is best reserved for those with ideal aortic anatomy or who are poor surgical candidates.

PATIENT SELECTION CRITERIA

Patients considered suitable for endovascular treatment of a thoracic aneurysm have a proximal and distal segment of relatively normal aorta for fixation with satisfactory seal. These regions are often referred to as "attachment/landing zones" or "aortic neck" and should ideally encompass >15 mm free of aortic wall atheroma or thrombus. Access vessels must be evaluated for size and tortuosity to accommodate the stent-graft delivery system. Patient renal function should be assessed and, if abnormal, precautions to prevent contrast-induced nephropathy

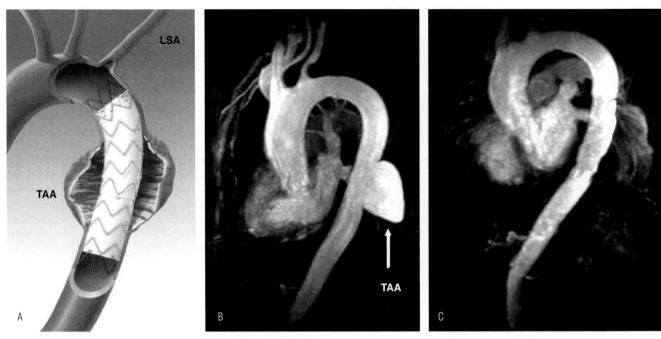

FIGURE 9-7.   **A:** Diagram of endovascular stent-graft implantation into a true aneurysm in the descending thoracic aorta. **B:** MR angiogram displaying a saccular aortic aneurysm. **C:** MR angiogram after stent-graft placement. The aneurysm is completely thrombosed and there is no evidence for any kind of endoleakage. *LSA,* left subclavian artery; *TAA,* true aortic aneurysm.

should be implemented. Features unfavorable for endovascular aortic repair (EVAR) in the thoracic aorta include severe aortic angulation or tortuosity, friable atheroma or thrombus lining the aortic wall (risk of embolization), and aneurysmal involvement of the ascending aorta or arch. The risk of postoperative paraplegia appears to be increased in patients with extensive thoracic aneurysms or aneurysms of both the thoracic and infrarenal aorta necessitating experimental side-branched devices. For aneurysms in the proximal segments of the descending aorta, proximity to the arch vessels makes placement of the endograft more difficult. The proximal attachment of the stent graft might necessitate intentional coverage of the ostium of the left subclavian artery. To minimize patient morbidity, it is vital to properly select patients without anomalous arch vessels (i.e., direct left vertebral branch from the aortic arch, lusorian artery) or a left internal mammary coronary bypass graft.[22] Thus, with appropriate precaution, overstenting of the LSA can be performed in most cases and vascular surgeries, if needed, can usually be performed later electively. Rarely, special surgical techniques are required *before* stent-graft deployment within the aortic arch (i.e., surgical transposition of left carotid and/or truncus brachiocephalicus).

ANATOMIC MEASUREMENTS BEFORE EVAR

The main features of the thoracic aorta derived from CT/MR scanning and other imaging include the shape and size of the thoracic aneurysm (diameter and length) and the condition of the aortic wall (atheroma, calcification, thrombus) as well as vascular angulation or tortuosity. Important measurements as part of preinterventional planning include length and maximal diameter of the TAA and length and diameter of the proximal and distal attachment zone. A diameter is measured in a horizontal plane perpendicular to the longitudinal axis of the aorta. One option is to measure to the external wall contour of the vessel in order to guarantee some degree of oversizing, which is considered desirable for prevention of type I endoleaks. An endoleak is a condition associated with endovascular stent grafts, defined by persisting blood flow outside the lumen of the stent graft but within the aneurysm sac or adjacent vascular segment being treated by the stent graft. An endoleak is evidence of incomplete exclusion of the aneurysm from the circulation and may resolve spontaneously. However, a proportion of those that do persist are associated with late aneurysm rupture.

An endoleak can be classified according to the time of occurrence. An endoleak first observed during the perioperative (<30 days) period is defined as a "primary endoleak," and one detected thereafter is termed a "secondary endoleak." Further categorization requires precise information regarding the course of blood flow in to the aneurysm sac:

A *Type I* endoleak is indicative of a persistent perigraft channel of blood flow caused by inadequate seal at either the proximal (Ia) or distal (Ib) stent-graft end or attachment zones.

A *Type II* endoleak is attributed to retrograde flow into the aneurysmal sac via aortic side branches.

A *Type III* endoleak is caused by component disconnection (IIIa) or fabric tear, fabric disruption, or graft disintegration (IIIb). A Type IIIb endoleak can be further stratified as minor (<2 mm) or major (>2 mm).

A *Type IV* endoleak is caused by blood flow through an intact but otherwise porous fabric, observed during the first 30 days after stent-graft implantation. This designation is not applicable to fabric-related endoleaks observed after the first 30-day period.

If an endoleak is visualized on imaging studies but the precise source cannot be determined, the endoleak is categorized as an endoleak of undefined origin. Endoleaks may be managed by (a) observation (especially type II and IV), (b) further endovascular procedure (e.g., balloon inflation and/or implantation of an additional stent graft, especially type I and III), or (c) conversion to open surgery (if further endovascular maneuvers fail to achieve complete exclusion of the aneurysm from circulation resulting in an increase of TAA diameter).

It has been observed that measurements of aortic diameter obtained from CT/MR scans are generally 10% to 30% larger than the corresponding measurement obtained from aortography. This is partly because the cross-sectional image will typically be measured to the adventitial surface of the vessel, whereas the angiographic measurement will show the luminal diameter. In addition, cross-sectional slices of the aorta will often transect the aorta obliquely, resulting in an ovoid shape, with two different diameters, the smaller of which is true. Computer programs are available that calculate a center line for the aorta and give a tangential plane through the aorta (aortic slice) to overcome potential errors. Calculation of these diameter measurements is aided by 3D reconstructions; regions of angulation and irregularity are shown more clearly, allowing realistic measurements of preferred sites for stent-graft placement. It is important that the operating interventionalist be directly involved in performing the correct anatomic measurements at the CT/MR work station. Magnetic resonance imaging and spiral CT scanning are equivalent for aortic imaging. However, there are certain contraindications for both techniques, which have been previously described.

DEVICE SIZING

There is a fundamental difference between thoracic endograft procedures and endoluminal procedures in the abdominal aorta, where it is generally considered best to line the entire aortic wall from just below the lowest renal artery down to the iliac artery bifurcations. For the thoracic aorta the intention is to fully exclude the aneurysm but not necessarily cover the entire aorta from the arch to the celiac trunk. It is generally agreed that the ends of an endovascular graft device should be oversized relative to the diameters of the proximal and distal landing zones, but no quantitative consensus has been reached so far. The instructions for use of commercial devices usually recommend oversizing around 10%. In some clinical reports of thoracic endograft series an oversizing of 20% to 30% was applied,[31,32] which may give a better seal, but can in rare instances set the stage for proximal device-induced dissection.[33–35] Moreover, imaging studies have demonstrated that with increased oversizing Gianturco stents cause greater infolding of the stent-graft material, which may leave furrows along the side of the graft, causing an endoleak or endotension. It is appreciated that a TAA can continue to enlarge after endovascular repair even in the absence of a detectable endoleak, and that this enlargement may lead to aneurysm rupture. This phenomenon is currently indicated as "endotension" and can be defined as a persistent or recurrent pressurization of the aortic aneurysm sac after endovascular repair. Currently the term *endotension* is still considered an investigative term because disagreement persists regarding its precise definition, appropriate usage, and current applicability.

Postdeployment ballooning creates more folds but of smaller size. Hooks and barbs in some devices may cause unequal distribution of folds.[36] In addition, if the neck is longer than the stent struts, a sufficient seal should be achieved at the end of the V-shaped end of the stent. However, if the neck is shorter, a direct communication may exist from above to the aneurysm sac. With increasing calcification of the aorta, oversizing will cause greater infolding of the Gianturco stent as opposed to a more compliant vessel.[36] Undersizing is also associated with prompt inadequate seal and possible loss of seal with neck expansion. The usual recommendation concerning the length of the attachment zones is a minimum of 15 mm, with lengths up to 30 to 40 mm in selected cases. Clinical experience with the Cook thoracic device has shown a higher incidence of complications when the attachment zone is shorter than 20 mm (personal communication). Similar results have also been reported with other devices.[37]

The length of device required might also depend on whether the length measurements are made along the greater or lesser curves of an angulated vessel. When two stent grafts are necessary in the overlapped or "telescope" technique, the amount of overlap should probably be a minimum of 30 mm in straight anatomic segments, and up to 50 mm or more in angulated or curved segments of the aorta. There is a tendency for the graft to move out toward the greater curve of the aneurysmatic aortic segment due to hemodynamic forces, which may result in distraction or migration of the modular component grafts. This may be a particular problem within large aneurysmatic aortic sacs.

ENDOVASCULAR TREATMENT OF COARCTATION IN ADULTS

INTRODUCTION

Coarctation of the aorta occurs in 8% of patients with congenital heart disease and is associated with higher morbidity due to coronary and cerebrovascular disease, thus limiting life expectancy to around 50 years of age if left untreated.[38–40] Surgical repair used to be the standard of care and surgically repaired coarctation of the aorta was regarded a benign condition with a definitive cure. Not even considering intraoperative mortality, it has been recognized, however, that morbidity and mortality tend to be premature in adolescent patients, who even after successful surgery reach only 38 years on average. Late postsurgical problems are caused by recoarctation, late aneurysm formation, potential rupture, and premature advanced vascular disease. With recoarctation ranging from 5% to 50%, resection of coarctation and end-to end repair became the method of choice in the young patient group,[41–43] whereas late formation of false aneurysm was often observed in adult patients undergoing any type of patch repair, in conjunction with a high likelihood of sustained and difficult-to-treat hypertension.[43–46]

Against this drawback interventional techniques were developed for transcatheter treatment of *simple* (without presence of other important intracardiac anomalies) and significant coarctation initially using simple balloon angioplasty.[47–51] One definition of *significant* coarctation requires a mean pressure gradient greater than 20 mm Hg across the coarctation site at angiography with or without proximal systemic hypertension. A second definition requires the presence of proximal hypertension in the company of echocardiographic or angiographic evidence of aortic coarctation (degree of stenosis >50%). Sustained removal of transcoarctation gradients requires disruption of both intimal and medial layers.[52] In about 5% to 20% of cases recoil following balloon dilatation may lead to aneurysm formation and occasionally to catastrophic full or contained rupture.[53] Nevertheless, long-term outcome appears similar to that after surgery.[47,54–56]

More recently, endovascular stents have been used to treat coarctation[57–66] in an attempt to overcome the elastic recoil properties of the aortic wall. A recent, detailed report emphasized the use of stents especially in discrete coarctation if plain balloon angioplasty failed to abolish the gradient completely.[63] The published experience provides ample evidence that stents may reduce trauma to the vessel wall by dispersing radial forces over a larger area, controlling small dissections, and avoiding aneurysm formation.[67] Generally excellent results have been reported with clinical success rates including abolished translesional gradients in >95% of cases, no significant restenosis rates, and no reported death. However, in a few cases emergency surgery was required. In addition, although short to mid-term results are excellent, the long-term outcome of stent placement in children and adolescents remains less certain. In the young the implanted stents could interfere with the normal growth and development of the aorta. Recently, successful primary use of newly designed balloon-expandable platinum stents to treat anatomically suitable aortic coarctation in the young was reported.[68] These new stents appear to provide uniform aortic wall scaffolding without vessel disruption, while allowing later postdilation if required during the aortic growth without significant stent shortening. If these initial results are confirmed, endovascular repair might become a viable alternative to open surgical repair even in children, with the acceptable drawback of minor interventions required to perform interim postdilations to accommodate the aortic growth. The potentials of the early endovascular repair hold promise not only to avoid late complications of hypertension but also to avoid surgical complications and reoperations.[30,63,69] Nevertheless, at present it appears that for tubular coarctation and hypoplastic arches surgery will likely remain the primary treatment option.

PATIENT SELECTION

The adverse natural history of untreated coarctation means that surgical or endovascular intervention is warranted in all but the mildest forms of coarctation. Hypertension is usually severe and unresponsive to medical therapy. The benefit and appropriate threshold for intervention is less clear in patients with moderate coarctation, which usually occurs in the context of previous surgical repair. Such patients often have significant resting hypertension or may only exhibit hypertension during exercise. Doppler assessment of the repair site usually demonstrates a high peak velocity, but only a mild or absent diastolic tail may be present. However, despite relatively normal peripheral blood pressures, a number of these patients have persistent left ventricular hypertrophy. Ambulatory blood-pressure monitoring may help to identify the true incidence of hypertension and loss of diurnal blood pressure variability, both being important negative prognostic indicators for late complications of hypertension. Therefore, the current reliance on peripheral blood pressure measurements must be considered a major limitation of current clinical practice.[70] In addition, Mahadevan et al. have recently demonstrated marked augmentation of the central systolic waveform in young patients with coarctation that significantly improves after stenting.[71] These observations seem to confirm O'Rourke's statement[72] that hypertension in patients with coarctation may be more harmful than in other hypertensive states.

Before endovascular management of aortic coarctation is considered, each patient requires a detailed assessment of the anatomy and physiology of the obstruction. In addition, intracardiac malformations and anomalies must be excluded. In our practice, standard clinical workup includes physical examination, blood pressure measurements in all four extremities, ambulatory blood pressure measurement, exercise stress test, detailed echocardiographic examination, and cardiac magnetic resonance scan including gadolinium enhanced angiography. A three-dimensional image reconstruction allows the operator to appreciate the alignment, tortuosity, and exact morphology of the narrowed segment as well as the topographic relationship to other vessels and surrounding structures (Fig. 9-8). In addition, the aortic size proximal and distal to the coarctation is accurately measured. Severity of the coarctation and presence of isthmus hypolasia do not contraindicate an endovascular

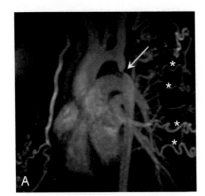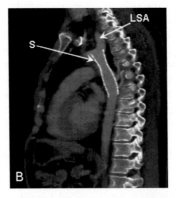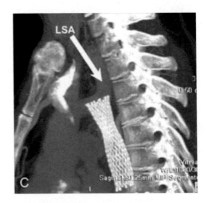

FIGURE 9-8. A: Preinterventional MRA (in maximum intensity projection) in a male patient with severe native aortic coarctation (*arrow*) and numerous large collateral vessels (*asterisks*). **B:** Reconstruction of postinterventional CT angiogram in sagittal plane shows a marked improvement in luminal diameter with no evidence of aortic dissection. **C:** Postinterventional CT angiogram (in maximum intensity projection) displays the implanted stent in detail. *C,* aortic coarctation; *LSA,* left subclavian artery; *S,* stent.

approach. However, in patients over 50 years old with calcified aorta, stenting may be technically difficult, particularly when the aorta is also extremely tortuous and malaligned. Close proximity to the left subclavian artery does not preclude stenting, and the proximal end of the stent may be positioned within the transverse segment of the aortic arch. However, placement of a covered stent across the ostium of the left subclavian artery should be avoided wherever possible. Although overstenting of the subclavian artery ostium has been frequently done in endovascular management of aortic aneurysms,[22] it might be contraproductive in patients with coarctation because of the presence of collaterals not affected by stent insertion.

EXECUTION OF THE PROCEDURE, RISKS, AND POTENTIAL COMPLICATIONS

As with all interventional procedures, careful planning and execution by experienced operators can reduce the risk of procedural complications. The procedure is usually performed using two arterial access sites: a right radial or brachial access with a 6F sheath for the placement of a pigtail catheter in the aortic arch, and a femoral access for insertion of the interventional devices. Accurate trans-stenotic gradient is measured and aortography is performed, usually in LAO 45-degree projection (no cranial/caudal angulation). The aortic anatomy before and after coarctation need to be carefully examined, and accurate sizing of the posterior arch can be done with a digital reference system using the baseline angiogram. If possible, we prefer primary placement of a self-expandable stent followed by balloon inflation within the stent segment. The balloon should only be gently inflated to low pressure values (4 to 6 bar). Relevant residual stenosis will eventually lead to further attempts to reduce the pressure gradient with bigger balloons. Finally, the postangioplasty gradient and a last aortic angiogram should be recorded.

The most important complications are acute rupture or extensive dissection of the aortic wall (some degree of dissection is inevitable). Although there were no deaths in the reported series, aortic rupture resulting in death of the patient has recently been reported from an experienced center.[73] In addition, two further cases of procedural deaths have been reported,[71] as well as a case where aortic rupture was successfully treated by immediate placement of a stent graft. Interestingly, in all these instances, postdilatation of the stent appears to have precipitated the rupture of the aorta with its attendant consequences. Patient's age appears to be an important risk factor for major complications, particularly if the aorta is calcified. Oversizing of balloons should be avoided, and our practice is not to try and flare the ends of the stent to fully oppose it to the aortic wall, as this often requires the use of a larger balloon. Whether an incomplete apposition of the stent at the proximal and distal ends will be of any long-term consequence is unknown at present. Balloon-expandable covered stents are currently being developed that might reduce procedural complications, although at the expense of additional complexity and larger sheath size. Although there are some data to show that redilatation of stents is feasible in young adults,[50] the safety of such procedures in older patients is not known. Other complications include stent displacement, particularly in patients with moderate coarctation and poor collateral formation. This can be minimized by use of stiff guidewires and rapid stent deployment under controlled hypotension. In

these patients, we would avoid the use of covered stents, which if displaced might occlude important visceral branches. The incidence of femoral artery complications has been reduced by using closure devices, and immediate hemostasis is almost always achieved even in heparinized patients.

The potential for major complications mandates that endovascular procedures for aortic coarctation should only be performed in major centers with appropriate institutional and operator experience. Appropriate Dacron-covered stent-grafts should be immediately available in the event of aortic rupture or dissection with on-site thoracic surgical backup.

LONG-TERM OUTCOME

More than 300 cases of stenting for aortic coarctation have now been reported in case series.[57–60,62,63,74–78] These series have all reported high rates of procedural success with almost complete abolition of resting gradients and improved hypertension control. Consistent with surgical series, a proportion of patients will still require antihypertensive medication. The actual proportion will depend on the target blood pressure and the vigor with which it is pursued. In our practice, we aim to achieve a blood pressure normal for the patient's age rather than using standard thresholds for treatment derived from older populations of patients with idiopathic hypertension. Although this is more effectively achieved following stenting, the majority of patients will still require antihypertensive medication. There are few data on the long-term outcome following endovascular management of aortic coarctation. Marshall et al.[59] reported a decrease in left ventricular end diastolic pressure after stenting for mild residual or recurrent aortic coarctation. However, this was in a small patient series, and further data are necessary to see whether these translate into prognostic benefit.

The importance of assessing the hemodynamic efficacy of different treatment strategies for aortic coarctation and the limitations of simple peripheral blood pressure measurements is emphasized by a recent animal study. Morita et al.[79] studied the effect of ligation of the aortic arch distal to the left subclavian and extra-anatomic ascending to descending aortic bypass with a noncompliant Dacron graft in six dogs. There was no change in cardiac output or mean blood pressure with a modest 25% increase in systolic blood pressure. However, impedance increased by 255%, suggesting a marked increase in systemic afterload. Interestingly, introduction of an air chamber into the graft, to increase its compliance, almost completely ameliorated the increase in impedance. These data emphasize the need to assess the overall hemodynamic performance of the repair as part of a coupled pulsatile system, and its impact on associated abnormalities of vascular function. This is particularly important for older patients undergoing endovascular stenting of coarctation, where the introduction of a rigid stent into the circulation might have adverse hemodynamic effects and potentially offset the short-term gain from a less invasive procedure. In healthy animals, Pihkala et al.[80] have reported no adverse impact of introduction of a rigid stent on vascular impedance, but this does not imply a satisfactory outcome in humans with aortic coarctation, where additional factors including, length of stent used, residual waist, hypoplasia of the transverse arch and isthmus, collaterals, and generalized abnormalities of vascular function will all determine the long-term effectiveness of this approach.

ENDOVASCULAR MANAGEMENT OF AORTIC ANEURYSM

Although restenosis does not appear to be a major concern, the development of aneurysms due to vascular damage may occur at the site of the stent implantation. In a recent series,[60] the incidence was as high as 17%, though our current experience suggests a much lower incidence. These aneurysms are generally small and do not progress. Neither plain radiography nor echocardiography have a high enough sensitivity to detect all aneurysms. We routinely perform a contrast-enhanced CT at 6 weeks with repeat angiography and magnetic resonance scan at 9 months poststenting. Large aortic aneurysms are more frequently encountered following surgical repair of aortic coarctation, particularly following angioplastic repairs utilizing a Dacron patch. The prognosis from these aneurysms appears to be poor, and they often will require reintervention. We and others have had some success in treating these using endovascular stent grafts.[30,81] These self-expanding devices are rapidly evolving but still require large introducer sheaths (up to 24F) necessitating surgical access. Although the endovascular approach may avoid the need for difficult thoracic surgery, the long-term durability of stent grafts is not known and their use in young patients, who may need an effective graft for 50 years or more, remains unproven at this stage.

REFERENCES

1. Ince H, Nienaber CA. The concept of interventional therapy in acute aortic syndrome. J Card Surg. 2002;17:135–142.
2. Nienaber CA, Fattori R, Lund G, et al. Nonsurgical reconstruction of thoracic aortic dissection by stent-graft placement. N Engl J Med. 1999;340:1539–1545.
3. Dake MD, Kato N, Mitchell RS, et al. Endovascular stent-graft placement for the treatment of acute aortic dissection. N Engl J Med. 1999;340:1546–1552.
4. Walkers PJ, Miller DC. Aneurysmal and ischemic complications of type B (type III) aortic dissections. Semin Vasc Surg. 1992;5:198–214.
5. Bossone E, Rampoldi V, Nienaber CA, et al. Usefulness of pulse deficit to predict in-hospital complications and mortality in patients with acute type A aortic dissection. Am J Cardiol. 2002;89:851–855.
6. Cambria RP, Brewster DC, Gertler J, et al. Vascular complications associated with spontaneous aortic dissection. J Vasc Surg. 1988;7:199–209.
7. Laas J, Heinemann M, Schaefers HJ, et al. Management of thoracoabdominal malperfusion in aortic dissection. Circulation. 1991;84:20–24.
8. Miller DC. The continuing dilemma concerning medical versus surgical management of patients with acute type B dissections. Semin Thorac Cardiovasc Surg. 1993;5:33–46.
9. Miller DC, Mitchell RS, Oyer PE, et al. Independent determinants of operative mortality for patients with aortic dissections. Circulation. 1984;70:153–164.
10. Elefteriades JA, Hartleroad J, Gusberg RJ, et al. Long-term experience with descending aortic dissection: the complication-specific approach. Ann Thorac Surg. 1992;53:11–20.
11. Walker PJ, Dake MD, Mitchell RS, et al. The use of endovascular techniques for the treatment of complications of aortic dissection. J Vasc Surg. 1993;18:1042–1051.
12. Fann JI, Sarris GE, Mitchell RS, et al. Treatment of patients with aortic dissection presenting with peripheral vascular complications. Ann Surg. 1990;212:705–713.
13. Yano H, Ishimaru S, Kawaguchi S, et al. Endovascular stent-grafting of the descending thoracic aorta after arch repair in acute type A dissection. Ann Thorac Surg. 2002;73:288–291.
14. Kato N, Shimono T, Hirano T, et al. Transluminal placement of endovascular stent-grafts for the treatment of type A aortic dissection with an entry tear in the descending thoracic aorta. J Vasc Surg. 2001;34:1023–1028.
15. Iannelli G, Piscione F, Di Tommaso L, et al. Thoracic aortic emergencies: impact of endovascular surgery. Ann Thorac Surg. 2004;77:591–596.
16. Saito S, Arai H, Kim K, et al. Percutaneous fenestration of dissecting intima with a transseptal needle. A new therapeutic technique for visceral ischemia complicating acute aortic dissection. Cathet Cardiovasc Diagn. 1992, 26:130–135.
17. Nienaber CA, Ince H, Petzsch M, et al. Endovascular treatment of thoracic aortic dissection and its variants. Acta Chir Belg. 2002;102:292–298.
18. Nienaber CA, Ince H, Weber F, et al. Emergency stent-graft placement in thoracic aortic dissection and evolving rupture. J Card Surg. 2003;18:464–470.
19. Beregi JP, Haulon S, Otal P, et al. Endovascular treatment of acute complications associated with aortic dissection: midterm results from a multicenter study. J Endovasc Ther. 2003;10:486–493.
20. Bortone AS, Schena S, D'Agostino D, et al. Immediate versus delayed endovascular treatment of post-traumatic aortic pseudoaneurysms and type B dissections: retrospective analysis and premises to the upcoming European trial. Circulation. 2002;106:234–240.
21. Knobelsdorff G, Hoppner RM, Tonner PH, et al. Induced arterial hypotension for interventional thoracic aortic stent-graft placement: impact on intracranial haemodynamics and cognitive function. Eur J Anaesthesiol. 2003;20:134–140.
22. Rehders TC, Petzsch M, Ince H, et al. Intentional occlusion of the left subclavian artery during endovascular stent-graft implantation in the thoracic aorta: risk and relevance. J Endovasc Ther. 2004;11:659–666.
23. Slonim SM, Nyman U, Semba CP, et al. Aortic dissection: percutaneous management of ischemic complications with endovascular stents and balloon fenestration. J Vasc Surg. 1996;23:241–251.
24. Shimono T, Kato N, Yasuda F, et al. Transluminal stent-graft placement for the treatments of acute onset and chronic aortic dissections. Circulation. 2002;106:241–247.
25. Pansini S, Gagliardotto PV, Pompei E, et al. Early and late risk factors in surgical treatment of acute type A aortic dissection. Ann Thorac Surg. 1998;66:779–784.
26. Isselbacher EM. Thoracic and abdominal aortic aneurysms. Circulation. 2005;111:816–828.
27. Davies RR, Goldstein LJ, Coady MA, et al. Yearly rupture or dissection rates for thoracic aortic aneurysms: simple prediction based on size. Ann Thorac Surg. 2002;73:17–28.
28. Dapunt OE, Galla JD, Sadeghi AM, et al. The natural history of thoracic aortic aneurysms. J Thorac Cardiovasc Surg. 1994;107:1323–1332.
29. Ellozy SH, Carroccio A, Minor M, et al. Challenges of endovascular tube graft repair of thoracic aortic aneurysm: midterm follow-up and lessons learned. J Vasc Surg. 2003;38:676–683.
30. Ince H, Petzsch M, Rehders T, et al. Percutaneous endovascular repair of aneurysm after previous coarctation surgery. Circulation. 2003;108:2967–2970.
31. Bergeron P, De Chaumaray T, Gay J, et al. Endovascular treatment of thoracic aneurysms. J Cardiovasc Surg. 2003;44:349–361.
32. Wyers MC, Fillinger MF, Schermerhorn ML, et al. Endovascular repair of abdominal aortic aneurysm without preoperative arteriography. J Vasc Surg. 2003;38:730–738.
33. Mohan IV, Laheij RJ, Harris PL, et al. Risk factors for endoleak and the evidence for stent-graft oversizing in patients undergoing endovascular aneurysm repair. Eur J Vasc Endovasc Surg. 2001;21:344–349.
34. Sternbergh W 3rd, Money SR, Greenberg RK, et al. Influence of endograft oversizing on device migration, endoleak, aneurysm shrinkage, and aortic neck dilation: results from the Zenith Multicentre Trial. J Vasc Surg. 2004;39:20–26.
35. Conners MS 3rd, Sternbergh WC 3rd, Carter G, et al. Endograft migration one to four years after endovascular abdominal aortic repair with the AneuRx device: a cautionary note. J Vasc Surg. 2002;36:476–484.
36. Schurink GW, Aarts NJ, van Baalen JM, et al. Stent attachment site-related endoleakage after stent graft treatment; an in vitro study of the effects of graft size, stent type, and atherosclerotic wall changes. J Vasc Surg. 1999;30:658–667.
37. Dake MD, Miller DC, Mitchell RS, et al. The "first generation" of endovascular stent-grafts for patients with aneurysms of the descending thoracic aorta. J Thorac Cardiovasc Surg. 1998;116:689–704.
38. Campbell M. Natural history of coarctation of the aorta. Br Heart J. 1970;32:633–640.
39. Fyler DC, Buckley LP, Hellenbrand WE, et al. Report of the New England regional infant cardiac program. Pediatrics. 1980;65:432–436.
40. Cohen M, Fuster V, Steele PM, et al. Coarctation of the aorta. Long-term follow-up and prediction of outcome after surgical correction. Circulation. 1989;80:840–845.
41. Mendelsohn AM, Lloyd TR, Crowley DC, et al. Late follow-up of balloon angioplasty in children with a native coarctation of the aorta. Am J Cardiol. 1994;74:696–700.
42. Presbitero P, Demarie D, Villani M, et al. Long term results (15–30 years) of surgical repair of aortic coarctation. Br Heart J. 1987;57:462–467.
43. Bouchart F, Dubar A, Tabley A, et al. Coarctation of the aorta in adults: surgical results and long-term follow-up. Ann Thorac Surg. 2000;70:1483–1488.
44. Aris A, Subirana MT, Ferres P, et al. Repair of aortic coarctation in patients more than 50 years of age. Ann Thorac Surg. 2000;70:1483–1488.
45. Hehrlein FW, Mulch J, Rautenburg HW, et al. Incidence and pathogenesis of late aneurysms after patch graft aortoplasty for coarctation. J Thorac Cardiovasc Surg. 1986;92:226–230.
46. Brouwer RM, Erasmus ME, Ebels T, et al. Influence of age on survival, late hypertension, and recoarctation in elective aortic coarctation in elective aortic coarctation repair. Including long-term results after elective aortic coarctation repair with a follow-up from 25 to 44 years. J Thorac Cardiovasc Surg. 1994;108:525–531.
47. Ovaert C, Benson LN, Nykanen D, et al. Acute and follow-up intravascular ultrasound findings after balloon dilation of coarctation of the aorta. Pediatr Cardiol. 1998;19:27–44.
48. Mendelsohn AM, Lloyd TR, Crowley DC, et al. Late follow-up of balloon angioplasty in children with a native coarctation of the aorta. Am J Cardiol. 1994;74:696–700.
49. Rao PS, Galal O, Smith PA, et al. Five- to nine-year follow-up results of balloon angioplasty of native aortic coarctation in infants and children. J Am Coll Cardiol. 1996;27:462–470.
50. Fletcher SE, Nihill MR, Grifka RG, et al. Balloon angioplasty of native coarctation of the aorta: midterm follow-up and prognostic factors. J Am Coll Cardiol. 1995;25:730–734.
51. Hijazi ZM, Fahey JT, Kleinman CS, et al. Balloon angioplasty for recurrent coarctation of aortic. Immediate and long term results. Circulation. 1991;84:1150–1156.
52. Sohn S, Rothman A, Shiota T, et al. Acute and follow-up intravascular ultrasound findings after balloon dilation of coarctation of the aorta. Circulation. 1994;90:340–347.
53. Kodolitsch YV, Aydin MA, Koschyk DH, et al. Predictors of aneurysm of formation after surgical correction of aortic coarctation. J Am Coll Cardiol. 2002;39:617–624.
54. Wells WJ, Prendergast TW, Berdjis F, et al. Repair of coarctation of the aorta in adults. Ann Thorac Surg. 1996;61:1168–1171.
55. Aydogan U, Dindar A, Gurgan L, et al. Late development of dissecting aneurysm following balloon angioplasty of native aortic coarctation. Cathet Cardiovasc Diagn. 1995;36:226–229.
56. Ovaert C, McCrindle BW, Nykanen D, et al. Balloon angioplasty of native coarctation: clinical outcomes and predictors of success. J Am Coll Cardiol. 2000;35:988–996.
57. Bulbul ZR, Bruckheimer E, Love JC, et al. Implantation of balloon-expandable stents for coarctation of the aorta: implantation data and short-term results. Cathet Cardiovasc Diagn. 1996;39:36–42.

58. Thanopoulos BD, Hadjinikolaou L, Konstadopoulou GN, et al. Stent treatment for coarctation of the aorta: intermediate term follow-up and technical considerations. *Heart.* 2000;84:65–70.

59. Marshall AC, Perry SB, Keane JF, et al. Early results and medium-term follow-up of stent implantation for mild residual or recurrent aortic coarctation. *Am Heart J.* 2000;139:1054–1060.

60. Harrison DA, McLaughlin PR, Lazzam C, et al. Endovascular stents in the management of coarctation of the aorta in the adolescent and adult: one year follow-up. *Heart.* 2001;85:561–566.

61. Mullen MJ. Coarctation of the aorta in adults: do we need surgeons? *Heart.* 2003;89:3–5.

62. Duke C, Qureshi SA. Aortic coarctation and recoarctation: to stent or not to stent? *J Intervent Cardiol.* 2001;14:283–298.

63. Zabal C, Attie F, Rosas M, et al. The adult patient with native coarctation of the aorta: balloon angioplasty or primary stenting? *Heart.* 2003;89:77–83.

64. Macdonald S, Thomas SM, Cleveland TJ, et al. Angioplasty or stenting in adult coarctation of the aorta? A retrospective single center analysis over a decade. *Cardiovasc Intervent Radiol.* 2003;26:357–364.

65. Johnston TA, Grifka RG, Jones TK. Endovascular stents for treatment of coarctation of the aorta: acute results and follow-up experience. *Cathet Cardiovasc Intervent.* 2004;62:499–505.

66. Pedra CAC, Fontes VF, Esteves CA, et al. Stenting vs. balloon angioplasty for discrete unoperated coarctation of the aorta in adolescents and adults. *Cathet Cardiovasc Intervent.* 2005;64:495–506.

67. Diethrich EB, Heuser RR, Cardenas JR, et al. Endovascular techniques in adult aortic coarctation: the use of stents for native and recurrent coarctation repair. *J Endovasc Surg.* 1995;2:183–188.

68. Haas NA, Lewin MAG, Knirsch W, et al. Initial experience using the NuMED Cheatham Platinum (CP) Stent for interventional treatment of coarctation of the aorta in children and adolescents. *Z Kardiol.* 2005;94:113–120.

69. Therrien J, Thorne SA, Wright A, et al. Repaired coarctation: a "cost-effective" approach to identify complications in adults. *J Am Coll Cardiol.* 2000;35:997–1002.

70. Swan L, Ashrafian H, Gatzoulis MA. Repair of coarctation: a higher goal? *Lancet.* 2002;359:977–978.

71. Mahadevan V, Mullen MJ. Endovascular management of aortic coarctation. *Int J Cardiol.* 2004;97(suppl 1):75–78.

72. Specific disease. In: O'Rourke MF, Nichols WW, eds. *McDonald's Blood Flow in Arteries: Theoretical, Experimental and Clinical Principles.* 4th ed. London: Edward Arnold, 1998:405–414.

73. Varma C, Benson LN, Butany J, et al. Aortic dissection after stent dilatation for coarctation of the aorta: a case report and literature review. *Cathet Cardiovasc Intervent.* 2003;59:528–535.

74. Ebeid MR, Prieto LR, Latson LA. Use of balloon-expandable stents for coarctation of the aorta: initial results and intermediate-term follow-up. *J Am Coll Cardiol.* 1997;30:1847–1852.

75. Suarez DL, Pan M, Romero M, et al. Immediate and follow-up findings after stent treatment for severe coarctation of aorta. *Am J Cardiol.* 1999;83:400–406.

76. Cheatham JP. Stenting of coarctation of the aorta. *Cathet Cardiovasc Intervent.* 2001;54:112–125.

77. Hamdan MA, Maheshwari S, Fahey JT, et al. Endovascular stents for coarctation of the aorta: initial results and intermediate-term follow-up. *J Am Coll Cardiol.* 2001;38:1518–1523.

78. Ledesma M, Alva C, Gomez FD, et al. Results of stenting for aortic coarctation. *Am J Cardiol.* 2001;88:460–462.

79. Morita S, Kuboyama I, Asou T, et al. The effect of extraanatomic bypass on aortic input impedance studied in open chest dogs. Should the vascular prosthesis be compliant to unload the left ventricle? *J Thorac Cardiovasc Surg.* 1991;102:774–783.

80. Pihkala J, Thyagarajan GK, Taylor GP, et al. The effect of implantation of aortic stents on compliance and blood flow. An experimental study in pigs. *Cardiol Young.* 2001;11:173–181.

81. Bell RE, Taylor PR, Aukett M, et al. Endoluminal repair of aneurysms associated with coarctation. *Ann Thorac Surg.* 2003;75:530–533.

Martin Köcher

Petr Utíkal

CHAPTER **10**

Abdominal Aortic Aneurysm

Infrarenal aneurysm of the abdominal aorta (AAA) afflicts 1% to 6% of the population >60 years of age, and its incidence is constantly rising.[1,2] When left untreated, AAA may be fatal. Within 1 year of establishment of the diagnosis, 50% of AAAs rupture, and within 5 years this number rises to 90%.[3]

Whereas the mortality of patients undergoing acute operations for the rupture of an aneurysm approaches 70%, that of elective operative treatment ranges up to 5% in most studies.[4–9] Efforts are thus concentrated on the elective treatment of all identified AAAs. The aim of AAA treatment is to prevent its rupture by shutting off the aneurysmal sack from the circulation.

The standard treatment of AAA is open surgical repair. The technique and strategy of resecting the AAA, replacing the aorta with an artificial vascular prosthesis, was developed and has been employed in clinical practice since the 1950s.[10,11]

However, open surgery is not a good option for patients with high surgical risk, since their mortality is 19% and morbidity 40%.[12,13] In fact, elective surgical procedure may even be contraindicated in some patients because of coexisting morbidities.

In 1991, Parodi et al.[14] introduced endovascular aneurysm repair (EVAR), which now represents a viable alternative to open surgery.

CLINICAL DESCRIPTION

ETIOLOGY AND EPIDEMIOLOGY OF ABDOMINAL AORTIC ANEURYSM

Dimensions of the normal supraceliac, suprarenal, and infrarenal aorta have been recently reviewed.[15] AAA is defined as a distension of the infrarenal aorta by >50% (or 1.5 times) compared with a corresponding healthy, age- and gender-matched population.[16]

AAA affects 1% to 6% of the population aged >60 years,[1,2] and the incidence rises by approximately 0.15% annually. The incidence may be also increasing because of aging populations and the greater availability of ultrasound screening.[17] The incidence ratio of AAA in men and women is 4–5:1.

According to its pathological morphology, AAA is considered a true aneurysm, because it comprises all layers of the arterial wall, most commonly forming into a fusiform shape. Aneurysms with a diameter <5 cm are considered small, and those >6.5 cm large.[15]

The most common cause of AAA is a dilation type of atherosclerosis (95%). Less common are AAAs of infectious or inflammatory origin, or those associated with connective tissue diseases.[18] The process of AAA formation is multifactorial. Apart from the general risk factors of atherosclerosis, genetic disposition, autoimmunity, and hemodynamic factors all play roles in its formation.[18] AAA is 1.5 times more frequent in hypertensive patients and in those with manifested atherosclerotic peripheral arterial disease.[19,20] A significantly higher incidence of AAA has been observed in smokers (eight times).[21] A common histopathologic element is the inflammatory reaction within the aortic wall that leads to the destruction of the intercellular matrix (particularly elastin) and the remodeling of collagen, which consequently leads to the loss of aortic wall elasticity and rigidity.[15]

CLINICAL SIGNS OF ABDOMINAL AORTIC ANEURYSM

In up to 75% of patients, AAA remains asymptomatic and presents acutely with ruptures.[22] In patients with clinical symptoms, the manifestation may be nonspecific; abdominal or back pain may be clinical signs of an already unstable or penetrating aneurysm. At present, the majority of aneurysms are discovered during examinations (e.g., ultrasonography, USG; computed tomography, CT; or magnetic resonance, MR, imaging) that were indicated for other reasons. According to their presentation, the aneurysms are classified as asymptomatic and symptomatic with or without a rupture.[15]

The prognosis of a patient with AAA is unfavorable. In men older than 55 years, AAA is the 10th most frequent cause of death. The rupture of an aneurysm is the most severe complication and, when untreated, it is usually lethal. Overall, of all sudden deaths in the age group 18–70 years, 4.2% in men and 1.2% in women are related to a ruptured AAA.[23] It is generally accepted that within 1 year of the established diagnosis, approximately half of the cases of AAA rupture and within 5 years this number rises to 90%. The average interval between an established diagnosis and the rupture of an untreated aneurysm has been reported to be 16 months.[3] The risk of rupture increases with the size of the AAA, with the transverse diameter of the AAA being the most powerful predictor of rupture. In small aneurysms (<5 cm) the yearly risk of rupture is 6%, in aneurysms with a diameter of 7 cm it is 23%, and in those >10 cm it is 60%.[24] According to other authors, the annual risk of rupture approaches 0% for aneurysms <4 cm in diameter, whereas for aneurysms with a diameter of 4 to 4.9 cm, 5 to 5.9 cm, 6 to 6.9 cm, 7 to 7.9 cm, and 8 cm and larger, the annual risk of rupture ranges from 0.5% to 5%, 3% to 15%, 10% to 20%, 20% to 40%, and 30% to 50%, respectively.[25–27]

However, there is not always a linear correlation between the size of an AAA and the risk of aneurysmal rupture. Even a small aneurysm can rupture.[28,29] Furthermore, 80% of aneurysms expand. Among these, 20% expand >0.5 cm per year, and this rapid growth also increases the risk of rupture.[30] Other risks of rupture include cigarette smoking,[31,32] hypertension,[32] positive family history,[33,34] chronic obstructive pulmonary disease,[32,35] female gender (the risk of rupture is three times higher in women than it is in men),[32] and a saccular shape of aneurysm.[36,37]

Patients with AAA are included in the group of so-called "vascular surgically ill" patients and the majority of these patients have a high operative risk. Operative risk factors include creatinine >1.8 mg/dL, congestive heart failure, evidence of myocardial ischemia on ECG, pulmonary dysfunction, age, and female gender.[38] In addition, 75% of AAA patients have at least two severe comorbidities, including peripheral arterial disease frequently associated with a generalized vascular disease involving the coronary, renal, and cerebral circulation. Coronary artery disease may be present in as many as 80% of patients. Most patients are smokers with respiratory disorders, hypertension, and diabetes mellitus. The presence of severe coexistent diseases significantly restricts the surgical options for AAA treatment and plays a significant role in the perioperative morbidity and mortality.[3,38]

TREATMENT STRATEGIES FOR ABDOMINAL AORTIC ANEURYSM

SURGICAL TREATMENT

The standard surgical treatment technique is resection of the aneurysmal sack and its replacement with an artificial vascular prosthesis that is sutured onto the aorta with vascular stitches.[10,11] This invasive procedure is associated with hemodynamic compromise due to opening the abdominal wall (laparotomy) and temporary clamping of the infrarenal aorta.[40]

The outcome of surgical treatment of AAA depends primarily on the emergency versus elective status of the procedure and on the morbidity of the patient. The reported mortality of emergency surgical treatment for ruptured AAA ranges between 23% and 70%. In contrast, the reported mortality of elective surgical treatment of AAA is approximately 2% to 8% at present.[4–9,16,41] Surgical AAA repair is associated with considerable morbidity, including cardiac morbidity ranging between 10% and 12%, pulmonary morbidity ranging between 5% and 10%, and renal morbidity ranging between 5% and 7%; these figures pertain to elective surgical AAA treatment in patients with a low operative risk. In patients with high operative risk, the mortality and cardiopulmonary morbidity is considerably higher, namely, 19% and 40%, respectively.[12,13] To improve the early outcome of elective AAA surgery, stricter selection criteria would be required. Prior to EVAR, this meant exclusion of a number of patients eligible for elective treatment.[42]

ENDOVASCULAR TREATMENT

EVAR is today considered an important alternative to open surgery for AAA.[43] The principle of EVAR is to shut off the aneurysm from the circulation by bridging it with a stent-graft prosthesis introduced and placed endoluminally. The stent-graft prosthesis is introduced in a folded state from a common femoral artery via the pelvic vessels into the aorta using a guidewire-based delivery system. In the aorta, the stent graft is released and anchored at the sites above and below the aneurysmal bulge into the nondilated, if possible healthy aorta and iliac artery. The proximal anchorage is the so-called "neck of the aneurysm." Compared with open surgery, the endovascular procedure is not only less invasive but also hemodynamically better tolerated because transient clamping of the subrenal aorta is not necessary. This technique of endovascular AAA repair using stent-graft prostheses was introduced into clinical practice following a series of experimental studies conducted independently by Volodos and Parodi in the late 1980s and early 1990s.[14,44,45]

MORPHOLOGY OF THE ABDOMINAL AORTIC ANEURYSM

The basic requirement for EVAR is suitable morphology of the AAA and iliac arteries allowing safe introduction and reliable expansion and anchoring of the stent graft. However, it should be noted that the morphologic criteria of EVAR change with time, corresponding to the evolution of endovascular techniques and technology. The morphology of AAA and iliac arteries is evaluated on the basis of imaging and the measurement of selected parameters of the infrarenal aorta with the aneurysm and iliac arteries (Fig. 10-1). In planning EVAR, the most critical part of the abdominal aorta is the region between the take off of the renal arteries and the bulge of the aneurysm—the so-called proximal neck of the aneurysm. The diameter, length, and shape of the proximal neck along with the presence of calcifications and thrombi are evaluated to determine the suitability of an individual pathoanatomic substrate for EVAR. The pathoanatomic quality of the proximal neck is also important for the long-term outcome and stability of the implanted stent graft. Furthermore, the aneurysmal sack and the region of

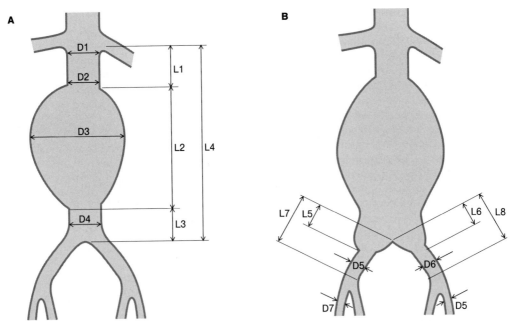

FIGURE 10-1. Schematic diagram of the method for measuring selected parameters of the infrarenal aorta with an aneurysmal and iliac vasculature. **A,B:** D1, aortic diameter (proximal aneurysmal neck) immediately under the outflow of the distally inserted renal arteries; D2, aortic diameter (proximal aneurysmal neck) immediately above the aneurysm; D3, aneurysmal diameter; D4, aortal diameter (distal neck, if present) under aneurysm; D5, diameter of the "healthy section" of the common iliac artery(CIA) under the aneurysm on the right; D6, diameter of the "healthy section" CIA under the aneurysm on the left; D7, diameter of the left external iliac artery (EIA); D8, diameter of right EIA; L1, length of the proximal neck of the aneurysm; L2, length of the aneurysmal sack; L3, length of the distal neck of the aneurysm (if present); L4, total length of the subrenal aorta; L5, length of the section of the right CIA affected by aneurysm; L6, length of the section of the left CIA affected by aneurysm; L7, length of the right CIA; L8, length of the left CIA.

bifurcation are measured to determine the diameter and length of the aneurysmal sack and evaluated to determine the presence of thrombus within the aneurysmal sack. An equally important parameter is the angle of the longitudinal axis of the aneurysm and the longitudinal axis of the aneurysmal neck, which should be <60 degrees. The availability of a distal neck, that is, a healthy section of the aorta below the aneurysm, determines the selection of the type of stent graft. In AAA without a distal neck, the diameter of the bifurcation determines whether sufficient space is available to pass through both sleeves of a bifurcation-type stent graft, which is appropriate for a given location. If the aneurysm extends distal to the bifurcation, the extent of the involvement of the iliac arteries is examined. The aneurysmal sack is further evaluated for the presence and number of patent vessels that arise from aneurysmal sack (i.e., lumbar arteries, inferior mesenteric artery, accessory renal arteries, internal iliac arteries). Depending on their number, these vessels may become the source of a clinically relevant retrograde flow into the aneurysmal sack, thus compromising the outcome.[46] The iliac arteries are evaluated with regard to dimensions (length and diameter), shape (tortuosity), and arterial wall quality (stenosis, patency, ulcerations, calcifications, mural thrombosis). In summary, the most critical parameters in determining the technical feasibility of EVAR include the length of the proximal neck and the degree of axial deviation of the infrarenal aorta. In standard procedures, that is, not considering the new and thus far experimental technical options (e.g., fenestrated stent graft, branched stent graft) or combined

endovascular-surgical methods, the minimal length of the proximal neck should be 15 mm and the axial deviation of the infrarenal aorta <60 degrees.

At present the morphology of the aneurysmal sack is determined and all EVAR-related measurements are preferably performed using computed tomography angiography (CTA). Although thin-cut (<3 mm) conventional dynamic CT scanning may be adequate, helical/spiral scanning with multiplanar reconstruction is preferable.[47] The measurement of the diameter must be performed at right angles to the longitudinal axis of the artery. The longitudinal measurements are done while taking into consideration the expected course of the stent graft within the aneurysm so as to exclude possible inaccuracies.[48] Alternatively, but less commonly, the preinterventional assessment of the AAA may be performed using abdominal aortic digital subtraction angiography (DSA) with a calibrated catheter in place to determine the length of the aneurysm and iliac arteries for selecting the optimum stent graft prosthesis for each individual patient (Tables 10-1 and 10-2).[47] The advantage of DSA is the exact definition of blood supply and vascular networks of the visceral organs, spine, and pelvis.

To improve treatment decisions, a morphological classification of AAA was introduced that is based on the evaluation of the extent of the aneurysm with respect to the presence and length of the upper and lower aortic neck. Systematic use of the classification allows better matching and selection of patients for EVAR and the specific types of stent grafts, and permits standard comparisons of outcomes to be made on the basis of

TABLE 10-1. Targets of Preinterventional Diagnostic Evaluations in Patients with Abdominal Aortic Aneurysm (AAA)

1. To detect or confirm the detection of the AAA.
2. To stage the AAA. Staging questions that need to be answered are:
   a. The maximal diameter and length of the AAA and its lumen;
   b. The diameter, length, and angulation of the proximal landing zone;
   c. The diameters, lengths, and angulation of all the distal landing zones;
   d. The diameter and angulation of the potential access routes;
   e. The total length of territory to be covered;
   f. The distance from the lowest renal artery to the aortic bifurcation;
   g. The distance from the lowest renal artery to each iliac bifurcation;
   h. The diameter of the aortic bifurcation;
   i. Relative location and extent of the AAA (where does it start and where does it stop in relationship to major branches and bifurcations);
   j. Presence of and location of thrombus in the AAA;
   k. Presence of rupture of the AAA or coexisting periaortic pathology (inflammatory AAA);
   l. Presence and location of coexisting aneurysmal disease (iliac, femoral, visceral);
   m. Presence and location of coexisting iliofemoral occlusive disease;
   n. Number and types of patent branches arising from the aneurysm sac;
   o. Patency and location of the SMA, IMA, and celiac;
   p. Quality of landing zones and potential access routes (calcification, atheroma);
   q. Presence of vascular anomalies (multiple renal arteries, early bifurcations, venous anomalies).

Reprinted with permission from Geller SC and the members of the Society of Interventional Radiology Device Forum. Imaging guidelines for abdominal aortic aneurysm repair with endovascular grafts. *J Vasc Intervent Radiol.* 2003;14:S263-S264.

the anatomic substrate. Schumacher and EUROSTAR morphological classifications are currently employed (Fig. 10-2).[49,50]

Indications for the Endovascular Treatment of Abdominal Aortic Aneurysm

According to the recently published ACC/AHA guidelines, patients with infrarenal or juxtarenal AAAs ≥5.5 cm in diameter should undergo repair and those with AAAs measuring 4.0 cm to 5.4 cm in diameter should be monitored by ultrasound or CT every 6 to 12 months (both class I evidence level A). In the latter group of patients, also, repair can be beneficial (class I evidence level B). In patients with AAAs <4.0 cm ultrasound examination every 2 to 3 years was recommended.[15]

Indications for elective EVAR are similar to those for open surgery and are guided by the presumed risk of rupture in an individual patient. Most patients with AAA are elderly (65 years of age and older) with multiple coexisting morbidities frequently associated with a high operative risk or even contraindications for open surgery repair. Specifically for these high-risk patients, with the operative risk level graded ASA III (American Society of Anesthesiology classification) and ASA IV,[51] EVAR currently represents an acceptable treatment of choice with clearly lower perioperative mortality and morbidity, and lower or at least noninferior short-term and mid-term results compared with open surgery.[13]

However, not all patients have a suitable pathoanatomy of the aortoiliac segment, thus restricting the indications for endovascular AAA treatment on grounds of technical feasibility.[52] Limiting factors include the extension of the aneurysm suprarenally, absence of a suitable proximal aneurysmal neck or its unsuitable

TABLE 10-2. Suggested Diagnostic Techniques to Evaluate Patients with Abdominal Aortic Aneurysm Considered for Endovascular Treatment

I. Thin-cut (<3 mm) conventional dynamic CT scanning, helical/spiral CT arteriography (CTA) with multiplanar reconstruction.
   1. A localizing scan should be performed first. This scan
      a. requires no oral and no intravenous contrast; and should be performed from the diaphragm to mid-intertrochanteric region;
      b. if done in helical/spiral mode can have 10-mm collimation, 2.0 pitch, 80–100 kV, 90–100 mA;
      c. should be used to localize the celiac origin level and femoral bifurcations. It is also useful to assess calcification and general issues.
   2. A CTA scan should then be performed. This scan
      a. should be a helical/spiral scan from celiac origin to the femoral bifurcation preferably in one or two breath holds. Total scan time should be about 40–50 s;
      b. should use 3-mm (or less) collimation, 2.0 pitch; 120 kV, 280 mA, 750-ms gantry rotation;
      c. should have a volume of 120–200 mL of low osmolar contrast administered via large-bore (18-gauge) antecubital vein at 2–5 mL/s with either a timed delay or a 20–30 s delay, depending on estimated circulation time.
   3. A reconstruction series (2 mm or less) can then be constructed from the above scan that includes the total table travel distance (usually 33–42 cm) and smaller field of view centered on aorta (18–20 cm). Most of the quantitative measurements and much of the qualitative information can be obtained from this data. This series needs to be evaluated on a work station capable of multiplanar reformation.

II. Catheter Angiography
Catheter angiography performed with a calibrated marker catheter that has radiopaque marks every 15 cm over at least a 20-cm segment is recommended. The angiogram should encompass the abdominal aorta from the celiac axis to the femoral bifurcations. The abdominal aorta should be imaged in at least two views (90 degrees apart, anteroposterior and lateral preferably). A view including the renal arteries to the iliac bifurcations on one image should be included in this series. The pelvic (iliofemoral) segment should be imaged in at least three views (anteroposterior, right anterior oblique, left anterior oblique) with the catheter positioned in the lower abdominal aorta. Digital imaging with or without subtraction or cut-film imaging is adequate. Additional appropriate views to ensure visualization of branch origins are necessary.

Computer tomographic angiography (CTA) and x-ray angiography performed as outlined should suffice in the vast majority of patients. In patients with contraindications to iodinated contrast agents, gadolinium-enhanced magnetic resonance angiography (MRA) combined with a noncontrast thin-cut CT or intravascular ultrasound (US) may considered instead.

Reproduced with permission from Geller SC and the members of the Society of Interventional Radiology Device Forum. Imaging guidelines for abdominal aortic aneurysm repair with endovascular grafts. *J Vasc Intervent Radiol.* 2003;14:S263-S264.

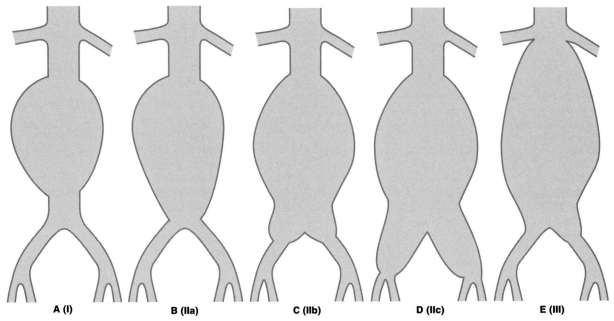

A (I)   B (IIa)   C (IIb)   D (IIc)   E (III)

FIGURE 10-2. Types of aneurysms, classified according to the EUROSTAR study (classification according to Schumacher). **A:** (I) proximal and distal aneurysmal necks present; (**B**) (IIa) aneurysm extends up to the bifurcation, distal neck not present; (**C**) (IIb) aneurysm also affects the proximal section of the common iliac artery on one or both sides; (**D**) (IIc) aneurysm also affects the proximal section of the common iliac artery on one or both sides in its entire extent; (**E**) (III) proximal neck of the aneurysm not present.

shape, extensive thrombus in the region of the proximal neck of the aneurysm, large axial deviation of the infrarenal abdominal aorta, and extremely tortuous, small, or stenotic pelvic arteries. According to strict morphological criteria, it has been reported that 30% to 50% of all AAAs are at present suitable for EVAR.[52] With the availability of customized stent-graft prostheses this percentage may be higher (40% to 80%),[53] and better designs and a greater selection of stent grafts continue to expand the indications for EVAR based on AAA pathoanatomy. However, disregard for the present morphologic criteria for EVAR indications may increase the incidence of primary technical failure, late complications, and secondary failure. Therefore, in patients with difficult AAA pathoanatomy, a combined endovascular and surgical approach is preferable.[54,55]

Whereas the indications for the EVAR in young patients, in patients with low operative risk, and in patients with a good long-term prognosis are uncertain because of the lack of long-term data, in patients with high surgical risk or severe coexisting diseases of the abdominal cavity or retroperitoneum, and in patients considered for nonvascular abdominal surgery, the endovascular treatment provides an important treatment option.

In addition, recent publications seem to indicate that acute rupture of AAA (RAAA) may be an important indication for EVAR. The mortality entailed in urgent surgical treatment of RAAA can reach 41% to 90%, depending on additional risk factors,[56,57] whereas EVAR for RAAA has a mortality rate ranging between 12% and 20%.[58,59]

The advantages of EVAR in emergency settings include avoidance of laparotomy, stable hemodynamics, lower cardiorespiratory distress, and less blood loss. The disadvantages include tedious preoperative diagnostics, CT or calibrated angiography, respectively, and at present limited availability of customized stent grafts.

Contraindications

Contraindications for EVAR are completely unsuitable morphology of the AAA, infected aneurysms, and aneurysms associated with connective tissue disorders. The only absolute contraindication for EVAR at present appears to be acute free AAA rupture in a patient unable to tolerate the required preinterventional diagnostic evaluations.

Stent Grafts

A stent graft (endovascular prosthesis) is a combination of a stent and a synthetic vascular prosthesis. The stent fulfills the function of an intraluminal fixator for vascular replacement. The body of the stent graft can be formed only by the actual vascular prosthesis, whose ends are connected to the stent. These allow fixation of the prosthesis to the vascular wall endoluminally (i.e., "stented graft"). The stent graft can also be formed over the entire surface by a metallic construction that is internally or externally lined by the vascular prosthesis (i.e., "grafted stent").

According to the type of stent skeleton used, the stent grafts are divided into self-expanding or balloon-expandable. Most stent grafts are constructed on the basis of a self-expanding stent. Their advantages lie in easier manipulation and their ability to mimic the changes in neck morphology with the passing of time. Balloon-expandable stents are utilized for fixation of prosthesis as a counterpart to "stented grafts."

According to their shape, stent grafts are divided into three basic types—tubular (aortoaortal), uni-iliac (aortoiliac), and bifurcated (aortobi-iliac) (Fig. 10-3). The type of stent graft used is based on the morphology of the aneurysm and the pelvic arteries. In aneurysms with suitable proximal and distal necks (>15 mm),

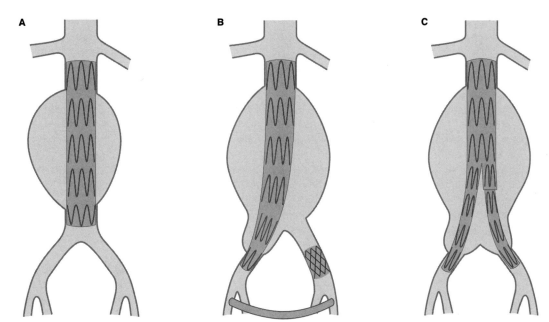

FIGURE 10-3. Types of stent grafts. **A:** Tubular (aortoaortal) stent graft; **(B)** uni-iliac (aortoiliac) stent graft femorofemoral crossover graft and left common iliac stent also shown; **(C)** bifurcational (aortobi-iliac) stent graft.

the implantation of a tubular type of stent graft is indicated. Aneurysms that are suitable from a morphological perspective for the implantation of a tubular stent graft are relatively rare. Tubular stent grafts are indicated in <10% of aneurysms. In aneurysms without a suitable distal neck, the type of stent graft depends on the morphology of the iliac arteries. The ideal solution is a monocomposite or multicomposite bifurcation stent graft that completely scaffolds the revascularized aortoiliac segment while preserving its function.[60] Introduction, placement, and positioning of bifurcation stent grafts require specialized techniques and instrumentation. The body and branches of the monocomposite bifurcation stent graft consist of a single piece. The placement of the contralateral branch is performed using the so-called crossover manipulation technique, which is technically demanding in most cases. In fact, the advantage of the one-piece graft usually does not outweigh the complex manipulation necessary to place the graft associated with the attending procedural risks, the risks of dislocation and imprecise placing. The multicomposite bifurcation stent graft is constructed from at least two pieces assembled endoluminally, namely, the aortoiliac and the contralateral iliac branch segments. Using both common iliac arteries for access, the iliac branches can be telescopically adjusted at both sides with the aid of additional extension segments, if needed. The implantation of multicomposite bifurcation stent grafts appears technically less demanding than that of monocomposite grafts, yet the iliac connection sites are a potential source of leakage and continued filling of the aneurysmal sack. The selection of the most suitable stent grafts and the choice of interventional strategy in individual patients are primarily determined by the given pathoanatomy, availability of the suitable prosthesis, and local expertise of the interventionist and the surgeon. For example, in patients with AAA and aneurysm without a suitable distal neck in the presence of a difficult bilateral iliac artery anatomy including small vessels, severe tortuosity, and

severe calcifications, the use of a uni-iliac monocomposite stent graft supplying the contralateral common iliac artery combined with revascularization of the other limb by an extra-anatomic femorofemoral crossover bypass probably represent the least traumatic therapy option.

For a successful, safe, and stable wall adaptation of the stent-graft, it is essential to precisely determine the dimensions and exact morphology of the aneurysm to allow for sufficient expansion of the extended stent-graft. The tightness and quality of sealing of the proximal and distal anastomosis are critically dependent on the correct diameter of the stent graft matching exactly the diameter of the aorta and the iliac artery, respectively. The preferred diameter of the stent-graft for the proximal and distal anastomosis is typically 15% to 20% greater than the true diameter of the aorta or artery at the anchoring sites. In order to support stent-graft stability and reduce the risk of its migration, metallic hooks or caudally orientated barbs are placed on the proximal parts of the stent-graft body.[61]

In aneurysms with a short proximal neck (<15 mm), a stent graft with an uncoated proximal segment should be selected. The implantation of an uncoated proximal segment across the ostia of the renal arteries improves the anchoring of the stent graft, even in aneurysms with a sufficiently long proximal neck, thus reducing the risk of migration and incidence of proximal perigraft endoleak.[62]

Endovascular Procedure

The actual endovascular procedure is performed with the patient under general, spinal, or local anesthesia. Considering the severity of the accompanying diseases in most patients, it is preferable to perform the procedure under spinal or local anesthesia. Local anesthesia is recommended particularly in EVAR of ruptured AAA, since it decreases the risk of acute hemodynamic compromise and abdominal wall atony.[63] However, at the outset of the intervention, patients must be prepared to undergo conversion to a standard open surgery procedure if the endovascular technique fails. At the beginning of the procedure 100 IU of unfractionated heparin/kg is administered and a broad-spectrum antibiotic is given. According to the type of sheath and considering its width, the stent graft is implanted using a single- or double-sided arteriotomy of the common femoral artery. If the width of the femoral or external iliac artery does not permit passage of the sheath, the stent graft may be implanted from an extraperitoneal approach via the common iliac artery. Using angiographic guidance and fluoroscopic control to locate the ostia of the renal arteries, the stent graft contained within the delivery system is introduced over an extra-stiff 0.035-in. guidewire (Back-up Meier, Boston Scientific, Watertown, MA, USA) onto the site of implantation. After precise placement, the stent graft is released from the delivery system. If a multicomposite bifurcation stent graft is used, the body of the released graft is traversed by a second stiff or super-stiff 0.035-in. guidewire introduced from the contralateral arteriotomy through the short limb. Subsequently, the contralateral limb is placed and docked onto the main body of the stent graft to complete the bifurcation reconstruction (Fig. 10-4). If the retrograde catheterization of the short branch proves difficult or impossible, a crossover technique from the ipsilateral femoral artery or antegrade technique from a brachial approach is used instead. Following full stent-graft deployment, in most cases definitive stent-graft adaptation to the aortic and arterial walls is accomplished using overlapping inflations of a large dilatation balloon. With perfect apposition of the stent graft, angiography, via a transfemoral or transbrachial access, is performed to

document the final results (Fig. 10-5). During the procedure typically several intermediary angiograms are acquired to assist correct placement and full deployment of the stent graft. The procedure is terminated with the operative closure of the arteriotomy sites in both common femoral arteries and suturing of the operative wounds. In the cases of uni-iliac stent grafts and extra-anatomic bypass revascularization of the contralateral limb, closure of the ipsilateral arteriotomy is preceded by surgical ligation of the contralateral common iliac artery and by placing an extra-anatomic femorofemoral crossover bypass (Fig. 10-6).

In aneurysms classified as IIc, safe anchor of the stent graft requires its implantation to the external iliac artery and covering the origin of the internal iliac artery on one or both sides. In order to prevent retrograde filling of the aneurysm, it is necessary to occlude the internal pelvic artery by ligation or prior embolization. In cases where it may become necessary to occlude both internal pelvic arteries, a step that is connected with a greater risk of intestinal ischemia, gluteal claudications, and in male patients vasculogenic erectile dysfunction, placement of a surgically created bypass onto one of the internal iliac arteries that then provides functionally fully adequate revascularization for the pelvic organs and gluteal muscles should be considered in all cases (Fig. 10-7).[55,64,65]

In an attempt to further minimize the invasiveness of the procedure, and probably allowing an additional reduction in periprocedural morbidity, percutaneous closure of the arterial access (up to 22F) or reduced diameter of the delivery system of the stent graft appear critical in the future. Although development of smaller stent-graft delivery systems appears currently not technically feasible, percutaneous closure of the arterial access sites has been shown to be feasible.[66,67]

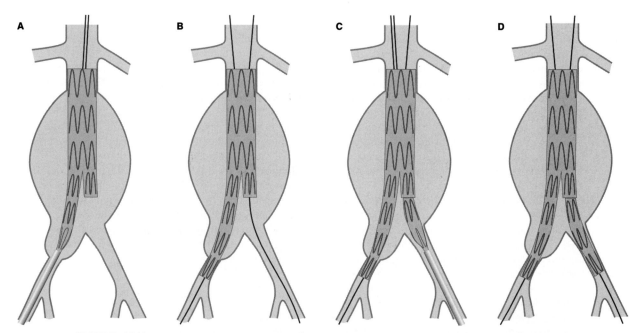

FIGURE 10-4. Schematic representation of the intraluminal construction of the bifurcational multicomposite types of prosthesis. **A:** Implantation of the aortoiliac component; (**B**) catheterization of the short branch of the aortoiliac component; (**C**) implantation of the contralateral iliac branch; (**D**) resultant bifurcation shape of the stent graft.

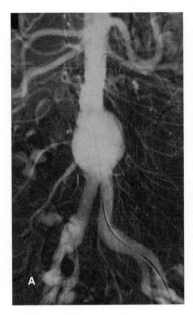 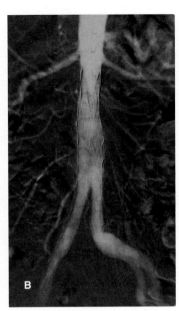

FIGURE 10-5. A 67-year-old man with an aneurysmal sack of the subrenal aorta type IIa indicated for the implantation of a bifurcation type of stent graft. **A:** Arteriography of the abdominal aorta and iliac vasculature prior to stent-graft implantation; **(B)** arteriography after stent-graft implantation: correctly placed patent stent graft without signs of endoleak.

Follow-Up

The main criterion for the early success of endovascular therapy is the complete exclusion of the aneurysm from the circulation, and the main criterion for the long-term success and effectiveness of endovascular treatment is the persistent isolation of the aneurysm from the circulation and the gradual reduction of the aneurysmal sack. The aim of follow-up examinations is to obtain information about the changes that occur to the actual stent graft and aneurysm and to promptly detect complications and eventual failure of EVAR. For this purpose, native x-rays of the abdomen, CTA, and Duplex ultrasound (DUS) are indicated. CT and DUS are performed prior to discharge, and 3, 6, and 12 months after implantation and every 12 months thereafter. Native x-rays of the abdomen are taken prior to discharge and then at yearly intervals. The diameter of the aneurysmal sack, the diameter of the proximal neck, the presence of endoleak, the patency of stent graft, the patency of the renal arteries in cases of suprarenal fixation, the patency of the iliac arteries, the position of the stent graft, and the configuration of

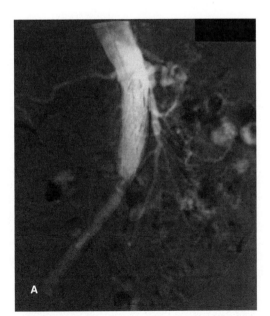 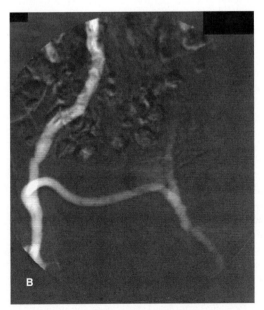

FIGURE 10-6. A 74-year-old man with an aneurysmal sack of the subrenal aorta type IIa and extremely tortuous and stenotic left iliac vasculature indicated for the implantation of a uni-iliac type stent graft. **A,B:** Arteriography after uni-iliac stent-graft implantation with the formation of a femorofemoral crossover bypass and the occlusion of the left common iliac artery.

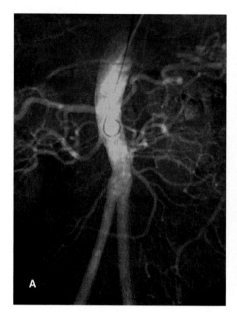

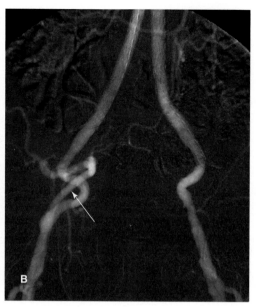

FIGURE 10-7. A 73-year-old man with a subrenal aneurysmal sack type IIc extending to both common iliac arteries in their entire extent. Patient indicated for the implantation of a bifurcation type of stent graft anchored to the external iliac arteries bilaterally and bypass to the right common iliac artery. **A:** Arteriography after the implantation of a bifurcation type of stent graft. **B:** Both iliac stent graft components and bypass from the right common femoral artery to the right internal iliac artery (*arrow*) are shown.

its skeleton are all examined. The main parameters monitored are the maximal diameter of the aneurysmal sack and the presence of blood flow within the aneurysmal sack outside the stent graft—so-called endoleak.

COMPLICATIONS

Apart from the complications that can be encountered in surgical procedures with the use of artificial vascular prostheses and in endovascular procedures (local access site, distant target site, and general systemic complications), EVAR carries its own specific complications.[68]

Clinically relevant nonspecific EVAR-related complications are listed in Table 10-3. The most severe are cardiopulmonary complications which occur in 6.9% as opposed to 19.6% of those undergoing surgery.[12,13,69] Symptomatic embolization into the periphery caused by manipulation in the aneurysmal sack occurs in up to 3%,[70] and renal failure after EVAR resulting either from administering iodinated contrast agents, particularly in patients with pre-existing chronic renal insufficiency, or as the result of embolization during instrumental endovascular manipulation occurs in 2% to 3% of patients. The incidence of complications associated with the iatrogenic occlusion of both internal iliac arteries, including gluteal claudications, vasculogenic erectile dysfunction, and pelvic discomfort, ranges between 12% and 40%.[71–73] In addition, with bilateral internal iliac artery occlusion the risk of intestinal and spinal ischemia also rises.

Specific EVAR-related complications are those directly related to the stent-graft prosthesis or to the delivery system. Complications related to the endoprosthesis include incorrect placement, occlusion, infection, persisting perfusion of the aneurysmal sack (so-called endoleak), kinking of the stent graft, its stenosis, migration from the original site of fixation, and damage to the skeleton and prosthesis of the stent graft. The most catastrophic specific complication of EVAR is the rupture of the

TABLE 10-3. Nonspecific Complications of Endovascular Treatment of Abdominal Aortic Aneurysm (EVAR)

Local (operative wound)	Hematoma
	Pseudoaneurysm
	Lymphatic fistula
	Infection
Distant	Thromboembolization into visceral arteries
	Thromboembolization into lower limb arteries
General	Cardiac
	Pulmonary
	Renal
	Cerebrovascular events
	Deep vein thrombosis
	Pulmonary embolism
	Colon ischemia
	Spinal ischemia
	Pelvic ischemia

aneurysmal sack. A rare specific complication of EVAR is *endotension*. Endotension is present when the size of the aneurysmal sack enlarges after EVAR, without any evidence of an endoleak and with ongoing or newly progressing pressure within the sack. This increasing pressure may also lead to the rupture of the aneurysmal sack, and its incidence has been reported at approximately 1.5%.[68] The cause of the endotension has not yet been clarified. Other rare procedural complications include dissection of aorta and pelvic arteries or its perforation.

Based on their occurrence in relation to the intervention, the complications can be divided into early (<30 days) or late (>30 days).[74]

The most common specific complication and also sign of incomplete exclusion of the aneurysmal sack from the circulation are endoleaks. This persistent flow of blood in the aneurysmal sack maintains pressure within the aneurysmal sack near to systemic levels and thus threatened rupture. According to its site, four types of endoleaks are recognized (Table 10-4; Fig. 10-8). Primary endoleaks are detected during the procedure or within 30 days after the procedure. Secondary endoleaks are diagnosed >30 days after a primarily successful procedure. An acceptable reported incidence of primary endoleaks is <10%.[75,76] Most endoleaks are type I or III (Fig. 10-9). The incidence of secondary endoleak ranges between 20% and 40%.[76–78] Secondary endoleak is usually of type II (Fig. 10-10).

Generally, type I and III endoleaks are known to be prognostically most adversely significant, because of the higher risk of aneurysmal sack rupture.[79,80] Therefore, type I and III endoleaks must be treated, in the majority of cases by endovascular means. Here, the leaking section is typically covered with extension segments. Type I endoleaks can sometimes be treated by so-called surgical banding, that is, placing an external ligature to seal the proximal neck of the aneurysm around the endoluminally implanted stent graft.[55,81] When a complication correction cannot be performed endovascularly, conversion to an open surgical procedure is required.

In type II endoleaks, the risk of aneurysmal sack rupture is low.[82–84] Therefore, hemodynamically insignificant type II endoleaks are usually not considered to be an EVAR failure.[74] Endoleaks type II should be treated only if they are hemodynamically significant, that is, connected with an ongoing enlargement of the aneurysmal sack.[85] The treatment of endoleak type II is performed by superselective embolization of the feeding branch of the sack (most commonly the lumbar artery or inferior mesenteric artery), in which the blood flow direction has been reversed because of the reversed pressure gradient following stent-graft implantation. However, superselective embolization of the feeder might be technically demanding, and in some cases it is not even feasible. In retrograde endoleak via the inferior mesenteric artery, it may be possible to laparoscopically clip the artery at its ostium rather than embolizing the artery. Another possible method of treatment of a retrograde flow is the percutaneous administration of thrombin directly into the aneurysmal sack at the site of the apparent endoleak. If despite endovascular treatment of endoleak type II, ongoing

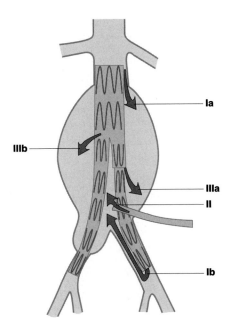

FIGURE 10-8. Types of endoleaks (see Table 10-4 for explanation).

enlargement of the aneurysmal sack is seen, conversion to an open surgical procedure is indicated.

RESULTS AND RECOMMENDATIONS

On the basis of published evidence, the primary success of endovascular treatment of AAA ranges between 48% and 93%.[69,70,86–88] The reported incidence of conversions into surgical treatment ranges between 0% and 16.5%, and 30-day mortality ranges between 1.5% and 7%,[70,86,87,89,90] which is comparable with surgical treatment. In patients with operative risk graded ASA III and ASA IV, the mortality of the endovascular procedure is clearly less than the mortality of the surgical procedure.[13] On

TABLE 10-4. Classification of Endoleak According to Cause and Site of Origin

TYPE I—PERIGRAFT ENDOLEAK—LEAKAGE AT THE SITE OF STENT GRAFT ANCHORING ("ANASTOMOSIS")

Ia	At the proximal end of the stent graft
Ib	At the distal end of the stent graft
Ic	Around an occluder in uni-iliac type of stent graft

TYPE II—RETROGRADE ENDOLEAK—RETROGRADE FLOW VIA A FREE BRANCH WITHIN THE ANEURYSMAL SACK

IIa	One branch into a blind space
IIb	Two and more with an inflow and outflow

TYPE III—LEAKAGE OF THE ACTUAL STENT GRAFT

IIIa	Loosening of a part of the stent graft
IIIb	Tear in the stent-graft material

TYPE IV—INCREASED PERMEABILITY OF UNDAMAGED MATERIAL UP TO 30 DAYS AFTER THE PROCEDURE

ENDOLEAK OF UNKNOWN ETIOLOGY—BLOOD FLOW CAN BE SEEN BUT SOURCE CANNOT BE ISOLATED

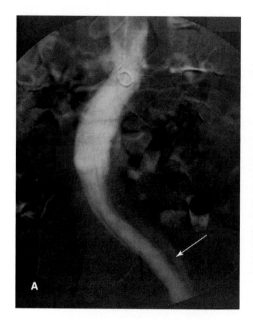

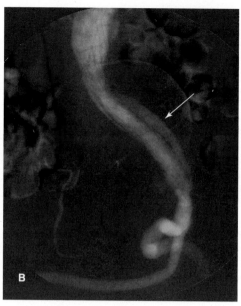

FIGURE 10-9. After the implantation of a uni-iliac type of stent graft. **A,B:** Endoleak type Ib (*arrow*).

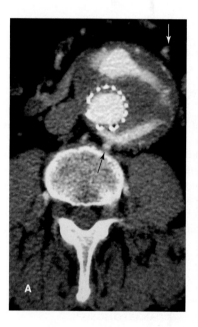

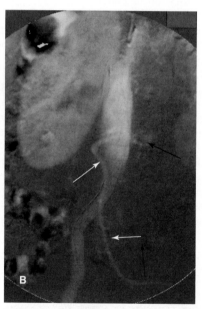

FIGURE 10-10. After the implantation of an uni-iliac type of stent graft. **A:** Computed tomography scan—endoleak type IIb. Inferior mesenteric artery (*white arrow*), lumbar artery (*black arrow*). **B:** Arteriography shows a retrograde flow in the inferior mesenteric artery (*white arrows*) and the flow in the sack of the aneurysm (*black arrows*).

the basis of the current published first randomized controlled trials, the 30-day mortality of patients suitable for EVAR and for open repair is lower in patients treated by EVAR, but reinterventions are required more frequently in EVAR treated patients. On 2-year follow-up, the cumulative survival rates seen in patients treated with EVAR, which were initially better, have not been maintained.[43,91,92]

The advantages of EVAR compared with standard surgical AAA repair include a significant reduction in perioperative morbidity and blood loss,[69,91,92] shorter hospitalization ranging between 1 and 12 days, and shorter length of stay in the intensive care unit, usually not exceeding 2 days. In addition, EVAR is associated with the patient's early return to normal life compared with open surgery.[93] Interestingly, although the quality of life during the first 3 months was better after EVAR than after open repair,[43,91,92] after 1 year it was equal[43] or even worse after EVAR.[91,92]

The single most important criterion for the long-term efficacy of the endovascular treatment is the definitive and persisting exclusion of the aneurysm from the circulation with an ensuing progressive reduction in the size of the thrombosed aneurysmal sack on follow-up (Fig. 10-11). The progressive reduction of the size of the aneurysm correlates with a reduction of pressure in the excluded aneurysmal sack.[94,95] This reduction in aneurysmal sack size occurs in 45% to 70% of patients treated by EVAR.[70,96,97] A significant reduction in the aneurysmal sack was noted by Blum et al. even after 24 months.[75]

In summary, on the basis of incomplete evidence, EVAR provides an important treatment option for selected patients with AAA, primarily those with high surgical risk. To choose the optimum management for an individual patient, consensus decisions between an interventionist and surgeon based on critical risk and benefit assessment as well as acknowledgment of strength and limitations of both procedures are required. To consider EVAR as an alternative to open surgery in the majority of patients with AAA in the future, improved stent grafts with lifelong longevity, documented in long-term trials, along with technical improvements including simpler implantation techniques and better control of endoleaks will be needed.[43,91,92,98]

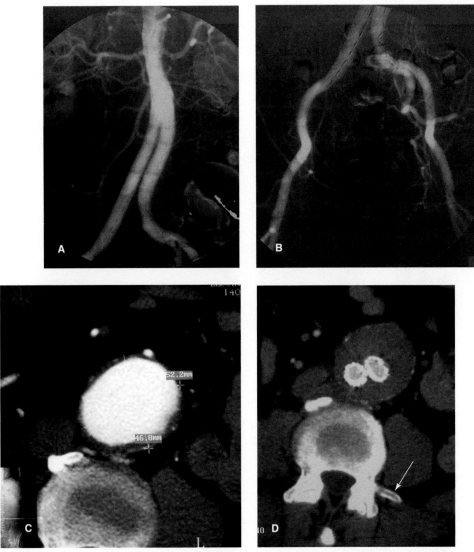

FIGURE 10-11. Evolution of aneurysmal sack size after endovascular treatment (EVT). A 65-year-old man with an aneurysmal sack of the subrenal aorta type IIc indicated for the implantation of a bifurcation type of stent graft. **A,B:** Arteriography after bifurcation type stent-graft implantation without signs of endoleak. Right branch stent graft anchored into the external iliac artery. Ligation of the right internal iliac artery. **C:** Computed tomography (CT) scan of the aneurysmal sack (52.2 × 46.8 mm cross-section diameters at this level) prior to EVT. **D–H:** CT scans at the same level (a severe ventrolateral osteophyte on the vertebral body is apparent) on the subsequent follow-up is demonstrated immediately after the stent graft implantation, and within 6, 12, 24, and 48 months. A significant reduction in aneurysmal sack size is apparent 1 year after the implantation of the stent graft (*arrow*), as its gradual shrinking (**F**). (*Continued*)

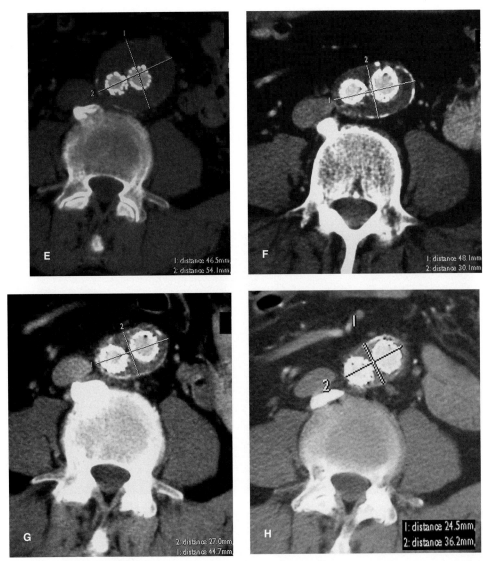

FIGURE 10-11. (*Continued*)

REFERENCES

1. Turk KAD. The post-mortem incidence of abdominal aortic aneurysms. *Proc R Soc Med.* 1965;58:869–870.
2. Scott RAP, Ashton HA, Kay DN. Abdominal aortic aneurysm in 4237 screened patients: prevalence, development and management over 6 years. *Br J Surg.* 1991;78:1122–1125.
3. Firt P, Hejnal J, Vanek I. *Cévní chirurgie.* Prague: Avicenum Publishing, 1991:148–159.
4. Ernst CB. Abdominal aortic aneurysm. *N Engl J Med.* 1993;328:1167–1172.
5. Walker SR, Macierewicz J, MacSweeney ST, et al. Mortality rates following endovascular repair of abdominal aortic aneurysms. *J Endovasc Surg.* 1999;6:233–238.
6. May J, White GH, Yu W, et al. Conversion from endoluminal to open repair of abdominal aortic aneurysms: a hazardous procedure. *Eur J Vasc Endovasc Surg.* 1997;14:4–11.
7. Blankensteijn JD, Lindenburg FP, Van der Graaf Y, et al. Influence of study design on reported mortality and morbidity rates after abdominal aortic aneurysm repair. *Br J Surg.* 1998;85:1624–1630.
8. Katz DJ, Stanley JC, Zelenock GB. Operative mortality rates for intact and ruptured abdominal aortic aneurysms in Michigan: an eleven-year statewide experience. *J Vasc Surg.* 1994;19:804–817.
9. Crawford ES, Saleh SA, Babb JW III, et al. Infrarenal abdominal aortic aneurysm: factors influencing survival after operation performed over 25-year period. *Ann Surg.* 1981;193:699–709.
10. Dubost C, Allary M, Oeconomos N. Resection of an aneurysm of the abdominal aorta: reestablishment of the continuity by a preserved human arterial graft, with result of five months. *Arch Surg.* 1952;64:405–408.
11. De Bakey ME, Cooley DA, Crawford ES, et al. Clinical application of a new flexible knitted Dacron arterial substitute. *Am Surg.* 1958;24:862–869.
12. May J, White GH, Yu W, et al. Concurrent comparison of endoluminal versus open repair in the treatment of abdominal aortic aneurysms: analysis of 303 patients by life-table method. *J Vasc Surg.* 1998;27:213–221.
13. Taufelsbauer H, Prusa AM, Wolff K, et al. Endovascular stent-grafting versus open surgical operation in patients with infrarenal aortic aneurysms. A propensity score-adjusted analysis. *Circulation.* 2002;106:782–787.
14. Parodi JC, Palmaz JC, Barone HD. Transfemoral intraluminal graft implantation for abdominal aortic aneurysms. *Ann Vasc Surg.* 1991;5:491–499.
15. Hirsch AT, Haskal ZJ, Hertzer NR, et al. ACC/AHA guidelines for the management of patients with peripheral arterial disease (lower extremity, renal, mesenteric, and abdominal aortic): Executive summary. A collaborative report from the American Association for Vascular Surgery/Society for Vascular Surgery, Society for Cardiovascular Angiography and Interventions, Society for Vascular Medicine and Biology, Society of Interventional Radiology, and the ACC/AHA Task Force on Practice Guidelines (Writing Committee to develop guidelines for the management of patients with peripheral arterial disease). www.cardiosource.com/guidelines/cguidelines/pad/pad_execsumm.pdf. Accessed May 25, 2006.
16. Krupski WC. Arterial aneurysm. In: Rutherford RB ed. *Vascular Surgery.* Vol. 2. Philadelphia: W B Saunders, 1995: 1025–1069.
17. Melton LJ, Bickerstaff LK, Hollier LH, et al. Changing incidence of abdominal aortic aneurysms: a population-based study. *Am J Epidemiol.* 1984;120:379–386.
18. Treska V, Valenta J, Bilek J, et al. Aneuryzmata abdominalni aorty. *Rozhl Chir.* 1997;76:176–180.

19. Allardice JT, Allwright GT, Wafula JMC, et al. High prevalence of abdominal aortic aneurysm in men with peripheral vascular disease: screening by ultrasonography. *Br J Surg.* 1988;75:240–242.
20. Williams IM, Winter RK, Hughes ODM, et al. Prevalence of abdominal aortic aneurysm in hypertensive population. *Ann R Coll Surg Engl.* 1996;78:501–504.
21. Lee AJ, Fowkes FGR, Carson MN, et al. Smoking, atherosclerosis and risk of abdominal aortic aneurysm. *Eur Heart J.* 1997;18:671–676.
22. Budd JS, Finch DRA, Carter PG. A study of the mortality from ruptured abdominal aortic aneurysms in a district community. *Eur J Vasc Surg.* 1990;11:1–6.
23. Samy AK, MacBain G. Abdominal aortic aneurysms: ten years hospital population in the city of Glasgow. *Eur J Vasc Surg.* 1993;7:561–566.
24. Estes JR Jr. Abdominal aortic aneurysm: a study of one hundred and two cases. *Circulation.* 1950;2:258–264.
25. Brown LC, Powell JT. Risk factors for aneurysm rupture in patients kept under ultrasound surveillance. UK Small Aneurysm Trial Participants. *Ann Surg.* 1999;230:289–296.
26. Brewster DC, Cronenwett JL, Hallett JW Jr., et al. Joint Council of the American Association for Vascular Surgery and Society for Vascular Surgery. Guidelines for the treatment of abdominal aortic aneurysms. Report of a subcommittee of the Joint Council of the American Association for Vascular Surgery and Society for Vascular Surgery. *J Vasc Surg.* 2003;37:1106–1117.
27. Reed WW, Hallett JW, Jr., Damiano MA, et al. Learning from the last ultrasound. A population-based study of patients with abdominal aortic aneurysm. *Arch Intern Med.* 1997;157:2064–2068.
28. Geroulakos G, Nicolaides A. Infrarenal abdominal aortic aneurysms less than five centimetres in diameter. The surgeon's dilemma. *Eur J Vasc Surg.* 1992;6:616–622.
29. May J, White GH, Yu W, et al. Concurrent comparison of endoluminal repair and no treatment for small abdominal aortic aneurysms. Presented at the Annual Meeting of the International Society for Vascular Surgery, Chicago, 1996.
30. Vardulaki KA, Prevost TC, Walker NM, et al. Growth rates and risk of rupture of abdominal aortic aneurysms. *Br J Surg.*1998;85:1674–1680.
31. Strachan DP. Predictors of death from aortic aneurysm among middle-aged men: the Whitehall study. *Br J Surg.* 1991;78:401–404.
32. Brown LC, Powell JT. Risk factors for aneurysm rupture in patients kept under ultrasound surveillance. UK Small Aneurysm Trial Participants. *Ann Surg.* 1999;230:289–296.
33. Darling RC 3rd, Brewster DC, Darling RC, et al. Are familial abdominal aortic aneurysms different? *J Vasc Surg.* 1989;10:39–43.
34. Verloes A, Sakalihasan N, Koulischer L, et al. Aneurysms of the abdominal aorta: familial and genetic aspects in three hundred thirteen pedigrees. *J Vasc Surg.* 1995;21:646–655.
35. Cronenwett JL, Sargent SK, Wall MH, et al. Variables that affect the expansion rate and outcome of small abdominal aortic aneurysms. *J Vasc Surg.* 1990;11:260–268.
36. Hunter GC, Smyth SH, Aguirre ML, et al. Incidence and histologic characteristics of blebs in patients with abdominal aortic aneurysms. *J Vasc Surg.* 1996;24:93–101.
37. Faggioli GL, Stella A, Gargiulo M, et al. Morphology of small aneurysms: definition and impact on risk of rupture. *Am J Surg.* 1994;168:131–135.
38. Steyerberg EW, Kievit J, de Mol van Otterloo JC, et al. Perioperative mortality of elective abdominal aortic aneurysm surgery. A clinical prediction rule based on literature and individual patient data. *Arch Intern Med.* 1995;155:1998–2004.
39. Becquemin JP, Chemla E, Chatellier G, et al. Perioperative factors influencing the outcome of elective abdominal aorta aneurysm repair. *Eur J Vasc Endovasc Surg.* 2000;20:84–89.
40. Giulini SM, Bonardelli S, Portolani N, et al. Suprarenal aortic cross-clamping in elective abdominal aortic aneurysm surgery. *Eur J Vasc Endovasc Surg.* 2000;20:286–289.
41. Blankensteijn JD. Mortality and morbidity rates after conventional abdominal aortic aneurysm repair. *Semin Intervent Cardiol.* 2000;5:7–13.
42. Utikal P., Köcher M, Koutna J, et al. AAA elective treatment indication tactics in EVAR era. *Biomed Pap Med Fac Univ Palacky Olomouc.* 2004; 148:183–187.
43. EVAR trial participants. Endovascular aneurysm repair versus open repair in patients with abdominal aortic aneurysm (EVAR trial 1): randomized controlled trial. *Lancet.* 2005;365: 2179–2186.
44. Volodos NL, Shekhanin VE, Karpovich IP, et al. Synthetic self-fixing prosthesis for endoprosthetics of the vessels. *Vestn Khir.* 1986;11:123–124.
45. Volodos NL, Karpovich IP, Troyan VI, et al. Clinical experience of the use of self-fixing synthetic prosthesis for remote endoprosthetics of the thoracic and abdominal aorta and iliac arteries through the femoral artery and as intraoperative endoprosthesis for aorta reconstruction. *VASA.* 1991;33(suppl):93–95.
46. Fan CM, Rafferty EA, Geller SC, et al. Endovascular stent-graft in abdominal aortic aneurysms: the relationship between patent vessels that arise from the aneurysmal sac and early endoleak. *Radiology.* 2001;218:176–182.
47. Geller SC and the members of the Society of Interventional Radiology Device Forum. Imaging guidelines for abdominal aortic aneurysm repair with endovascular grafts. *J Vasc Intervent Radiol.* 2003;14:S263–264.
48. Semba PC, Razavi MK, Kee ST, et al. Applications of spiral CT in endovascular aortic interventions. *Semin Intervent Radiol.* 1998;15:179–187.
49. Schumacher H, Allenberg JR, Eckstein HH. Morphological classification of abdominal aortic aneurysm in selection of patients for endovascular grafting. *Br J Surg.* 1996; 83:949–950.
50. Harris PL, Buth J, Miahle C, et al. The need for clinical trials of endovascular abdominal aortic aneurysm stent-graft repair: The EUROSTAR project. *J Endovasc Surg.* 1997;4:72–77.
51. Herold I. Metodick_ návod k provád_ní vy_et_ení nemocn_ch p_ed opera_ními a diagnostick_mi v_kony v celkové a svodné anestezii. *Anest Neodkl Pé_e.* 1995;6:12–15.
52. Ferko A, Krajina A, Lojik M, et al. Endovaskularni lecba aneuryzmat abdominalni aorty. Morfologie aneuryzmatu jeden z rozhodujicich momentu v indikaci. *Rozhl Chir.* 1997;76: 589–593.
53. Ohki T, Veith FJ. Patient selection for endovascular repair of abdominal aortic aneurysms: changing the threshold for intervention. *Semin Vasc Surg.* 1999;12:226–234.
54. Utikal P, Köcher M, Bachleda P, et al. Lecba AAA na prelomu tisicileti—stentgrafting—role cevniho chirurga. *Prakt Flebol.* 2001;10:111–113.
55. Utikal P, Köcher M, Koutna J, et al. Combined strategy in AAA elective treatment. *Biomed Pap Med Fac Univ Palacky Olomouc.* 2005;149:159–163.
56. Noel A, Gloviczki P, Cherry KJ Jr., et al. Ruptured abdominal aortic aneurysms: the excessive mortality rate of conventional repair. *J Vasc Surg.* 2001;34:41–46.
57. Brown MJ, Sutton AJ, Bell PRF, et al. A meta analysis of 50 years of ruptured abdominal aortic aneurysm repair. *Br J Surg.* 2002;89:714–730.
58. Lee WA, Hirneise CM, Tayyarah M, et al. Impact of endovascular repair on early outcomes of ruptured abdominal aortic aneurysms. *J Vasc Surg.* 2004;40:211–215.
59. Castelli P, Carrono R, Piffaretti, et al. Ruptured abdominal aortic aneurysm: endovascular treatment. *Abdom Imaging.* 2005;30:263–269.
60. May J, White GH, Yu W, et al. Importance of graft configuration in outcome of endoluminal aortic aneurysm repair: a 5 year analysis by the life table method. *Eur J Vasc Endovasc Surg.* 1998;15:406–411.
61. Malina M. Will stents with hooks and barbs prevent stent-graft migration? In: *Endovascular Repair of Abdominal Aortic Aneurysms—Aspects on a Novel Technique.* Lund, Sweden: Studentlitteratur, 1998:121–131.
62. Marin ML, Parsons RE, Hollier LH, et al. Impact of transrenal aortic endograft placement on endovascular graft repair of abdominal aortic aneurysms. *J Vasc Surg.* 1998;28:638–646.
63. Lachat ML, Pfammatter T, Witzke HJ, et al. Endovascular repair with bifurcated stent-graft under local anesthesia to improve outcome of ruptured aortoiliac aneurysms. *Eur J Vasc Endovasc Surg.* 2002;23:528–536.
64. Köcher M, Utikal P, Buriankova E, et al. Ctyrlete zkusenosti se stentgraftem Ella v endovaskularni lecbe AAA. *Ces Radiol.* 2001;55:159–166.
65. Utikal P, Köcher M, Bachleda P, et al. Femoral - internal iliac bypass in aortoiliac aneurysms endovascular repair. *Biomed Pap Med Fac Univ Palacky Olomouc.* 2004;148:91–93.
66. Howell M, Villareal R, Krajcer Z. Percutaneous access and closure of femoral artery access sites associated with endoluminal repair of abdominal aortic aneurysms. *J Endovasc Ther.* 2001;8:68–74.
67. Köcher M, Utikal P, Koutna J, et al. Kompletni perkutanni lecba aneuryzmatu abdominalni aorty. Popis metody a prvni zkusenosti. *Ces Radiol.* 2003;57:147–151.
68. White GH, May J, Petrasek P. Specific complications of endovascular aortic repair. *Semin Intervent Cardiol.* 2000;5:35–46.
69. Zarins CK, White RA, Schwarten D, et al. AneuRx stent-graft versus open surgical repair of abdominal aortic aneurysms: multicentre prospective clinical trial. *J Vasc Surg.*1999;29: 292–308.
70. Blum U, Voshage G, Lammer J, et al. Endoluminal stent-grafts for infrarenal abdominal aortic aneurysms. *N Engl J Med.* 1997;336:13–20.
71. Razavi MK, De Groot M, Olcott C, et al. Internal iliac artery embolization in the stent-graft treatment of aortoiliac aneurysms: analysis of outcomes and complications. *J Vasc Intervent Radiol.* 2000;11:561–566.
72. Schoder M, Zaunbauer L, Holzenbein T, et al. Internal iliac artery embolization before endovascular repair of abdominal aortic aneurysm: frequency, efficacy, and clinical results. *AJR Am J Roentgenol.* 2001;177:599–605.
73. Yano OJ, Morrisey N, Eisen L, et al. Intentional internal iliac artery occlusion to facilitate endovascular repair of aortoiliac aneurysm. *J Vasc Surg.* 2001;34:204–211.
74. Chaikoff EL, Blankenstein JD, Harris, et al. Reporting standards for endovascular aortic aneurysm repair. *J Vasc Surg.* 2002;35:1048–1060.
75. Blum U, Langer M, Spillner G, et al. Abdominal aortic aneurysms: preliminary technical and clinical results with transfemoral placement of endovascular self-expanding stent-grafts. *Radiology.* 1996;198:25–31.
76. Parent FN, Meier GH, Godziachvili V, et al. The incidence and natural history of type I and type II endoleak: a 5-year follow-up assessment with color duplex ultrasound scan. *J Vasc Surg.* 2002;35:474–481.
77. White GH, Yu W, May J, et al. Endoleak as a complication of endoluminal grafting of abdominal aortic aneurysms: classification, incidence, diagnosis, and management. *J Endovasc Surg.* 1997;4:152–168.
78. Raithel D, Heilberger P, Ritter W, et al. Secondary endoleaks after endovascular aortic reconstruction. *J Endovasc Surg.* 1998;5:126–127.
79. Alimi YS, Chakfe N, Rivoal E, et al. Rupture of an abdominal aortic aneurysm after endovascular graft placement and aneurysm size reduction. *J Vasc Surg.* 1998;28:178–183.
80. van Marrewijk C, Buth J, Harris PL, et al. Significance of endoleaks after endovascular repair of abdominal aortic aneurysms: the EUROSTAR experience. *J Vasc Surg.* 2002;35: 461–473.
81. Utikal P, Köcher M, Bachleda P, et al. Banding in aortic stent-graft fixation in EVAR. *Biomed Pap Med Fac Univ Palacky Olomouc.* 2004;148:175–178.
82. Resch T, Ivancev K, Lindh M, et al. Persistent collateral perfusion of abdominal aortic aneurysm after endovascular repair does not lead to progressive change in aneurysm diameter. *J Vasc Surg.* 1998;28:242–249.
83. Hinchliffe RJ, Singh-Ranger R, Davidson IR, et al. Rupture of an abdominal aneurysm secondary to type II endoleak. *Eur J Vasc Endovasc Surg.* 2001;22:563–565.
84. Dattilo JB, Brewster DC, Fan CM, et al. Clinical failures of endovascular abdominal aortic aneurysm repair: incidence, causes, and management. *J Vasc Surg.* 2002;35:1137–1144.
85. Parry DJ, Kessel DO, Robertson I, et al. Type II endoleaks: predictable, preventable, and sometimes treatable? *J Vasc Surg.* 2002;36:105–110.
86. Hausegger KA, Mendel H, Tiessenhausen K, et al. Endoluminal treatment of infrarenal aortic aneurysms: clinical experience with the Talent stent-graft system. *J Vasc Intervent Radiol.* 1999;10:267–274.
87. Pfammatter T, Lachat ML, Kunzli A, et al. Short-term results of endovascular AAA repair with the Excluder bifurcated stent-graft. *J Endovasc Ther.* 2002;9:474–480.
88. Köcher M, Utikal P, Koutna J, et al. Endovascular treatment of abdominal aortic aneurysms—six years of experience with Ella Stent-graft Systém. *Eur J Radiol.* 2004;51:181–188.

89. Kato N, Dake MD, Semba CP, et al. Treatment of aortoiliacal aneurysms with use of single-piece tapered stent-grafts. *J Vasc Intervent Radiol.* 1998;9:41–49.

90. Hill BB, Wolf YG, Lee WA, et al. Open versus endovascular AAA repair in patients who are morphological candidates for endovascular treatment. *J Endovasc Ther.* 2002;9:255–261.

91. Prinssen M, Verhoeven ELG, Buth J, et al. A randomized trial comparing conventional and endovascular repair of abdominal aortic aneurysm. *N Engl J Med.* 2004;351:1607–1618.

92. Blankensteijn JD, de Jong SECA, Prinssen M, et al. Two-year outcomes after conventional or endovascular repair of abdominal aortic aneurysms. *N Engl J Med.* 2005; 352:2398–2405.

93. Utikal P, Köcher M, Bachleda P, et al. Trilete zkusenosti se stentgraftingem AAA ve FN UP v Olomouci. *Prakt Flebol.* 2000;9:175–179.

94. Rhee RY, Eskandari MK, Zajko AB, et al. Long-term fate of the aneurysmal sac after endoluminal exclusion of abdominal aortic aneurysma. *J Vasc Surg.* 2000;32:689–696.

95. Dias NV, Ivancev K, Malina M, et al. Intra-aneurysm sac pressure measurements after endovascular aneurysm repair: differences between shrinking, unchanged and expanding aneurysms with and without endoleaks. *J Vasc Surg.* 2004;39:1229–1235.

96. Matsumura JS, Pearce WH, McCarthy WJ, et al. Reduction in aortic aneurysm size: early results after endovascular graft placement. *J Vasc Surg.* 1997;25:113–123.

97. Ricco JB, Letort M, Magnan PE, et al. Endovascular repair of abdominal aortic aneurysm: one-year results of the French AneuRx trial. *Ann Vasc Surg.* 2002;16:685–692.

98. Lederle FA. Endovascular repair of abdominal aortic aneurysm-round two. *N Engl J Med.* 2005;352:2443–2445.

Peter Lanzer
Ralf Weser

CHAPTER **11**

Renal Arteries

RENAL ARTERY DISEASE

Renal artery diseases comprise a wide range of systemic and local disorders that may affect directly or indirectly both the large and small vessels of the kidneys. The most frequent cause of renal artery diseases is atherosclerosis, followed by fibromuscular dysplasia. Less frequent causes include vasculitides such as Takayasu's arteritis, arteriovenous malformations, aneurysms, renal venous diseases, extrinsic vascular compression or damage by cysts or tumors, renovascular radiation injuries, neurofibromatosis lesions, retroperitoneal fibrosis, thromboembolic disease, traumata, and a number of renal parenchymal diseases. Several diseases, notably diabetes mellitus and systemic hypertension, may affect both the renal parenchyma and the renal vasculature at the same time (for review, see references 1 and 2).

RENAL ARTERY STENOSIS

Renal artery stenosis (RAS) appears to be a common cause of renovascular hypertension (RVH), hypertensive nephropathy (HTN), ischemic nephropathy (IN), and renal insufficiency, including end-stage renal disease (ESRD) (for review, see reference 3).

The recognition that RAS and systemic hypertension[4,5] were associated with each other, as were RVH and activation of the renin-angiotensin-aldosterone system (RAAS),[6] was an important step toward understanding the pathophysiologic links between renovascular disease and systemic hypertension. RAS-related reduction in renal perfusion, autoregulatory vasodilatation of the afferent (precapillary) arterioles (mediated by tubuloglomerular feedback and by direct myogenic responses with consecutive renin release triggering RAAS activation), angiotensin II release leading to vasoconstriction of the efferent (postcapillary) arterioles, an increase in intraglomerular pressure, and the systemic effects of RAAS activation have become widely recognized as critical pathogenetic principles involved not only in regulation of renal perfusion but also in preservation of glomerular filtration and development of RVH. Thus, sustained hypertension may induce structural renovascular changes triggering a vicious circle that may result in the development of HTN.[7] Nevertheless, the relationship between the severity of RAS and the degree of blood pressure elevation does not appear to be linear[8] and the specific factors responsible for the development of HTN have yet to be identified.

RAS may also cause global chronic renal ischemia, which, if sustained, may result in progressive interstitial fibrosis, and the glomerular and intrarenal vascular nephrosclerosis associated with IN (for review, see reference 9). However, the relationship between the severity of RAS and IN remains uncertain. On the basis of the definition of critical ischemia, RAS covering more than 70% to 80% of the cross-sectional area (or 45% to 56% of the diameter) has been considered hemodynamically significant.[10] Besides causing global chronic renal ischemia, atherosclerotic RAS (ARAS) also appears to be a potential source of atheroembolism causing regional renal ischemic defects and microrinfarcts; this has been documented by histology in patients with IN.[11] However, the importance of thromboembolism associated with RAS in the pathogenesis of IN still remains to be elucidated.

Finally, RAS appears to be associated with chronic renal insufficiency defined as renal failure (glomerular filtration rate, GFR 5 to 25 mL/min) and ESRD (GFR <5 mL/min) (for review, see references 9 and 12). Yet, chronic renal insufficiency represents a common final pathway of numerous disorders including hypertension, diabetes, interstitial nephritis, glomerulonephritis, acute tubular necrosis, immune-related disorders, and tubulopathies, and the specific relevance of RAS has yet to be explored. Interestingly, systematic renal biopsies performed in a well-defined population of patients with ESRD showed that hypertension-ischemia-induced nephropathy was the most frequent etiology (12.9%) followed by diabetic (10.4%), immunoglobulin-A (IgA) (9.1%), and thin-membrane (8.5%) renal diseases.[13]

In most cases, RAS is caused by renal artery atherosclerosis (up to 90% of proximal RAS) and renal artery fibromuscular dysplasia (up to 10% of proximal RAS).

ATHEROSCLEROTIC RENAL ARTERY STENOSIS

Atherosclerotic renal artery stenosis (ARAS) is a frequent manifestation of systemic atherosclerosis,[14] yet its true incidence and prevalence remain uncertain. In a recent study the estimated incidence of ARAS in people 65 years of age and older was 6.8%[15] and it was substantially higher in patients with atherosclerotic disease in other vascular beds (for review, see reference 16).

Although the causal relationship between ARAS and systemic hypertension, HTN, IN, and chronic renal insufficiency including ESRD appears likely, still much has to be learned about the true nature of the assumed pathogenetic links in individual patients. For example, it is well-recognized that RAS may or may not be associated with hypertension; in fact, in one of the early studies hypertension was present only in 50% of patients presenting with RAS.[17] Similarly, the severity of RAS does not appear to correlate with the degree of the associated renal dysfunction.[18] Some of the variability could be related to differences in biological dignity of atherosclerotic lesions underlined to ARAS, expressed for example in the embolic activity, biological and mechanical stability, and other factors. In addition, the frequent anatomic variants in renal blood supply (see below) and special renal hemodynamics could modify the functional impact, including:

- *High blood flow rates*: The kidney receives approximately 1.0 to 1.2 L blood/min, corresponding to approximately 20% of the resting cardiac output; this makes the kidney the organ with the highest blood flow per gram of tissue of the body (approximately 400 mL/min/100 g tissue vs., e.g., liver with 20 mL/min/100 g tissue)
- *Low oxygen extraction rates*: For example, oxygen delivery is approximately 84.0 mL/min/100 g, while oxygen consumption is approximately 6.8 mL/min/100 g; this corresponds to an extraction rate of 8.1%
- *High oxygen demand*: At a rate of 11.9 O_2 mL/min/100 g, this is second only to the heart
- *High glomerular capillary pressure compared with other capillary beds in the body*: 60 versus 13 mm Hg;
- *Precise autoregulation* [19]
- *Near maximum flow conditions at rest implying near maximum peripheral dilatation*: This corresponds to an approximately twofold flow reserve compared with an approximately 20-fold flow reserve in skeletal muscle (see Chapter 2).

Therefore, it appears likely that the severity of ARAS may be modified by numerous other factors acting in concert and participating in the pathogenesis of endorgan damage and injury. Thus, pathogenetic synergism between thromboembolic events and sustained hypercholesterolemia has been previously discussed.[20]

ARAS usually involves the proximal third of the artery, frequently (in about 75% of cases) including the ostia. In up to 30%

of cases, both renal arteries may be stenosed. In severe cases more distal arterial segments may also be narrowed. The reason for the susceptibility of the ostia to atherosclerosis has not been clarified, yet it may be related to altered mechanical properties due to differences in the histological architecture of the transitional zone between the elastic aorta and muscular renal artery.[21] The rate of progression of ARAS is a matter of debate. In one study using duplex classification of renal stenosis severity, the cumulative rates of progression from normal to <60% narrowing at 1, 2, and 3 years were 0%, 0%, and 8%, and those from <60% to >60% were 30%, 44%, and 48%, respectively.[22] Similar rates of progression were reported more recently, with the risk of progression being highest in individuals with a pre-existing RAS in either one of the renal arteries, elevated systolic blood pressure, and diabetes.[23] Progression of ARAS appears to be associated with a progressive loss of renal tissue.[24]

FIBROMUSCULAR DYSPLASIA

Fibromuscular dysplasia (FMD), first described in 1938,[25] is a vascular disease of unknown origin that most frequently affects the renal arteries (in 60% to 75% on one side only, in 35% bilaterally) and internal carotid arteries (25% to 30%). However, any artery and, rarely, even veins may be involved. FMD predominates in women (female-to-male ratio 3:1), and the typical age of presentation is 25 to 50 years. Hypertension, thromboembolism, and hemorrhage are typical presenting symptoms. Depending on the location of FMD lesions, medial, perimedial, intimal, and adventitial disease types may be distinguished (for review, see references 26 and 27).

On the basis of appearance, three angiographic types have commonly been distinguished:

- Type 1 angiography is described as a "string of beads," affects about 80% of cases, and mostly represents medial FMD. This type reveals a typical beading pattern with alternating segments of strictures and dilations, most frequently located in the middle-to-distal segment of the renal artery. The dilated segments are larger than the nominal diameter of the vessel. The differential diagnosis includes atherosclerotic disease, arteritis, and vasospasms.
- Type 2 angiography is "diffuse," affecting about 10% of cases, and mostly involves intimal but also perimedial locations. It presents as a long tubular stenosis. The differential diagnosis includes dissections, arteritis, congenital dyplasias, compression from outside, vasospasm, and functional narrowing due to decreased flow secondary to proximal or distal stenotic lesions.
- Type 3 angiography is described as "solitary," affecting about 5% of cases, and is frequently intimal FMD. It is associated with focal concentric lesions that may be difficult to distinguish from atheroma or pseudoaneurysm by angiography.

DIAGNOSIS OF RENAL ARTERY STENOSIS

Clinical findings suggestive of RAS include:

- Sudden onset or sudden worsening of a severe and refractory hypertension[28]
- Rapid elevation of serum creatinine, particularly if associated with institution of angiotensin-converting enzyme

(ACE) inhibitor treatment (due to the abolition of compensatory vasoconstriction of the efferent arterioles)[29]

- Hypertension associated with small kidneys
- Different-sized kidneys
- Hypertension in patients with severe systemic atherosclerosis[30]
- Recurrent flash pulmonary edema[31]

In addition, hyponatremia may be more common.[32] However, in the majority of cases RAS remains clinically silent.

According to the recent ACC/AHA guidelines,[16] diagnostic evaluations for RAS are indicated in patients with the onset of hypertension before the age of 30 years, patients with the onset of severe hypertension after the age of 55 years (both class I evidence level B), those with accelerated hypertension or drug-resistant hypertension or malignant hypertension (class I evidence level C), patients with azotemia or worsening renal function associated with administration of ACE inhibitors, unexplained renal atrophy or size difference between the two kidneys >1.5 cm, and finally those with unexplained "flush" pulmonary edema (all class I evidence level B). Class IIa evidence level B indications include patients with unexplained renal failure, and Class IIb evidence level B and C concerns patients with multivessel coronary artery disease or peripheral arterial disease at the time of arteriography and patients with unexplained congestive heart failure or refractory angina, respectively.

Noninvasive screening for RAS includes duplex ultrasonography, magnetic resonance angiography, and CT angiography (all ACC/AHA class I evidence level B).[16] Given a high level of suspicion or inconclusive noninvasive tests, selective arterial digital subtraction angiography (DSA) is recommended to establish the diagnosis (ACC/AHA class I evidence level B). Despite progress in noninvasive imaging methods, DSA still represents the gold standard and reference technique to provide a definitive RAS diagnosis and to allow an anatomically precise road map for revascularization (for review, see reference 33). A captopril renogram, for which 25 to 50 mg captopril PO is administered before radioisotope scanning and usually using ^{99m}Tc-DTPA as a tracer, may allow identification of an angiotensin-II-dependent kidney; in such cases, following captopril administration there is a decrease in GFR (perfusion decreased by >40%), a delayed peak uptake in the ipsilateral kidney, and—frequently—enhanced compensatory perfusion in the contralateral kidney.[34,35] However, because of the rather low sensitivity and specificity, captopril renography has been largely abandoned. Similarly, measurements of renin plasma activity at baseline and following captopril challenge,[36] side-selective renal vein renin determinations where the ipsilateral kidney stimulates renin production while the contralateral kidney suppresses it[37] are rarely employed.

In peri-interventional settings, DSA represents the only method allowing reliable assessment of the lesion and of the progress of the intervention.

Peri-interventional RAS DSA should unequivocally determine the severity and morphology of the target lesion and the complete ipsilateral renal blood supply. The anatomy of the renal artery and its branches, clinical x-ray anatomy of the variants, the renal collateral circulation (capsular, peripelvic, and periureteric systems),[38,39] and the principles of diagnostic renal arteriography have been covered extensively in the literature.[40]

Radiographic evaluation of RAS consists of abdominal aortic DSA and, if needed, selective renal DSA, both performed as breath-hold imaging (shallow inspiration). First, the pigtail catheter is positioned just above or at the level of the presumed take-off of the renal arteries (lumbar vertebra L1 or L2, right higher than left). Then, a DSA sequence is taken that is long enough to cover at least the arterial but preferably also the nephrogenic and venous phases of contrast-agent passage using an automatic injector. In evaluating the arterial phase, the origin, number, size, course, and branching pattern of the renal arteries are determined. Usually the main renal artery, its segmental branches, and the interlobar and arcuate arteries can be differentiated. Interlobular arteries and arterioles, however, cannot be clearly distinguished. In the nephrogenic phase, the cortical arteriogram, glomerulogram, cortical nephrogram, and complete nephrogram are displayed in a short sequence, with a complete washout of contrast agent taking 20 seconds and

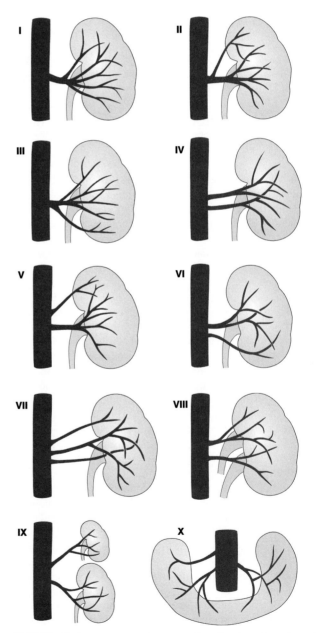

FIGURE 11-1. Variations of patterns of ramification of renal arteries. (Modified from Lusza G. *X-ray Anatomy of the Vascular System.* Philadelphia: JB Lippincott, 1964:227–231.)

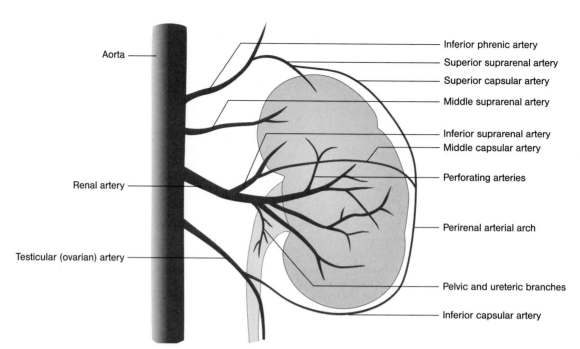

FIGURE 11-2.   Intrarenal and extrarenal collateral circulation of the renal artery. (Modified from Lusza G. *X-ray Anatomy of the Vascular System.* Philadelphia: JB Lippincott, 1964:227–231.)

longer. The venous phase partially overlaps the nephrogenic phase, starting about 3 seconds after the entry of the contrast agent into the renal artery and peaking at about 8 seconds. Because of the overlapping vascular structures, intrarenal vein structures can barely be distinguished and only some parts of the extrarenal veins can be evaluated.[40] Figure 11-1 shows pattern variations in the ramification of renal arteries. In Figure 11-2, the principal collateral pathways of the renal artery are shown.

In patients with suspect anatomy in the overview DSA aortograms, side-selective renal arteriograms using preshaped catheters are required. Because of the vulnerability of the ostia care must be taken to avoid injury, and gentle "puff" injections of the contrast agent are used for localization of the ostia. Because of the variable laterality of the origin of the renal arteries and variable diameter of the abdominal aorta, different oblique angulations may be required in individual patients to visualize the true profile of the ostia and of the proximal segment free of overlap with the adjacent aorta. Based on extensive CT-based measurements, anteroposterior (AP) and 20-degree left anterior oblique (LAO) projections (combined successfully in 86% of cases) for the left renal artery and 20-degree LAO, 40-degree LAO, and AP projections (combined successfully in 93% to 95% of cases) for the right renal artery have been recommended. The largest yield of orthogonal ostial projections on either side was achieved using a 20-degree LAO projection. Deviation from the optimal degree of angulation by ±10% may be responsible for 5-mm proximal foreshortening, thus hiding the ostium from adequate visualization. On the basis of this data, the combination of AP, 20-degree, and 40-degree LAO projections allows adequate angiographic definition of both ostia in both genders in the vast majority (92%) of all individuals.[41]

In patients with RAS, the location, severity, and morphology of the target lesion should be documented. Typically, ostial stenoses

(≤5 mm from the orifice), nonosteal stenoses (>5 mm from the orifice), branch stenoses, and angiographic lesions of less than and at least 50% diameter are distinguished. The degree of RAS can be calculated using the edge detection or densitometry-based quantitative angiography programs as 1 minus the ratio of the diameter of the lumen at the stenosis to the diameter of the lumen of the uninvolved renal artery distal to the stenosis multiplied by 100. Stenoses of at least 50% diameter are considered hemodynamically significant. In addition, the minimal luminal diameter (MLD), measured in millimeters across the stenosis, should be reported.[42]

In patients with angiographically indeterminate or borderline lesions (typically 50% to 70% diameter stenoses), translesional blood-pressure measurements may be required. However, if pressure wire has not been used, invasive measurements require crossing the lesion with the guidewire and usually a curved catheter with the attending risk of injury; for this reason, invasive pressure measurements should be performed with care and only in selected cases. In the absence of any documented evidence, some investigators consider a 20 mm Hg peak-to-peak systolic pressure gradient between the abdominal aorta and distal renal artery to be hemodynamically relevant, whereas others consider a resting peak systolic pressure gradient of 10 mm Hg at baseline conditions or a pressure gradient of 20 mm Hg after vasodilatation significant (for review, see reference 43). These and other threshold values have been considered as indications for revascularization in the presence of borderline lesions. Translesional gradients should preferably be measured using 0.0014-in. pressure wires; however, in current clinical practice, the majority of measurements are performed using two different fluid-filled catheters with the tip at the ostium and distal to the lesion, respectively. The accuracy, that is, proximity to the true value, and precision, that is, reproducibility of measurements, depend on a number of factors including the coaxial position of the tip, the luminal diameters of the catheters, the position of the orifices (end-hole catheters measure higher intraluminal pressure because of additional conversion of the kinetic energy into pressure), and the catheter material (for review, see reference 43). To obtain reliable data, standardized and carefully performed measurements are required.

The morphology of target RAS lesions has not yet been systematically evaluated, yet the presence of thrombus definitely increases the risk of distal embolization, and other lesion characteristics such as ulcerations probably deserve further study. In addition to the renal artery, evaluation of the ostium and the adjacent aortic walls is important. Angulation of the renal artery take-off, the degree of calcification, and the presence of plaques should be noted.

Since the risks of contrast-induced nephropathy (CIN) are greater in patients with pre-existing renovascular disease, strict adherence to the established standard of iodinated contrast agent administration is required. CIN can be defined as serum creatinine elevation of $\geq$0.5mg/dL (44 μmol/L) with baseline creatinine of $\geq$2.0 mg/dL (176 μmol/L), or as serum creatinine elevation of $\geq$1.0 mg/dL (88 μmol/L) with baseline creatinine of $\geq$2.0 mg/dL (176 μmol/L) occurring within 48 hours after contrast exposure[44,45]; however, other definitions are also available in the literature.

Recommendations for CIN prevention have recently been summarized and include:

- Careful risk-benefit assessment, particularly in patients with pre-existing renal dysfunction
- Avoidance of volume depletion, and adequate hydration with intravenous saline before and after the procedure (a note of warning: particular care must be taken here in patients with heart failure)
- The use of low or iso-osmolal nonionic contrast agents (low-osmolar contrast media, LOCM)
- The use of the lowest possible dose of the iodinated contrast agent
- Avoidance of nephrotoxic agents
- Oral administration of the antioxidant *N*-cetylcysteine (600 mg b.i.d.) on the day of angiography and the day after (for review, see references 46–47).

The benefits of administering other agents such as diuretics, calcium antagonists, or theophylline are questionable, and their use is not recommended. To reduce contrast agent exposure, carbon dioxide might be considered for diagnostic evaluations below the diaphragm, yet experience in peri-interventional settings has been limited.[48] Suggested indications for invasive angiography in patients with RAS are summarized in Table 11-1.[49] Suggested indications for RAS revascularization based on a traditional approach are provided in Table 11-2.[50] In Table 11-3, predictors of clinical success with regard to renal function are summarized. Table 11-4 gives suggested indications for surgical RAS revascularization.

REVASCULARIZATION OF RENAL ARTERY STENOSIS

RAS has been treated surgically since 1973[51] and, at present, essentially three different surgical approaches of revascularization are available, namely, aortorenal bypass, thromboendarterectomy, and reimplantation (for review, see reference 52).

TABLE 11-1. Suggested Indications for Invasive X-ray Angiography for Evaluating Renal Artery Stenosis; Criteria Society of Interventional Radiology

Clinical signs of renovascular hypertension, ischemic nephropathy, or a cardiac disturbance syndrome are present and at least one of the following:

1. Noninvasive vascular imaging is suggestive that a renal artery stenosis of more than 50% is present,
2. Progression of a hemodynamically significant renal artery stenosis is indicated by noninvasive vascular imaging,
3. Noninvasive vascular imaging is technically inadequate, equivocal or cannot be obtained,
4. Onset of hypertension occurs in a patient less than 30 years of age,
5. Renal artery fibromuscular dysplasia is suspected as the etiology of renal artery stenosis,
6. There is recent onset of hypertension in a patient 60 years of age or older,
7. There is loss of renal mass or deterioration of renal function while hypertension is being controlled medically, especially when being treated with ACE inhibitors or angiotensin II receptor blockers.

Note. The threshold for the presence of the indications for renal angiography is 95%.

Reproduced with permission from Martin LC, Rundback JH, Sacks D, et al. Quality improvement guidelines for angiography, angioplasty, and stent placement in the diagnosis and treatment of renal artery stenosis in adults. *J Vasc Intervent Radiol.* 2003;14:S297-S310.

Although the published short- and long-term results of RAS revascularization have been satisfactory (for review, see reference 53), the use of surgery for isolated RAS has rapidly declined with the availability of endovascular treatment options.

Renal artery angioplasty was introduced by Grüntzig et al. in 1978.[54] In early series[55,56] the reported technical success rates ranged between 73% and 100% in patients with FMD, and between 75% and 100% in patients with nonstial ARAS. The corresponding rates of medical cure and improvement were 25% to 63% and 13% to 63% for FMD, and 7% to 47% and 31% to 60% for nonstial ARAS, respectively (for review, see references 57 and 58). The introduction of stent-supported renal artery angioplasty in the early 1990s[59] markedly improved the safety of the intervention and extended the spectrum of indications to include the treatment of ostial lesions.[60] Thus, for example, in the series reported by Blum et al.,[60] technical success (defined as residual stenosis of <50% according to angiography and a trans-stenotic pressure gradient of <20 mm Hg) was achieved in 96% of all treated lesions (71 of 74). At 5-year follow-up, a sustained improvement in mean arterial blood pressure and no significant changes in serum creatinine were observed. In published uncontrolled series, the combined success rate (cure or improvement of hypertension) was 65% to 80%, and in-stent restenosis ranging between 11% and 17% was reported. In addition, a variable improvement or stabilization of plasma creatinine concentration has been reported (for review, see reference 58). Selected early results of stent-supported renal artery angioplasty for RAS treatment are provided in Tables 11-5 to 11-8.[61]

Marked improvements in endovascular instrumentation have allowed downsizing of the interventional systems: 0.035-in. guidewires have been replaced by 0.0014-in. ones; bulky peripheral over-the-wire dilatation balloon catheters have been replaced by low-profile rapid-exchange balloon catheters; and stent delivery

TABLE 11-2. Suggested Indications for Renal Artery Stenosis (RAS) Revascularization Based on a Traditional Approach

RAS Characteristics	Indications
Bilateral	Bilateral revascularization regardless of renal function
Solitary functional kidney	Revascularization regardless of renal function
Ipsilateral	
Normal renal function	Prevention of renal insufficiency in patients with severe RAS (≥80%)
	Prevention of renal insufficiency in patients with RAS 50% to 80% and positive captopril-enhanced nephrogram
Impaired renal function	Recovery of renal function or stabilization of renal insufficiency, when serum creatinine >4 mg/dL, but recent rental vein thrombosis possible or documented with additional criteria RAS ≥80% or RAS 50% to 80% and positive captopril-enchanced nephrogram
Clinical characteristics	
Flash pulmonary edema ESRD, reversible azotemia associated with administration of ACE inhibitors and angiotensin receptor antagonists	Bilateral or ipsilateral revascularization

ESRD, end-stage renal disease; ACE, angiotensin-converting enzyme.
Based on Spinowitz BS, Rodriquez J. Renal artery stenosis. Available at: www.emedicine.com/med/topic2001.htm. Accessed December 27, 2005.

TABLE 11-3. Potential Predictors of Clinical Success with Regard to Renal Function

Collateral circulation and nephrogram on angiography
- Renal length > 9 cm
- Lateralization of renin secretion in side-selective renal vein measurements
- Differential concentration of urine on side-split-function studies
- Viable nephrons on biopsy tissue examination

Modified from Spinowitz BS, Rodriquez J. Renal artery stenosis. Available at: www.emedicine.com/med/topic2001.htm. Accessed December 27, 2005.

TABLE 11-4. Suggested Definitive and Optional Indications for Surgical Renal Artery Stenosis (RAS) Repair

- Presence of abdominal aortic aneurysm
- Ipsilateral renal artery aneurysm
- Renal artery occlusion (with unsuccessful thrombolysis)
- Renal artery rupture
- RAS secondary to kinking (optional)
- Peripheral multifocal stenosis (optional)
- Unsuccessful stent-supported angioplasty

Modified from Spinowitz BS, Rodriquez J. Renal artery stenosis. Available at: www.emedicine.com/med/topic2001.htm. Accessed December 27, 2005.

systems with distal protection devices have been introduced.[62] All these have transformed RAS revascularization into a less complex and safer procedure, similar to a coronary intervention. Accordingly, the coronary-like approach to RAS intervention can be defined by the use of small size introductory sheath, typically 6F, to reduce trauma, pre-shaped guiding catheters to improve seating and steering of the instrumentation, coronary 0.014-in. guidewires, low-profile dilatation balloon catheters, and/or stent-delivery devices with rapid-exchange design to facilitate each interventional step.

TABLE 11-5. Technical Success of Stent-supported Renal Angioplasty: Early Experiences

Study Series	Study Period	Arteries, n	Stent Type	Ostial Lesion, %	Success Definition	Technical Success, %
Rodriguez-Lopez et al.	1993–1996	125	Palmaz	66	No RS/dissection	98
van de Ven et al.	1993–1997	52	Palmaz	100	RS 50%	90
Henry et al.	—	104	AVE[†]	77	RS 20%	99
Rocha-Singh et al.	1993–1995	180	Palmaz	43	PG 5 mm Hg	98
Tuttle et al.	1991–1996	148	Palmaz	100	RS 30%	98
Dorros et al.	1990–1995	202	Palmaz	—	RS 50%	99
Rundback et al.	—	54	Palmaz	—	RS 30%	94
White et al.	1992–1994	133	Palmaz	81	RS 30%	99
Harden et al.	1992–1995	32	Palmaz	75	RS 10%	100
Blum et al.	1989–1996	74	Palmaz	100	RS 50%	100
Henry et al.	1990–1994	64	Palmaz	53	RS 20%	100
Iannone et al.	1992–1993	83	Palmaz	78	RS 30%	99
Hennequin et al.	1987–1991	21	Wallstent	33	—	100
Rees and Snead	1988–1992	296	Palmaz	100	RS 30%	98

Palmaz: Cordis, Miami, FL.
RS, residual stenosis; PG, pressure gradient.
Reproduced with permission from Lim ST, Rosenfield K. Renal artery stent placement: indications and results. *Curr Intervent Cardiol Rep.* 2000;2:130–139.

TABLE 11-6.   Effect of Stent-supported Renal Angioplasty on Hypertension: Early Experiences

Study series	Patients, n	Blood Pressure, mm Hg Present	Last follow-up	Average Drugs Present	Last follow-up	Blood Pressure Trend Cured	Improved	Cured or improved
Rodriguez-Lopez et al.	108	—	—	—	—	11	55	66
van de Ven et al.	40	180/105	160/90	1.8	1.5	—	—	58
Henry et al.	94	—	—	—	—	20	60	80
Rocha-Singh et al.	140	MAP = 110	MAP = 98	2.9	1.9	6	50	56
Tuttle et al.	129	158/84	135/79	2.2	2.1	0	55	55
Dorros et al.	163	166/86	148/80	2.2	1.8	1	42	43
White et al.	100	175/98	140/73	2.6	2	—	—	—
Harden et al.	32	169/95	164/87	1.6	1.4	0	—	—
Blum et al.	68	188/105	—	2.9	—	16	62	78
Rundback et al.	20	179/86	143/78	2.4	1.8	0	63	63
Henry et al.	59	172/98	144/81	1.8	1.4	18	57	73
Iannone et al.	63	160/80	148/78	2.5	2.2	4	35	39
Hennequin et al.	21	182/107	138/78	—	—	14	86	100
Rees and Snead	263	—	—	—	—	3	58	61

MAP, mean arterial pressure.
Reproduced with permission from Lim ST, Rosenfield K. Renal artery stent placement: indications and results. *Curr Intervent Cardiol Rep.* 2000;2:130–139.

TABLE 11-7.   Effect of Stent-supported Renal Angioplasty on Renal Function

Study Series	Patients, n	Renal Function Improved, %	Stable, %	Deteriorated, %
van de Ven et al.	42	12	62	26
Rocha-Singh et al.	150	22	70	8
Tuttle et al.	129	15	81	4
Dorros et al.	163	18	48	34
Rundback et al.	45	20	47	33
Harden et al.	32	34	38	28
Weighted average		19	62	19

Reproduced with permission from Lim ST, Rosenfield K. Renal artery stent placement: indications and results. *Curr Intervent Cardiol Rep.* 2000;2:130–139.

TABLE 11-8.   Effect of Stent-supported Renal Angioplasty in Patients with Baseline Renal Impairment

Study Series	Patients, n	Renal Function Improved, %	Stable, %	Deteriorated, %
van de Ven et al.	29	17	55	28
Rocha-Singh et al.	71	28	59	13
Rundback et al.	45	20	47	33
Harden et al.	32	34	38	28
Blum et al.	20	0	100	0
Henry et al.	10	20	60	20
Iannone et al.	29	36	46	18
Dorros et al.	29	28	28	45
Hennequin et al.	6	17	50	33
Rees and Snead	124	37	37	26
Weighted average		28	48	24

Reproduced with permission from Lim ST, Rosenfield K. Renal artery stent placement: indications and results. *Curr Intervent Cardiol Rep.* 2000;2:130–139.

STENT-SUPPORTED ANGIOPLASTY OF RENAL ARTERY STENOSIS: THE CORONARY-LIKE APPROACH

Stent-supported renal artery angioplasty using the coronary-like approach has markedly facilitated RAS interventions, since it allows revascularization of lesions formerly considered "hostile" at much lower procedural risk. Facile and safe use of the coronary-like RAS revascularization represents a critical step toward evaluations of clinical benefits of the endovascular RAS repair in well-controlled studies using standard protocols.[42,49,63] Examples of standardized RAS definitions are provided in Table 11-9. An example of suggested indications for coronary endovascular RAS treatment is provided in Table 11-10. Figures 11-3 to 11-6 provide typical examples of RAS interventions using the coronary approach.

EVIDENCE

In a prospective study involving 215 patients with 277 renal ostial stenoses treated between October 1996 and October 2000 using stent-supported angioplasty with stents of various designs, the technical success rate defined as residual stenosis ≤30% diameter was 100%. Six patients (2.8%) suffered severe procedure-related complications (renal artery rupture requiring surgery in one patient, progression from preterminal renal failure to terminal renal failure caused by renal embolism or dye-induced nephropathy in four patients, and occlusion of the common femoral artery after sheath removal requiring surgery in one patient). In addition, in five patients (2.3%) clinically unapparent complications were observed (one dissection of the descending aorta with spontaneous thrombosis of the false lumen, one guidewire-induced renal artery dissection with a persistent occlusion of a side branch, two stent displacements requiring the placement of a second stent, and one wire-induced perforation of a segment artery with spontaneous sealing of the leakage). Furthermore, four false aneurysms (1.8%) had to be treated with duplex-guided compression therapy. No procedure-related deaths or subacute stent thromboses were reported. The in-stent restenosis rate (stenosis of ≥70% diameter estimated visually) was 9.6% at 6 months and 11.2% at 12 months. At 1-year follow-up, median serum creatinine concentration dropped significantly from 1.21 mg/dL (quartiles: 0.92, 1.60 mg/dL) at baseline to

TABLE 11-9. Definition of Standard Criteria Pertaining to Percutaneous Treatment of Renal Artery Stenosis

Renal artery stenosis

Narrowing of the renal artery lumen by 50% or greater, expressed as a percentage of the diameter of a normal renal vessel (i.e., % renal artery stenosis = 100 × 1 − [diameter of the narrowed lumen/the normal vessel diameter]). In the presence of an angiographically visible dissection at the treatment site, the residual lumen is measured from the widest opacified lumen, including intimal crack depth, knowing that the true lumen is difficult to measure accurately in this situation.

Ostial renal artery stenosis

Narrowing of the renal artery at its origin from the aorta, generally considered to be within 5 mm but may be extended to within 10 mm if confirmed by computed tomographic angiography.

Truncal renal artery stenosis

Nonostial renal artery stenosis occurring proximal to renal artery branching (i.e., segmental arteries).

Technically successful renal revascularization

Less than 30% residual stenosis measured at the narrowest point of the vascular lumen and restoration of the pressure gradient to less than the selected threshold for intervention. In the presence of an angiographically visible dissection at the treatment site, the residual lumen is measured from the widest opacified lumen regardless of intimal dissections, knowing that the true lumen is difficult to measure in this situation. (Comment: in "coronary" approach stenting of all relevant dissections is indicated,)

Indicator threshold

Specific level of an indicator that should prompt a review (applicable to indications, success rates, complications).

Modified from Rundback JH, Sacks D, Kent C, et al. for the American Heart Association Council on Cardiovascular Radiology, High Blood Pressure Research, Kidney in Cardiovascular Disease, Cardio-Thoracic and Vascular Surgery, and Clinical Cardiology, and the Society of Interventional Radiology FDA Device Forum Committee. Guidelines for the reporting of renal artery revascularization in clinical trials. *Circulation.* 2002;106:1572–1585; and Martin LC, Rundback JH, Sacks D, et al. Quality improvement guidelines for angiography, angioplasty, and stent placement in the diagnosis and treatment of renal artery stenosis in adults. *J Vasc Intervent Radiol.* 2003;14:S297–S310.

TABLE 11-10. Suggested Indications for Endovascular Therapy Using a "Coronary" Approach of a Hemodynamically Significant Renal Artery Stenosis

1. Hypertensive control
   a. A reasonable likelihood of cure of renovascular hypertension.
      i. Onset of hypertension before age 30,
      ii. Recent onset of hypertension after age 60,
      iii. Stenosis is caused by fibromuscular hyperplasia.
   b. Hypertension is refractory to medical control with at least three medications of different classes including a diuretic.
   c. Hypertension is accelerated (i.e., there is sudden worsening of previously controlled hypertension).
   d. Hypertension is malignant (i.e., is associated with endorgan damage such as left ventricular hypertrophy, congestive heart failure, visual or neurological disturbance, grade III–IV retinopathy).
   e. The patient is intolerant or noncompliant with antihypertensive medical treatment.

2. Renal salvage
   a. Unexplained worsening of renal function.
   b. Loss of renal mass, especially while under surveillance during medical antihypertensive treatment.
   c. Impairment of renal function or acute renal failure secondary to antihypertensive medication, particularly with an angiotensin converting enzyme inhibitor.
   d. Progression of a hemodynamically significant renal artery stenosis while under surveillance.

3. Cardiac and coronary indications
   a. Recurrent "flash" pulmonary edema secondary to impaired left ventricular function.
   b. Unstable angina.

Note. For indications for angioplasty of a hemodynamically significant renal artery stenosis, the threshold is 95%.

Reproduced with permission from Martin LC, Rundback JH, Sacks D, et al. Quality improvement guidelines for angiography, angioplasty, and stent placement in the diagnosis and treatment of renal artery stenosis in adults. *J Vasc Intervent Radiol.* 2003;14:S297–S310.

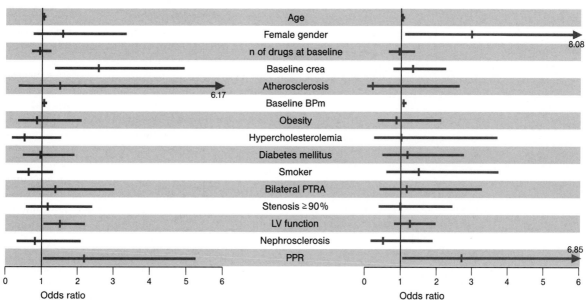

FIGURE 11-3. Predictors of improved serum creatinine concentration (*left*) or improved mean arterial blood pressure (*right*) by multivariate logistic regression analysis. Graphs show odds ratios and their 95% CIs. BPm, mean arterial blood pressure; crea, creatinine; PTRA, percutaneous transluminal renal angioplasty; LV, left ventricle function; PPR, parenchymal/pelvic ratio. (Redrawn from Zeller T, Frank U, Müller C, et al. Predictors of improved renal function after percutaneous stent-supported angioplasty of severe atherosclerotic ostial renal artery stenosis. *Circulation.* 2003;108:2244–2249.)

1.10 mg/dL (quartiles: 0.88, 1.50 mg/dL) at 1 year (*p* = 0.047). Mean arterial blood pressure decreased significantly, from 102 ± 12 mm Hg (mean ± SD) at baseline to 92 ± 10 mm Hg at 1 year (*p* <0.001).[64] Figure 11-3 shows some predictors of improved serum creatinine concentration (*left*) or improved mean arterial blood pressure (*right*) according to multivariate logistic regression analysis, and Figure 11-4 shows the time course of systolic, mean, and diastolic blood pressure and number of drugs during 1 year as determined in a nonrandomized prospective trial.[64]

In a prospective nonrandomized study, 208 patients were treated for ostial renal artery stenoses at 23 U.S. medical centers between December 1997 and May 1999, using stent-supported angioplasty with the Palmaz balloon-expandable stent (Cordis, Miami Lakes, FL, USA). For critical lesions (defined as ≥70% de novo lesions, restenotic atherosclerotic stenoses, a persistent peak-to-peak translesional pressure gradient of ≥20 mm Hg, flow-limiting dissections, or residual ≥50% stenoses after percutaneous transluminal renal angioplasty, PTRA), the technical success rate was 80.2% (residual stenosis ≤50% diameter). Procedural complications included major embolic events (1.4%), stent thrombosis (0.5%), major hemorrhage (1.0%), and combined vascular events other than hemorrhage (2.4%). At 9 months, the restenosis rate (defined as stenosis of ≥50% diameter) was 17.4%. Also at 9-month follow-up, systolic/diastolic blood pressure decreased from 168 ± 25/82 ± 13 mm Hg (mean ± standard deviation) at baseline, to 149 ± 24/77 ± 12 mm Hg (*p* <0.001 vs. baseline) and 149 ± 25/77 ± 12 mm Hg at 24 months (*p* <0.001 vs. baseline). Mean serum creatinine concentration was unchanged from baseline values at 9- and 24-month follow-up.[65] In our own evaluation of the coronary-like management of RAS technical

success defined as residual stenosis ≤30% was achieved in 178 (98.3%) of patients. In one patient each, the target ARAS could not be crossed, large plaque burden prevented full stent expansion, or residual stenosis was >30%. No major adverse cardiac and cerebral effects were observed. In 3.9% of patients, minor local complications of the access site occurred; 4 (2.2%) inguinal hematoma, 3 (1.1%) pseudoaneurysm.[66]

The large-scale National Heart, Lung, and Blood Institute (NHLBI) sponsored CORAL (Cardiovascular Outcomes in Renal Atherosclerotic Lesions) multicenter trial is designed to determine the effect of optimum medical therapy alone versus optimum medical therapy with stent angioplasty on composite cardiovascular and renal endpoints. These include cardiovascular or renal death, myocardial infarction, hospitalization for congestive heart failure, stroke, doubling of serum creatinine level, and the need for renal replacement therapy. The results will become available in 2010.

INSTRUMENTATION

In the majority of cases, renal artery stent-supported angioplasty can be performed using a preformed guiding catheter and standard coronary interventional instrumentation. Typically, 6F systems are used. Choice of the access site and the angulation of the renal artery take-off determine the length and the form of the guiding catheter (transfemoral 50 cm long, renal double curve, RDC; transbrachial 100 cm, Judkins right or hockey stick). To navigate the ostium and to cross the lesion, coronary 0.014-in., floppy-tip, stiff-shaft guidewires are utilized. To facilitate steering and to improve backup, a 5F diagnostic catheter is usually employed in a telescopic coaxial manner to reinforce the guiding catheter. In standard revascularizations,

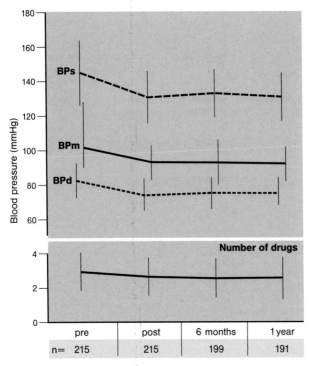

FIGURE 11-4. Time course of systolic (BPs), mean (BPm), and diastolic blood pressure (BPd) and number of drugs during 1 year. Graph shows mean and SD. *P* <0.001 for each comparison between preinterventional and postinterventional; *n*, number of patients. (Adapted from Zeller T, Frank U, Müller C, et al. Predictors of improved renal function after percutaneous stent-supported angioplasty of severe atherosclerotic ostial renal artery stenosis. *Circulation.* 2003;108:2244–2249.)

0.035-in., hydrophilic, stiff guidewires are not required. Because of low-profile technology, most RASs may be stented directly using dedicated (high radial force) peripheral balloon-expansible 4 to 7-mm-diameter and 12 to 18-mm-long stents. A manual inflation device and, in rare cases, a distal embolic protection device complete the set.

The basic structure of coronary-like RAS revascularization is similar to that of any percutaneous intervention, consisting of initialization, main interventional cycle, and termination driven by continuous risk-benefit analysis with each individual step interlinked by iterations.

INITIALIZATION

Intialization begins with establishing the vascular access and ends with providing direct access to the interventional site by seating the tip of the guiding catheter at the ostium of the target vessel. In planning RAS interventions, there are several important considerations. Choice of the access site (femoral vs. brachial) depends on the operator's estimate of the accessibility and crossability of the target lesion. To allow optimum transmission of the pushing force, the transition between the distal curve of the guide and the proximal segment of the renal artery should be smooth and flat, forming a shallow arch. Choice of system size is primarily determined by the required stability and backup of the system. In most cases, 6F systems are preferable. In selecting guidewires, the stiffness of the shaft, softness of the tip, and short, soft tip segments are important. In selecting stents and balloon catheters, high mobility of the renal artery with breathing and stretching on instrumentation, elongations, tortuosities, and poststenotic dilatations should be considered.

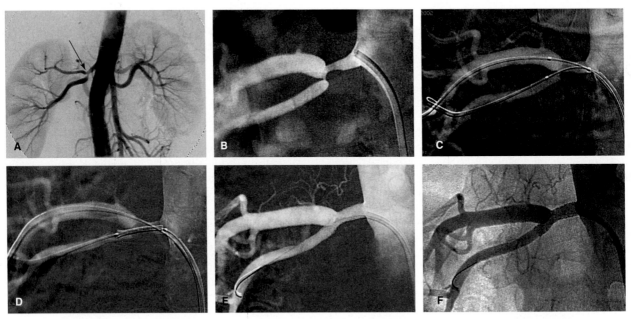

FIGURE 11-5. Bifurcation stenosis. **A:** Diagnostic aortography. High-grade bifurcation stenosis of the right renal artery is documented (*arrow*). The origin of the left renal artery has not been clearly visualized in straight anterior-posterior projection. **B:** Preinterventional angiography, right renal artery. Definition of the target bifurcation lesion. **C:** Kissing balloon angioplasty. Shown are both catheters in place before inflation. **D:** Following kissing balloon predilatation positioning of the stent (6 ×18 mm Herculink, Guidant). Stent placement into the lower branch because the major plaque burden and recoil were present in this branch. **E:** Final result. Post-stent-deployment ostial dilatation with a larger balloon was used to improve strut-to-aortic wall adaptation. **F:** Final result. To improve definition of the ostium and of the take-off of the upper branch, DSA mask was removed. Intact stent and intact upper (main) branch are demonstrated.

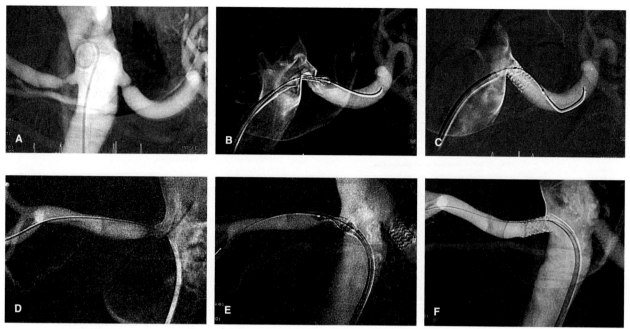

FIGURE 11-6. Bilateral renal artery stenosis. **A:** Diagnostic aortography. Bilateral renal artery stenosis is demonstrated. **B:** Left renal artery. Stent positioning. Direct stent placement (no predilatation). Positioning of the stent using partial balloon inflation (shown are the proximal and distal shoulders of the partially inflated balloon). In the next step (not shown) the entire system was slightly pushed cranially to allow exact alignment between the proximal renal artery and the delivery system for exact stent positioning across the lesion and in respect to the ostium. **C:** Left renal artery control angiography post stent placement. Exact lesion coverage of the target lesion is shown. **D:** Right renal artery. Using the same material, the guidewire was placed across the lesion. **E:** Right renal artery. Direct stent placement (no predilatation). Positioning of the stent using partial balloon inflation (shown are the proximal and distal shoulders of the partially inflated balloon). In the next step (not shown) the entire system was pushed gently cranially to allow exact stent positioning across the lesion and in respect to the ostium. **F:** Final result. Symmetrical strut apposition and zero residual stenosis are documented. Exact stent positioning across the lesion with one ring protrusion into the aorta is shown.

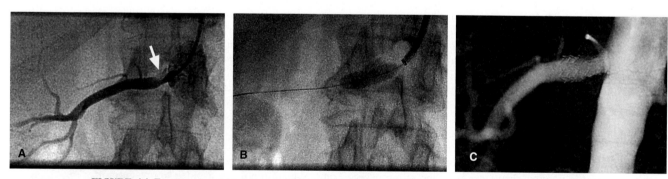

FIGURE 11-7. Transbrachial access, partial stent recoil due to major plaque burden and aortic wall lesion. **A:** Preinterventional selective angiogram, right renal artery. Ostial high-grade lesion secondary to a massive calcified plaque. **B:** Right renal artery, stent deployment. Following multiple predilatations, stent was positioned and inflated at high pressure. Full balloon expansion was achieved. **C:** Right renal artery, control angiography following the stent deployment. Partial collapse of the proximal stent segment due to the recoil of the aortic wall is shown. Because of the massive plaque burden and lack of a significant translesional gradient, the functional result was accepted.

Following sheath placement using the Seldinger technique, the interventional system—typically consisting of a preshaped guiding catheter and usually reinforced by a diagnostic catheter—is advanced to engage the target ostium. Depending on the angle of the take-off, the distal end of the guide can be stretched to a greater or lesser extent by advancing or withdrawing the diagnostic catheter within it below, at the level of, or above the ostium, to allow smooth engagement. Subsequently, angiograms are taken and stored on the monitor to guide the intervention.

MAIN INTERVENTIONAL CYCLE: ASSESS, INTERVENE, REPEAT

The main interventional cycle begins with the exploration and crossing of the target lesion, and it ends with achieving the final result. Following acquisition of the preinterventional angiograms, the guidewire tip is shaped to accommodate the ostium and carefully maneuvered into the ostium and across the target lesion. Following safe crossing, the guidewire tip is placed in one of the

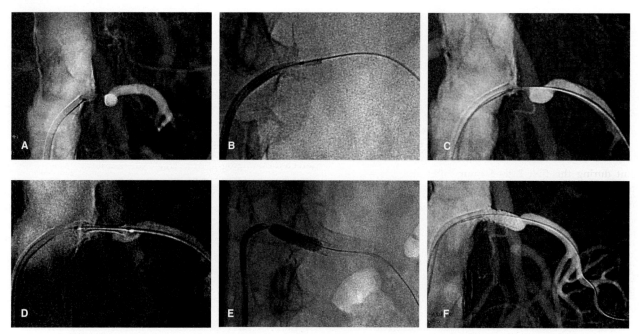

FIGURE 11-8.   Hard lesion, subtotal occlusion, left renal artery. **A:** Preinterventional angiogram. Following contrast agent injection, the residual lumen of the target stenosis has not been delineated. Postlesional segment appears ectatic and elongated with a slow flow. Aortic wall is highly irregular with large plaques. **B:** Dilatation. Following 0.014-in. guidewire passage, low-profile 1.5-mm balloon predilatation was performed. **C:** Postdilatation angiography. High-grade ostial lesion was demarcated. **D:** Stent positioning. Using similar technique as described in Figure 11-6, stent placement was performed. Note the positioning of the distal stent end in regard to vessel elongation by the guidewire. Following stent deployment and guidewire withdrawal, normally the vessel shortens to the original length bearing the risk of endothelial injury by the distal struts if a longer stent was selected. **E:** Afterdilatation. To improve stent strut apposition, the balloon was partially withdrawn to avoid distal injury and a high-pressure dilatation was performed. **F:** Final result. Exact stent positioning in respect to the poststenotic ectasia and elongation is shown. The original anatomy of the renal artery has been restored; minimal recoil of the proximal stent segment can be appreciated.

segmental arteries and remains in that position throughout the procedure. To prevent distal injury, the guidewire tip must not be moved forward. The diagnostic catheter inside can be removed before or after guidewire placement.

The evaluation of angiograms determines whether predilatation is needed. Only in severe or highly calcified lesions, particularly if they are associated with poor seating of the guide, is undersized predilatation with a low-profile 2.0 to 3.0-mm rapid-exchange coronary balloon catheter required. In all other cases, direct stenting is performed. Precise positioning of the stent is critical, particularly in ostial lesions. Stents usually sized to the nominal diameter of the target artery are placed to completely cover the lesion; lesion overreach by 1 to 2 mm at both ends is permissible. In ostial lesions, the proximal end of the stent should match or slightly overreach the endoluminal interface of the aortic wall (by about 1 mm). To allow precise placement, stable positioning of the guide, shallow breathing, and strictly orthogonal ostial projection are required. Once the stent has been positioned, the stent delivery system may be raised slightly to align it with the plane of the proximal target artery segment and rapidly inflated. After high-pressure stent deployment (about 14 bar), DSA images are taken to assess the results. Post-stent-deployment angiograms are assessed to determine the geometric precision of stent placement, the strut structure (indicating complete deployment and apposition), distal runoff vessels, the renal artery ostium, and the aortic wall. If the angiograms show satisfactory results,

the intervention can be terminated. Where there is focal strut recoil or partial collapse, careful postdilatations are required with a rapid-exchange balloon a nominal size shorter than the stent. Using higher inflation pressures or larger balloons, if needed, corrections in luminal size of up to 1 mm may be achieved. Dilatations distal to the stent should be avoided. In ostial lesions, the proximal end of the stent should be adapted to the aortic wall. To achieve a funnel-like shape, inflations with a slightly oversized balloon in up-and-down and left-to-right directions are performed. Although in most cases high-pressure inflations are required to fully expand the stent, excessive manipulation must be avoided to prevent injury.

In lesions with massive plaque burden, attempts to achieve zero-degree residual stenoses may be associated with undue risk and should be abandoned in favor of debulking or, in extreme cases, open surgery if acceptable anatomic results can not be achieved (residual stenosis ≤30% diameter).

TERMINATION

Termination begins with angiographic documentation of final results and ends with sheath removal. Intervention is terminated when the target of the intervention has been achieved or, rarely, when the actional risk of continuing the procedure exceeds the predictable benefits. In some cases, a staged procedure may be required, such as in order to use different equipment, or for a high-volume load. Following a complete retraction of the instrumentation, a selective ipsilateral renal angiogram is acquired to document the final result followed by sheath removal and hemostasis.

PERI-INTERVENTIONAL PATIENT CARE AND FOLLOW-UP

During the intervention, ECG and blood pressure monitoring are routinely performed.

Following the intervention, blood pressure and renal function are monitored. Unstable hemodynamics are particularly frequent during the first 2 to 4 hours after the procedure; hypotension and bradycardia can be treated efficiently with intravenous atropine and volume substitution. During the following approximately 2 weeks of neurohumoral adaptation, frequent blood-pressure controls and readjustment of antihypertensive medication are required.

To monitor renal function, serum creatinine is measured, and if needed, creatinine clearance is calculated. Usually, the first control is performed 2 to 4 hours after the procedure and then twice at 12-hour intervals daily until the baseline steady state is achieved. In uncomplicated cases, three intial successive documentations of normal renal function usually suffice. After discharge, weekly controls are recommended for 4 weeks.

Duplex ultrasonography of the ipsilateral kidney and renal artery is recommended at 2 and 6 weeks, at 6 months, and then yearly following the procedure. Angiography is usually performed again at 12 months.

ADJUVANT MEDICATION

Prior to the procedure, 5000 to 10000 U unfractionated heparin are administered intravenously or as an intra-arterial bolus. In standard interventions, measurement of the activated clotting time (ACT) is not required. However, in complex procedures, close ACT monitoring is mandatory. In all patients lifelong treatment with acetylsalicylic acid (usually 100 mg/day) is required.

MANAGING COMPLICATIONS

Using the coronary-like approach, the complication rates are exceedingly low and the technical success rate was 98.3%. Similar results were reported by others.[66] In other series using low-profile instrumentation, the reported technical success rate was 95% and the major complication rate, 6.1%.[67]

In earlier studies, a number of rare but severe complications were reported, including renal artery and renal parenchymal perforation, perinephric and retroperitoneal bleeding, atheroembolization, stent thrombosis, vessel closure, extensive renal artery dissection, type B Stanford classification aortic dissections, and acute renal failure requiring hemodialysis.[61,68,69] Table 11-11 shows examples of such complications reported previously in RAS interventions. Table 11-12 shows suggested complication thresholds in patients with RAS interventions.

Dissection and Rupture of the Renal Artery

Renal artery wall dissection and rupture are rare events using the coronary-like approach. However, even using low-profile instrumentation they may occur and are usually associated with distal guidewire manipulation or postdilatations outside the stent margins. In both cases, prompt angiographic definition of the lesion and immediate stent coverage are required. In some cases, smaller dissections or even covered ruptures may escape angiographic detection, with the patient presenting several hours later with blood pressure fluctuation, lumbar pain, or hemodynamic instability. In these patients, immediate renal ultrasound and, preferably, CT of the abdomen are performed to establish the diagnosis, to define the extent of the bleeding, and to document the integrity of the aortic wall followed by emergency reangiography. The site of active bleeding may be detected on angiography as free extravasation or as a pseudoaneurysmic deformation of the renal artery wall. In most cases, capsular or retroperitoneal bleeding is present. If distal extravasation is present, a superselective distal embolization is usually required. The primary goal of the interventional therapy is to stop the bleeding and preserve the organ, which is not always possible with surgical treatment. Preventive measures include the use of soft-tip guidewires, avoidance of very distal placement of the tip, and, particularly, avoidance of any forward guidewire motion after the final placement. Using the coronary approach, the need for a surgical repair has become exceedingly rare.

Dissection and Rupture of the Abdominal Aorta

Ostial lesions are present in ≥75% of RAS interventions. According to the origin of the plaque, renal artery and abdominal aortic ostial lesions may be distinguished.[70] A large aortic atheroma partially occluding the ostium may be extremely resistant to dilatation, thus preventing adequate stent deployment. Because it is sometimes difficult to seat the guiding catheter properly or to navigate the guidewire through the ostium and because high pressures are required to "crack" the lesion, the risk of ostial dissections and tears is increased in these patients. In cases with small-scale intramural staining, a conservative approach, close monitoring, and next-day CT control may suffice. In most cases, CT documents restored stability and integrity of the aortic wall, although a persisting aortic dissection has been reported.[69]

Distal Embolization

Thrombotic RAS or acute thrombosis associated with the interventional therapy may cause spontaneous or iatrogenic distal embolizations of thrombus particles, whereas ulcerated RAS with a diffuse atherosclerosis is more likely to cause spontaneous or iatrogenic embolization of cholesterol crystals or broken-off plaque debris. Depending on the type (thrombotic vs. atherosclerotic), size, and number of emboli, total or subtotal, segmental and subsegmental, or multiple, peripheral, or diffuse microcirculatory obstructions may occur.

In most cases of partial or total thrombotic occlusions, the thrombus is superimposed on a ruptured atherosclerotic plaque or, in rare cases, on traumatic or spontaneous intimal tears. However, thrombotic renal artery occlusions are far less frequent than renal emboli due to left atrial thrombi secondary to atrial fibrillation; left ventricular thrombi secondary to myocardial infarction; septic emboli due to cardiac valve endocarditis; cholesterol plaque and debris emboli from aortic plaques; paradox emboli from the venous circulation; and, much less frequently, tumor particles or fat emboli.

TABLE 11-11.   Complications of Stenting for Atherosclerotic Renovascular Disease
in Earlier Studies

Study Series	Patients, n	Procedure-related Mortality, n (%)	Other Complications
Rodriguez-Lopez et al.	108	4 (4)	2 perinephric hematoma, 1 retroperitoneal hematoma, 1 pseudoaneurysm
van de Ven et al.	40	0 (0)	4 cholesterol embolism, 3 renal artery injury, 3 FA aneurysm, 8 major bleeding
Rocha-Singh et al.	150	2 (1.3)	2 kidney perforation, 1 massive GI bleed, 7 ARF with 2 needing dialysis
Tuttle et al.	129	0 (0)	1 perirenal hematoma, 1 acute stent thrombosis, 2 atheroembolism, 9 groin hematoma, 15 ARF
Dorros et al.	163	1 (0.6)	21 ARF, 2 retroperitoneal hematoma
Rundback et al.	45	2 (4.4)	1 acute stent thrombosis, 1 needing dialysis
White et al.	100	0 (0)	1 subacute stent thrombosis, 2 ARF, 7 access site complications
Harden et al.	32	1 (3)	3 bleeding, 3 FA pseudoaneurysm
Beek et al.	50	0 (0)	5 cholesterol embolism, 1 kidney perforation, 1 femoral pseudoaneurysm, 1 groin hematoma needing transfusion
Blum et al.	75	0 (0)	3 minor groin hematoma
Henry et al.	59	0 (0)	1 acute stent thrombosis, 1 renal artery perforation
Iannone et al.	63	1 (1.6)	8 ARF, 2 needing dialysis; 7 perinephric hematoma; 1 retroperitoneal hematoma; 3 renal artery perforation; 1 FA pseudoaneurysm; 6 minor groin hematoma; 1 peripheral embolism
Hennequin et al.	21	0 (0)	1 distal embolism, 1 renal artery perforation, 1 acute closure, 1 ARF
Total	1035	11 (1.1)	

FA, femoral artery; ARF, acute renal failure; GI, gastrointestinal.

Reproduced with permission from Lim ST, Rosenfield K. Renal artery stent placement: indications and results. *Curr Intervent Cardiol Rep.* 2000;2:130–139.

Sudden embolic-thrombotic or local thrombotic occlusions of the renal artery or its branches may lead to complete or segmental renal infarctions. These patients typically present with acute onset of nausea and vomiting, flank, lower back, or abdominal pain and fever, and possibly signs of extrarenal embolizations.[71] However, the presenting symptoms are variable and, in patients with slowly developing, complete or incomplete, thrombotic occlusions may even be absent entirely. Laboratory findings are mostly nonspecific and may include elevated white blood cell count and plasma creatinine concentration in large infarcts. Gross or microscopic hematuria may also be present.[72] A sudden marked rise in plasma lactate dehydrogenase (LDH) without a concomitant increase in plasma transaminases may suggest renal infarction.[72] In patients with suspected renal infarction, contrast-enhanced CT of the abdomen provides a definite diagnosis in most cases.[71] In patients with CT-documented renal infarction, DSA is required to determine the cause. In patients presenting with complete or incomplete renal artery occlusion shortly after the initiating event, surgical or percutaneous revascularization should be considered. This interventional window usually corresponds to the ischemic tolerance of renal tissue (up to 3 hours).[73] In patients presenting with occlusions of segmental branches and smaller arteries, conservative management including anticoagulation using heparin followed by warfarin is indicated.

Embolization of cholesterol crystals and plaque debris occur mostly in older patients and may cause acute renal failure in extreme cases.[74,75] In contrast to thromboembolic and sudden thrombotic occlusions, atherosclerotic emboli more frequently produce incomplete occlusions, associated with atrophy related to chronic ischemia and tissue proliferation resulting from a foreign body reaction, both of which are associated with a progressive decline in renal function.[76,77] Depending on the severity and extent of distal renal embolization, the patient presents with marked and sudden deterioration of renal excretory function, progressively deteriorating renal function that worsens with each new embolic episode, or stable renal insufficiency.

TABLE 11-12. Complications of Renal Artery Stenosis Revascularizations and Suggested Complication Thresholds

Complication	Reported Rate (%)	Threshold (%)
30-day mortality	1	1
Secondary nephrectomy	<1	1
Surgical salvage operation	1	2
Symptomatic embolization	3	3
Main renal artery occlusion	2	2
Branch renal artery occlusion	2	2
Access site hematoma requiring surgery, transfusion, or prolonged hospital stay	5	5
Acute renal failure	2	2
Worsening of chronic renal failure requiring an increase in the level of care	2	5

Note. Published rates for individual types of complications are highly dependent on patient selection and are based on series comprising several hundred patients, which is a volume larger than most individual practitioners are likely to treat. Therefore, it is recommended that complication-specific thresholds usually should be set higher than the complication-specific reported rates listed in this table. It is also recognized that a single complication can cause a rate to cross above a complication-specific threshold when the complication occurs in a small volume of patients (e.g., early in a quality-improvement program). In this situation, the overall procedure threshold is more appropriate for use in a quality-improvement program. All values were supported by the weight of literature evidence and panel consensus.
Reproduced with permission from Martin LC, Rundback JH, Sacks D, et al. Quality improvement guidelines for angiography, angioplasty, and stent placement in the diagnosis and treatment of renal artery stenosis in adults. *J Vasc Intervent Radiol.* 2003;14:S297-S310.

Laboratory findings are nonspecific and may include cells or casts, rarely hematuria and red cell casts (in cases of acute glomerulonephritis or vasculitis) in urine sediment, proteinuria, and transient eosinophilia and hypocomplementemia (lasting approximately 1 week). In uncertain cases, to achieve a definitive diagnosis renal tissue biopsy may be required (for review, see reference 78). In patients with documented atheroembolic disease, the source of the embolization should be identified and treated, while the secondary renal disease is treated conservatively.

The presence of a thrombus associated with the target lesion increases the procedural risk, primarily because of the possibility of distal embolic complications. In such cases, the options are mechanical thrombus extraction using one of the available thrombectomy devices, deployment of the distal protection device, or direct stenting to "tack on" the thrombus. In addition, to prevent appositional thrombus growth and secondary embolizations, optimum anticoagulation is required (ACT 250 to 300 seconds). Since the pre-existing thrombi are usually older, fibrinolytic pharmacotherapy is not recommended. In de novo thrombi associated with the interventional procedure, empirical pharmacotherapy using GP IIb/IIIa receptor inhibitors might be attempted.

The presence of ulcerated target lesions in diffuse atherosclerosis settings predisposes to atheroembolic complications, making a careful atraumatic interventional approach ("notouch" technique) mandatory.

In patients with a progressive deterioration of renal function following RAS intervention and no angiographic signs of peripheral renal embolization, it may be difficult to distinguish between thrombus- or atheroma-related embolic disease and CIN. Although the deterioration of the renal function follows the intervention closely in both cases, in patients with CIN but without any pre-existing renal dysfunction, a full recovery may be expected usually within 3 weeks, whereas in patients with a significant embolic disease, the recovery of renal function (or its stabilization in patients with pre-existing renal dysfunction) might be more gradual and usually remains incomplete. In patients with CIN and pre-existing renal dysfunction, a definitive distinction between the two etiologies may not be possible on clinical grounds and could require renal tissue biopsy if necessary.

Contrast-Induced Nephropathy and Worsening Renal Failure

RAS interventions using the coronary-like approach may be straightforward, yet in patients with difficult anatomy, much longer procedures might be required, which usually increase the use of contrast agents. In our own series in uncomplicated cases, the average amount of contrast agent used in RAS interventions using the coronary-like approach was about 60 mL but in complex cases it could be as high as 200 mL. As there is a high percentage of patients with overt pre-existing renal dysfunction among patients undergoing RAS interventions (about 25% in own series), the issue of CIN appears particularly critical in patients undergoing RAS interventions.

Besides pre-existing renal dysfunction, the incidence of CIN is higher in patients with heart failure and hypovolemia. In addition, a high dose of contrast agent carries a higher risk of CIN, probably in a dose-dependent manner,. Although, a low dose of contrast agent (~ ≤100 mL) appears safe in most patients, even a much lower dose (20 to 30 mL) might trigger acute renal failure (ARF) in susceptible patients.

Following administration of the contrast agent, a small increase in plasma creatinine concentration (~0.2 mg/dL) is common. More pronounced deterioration in renal function (>50% above baseline or >1 mg/dL) may occur immediately after exposure, but usually resolves on treatment within several days. However, in high-risk patients, particularly in those with pre-existing advanced renal dysfunction, renal failure requiring hemodialysis and prolonged treatment may develop. Among these patients, irreversible renal failure may also develop rarely.

Prevention of CIN includes the use of low-dose contrast agent with low nephrotoxicity, avoidance of contrast-agent exposure at close intervals, avoidance of volume depletion, discontinuation of any nephrotoxic agents in peri-interventional settings, prophylactic volume supplementation (intravenous normal saline), and acetylcysteine administration. It has been reported that iodixanol (iso-osmolality nonionic contrast agent) may lower the incidence of CIN in diabetic patients with renal dysfunction compared with iohexol (low-osmolality nonionic contrast agent).[79] The prophylactic value of hemofiltration and hemodialysis in preventing CIN in high-risk patients has not been unequivocally proven, and their value remains uncertain (for review, see reference 80).

TABLE 11-13.   Restenosis Rate of Renal Stent-supported Angioplasties Reported in Earlier Studies

Study Series	Arteries, n	Arteries Evaluated (Original Total Arteries, %)	Ostial Lesion, %	Stent Type	Method of Evaluation	Average Time to Evaluation, mo	Restenosis of Artery Evaluated, %
van de Ven et al.	52	50 (95)	100	Palmaz	Angio	6	21
Rocha-Singh et al.	180	158 (88)	43	Palmaz	Duplex angio	13	12
Tuttle et al.	148	49 (33)	100	Palmaz	Angio	8	14
Rundback et al.	54	28 (52)	—	Palmaz	Angio Spiral CT	12	26
White et al.	133	80 (60)	81	Palmaz	Angio	9	19
Harden et al.	32	24 (75)	75	Palmaz	Angio	6	12
Blum et al.	74	74 (100)	100	Palmaz	Angio	24	11
Henry et al.	64	54 (84)	53	Palmaz	Angio	14	9
Iannone et al.	83	69 (85)	78	Palmaz	Duplex	11	14
Dorros et al.	92	56 (61)	100	Palmaz	Angio	7	25
Hennequin et al.	21	20 (95)	33	Wallstent	Angio	29	20
Rees and Snead	296	150 (51)	100	Palmaz	Angio	7	33
Weighted average						10	20

Palmaz: Cordis, Miami, FL.

Wallstent: Boston Scientific Corp., Natick, MA.

Angioprotocol-specified angiographic follow-up: duplex ultrasonography.

Reproduced with permission from Martin LC, Rundback JH, Sacks D, et al. Quality improvement guidelines for angiography, angioplasty, and stent placement in the diagnosis and treatment of renal artery stenosis in adults. *J Vasc Intervent Radiol.* 2003;14:S297-S310.

To avoid renal complications in patients undergoing RAS interventions, routine measurements of serum creatinine at baseline and following the intervention represent a standard of care. As stated above, the controls are usually performed 2 to 4 hours after the procedure and then at 12-hour intervals daily until the baseline steady state is achieved. In high-risk patients for CIN and in patients with pre-existing chronic renal insufficiency, in addition to serum creatinine and urea measurements, the glomerular filtration rate, which represents the most comprehensive clinical index of renal function, should be calculated according to the Cockcroft-Gault formula [creatinine clearance = $(140 - \text{age}) \times$ kg body weight/$72 \times$ creatinine serum concentration in mg/100 mL].[81]

Restenosis and In-Stent Restenosis

In RAS interventions, stent-supported angioplasty has nearly completely replaced plain balloon angioplasty; at present, the vast majority of RAS interventions employ unconditional stenting. As in other vascular beds, renal artery in-stent restenosis has been reported in recent series to occur in up to approximately 20% of cases, yet its impact on clinical outcome may not be critical.[82] Predictors of renal artery in-stent restenosis include small vessel size (≤ 4 mm/4.5 mm) and possibly cigarette smoking.[82–84] Interestingly, partial stent recoil, which was observed in 6% of patients in one study, did not seem to predict restenosis.[84] In earlier studies, higher restenosis rates were reported (Table 11-13).

Restenosis may be detected during follow-up using duplex ultrasonography or DSA, and annual ultrasound examination of the renal arteries in patients who have undergone RAS interventions is recommended.

As in other vascular beds, renal artery in-stent restenosis can be treated using repeat dilatation, preferably using a cutting balloon,[85] in-stent stenting,[86] and brachytherapy.[87] However, no systematic evaluation of any of these techniques is available. The use of drug-eluting stents to prevent in-stent restenosis in renal arteries has not yet been reported.

The technique of reintervention is similar to that for de novo lesions. One important distinction is the initial guidewire exploration of the interventional site. Since the strut frequently protrudes slightly into the aorta, the risk of substrut placement with consecutive dissection is increased. To avoid this complication, careful seating of the tip of the guiding catheter in multiple projections within the ostial circumference of the stent with subsequent careful guidewire exploration appears critical. Correct positioning of the guidewire within the true lumen of the artery and within the stent boundaries is usually confirmed by the smooth passage of a low-profile deflated balloon catheter. Following secure dilatation balloon positioning, high-pressure nominal-size balloon dilatation may be securely performed. In the absence of systematic data, revascularization of in-stent restenosis may involve any of the established techniques (see earlier discussion); however, in most cases redilatations are performed with re-expansion of the deployed stent. In cases of incomplete lesion coverage, placement of a second stent may be required.

REFERENCES

1. Lappin DWP, Brady HR. Renal vascular diseases. In: Lanzer P, Topol EJ, eds. *PanVascular Medicine: Integrated Clinical Management.* New York: Springer, 2002:1751–1786.
2. Baum S, ed. *Abram's Angiography.* Vol 2. 4th ed. Boston: Little, Brown and Company, 1997:1101–1351
3. Textor SC, Wilcox CS. Renal artery stenosis: a common, treatable cause of renal failure? *Ann Rev Med.* 2001;52:421–442.
4. Goldblatt H, Lynch J, Hanzal RF, et al. Studies on experimental hypertension: I: The production of persistent elevation of systolic blood pressure by means of renal ischemia. *J Exp Med.* 1934;59:347–379.

5. Goldblatt H. The renal origin of hypertension. *Physiol Rev.* 1947;27:120–162.
6. Hall JE, Guyton AC, Jackson TE, et al. Control of glomerular filtration rate by renin-angiotensin system. *Am J Physiol.* 1977;233:F366-F388.
7. Anderson WP, Kett MM, Stenvenson KM, et al. Renovascular hypertension. Structural changes in the renal vasculature. *Hypertension.* 2000;36:648–652.
8. Anderson WP, Korner P, Angus J, et al. Contribution of stenosis resistance to the rise in total peripheral resistance during experimental renal hypertension in conscious dogs. *Clin Sci.* 1981;61:663–670.
9. Textor SC. Ischemic nephropathy: Where are we now? *J Am Soc Nephrol.* 2004;15:1974–1982.
10. Textor SC, Novick A, Tarazi RC, et al. Critical perfusion pressure for renal function in patients with bilateral atherosclerotic renal vascular disease. *Ann Intern Med.* 1985;102:309–314.
11. Novick AC. Patient selection for intervention to preserve renal function in ischemic renal disease. In: Novick AC, Scoble J, Hamilton G, eds. *Renal Vascular Disease.* London: HBJ College & School Division, 1996:323–337.
12. Rose BD, Mailloux LU, Kaplan NM. Chronic kidney disease due to ischemic renovascular disease. Available at: www.patients.uptodate.com/print.asp?=true/18690. Accessed December 27, 2005.
13. Ball S, Lloyd J, Cairns T, et al. Why is there so much end-stage renal failure of undetermined cause in UK Indo-Asians? *Q J Med.* 2001;94:187–193.
14. Kalra PA, Guo H, Kausz AT, et al. Atherosclerotic renovascular disease in United States patients aged 65 years or older: risk factors, revascularization and prognosis. *Kidney Int.* 2005;86:293–297.
15. Hansen KJ, Edwards MS, Craven TE, et al. Prevalence of renovascular disease in the elderly: a population-based study. *J Vasc Surg.* 2002;36:443–451.
16. Hirsch AT, Haskal ZJ, Hertzer NR, et al. ACC/AHA guidelines for the management of patients with peripheral arterial disease (lower extremity, renal, mesenteric, and abdominal aortic): Executive summary. A collaborative report from the American Association for Vascular Surgery/Society for Vascular Surgery, Society for Cardiovascular Angiography and Interventions, Society for Vascular Medicine and Biology, Society of Interventional Radiology, and the ACC/AHA Task Force on Practice Guidelines (Writing Committee to develop guidelines for the management of patients with peripheral arterial disease). Available at: www.cardiosource.com/guidelines/cguidelines/pad/pad_execsumm.pdf. Accessed May 25, 2006.
17. Dustan HP, Humphries AW, de Wolfe VG, et al. Normal arterial pressure in patient with renal arterial stenosis. *JAMA.* 1964;187:1028.
18. Suresh M, Laboi P, Mamtora H, et al. Relationship of renal dysfunction to proximal arterial disease severity in atherosclerotic renovascular disease. *Nephrol Dial Transplant.* 2000;15:631–636.
19. Coritsidis GN. Renal blood flow-glomerular filtration rate. Available at: www.uhmc.sun-ysb.edu/internetmed/nephro/webpages/Part_A.htm. Accessed November 19, 2005.
20. Chade AR, Rodriguez-Procel M, Grande JP, et al. Distinct renal injury in early atherosclerosis and renovascular disease. *Circulation.* 2002;106:1165–1171.
21. Janzen J, Lanzer P, Rothenberger-Janzen K, et al. The transitional zone in the tunica media of renal arteries has a maximum length of 10 millimeters. *VASA.* 2000;29:168–172.
22. Zierler RE, Bergelin RO, Davidson RC, et al. A prospective study of disease progression in patients with atherosclerotic renal artery stenosis. *Am J Hypertens.* 1996;9:1055–1061.
23. Caps MT, Perissinotto C, Zierler RE, et al. Prospective study of atherosclerotic disease progression in the renal artery. *Circulation.* 1998;98:2866–2872.
24. Strandness ED Jr. Natural history of renal artery stenosis. *Am J Kidney Dis.* 1994;24:630–635.
25. Leadbetter WF, Burkland CE. Hypertension in unilateral renal disease. *J Urol.* 1938;39:611–626.
26. Slovut DP, Olin JW. Fibromuscular dysplasia. *N Engl J Med.* 2004;350:1862–1871.
27. Harrison EG Jr, McCormack LJ. Pathologic classification of renal arterial disease in renovascular hypertension. *Mayo Clin Proc.* 1971;46:161–167.
28. Mann SJ, Pickering TG. Detection of renovascular hypertension. State of the art: 1992. *Ann Intern Med.* 1992;117:845–890.
29. van de Ven PJ, Beutler JJ, Kaatee R, et al. Angiotensin converting enzyme inhibitor-induced renal dysfunction in atherosclerotic renovascular disease. *Kidney Int.* 1998;53:986–992.
30. Rimmer JM, Gennari FJ. Atherosclerotic renovascular disease and progressive renal failure. *Ann Intern Med.* 1993;118:712–720.
31. Gandhi SK, Powers JC, Nomeir AM, et al. The pathogenesis of acute pulmonary edema associated with hypertension. *N Engl J Med.* 2001;344:17–22.
32. Agarwal M, Lynn KL, Richards AM, et al. Hyponatremic-hypertensive syndrome with renal ischemia: An underrecognized disorder. *Hypertension.* 1999;33:1020–1025.
33. Kaplan NM, Rose RD. Screening for renovascular hypertension. Available at: www.patients.uptodate.com/topic.asp?file=hyperten/12756. Accessed December 27, 2005.
34. Setaro JF, Saddler MC, Chen CC, et al. Simplified captopril renography in diagnosis and treatment of renal artery stenosis. *Hypertension.* 1991;18:289–306.
35. Elliott WJ, Martin WB, Murphy MB. Comparison of two noninvasive screening tests for renovascular hypertension. *Arch Intern Med.* 1993;153:755–81.
36. Wilcox CS. Use of angiotensin-converting-enzyme inhibitors for diagnosing renovascular hypertension. *Kidney Int.* 1993;44:1379–1384.
37. Derkx FH, Schalekamp MA. Renal artery stenosis and hypertension. *Lancet.* 1994;344:237–242.
38. Lusza G. *X-ray Anatomy of the Vascular System.* Philadelphia: JB Lippincott, 1964:227–231.
39. Uflacker R. *Atlas of Vascular Anatomy: An Angiographic Approach.* Philadelphia: Lippincott Williams & Wilkins, 1997.
40. Boijen E. Renal angiography: techniques and hazards; anatomic and physiologic considerations. In: Baum S, ed. *Abram's angiography.* Vol 2. 4th ed. Boston: Little, Brown and Company, 1997;1101–1131.
41. Verschuyl E-J, Kaatee R, Beek FJA, et al. Renal artery origins: best angiographic projection angles. *Radiology.* 1997;205:115–120.
42. Rundback JH, Sacks D, Kent C, et al. for the American Heart Association Council on Cardiovascular Radiology, High Blood Pressure Research, Kidney in Cardiovascular

Disease, Cardio-Thoracic and Vascular Surgery, and Clinical Cardiology, and the Society of Interventional Radiology FDA Device Forum Committee. Guidelines for the reporting of renal artery revascularization in clinical trials. *Circulation.* 2002;106:1572–1585.
43. McWilliams RG, Robertson I, Smye SW, et al. Sources of error in intra-arterial pressure measurements across a stenosis. *Eur J Endovasc Surg.* 1998;15:535–540.
44. Katzberg RW. Urography into the 21st century: new contrast media, renal handling, imaging characteristics, and nephrotoxicity. *Radiology.* 1997;204 : 297–312.
45. Barrett BJ, Parfrey PS. Prevention of nephrotoxicity induced by radiocontrast agents. *N Engl J Med.* 1994;331:1449–1450.
46. Gleeson TG, Bulugahapitiya S. Contrast-induced nephropathy. *AJR Am J Roentgenol.* 2004;183(6):1673–1689.
47. Parfrey PS, Griffiths SM, Barrett BJ, et al. Contrast material-induced renal failure in patients with diabetes mellitus, renal insufficiency, or both. *N Engl J Med.* 1989;320:143–153.
48. Beese RC, Bees NR, Belli AM. Renal angiography using carbon dioxide. *Br J Radiol.* 2000;73(865):3–6.
49. Martin LC, Rundback JH, Sacks D, et al. Quality improvement guidelines for angiography, angioplasty, and stent placement in the diagnosis and treatment of renal artery stenosis in adults. *J Vasc Intervent Radiol.* 2003;14:S297-S310.
50. Spinowitz BS, Rodriquez J. Renal artery stenosis. Available at: www.emedicine.com/med/topic2001.htm. Accessed December 27, 2005.
51. Freeman N. Thromboendarterectomy for hypertension due to due to renal artery occlusion. *JAMA.* 1973;157:1077–1083.
52. Stanley JC. Renal vascular diseases: Surgical therapy. In: Lanzer P, Topol EJ, eds. *PanVascular Medicine: Integrated Clinical Approach.* New York: Springer-Verlag, 2002:1798–1808.
53. Hasen JK, Dean RH. Renovascular disease. In: Moore WS, ed. *Vascular Surgery: A Comprehensive Review.* 6th ed. Philadelphia: WB Saunders, 2002:548–569.
54. Grüntzig A, Kuhlmann U, Vetter W. Treatment of renovascular hypertension with percutaneous transluminal dilatation of a renal artery stenosis. *Lancet.* 1978;1: 801–802.
55. Schwarten DE, Yune HY, Klatte EC, et al. Clinical experience with percutaneous transluminal angioplasty (PTA) of stenotic renal arteries. *Radiology.* 1980;135:601–604.
56. Tegtmeyer CJ, Ayers CA, Wellons HA. Axillary approach to percutaneous renal artery dilatation. *Radiology.* 1980;135:775–776.
57. Trost DW, Sos TA. Renal artery angioplasty and stent placement: indications and results. In: Perler BA, Becker GJ, eds. *Vascular Intervention: A Clinical Approach.* New York: Thieme Medical Publishers;1998:575–583.
58. Kaplan NM, Rose BD. Treatment of unilateral renal artery stenosis. Available at: http://patients.uptodate.com/topic.asp?file=hyperten/16017&title=Renal+artery+Stenting. Accessed December 28, 2005.
59. Dorros G, Prince C, Mathiak L. Stenting of renal artery stenosis achieves better relief of the obstructive lesion than balloon angioplasty. *Cathet Cardiovasc Diagn.* 1993;29:191–198.
60. Blum U, Krumme B, Flügel P, et al. Treatment of ostial renal artery stenosis with vascular endoprosthesis after unsuccessful balloon angioplasty. *N Engl J Med.* 1997;336: 459–465.
61. Lim ST, Rosenfield K. Renal artery stent placement: indications and results. *Curr Intervent Cardiol Rep.* 2000;2:130–139.
62. Henry M, Henry I, Klonaris C, et al. Renal angioplasty and stenting under protection: the way for the future? *Cathet Cardiovasc Intervent.* 2003;60:299–312.
63. Zalunardo N, Tuttle K. Atherosclerotic renal artery stenosis: current status and future directions. *Curr Opin Nephrol Hypertens.* 2004;13:613–621.
64. Zeller T, Frank U, Müller C, et al. Predictors of improved renal function after percutaneous stent-supported angioplasty of severe atherosclerotic ostial renal artery stenosis. *Circulation.* 2003;108:2244–2249.
65. Rocha-Singh K, Jaff MR, Rosenfield K for the ASPIRE-2 Investigators. Evaluation of safety and effectiveness of renal artery stenting after unsuccessful balloon angioplasty: the ASPIRE-2 Study. *J Am Coll Cardiol.* 2005;46:776–832.
66. Lanzer P, Weser R, Prettin C. Coronary-like revascularization for atherosclerotic renal artery stenosis; results in 181 consecutive patients. *Clin Res Cardiol.* 2006;95:965–972.
67. Nolan BW, Schermerhorn ML, Rowell E, et al. Outcomes of renal artery angioplasty and stenting using low-profile systems. *J Vasc Surg.* 2005;41:46–52.
68. Beek FJA, Kaatee R, Beutler JJ, et al. Complications during renal artery stent placement for atherosclerotic ostial stenosis. *Cardiovasc Intervent Radiol.* 1997;20:184–190.
69. Bloch MJ, Trost DW, Sos TA. Type B aortic dissection complicating renal artery angioplasty and stent placement. *J Vasc Intervent Radiol.* 2001;12:517–520.
70. Cicuto KP, McLean GK, Oleaga JA, et al. Renal artery stenosis: Anatomic classification for percutaneous transluminal angioplasty. *Am J Radiol.* 1981;137:599–601.
71. Hazanov N, Somin M, Attali M, et al. Acute renal embolism. Forty-four cases of renal infarction in patients with atrial fibrillation. *Medicine (Baltimore).* 2004;83:292–301.
72. Lessman RK, Johnson SR, Coburn JW, et al. Renal artery embolism: clinical features and long-term follow-up of 17 cases. *Ann Intern Med.* 1978;89:477–482.
73. Blum U, Billman P, Krause T, et al. Effect of local low-dose thrombolysis on clinical outcome in patients with acute embolic renal artery occlusion. *Radiology.* 1993;189:549–554.
74. Scolari F, Ravani P, Pola A, et al. Predictors of renal and patient outcomes in atheroembolic renal disease: a prospective study. *J Am Soc Nephrol.* 2003;14:1584–1591.
75. Haas M, Spargo BH, Wit EJ, et al. Etiologies and outcome of acute renal insufficiency in older adults: a renal biopsy study of 259 cases. *Am J Kidney Dis.* 2000;35:433–471.
76. Thadhani RI, Camargo CA Jr, Xavier RJ, et al. Atheroembolic renal failure after invasive procedures. Natural history based on 52 histologically proven cases. *Medicine (Baltimore).* 1995;74:350–356.
77. Mannesse CK, Klankestijn PJ, Man in't Veld AJ, et al. Renal failure and cholesterol crystal embolization: a report of 4 surviving cases and a review of the literature. *Clin Nephrol.* 1991;36:240–248.
78. Rose BD, Tunick PA. Clinical characteristics of renal atheroemboli. Available at: http://patients.upload.com/topic.asp?file=renldis/16306&title=Renal+atheroemboli. Accessed December 30, 2005.

79. Aspelin P, Aubry P, Fransson SG, et al. Nephrotoxic effects in high-risk patients undergoing angiography. *N Engl J Med.* 2003;348:491–499.

80. Rudnick MR, Rose BD. Radiocontrast media-induced acute renal failure. Available at: http://patients.uptodate.com/topic.asp? file=renlfail/9576 &title=Contrast+induced+renal+failure. Accessed December 30, 2005.

81. Cockcroft DW, Gault MH. Prediction of creatinine clearance from serum creatinine. *Nephron.* 1976;16:31–41.

82. Perkovic V, Thomson KR, Mitchell PJ, et al. Treatment of renovascular disease with percutaneous stent insertion: long-term outcomes. *Australas Radiol.* 2001;45:438–443.

83. Lederman RJ, Mendelsohn FO, Santos R, et al. Primary renal artery stenting: characteristics and outcomes after 363 procedures. *Am Heart J.* 2001;142:314–323.

84. Shammas NW, Kapalis MJ, Dipple EJ, et al. Clinical and Angiographic Predictors of Restenosis Following Renal Artery Stenting. *J Invasive Cardiol.* 2004;16:10–13.

85. Munnecke GJ, Engelke C, Morgan RA, et al. Cutting balloon angioplasty for renal artery in-stent restenosis. *J Vasc Intervent Radiol.* 2002;13:327–331.

86. Bax L, Mali WPTM, van de Ven PJG, et al. Repeated intervention for in-stent restenosis of the renal arteries. *J Vasc Intervent Radiol.* 2002;13:1219–1224.

87. Chrysant GS, Goldstein JA, Casserly IP, et al. Endovascular brachytherapy for treatment of bilateral renal artery in-stent restenosis. *Cathet Cardiovasc Intervent.* 2003;59:251–254.

Peter Lanzer
Ralf Weser

CHAPTER **12**

Abdominal Aorta, Iliac, and Lower Extremity Arteries

PERIPHERAL ARTERIAL DISEASE

The term peripheral arterial disease (PAD) means different things to different people. For example, in the recent joint ACC/AHA publication, PAD definition included the infradiaphragmatic arteries, i.e., abdominal aorta, renal arteries, mesenteric arteries, and arteries of the lower extremities.[1] In the context of this textbook peripheral arterial disease (PAD) comprises diseases of the distal abdominal aorta, iliac (aortoiliac segment), and infrainguinal arteries, divided into a femoropopliteal and infrapopliteal segment. Arterial diseases of the upper arm have not been included primarily because in that vascular bed percutaneous revascularization is rarely applied and, if needed, it follows similar principles to those presented. Because of the continuity of peripheral vessels from proximal to distal, disease of the proximal vessels always affects all downstream vessels (run-in effect). Conversely, any disease of the downstream vessels adversely affects the upstream circulation (runoff effect). Therefore, from the pathophysiological standpoint, vessels distal to the distal abdominal aorta form a complex functional unity of interacting vascular segments. However, for the purposes of endovascular therapy, separation of the peripheral vascular bed into vascular segments and territories is useful, mainly because of differences in vessel structure and morphology that prescribe different interventional strategies. Figure 12-1 shows the anatomic and functional continuity of the peripheral arterial vascular bed and its endovascular partition.

PAD is caused in the vast majority of patients by atherosclerosis and diabetic vasculopathy.[2] Other causes, including vasculitides[3] and obliterating thrombangitis of Winiwarter and Buerger,[4] are rare by comparison. In specific vascular beds other etiologies must be considered in differential diagnostics. For example, in the popliteal artery, an entrapment syndrome may occur due to outside compression of the artery by the gastrocnemius, popliteus, or soleus muscles,[5,6] as may aneurysms[7] and cystic adventitial disease (compression of the artery by mucoid adventitia-derived cysts).[8,9] In all cases of suggested PAD, nonvascular causes of symptoms (pseudoclaudication) such as nerve root compression, spinal stenosis, hip arthritis, and others must be considered and excluded.[10]

Atherosclerotic PAD may be one of the most frequently undetected, chronic, debilitating disorders, and it is certainly the most frequently unrecognized atherosclerotic cardiovascular disease (CVD). This is surprising given the availability of a highly sensitive (95%) and highly specific (100%) screening test, namely, the ankle-brachial index (ABI).[11]

Depending on the population studied and the method of detection utilized, the prevalence and the incidence of PAD reported in the literature vary widely. Table 12-1 provides an example of prevalence reported in individual studies[12]; Figures 12-2 and 12-3 show the summary incidence and prevalence from large population-based studies.[13] Using objective criteria for evidence of PAD (ABI measurements) and CVD, defined as a history of atherosclerotic coronary, cerebral, and abdominal aortic aneurysmal disease in a selected population of patients (>70 years and 50 to 69 years with diabetes and/or cigarette smoking ≥10 pack years), the overall prevalence of PAD was 29%! The prevalence of isolated PAD was 13%; that of PAD associated with CVD was 16%. Newly detected, that is, previously unrecognized, PAD was present in 13% of patients (7% in the

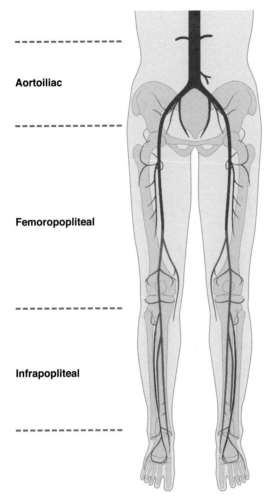

Aortoiliac

Femoropopliteal

Infrapopliteal

FIGURE 12-1. Anatomic and functional continuity of the peripheral arterial vascular bed and its endovascular partition into aortoiliac, femoropopliteal, and infrapopliteal segments.

isolated PAD group and 6% in the combined PAD and CVD group), suggesting that in this selected population, 45% of the patients with PAD were not aware of its presence![14]

Major modifiable risk factors for PAD include diabetes and cigarette smoking (Fig. 12-4). An example of the incidence of cardiovascular risk factors in individuals with and without PAD is shown in Table 12-2.[15] Critical prognosis of PAD, primarily as a harbinger of CVD morbidity and mortality has been well documented[16] and widely recognized.[11] Figure 12-5 compares the 10-year survival of patients with and without PAD.

The pace of clinical progression of PAD remains a matter of debate; earlier reports suggested a rather benign course[17,18] with approximately 25% of patients progressing from claudication to intervention (for review, see reference 13), but in a more recent study, marked progression was noted in individuals with ABI <0.50.[19] Risk factors of progression appear identical to those of PAD (for review, see reference 13).

Depending on the severity of the lower leg ischemia, PAD may be associated with the clinical symptom of intermittent claudication (buttocks, hips, thighs, calves, and feet) or in more advanced cases with rest pain. However, in a large number of patients, PAD may remain asymptomatic or it may present with nonspecific and atypical symptoms. To stress the critical importance of revascularization in patients with advanced PAD associated with threat to the limb, the syndromes of chronic and chronic critical or acute lower extremity ischemia have been introduced as specific entities. To classify the patient properly thorough history including documentary as to the nature, duration, and temporal course of symptoms is absolutely critical.

On the basis of clinical symptoms, the Fontaine classification[20] in modified form (replacing stage IV for stages IVa and IVb and introducing stages IIa and IIb)[21] distinguishes four different stages of severity of chronic leg ischemia (Table 12-3). A similar classification of chronic leg ischemia based on clinical findings and blood pressure measurements at rest and during exercise, has been proposed by Rutherford et al. (Table 12-4) and implemented in clinics.[22–25]

TABLE 12-1. Prevalence of Peripheral Arterial Disease, Claudication, and Concomitant Cardiovascular Disease in Selected Studies

Study	No. of Subjects	Age (yr)	Sex	Prevalence of Peripheral Arterial Disease	Prevalence of Claudication(%)	Prevalence of Clinical Cardiovascular Disease
Schroll and Munck	666	>60	M	16	6	—
			F	13	1	—
Meijer et al.	7,715	>55	M	17	2	48
			F	21	1	33
Fowkes et al.	1,509	55–74	Both	18	5	54
Newman et al.	190	>60	Both	27	6	47
Newman et al.	5,084	>65	M	14		56
			F	11	2	40
Zheng et al.	15,792	45–64	M	3	1	21
			F	3	1	5

Ankle-brachial index value of less than 0.90 was considered diagnostic of peripheral arterial disease in all the studies. Dashes indicate that no data were presented.

Reproduced with permission from Hiatt WR. Medical treatment of peripheral arterial disease and claudication. *N Engl J Med.* 2001;344:1608–21.

Besides history and physical examination, ABI represents the single most important test in diagnosing PAD. Figure 12-6 shows the definition of points of ABI measurement and the interpretation of findings. In patients with peripheral artery calcifications (ABI >1.1), toe blood pressure and toe/brachial index may be used to distinguish between PAD and nonobstructive arterial wall hardening.[26]

Noninvasive diagnostic techniques applicable to the assessment of PAD have been reviewed in the literature.[1,27,28] Magnetic resonance angiography (MRA) of peripheral arteries provides a

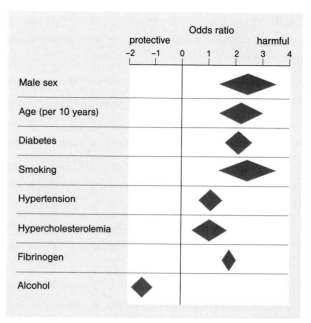

FIGURE 12-4. Nonmodifiable and modifiable major risk factors for peripheral arterial disease with range of odds ratios, Redrawn from TransAtlantic Inter-Society Consensus (TASC). Management of peripheral arterial disease (PAD). *J Vasc Surg.* 2000;31(suppl):1–296.

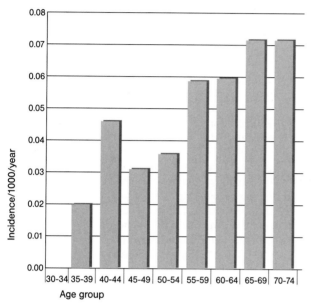

FIGURE 12-2. Incidence of intermittent claudication in the age group 35–74 years. Redrawn from TransAtlantic Inter-Society Consensus (TASC). Management of peripheral arterial disease (PAD). *J Vasc Surg.* 2000;31(suppl):1–296.

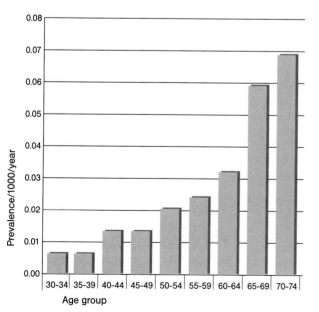

FIGURE 12-3. Prevalence of intermittent claudication in the age group 35–74 years. Redrawn from TransAtlantic Inter-Society Consensus (TASC). Management of peripheral arterial disease (PAD). *J Vasc Surg.* 2000;31(suppl):1–296.

TABLE 12-2. Cardiovascular Disease Risk Factors among Persons with and without Prevalent Peripheral Arterial Disease (PAD)

	Prevalent PAD (n = 141), % (SE)	No PAD (n = 2033), % (SE)
Mean age, years	68.7 (1.5)	55.7 (0.4)
Male, %	46.2 (5.8)	48.2 (0.8)
Hypertension, %	73.6 (4.7)	45.4 (1.7)
Hypercholesterolemia, %	60.6 (4.5)	44.9 (1.5)
Diabetes, %	26.4 (8.4)	10.1 (1.5)
Current smoking, %	32.8 (5.5)	20.3 (1.4)
Hypertension, hypercholesterolemia, diabetes, or current smoking, %	95.2 (2.7)	75.7 (1.4)
Mean BMI, kg/m²	27.1 (0.6)	28.2 (0.3)
Mean GFR, mL min⁻¹ 1.73 m⁻²	77.0 (2.9)	89.2 (0.8)
Mean CRP, mg/L	7.4 (1.1)	4.6 (0.2)
Geometric mean CRP, mg/L	3.8 (0.4)	2.3 (0.1)
Mean fibrinogen, mg/dL	398.8 (10.1)	353.8 (3.0)
Self-reported history of coronary heart disease, %	24.0 (4.4)	7.1 (0.7)
Self-reported history of stroke, %	11.2 (3.5)[a]	2.9 (0.5)
Self-reported history of congestive heart failure, %	5.3 (2.2)[a]	2.6 (0.5)
Self-reported history of any cardiovascular disease, %	33.1 (4.8)	10.2 (1.0)

Adults aged 40 years and older, United States, 1999–2000 (n = 2174)
[a]Estimate has a relative standard error >30%

Reproduced with permission from Selvin E, Erlinger TP. Prevalence of and Risk Factors for Peripheral Arterial disease in the United States Results From the National Health and Nutrition Examination Survey, 1999–2000. *Circulation.* 2004;110:738–743.

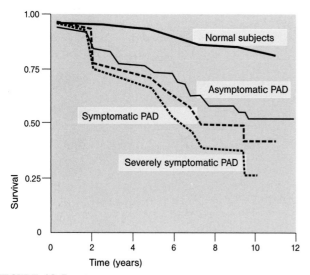

FIGURE 12-5. Comparison of 10-year survival of patients with and without peripheral arterial disease (PAD), based on the study population from Criqui MH, Langer RD, Fronek A, et al. Mortality over a period of 10 years in patients with peripheral artery disease. *N Engl J Med.* 1992;326:381–386. Redrawn from Belch JJ, Topol EJ, Agnelli G, et al. Critical issues in peripheral arterial disease detection and management. *Arch Intern Med.* 2003;163:884–892.

TABLE 12-3. Intermittent Claudication, Modified Fontaine Classification

Stage	Symptoms
I	Asymptomatic
II	Intermittent claudication
IIa	Pain-free, claudication walking >200 m
IIb	Pain-free, claudication walking <200 m
III	Rest/nocturnal pain
IV	Necrosis/gangrene

useful road map for targeting endovascular interventions[29] and may become an important adjunct in specific settings.[30] However, in peri-interventional settings, digital subtraction angiography (DSA) continues to be uniquely positioned to provide a road map and to guide peripheral catheter-based interventions.

CRITICAL LIMB ISCHEMIA

The term *critical ischemia* was originally introduced to designate ischemia requiring successful revascularization to avoid amputation.[31] The originally proposed objective criteria to define critical ischemia (ankle pressure <40 mm Hg; resting pain and <60 mm Hg; ulceration) were later modified, and the term *chronic critical limb ischemia* (CLI) has been coined to denote a condition with "chronic ischemic rest pain, ulcers, or gangrene attributable to objectively proven arterial occlusive disease." Furthermore the "term critical limb ischemia implies chronicity and is to be distinguished from acute limb ischemia. In most cases a major amputation would be expected within the next 6 months to a year in the absence of a significant hemodynamic improvement" (for review, see reference 13). Table 12-5 summarizes the proposed objective criteria required for establishing the diagnosis of CLI.

Patients presenting with CLI typically have rest pain in the affected limb requiring narcotic medication for analgesia. The pain may improve with dependency and worsens if the patient is in the supine position. The immediate objectives of the diagnostic evaluations include confirmation of the diagnosis and precise anatomic definition of the status of the frequently multilevel PAD allowing definite decisions as to the feasibility, timing, and strategy of revascularization.

The choice of diagnostic modalities and interim management options depends on a number of factors including presence of coexistent morbidities, status of the cardiac and renal function, and other factors, and this choice must be tailored to the needs of individual patients. In all cases, a thorough risk and benefit analysis by a team consisting of vascular specialists, interventionists, and vascular surgeons is required.

TABLE 12-4. Clinical Categories of Chronic Lower Limb Ischemia According to Rutherford et al.

Grade	Category	Clinical Description	Objective Criteria
0	0	Asymptomatic—not hemodynamically significant	Normal treadmill/stress test
I	1	Mild claudication	Completes treadmill exercise,[a] AP after exercise <50 mm Hg but >25 mm Hg less than BP.
	2	Moderate claudication	Between categories 1 and 3.
	3	Severe claudication	Cannot complete treadmill exercise and AP after exercise <50 mm Hg.
II	4	Ischemic rest pain	Resting AP <40 mm Hg, flat or barely pulsatile ankle or metatarsal PVR; TP <30 mm Hg.
III	5	Minor tissue loss—nonhealing ulcer, focal gangrene with diffuse pedal ischemia	Resting AP <60 mmHg, ankle metatarsal PVR flat or barely pulsatile; TP <40 mm Hg.
IV	6	Major tissue loss—extending above TM level, functional foot no longer salvageable	Same as category 5.

AP, ankle pressure; BP, blood pressure; PVR, pulse volume recording; TP, toe pressure; TM, transmetatarsal.

[a]5 min at 2 mph on a 12% incline.

Based on Rutherford RB, Flanigan DP, Gupta SK, et al. Suggested standards for reports dealing with lower extremity ischemia. *J Vasc Surg.* 1986;4:80–94.

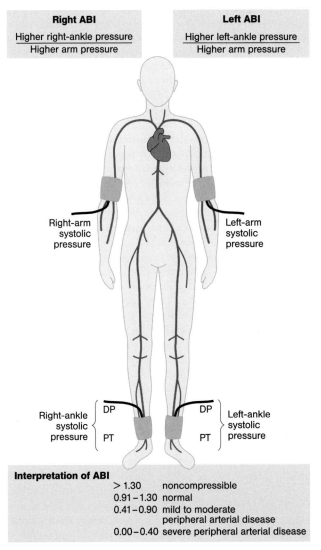

FIGURE 12-6. Ankle-brachial index: definition of points of measurement and interpretation. Redrawn from Hiatt WR. Medical treatment of peripheral arterial disease and claudication. *N Engl J Med.* 2001;344:1608–1621.

TABLE 12-5. Suggested Criteria of Chronic Critical Limb Ischemia by TransAtlantic Inter-Society Consensus (TASC)

Suggested Objective Criteria	Measurement
Ankle pressure	<50–70 mm Hg or
Toe pressure	<30–50 mm Hg or
TcPO2	<30–50 mm Hg

TcPO2, transcutaneous partial oxygen pressure.

Adapted from Trans Atlantic Inter-Society Consensus (TASC). Management of peripheral arterial disease (PAD). *J Vasc Surg.* 2000;31 (suppl);1–296.

ACUTE LIMB ISCHEMIA

Acute limb ischemia (ALI) has been defined as "any sudden decrease or worsening in limb perfusion causing a potential threat to extremity viability."[13] More recently ALI was defined as "any sudden decrease in or worsening of limb perfusion causing a threat to extremity mobility and viability that has been present for less than 14 days."[32] Although ALI due to acute thrombosis or embolization, often without a critical PAD, and CLI often due to decompensation of advanced PAD, sometimes associated with thrombotic occlusions, represent distinct pathogenetic entities in clinical practice, their differentiation can be difficult. A detailed history as to the timing and time course of the symptoms and clinical and laboratory examinations focusing on the detection of the presence and severity of the underlying PAD usually will provide clues to allow the distinction. To plan treatment, most importantly a definite anatomic definition of the involved vascular bed including the status of the run-in and runoff vessels and the status of the extremity with regard to the severity of ischemia, potential reversibility, threat to viability, and risk of ischemia-reperfusion injury must be established. However, the frequently protracted course and great variability of ischemic tolerance of the peripheral skeletal muscle in individual patients make the assessment of viability and prognostication of reversibility and reperfusion injury difficult, occasionally even for experienced physicians with access to a complete vascular diagnostic battery. Table 12-6 summarizes some of the findings associated with ischemic injury in patients presenting with ALI.

TABLE 12-6. Reversibility of Ischemic Injury in Patients Presenting with Acute Limb Ischemia (ALI)

Category	Description	Capillary Return	Muscle Weakness	Sensory Loss	Doppler Signals Arterial	Venous
Viable	Not immediately threatened	Intact	None	None	Audible (AP >30 mm Hg)	Audible
Threatened	Salvageable if promptly treated	Intact, slow	Mild, partial	Mild, incomplete	Inaudible	Audible
Irreversible	Major tissue loss, amputation regardless of treatment	Absent (marbling)	Profound, paralysis (rigor)	Profound, anesthetic	Inaudible	Inaudible

AP, ankle pressure.

Reproduce with permission from Rajan JK, Patel NH, Valji K, et al. Quality improvement guidelines for percutaneous management of acute limb ischemia. *J Vasc Intervent Radiol.* 2005;16:585–595.

DIAGNOSTIC AND PERI-INTERVENTIONAL AORTOILIAC AND PERIPHERAL ARTERIOGRAPHY

With the advances made in noninvasive computed tomography (CT) and magnetic resonance (MR) peripheral angiography and its increasing ability to localize and to define disease,[33,34] the indications for diagnostic x-ray digital subtraction angiography (DSA) have now become limited to specific settings, frequently depending on the actual quality and validity of noninvasive studies in individual patients. To allow definitive decisions on the need for and technical feasibility of peripheral arterial revascularization, diagnostic arteriography should provide a full anatomic and morphologic definition of arteries and lesions from the infrarenal abdominal aorta down to the arteries of the feet. Depending on the findings such as presence of stenoses, status of collateral vessels, and vascular anomalies, additional series of specific vascular regions might be required. In cases where the noninvasive diagnostic MR or CT angiography provides all required information, x-ray angiography is used only during the intervention. In cases with suboptimal MR or CT image quality or incomplete vascular definition, diagnostic x-ray angiography is prescribed to complete the study and to allow definitive statements. In patients with complex multilevel PAD, diagnostic x-ray angiography might be preferable, allowing a single-stage definitive assessment and treatment decisions. Peripheral DSA studies may be performed using either automated preprogrammed series of DSA images timed to the progress of the contrast agent downstream in the peripheral arteries (bolus-chase peripheral DSA angiography) or static DSA with manual adjustment of every subsequent imaging level. Since image quality is better when static masks are used for subtraction[35] and because of frequent disparities between the speed of travel of the contrast agent between the left and right leg, static DSA peripheral arteriography is preferable in most cases.

To perform a full diagnostic evaluation of the peripheral vasculature using DSA, the patient is securely positioned on the table with his legs brought together, resting quietly and fastened to avoid motion. When a standard femoral or brachial access has been established, a pigtail catheter is positioned proximally (suprarenal aortography) or distally (infrarenal aortography) to the take-off of the renal arteries and sequential DSA series are acquired using preprogrammed set of image acquisition parameters, spanning the entire region of interest in anteroposterior projection. Examples of standard imaging protocols are provided in Table 12-7.[36] Adjustments of individual imaging parameters might be required to account for variable regional pathoanatomy and hemodynamics. To improve the distal peripheral inflow after the acquisition of abdominal aortic angiograms, the pigtail catheter is repositioned just above the aortic bifurcation to acquire peripheral runoff angiograms. In patients with disparate velocity of blood flow between the two legs and complex multilevel disease, side-selective or additional segmental peripheral angiograms might be needed to fully define the peripheral arterial pathoanatomy. In patients with a severe distal disease, additional DSA series via antegrade fine-needle or small-size sheath (3F) access might be required.

To open up the left common iliac artery and the right common femoral artery bifurcations, an additional right anterior oblique projection acquired at the appropriate level may be useful, as is the case with an additional left anterior oblique projection to define the bifurcations of the right common iliac artery and the left common femoral artery. To visualize stenotic lesions a second projection, preferably perpendicular to the anteroposterior (AP) projection (lateral projection), should be acquired. During the imaging at the ankle level, the feet should be rotated externally to allow a better separation of the three infrapopliteal vessels. To improve visualization of the distal runoff vessels, reactive hyperemia following inflation of the blood pressure cuff at the thigh (20 mm Hg above systolic pressure for 3 to 5 minutes) or intra-arterial administration of a vasoactive agent such as calcium channel blockers (e.g., diltiazem 5 mg) might be helpful. However, the patient's tolerance of ischemic pain associated with blood pressure cuff inflation might limit the clinical applicability of this approach. In patients with severe obstructions of the pelvic arteries or common femoral disease, preferably the left brachial access should be selected.

TABLE 12-7. Examples of Standard Imaging Protocols for Peripheral Digital Subtraction Angiography (DSA)

Vascular Territory	DSA Frame Rate (frames/sec)	Contrast Agent Dose (mL)	Contrast Agent Flow Rate (mL/sec)	Additional Projections
SPECIFIC VASCULAR BEDS				
Infrarenal aorta	2	15	10	
Common iliac artery	2	10	6	Contralateral oblique 30–45 degrees;
Internal iliac artery	2	6	3	Ipsilateral oblique 30 degrees;
Pudendal artery	1	5	2	Ipsilateral oblique 30 degrees;
PERIPHERAL RUNOFF				
Suprarenal aorta	2	10	15	
Iliac arteries	2	15	10	Contralateral oblique 30–45 degrees;
Proximal femoral arteries	1	15	10	Ipsilateral oblique 15–30 degrees;
Distal femoral arteries	1	15	10	
Popliteal and proximal infrapopliteal arteries	0.5–1	15	10	Lateral
Distal infrapopliteal arteries	0.5	20	15	Lateral

Adapted from Pattynama PMT. X-ray peripheral and visceral angiography. In Lanzer P, Topol EJ, eds. *PanVascular Medicine: Integrated Clinical Management.* New York: Springer-Verlag, 2002:636–658.

Exact knowledge of peripheral vascular anatomy is required for optimum image acquisition and interpretation. A simplified schema of the clinical vascular anatomy of the peripheral circulation is shown in Figure 12-7. In addition, the interventionist must know the principal peripheral collateral pathways and must recognize their functional significance in individual patients in order to understand the numerous potential steal and flow-reversal phenomena, particularly in cases considered for catheter-based and/or surgical revascularizations or those with previous peripheral artery bypass surgeries or interventions. Figure 12-8 shows the principal collateral pathways in the presence of occlusions in the aortoiliac and iliofemoral segments.[37] Figure 12-9 demonstrates the principal collateral pathways of the femoropopliteal segment.[38] Because of its importance as a natural collateral channel, the anatomy of the deep femoral artery and its branches should be clearly depicted and visualized. Taking off from the posterolateral border of the common femoral artery, usually 3 to 4 cm distal to the inguinal ligament, it usually provides medial and lateral branches

supplying the adjacent muscles and the head of the femur, along with four perforating branches that perforate the dorsal muscle and are a rich source for intra- and interarterial collateralization between the common femoral and the popliteal arteries.

The popliteal artery extends from the inferior border of the adductor canal up to the take-off of the anterior tibial artery. Its course may be conveniently divided into three parts, proximal (part I) between the distal end of the adductor channel and the inlet into the tunnel of the gastrocnemius, middle (part II) up to the horizontal plane of the proximal border of the knee cleft, and distal (part III) up to the take-off of the anterior tibial artery, segments (Figure 12-10).[39] Variations in the division of the popliteal artery are shown in Figure 12-11.

With increasing ability to treat infrapopliteal disease using a coronary-like approach to peripheral interventions, the functional anatomy of the three principal lower leg arteries, namely, the posterior and anterior tibial and fibular (peroneal) arteries, must also be clearly understood. The anterior tibial artery

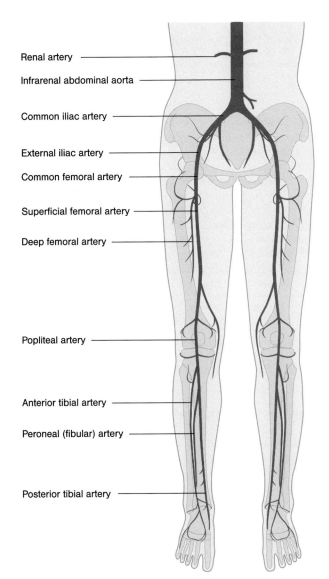

FIGURE 12-7. Clinical anatomy of the principal peripheral arteries relevant to the peripheral arterial interventions.

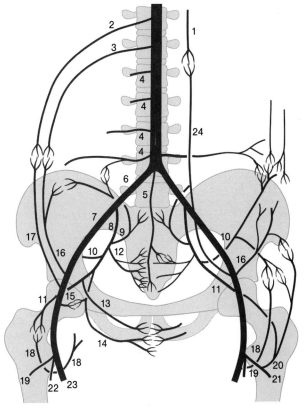

FIGURE 12-8. Essential collateral pathways in the presence of occlusions in the aortoiliac and iliofemoral segments. Arabic numbers denote individual arteries: *1*, superior epigastric; *2*, intercostals; *3*, subcostal; *4*, lumbar; *5*, middle sacral; *6*, common iliac; *7*, external iliac; *8*, internal iliac; *9*, iliolumbar; *10*, superior gluteal; *11*, inferior gluteal; *12*, lateral sacral; *13*, obturator; *14*, internal pudendal; *15*, external pudendal; *16*, deep iliac circumflex; *17*, superficial iliac circumflex; *18*, medial iliac circumflex; *19*, lateral femoral circumflex; *20*, lateral ascending branch; *21*, lateral descending branch; *22*, profunda femoris; *23*, superficial femoral; *24*, inferior epigastric. Note the intersegmental character of the individual vascular bridges. Redrawn from Hallisey MJ, Meranze SG. The abnormal abdominal aorta. Arteriosclerosis and other diseases. In: Baum S, ed. *Abram's Angiography.* Vol 2. 4th ed. Boston: Little, Brown and Company, 1997:1052–1072.

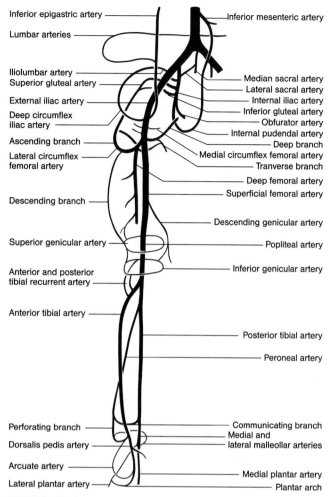

Inferior epigastric artery
Lumbar arteries
Iliolumbar artery
Superior gluteal artery
External iliac artery
Deep circumflex iliac artery
Ascending branch
Lateral circumflex femoral artery
Descending branch
Superior genicular artery
Anterior and posterior tibial recurrent artery
Anterior tibial artery
Perforating branch
Dorsalis pedis artery
Arcuate artery
Lateral plantar artery

Inferior mesenteric artery
Median sacral artery
Lateral sacral artery
Internal iliac artery
Inferior gluteal artery
Obfurator artery
Internal pudendal artery
Deep branch
Medial circumflex femoral artery
Tranverse branch
Deep femoral artery
Superficial femoral artery
Descending genicular artery
Popliteal artery
Inferior genicular artery
Posterior tibial artery
Peroneal artery
Communicating branch
Medial and lateral malleollar arteries
Medial plantar artery
Plantar arch

FIGURE 12-9. Essential collateral pathways of the lower extremity (right leg shown). Note the intersegmental character of the individual vascular bridges. Redrawn from Lusza G. *X-ray Anatomy of the Vascular System.* Philadelphia: JB Lippincott, 1963.

perforates the interosseus membrane between the tibia and fibula and courses distally between the extensor muscles of the lower leg to become the dorsalis pedis artery at the dorsum of the foot; this gives off the arcuate artery, which runs forming an arch to the level of the tarsometarsal line. The five dorsal metatarsal arteries arising from the arcuate artery continue as the dorsal digital arteries to the toes. The other terminal branch of the popliteal artery, the posterior tibial artery, descends straight toward the medial malleolus, while the peroneal (fibular) artery descends toward the lateral malleolus. The larger of the two terminal branches of the posterior tibial artery, the lateral plantar artery, forms the plantar arch at the base of the metatarsal bones; this in turn forms the plantar metatarsal arteries for the second, third, and fourth toes, becoming the common and proper plantar digital arteries. The lateral side of the fifth toe is usually supplied by an artery directly arising from the lateral plantar artery, whereas the first toe is largely supplied by the usually smaller medial plantar artery. Thus, the arterial blood supply to the feet is mainly provided by the arcuate artery of the anterior tibial (dorsal supply) and plantar arch of the posterior tibial (plantar supply). However, the peroneal artery might become an important

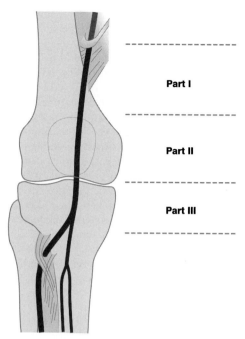

Part I

Part II

Part III

FIGURE 12-10. Division of the popliteal artery into segments, parts I–III. Redrawn from Diehm C, Allenberg J-R, Numura-Eckert K. *Farbatlas der Gefäßkrankheiten.* Berlin: Springer, 1999.

supplier of collaterals to the feet in the presence of tibial artery obstructions. Figure 12-12 shows the anatomy of the arterial supply of the feet.

Besides understanding normal vascular anatomy, including the most common vascular anomalies[40] and pathoanatomy of atherothrombotic peripheral artery disease,[38,41] specific findings relevant to percutaneous interventions should also be recognized. Thus, in patients with documented aneurysms and pseudoaneurysms, angiographic definition of the site—size (small to giant), form (saccular or berry; fusiform), and neck (width, spatial orientation)—is also required. In patients with documented abnormal connections between the arteries and

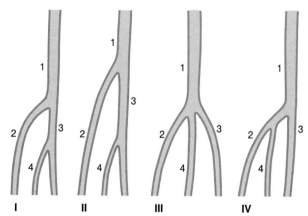

I   II   III   IV

FIGURE 12-11. Variations in the patterns of division of the popliteal artery. Type I, normal type; type II, high division; type III, trifurcation; type IV, peroneal artery arises from the anterior tibial artery; *1,* popliteal artery; *2,* anterior tibial artery, *3,* posterior tibial artery; *4,* peroneal (fibular) artery. Redrawn from Lusza G. *X-ray Anatomy of the Vascular System.* Philadelphia: JB Lippincott, 1963.

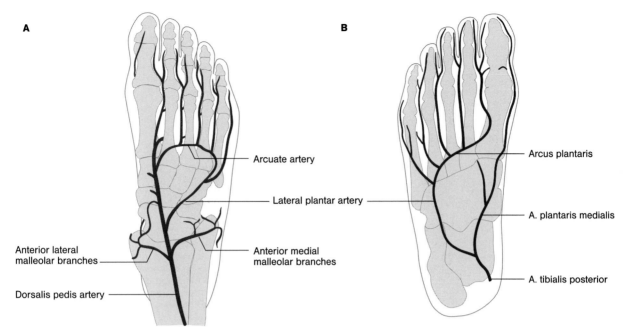

FIGURE 12-12. Arterial circulation of the foot, dorsal (**A**) and plantar (**B**) views.

veins of the leg, an effort should be made to distinguish between the congenital and acquired forms, the latter being in most cases due to injuries associated with simultaneous penetration of neighboring arteries and veins. Arteriographic definition of arteriovenous fistulas includes definition of the feeding arteries and connecting channels as well as distal venous and arterial circulation, and bridging collateral circulation. Arteriographic definition of arteriovenous congenital malformations must provide a complete road map to allow treatment considerations if required (not considered in this chapter). The angiographic appearance of obliterating thrombangitis of Winiwarter and Buerger (a corkscrew appearance in the bridging collaterals and paucity of the typical signs of diffuse atherosclerosis) should be recognized (for review, see references 38, 41, and 42).

In patients with indeterminate or borderline angiographic lesions on standard angiograms, additional projections should be acquired. In addition, measurements of translesional pressure gradients may be helpful, although numerous cutoff values of systolic and mean pressure gradients measured at rest and after vasodilatation indicative of the hemodynamic significance of a stenotic lesion have been reported in the literature (for review, see references 43 and 44). Despite the fact that the most accurate measurements of translesional pressure gradients can be achieved using the flow/pressure-wire technology,[45] in the clinical environment the majority of measurements are performed using the traditional fluid-filled systems. Here, diagnostic catheters or sheaths of various designs are applied employing various techniques such as simultaneous measurements using a single catheter with two ports, continuous measurements using a single catheter with one port during withdrawal, and simultaneous measurements obtained from the catheter tip and introductory sheath.[43] According to the recommendations of the TransAtlantic Inter-Society Consensus (TASC), stenoses with resting mean pressure gradients greater than 5 to 7 mm Hg (bar)

or postvasodilatation gradients greater than 10 to 15 mm Hg (bar) should be considered hemodynamically significant and indicative for revascularization.[3]

Because of the high percentage of interventions performed in patients with previous reconstructive vascular surgery, knowledge of the principal bypass channels is also required. Thus, the course and the proximal and distal anastomoses of the inter- and intrasegmental grafts—aortoiliac, iliofemoral, proximal and distal femoropopliteal, femorocrural, popliteocrural, crurocrural, axillofemoral, crossover femorofemoral, and other variants—and their functional importance for blood supply to the lower extremity must be clearly understood.

During procedures on the aortoiliac, femoropopliteal, and infrapopliteal (tibioperonal) arteries, only arterial DSA and fluoroscopy is sufficiently accurate to guide the interventions.

In DSA angiography-guided peripheral interventions, standard imaging protocols are implemented, consisting of selected projections of the interventional site and the distal runoff to document the baseline (preinterventional), intermediate (interventional), and final (postinterventional) findings. Pre- and postinterventional angiograms must include documentation of the peripheral runoff vessels. During the procedure, road mapping and fluoroscopy are used to guide the individual steps of the interventional cycle. Interventionists performing peripheral arterial interventions must be familiar with the angiographic representation of changing vessel wall morphology after interventions due to acute remodeling associated with plaque shifts, dissections, and perforations. Total fluoroscopy time and the amount of contrast agent used reflect on several variables including complexity of the disease, extent of the intervention, level of technical difficulty, and the quality of the procedure. Tables 12-8 and 12-9 provide examples of indications and relative contraindications for diagnostic peripheral arteriography.[46] Table 12-10 provides an example of suggested complication thresholds for diagnostic peripheral arteriography.[46]

TABLE 12-8. Example of Suggested Indications for Diagnostic Peripheral Arteriography

Aortography	*Pelvic Arteriography*	*Extremity Arteriography*
Intrinsic abnormalities, including transection, dissection, aneurysm, occlusive disease, aortitis, and congenital anomaly	Atherosclerotic aortoiliac disease	Atherosclerotic vascular disease, including aneurysms, emboli, occlusive disease, and thrombosis
Evaluation of aorta and its branches before selective studies	Gastrointestinal or genitourinary bleeding	Vascular trauma
Before interventional procedures	Trauma	Preoperative planning and postoperative evaluation for reconstructive surgery
	Primary vascular abnormalities, including aneurysms, vascular malformations, and vasculitis	Evaluation of surgical bypass grafts and dialysis grafts and fistulas
	Male impotence caused by arterial occlusive disease	Other primary vascular abnormalities, including vascular malformations, vasculitis, entrapment syndrome, thoracic outlet syndrome, etc.
	Pelvic tumors	Tumors
	Before interventional procedures	Before interventional procedures

Modified from Singh H, Cardella JF, Cole PE, et al. Quality improvement guidelines for diagnostic arteriography. *J Vasc Intervent Radiol.* 2002;13:1–6.

TABLE 12-9. Example of Suggested Relative Contraindications for Diagnostic Peripheral Arteriography

Severe hypertension
Uncorrectable coagulopathy
Clinically significant iodinated contrast material sensitivity
Renal insufficiency
Congestive heart failure
Certain connective tissue disorders (reported complications at the puncture site)

Reproduce with permission from Singh H, Cardella JF, Cole PE, et al. Quality Improvement Guidelines for Diagnostic Arteriography. *J Vasc Intervent Radiol.* 2002;13:1–6.

TABLE 12-10. Indicators and Thresholds for Complications in Diagnostic Peripheral Arteriography

Department Indicators	*Reported Rates (%)*	*Major Adverse Event Threshold (%)*
PUNCTURE SITE COMPLICATIONS		
Hematoma (requiring transfusion, surgery, or delayed discharge)	0.0–0.68	0.5
Occlusion	0.0–0.76	0.2
Pseudoaneurysm/arteriovenousfistula	0.04–0.2	0.2
CATHETER-INDUCED COMPLICATIONS (OTHER THAN PUNCTURE SITE)		
Distal emboli	0.0–0.10	0.5
Arterial dissection/subintimal passage	0.43	0.5
Subintimal injection of contrast	0.0–0.44	0.5
Major contrast reactions	0.0–3.58	0.5
Contrast-media-associated nephrotoxicity	0.2–1.4	0.2

Reproduced with permission from (from Singh H, Cardella JF, Cole PE, et al. Quality improvement guidelines for diagnostic arteriography. *J Vasc Intervent Radiol.* 2002;13:1–6).

PERIPHERAL VASCULAR INTERVENTIONS: BASIC CONSIDERATIONS

The first evidence for clinical potentials of endovascular interventions in femoropopliteal atherosclerotic disease was provided by Charles Dotter and Melvin Judkins, both radiologists at the Oregon Health Sciences University in Portland, Oregon, in their in 1964 published report.[47] These interventions were performed using coaxial Teflon dilating catheters; later, double-lumen balloon catheters with a caged ("Korsett") design were proposed,[48] and finally low-compliance poly(vinyl chloride) balloons[49] were implemented. In 1983, Dotter introduced the term *stent* for a coiled wire implant to scaffold a femoral artery in animal experiments[50]; the first peripheral stents for human use were introduced in the mid-1980s.[51]

Following the pioneering work of Charles Dotter, Andreas Grüntzig, and other "torch bearers,"[52] peripheral vascular interventions were performed throughout the 1980s and early 1990s by interventional radiologists. The radiology-based approach to peripheral interventional procedures typically employed large- size sheaths (7–8F), 0.035-in. guidewires, and high-profile, over-the-wire (OTW) instrumentation. By contrast, the more recent coronary-like approach to peripheral interventions increasingly employed smaller systems (5F to 6F), 0.014-in. guidewires, and low-profile rapid exchange devices, all critically instrumental to the integrated coaxial telescopic interventional approach. Using the more facile and less traumatic instrumentation enabled broader indications for endovascular therapy and has led to proliferation and expansion of coronary and coronary-like techniques in noncoronary vascular territories including the renal, carotid, femoral, and infrapopliteal arterial interventions. At present these peripheral arterial interventions are performed by interventional radiologists, vascular surgeons, and, in rapidly increasing numbers, by interventional cardiologists. With increasing convergence of endovascular techniques, the new specialty of vascular (excluding coronary arteries) and panvascular (all vascular beds included) medicine has began to emerge. Because of the present heterogeneity of the field, the standards of practice and the criteria for training, performance, outcome, and quality assurance of peripheral interventions also vary among the involved professional societies. Selected issues relevant to the performance of peripheral interventions are briefly reviewed in the subsequent sections.

TRAINING REQUIREMENTS

Current recommendations for standard requirements include the joint statements of the American College of Cardiology, American College of Physicians, Society for Cardiovascular Angiography and Interventions, Society for Vascular Medicine and Biology, Society for Vascular Surgery (ACC/ACP/SCAI/SVMB/SVS) panel,[53] and the older Society of Interventional Radiology (SIR) guidelines.[54–56] Tables 12-11 to 12-13 present summaries of the requirements on competence in catheter-based peripheral vascular interventions proposed by the joint ACC/ACP/SCAI/SVMB/SVS panel. To achieve this broad competence in vascular interventions as proposed by the panel, centers of broad vascular or panvascular expertise will first need to be established. At present, only a very few selected centers would qualify to provide a fully comprehensive vascular or panvascular interventional training and education.

TABLE 12-11.   Minimal Knowledge and Skills Required for Competence in Peripheral Catheter-based Interventions

The vascular interventionalist should be knowledgeable about each of the following:

- Mechanisms that regulate blood vessel function and hemostasis
- Pathophysiology, clinical manifestation, natural history, evaluation, and treatment of peripheral arterial disease, renal artery stenosis, mesenteric ischemia, extracranial cerebrovascular disease, aneurysmal disease, arterial dissection, and arterial and venous thromboembolism
- Noninvasive vascular tests such as segmental blood pressure measurements, arterial and venous duplex ultrasonography, and computed tomographic and magnetic resonance angiography
- Accuracy and limitations of diagnostic tests
- Radiation physics, safety, and radiographic imaging equipment
- Principles of image acquisition and display
- Advantages, disadvantages, and potential complications of iodinated and noniodinated contrast agents
- Advantages, disadvantages, potential outcomes, and complications of interventional procedures
- Indications, alternatives, and contraindications for catheter-based interventions

The vascular interventionalist should have the following technical skills:

- Ability to safely gain vascular access from multiple sites (femoral, popliteal, and upper extremity arteries, as well as femoral, upper extremity, and neck veins)
- Ability to obtain hemostasis including application of compression and vascular closure devices
- Ability to manipulate guidewires and catheters
- Ability to place and deploy angioplasty equipment (e.g., balloons, atherectomy devices, stents, distal protection devices)
- Ability to recognize and treat procedure-related complications (e.g., dissection, pseudoaneurysms, embolism, vessel perforation or occlusion, stent thrombosis, adverse hemodynamic events)
- Ability to perform catheter-directed thrombolysis/thrombectomy
- Ability to perform vascular interventions in each of the following: aorta and lower extremity arteries, brachiocephalic and upper extremity arteries, mesenteric and renal arteries, central and peripheral veins, and pulmonary arteries

Reproduced with permission from Creager MA, Goldstone J, Hirschfeld JW Jr., et al. for the Writing Committee Members. ACC/ACP/SCAI/SVMB/SVS Clinical Competence Statement on vascular medicine and catheter-based peripheral vascular interventions. *J Am Coll Cardiol.* 2004;44:941–957.

TABLE 12-12. Formal Training to Achieve Competence in Peripheral Catheter-based Interventions

Training requirements for cardiovascular physicians
- Duration of training[a]—12 months
- Diagnostic coronary angiograms[b]—300 cases (200 as the primary operator)
- Diagnostic peripheral angiograms—100 cases (50 as primary operator)
- Peripheral interventional cases[c]—50 cases (25 as primary operator)

Training requirements for interventional radiologists
- Duration of training[d]—12 months
- Diagnostic peripheral angiograms—100 cases (50 as primary operator)
- Peripheral interventional cases[c]—50 cases (25 as primary operator)

Training requirements for vascular surgeons
- Duration of training—12 months[e]
- Diagnostic peripheral angiograms[f]—100 cases (50 as primary operator)
- Peripheral interventional cases[c]—50 cases (25 as primary operator)
- Aortic aneurysm endografts—10 cases (5 as primary operator)

This table is consistent with current Residency Review Committee requirements.

[a]After completing 24 months of core cardiovascular training and 8 months of cardiac catheterization.

[b]Coronary catheterization procedures should be completed prior to interventional training.

[c]After completing general radiology training

[d]The case mix should be evenly distributed among the different vascular beds. Supervised cases of thrombus management for limb ischemia and venous thrombosis, utilizing percutaneous thrombolysis or thrombectomy, should be included.

[e]In addition to 12 months of core vascular surgery training.

[f]In addition to experience gained during open surgical procedures.

Reproduced with permission from Creager MA, Goldstone J, Hirschfeld JW Jr., et al. for the Writing Committee Members. ACC/ACP/SCAI/SVMB/SVS Clinical Competence Statement on vascular medicine and catheter-based peripheral vascular interventions. *J Am Coll Cardiol.* 2004;44:941–957.

TABLE 12-13. Alternative Routes to Achieving Competence in Peripheral Catheter-based Intervention

1. Common requirements
   a. Completion of required training within 24-month period
   b. Training under proctorship of formally trained vascular interventionalist competent to perform full range of procedures described in this document
   c. Written curriculum with goals and objectives
   d. Regular written evaluations by proctor
   e. Documentation of procedures and outcomes
   f. Supervised experience in inpatient and outpatient vascular consultation settings
   g. Supervised experience in a noninvasive vascular laboratory

2. Procedural requirements for competency in all areas
   a. Diagnostic peripheral angiograms—100 cases (50 as primary operator)
   b. Peripheral interventions—50 cases (25 as primary operator)
   c. No fewer than 20 diagnostic/10 interventional cases in each area, excluding extracranial cerebral arteries[a]
   d. Extracranial cerebral (carotid/vertebral) arteries—30 diagnostic (15 as primary operator)/25 interventional (13 as primary operator)
   e. Percutaneous thrombolysis/thrombectomy—5 cases

3. Requirements for competency in subset of areas (up to 3, excluding carotid/vertebral arteries)
   a. Diagnostic peripheral angiograms per area—30 cases (15 as primary operator)
   b. Peripheral interventions per area—15 cases (8 as primary operator)
   c. Must include aortoiliac arteries as initial area of competency

The fulfillment of requirements via an alternative pathway is only appropriate if the candidate physician has the cognitive and technical skills outlined in Table 12-11 and is competent to perform either coronary intervention, interventional radiology, or vascular surgery. These alternative routes for achieving competency are available for up to 5 years following publication of this document.

[a]Vascular areas are: (1) aortoiliac and brachiocephalic arteries; (2) abdominal visceral and renal arteries; and (3) infrainguinal arteries

Reproduced with permission from Creager MA, Goldstone J, Hirschfeld JW Jr., et al. for the Writing Committee Members. ACC/ACP/SCAI/SVMB/SVS Clinical Competence Statement on vascular medicine and catheter-based peripheral vascular interventions. *J Am Coll Cardiol.* 2004;44:941–957.

DOCUMENTATION AND REPORTING

On the basis of early reports,[54,55] the need for the development of standards in documenting and reporting the outcomes of peripheral interventions has been recognized, and guidelines and recommendations that permit comparisons of data and comparison-based benchmarking have been successively developed.[56,57] Although some of the definitions proposed in these documents may no longer apply, may be too cumbersome, or may be in need of revision, their essential parts are reproduced to illustrate these efforts, to encourage their adoption where applicable, or to stimulate their improvement where necessary. In Tables 12-14 to 12-18, the definition of patency, success, clinical improvement, complications, and length of follow-up periods are provided. In Tables 12-19 to 12-21, suggested standards for notes and reporting are reviewed, whereas Table 12-22 provides a suggested checklist for study protocols relevant to PAD.

CRITERIA FOR INDICATIONS

The criteria for indications for peripheral interventions are subject to change as progress is made in understanding the pathogenesis of the peripheral arterial disease and the perceived utility of competing and complementary treatments. In addition, the local expertise and availability of resources are decisive factors. In essence, however, the decisions to treat a patient with PAD by catheter-based interventions should be based on the

---

TABLE 12-14.   Definition of Patency in Peripheral Arterial Interventions

---

Patency

Lack of occlusion of the treated segment determined by the presence of any one or more of the following criteria:

1. Demonstrably open with vascular imaging (arteriography, duplex Doppler, or magnetic resonance imaging)
2. Maintenance of achieved improvement in the appropriate segmental limb pressure index (i.e., ABI or thigh/brachial index must have increased by more than 0.10 initially and not deteriorated by more than 0.15 from the maximum early postprocedure level.
3. Pulse volume recording distal to the treated segment maintained at 5 mm above preoperative tracing (only for diabetic patients with incompressible arteries)
4. Palpable pulse or biphasic or triphasic Doppler waveform measured at two points directly over a superficially placed graft
5. Direct observation at operation or post mortem

Primary patency

Uninterrupted patency with no procedures performed on or at the margins of the treated segment. Only procedures performed proximal or distal to the initially treated segment to treat progression of disease in an adjacent native vessel are exempted. If any procedure is performed before thrombosis that might prevent eventual failure (as well as any procedure that restores patency after thrombosis, primary patency is lost).

Assisted primary patency

Any procedure performed in the treated segment before thrombosis that might prevent eventual failure

Secondary patency

Any procedure that restores patency after thrombosis. The flow should be restored through most of the original graft or treated segment of native vessel and in the case of grafts, at least one of the original anastomoses

---

ABI, ankle-brachial index.
Reproduced with permission from Sacks D, Marinelli DL, Martin LG, et al. Reporting standards for clinical evaluation of new peripheral arterial revascularization devices. *J Vasc Intervent Radiol.* 1997;8:137–149.

TABLE 12-15.   Definition of Success in Peripheral Arterial Interventions.

Technical Success	*Clinical*
Meets the criteria for both anatomic and hemodynamic success in the immediate postprocedure period **A. Anatomic:** <30% final residual stenosis measured at the narrowest point of the vascular lumen. Continued anatomic: <50% recurrent stenosis **B. Hemodynamic:** ABI or thigh/brachial index improved by 1.0 or greater above baseline and not deteriorated by >0.15 from the maximum early postprocedure level, or pulse volume recording distal to the reconstruction maintained at 5 mm above the preoperative tracing (only for patients with incompressible vessels)	Immediate improvement by at least 1 clinical category. Sustained improvement by at least 1 clinical category. Patients with tissue loss (categories 5 and 6) must move up at least 2 categories and reach the level of claudication to be considered improved

---

ABI, ankle-brachial index.
Reproduced with permission from Sacks D, Marinelli DL, Martin LG, et al. Reporting standards for clinical evaluation of new peripheral arterial revascularization devices. *J Vasc Intervent Radiol.* 1997;8:137–149.

TABLE 12-16. Definition of Clinical Improvement in Peripheral Arterial Interventions

Grade	Clinical Description
+3	Markedly improved: symptoms gone or markedly improved; ankle/brachial index increased to more than 0.90.
+2	Moderately improved: still symptomatic, but at least single category improvement; ankle/brachial index increased by more than 0.10 but not normalized.
+1	Minimally improved: greater than 0.10 increase in ankle/brachial index but no categorical improvement, or vice versa (i.e., upward categorical shift without an increase in ankle/brachial index of more than 0.10).
0	No change: no categorical shift and less than 0.10 change in ankle/brachial index
−1	Mildly worse: no categorical shift but ankle/brachial index decreased more than 0.10, or downward categorical shift with ankle/brachial index decreases less than 0.10.
−2	Moderately worse: one category worse or unexpected minor amputation.
−3	Markedly worse: more than one category worse or unexpected major amputation.

Reproduced with permission from Sacks D, Marinelli DL, Martin LG, et al. Reporting standards for clinical evaluation of new peripheral arterial revascularization devices. *J Vasc Intervent Radiol.* 1997;8:137–149.

TABLE 12-17. Definition of Complications in Peripheral Arterial Interventions

Minor
- A. No therapy, no consequence, or
- B. Nominal therapy, no consequence; includes overnight admission for observation only

Major
- C. Require therapy, minor hospitalization (<48 h)
- D. Require major therapy, unplanned increase in level of care, prolonged hospitalization (>48 h),
- E. Have permanent adverse sequelae, or
- F. Result in death

Reproduced with permission from Sacks D, Marinelli DL, Martin LG, et al. Reporting standards for clinical evaluation of new peripheral arterial revascularization devices. *J Vasc Intervent Radiol.* 1997;8:137–149.

TABLE 12-18. Suggested Definitions of the Length of Follow-up Periods

Follow-up Period	Months of Observation
Immediate	0–1 month
Short-term	1–12 months
Long-term	>12 months

Reproduced with permission from Sacks D, Marinelli DL, Martin LG, et al. Reporting standards for clinical evaluation of new peripheral arterial revascularization devices. *J Vasc Intervent Radiol.* 1997;8:137–149.

TABLE 12-19. Suggested Preprocedural Documentation for Peripheral Arterial Interventions.

Indication for procedure and brief history

Physical examination findings

Laboratory findings (including noninvasive)

Risk stratification, such as the American Society of Anesthesiologists Class

Documentation that informed consent, including risks, benefits, and alternatives, was obtained, or in the case of an emergency, that this was an emergency medical procedure

The diagnostic and/or anticipated treatment plan for each procedure to be performed

Reproduced with permission from Omary RA, Bettmann MA, Cardella JF, et al. Quality improvement guidelines for the reporting and archiving of interventional radiology procedures. *J Vasc Intervent Radiol.* 2003; 14:S293–S295.

TABLE 12-20. Suggested Immediate Procedure Note for Peripheral Arterial Interventions

Identification and brief description of procedure

Operator(s)

Results

Complications

Postprocedure monitoring/treatment plan

Reproduced with permission from Omary RA, Bettmann MA, Cardella JF, et al. Quality improvement guidelines for the reporting and archiving of interventional radiology procedures. *J Vasc Intervent Radiol.* 2003; 14:S293–S295.

TABLE 12-21. Suggested Final Report for Peripheral Arterial Interventions

Goals and Objectives
1. To transmit procedural information to all members of health care community who may participate in subsequent care of the patient
2. For legal purposes
3. For reimbursement

Specific information

Depend on the procedure

Recommend elements include procedure; Date; Operator(s); Indication; Procedure/technique: a technical description of procedure. This information should include access site (and all attempted access sites), guidance modalities, catheters/guide wires/needles, vessels or organs catheterized, technique, and hemostasis. Each major vessel catheterized for imaging or intervention should be noted specifically. If informed consent was obtained, this should be stated; Complications; Results/findings; Conclusion; Plan, if appropriate

Modified from Omary RA, Bettmann MA, Cardella JF, et al. Quality improvement guidelines for the reporting and archiving of interventional radiology procedures. *J Vasc Intervent Radiol.* 2003; 14:S293–S295.

documentation of presumably greater benefits compared with medical or open surgery treatment. This documentation of presumably greater benefits should be based on objective evidence and local expertise required for successful treatment, and should result from a thorough risk and benefit analysis in a given patient.

The decision on an optimum strategy may be relatively straightforward in "simple" cases, yet it may be difficult in complex ones. Similar to interventions in other vascular territories a thorough evaluation of the relevant patient-, PAD-, and target lesion-related

TABLE 12-22. Suggested Checklist for Reporting of Data in Clinical Studies Pertaining to Peripheral Arterial Interventions

Data	Required	Highly Recommended	Recommended
PRETREATMENT EVALUATION			
Risk factors/comorbidities	X		
MEASURES OF DISEASE SEVERITY			
Stenosis of treated site	X		
Runoff grade	X		
Eccentricity			X
Noninvasive indices (ABI, TBI, PVR)	X		
Treadmill (claudicants)	X	X	
Graded treadmill			
Functional status		X	
Quality of life		X	
TREATMENT DESCRIPTION	X		
Post-treatment evaluation			
Follow-up angiogram		X	
Technical success			
Anatomic			
Stenosis	X		
Luminal gain		X	
Hemodynamic			
Noninvasive (ABI, TBI, PVR)	X		
Intravascular pressures		X	
Clinical success			
Improvement category	X		
Functional status		X	
Quality of life		X	
Treadmill (claudicants)	X		
Graded treadmill (claudicants)		X	
Separate life-tables for anatomic, hemodynamic, and clinical data	X		
Complications	X		
Compliance		X	
COSTS			
Gross estimate (equipment, length of stay, ICU days, number of encounters)		X	
Detailed			X

ABI, ankle-brachial index; TBI, thigh-brachial index; PVR, pulse-volume recording; ICU, intensive care unit

Modified from Sacks D, Marinelli DL, Martin LG, et al. Reporting standards for clinical evaluation of new peripheral arterial revascularization devices. *J Vasc Intervent Radiol.* 1997;8:137–149.

factors is critical to objective judgments. Critical decision criteria include presence of coexistent morbidities, in particular heart failure, renal dysfunction, and diabetes; vascular multimorbidity, in particular coronary and cerebrovascular disease; and severity and extent of the targeted PAD. In patients with PAD considered for catheter-based interventions, access to the target lesion, technical feasibility, and the expected long-term (!) outcome are also decisive. With the rapidly evolving coronary-like techniques applicable to infrainguinal interventions, and with better skills and instrumentation, the factors concerning technical feasibility are becoming less important, whereas considerations of clinical outcome, efficacy, costs, and available expertise are now decisive. Thus, although the primarily target lesion based criteria devised in the 1990s remain practical, their clinical validity and interpretation are increasingly subject to re-evaluation depending on the availability of locally available expertise and state of steadily improving peripheral endovascular instrumentation. Standard target lesion decision indicators are summarized in Table 12-23.[58] However, rigid interpretations of these guidelines[13,58] in clinical settings of aortoiliac, femoropopliteal, and infrapopliteal interventions appear no longer appropriate. Instead, experienced operators have learned to integrate this existing framework into far more comprehensive risk and benefit evaluations in individual patients. Indeed, in experienced centers increasing numbers of category 3 and 4 lesions (see Table 12-23) are now reasonable candidates for catheter-based therapy. To improve outcomes particularly in "complex cases," that is, in patients with complex PAD and multiple coexisting morbidities,

TABLE 12-23. Definition of Categories of Target Lesions and Proposed Means of Treatment

Category 1	Category 2	Category 3	Category 4
Lesions for which percutaneous transluminal angioplasty alone is the procedure of choice. Treatment of these lesions will result in a high technical success rate and will generally result in complete relief of symptoms or normalization of pressure gradients.	Lesions that are well suited for percutaneous transluminal angioplasty. Treatment of these lesions will result in complete relief or significant improvement in symptoms, pulses, or pressure gradients. This category includes lesions that will be treated by procedures to be followed by surgical bypass to treat multilevel vascular disease.	Lesions that may be treated with percutaneous therapy, but because of disease extent, location, or severity have a significantly lower chance of initial technical success or long-term benefit than if treated with surgical bypass. However, percutaneous transluminal angioplasty may be performed, generally because of patient risk factors or because of lack of suitable bypass material.	Extensive vascular disease, for which percutaneous therapy has a very limited role because of low technical success rate or poor long-term benefit. In very-high-risk patients, or in those for whom no surgical procedure is applicable, percutaneous transluminal angioplasty may have some place.

Reproduced with permission from Pentecoast MJ, Criqui MH, Dorros G, et al. Guidelines for peripheral percutaneous transluminal angioplasty of the abdominal aorta and lower extremity vessels. A statement for health professionals from a Special Writing Group of the Councils on Cardiovascular Radiology, Arteriosclerosis, Cardio-thoracic and Vascular Surgery, Clinical Cardiology, and Epidemiology and Prevention, American Heart Association. *Circulation.* 1994;89:511–531.

interdisciplinary consensus decisions between interventionists and vascular surgeons and case-customized design of complementary revascularization strategies represent the best approach.

To allow sensible assessments of risks and benefits in individual patients, unequivocal definitions of risks, benefits, and clinical outcomes associated with catheter-based interventions are required. In peripheral interventions, as in interventions in other vascular territories, risks may be divided into the broad categories comprising the local access site complications, proximal and distal complications pertaining to the intervention site, and systemic complications (Table 12-24).[58] Systemic complications are frequently termed major adverse cardiac (and cerebrovascular) events (MAC(C)E) and typically include death, myocardial infarction, cerebrovascular accidents, and target vessel failure or target vessel revascularization. Adverse outcomes may be differentiated on the basis of severity, as shown in Table 12-17. Complication rates are relative values and may change with the selection of patients (patient bias) and the skills of the operator (operator bias). Objective criteria to define benefits in peripheral vascular interventions may be difficult to obtain; Table 12-16 provides an example of outcome assessment. Other means include quality-adjusted survival/life expectancy and generic health status (for review, see reference 13).

PERIPHERAL VASCULAR INTERVENTIONS: BASIC STRUCTURE

The basic structure of endovascular interventions exemplified by coronary interventions has been provided in Chapter 4. Thus, the individual steps of peripheral vascular interventions can be divided into the three basic stages of initialization, main interventional cycle, and termination.

Consequently, initialization includes indication, definition of initial strategy of the intervention, establishment of the vascular access, placement of the guiding catheter or sheath to allow access to the target lesion, and ends with the acquisition of the preinterventional angiograms.

TABLE 12–24. Incidence of Complications of Peripheral Arterial Interventions, Data Based on Early Evidence

Complication	Incidence (%)
PUNCTURE SITE (TOTAL)	4.0
Bleeding	3.4
False aneurysm	0.5
Arteriovenous fistula	0.1
ANGIOPLASTY SITE (TOTAL)	3.5
Thrombus	3.2
Rupture	0.3
DISTAL VESSEL (TOTAL)	2.7
Dissection	0.4
Embolization	2.3
SYSTEMIC (TOTAL)	0.4
Renal failure	0.2
Myocardial infarction (fatal)	0.2
Cerebrovascular accident (fatal)	0.55
CONSEQUENCES	
Surgical repair	2.0
Limb loss	0.2
Mortality	0.2

Reproduced with permission from Pentecoast MJ, Criqui MH, Dorros G, et al. Guidelines for peripheral percutaneous transluminal angioplasty of the abdominal aorta and lower extremity vessels. A statement for health professionals from a Special Writing Group of the Councils on Cardiovascular Radiology, Arteriosclerosis, Cardio-thoracic and Vascular Surgery, Clinical Cardiology, and Epidemiology and Prevention, American Heart Association. *Circulation.* 1994;89:511–531.

The main procedural cycle consists of individual repetitive cycles (IRC) that comprise assessment, interventional action, and reassessment IRCs are iterations towards the set goal of the intervention, ideally 100% success with 0% complications. The number of IRC is indicative of the complexity, but also of the quality of the intervention. Typically, the lower number of IRCs required to successfully complete the intervention (the ideal number of IRCs is 1) is indicative of lower complication rates and lower costs.

On the basis of the reassessment, the next cycle is initiated or the procedure is terminated. Termination includes retraction of all endovascular instrumentation from the target vessel, acquisition of the final postprocedural angiograms, sheath removal, and hemostasis. Establishing arterial access and hemostasis are common to all peripheral interventions and will be addressed in the following sections.

ACCESS

The first initializing step of any percutaneous vascular intervention is establishment of the arterial access. The Seldinger percutaneous technique[59] has become a principal means to establish vascular access for endovascular interventions. Possible access sites include the common femoral, brachial, radial, axillary, and popliteal arteries, and for diagnostic peripheral arteriography also the lumbar aorta. Selection of the arterial access site depends primarily on the availability of the access artery, required size of the system, and location of the target vascular region with regard to the access site; for the majority of peripheral interventions, more than one access site is available.

The availability of an access artery depends on the presence of the disease at the site of the arterial puncture and distribution of the disease in the adjacent proximal and distal segments. In addition, the size of the artery must be compatible with the size of the system required to perform the intervention. Transfemoral access is by far the most flexible and accessible for percutaneous intervention; depending on the constitution of the patient, systems of up to 20F in size can be employed. By contrast, access via the brachial and axillary arteries is limited up to 6F to 7F, in the radial artery up to 6F, and in the popliteal artery up to 7F system sizes.

An important criterion for the selection of the access site is the accessibility of the target lesion. In most cases, a short, but not too short, distance to the target vascular site is preferable. However, although a short distance between the access site and target lesion is desirable, it cannot be achieved in coronary or brachiocephalic interventions and may need to be sacrificed also in peripheral interventions in the presence of other, more important considerations such as safety. In patients with a longer vascular pathway with several branching points between the access site and the target lesion, atraumatic passage of the instrumentation through the vascular system must be ensured. This goal is served by careful guidewire passage beyond the target lesion and establishing a working channel by placing a long sheath or guiding catheter proximal to the target site. To provide optimum working conditions, the working channel should be seated stably and the ostium of the guide should be close to the target lesion. In infrainguinal interventions, frequently the direct access to the lesion is sacrificed and the crossover approach from the contralateral side is established to reduce the risk of proximal and distal complications associated with hemostasis and compromise in run-in blood flow. Before selecting the crossover approach, the pathoanatomy of both iliac arteries and aortic bifurcation must be considered with regard to the presence of stenoses, tortuosities, ectasia, and elongations, as

well as the axial angle of the bifurcation. In selecting antegrade transfemoral access, the status, the length and width of the ipsilateral common femoral artery, the topographic location of the femoral artery bifurcation, and the distance from the entry site to the target lesion should be considered on the basis of diagnostic angiograms. In addition, the constitution of the patient should be taken into account. In the presence of adverse conditions such as excessive obesity, an alternative access should be selected. Interventions involving the aorta and aortic bifurcation usually require bilateral transfemoral access with the "better" side selected for the introduction of the larger system. Alternatively, in aortic bifurcation interventions, the smaller protection balloon can be introduced using the, mostly left, brachial access. The popliteal retrograde access remains a rarity; yet because of the great force it allows to be transmitted directly onto the instrumentation, it can be beneficial in selected cases of chronic total superficial femoral artery occlusions and previously failed interventions. Downsides include difficult hemostasis and a greater risk of hemorrhage and phlebothrombosis.

It should be kept in mind that complications of the access site are a major source of morbidity and a considerable cost factor associated with percutaneous interventions; therefore, meticulous technique of arterial puncture and thorough hemostasis are a high priority. To avoid damage of the dilator or the sheath during skin and tissue penetration potentially associated with arterial injury, a short transverse cut of the skin, and if needed, upsizing predilatation of the subcutaneous channel with stiff dilatators may be required, in hostile settings such as excessive scarring of the subcutaneous tissues, heavy vessel wall calcification or obesity, present singly or combined, even when low-profile introductory sets have been used. For safe puncture, the operator must practice palpation of the arterial pulse with measured pressure to allow identification of the point of maximum impulse, while stabilizing the artery against the background tissues. The needle is typically angulated at approximately 45 degrees to the skin surface and introduced from the skin penetration site to the site of the arterial puncture on the straightest path. After the skin has been penetrated, which is usually 1 to 3 cm downstream (retrograde puncture) or upstream (antegrade puncture) from the site of the arterial front wall penetration, the direction of the injection should not be changed. If a second attempt is needed, the needle should be withdrawn and redirected. Only the front wall of the artery should be penetrated. The quality and intensity of the jet of returning blood provides information on the position of the needle tip within the lumen. A strong and pulsatile jet is indicative of a secure intraluminal position. In patients with severe peripheral disease, only weak blood return is frequent, despite an optimal intraluminal needle position. In these cases, a particularly meticulous handling of the introductory guidewire is required. Individual access sites are briefly reviewed in the following.

The common femoral artery can be cannulated using the standard retrograde or the antegrade approach. The common femoral artery is a direct continuation of the external iliac artery, just below the inguinal ligament. It has a short stem before it bifurcates into the superficial and deep femoral arteries. The clinical anatomy of the inguinal region is helpful to determine the optimum site of skin and artery wall penetration. Ideally, the point of artery wall penetration should be about 1 cm distal to the inguinal ligament. The anatomic position of the ligament corresponds to the line between the symphysis pubis and the anterior superior iliac spine. The common femoral artery passes under the ligament at the midline between the two anatomic landmarks just above the head of the femur. The corresponding nerve is on the lateral side, and the vein on the medial side to the artery, with the lymphatic nodes occupying the most medial position (N-erve, A-rtery, V-ein, L-ymphatic). The skin fold is an unreliable marker, because of the large variation found. The point of entry of the needle through the skin is typically 2 to 3 cm below the crossing between the line of the ligament and femoral artery. If the arterial wall puncture is too high (above or into the ligament), it is associated with greater risk of bleeding; if it is too low (below the bifurcation), it may be associated with injury to the deep femoral artery. In patients with severe bilateral iliofemoral or distal aortic disease, an alternative access site should be selected. Puncture of synthetic grafts should be avoided, despite the difference in opinion in the literature, because of difficult hemostasis due to the extensive scar tissue formation, the inability to use closure devices and appreciable risk of graft damage. In difficult cases, fluoroscopy may be helpful in guiding the arterial puncture in the presence of vessel wall calcifications; rarely, ultrasound guidance is needed. Retrograde femoral access is the most frequently used site for ipsilateral aortoiliac, contralateral iliofemoral, femoropopliteal, and also coronary and renal interventions, and it is the only side available for brachiocephalic interventions. Antegrade transfemoral access with the patient turned by 180 degrees on the table is technically more demanding because of the limited space above the patient's abdomen, particularly in obese patients. To allow safe puncture, the level of femoral bifurcation in respect to the anatomic landmarks is noted based on diagnostic angiography and marked using a radiopaque pointer that is firmly attached to the draping covering the patient. The finger tip palpating the femoral pulse must be placed at or slightly cranial to the marked bifurcation level to allow common femoral artery puncture. Arterial puncture above the bifurcation allows the introductory guiding catheter to be directed into the superficial femoral artery (SFA). Antegrade femoral access may be used for ipsilateral mid- and distal femoral, popliteal and infrapopliteal interventions. Figure 12-13A shows the topographic anatomy of the inguinal region relevant to retrograde and antegrade femoral access.

The brachial artery is the second most frequently used access site for endovascular interventions. In peripheral interventions the left brachial artery is preferred because manipulation across the aortic with its attending risk of intracranial embolization is avoided, and the intravascular pathway is shortened. With the patient in a supine position, the arm is placed on an extension board at 45 to 60 degrees to the main axis of the body, supinated, and externally rotated to fully expose the lower upper arm and the antecubital fossa. The skin is punctured just above the antecubital fossa to reach the artery before it "dives" between the biceps and brachial muscles. At this level, "rolling" can be prevented by applying gentle pressure onto the artery against the head of the humerus. To navigate the guidewire from the subclavian artery into the descending aorta, a pigtail catheter or catheters with a longer distal curve are usually required. Brachial access may be used for interventions involving the aortoiliac and femoropopliteal segments; in short individuals, even the infrapopliteal segment may be reached.

In contrast to coronary interventions, the radial artery is a rare access site for peripheral interventions. Before selecting the radial artery for arterial puncture, the collateral circulation to the hand should be evaluated. To be sure of patency of the radial and ulnar arteries and adequate collateral blood supply to the hand, the Allen test and preferably duplex or Doppler imaging of both forearm arteries is required.[60] The distal radial artery may be palpated proximal to the wrist above the styloid process at the lateral side of the radius. Because of the small size of the artery, only the very tip of the finger and gentle pressure should be used to identify the point of maximum impulse of the pulse. The skin should be punctured about 2 to 3 cm above the styloid process and slowly advanced to avoid double puncture of the walls. As the blood return is frequently only a trickle, the introductory guidewire must be introduced gently and carefully to avoid dissections. Figure 12-13B shows the topographic anatomy relevant to the retrograde brachial and radial access.

Retrograde transaxillary or high brachial access is rarely used for percutaneous interventions. The axillary artery is the direct continuation of the subclavian artery on its entrance into the axilla, and it ends on entering the upper arm, at a point that projects over the inferior border of the teres major muscle. The axillary artery is anatomically divided into three segments by the pectoralis minor muscle, which crosses it in front. Together with the vein and the nerve, the artery is surrounded by the axillary sheath. With the patient in a supine position, preferably the left arm is placed under the patientís head turned to the contralateral side. The axillary artery is palpated at the lateral edge of the major pectoral muscle, and its direction is ascertained. Fixed between the index and middle fingertip to avoid rolling, the skin is penetrated at the lateral aspect of the axilla to puncture the artery as far laterally (downstream) as possible. If the brachial plexus has been touched, the patient experiences "electric shock" and twitches; in this case, needle withdrawal and redirection is necessary. If bleeding into the neurovascular sheath occurs, prompt surgical decompression might be necessary to avoid permanent neural injury.[61] Because of greater risk of neural damage and more difficult hemostasis, axillary/high brachial access is rarely used in most interventional centers. Figure 12-13C shows the topographic anatomy relevant to the transaxillary vascular access.

Retrograde transpopliteal access is also termed the "back door" to the SFA. First retrograde transfemoral access is established using a 4F sheath for contrast agent administration. Subsequently, the patient is brought into a prone position; using a road-map technique, the topographic course of the popliteal artery is visualized, and the puncture site selected. Taking the vascular anatomy within the popliteal fossa into consideration (where the popliteal vein takes a more lateral and mostly posterior course than the artery), the skin is typically penetrated 1 cm medial to the midline of the popliteal fossa, about 3 to 4 cm above the level of the femoropopliteal joint, as determined by fluoroscopy. To avoid transvenous arterial puncture, the needle is directed from medial to lateral to enter the artery about 6 to 7 cm cranial to the level of the femorotibial joint.[62] Figure 12-13D shows the topographic anatomy relevant to the transpopliteal access.

Aortic lumbar (antegrade) access was introduced in 1929[63] and allows direct access to the distal abdominal aortic and peripheral circulation; it has never had any role in interventional therapy, and the importance of this access site for peripheral angiography has been greatly reduced because of the wide availability of noninvasive MR and CT angiographic techniques.

ultrasound-guided compression of the neck, with or without local injection of thrombin, collagen, or other thrombogenics into the pseudoaneurysm cavity. Larger (>2 cm) and particularly expanding aneurysms may require surgical revision (for review, see reference 66).

In transvenous arterial punctures, the puncture canal may persist, resulting in formation of an arteriovenous fistula. Late fistula formation by erosion of the adjacent venous wall during the healing process following bleeding complications is also possible. Arteriovenous fistulas may be recognized by the presence of a continuous bruit at the former cannulation site; duplex imaging defines the anatomy, and angiographic definition is only rarely required. In small fistulas, no treatment is required, but larger fistulas require transcatheter closure or surgical revision.

Arterial closure during the course of or following the intervention may be associated with acute thrombosis, distal embolization, or other mechanical obstruction, such as dissection. The resulting ALI requires immediate angiography and frequently surgical revision.

AORTOILIAC AND ILIAC INTERVENTIONS

Abrupt occlusion of the distal abdominal aorta is rare and almost always caused by embolizations. Acute symptoms include sudden onset of pain, pallor, paralysis, and coldness of both legs, associated with a variable degree of hemodynamic compromise and frequently circulatory shock. Emergency CT or brachial access abdominal angiography-guided embolectomy may be lifesaving.

Chronic occlusion of the aortic bifurcation may remain asymptomatic in the presence of functionally adequate collateralization. In individuals with absent collaterals, the full clinical picture of the Leriche syndrome develops, consisting of buttock claudication, lower extremity weakness, global atrophy without trophic changes of the skin or nails, complete distal pulselessness, persistent foot and leg pallor that is unchanged if the legs are hanging down, and vasculogenic impotence. In the original description of Leriche, the syndrome was reported to be more common in young adult males.[67]

In the majority of patients, atherothrombosis of the distal abdominal aorta and proximal iliac arteries represents a morphologic continuum. Severe PAD with associated clinical symptoms results in most patients. Abdominal aortic aneurysms and their management are reviewed in Chapter 10. Nonatherosclerotic causes of the aortoiliac disease are rare and include coarctation and inflammatory disorders such as Takayasu arteritis and syphilis. Atherosclerosis of the infrarenal abdominal aorta may be associated with acute and chronic syndromes of any of the paired and unpaired visceral arteries. Involvement of spinal arteries is also possible; however, because of usually adequate collateralization, spinal ischemia and infarcts are rare. Nevertheless, simultaneous involvement of several spinal arteries due to abdominal aortic dissections or systemic vasculitides might cause spinal infarcts.

In patients with aortoiliac disease, isolated proximal disease is rare, and in most cases diffuse disease of the entire downstream iliac and lower leg circulation is present. Among various topographic distributions of PAD, diffuse aortoiliac, femoropopliteal, and infrapopliteal involvement was found to be the third most frequent pattern (Fig. 12-14).[68] On the basis

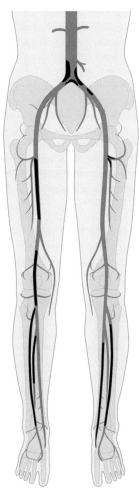

FIGURE 12-14. Topography of peripheral arterial disease. Aortoiliac disease associated with peripheral femoropopliteal and infrapopliteal disease. Redrawn from Haimovici H. Patterns of arteriosclerotic lesions of the lower extremity. *Arch Surg.* 1967;95:918–933.

of the length and complexity of lesions, four grades of the aortoiliac disease and four grades of the iliac disease may be distinguished (Tables 12-15 and 12-16).[58] Although aortoiliac bypass surgery remains the principal means of revascularization,[69] the availability of balloon angioplasty since the 1980s and later stent-supported angioplasty has provided increasingly important treatment options in selected patients.[70–73]

INDICATIONS FOR AORTOILIAC INTERVENTIONS

Indications for catheter-based versus surgical revascularization of an isolated or combined multilevel aortoiliac and distal run-off disease as opposed to the conservative PAD management have not been well-defined. In general, patients in whom conservative management has failed and significant symptoms persist are considered candidates for revascularization. In most vascular centers with endovascular and surgery services, the selection of patients depends primarily on patient-related factors such as symptoms, coexisting morbidities, surgical risk, patient's preference, life expectancy, and other, lesion-related factors such the morphology and technical accessibility of the target lesion and the status of the inflow, outflow, and collateral vessels. Although according to the TASC recommendations bypass surgery may represent the strategy of choice in patients with multilevel diffuse disease associated with type D (corresponding to Pentecoast category 4 lesions, Table 12-23) and frequently intermediary types C and B lesions (corresponding to Pentecoast category 3 and 2 lesions, Table 12-23) in real-life clinical practice even in these frequently multimorbid patients, catheter-based revascularizations alone or in context with hybrid strategies consisting of combination of open surgical and endovascular revascularization procedures should also be considered. Thus, in experienced centers, treatment decisions are customized to the needs of individual patients while utilizing the individual or combined strength of endovascular intervention and open surgery. In patients with isolated aortoiliac disease and preferably type A lesions (corresponding to Pentecoast category 1 lesions, Table 12-23), catheter-based therapy is recommended. Table 12-25 provides an example of aortoiliac lesions based on morphology.

INDICATIONS FOR ILIAC INTERVENTIONS

Early classification of iliac artery lesions (Table 12-26) was provided by Pentecoast, et al. in 1994.[58] According to the 1999 TASC panel recommendations,[13] the detailed anatomy of the target iliac artery lesion was the most important indicator for the selection of revascularization strategy in individual patients. Type A lesions were considered primarily suitable for catheter-based treatments and type D lesions were considered primarily a surgical disease. Intermediary B and C types lesions, were open to individual decisions (Table 12-27). Although the TASC recommendations still provide a useful framework for decision making in experienced vascular centers, the treatment decisions are based on a comprehensive evaluation of individual patients including multiple aspects of the target vessel and target lesion anatomy. Available interventional and surgical expertise plays an important role in risk and benefit analysis and treatment decisions.

TABLE 12-25. Classification of Aortoiliac Lesions

Category 1

Short-segment stenosis of the infrarenal abdominal aorta (less than 2 cm) with minimal atherosclerotic disease of the aorta otherwise.

Category 2

Medium-length stenosis of the infrarenal abdominal aorta (2–4 cm) with mild atherosclerotic disease of the aorta otherwise

Category 3

(1) Long segment (>4 cm) stenosis of the infrarenal abdominal aorta; (2) aortic stenosis with atheroembolic disease (blue toe syndrome); or (3) medium-length stenosis of the infrarenal abdominal aorta (2–4 cm) with moderate to severe atherosclerosis of the aorta otherwise

Category 4

(1) Aortic occlusion or (2) aortic stenosis associated with an abdominal aortic aneurysm

Reproduced with permission from Pentecoast MJ, Criqui MH, Dorros G, et al. Guidelines for peripheral percutaneous transluminal angioplasty of the abdominal aorta and lower extremity vessels. A statement for health professionals from a Special Writing Group of the Councils on Cardiovascular Radiology, Arteriosclerosis, Cardio-thoracic and Vascular Surgery, Clinical Cardiology, and Epidemiology and Prevention, American Heart Association. *Circulation.* 1994;89:511–531.

TABLE 12-26. Classification of Iliac Lesions

Category 1

Stenosis is less than 3 cm in length and concentric and noncalcified.

Category 2

(1) Stenosis is 3–5 cm in length or (2) calcified or eccentric and less than 3 cm in length.

Category 3

(1) Stenosis is 5–10 cm in length or (2) occlusion is less than 5 cm in length after thrombolytic therapy with chronic symptoms.

Category 4

(1) Stenosis is greater than 10 cm in length, (2) occlusion is greater than 5 cm in length, after thrombolytic therapy and with chronic symptoms, (3) there is extensive bilateral aortoiliac atherosclerotic disease, or (4) the lesion is an iliac stenosis in a patient with abdominal aortic aneurysm or another lesion requiring aortic or iliac surgery.

Reproduced with permission from Pentecoast MJ, Criqui MH, Dorros G, et al. Guidelines for peripheral percutaneous transluminal angioplasty of the abdominal aorta and lower extremity vessels. A statement for health professionals from a Special Writing Group of the Councils on Cardiovascular Radiology, Arteriosclerosis, Cardio-thoracic and Vascular Surgery, Clinical Cardiology, and Epidemiology and Prevention, American Heart Association. *Circulation.* 1994;89:511–531.

TABLE 12-27. TransAtlantic Inter-Society Consensus (TASC) Classification of Aortoiliac Lesions

Type A	*Type B*	*Type C*	*Type D*
CIA or EIA stenosis <3 cm unilateral or bilateral	Single stenosis 3–10 cm long not extending into the CFA; Total of two stenosis <5 cm long in the CIA and/or EIA, not extending into the CFA; Unilateral CIA occlusion	Bilateral 5–10cm long stenosis of the CIA and/or EIA, not extending into the CFA; Unilateral EIA occlusion not extending into CFA; Unilateral EIA stenosis extending into CFA; Bilateral CIA occlusion	Diffuse multiple unilateral stenoses involving the CIA, EIA, and CFA— usually >10 cm; Unilateral occlusion involving both the CIA and EIA, bilateral EIA occlusions; Diffuse disease involving the aorta and both iliac arteries; Iliac stenoses in a patient with an abdominal aortic aneurysm or other lesion requiring aortic or iliac surgery

CIA, common iliac artery; EIA, external iliac artery; CFA, common femoral artery.
Modified from TransAtlantic Inter-Society Consensus (TASC). Management of peripheral arterial disease (PAD). *J Vasc Surg.* 2000;31(suppl):1–296.

INSTRUMENTATION

Aortoiliac interventions are performed using 6F to 7F systems, stiff or superstiff 0.035-in. mostly hydrophilic guidewires, and variably long up to 20-mm dilatation balloon catheters and balloon-expandable stents.

Iliac interventions are performed using 5F to 6F systems, stiff 0.035-in. mostly hydrophilic guidewires, and variably long, up to 10-mm diameter dilatation balloon catheters and mostly balloon-expandable stents. Guiding catheters are not required.

BASIC STRUCTURE OF AORTOILIAC AND ILIAC ARTERY INTERVENTIONS

All aortoiliac and iliac artery interventions are guided by DSA. Angiographic distribution and morphology of target lesions determine the access site, selection of instrumentation, and strategy of the intervention.

Initialization

Except for cases with chronic total unilateral occlusions of the iliac arteries, two access sites are required for aortoiliac interventions; bilateral femoral access or alternatively unilateral femoral and brachial access are typically selected. Even in unilateral treatments in the presence of patent iliac arteries, a second access is needed to ensure protection of the contralateral side. Following sheath placement, a pigtail catheter is placed into the distal abdominal aorta and baseline DSA angiograms are acquired to guide the intervention and to document the status of the runoff vessels.

For proximal uni- and bilateral common iliac artery lesions, two access sites are required to accommodate the kissing-balloon technique to reducing the risk of major plaque shifts and distal embolizations. For lesions that include the distal common iliac artery and uni- or bilateral external iliac lesions, single access designed for crossover access to the contralateral lesions or ipsilateral retrograde access is established. With the sheath in place with the tip just proximal to the target lesion, preinterventional DSA angiograms of the interventional site and the runoff vessels are acquired. Because the placement of the sheath frequently requires crossing of the target lesion by the guidewire, utmost care is needed to avoid dissection or vessel closure.

Main Interventional Cycle: Assess, Intervene, Repeat

The main interventional cycle begins with the introduction, crossing of the target lesion, and distal placement of the tip of the 0.035-in. guidewire. Aortoiliac and iliac artery stenoses are usually easier to pass from the caudocranial direction because the distance to the target lesion is shorter, allowing for better steering of the guidewire and greater push. In contrast, aortoiliac and iliac occlusions are often easier to recanalize by an antegrade approach from the contralateral side using a crossover maneuver or from the brachial access, both frequently in combination with the wire-loop technique.[74] In all aortoiliac and bilateral proximal common iliac and in most unilateral proximal common iliac artery interventions, simultaneous protection balloon and expandable-stent inflations using the kissing technique are employed to reduce the risk of proximal and distal complications (due to plaque shifts and embolizations). In aortoiliac lesions, unconditional bilateral stenting with reconstruction of the aortic bifurcation is required in nearly all cases. In iliac lesions, provisional stenting based on the results of the balloon dilatation is the preferred approach. Because of the typically downstream direction of dissections and consequently a greater risk of vessel closure, lesions with relevant postangioplasty dissections that were approached from the craniocaudal direction should be stented, regardless of the angiographic results. In patients with extensive diffuse disease and those with a large focal plaque burden, stenting is required in nearly all cases. Although conditional stenting appears the preferable strategy in a large number of patients, direct stenting might be considered in eccentric and moderately severe (50% to 75%) lesions; however, initial dilatation is suggested in moderately severe, heavily calcified lesions and in lesions with a large plaque burden to document their dilatability. In patients with stentlike results (residual stenosis <30%) following plain balloon angioplasty, stenting may be omitted. Intervention is terminated when the optimum angiographic result has been achieved and distal and systemic complications have been excluded.

Termination

The concluding steps of the aortoiliac or iliac artery intervention include retraction of the instrumentation and final angiograms documenting the interventional site and the runoff vessels, followed by sheath removal and hemostasis. Figures 12-15 to 12-17

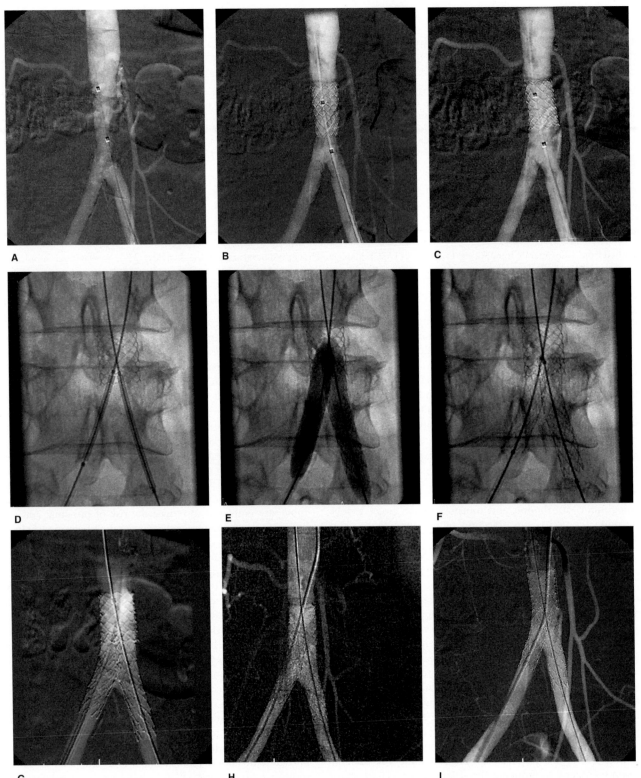

FIGURE 12-15. A 50-year-old woman presenting with a subacute occlusion of the left superficial femoral artery (not shown). Spontaneous aortic plaque dissection and aortic bifurcation reconstruction. **A:** Large semicircular plaque of the distal abdominal aorta with longitudinal spontaneous plaque rupture extending proximally up to the take-off of the inferior iliac artery and distally up to the take-off of the left common iliac artery, causing an embolic occlusion of the left superficial femoral artery (not shown). Stent delivery system in place before direct stenting. **B:** Direct stenting, balloon-expandable stent with shortening, following deployment and incomplete distal coverage of the aortic lesion. Semicircular horizontal plaque tear at the proximal stent end; plaque involves the inferior mesenteric artery. **C:** Distal postdilatation with an extensive dissection of the distal aorta involving the left common iliac artery. **D:** Stent positioning before deployment. Reconstruction of the aortic bifurcation using kissing stent implantation technique. The left and right stents both overlap the aortic stent by one and a half rings. **E:** Simultaneous inflation of both stent delivery systems. **F:** Bifurcation prosthesislike adaptation of both distal stents onto the aortic stent, native image. **G:** Angiographic control, demonstrating the patency of the reconstructed aortic bifurcation and proximal and distal stent adaptation. **H:** Final control in the "working" anterior-posterior projection, showing a satisfactory proximal aortic plaque coverage and excellent result of aortic bifurcation reconstruction with fully deployed stents. **I:** Right anterior oblique projection shows patent mesenteric inferior artery, full coverage of the dissection, and no additional plaque instability.

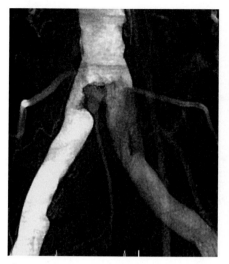
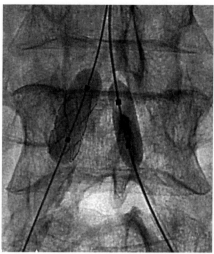
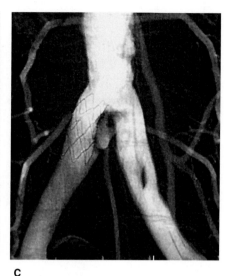

A   **B**   **C**

FIGURE 12-16. A 65-year-old man presenting with peripheral arterial disease, presenting with a right-sided intermittent claudication Fontaine IIb. Digital subtraction angiography (DSA) of the aortic bifurcation and partial bifurcation reconstruction. **A:** Complex aortic bifurcation lesions with a high-grade eccentric stenosis of the right proximal common iliac artery and clinically asymptomatic chronic plaque dissection involving the left common iliac artery. **B:** Kissing balloon inflation: a balloon-expandable stent delivery system on the right and a smaller protection balloon on the left for plaque shift and embolization prevention. **C:** Final result. Right excellent stent adaptation and complete coverage of the lesion; left unchanged baseline findings with a stable chronic dissection and excellent antegrade flow.

show representative examples of catheter-based aortoiliac revascularizations. Figure 12-18 to 12-20 demonstrate examples of iliac artery catheter-based interventions.

Aftercare and Follow-up

In the majority of patients, the sheaths are removed in the catheterization laboratory, and the access site is closed using a closure device. In patients with a heavily calcified access artery, local infections, thrombotic lesions, and other local complicating factors, the use of a closure device may be contraindicated and manual compression is suggested. Postinterventional care includes careful monitoring of the arterial access and of the dependent ipsilateral extremity, early mobilization, frequent blood pressure measurement, and up to 12 hours monitoring. Measurement of the ABI prior to discharge and duplex ultrasound studies at 3 and 6 months, with regular follow-up thereafter, are customary. Acetylsalicylic acid (100 to 300 mg per day) and usually statins and angiotensin-converting enzyme (ACE) inhibitors are important components of the patient's medication.

Complications

Procedural complications associated with the access site were reviewed earlier in this chapter. The use of smaller systems and a meticulous technique of arterial puncture and sheath placement radically reduce the incidence of local complications. The overall reported complications rates of stent-supported angioplasties range between 0% and 17% (average 7.6%), with 0% to 17% (average 3.1%) of these complications requiring surgery.[75] Other procedural complications include major dissections, perforations and ruptures, distal embolizations, and device-related misadventures. Procedure-related rupture of the aortoiliac axis is a rare complication, but one with potentially devastating

consequences. In one study, a 0.8% incidence of vessel rupture of iliac interventions was reported; the procedure-related risk factors included calcified vessels, total occlusions, oversizing, and recent endarterectomy.[76] Emergency treatment consists of proximal balloon tamponade, covered stent deployment, and reversal of anticoagulation. In the case of failure—which is mainly due to the inability to deliver or deploy the bulky covered stent across a dissecting closure or previously deployed stents—emergency surgical repair may be lifesaving. Symptomatic distal embolization may complicate up to 24% of iliac interventions,[77] with an average risk of about 4%[78] depending on case selection bias, skills of the operator, and other factors. Interventions for chronic total occlusions and primarily unstable lesions associated with spontaneous embolic events increase the risk. In distal embolizations associated with a retrograde approach to the lesion, access to the distal emboli may be difficult, and surgical endarterectomy might be required. However, in the majority of cases, percutaneous thrombectomy will suffice to restore the antegrade blood flow. Complete angiographic documentation of the final results is always required. Stent-related complications include stent migration, particularly in self-expandable stents, which is mainly due to undersizing or large differences in the vessel caliber within the stented segment, and, rarely, stent infection and secondary aneurysm formation. In cases of stent migration, percutaneous stent extraction is preferable; in some cases stent deployment in a nontarget location may be required. Incomplete coverage of the target lesion, malappositions, and edge dissections are usually easily correctable technical complications.

Long-term Patency

Reported calculated mean patency rates for iliac angioplasty were 81% at 2 years and 72% at 5 years.[79] Patency rates were higher in patients with angioplasties for claudication than for

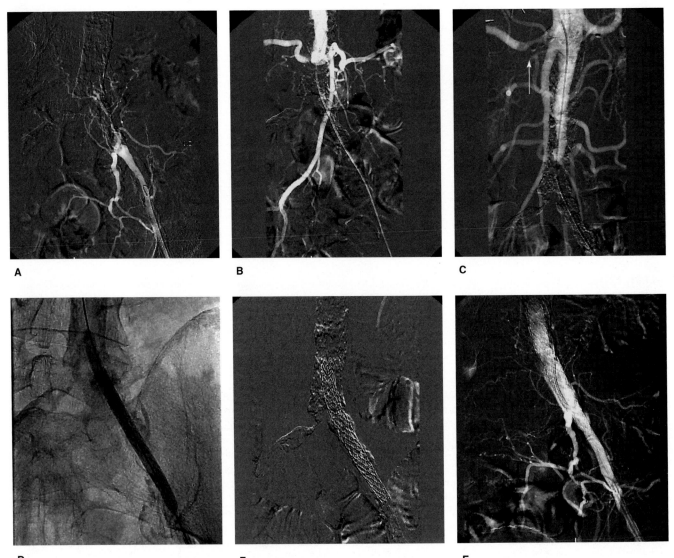

FIGURE 12-17. A 64-year-old multimorbid man presenting with an incomplete Leriche syndrome and bilateral intermittent claudication Fontaine IIb . Digital subtraction angiography (DSA) of the aortic bifurcation, complete distal aortic occlusion, and palliative, bifurcation recanalization. **A:** Complete chronic occlusion the distal abdominal aorta. Massive calcification and sclerosis of the distal abdominal aorta and both common iliac arteries, and the patent left external iliac artery, are shown. **B:** Following hydrophilic guidewire recanalization of the left common iliac artery and placement of a 4F diagnostic catheter into the distal abdominal aorta, angiography revealed a markedly narrowed distal aorta, patent up to the level of the take-off of the mesenteric inferior artery, and a distal pair of the lumbar arteries serving as collaterals. Intraluminal placement of the catheter is ascertained. **C:** An abdominal aortogram was acquired to document the integrity of the aortic wall, the width of the residual lumen of the aorta for sizing, and the extent of the collateral circulation via the lumbar and inferior mesenteric arteries. Angiographic documentation of the collateral vessels is important to prevent injury during intervention. Right renal artery stenosis was also documented (*arrow*). **D:** Placement of a long balloon dilatation catheter, sized to the nominal residual lumen with multiple successive dilatations. **E:** DSA without contrast agent shows three, overlapping, fully deployed stents with symmetrical strut apposition and preserved stent architecture. Absence of any local recoil hints at an excellent radial stability of the stent. **F:** Palliative recanalization and reconstruction of the left aortoiliac segment with normal runoff. Because of a high surgical risk due to major coexistent morbidities, revascularization of the right leg was subsequently performed using a femorofemoral crossover bypass (not shown).

limb salvage.[80] In stent-supported angioplasty, the reported patency rates at 1 year, 3 years, and 5 years were 78% to 95%, 53% to 88%, and 58% to 82%, respectively, with a weighted average not based on life-table analysis of 86%, 74%, and 73%. The corresponding secondary patency rate ranges were 86% to 98%, 81% to 94%, and 78% to 91%, respectively, with weighted averages of 92%, 87%, and 85% (for review, see reference 75). Trends toward lower patency rates were associated with recanalization of chronic total occlusions versus stenotic lesions, with patency rates being similar between common iliac artery and external iliac artery interventions, and between interventions for claudication and limb salvage.[81]

FEMOROPOPLITEAL INTERVENTIONS: CORONARY-LIKE APPROACH

Femoropopliteal atherosclerotic disease is rarely isolated; in most cases it is part of a multilevel disease.[68,82] The pathogenetic principle responsible for the marked vulnerability of

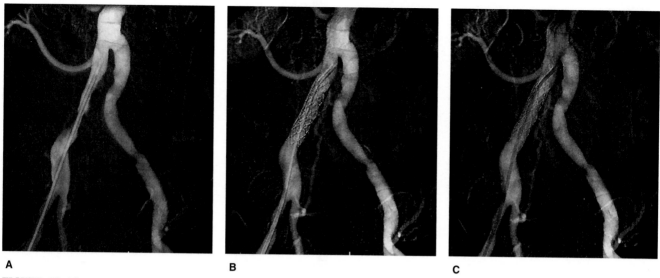

FIGURE 12-18. A 42-year-old man presenting with intermittent claudication Fontaine IIb of the right lower extremity. **A:** Digital subtraction angiography (DSA) revealed bilateral stenoses of the external iliac artery, complete occlusions of both internal iliac arteries, and a right accessory lower pole renal artery with a take-off from the right common iliac. **B:** Direct stenting of the right-sided lesion revealed an excellent anatomic and functional result. **C:** Oblique projection confirms excellent anatomic and functional result and an intact accessory lower pole renal artery.

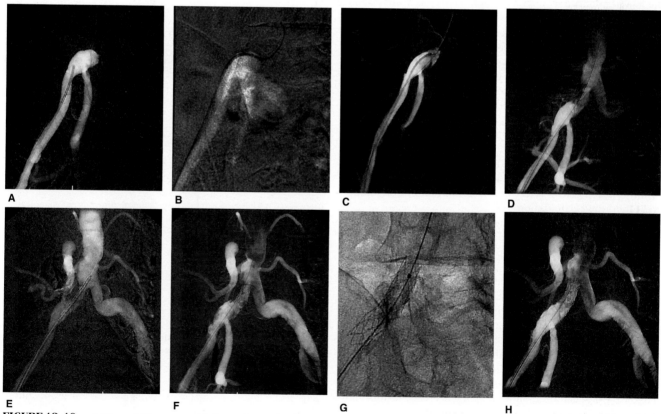

FIGURE 12-19. A 64-year-old woman with intermittent claudication Fontaine IIb of the right leg. **A:** Retrograde selective digital subtraction angiography (DSA) revealed a complete occlusion of the right common iliac artery. **B:** Because of the pouch formation and ectasia of the proximal external iliac artery, a retrograde guidewire recanalization attempt failed. **C:** Using a left transbrachial access and a long 0.035-in. hydrophilic guidewire, a common iliac occlusion was successfully recanalized in an antegrade fashion. **D:** Using the wire-loop technique, the brachial guidewire tip was extracted using the femoral access and exchanged for a femoral guidewire via a diagnostic catheter from the femoral access. Subsequently, predilatation was performed, revealing a major dissection. **E:** Balloon-expandable stent was placed across the lesion and positioned. **F:** Stent was deployed; angiography revealed a gross mismatch between the stent and the size of the poststenotic dilatation of the proximal external iliac artery segment and the distal part of the deployed stent. **G:** Using an oversized balloon distal stent, postdilatation was performed, allowing improved stent–vessel wall adaptation. **H:** Final control angiogram revealed fully reconstructed right common and external iliac anatomy. Poststenotic dilatation can be appreciated.

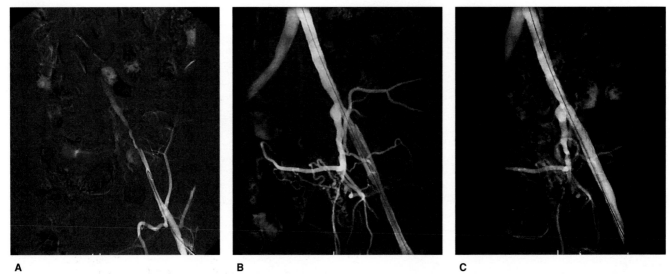

A   **B**   **C**

FIGURE 12-20.   A 51-year-old man with intermittent claudication Fontaine IIb of the left leg. **A:** Digital subtraction angiography (DSA) revealed a subtotal occlusion of the left external iliac artery. **B:** Following guidewire recanalization and balloon dilatation, a large subtotally occlusive spiral dissection was documented. **C:** Following provisional stenting and postdilatation, an excellent anatomic and functional result was documented.

the femoropopliteal segment for atherosclerosis remains poorly understood; a mechanically hostile environment (two flexing points, adductor canal, exposure to outside pressures and compressions), disturbed flow dynamics with leg exercise, but also low flow at rest are potential causes. Among the various topographic patterns of distribution the combination of femoropopliteal and infrapopliteal disease appears most typical in diabetic and nondiabetic patients (Fig. 12-21). Superficial femoral artery, SFA, obstructions located distal to the take-off of the profunda femoral artery and proximal to the distal reconstitution of the SFA via profunda collaterals may remain asymptomatic for an extended period of time, sometimes even for decades. In contrast, occlusions of the distal SFA involving the popliteal artery may result in rapidly developing and progressing claudication.

Two main indications for femoropopliteal interventions include claudication ≥Fontaine IIb and limb salvage. Prophylactic indications in asymptomatic patients with PAD and in patients without significant translesional pressure gradient despite augmentation with vasodilators have been considered contraindicated based on the ACC/AHA guidelines (class III, evidence level C).[1] Indications for revascularization in patients with claudication Fontaine IIa or atypical presentation and in patients with markedly accelerated disease are matters of debate. Particularly in these individuals, thorough benefit and risk analysis based on comprehensive, preinterventional evaluation including assessment of occupational needs and hazards, lifestyle, and level of physical activity along with all lesion-related factors and the available interventional expertise is required.

Indications for catheter-based versus surgical revascularization as opposed to the conservative PAD management are subject to evolving concepts concerning the optimum PAD management. As in the aortoiliac segment, treatment decisions are based on patient- and target vessel-related factors. In cases with comparable risk and benefit estimates for the interventional and surgical treatments, the least invasive strategy is selected.

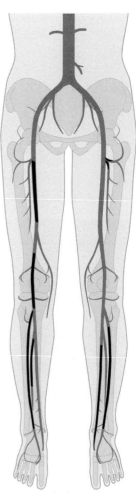

FIGURE 12-21.   Topography of peripheral arterial disease. Typical pattern of distribution of peripheral femoropopliteal and infrapopliteal disease. Redrawn from Haimovici H. Patterns of arteriosclerotic lesions of the lower extremity. *Arch Surg.* 1967;95:918–933.

Among the target lesion-related factors, the lesion's morphology requires particular consideration. Two available classifications of femoropopliteal lesions are given in Tables 12-28 and 12-29. According to the TASC recommendations,[13] type A lesions were recommended for catheter-based treatments and type D lesions for surgical revascularization. For the intermediary B lesions, catheter-based surgery and for the C lesions, surgery was preferred. In real-life clinical practice target lesion morphology is embedded in a broader context of complementary factors.

Femoropopliteal percutaneous transluminal angioplasty (PTA) has been associated with a high technical success (range: 82% to 96%), with acceptable primary patency rates at 1 year, 2 years, and 3 years ranging at 50% to 86%, 42% to 60% and 38% to 58%, respectively and acceptable overall complication rates (2.5% to 6.3%).[13] In a representative single center, long-term study patency rates at 1, 3, and 5 years were 81%, 61%, and 58%, respectively, with nearly a linear progression of reocclusion rates up to 10 years. Target lesion–related factors associated with reocclusion were long, eccentric lesions and suboptimal angiographic post-PTA results. Patient-related predictors of reocclusion included type II diabetes, diffuse atherosclerotic disease, and threatened

limb loss.[83] However, the length of the lesion and the presence of occlusions might not be such strong predictors of outcome as shown in the earlier data.[84,85]

Diffuse, eccentric, and calcified lesions, and lesions with high elastic recoil such as graft anastomoses have been considered potential candidates for stenting, in addition to bailout in threatened or actual vessel closure in failed angioplasty. However, initial experience with primary stenting was rather sobering. Although the reported technical success rates were high (range: 93% to 100%) the reported 1-year patency rates were not (range: 22% to 81%).[13] The disappointingly high rates of in-stent restenosis and stent failures of up to 80% in the femoropopliteal segment in some series[83,86] have resulted in controversies on indications and strategies.

Using the Palmaz stent (Johnson & Johnson Medical Devices, New Brunswick, NJ, USA), the 6-month patency rate at the >50% diameter level was 11% for the femoral and 20% for the popliteal arteries. The 4-year primary patency rate was 65% ±7.5% for the femoral and 50% ±17.7% for the popliteal arteries. In addition, the relationships between the type of the obstruction (stenosis vs. obstruction), length of the lesion, and number of stents, and patency were observed (Table 12-30).[87] A

TABLE 12-28. Classification of Femoropopliteal Lesions

Category 1

Single stenosis up to 5 cm in length that is not at the superficial femoral origin or distal portion of the popliteal artery, or (2) single occlusion up to 3 cm in length not involving the superficial femoral origin or distal portion of the popliteal artery.

Category 2

(1) Single stenosis 5 to 10 cm in length, not involving the distal popliteal artery, (2) single occlusion 3 to 10 cm in length, not involving the distal popliteal artery, (3) heavily calcified stenosis up to 5 cm, (4) multiple lesions, each less than 3 cm, either stenoses or occlusions, or (5) single or multiple lesions where there is no continuous tibial runoff to improve inflow for distal surgical bypass.

Category 3

(1) Single occlusion 3 to 10 cm in length, involving the distal popliteal artery, (2) multiple focal lesions, each 3 to 5 cm (may be heavily calcified), or (3) single lesion, either stenosis or occlusion, with a length of more than 10 cm.

Category 4

(1) Complete common and/or superficial femoral occlusions, (2) complete popliteal and proximal trifurcation occlusions, or (3) severe diffuse disease with multiple lesions and no intervening normal vascular segments.

Reproduced with permission from Pentecoast MJ, Criqui MH, Dorros G, et al. Guidelines for peripheral percutaneous transluminal angioplasty of the abdominal aorta and lower extremity vessels. A statement for health professionals from a Special Writing Group of the Councils on Cardiovascular Radiology, Arteriosclerosis, Cardio-thoracic and Vascular Surgery, Clinical Cardiology, and Epidemiology and Prevention, American Heart Association. *Circulation.* 1994;89:511–531.

TABLE 12-29. TransAtlantic Inter-Society Consensus (TASC) Classification of Femoropopliteal Lesions

Type A	*Type B*	*Type C*	*Type D*
Single stenosis<3 cm (unilateral/bilateral)	Single stenosis 3–10 cm in length not involving the distal popliteal artery; Heavily calcified stenosis <3 cm in length; Multiple lesions, each<3 cm in length (stenoses or occlusions); Single or multiple lesions in the absence of continuous tibial runoff to improve inflow for distal surgical bypass	Single stenosis or occlusion >5 cm; Multiple stenoses or occlusion, each 3–5 cm, with or without heavy calcification	Complete common femoral artery or superficial femoral artery occlusions or complete popliteal and proximal trifurcation occlusions.

Reproduced with permission from TransAtlantic Inter-Society Consensus (TASC). Management of peripheral arterial disease (PAD). *J Vasc Surg.* 2000;31(suppl):1–296.

TABLE 12-30. Dependence of Patency Rates on Type of Obstruction, Length of the Lesion and Number of Deployed Stents in Femoropopliteal Stent-Supported Percutaneous Transluminal Angioplasty (PTA)

Feature	Primary Patency (%)	Secondary Patency (%)
Stenoses	80	94
Occlusions	39	86
Lesions <3 cm	82	94
Lesions >3 cm	69	87
1 stent	82	93
>1 stent	70	91

Adapted from Henry M, Amor M, Ethevenot G, et al. Palmaz stent placement in iliac and femoropopliteal arteries: primary and secondary patency in 310 patients with 2–4 year follow-up. *Radiology.* 1995;197:167–174.

representative example of long-term results using a self-expandable nitinol stent (Intracoil stent, Sulzer IntraTherapeutics) in the femoropopliteal segment is provided in Table 12-31.[88] Data from more recent trials—including the Bilateral Lower Arterial Stenting Employing Reopro (BLASTER) and SCIROCCO II trials, which used the second-generation, self-expanding nitinol coil and nitinol mesh stents—suggest a better outcome compared with the results achieved with the earlier generations of stents (Figure 12-22).[89] Nevertheless, because of the higher costs and still uncertain benefits involved, the strategy of primary

stenting has not been recommended,[90] and it was considered contraindicated in recent ACC/AHA guidelines (class III, evidence level C).[1] In addition, the high incidence (25.4%) of minor, moderate, and severe strut fractures associated with longer stents and stent overlaps, and worse clinical outcome (higher rates of restenosis and reocclusion) (Figure 12-23) recently reported from a registry study of three different self-expanding stents deployed in the SFA and the first popliteal segment[91] supports the current recommendations for use of stents in femoropopliteal segment restricted to conditional bailout situations (ACC/AHA class IIa, evidence level C).[1]

Attempts to improve the results and to reduce the incidence of restenosis following femoropopliteal interventions have included the use of conventional stents, covered stents, brachytherapy, and, most recently, drug-eluting stents. The use of conventional stent did not convincingly reduced the restenosis rates in all studies,[13] making the prognostic indication for stenting in the femoropopliteal an unlikely proposition. The use of covered stents (endografts) showed some promising results (cumulative primary and secondary patency rates at 12 months 73% and 83%, even when long lesions were treated)[92] and some less favorable results (cumulative primary and secondary patency rates at 12 months of 58% and 73%).[93] Although endografts do seem to reduce restenosis rates compared with plain balloon angioplasty, their clinical relevance remains uncertain.[94] Primary brachytherapy appears to reduce the cumulative angiographic restenosis at 6 and 12 months,[95] yet it is not widely available. Initial experience with drug-eluting stent devices suggested reduction in restenosis rates compared

TABLE 12-31. Three-year Primary and Secondary Patency Rates Using the Nitinol Intracoil Stent

Location	Primary Patency Rate (%)	Secondary Patency Rate (%)
All lesions	62.1	72.4
Stenoses	69.6	79.8
Occlusions	49	60.4
Common femoral artery	87.9	93.3
Superficial femoral artery, proximal third	48.4	60.9
Superficial femoral artery, middle third	59.9	72.7
Superficial femoral artery, distal third	65.5	74.1
Lesions ≥4 cm	79.9	86.1
Stenoses	84.4	94.5
Occlusions	59.2	55.4
Lesions ≤8 cm	66.4	76.9
Stenoses	69.8	80.6
Occlusions	55.7	67.2
Lesions >8 cm	36.4	48
Stenoses	66.7	66.7
Occlusions	31	45.8
Popliteal artery, all lesions	66.1	78.6
Popliteal artery, stenoses	67.3	78.4
Popliteal artery, occlusions	62.5	81.8

Adapted from Henry M, Henry I, Klonaris C, et al. Percutaneous endovascular treatment of femoropopliteal occlusive disease. In: Heuser RR, Henry M, eds. *Textbook of Peripheral Vascular Interventions.* London: MD Martin Dunitz, 2004:243–262.

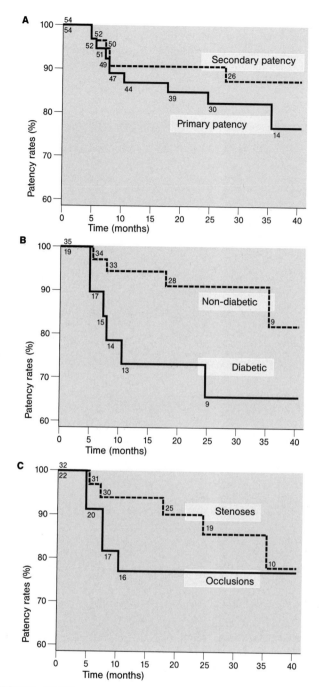

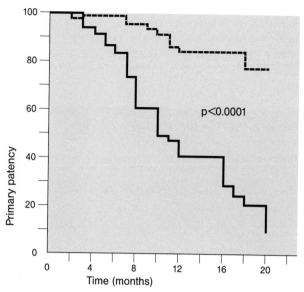

FIGURE 12-23.   Primary stent patency rates for fractured and non-fractured stents. *Dotted line*, no stent fracture; *solid line*, stent fracture. Adapted from Scheinert D, Scheinert S, Sax J, et al. Prevalence and clinical impact of stent fractures after femoropopliteal stenting. *J Am Coll Cardiol.* 2005;45:312–315.

FIGURE 12-22.   Outcome of femoropopliteal stent-supported angioplasty. Life-table analyses according to the Kaplan-Meier method. **A:** Analysis shows patency rates for 54 arteries (superficial femoral and popliteal arteries) in which stents were placed. *Solid line*, primary patency; *dotted line*, secondary patency. Numbers indicate extremities at risk. **B:** Analysis shows patency rates for diabetic patients (*solid line*) and nondiabetic patients (*dotted line*). Numbers indicate extremities at risk. The difference between patency rates over time was borderline significant (*P* = 0.08). **C:** Analysis shows patency rates for treated stenoses (*dotted line*) and treated occlusions (*solid line*). Numbers indicate extremities at risk. The difference between patency rates over time was not statistically significant (*P* = 0.70). Redrawn from Lugmayer HF, Holzer H, Kastner M, et al. Treatment of complex arteriosclerotic lesions with nitinol stents in the superficial femoral and popliteal arteries: a midterm follow-up. *Radiology.* 2002;222:37–43.

with plain balloon angioplasty,[96] results still to be confirmed by other trials such as the ongoing Zilver Nitinol Stent Trial.

In summary, based on the available incomplete evidence, the present suggested indications for stenting in femoropopliteal disease include a bailout situation of threatened or actual vessel closure, and conditional stenting in cases with suboptimal angiographic results after plain balloon angioplasty. Preferably, the new generation nitinol stents should be used in these cases. To define the role of stent-supported angioplasty in femoropopliteal interventions, more data are needed to document long-term clinical and angiographic outcome. In contrast to applications of drug-eluting stents in treatment of coronary artery disease, antiproliferative stents alone may not decisively improve the outcome in patients with PAD. Combination with a greater mechanical stability of stents preserving their integrity, not only in straight vascular segments but also across the inquinal and popliteal flexing points and articulations, might be required. In the future, bioabsorbable stents possibly combined with antiproliferative drug elution might consolidate the clinical role of stenting in femoropopliteal disease.

STRATEGY OF INTERVENTION

Adaptation to the coronary-like approach has markedly facilitated femoropopliteal interventions. In principle, the access to the target lesion can be established from the contralateral common femoral artery using the cross-over technique, ipsilateral common femoral artery using the antegrade approach, or less frequently brachial or popliteal artery using the retrograde approach. Sheaths, guidewires, and catheters are employed using the coaxial telescopic principle and technique. Typically, following the sheath placement over a 0.035-in. guidewire with the tip just proximal (in popliteal access just distal) to the target lesion, direct access to the interventional site is established and from then on coronary instrumentation based on 0.014-in. technology is implemented. In general, craniocaudal crossover access to the target lesion appears to be associated with a reduced risk of ipsilateral local and distal vascular complications while providing safer access to peripheral sites in case of complications.

Placement of the tip of the sheath close to the target region compensates, at least in part, for the longer distance from the access site. The principle of the coaxial telescopic technique employed in a crossover approach to the contralateral distal SFA lesion is shown in Figure 12-24.

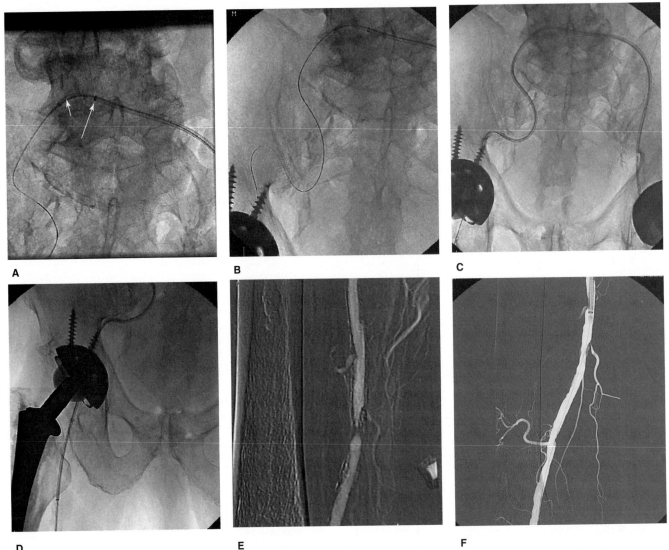

A   **B**   **C**

D   **E**   **F**

FIGURE 12-24.   Crossover approach and co-axial telescopic technique. **A:** Coaxial system consisting of a 0.035-in., stiff hydrophilic guidewire, preformed (pigtail, shepherd's crook, sidewinder) diagnostic catheter, and long introductory sheath (mostly 5F to 6F; Arrow, Arrow International, Reading, PA, USA) is assembled. Diagnostic catheter is advanced via the 0.035-in. guidewire up to the aortic bifurcation, and the tip is directed to face the ostium of the contralateral iliac artery. Subsequently, the 0.035-in. guidewire is passed downstream, followed by the diagnostic catheter. The image shows the 0.035-in. guidewire in the common femoral artery; diagnostic catheter has just passed the aortic bifurcation (*small arrow*) with the tip of the sheath just below the bifurcation still on the ipsilateral side (*large arrow*). **B:** To improve the tracking support, the 0.035-in. stiff guidewire has been advanced further downstream into the superficial femoral artery. The tips of the diagnostic catheter and of the sheath retained the same position; the more upward and horizontal orientation of the sheath is indicative of the failed attempt to advance the sheath across the aortic bifurcation, requiring more distal placement of the guidewire. **C:** With the 0.035-in. guidewire securely placed, and the diagnostic catheter positioned on the contralateral side, successive alternating advancement of the diagnostic catheter and the sheath allows the adverse anatomy (elongation, tortuosity, plaques) to be overcome in small steps. The tip of the diagnostic catheter is hidden behind the structure of the artificial right hip; the tip of the sheath is ready to move beyond a distal external iliac elongation. **D:** To prepare for an intervention, the tip of the sheath is positioned in the proximity of the target lesion without limiting the antegrade blood flow. In preparation for the ensuing superficial femoral artery (SFA) intervention, the tip of the introductory sheath has been positioned in the proximal SFA, in this case beyond the level of the profunda femoris take-off. For infrapopliteal interventions, the tip of the sheath is advanced even more distally; to improve the distal steerability and support, a guiding catheter may be introduced into the sheath and positioned as close as possible to the target lesion. With this arrangement, 0.014-in. guidewires and low-profile coronary dilatation balloon catheters may replace the 0.035-in. guidewire-based system. **E:** Subtotal occlusion of the distal SFA and spontaneous spiral retrograde dissection are shown. **F:** To improve distal control, the tip of the introductory sheath was advanced distally closer to the lesion, and a coronary system was used for dilatation. A 0.014-in. guidewire was placed downstream the target lesion, and a satisfactory postdilatation result and distal placement of the tip of the sheath are shown.

INSTRUMENTATION

For femoropopliteal interventions, usually 5F to 6F (range 4F to 7F) systems are employed. For the crossover maneuver, either a long sheath (≥45 cm) or coronary guiding catheter (usually Judkins right 4), with high flexibility and optimum radial stability are employed in conjunction with a curved diagnostic catheter (e.g., sidewinder).

The 0.035-in. hydrophilic guidewires with a shapeable, floppy tip, and stiff shaft are employed to accomplish the maneuver and to reach the interventional site, whereas 0.014-in. coronary guidewires with shapeable hydrophilic tip and stiff shaft are used to perform the intervention.

Dilatation balloon catheters with rapid-exchange design are preferred; however, the limited selection available (up to 5 mm and 40 mm length) necessitates the use of standard peripheral dilatation balloon catheters (up to 7 mm and 100 mm length), mostly OTW design.

For stenting in bailout situations, one of the current generation of self-expandable 4- to 7-mm-diameter nitinol stents is most frequently employed. Balloon-expandable stents are contraindicated in stenting vessels across articulations.

BASIC STRUCTURE OF FEMOROPOPLITEAL INTERVENTIONS

As in other vascular beds, femoropopliteal interventions consist of initialization, main interventional cycle, and termination.

Initialization

On the basis of a review of the diagnostic MR, CT, or x-ray angiograms of the interventional site and the inflow and runoff vessels, the site of the access and the size of the system are determined. In chronic total SFA occlusions, alternative techniques such as peripheral excimer laser angioplasty (PELA)[97] and percutaneous intentional extraluminal revascularization (PIER)[98] should be considered. Using these techniques, high primary procedural success rates, even in long chronic total SFA occlusions (85%),[99] and high limb salvage success rates (66%)[100] have been reported. When the arterial access has been established, preinterventional angiograms of the interventional site and the runoff vessels are acquired; images defining the target lesion best are stored on the monitor to guide the intervention.

Main Interventional Cycle: Assess, Intervene, Repeat

With the tip of the sheath or the guiding catheter at close range to the target lesion, the tip of the 0.014-in. or 0.035-in. hydrophilic guidewire is advanced, and steered across the lesion. After crossing the target lesion, the tip of the guidewire is parked in the popliteal artery, and control angiography is performed to confirm the safe placement of the guidewire within the lumen of the target vessel. The guidewire tip should not pass distal to part II of the popliteal artery to avoid distal injury. Then, a dilatation balloon catheter matching the nominal size of the target vessel is selected, placed across the lesion, and inflated. Following deflation and withdrawal of the dilatation catheter, a control angiogram is acquired. On the basis of the results, the next interventional cycle is resumed or the intervention is terminated. In patients with threatened closure or suboptimal results of plain balloon angioplasty, self-expandable nitinol stents are typically sized to the nominal size of the target vessel, or they are slightly oversized (up to 10%). The stent length is selected to fully cover the lesion accounting for the axial shortening. If a stent was used, high-resolution angiograms should document the full stent apposition and exclude any edge defects. Afterdilatations are frequently required to improve the vessel strut adaptation.

In patients with chronic total occlusions of the SFA, the PIER technique of recanalization may be employed. Using this technique, a steerable guidewire is advanced to engage the proximal cap of the occlusion; then an angled 5F diagnostic catheter is advanced to the level of the proximal end of the occlusion and firmly seated at the site of the cap penetration. Subsequently, using the road-map image for guidance, the guidewire tip is allowed to form a proximal loop and successively advanced and steered to reach the proximal end of the distally reconstituted vessel. The point of re-entry into the vessel lumen and intraluminal guidewire placement is documented in two angiographic projections. Once the intraluminal guidewire placement has been confirmed, a small-diameter dilatation balloon catheter is advanced and inflated to open up a new channel successively enlarged by consecutive upsizing dilatations.

Termination

Technical success is achieved and intervention can usually be terminated when residual stenosis of <30% following plain balloon angioplasty and of <20% following stenting has been achieved. In addition, optimum runoff should be present for long-term procedural benefit. The termination criteria may be modified in patients undergoing palliative interventions (improvement of collateral circulation) as opposed to curative interventions (reconstitution of the vascular anatomy). Retraction of the instrumentation should be performed carefully using fluoroscopy guidance to avoid damage to the target lesion or deployed stent. Figures 12-25 to 12-32 provide representative examples of femoropopliteal interventions.

Aftercare and Follow-up

In most patients, the sheath is removed and the access site is closed using a closure device in the catheterization laboratory. Postprocedural monitoring depends on the outcome of the intervention and the status of the access site. In uncomplicated cases and retrograde arterial puncture, immediate mobilization and 2 to 4 hours of postprocedural monitoring are required. If antegrade transfemoral access is used, particularly in combination with a potent antithrombotic pharmacotherapy (e.g., GP IIb/IIIa receptor inhibitors), gradual mobilization and extended postprocedural monitoring for a minimum of 12 hours is recommended. Prior to discharge, the ABI should be measured. Duplex ultrasound studies of the interventional site and the downstream circulation are scheduled at 3 and 6 months; thereafter, regular follow-up is customary. Acetylsalicylic acid (100 to 300 mg per day) and usually statins and ACE inhibitors are important components of the patient's medication.

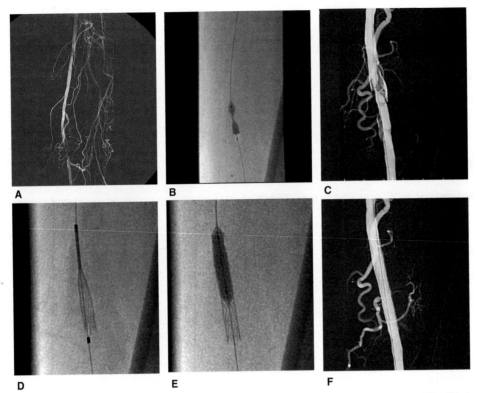

FIGURE 12-25.   A 62-year-old woman with Fontaine IIb claudication. Diagnostic angiography revealed a subtotal occlusion of the left distal superficial femoral artery. **A:** Subtotal, chronic, richly collateralized occlusion of the left distal superficial femoral artery in the preinterventional angiogram. **B:** Demarcation of the target lesion marked by the incomplete expansion of the dilatation balloon at nominal pressure. High pressure was required to fully open the lesion. **C:** Postdilatation severe spiral dissection with vessel-wall instability at higher magnification. **D:** Partial deployment of a self-expanding nitinol stent. **E:** Postdilatation was required because of the partial stent collapse in the proximal segment. **F:** Final result.

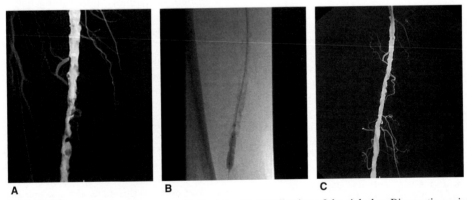

FIGURE 12-26.   A 60-year-old woman with Fontaine IIb claudication of the right leg. Diagnostic angiography revealed diffuse heavily calcified stenosis of the distal superficial femoral artery. **A:** Massively calcified plaques in the distal superficial femoral artery documented by preinterventional angiography. **B:** Multiple overlapping dilatations with a nominal-size balloon to avoid dissections. **C:** Final result with focal plaque recoils, excellent runoff.

Complications

Typical procedural complications include unintentional subintimal guidewire passage with extensive dissections, extraluminal angioplasty due to extravasation of the guidewire, guidewire perforation of the runoff vessel, and distal thromboembolization. Although occasionally technically demanding, the majority of complications can be treated percutaneously by combination of fibrinolysis and dilatation; in rare cases, particularly in patients with one last remaining infrapopliteal vessel and a threatened limb, surgery might be required. Complications of the access site in femoropopliteal interventions have been reviewed in the literature (Table 12-32).[101]

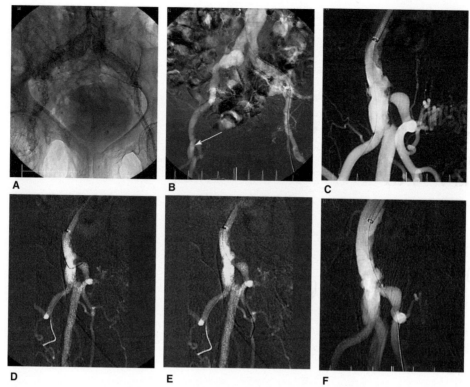

FIGURE 12-27. An 85-year-old woman with bilateral peripheral artery disease and residual pain in the right leg and preceding bilateral iliac artery interventions. Palliative revascularization. **A:** Native film of the pelvis shows heavy diffuse calcifications of both common and external iliac arteries. Diagnostic catheter is placed in the left external iliac artery. **B:** Digital subtraction angiography (DSA) in the left anterior oblique projection shows high-grade diffuse atherosclerosis of both elongated, tortuous, and partially ectatic common and external iliac arteries. Stent-corrected stenoses of the left middle external iliac and right proximal and right distal external iliac artery are poorly visualized. In the presence of chronic total occlusion of the right superficial femoral artery, the culprit lesion documented by angiography was a high-grade ostial lesion of the right profunda femoris artery (*arrow*). Because of coexistent morbidities, poor vascular status, and age, the patient was not considered a candidate for surgery. Extremely difficult vascular anatomy represented a difficult anatomic substrate for the crossover technique. **C:** Appropriate material selection and careful use of the telescopic technique (Fig. 12-24) overcome the hostile vascular status allowing, atraumatic stent passage, and sufficient maneuverability at the site of intervention. Following a successful crossover maneuver, the culprit lesion of the first profunda branch is shown. For better support and profunda protection, the guidewire was placed into the second profunda branch. **D:** Exploration of the ostial lesion of the first profunda branch with a second guidewire. **E:** Successful passage of the second guidewire downstream of the target artery. **F:** View of the interventional site demonstrating an acceptable palliative result following multiple upsizing balloon inflations.

Long-term Patency

The long-term patency of the femoropopliteal segment is significantly lower than in aortoiliac disease. Using plain balloon angioplasty, patency rates of 69.8%/50.3% and 62.4%/43.1% were reported for the femoropopliteal lesions at 1 and 3 years (for review, see reference 101). Using nitinol stent-supported angioplasty for the femoropopliteal lesions, a 3-year primary patency rate of 62.1% and secondary patency rate of 72.4% were reported.[88]

INFRAPOPLITEAL INTERVENTIONS

Infrapopliteal distribution of PAD is more frequent in patients with type II diabetes and diabetic vasculopathy[102] and in patients with an advanced multilevel PAD.[68] Distal to the trifurcation, the anterior tibial artery is most frequently involved, followed by the posterior tibial and the peroneal arteries. Depending on the degree of collateralization, segmental occlusions of one, two, and even all three infrapopliteal arteries may remain asymptomatic for an extended period of time until the symptoms of foot claudication appear. Thus, foot claudication is nearly always associated with severe diabetic macro- and microangiopathy or extensive multilevel disease. In the majority of patients with CLI or lifestyle-limiting claudication, a single popliteal vessel with a de novo lesion is documented on angiography, or multiple stenoses or occlusions in all three infrapopliteal vessels with rich but decompensating collateralization are present. Patients presenting with infrapopliteal disease are usually older and sicker than patients with more proximal PAD. In addition, infrapopliteal disease is usually multifocal or diffuse, frequently involving all three vessels to a variable degree. Table 12-33 provides an example of infrapopliteal lesion classification.

Although the technical feasibility and acceptable clinical utility of infrapopliteal angioplasty were documented early on[103–107] and performed by accomplished interventional radiologists, even today infrapopliteal interventions remain challenging procedures in real-life settings. However, the coronary-like approach to infrapopliteal interventions and consequent revascularizations of inflow vessels have improved clinical outcome in experienced centers. Thus, in patients with CLI, primary angiographic success rates of 84% and 61%, respectively, were reported for stenoses and occlusions, corresponding to a

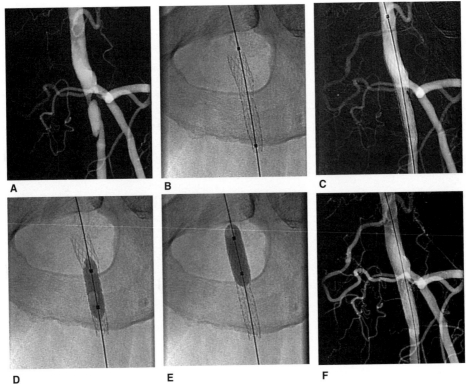

FIGURE 12-28. A 57-year-old man presenting with an acute onset Fontaine IIb claudication in the left leg. Diagnostic angiography revealed a high-grade ostial stenosis of the left superficial femoral artery. **A:** Preinterventional angiogram confirmed a complex high-grade ostial stenosis of the left superficial femoral artery (SFA). **B:** Predilatation resulted in threatened closure (not shown) requiring stent placement. A nitinol self-expandable stent was deployed. **C:** Control angiography showed suboptimal stent deployment and poor vessel wall adaptation. **D:** Postdilatation to improve distal stent–vessel wall adaptation with a dilatation balloon sized to the nominal size of the SFA plus 10%. **E:** Postdilatation to improve distal stent–vessel wall adaptation with a dilatation balloon sized to the nominal size of the common femoral artery plus 10%. **F:** Final result with excellent morphologic stent–vessel wall adaptation. No plaque shift into the profunda femoral artery.

primary clinical success rate of 63% and respective restenosis rates of 32% and 52% at 10 months. At 18-month follow-up, primary and secondary patency rates were 48% and 56%, with a cumulative limb salvage of 80% reported (Fig. 12-33).[108] In another study of patients with infrapopliteal interventions for CLI, the primary technical success rate was 98% for stenoses and 73% for occlusions, and at 5-year follow-up, the rate for limb salvage was 91%.[109] The status of the inflow vessel and the need for proximal revascularization, periprocedural complication rates, and 5-year clinical outcome data of this important study are provided in Tables 12-34 to 12-36. In the first study, which included 32% claudicants in addition to 68% patients with CLI, the primary technical success rate of stent and GP IIb/IIIa receptor inhibitor–supported infrapopliteal angioplasty was 94%; improved clinical status was reported in 45% of patients with CLI and in 37% of patients with lifestyle-limiting claudication at 1-year follow-up.[110] Despite this encouraging report, the long-term outcome of infrapopliteal stenting remains guarded and further studies are needed to confirm these results in larger populations. Because of the less impressive clinical results in advanced PAD and potentially more grave consequences from complications, including threatened limb loss, infrapopliteal interventions are usually considered only in patients with CLI and threat of amputation. More recently, in highly experienced centers, the interventional therapy has also

been offered to patients with severe lifestyle-limiting claudication. The high prevalence of critical limb ischemia, complex anatomy frequently associated with multilevel PAD, and coexistent morbidities markedly increase the risk in a large number of patients considered for infrapopliteal interventions. Therefore, in all patients the risks associated with the procedure must be carefully weighed against the potential short-term (e.g., healing of an ulcer) and long-term (e.g., relief of rest pain, better ambulation) benefits.

In patients considered for infrapopliteal interventions, realistic targets should be identified, and the most promising and the least traumatic approach should be selected. Selection of interventional targets is based primarily on the status of the anatomic substrate. Thus, morphology of the target lesions and the status of the inflow, outflow, and collateral vessels determining the outlook for successful opening of new vascular channels are weighed against the risks of damaging the existing frequently elaborate and complex blood supply of the lower extremity. Experienced interventionsts plan the procedures by integrating angiographic findings with the clinical picture, always accounting for the available interventional expertise. Infrapopliteal interventions by novice interventionists are contraindicated.

In selected patients with indeterminate angiographic findings, *explorative interventions* might be required. These interventions

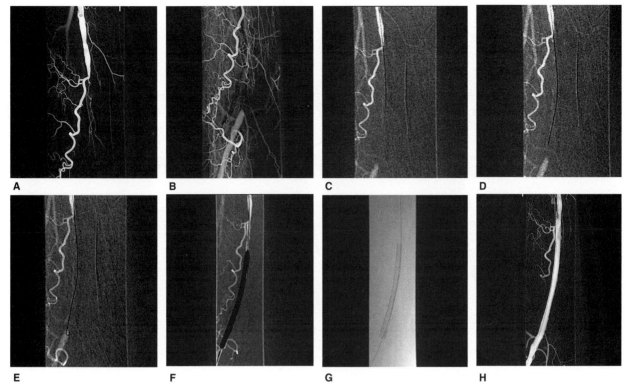

FIGURE 12-29. A 52-year-old man with Fontaine IIb claudication of the right calf. Diagnostic angiography revealed a long chronic total occlusion of the right superficial femoral artery. Intervention was performed via antegrade ipsilateral access using a 5F sheath and peripheral excimer laser angioplasty (PELA). **A:** Chronic total occlusion (CTO) of the proximal superficial femoral artery (SFA). Single collateral vessel from the distal SFA stump. **B:** Distal SFA reconstitution via collaterals. **C:** Stepwise PELA recanalization using a road-map guidance, proximal segment. **D:** Stepwise PELA recanalization using a road-map guidance, distal segment. **E:** Complete CTO recanalization; guidewire tip reaches the reconstituted lumen of the SFA. **F:** Passage of a long balloon catheter and dilatation. **G:** Nitinol self-expanding stent implantation due to recoil and vessel wall instability following PELA and balloon dilatation. **H:** Final result after stent deployment.

serve to identify suitable targets by careful guidewire exploration of the critical vascular sites. Because of attending risks, explorative infrapopliteal interventions are reserved for expert interventionists familiar with the delicate divide between reasonable last-resort attempts and heroic harmful actions.

In highly selected patients with chronic critical limb ischemia and segmental occlusions of all three infrapopliteal vessels, palliative last-resort reconstruction via collaterals might be considered. However, in these cases, worsening of the already tenuous blood supply of the lower leg may lead to irreversible injuries and consecutive limb loss. Therefore, the interventionist must be keenly aware of the delicate status of the lower leg circulation and the need to avoid harm. The clinical value of angiogenic growth factors[111] in the treatment of distal PAD remains at present uncertain (for review, see reference 112) and should be reserved for placebo-controlled trials (ACC/AHA recommendation class IIb, level of evidence C).[1]

STRATEGY OF INTERVENTION

The strategy of infrapopliteal interventions depends on the functional and anatomic morphology of the target vascular bed and patient-related factors. Functionally, the most critical and technically the most approachable lesions are identified and addressed.

Depending on patient's size, contralateral retrograde or ipsilateral antegrade common femoral artery access is selected. Selection of small size systems allowing lower limb perfusion throughout the procedure, gentle meticulous deliberate and atraumatic technique, and short procedural times are the best means to prevent complications.

INSTRUMENTATION

The majority of infrapopliteal interventions is performed using a 4F to 5F introductory sheath, or rarely, a 6F sheath; 0.035-in. guidewires are used to place the sheath and 0.014-in. floppy or intermediated tip coronary guidewires and 2.5- to 3.5-mm-diameter rapid-exchange or OTW coronary dilatation balloon catheters are employed for interventions. The use of stents should be avoided; if needed, nitinol self-expandable stents, or less frequently chromium/cobalt stents sized to the nominal size of the target segment, are used.

BASIC STRUCTURE OF INFRAPOPLITEAL INTERVENTIONS: CORONARY-LIKE APPROACH

Approach to infrapopliteal interventions is similar to that of femoropopliteal interventions consisting of initialization, main interventional cycle, and termination. Optimal anticoagulation

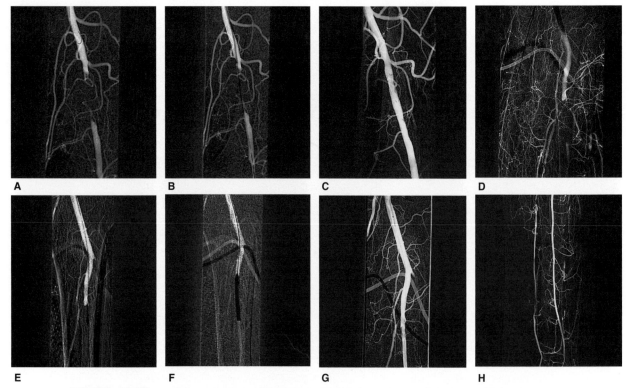

FIGURE 12-30. A 74-year-old man with accelerated Fontaine IIb claudication of the left lower leg. Diagnostic angiography revealed a 4-cm-long chronic total occlusion (CTO) of the distal superficial femoral artery (SFA), and segmental occlusions of both tibial arteries. **A:** Preinterventional angiogram. CTO of the distal SFA, likely appositional thrombotic, recanalization guidewire in place. **B:** Successful guidewire recanalization. **C:** Angiogram following deployment of a nitinol self-expandable stent. **D:** Runoff angiogram reveals complete embolic occlusion of the left trifurcation. **E:** Because diagnostic angiography identified the fibular artery to be the main supplier of the left foot, the guidewire was passed down this vessel and mechanical thrombectomy using the X-sizer catheter (EndiCOR Medical Inc., San Clemente, CA, USA) was resumed. **F:** Postdilatation following thrombectomy. **G:** Final result documenting complete recanalization of the fibular artery, proximal segment. **H:** Distal fibular artery is patent and provides collaterals to the distal tibial posterior artery, securing the blood supply to the foot. Segmental filling of the anterior tibial artery is also shown.

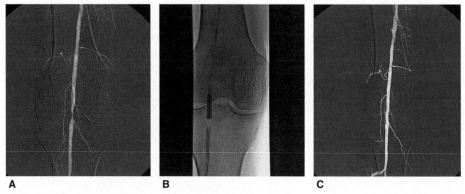

FIGURE 12-31. A 71-year-old woman with Fontaine IIb claudication of the right leg. Diagnostic angiography revealed a subtotal occlusion of the right popliteal artery, part II. Contralateral femoral access, 5F, crossover and telescopic technique. **A:** Preinterventional angiography revealed subtotal occlusion of the right popliteal artery, part II. **B:** Coronary, 0.014-in., floppy tip, stiff-shaft, hydrophilic guidewire crossed the lesion and a rapid-exchange, low-profile, coronary dilatation balloon was inflated. **C:** Final result with excellent morphologic result, prompt runoff. No stent was used.

using preferably 5000 U intravenous bolus of unfractionated heparin into the target artery, maintenance of antegrade blood flow and lower limb perfusion throughout the procedure, and meticulous technique are the best means to avoid complications.

Employing the contralateral access, the crossover maneuver using the coaxial telescopic technique, or less frequently the ipsilateral access using the antegrade approach, the tip of the sheath or the guiding catheter is brought into the close proximity of the

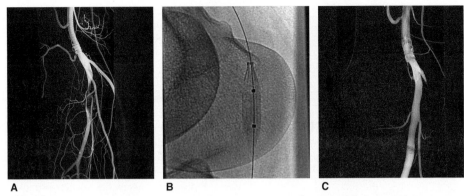

FIGURE 12-32. A 37-year-old man with sudden-onset Fontaine IIb claudication of the right lower leg. Diagnostic angiography showed spontaneous dissection and subtotal occlusion of the popliteal artery, part II, likely secondary to adventitial cyst. **A:** Preinterventional angiogram confirmed the diagnosis. Subtotal occlusion of the second popliteal segment secondary to dissections or adventitial cyst. **B:** Peripheral cutting balloon angioplasty following immediate recoil after conventional plain balloon dilatation. **C:** Final result with complete revascularization. Use of stent was avoided.

target lesion, usually part I or II popliteal artery, allowing a close-range access to the target site and optimal steering of the coronary instrumentation.

In patients with a significant inflow disease all proximal lesions are addressed first (ACC/AHA recommendation class I, evidence level C).[1] It is critical during this initiating stage to minimize the risk of distal embolizations by avoiding excessive

TABLE 12-32. Ranges of Complication Rates and (Not Weighted) Average in Percent (%) of the Access Site Reported in the Literature for Femoropopliteal Interventions

Hematoma—hemorrhage	0.8–8.6 (3.0)
Thrombosis	0.6–3.8 (2.0)
Embolization	0.8–10.0 (2.9)
Pseudoaneurysm	0.4–1.5 (0.9)
Arteriovenous fistula	0.5–1.5 (0.9)

Reproduced with permission from Murray RR Jr., Lutz JD. Femoropopliteal angioplasty and stents: patient selection and results. In Perler BA, Becker GJ, eds. *Vascular intervention: A Clinical Approach.* New York: Thieme Medical Publishers, 1998:169–176.

manipulations and the risk of distal dissection by strict control of the guidewire tip. In addressing the infrapopliteal lesions, high-quality road-map images acquired from a securely immobilized limb and firm control of the guidewire tip reinforced by the tip of the dilatation catheter at close range (1 to 2 cm) allow smooth probing advancement of the straight or looped guidewire tip across the target lesion or stepwise recanalization of the occluded segment. The use of stents should be avoided whenever possible; therefore prolonged dilatations to "tack on" intimal flaps, and in presence of adequate runoff, residual stenoses ≤50% diameter represent acceptable results. However, in cases with major dissections and threatened closure use of stents may represent the only available bail-out option (ACC/AHA class IIa, evidence level C recommendation).[1] To avoid proximal injury and distal embolizations following the revascularization, the coaxial telescopic system should be carefully retracted under fluoroscopy guidance over a guidewire. To avoid prolonged proximal compression of the target artery, liberal use of closure devices should be encouraged. GP IIb/IIIa receptor inhibitors might prove a beneficial adjunct to mechanical interventions, yet before their routine use in infrapopliteal procedures can be recommended, greater experience, preferably

TABLE 12-33. Classification of Infrapopliteal Lesions

Category 1

Single focal stenosis, 1 cm or less, of tibial or peroneal vessels.

Category 2

(1) Multiple focal stenoses, each 1 cm or less, of tibial or peroneal vessels, (2) one or two focal stenoses, 1 cm or less, of tibial trifurcation, or (3) tibial or peroneal stenosis dilated in combination with femoral popliteal bypass.

Category 3

(1) Moderate-length stenosis (1–4 cm) or moderate-length (1–2 cm) occlusion of tibial or peroneal vessel or (2) extensive stenosis of tibial trifurcation.

Category 4

(1) Tibial or peroneal occlusions longer than 2 cm or (2) diffusely diseased tibial or peroneal vessels.

Reproduced with permission from Pentecoast MJ, Criqui MH, Dorros G, et al. Guidelines for peripheral percutaneous transluminal angioplasty of the abdominal aorta and lower extremity vessels. A statement for health professionals from a Special Writing Group of the Councils on Cardiovascular Radiology, Arteriosclerosis, Cardio-thoracic and Vascular Surgery, Clinical Cardiology, and Epidemiology and Prevention, American Heart Association. *Circulation.* 1994;89:511–531.

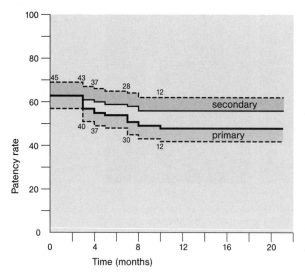

FIGURE 12-33. Results of survival analysis (Kaplan-Meier method) of the primary and secondary clinical patency rates for the 72 treated limbs. Initial failures are included. *Solid lines,* estimated patency rate; *dotted lines,* estimated patency rate plus or minus standard error. Numbers indicate number of cases remaining under evaluation as a function of time since angioplasty. Redrawn from Söder HK, Manninen HI, Jaakkola P, et al. Prospective trial of infrapopliteal artery balloon angioplasty for critical limb ischemia: Angiographic and clinical results. *J Vasc Intervent Radiol.* 2000;11:1021–1031.

in prospectively controlled studies, is required. Figures 12-34 and 12-35 show examples of infrapopliteal interventions using the coronary-like approach.

COMPLICATIONS, AFTERCARE, AND FOLLOW-UP

Complications include distal spasms that usually resolve on retraction of the instrumentation. Guidewire dissections and perforation should be relieved by prolonged dilatations rather than by stenting. Distal embolizations and local thrombosis are accessible to mechanical percutaneous thrombus extraction, usually using aspiration thrombectomy.

Following successful infrapopliteal interventions, angiographic documentation followed by sheath removal and hemostasis, preferably using a closure device are performed. In uncomplicated procedures, early mobilization and up to 12 hours of monitoring is recommended. Prior to discharge, the ipsilateral extremity is examined and the ABI measured. Duplex examinations are typically scheduled at 3 and 6 months, with further follow-up based on the status of the disease and the patient's clinical symptoms. Basic medication typically includes an antiplatelet agent, usually acetylsalicylic acid statins, ACE inhibitors, and, if needed, medication to control diabetes, and—less frequently—anticoagulants. Intensive follow-up in all patients is the key requirement to ensure beneficial long-term outcome.

TABLE 12-34.   Incidence of Inflow Lesions Dilated or Opened before Tibioperoneal Vessel Angioplasty (TPVA)

	CLI Group	*Class III Patients*	*Class IV Patients*
Inflow lesions dilated to allow access to infrapopliteal (TPV) lesions, *n* (%)			
Iliofemoral	11/11 (100)	11/11 (100)	4/4 (100)
SFA—popliteal	322/322 (100)	201/201 (100)	121/121 (100)
TPV (ipsilateral)	486/529 (92)	294/317 (93)	192/212 (91)
Patients, *n* (%) (No iliofemoral or SFA lesions dilated before TPV-PTA, limbs = 115)			
Iliofemoral	0	0	0
SFA—popliteal	0	0	0
TPV	136/152 (89)	77/84 (92)	59/68 (87)
Iliofemoral lesions, no SFA lesions (limbs = 2)			
Iliofemoral	2/2 (100)	2/2 (100)	0
SFA—popliteal	0	0	0
TPV	2/2 (100)	2/2 (100)	0
No iliofemoral lesions and only SFA popliteal lesions (limbs = 154)			
Iliofemoral	0	0	0
SFA—popliteal	308/308 (100)	192/192 (100)	116/116 (100)
TPV	335/362 (93)	206/222 (93)	129/140 (92)
Iliofemoral lesions and SFA popliteal lesions (limbs = 13)			
Iliofemoral	13/13 (100)	9/9 (100)	4/4 (100)
SFA-popliteal	14/14 (100)	9/9 (100)	5/5 (100)
TPV	13/13 (100)	9/9 (100)	4/4 (100)

PTA, percutaneous transluminal angioplasty; CLI, critical limb ischemia; Class III and IV, based on Fontaine classification; iliofemoral, common iliac, external iliac, and common femoral arteries; SFA, superficial femoral and popliteal arteries; and TPV (ipsilateral), tibioperoneal vessels on the same side (ipsilateral) as the iliofemoral or SFA—popliteal lesions

Reproduced with permission from Dorros G, Jaff MR, Dorros AM, et al. Tibioperonal (outflow lesion) angioplasty can be used as primary treatment in 235 patients with critical limb ischemia: Five-year follow-up. *Circulation.* 2001;104:2057–2062.

TABLE 12-35. Significant Procedural Complications

Significant Complications, n (%)	CLI	Class III	Class IV
In-hospital deaths	2 (0.7)	0	2 (1.7)
Procedurally related	1 (0.4)	0	1 (0.8)
Emergency vascular surgery	3 (1)	2 (1)	1 (0.8)
Arterial access repair	2 (0.7)	2 (1)	—
Bypass	0	—	—
Amputation	1 (0.4)[*]	—	1 (0.8)
Major infection	1 (0.4)	1 (1)	—
Compartment syndrome	1 (0.4)	—	1 (0.8)
Acute renal failure	20 (7.0)	5 (3)	15 (13)
Transfusion	1 (0.4)	1 (1)	—

CLI, critical limb ischemia, Class III and IV, based on Fontaine classification; amputation followed failed popliteal-tibial graft.

Reproduced with permission from Dorros G, Jaff MR, Dorros AM, et al. Tibioperonal (outflow lesion) angioplasty can be used as primary treatment in 235 patients with critical limb ischemia: Five-year follow-up. *Circulation.* 2001;104:2057–2062.

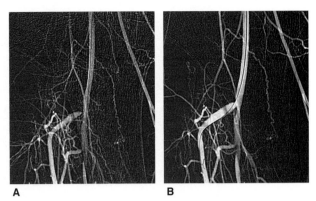

FIGURE 12-34. A 59-year-old patient with Fontaine IIb claudication of the right lower leg. Diagnostic angiography revealed a subtotal ostial occlusion of the right anterior tibial artery and high-grade proximal superficial femoral artery stenosis. Contralateral femoral access, 5F, crossover and telescopic technique. **A:** Preinterventional angiogram confirmed a high-grade filiform stenosis of the ostium of the right anterior tibial artery. **B:** Final result following coronary 0.014-in. guidewire crossing of the lesion and dilatation using a low-profile, coronary dilatation balloon with rapid-exchange design.

TABLE 12-36. Tibioperoneal Vessel Angioplasty: 5-year Clinical Follow-up

	All Patients	Class III	Class IV	P
Patients, n (%)	215	128 (60%)	87 (40%)	—
Limbs, n (%)	266	160 (60%)	106 (40%)	—
Age, years	67 ± 9 (37–86)	68 ± 8 (46–83)	67 ± 10 (37–86)	NS
Mean follow-up, months	34 ± 33	39 ± 34	30 ± 30	NS
Adverse events, n (%)				
Bypass	21 (8)	4 (3)	17 (16)	<0.05
AKA	5 (2)	1 (1)	4 (4)	<0.05
BKA	18 (7)	5 (3)	13 (12)	<0.05
Transmetatarsal	23 (9)	1 (<1)	22 (21)	<0.05
Survival, %				
1 year	90	94	75	<0.05
2 years	86	89	60	<0.05
3 years	78	79	41	<0.05
4 years	63	69	37	<0.05
5 years	56	58	33	<0.05
Event-free survival	31	43	26	<0.05

Class III and IV, based on Fontaine classification; *Bypass* indicates femoropopliteal or popliteal-tibial; AKA, above-knee amputation; BKA, below-knee amputation; and transmetatarsal, transmetatarsal amputation.

AKA, BKA, transmetatarsal: percentages refer to limbs, not patients

Reproduced with permission from Dorros G, Jaff MR, Dorros AM, et al. Tibioperonal (outflow lesion) angioplasty can be used as primary treatment in 235 patients with critical limb ischemia: Five-year follow-up. *Circulation.* 2001;104:2057–2062.

BYPASS GRAFT INTERVENTIONS

The surgical grafts for PAD are conduits employed to bypass obstructed native arterial segments providing the blood flow to the distal arteries of the ischemic limb. Vascular grafts can be classified on the basis of the anatomic or extra-anatomic location of the proximal and distal anastomosis or the graft material. Anatomic peripheral bypasses span any segmental level between the abdominal aorta and crural arteries. Extra-anatomic peripheral bypasses span the axillo-femoral and femoro-femoral vascular beds. Typical graft materials include autogenous vein grafts and less frequently arterial conduits (patient's own tissue),

harvested allografts (same species), or xenografts (different species), and synthetic grafts made usually from Dacron or expanded polytetrafluoroethylene (ePTFE). Typical complications of peripheral vascular grafts include occlusions, and less frequently formation of aneurysms at the anastomotic sites, distal embolizations, infections, and inflammatory erosions into adjacent structures, including fistula formation. Complication rates depend on technical factors, anatomical location, graft material, and skills of the operator.

The term "failing graft" designates a state of diminished function of a patent graft due to an impaired inflow, poor runoff secondary to progression of the native disease, or graft-associated

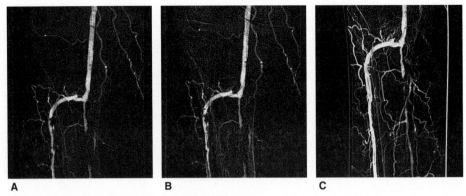

FIGURE 12-35. An 82-year-old woman with Fontaine III peripheral arterial disease of the right leg. Diagnostic angiography showed a single infrapopliteal vessel with proximal occlusion of the posterior tibial and peroneal arteries. Contralateral femoral access, 5F, crossover and telescopic technique. **A:** Anterior tibial artery with proximal diffuse disease and two highly eccentric focal stenoses. **B:** Crossing the lesions with a coronary 0.014-in., floppy-tip guidewire and low-profile, long coronary dilatation balloon of rapid-exchange design spanning both lesions. **C:** Final angiogram post dilatation shows excellent anatomic and functional result. Use of a stent was avoided.

problems; "failed" graft designates a complete graft occlusion.[13] The leading cause of graft failure is short-term graft thrombosis (i.e., within 30 days of surgery). In the majority of cases, graft thrombosis is associated with technical problems such as anastomosis defects, kinking, external compression, and incomplete valve lysis. Other causes include possible misjudged indications (poor target vessel, poor inflow or runoff, or irreversible peripheral tissue damage) and rarely hypercoagulable states and infections. Midterm graft failure (within 12 to 18 months) in autogenous vein grafts is usually due to myointimal proliferation and late defects due to suture dehiscence and the formation of aneurysms. Long-term graft failure (>18 months) is mostly due to progression of the native disease and graft material fatigue. Reported primary and secondary patency rates for infrainguinal bypass grafts range greatly, depending on the selection of patients, the location of the distal anastomosis, the selection of bypass materials, surgical techniques, and other factors (for review, see reference 113). Prevention of short-term graft failure includes immaculate graft preparation and expert surgical technique; prevention of mid- and long-term graft failure includes consequent graft surveillance (detection of failing grafts) and antiplatelet and antiatherosclerotic therapy.[13] The importance of failing graft detection and management is emphasized by the better outcome compared with the treatments of failed grafts. ACC/AHA recommendations regarding the surveillance of specific peripheral grafts based on evidence and interdisciplinary consensus are now available.[1]

In patients with documented failing grafts, therapy options include reoperation[113] or endovascular treatment (for review, see reference 114).

In patients presenting with acute or protracted bypass failure, the initial treatment depends on the symptoms and findings. In the majority of cases, peripheral x-ray angiography is indicated to define the anatomical substrate precisely. Depending on the findings, initial treatment may include surgical embolectomy, thrombectomy, bypass revision or replacement, and—in patients with reperfusion injury—fasciotomy[115] or endovascular therapy including fibrinolysis, mechanical thrombectomy, and plain or stent-supported angioplasty.[114] Limited evidence seems to suggest that balloon angioplasty may be most beneficial in patients with short lesions and graft occlusion within 3 months. Table 12-37 reviews the standard classification of graft lesions. Experience with stenting of the graft lesions is too limited to provide evidence-based guidance. In patients presenting with

TABLE 12-37. Classification of Bypass Graft Lesions

Category 1
Focal stenosis of the distal anastomosis of a femoral popliteal or femoral-tibial vein bypass.

Category 2
(1) Focal stenosis of the proximal anastomosis of a saphenous vein femoral-popliteal or femoral-tibial bypass, (2) short-segment (up to 3 cm) stenosis occurring within vein bypasses, (3) stenosis associated with aortobifemoral or aortobiiliac bypasses, or (4) stenosis associated with prosthetic extra-anatomic bypasses.

Category 3
Moderate-length stenosis (more than 3 cm) of venous bypass grafts.

Category 4
(1) Long-segment stenosis (more than 10 cm) in vein bypass grafts or (2) stenosis associated with anastomotic aneurysms.

Reproduced with permission from Pentecoast MJ, Criqui MH, Dorros G, et al. Guidelines for peripheral percutaneous transluminal angioplasty of the abdominal aorta and lower extremity vessels. A statement for health professionals from a Special Writing Group of the Councils on Cardiovascular Radiology, Arteriosclerosis, Cardio-thoracic and Vascular Surgery, Clinical Cardiology, and Epidemiology and Prevention, American Heart Association. *Circulation.* 1994;89:511–531.

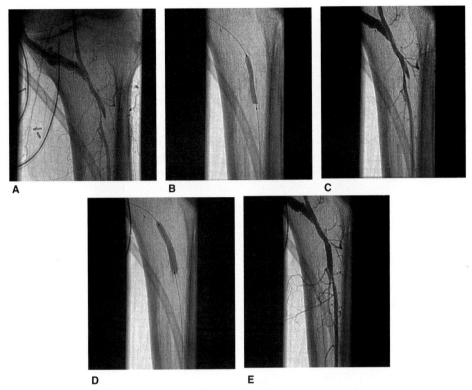

FIGURE 12-36. An 80-year-old man with bilateral peripheral arterial disease and right femoropopliteal (part III) bypass using a distal anastomosis venous graft. **A:** Immediate postbypass angiography revealed subtotally occlusive dissection of the fibular artery (last remaining vessel) distal to distal popliteal part III anastomosis. **B:** Crossing of the dissection with a 0.014-in. coronary guidewire and dilatation using a low-profile coronary dilatation balloon in an attempt to tack on the dissection. **C:** Recoil. **D:** Postdilatation following placement of a self-expandable nitinol stent. **E:** Final result with complete coverage of the dissection. Spasm distal to the stent.

early graft failure, surgical revision is usually required. In patients presenting early after occlusion of older grafts, initial fibrinolysis might be a useful first step, unless it is contraindicated or surgery for limb salvage is imminent, to improve definition of the site and to determine the strategy of definite revascularization. If endovascular repair has been selected, plain balloon angioplasty and the restrictive use of stents are employed. The techniques of graft lesion revascularization must take into account the differences in graft size and diameter of the native vessels, access to the target lesion, and differences in plaque structure according to the age of the lesion and degree of graft degeneration. Patients with chronic graft occlusions are referred for surgical revision following angiographic definition of the target vascular site. Aneurysms of the anastomosis may be treated by stent reconstruction and exclusion. Concurrent treatment of the inflow and outflow vessels is important to improve the long-term outcome. Figure 12-36 shows an example of an emergency postbypass intervention that was unresponsive to plain balloon angioplasty and required stent placement.

EMERGENCY AND URGENT INTERVENTIONS ON LOWER EXTREMITY ARTERIES

Emergency and urgent interventions in patients with PAD are performed in patients with ALI and CLI. ALI interventions usually account for <10% of all peripheral interventions in tertiary

vascular centers. Patients with ALI present with a broad spectrum of symptoms ranging from life-threatening hemodynamic compromise to poorly defined peripheral symptoms.

Although CLI represents a distinct pathogenetic entity, the clinical presentation may be similar. While CLI management usually does not represent an emergency, it certainly does represent medical urgency. Efficacious ALI and CLI management requires the availability of experienced interdisciplinary vascular teams and established clinical pathways.

ACUTE LIMB ISCHEMIA

In a vast majority of patients, ALI is caused by occlusive embolization or sudden occlusive thrombosis. Less frequently spontaneous dissections, vascular injury, or inflammatory changes are involved. Peripheral embolization is related to cardiac or proximal arterial diseases, including atrial fibrillation associated with left atrial thrombus formation, myocardial infarction, or dysfunction associated with left ventricular thrombus; patent foramen ovale associated with deep leg vein or systemic vein thrombosis; and proximal artery or aortic atherothrombosis.

The clinical presentation of ALI depends mainly on the anatomic location of vessel occlusion, the presence of preformed collaterals, and the ischemic tolerance of the dependent musculature. In general, the severity of presenting symptoms increases with more proximal sites and a lesser degree of pre-existent PAD. By contrast, in patients with advanced PAD and pre-existent collaterals, the clinical symptoms tend to be less severe. In addition, the severity of hemodynamic compromise is usually greater in more proximal occlusions, whereas the severity of local ischemic syndromes tends to be greater in more distal occlusions.

In patients admitted with suspected ALI the immediate history, vital sign assessment, and physical examination should determine the degree of the systemic hemodynamic compromise and severity of lower extremity ischemia, viability, reversibility of ischemic damage, and the risk of ischemia/reperfusion injury (Table 12-6). Subsequently, to confirm the diagnosis and to determine the anatomic level and, if possible, the nature of the occlusion and the status of the inflow, outflow, and collateral vessels, emergency angiography should be performed. In patients without life- or limb-threatening symptoms, noninvasive vascular imaging studies may be considered.

Once the anatomic substrate has been defined the treatment decision depends on clinical presentation in individual patients. Primary surgical revision is usually reserved for cases with immediate life- or limb-threatening symptoms that require immediate reperfusion; in all other cases, explorative endovascular intervention from the contralateral side or from another alternative access should be considered.

Based on ACC/AHA recommendations, catheter-based thrombolysis is indicated for patients presenting with ALI (Rutherford categories I and IIa) of <14 days' duration (class I, evidence level A). Furthermore, thrombolysis or thrombectomy may be considered for patients with ALI (Rutherford category IIb) of >14 days' duration (class IIb, evidence level B).[1]

In clinical practice, the endovascular approach typically includes atraumatic exploration of the culprit lesion with a 0.035-in. (aortoiliac vessels) or 0.0.14-in. (infrainguinal vessels) guidewire ("guidewire traversal test")[116] to estimate the probability of success of fibrinolyis; successful guidewire passage of the occlusion suggests fresh thrombus and increases the probability of successful fibrinolysis. Then, in absence of contraindications (Table 12-38), in most cases regional, selective intra-arterial thrombolysis using any of the established methods (Table 12-39), mostly employing urokinase, and less frequently employing other fibrinolytics with the exception of streptokinase (Table 12-40),[117] should be performed to uncover the culprit lesion and, if possible, to achieve revascularization. Standards for the conduct and documentation of peripheral fibrinolyis have been established and are given in Tables 12-41 and 12-42.[32,118] In patients with contraindications for thrombolysis, mechanical thrombectomy should be considered.[32]

In patients in whom revascularization was incomplete following fibrinolysis, depending on the severity of the uncovered residual stenosis, the status of the target vessel or graft, and the patient's symptoms, same-day or staged surgical or catheter-based mechanical revascularization should be performed. In patients with adequately restored antegrade flow and a morphologically

TABLE 12-38. Contraindications for Fibrinolysis in Patients with Acute Limb Ischemia

Absolute Contraindications	Relative Contraindications
Active clinically significant bleeding; Intracranial hemorrhage; Presence or development of compartment syndrome	Cardiopulmonary resuscitation within past 10 days; Major nonvascular surgery or trauma within past 10 days; Uncontrolled hypertension: >180 mm Hg systolic or >110 mm Hg diastolic blood pressure; Puncture of noncompressible vessel; Intracranial tumor; Recent eye surgery; Neurosurgery (intracranial, spinal) within past 3 months; Intracranial trauma within 3 months; Recent gastrointestinal bleeding (<10 days); Established cerebrovascular event (including transient ischemic attacks within past 2 months); Recent internal or noncompressible hemorrhage; Hepatic failure, particularly in cases with coagulopathy; Bacterial endocarditis; Pregnancy and immediate postpartum status; Diabetic hemorrhagic retinopathy; Life expectancy <1 year.

Reproduced with permission from Thrombolysis in the management of lower limb peripheral arterial occlusion—a consensus document. Working party on Thrombolysis in the Management of Limb Ischemia. *Am J Cardiol.* 1998;81:207–218.

TABLE 12-39. Strategies of Intra-arterial Pharmacological Thrombolysis for Acute Limb Ischemia

Intrathrombus infusion

In intrathrombus infusion, the thrombolytic agent is delivered by an intra-arterial catheter embedded within the thrombus. This position maximizes the concentration of the drug within the thrombus and delivers the drug to the region of thrombus-bound plasminogen.

Intrathrombus "bolusing" or "lacing"

The term "bolusing" has been used interchangeably with "lacing." These terms refer to the initial intrathrombic delivery of a concentrated thrombolytic agent with a view toward saturating the thrombus with the plasminogen activator before infusion. During this portion of the procedure, a catheter (with an end hole or multiple side orifices with or without a tip-occluding wire) is positioned in the most distal part of the thrombus. It is retracted proximally as the thrombolytic agent is delivered along the entire length of the thrombus.

Stepwise infusion

Stepwise infusion entails placing the tip of the catheter within the proximal thrombus and infusing a fixed dose of thrombolytic agent over a short period of time. As thrombus dissolves, the catheter is advanced.

Continuous infusion

Continuous infusion is infusion of thrombolytic agent at a constant rate (i.e., steady flow).

Graded infusion

Graded infusion entails periodic tapering of the infusion rates, with the highest doses given within the first few hours.

Forced periodic infusion

Forced periodic infusion (i.e., pulse-spray) entails forcefully injecting the thrombolytic agent into the thrombus to fragment it and increase the surface area available for thrombolytic action.

Reproduced with permission from Thrombolysis in the management of lower limb peripheral arterial occlusion—a consensus document. Working party on Thrombolysis in the Management of Limb Ischemia. *Am J Cardiol.* 1998;81:207–218.

TABLE 12-40. Dosage Regimen of Thrombolytic Agents for the Treatment of Acute Limb Ischemia

Agent	*Regimen*
STEPWISE INFUSION:	
SK	1000–3000 IU every 2, 3, 5–15 min
UK	3000–4000 IU every 3–5 min
CONTINUOUS INFUSION:	
SK	5000 IU/hr (rarely with initial loading dose of 20,000 or 40,000 IU over 20 min)
	10,000 IU/hr
UK	
Low-dose technique	Variable schemes up to 100,000 IU/hr (occasionally with variable loading dose)
High-dose technique	Mainly graded infusion (see below)
rtPA	0.25, 0.5, 1, or 2.5 mg/hr
	0.5 mg/hr
	0.5, 1, 3, or 10 mg/hr
	3, 5, or 10 mg/hr
	10 mg/hr (max. 30 mg)
	0.025 or 0.05 mg/kg per hour
	0.05 mg/kg per hour
	0.05 or 0.1 mg/kg per hour
GRADED INFUSION:	
UK	4000 IU/min up to anterograde flow
	1000 IU/min up to complete lysis
Modifications	4000 IU/min up to anterograde flow
	1000 to 2000 IU/min to complete lysis
	4000 IU/min for 2 hr
	2000 IU/min for next 2 hr
	1000 IU/min for remainder
	250,000 IU followed by 4000 IU/min for 4 hr and 2000 IU/min up to 36 hr
	4000 IU/min for 4 hr
	2000 IU/min for up to 48 hr
INTRATHROMBUS BOLUSING OR LACING	
UK	120,000 to 250,000 IU lacing dose
	60,000 IU lacing dose followed by McNamara's scheme
	250,000 IU lacing dose followed by 50,000 IU/hr
rtPA	3 × 5 mg (5–10 min interval) followed by 0.05 mg/kg per hour
	0.33 mg/mL 0.2 mL every 15 sec for 15 min, every 30 sec thereafter
FORCED PERIODIC (PULSE SPRAY) INFUSION	
UK	25,000 IU/mL
	0.2 mL every 30 sec for 20 min, every 60 sec thereafter
	20,000 IU/cm occlusion length (microhole balloon catheter)
	25,000 IU/10 cm thrombus followed by graded infusion
rtPA	0.5 mg/mL
	0.2 mL every 30 sec for 20 min, every 60 sec thereafter
	0.5 to 1 mg/cm occlusion length (microhole balloon catheter)
INTRAOPERATIVE THROMBOLYSIS	
SK	50,000 to 150,000 IU slow bolus or infusion over 30 min
UK	250,000 to 500,000 IU bolus in distal outflow vessel
	1000 to 2000 IU/min into distal thrombus
	250,000 IU over 30 min (with inflow occluded)
	375,000 IU over 30 min (with inflow occluded)
rtPA	3 × 5 mg bolus over 30 min

SK, streptokinase; UK, human-derived urokinase,; rtPA, recombinant tissue plasminogen activator.

Reproduced with permission from Patel N, Sacks D, Patel RI, et al. SIR reporting standards for the treatment of acute limb ischemia with the use of transluminal removal of arterial thrombus. *J Vasc Intervent Radiol.* 2003; (suppl):S453–S465.

TABLE 12-41. Recommended Scale to Judge the Clinical Success of Thrombolysis

Score	Description
−1	Ischemia is worse (by at least one major or minor category from SVS/ISCVS Clinical Categories of Acute Limb Ischemia)
0	No change (failure)
+1	Ischemia improved
	(a) Revascularization with thrombolytic methods alone
	(1) Amputation necessary but at a lesser level[a]
	(b) Adjunctive surgical revascularization necessary but at a lesser level°
	(1) Amputation necessary but at a lesser level[a]
	(c) Adjunctive endovascular revascularization necessary (e.g., angioplasty, stent, atherectomy)
	(1) Amputation necessary but at a lesser level[a]

Overall clinical success

Overall clinical success is defined as relief of the acute ischemic symptoms and return of the patient to at least his/her preocclusive clinical baseline level after the removal of thrombus and performance of adjunctive procedures (threshold, 75%).

Technical success

Technical success is defined as restoration of antegrade flow with complete or at least 95% thrombolysis of the thrombus or embolus (threshold, 70%).

Note. Categories a, b, c do not imply greater or lesser degrees of success.

[a]Levels of amputation: 1, above the knee; 2, below the knee; 3, transmetatarsal; and 4, toe.

°Levels of surgical revascularization: 1, Major: insertion of new bypass graft, replacement of an existing bypass graft, or excision or repair of an aneurysm. 2, Moderate: graft revision, patch angioplasty, endarterectomy, or profundaplasty. 3, Minor: thrombectomy/embolectomy or fasciotomy. SVS/ISCVS Society of Vascular Surgery/International Society of Cardiovascular Surgery

Reproduced with permission from McNamara TO, Fischer JR. Thrombolysis of peripheral arterial and graft occlusions: improved results using high-dose urokinase. *AJR Am J Roentgenol.* 1985;144:769–775, and Wolfe JHN, Porter JM. Basic treatment for critical limb ischemia. *J Vasc Srug.* 2000;31:Al.

TABLE 12-42. Complication Rates and Suggested Thresholds of Major and Minor Complication of Fibrinolysis

Specific Major Complications for Thrombolysis of Acute Limb Ischemia	*Reported Rate (%)*	*Suggested Threshold (%)*
PHARMACOLOGIC		
Intracranial hemorrhage	0–2.5	2
Major bleeding requiring transfusion and/or surgery	1–20	10
Compartment syndrome	1–10	4[a]
Distal embolization not corrected with thrombolysis	1–5	5
MECHANICAL		
Distal embolization (mechanical thrombectomy/ aspiration)	1.8	2

[a]Determined based on the weight of the majority of studies presented in the evidence table, excluding a single study in which the observed complication rate was 9.8%.

Reproduced with permission from McNamara TO, Fischer JR. Thrombolysis of peripheral arterial and graft occlusions: improved results using high-dose urokinase. *AJR Am J Roentgenol.* 1985;144:769–775, and Wolfe JHN, Porter JM. Basic treatment for critical limb ischemia. *J Vasc Surg.* 2000;31:A1.

stable-looking target lesion who were selected for angioplasty, a staged procedure is usually preferred to avoid fibrinolysis-induced thrombotic complications. The strategy of the intervention follows the identical principles applicable to elective procedures. Immediate postprocedural management includes intensive monitoring of the patient and the limb, including the assessment of ischemia-reperfusion injury with special attention to the signs of developing acute compartment syndrome in intensive care settings.

CHRONIC CRITICAL LIMB ISCHEMIA AND LIMB SALVAGE

Chronic critical limb ischemia (CLI) usually results from a multilevel PAD associated with long-term underperfusion and ischemic damage to peripheral tissues and distal vasculature. In patients presenting with CLI, the PAD is frequently an expression of a systemic panvascular syndrome involving more than one major vascular territory and structural disease of multiple endorgans. Vascular anatomy in patients with CLI is characterized by multiple obstructions and lesions distributed across the peripheral arterial system, partially compensated by bridging collateral vessels. The chronic course of CLI with slow deterioration of peripheral blood supply and increasing peripheral tissue ischemia and damage is frequently punctuated by intercurrent events associated either with sudden decompensation of the pre-existent and developed collateral circuits due to progression of the PAD or with increased external nutritional and oxygen demands due to tissue injury or infection. Thorough history and examination of the patient are needed to establish the likely cause of decompensation and the ischemic status of the limb. Only patients with likely reversible ischemic changes and sufficient outlook for revascularization, usually based on duplex ultrasound studies, are considered candidates for invasive diagnostic workup.

In candidates for angiography, evaluation of the renal and cardiac function is critical to prevention of complications and endorgan failure. To determine strategy of treatment usually the entire lower extremity blood supply including the distal abdominal aorta and pelvic arteries should be visualized. The quality of angiograms should allow definitive diagnosis based on the full anatomic and morphologic definition of all relevant vascular segments. To prevent complications, particularly in patients with renal and cardiac dysfunction, the least traumatic option of angiography should be selected. To visualize the entire peripheral vasculature along with detailed definition of the potential targets for revascularization, typically a combination of magnetic resonance and x-ray angiography exploiting the advantages of both techniques is required. Acquired peripheral angiograms are assessed to identify the likely critical and culprit vascular segments and to determine their accessibility to interventional or surgical revascularization. In patients with threatened limb loss, in addition the prospective level of amputation based on available blood supply should be assessed. In patients with concurrent critical vascular disease in other vascular beds, additional vascular studies including panvascular diagnostic imaging might be required in some cases to determine procedural risks and the sequence and strategy of the interventions.

In patients with established diagnosis of CLI (Table 12-5) who are candidates for revascularization procedures the strategy decisions should be based on consensus among vascular specialists, interventionists, and surgeons. The method of revascularization is selected according to expected risks, technical success, and mid- to long-term outcome. Decision criteria regarding preferred therapy options include considerations of lesion morphology, peripheral and general vascular status, presence of coexisting morbidities, previous peripheral procedures, patient's life expectancy, grade of ambulation and lifestyle, and, most importantly, local expertise and experience with prospective interventional or surgical procedures. As in other vascular therapeutic decisions, it appears even more critical in patients with CLI to consider the interventional and surgical revascularization techniques as complementary. In periprocedural settings, a multidisciplinary team approach to address the multitude of clinical issues present including ischemic pain control, foot care, including treatment of ulcers and gangrene, treatment of important coexistent morbidities, in particular diabetes, hypertension, heart failure, pulmonary and renal insufficiency, and associated risk factors is required (for review, see reference 119).

REFERENCES

1. Hirsch AT, Haskal ZJ, Hertzer NR, et al. ACC/AHA 2005 practice guidelines for the management of patients with peripheral arterial disease (lower extremity, renal, mesenteric, and abdominal aortic). A collaborative report from the American Association for Vascular Surgery/Society for Vascular Surgery, Society for Cardiovascular Angiography and Interventions, Society for Vascular Medicine and Biology, Society of Interventional Radiology, and the ACC/AHA Task Force on Practice Guidelines (Writing Committee to develop guidelines for the management of patients with peripheral arterial disease). Endorsed by the American Association of Cardiovascular and Pulmonary Rehabilitation, National Heart, Lung, and Blood Institute, Society for Vascular Nursing, TransAtlantic Inter-Society Consensus, and Vascular Diseases Foundation. Available at: http://circ.ahajournals.org/cgi/reprint/113/11/e463. Retrieved May 30, 2006.
2. Kannel WB, Skinner JJ, Schwartz MJ, et al. Intermittent claudication. Incidence in the Framingham Study. *Circulation.* 1970;41:875–883.
3. Hoffmann GS, Weygand CM, eds. *Inflammatory Diseases of Blood Vessels.* New York: Marcel Dekker Inc., 2002.
4. Buerger L. *The Circulatory Disturbances of the Extremities.* Philadelphia: WB Saunders, 1924.
5. Stuart TP. Note on a variation in the course of the popliteal artery. *J Anat Physiol.* 1879; 13:162.
6. Fowl RJ, Kempczinski RF. Popliteal artery entrapment. In: Rutherford RB, ed. *Vascular Surgery.* 5th ed. Philadelphia: WB Saunders, 2000:1087–1093.
7. Duffy St, Colgan MP, Sultan S, et al. Popliteal aneurysms: a 10-year experience. *Eur J Vasc Endovasc Surg.* 1998;16:218–222.
8. Atkins HJ, Key JA. A case of myxomatous tumor arising in the adventitia of the left external iliac artery. *Br J Surg.* 1947;34:426.
9. Jasinski RW, Masselink BA, Partridge RW, et al. Adventitial cystic disease of the popliteal artery. *Radiology.* 1987;163:153–155.
10. Davis SM. Pseudoclaudication. A review of etiology, diagnosis, and treatment. *Clin Geriatr Med.* 1985;1:373–380.
11. Belch JJ, Topol EJ, Agnelli G, et al. Critical issues in peripheral arterial disease detection and management. *Arch Intern Med.* 2003;163:884–892.
12. Hiatt WR. Medical treatment of peripheral arterial disease and claudication. *N Engl J Med.* 2001;344:1608–1621.
13. TransAtlantic Inter-Society Consensus (TASC). Management of peripheral arterial disease (PAD). *J Vasc Surg.* 2000; 31(suppl):1–296.
14. Hirsch AT, Criqui MH, Treat-Jacobson D, et al. Peripheral arterial disease detection, awareness, and treatment in primary care. *JAMA.* 2001;286:1317–1324.
15. Selvin E, Erlinger TP. Prevalence of and risk factors for peripheral arterial disease in the United States. Results from the National Health and Nutrition Examination Survey, 1999–2000. *Circulation.* 2004;110:738–743.
16. Criqui MH, Langer RD, Fronek A, et al. Mortality over a period of 10 years in patients with peripheral artery disease. *N Engl J Med.* 1992;326:381–386.
17. Boyd AM. The natural course of arteriosclerosis of the lower extremities. *Proc R Soc Med.* 1962;55:591–593.
18. Imparato Am, Kim GE, Davidson T, et al. Intermittent claudication: its natural course. *Surgery.* 1975,78:795–799.
19. McDermott MM, Liu K, Greenland P, et al. Functional decline in peripheral arterial disease. Associations with the ankle brachial index and leg symptoms. *JAMA.* 2004;292:453–461.
20. Fontaine R, Kim M, Kieny R. Die chirurgische Behandlung der peripheren Durchblutungsstörungen. *Helv Chir Acta.* 1954:21:499–533.
21. Bollinger A. *Funktionelle Angiologie.* Stuttgart: Thieme Medical Publishers, 1979:57–84.
22. Rutherford RB, Flanigan DP, Gupta SK, et al. Suggested standards for reports dealing with lower extremity ischemia. *J Vasc Surg.* 1986;4:80–94.
23. Rutherford RB, Becker GJ. Standards for evaluating and reporting results of surgical and percutaneous therapy for peripheral arterial disease. *J Vasc Intervent Radiol.* 1991;2:169–74.
24. Rutherford RB, Baker JD, Ernst C, et al. Recommended standards for reports dealing with lower extremity ischemia: revised version. *J Vasc Surg.* 1997;26:517–38, 19–21.
25. Pentecoast MJ, Criqui MH, Dorros G, et al. Guidelines for peripheral percutaneous transluminal angioplasty of the abdominal aorta and lower extremity vessels. A statement for health professionals from a Special Writing Group of the Councils on Cardiovascular Radiology, Arteriosclerosis, Cardio-thoracic and Vascular Surgery, Clinical Cardiology, and Epidemiology and Prevention, American Heart Association. *Circulation.* 1994;89:511–531.
26. Ramsey De, Manke DA, Sumner DS. Toe blood pressure. A valuable adjunct to ankle pressure measurement for assessing peripheral arterial disease. *J Cardiovasc Surg.* 1983;24:43–48.
27. Hiatt WR, Regensteiner J, Hirsch AT, eds. *Peripheral Arterial Disease.* Boca Raton: CRC Press, 2001.
28. Moore WS, ed. *Vascular Surgery: A Comprehensive Review.* 6th ed. Philadelphia: WB Saunders, 2002:523–569.
29. Schneider G, Prince MR, Meaney JFM, et al. *Magnetic Resonance Angiography: Techniques, Indications and Practical Applications.* New York: Springer-Verlag, 2005.
30. Meissner OA, Rieger J, Weber C, et al. Critical limb ischemia: hybrid MR angiography compared with DSA. *Radiology.* 2005;235:308–318.
31. Jamieson C. The definition of critical ischemia of a limb. *Br J Surg* 1982;69(Suppl):S1).
32. Rajan JK, Patel NH, Valji K, et al. Quality improvement guidelines for percutaneous management of acute limb ischemia. *J Vasc Intervent Radiol.* 2005; 16:585–595.
33. Koelemay MJW, Lijmer JG, Stoker J, et al. Magnetic resonance angiography for the evaluation of lower extremity arterial disease; a meta-analysis. *JAMA.* 2001;285:1338–1345.
34. Adriaensen M, Kock CJM, Stijnen T, et al., Peripheral arterial disease: therapeutic confidence of CT versus digital subtraction angiography and effects on additional imaging recommendations. *Radiology.* 2004;233:385–391.

35. Walsh C, Murphy D, O'Hare N. Development of a quality assurance protocol for peripheral subtraction imaging applications. *Phys Med Biol.* 2002;47:N91–N97.
36. Pattynama PMT. X-ray peripheral and visceral angiography. In: Lanzer P, Topol EJ, eds. *PanVascular Medicine: Integrated Clinical Management.* New York: Springer-Verlag, 2002: 636–58.
37. Hallisey MJ, Meranze SG. The abnormal abdominal aorta. Arteriosclerosis and other diseases. In: Baum S, ed. *Abramsi' Angiography.* Vol 2. 4th ed. Boston: Little, Brown and Company, 1997:1052–1072.
38. Lusza G. *X-ray Anatomy of the Vascular System.* Philadelphia: JB Lippincott, 1963.
39. Diehm C, Allenberg J-R, Numura-Eckert K. *Farbatlas der Gefäßkrankheiten.* Berlin: Springer, 1999.
40. Lippert H, Pabst R. *Arterial Variations in Man.* Munich: JF Bergman, 1985.
41. Uflacker R. *Atlas of Vascular Anatomy: An Angiographic Approach.* Philadelphia: Lippincott Williams & Wilkins, 1997.
42. Baum S, ed. *Abrams' Angiography.* 4th ed. Boston: Little, Brown and Company, 1997.
43. McWilliams RG, Robertson I, Smye SW, et al. Sources of error in intra-arterial pressure measurements across a stenosis. *Eur J Endovasc Surg.* 1998;15:535–540.
44. Bonn J. Percutaneous vascular intervention: value of hemodynamic measurements. *Radiology.* 1996;201:18–20.
45. De Bruyne B, Pijls HJ, Barbato E, et al. Intracoronary and intravenous adenosine 5'-triphosphate adenosine, papaverine, and contrast medium to assess fractional flow reserve in humans. *Circulation.* 2003;107:1877–1883.
46. Singh H, Cardella JF, Cole PE, et al. Quality improvement guidelines for diagnostic arteriography. *J Vasc Intervent Radiol.* 2002;13:1–6.
47. Dotter CT, Judkins MP. Transluminal treatment of arteriosclerotic obstruction. Description of a new technic and a preliminary report of its application. *Circulation.* 1964; 30:654–670.
48. Porstmann W. Ein neuer Korsett-Ballonkatheter zur transluminalen Rekanalisation nach Dotter unter besonderer Berücksichtigung von Obliterationen and den Beckenarterien. *Radiol Diagn.* 1973;14:239–244.
49. Grüntzig A, Hopff H. Perkutane Rekanalisation chronischer arterieller Verschlüsse mit einem neuen Dilatationskatheter. *Dtsch Med Wochenschr.* 1974;99:2502–2505.
50. Dotter CT, Buschmann RW, McKinney MK, et al. Transluminal expandable nitinol coil stent grafting: preliminary report. *Radiology.* 1983;147:259–260.
51. Palmaz JC, Sibbitt RR, Tio FO, et al. Expandable intraluminal vascular graft: a feasibility study. *Surgery.* 1986;99:199–205.
52. Rösch J. Historic highlights of interventional radiology. Available at: http://miit.com/PDF/MIIT%202002/Historic%20Highlights%20of%20Interventional%20Radiology.pdf. Accessed January 8, 2006.
53. Creager MA, Goldstone J, Hirschfeld JW Jr., et al. for the Writing Committee Members. ACC/ACP/SCAI/SVMB/SVS Clinical Competence Statement on vascular medicine and catheter-based peripheral vascular interventions. *J Am Coll Cardiol.* 2004;44:942–957.
54. Rutherford RB, Flanigan DP, Gupta SK, et al. Suggested standards for reports dealing with lower extremity ischemia. *J Vasc Surg.* 1986;4:80–94.
55. Rutherford RB, Becker GJ. Standards for evaluating and reporting results of surgical and percutaneous therapy for peripheral arterial disease. *J Vasc Intervent Radiol.* 1991;2: 169–174.
56. Sacks D, Marinelli DL, Martin LG, et al. Reporting standards for clinical evaluation of new peripheral arterial revascularization devices. *J Vasc Intervent Radiol.* 1997;8:137–149.
57. Omary RA, Bettmann MA, Cardella JF, et al. Quality improvement guidelines for the reporting and archiving of interventional radiology procedures. *J Vasc Intervent Radiol* .2003;14: S293–S295.
58. Pentecoast MJ, Criqui MH, Dorros G, et al. Guidelines for peripheral percutaneous transluminal angioplasty of the abdominal aorta and lower extremity vessels. A statement for health professionals from a Special Writing Group of the Councils on Cardiovascular Radiology, Arteriosclerosis, Cardio-thoracic and Vascular Surgery, Clinical Cardiology, and Epidemiology and Prevention, American Heart Association. *Circulation.* 1994;89:511–531.
59. Seldinger SI. Catheter placement of the needle in percutaneous arteriography. *Acta Radiol [Diagn] (Stockh).* 1953;39:368–376.
60. Jarvis MA, Jarvis CL, Jones PR, et al. Reliability of Allen's test in selection of patients for radial artery harvest. *Ann Thorac Surg.* 2000;70:1362–1365.
61. Lipchik EO, Sugimoto H. Percutaneous brachial artery catheterization. *Radiology.* 1986;160:842–843.
62. Trigaux J-P, Van Beers B, De Wispelaere J-F. Anatomic relationship between the popliteal artery and vein: a guide to accurate angiographic puncture. *AJR Am J Roentgenol.* 1991;157:1259–1262.
63. dos Santos R, Lamas A, Pereira-Caldas J. L'arteriographie des members de l'aorte et de ses branches abdominals. *Soc Nat Chir Bull Mem.* 1929;55:587–596.
64. Koreny M, Riedmuller E, Nikfardjam M, et al. Arterial puncture closing devices compared with standard manual compression after cardiac catheterization: systematic review and meta-analysis. *JAMA.* 2004; 291:350–357.
65. Nikolsky E, Mehran R, Halkin A, et al. Vascular complications associated with arteriotomy closure devices in patients undergoing percutaneous coronary procedures: a meta-analysis. *J Am Coll Cardiol.* 2004; 44:1200–1207.
66. Baim DS, Carozza JP. Complications of diagnostic cardiac catheterization. Available at: http://patients.uptodate.com/topic.asp?file=chd/13240. Accessed January 11, 2006.
67. Leriche R. Des obliterations arterielles hautes (obliteration de la terminaison de l'aorte) commes causes des insuffiances circulatoires des membres inferieurs. *Bull Med Soc Chir Paris.* 1923;49:1404–7.
68. Haimovici H. Patterns of arteriosclerotic lesions of the lower extremity. *Arch Surg.* 1967;95:918–933.
69. de Vries SO, Hunink MGM. Results of aortic bifurcation grafts for aortoiliac occlusive disease: a meta-analysis. *J Vasc Surg.* 1997;26:558–569.
70. Tegtmeyer CJ, Wellons HA, Thompson RN. Balloon dilatation of the abdominal aorta. *JAMA.* 1980;244:2626–2637.
71. Yakes WF, Kumpe DA, Brown SB, et al. Percutaneous transluminal aortic angioplasty: techniques and results. *Radiology.* 1989; 172: 965–970.
72. Ravimandalam K, Rao VR, Kumar S, et al. Obstruction of the infrarenal portion of the abdominal aorta: results of treatment with balloon angioplasty. *AJR Am J Roentgenol.* 1991;156:1257–1260.
73. Scheinert D, Schröder M, Balzer JO, et al. Stent-supported reconstruction of the aortoiliac bifurcation with the kissing balloon technique. *Circulation.* 1999;100(suppl II):II295–II300.
74. Gaines PA, Cumberland DC. Wire-loop technique for angioplasty of total iliac artery occlusions. *Radiology.* 1988;168:275–276.
75. Murphy TP. The role of stents in aortoiliac occlusive disease. In: Perler BA, Becker GJ, eds. *Vascular Intervention: A Clinical Approach.* New York: Thieme Medical Publishers, 1998:111–136.
76. Allaire E, Melliere D, Poussier B, et al. Iliac artery rupture during balloon dilatation: what treatment? *Ann Vasc Surg.* 2003;17:306–314.
77. Funovics MA, Lackner B, Cejna M, et al. Predictors of long-term results after treatment of iliac artery obliteration by transluminal angioplasty and stent deployment. *Cardiovasc Intervent Radiol.* 2002;5:397–402.
78. Mouanoutoa M, Maddikunta R, Allaqaband S, et al. Endovascular intervention of aortoiliac occlusive disease in high-risk patients using the kissing stents technique: long-term results. *Cathet Cardiovasc Intervent.* 2003;60:327–328.
79. Becker GJ, Katzen BJ, Dake MD. Noncoronary angioplasty. *Radiology.* 1989;170:403–412.
80. Spence RK, Freiman DB, Gatenby R, et al. Long- term results of transluminal angioplasty of the iliac and femoral arteries. *Arch Surg.* 1981;116:1377–1386.
81. Murphy TP, Webbs MS, Lambiase RE, et al. Percutaneous revascularization of complex iliac artery stenoses and occlusions using Wallstents: 3-year experience. *J Vasc Intervent Radiol.* 1996;7:21–27.
82. Rudofsky G. Peripheral arterial disease: chronic ischemic syndromes. In: Lanzer P, Topol EJ, eds. *PanVascular Medicine: Integrated Clinical Management.* New York: Springer-Verlag, 2002:1363–1422.
83. Capek P, McLean GK, Berkowitz HD. Femoropopliteal angioplasty. Factors influencing long-term success. *Circulation.* 1991;83(suppl 2):I70-I80.
84. Currie IC, Wakeley CJ, Cole SE, et al. Femoropopliteal angioplasty for severe limb ischemia. *Br J Surg.* 1994;81:191–193.
85. Murray JG, Apthorp LA, Wilkins RA. Long-segment ($\geq$10 cm) femoropopliteal angioplasty: improved technical success and long-term patency. *Radiology.* 1995;195:158–162.
86. Gray BH, Sullivan TM, Childs MB, et al. High incidence of restenosis/reocclusion of stents in the percutaneous treatment of long- segment superficial femoral artery disease after suboptimal angioplasty. *J Vasc Surg.* 1997;25:74–83.
87. Henry M, Amor M, Ethevenot G, et al. Palmaz stent placement in iliac and femoropopliteal arteries: primary and secondary patency in 310 patients with 2–4 year follow-up. *Radiology.* 1995;197:167–174.
88. Henry M, Henry I, Klonaris C, et al. Percutaneous endovascular treatment of femoropopliteal occlusive disease. In: Heuser RR, Henry M, eds. *Textbook of Peripheral Vascular Interventions.* London: MD Martin Dunitz, 2004:243–262.
89. Lugmayer HF, Holzer H, Kastner M, et al. Treatment of complex arteriosclerotic lesions with nitinol stents in the superficial femoral and popliteal arteries: a midterm follow-up. *Radiology.* 2002;222:37–43.
90. Greenberg B, Rosenfield K, Garcia LA, et al. In-hospital costs of self-expanding nitinol stent implantation versus balloon angioplasty in the femoropopliteal artery (the VascuCoil Trial). *J Vasc Intervent Radiol.* 2004;15:1065–1069.
91. Scheinert D, Scheinert S, Sax J, et al. Prevalence and clinical impact of stent fractures after femoropopliteal stenting. *J Am Coll Cardiol.* 2005;45:312-315.
92. Bauermeister G. Endovascular stent-grafting in the treatment of superficial femory artery occlusive disease. *J Endovasc Ther.* 2001;8:315–320.
93. Bray PJ, Robson WJ, Bray AE. Percutaneous treatment of long superficial femoral artery occlusive disease: efficacy of the Hemobahn stent-graft. *J Endovasc Ther.* 2003; 10:619–628.
94. Saxon RR, Coffmann JM, Gooding JM, et al. Long-term results of ePTFE stent-graft versus angioplasty in the femoropopliteal artery: single center experience from a prospective, randomized trial. *J Vasc Intervent Radiol.* 2003;14:303–311.
95. Minar E, Pokrajac B, Maca T, et al. Endovascular brachytherapy for prophylaxis of restenosis after femoropopliteal angioplasty. Results of a prospective randomized study. *Circulation.* 2000;102:2694–2699.
96. Duda SH, Pusich B, Richter G, et al. Sirolimus- eluting stents fort he treatment of obstructive superficial femoral artery disease: six month results. *Circulation.* 2002;106:1505–1509.
97. Litvack F, Grundfest WS, Segalowitz J, et al. Interventional cardiovascular therapy by laser and thermal angioplasty. *Circulation.* 1990;81:1099–1116.
98. Bolia A, Miles KA, Brennan J, et al. Percutaneous transluminal angioplasty of occlusions of the femoral and popliteal arteries by subintimal dissection. *Cardiovasc Intervent Radiol.* 1990;13:357–363.
99. Scheinert D, Biamino G. Femoropopliteal occlusions: experience with peripheral excimer laser angioplasty. *Curr Intervent Cardiol Rep.* 2001;3:130–138.
100. Spinosa DJ, Leung DA, Matsumoto AK, et al. Percutaneous intentional extraluminal recanalization in patients with chronic limb ischemia. *Radiology.* 2004;232:499–507.
101. Murray RR Jr., Lutz JD. Femoropopliteal angioplasty and stents: patient selection and results. In: Perler BA, Becker GJ, eds. *Vascular Intervention: A Clinical Approach.* New York: Thieme Medical Publishers, 1998:169–176.
102. Lanzer P. Topographic distribution of peripheral arteriopathy in non-diabetics and type 2 diabetics. Z Kardiol 90:99–102, 2001-04-22.
103. Greenfield A. Femoral, popliteal and tibial arteries: percutaneous transluminal angioplasty. *AJR Am J Roentgenol.* 1980;135:927–935.

104. Schwarten DE, Cutcliff WB. Arterial occlusive disease below the knee: treatment with percutaneous transluminal angioplasty performed with low-profile catheters and steerable guide wires. *Radiology.* 1988;169:71–74.

105. Bakal CW, Sprayregen S, Scheinbaum K, et al. Percutaneous transluminal angioplasty of the infrapopliteal arteries: results in 53 patients. *AJR Am J Roentgenol.* 1990;154:171–174.

106. Brown KT, Schoenberg NY, Moore ED, et al. Percutaneous transluminal angioplasty of infrapopliteal vessels: preliminary results and technical considerations. *Radiology.* 1988;169:75–78.

107. Schwarten DE. Clinical and anatomical considerations for nonoperative therapy in tibial disease and the results of angioplasty. *Circulation.* 1991;83:186–190.

108. Söder HK, Manninen HI, Jaakkola P, et al. Prospective trial of infrapopliteal artery balloon angioplasty for critical limb ischemia: angiographic and clinical results. *J Vasc Intervent Radiol.* 2000;11:1021–1031.

109. Dorros G, Jaff MR, Dorros AM, et al. Tibioperoneal (outflow lesion) angioplasty can be used as primary treatment in 235 patients with critical limb ischemia: five-year follow-up. *Circulation.* 2001;104:2057–2062.

110. Feiring AJ, Wesolowski AA, Lade S. Primary stent-supported angioplasty for treatment of below-knee critical limb ischemia and severe claudication. *J Am Coll Cardiol.* 2004;44:2307–2314.

111. Folkman J. Therapeutic angiogenesis in ischemic limbs. *Circulation.* 1998;97:1108–1110.

112. Annex BH. Therapeutic angiogenesis for PAD. *Endovasc Today.* 2004; suppl (October):17–19.

113. Hunter GC, Westerband A. Noninfectious complications in vascular surgery. In: Moore WS, ed. *Vascular Surgery: A Comprehensive Review.* 6th ed. Philadelphia: WB Saunders, 2002:751–782.

114. Krajcer Z, Levy M. Endovascular treatment for lower extremity bypass failure. In: Heuser RR, Henry M, eds. *Textbook of Peripheral Vascular Interventions.* London: MD Martin Dunitz, 2004:269–276.

115. Angle N, Quinones-Baldrich WJ. Acute arterial and graft occlusion. In: Moore WS, ed. *Vascular Surgery: A Comprehensive Review.* 6th ed. Philadelphia: WB Saunders, 2002:697–718.

116. McNamara TO, Fischer JR. Thrombolysis of peripheral arterial and graft occlusions: improved results using high-dose urokinase. *AJR Am J Roentgenol.* 1985;144:769–775.

117. Thrombolysis in the management of lower limb peripheral arterial occlusion—a consensus document. Working Party on Thrombolysis in the Management of Limb Ischemia. *Am J Cardiol.* 1998;81:207–218.

118. Patel N, Sacks D, Patel RI, et al. SIR reporting standards for the treatment of acute limb ischemia with the use of transluminal removal of arterial thrombus. *J Vasc Intervent Radiol.* 2003;(suppl):S453-S465.

119. Wolfe JHN, Porter JM. Basic treatment for critical limb ischemia. *J Vasc Surg.* 2000;31:A1. Available at: http://www.lava.med.br/mestrado/vascular/2003/Artigos_16_Otacilio_Figueiredo/D_4_Treatment_of_critical_limb_ischemia.htm. Accessed January 17, 2006.

Dierk Vorwerk

CHAPTER **13**

Hemodialysis Shunts

Percutaneous procedures for hemodialysis shunts are becoming increasingly important for interventional radiologists. A growing number of patients with renal insufficiency are enrolled in dialysis programs, the majority of them undergoing hemodialysis. In the West, this affects some 150 to 200 persons per million inhabitants.

Given the increase in patients' life expectancy, maintaining access to the vascular system continues to be a problem.[1] For example, the number of long-term functioning shunts is estimated to be 15%.[1] Primary patency of hemodialysis shunts is low: Approximately 65% of Brescia-Cimino shunts and 50% of polytetrafluoroethylene (PTFE)-covered shunts exhibit primary patency after 1 year, and the numbers sink after 2 and 4 years to 60% and 45% for the Brescia-Cimino shunts and to 43% and 10% for the PTFE-covered shunts.[2]

In Europe, arteriovenous Brescia-Cimino shunts are the preferred primary shunts, used in conjunction with the radial artery and veins of the lower arm. Autologous veins in the proximal lower arm and elbow region are generally preferred, even for renewed shunt application. PTFE-covered shunts, utilizing foreign-body implants such as Gore-Tex segments, are mainly used where the vascular conditions are very complicated and unfavorable. In the United States, in contrast, PTFE-covered shunts are used much more frequently as primary shunts, often accounting for the majority of shunts in a given patient population.

The choice of access site, the indications, and the interventional technique employed depend on the nature and location of the shunt, the site of the lesion, and the nature of the obstruction. As a rule, the presence of a stenosis or a thrombus, the type of shunt, and the location of the obstruction determine the type of technique used.

The objective of this chapter is to describe the technical options for percutaneous interventions for different types of shunt problems. The surgical alternatives are not discussed. It is important to mention, however, that comparative studies have not produced any indication of significant differences between surgical and percutaneous procedures with regard to immediate or long-term outcome.

DIAGNOSIS OF SHUNT PROBLEMS

Sufficient diagnosis to classify the location and nature of the disturbance is necessary before performing any intervention on hemodialysis shunts. Simple palpation of the brachial and radial arteries and the shunt veins with and without stasis provides important information about the condition of the veins and the presence of stenotic or thrombotic segments.[3]

High-quality, noninvasive, morphologic diagnosis and, to a lesser extent, functional diagnosis of hemodialysis shunts can be achieved with various sonographic methods. Real-time sonography and color-coded duplex sonography are superior to angiography in detecting thromboses and should be employed for shunt thromboses in order to image the extent of the clot.[4]

Angiographic study is, however, essential in the actual planning of an intervention. It always consists of complete representation of the supplying arteries (as far as possible), and of the draining veins up to the superior vena cava. The purpose of complete representation is to rule out the existence of multiple lesions.

TRANSBRACHIAL FINE NEEDLE ANGIOGRAPHY

Transbrachial angiography (Fig. 13-1 A, B) provides the best access to all shunt connections from the brachial artery distal to the elbow or any of its branches. It can be employed for almost all

Brescia-Cimino shunts and some PTFE-implant shunts. Under local anesthesia, a retrograde puncture of the palpable brachial artery is performed using a fine 22-gauge puncture needle with a plastic cover according to the Seldinger technique at elbow level where the artery passes under the aponeurosis of the biceps muscle. The plastic cover is best inserted into the artery as far as the Luer connector in order to reach a safe position. This occasionally makes it necessary to use an 0.018-in. guidewire. The synthetic needle is then fixed with sterile adhesive tape, and a thin extension tube with lock fitting (e.g., Perfusor tubing, Braun, Melsungen, Germany) is attached for contrast medium administration. Subsequently, a diluted solution of contrast medium is manually injected to permit visualization of the entire course of the shunt and long sections of the brachial artery using retrograde, digital subtraction angiography (one to two images per second). As a rule, 20 to 40 mL contrast medium (saline: contrast 1:1) is sufficient.

This procedure is simple, is infrequently associated with complications, and can be performed on an outpatient basis. Access to the artery can be maintained if a subsequent intervention is planned, in order to monitor the success of the intervention. Care should be taken that a puncture performed prior to the intervention does not puncture the artery in the immediate vicinity of the basilic vein, which is often adjacent, to avoid damage to the potential venous access.

TRANSFEMORAL ANGIOGRAPHY

Transfemoral selective brachial angiography via the subclavian artery is performed only in exceptional cases, including cases with high proximal arterial stenoses which cannot be adequately assessed by the retrograde brachial approach or duplex sonography or cases considered for angioplasty. As a rule, the transfemoral approach should not be performed on an outpatient basis.

SHUNT IMAGING (SHUNTOGRAM)

Direct puncture of the venous portion of the shunt for diagnostic purposes can be performed in PTFE-covered shunts with anastomosis to the brachial artery or above the elbow joint and for any type of shunt in the upper arm (Fig. 13-1 C,D). Using the fine-needle approach, the PTFE-implant loop or the vein is best punctured in the direction of flow, since the access can be also used for intervention. The arterial shunt portion can then be imaged using retrograde overflow angiography after compression of the venous drainage. Puncture should not be made too far from the arterial anastomosis to allow high quality imaging of the arterial shunt arm and to avoid complications.

In cases considered for a subsequent intervention, however, the puncture site should not be too close to the site of the intervention to allow secure sheath placement and endovascular instrumentation.

Diagnostic angiography should not be performed in patients with thrombosis of a PTFE-covered shunt since there is always complete closure of the shunt ranging from the arterial to the venous anastomosis.

Imaging of native upper arm shunts is best done in an antegrade direction in the section of the vein near the anastomosis where the pulse is still palpable, such that this access can be

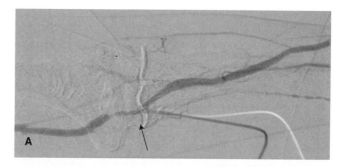

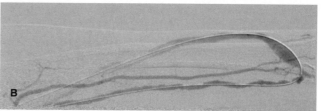

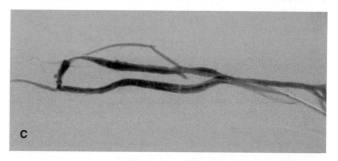

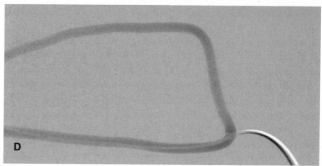

FIGURE 13-1. Transbrachial fine needle angiography. **A:** Retrograde fine-needle puncture at the elbow level (*arrow*). **B:** Imaging of the feeding artery, the anastomotic region with a stenosis, and the draining vein. **C:** Shuntogram with venous catheter placed into the feeding artery. **D:** Shuntogram with apex puncture of a loop implant shunt. Here the catheter has been advanced into the arterial limb to achieve a downstream angiography of the dialysis shunt.

enlarged and used for the subsequent intervention, if needed. In these cases, any puncture of the brachial artery should be avoided altogether.

OTHER IMAGING TECHNIQUES

Although other imaging modalities such as MR and CT angiography also allow shunt monitoring, they are too cumbersome and too expensive to become widely used for shunt diagnostics in real-life clinical practice. In cases with difficult puncture, sonography may be helpful.

ACCESS

The location and the type of shunt determine which access is appropriate.

NATIVE LOWER ARM SHUNTS

As a rule, venous access is chosen for Brescia-Cimino shunts. The shunt vein is punctured with the patient wearing a compression bandage. A large-bore cannula and a regular 0.035-in. guidewire should be used in large veins. In small and poorly palpable veins, the micropuncture is recommended using a 22-gauge needle and a 0.018-in. guidewire. Following the successful puncture, a 16-gauge plastic cannula can be easily inserted over the guidewire into the shunt vein and advanced while being carefully rotated. Imaging must confirm that the thin wire has not been kinked to prevent breaking. Once correct intraluminal position of the plastic cannula has been confirmed, the stylet and guidewire should be replaced by a 0.035-in. guidewire, preferably hydrophilically coated. Retrograde venous puncture is performed in lesions near anastomoses (i.e., distal venous lesions), stenotic anastomoses, and distal arterial stenoses.

Transbrachial arterial access may be necessary in exceptional cases if the operator does not succeed in crossing a stenosis near the anastomosis from the venous access. In these cases, the brachial artery is punctured in an antegrade fashion at the height of the elbow joint and, after careful probing of the artery supplying the shunt — normally the radial artery — a 4F catheter is inserted. The stenosis is probed using the guidewire reinforced by a dilatation catheter. Once the stenosis has been crossed the guidewire tip is caught by a snare introduced from the vein and guided out via the venous access. To minimize the risk of arterial injury the intervention is performed from the venous access.

For stenoses in the proximal segments of the draining veins, the shunt vein is punctured in an antegrade fashion at a more peripheral puncture site. If such a proximal stenosis cannot be probed and crossed from the peripheral site or probing is prevented by complicating dissections or perforations, then the crossing should be tried by approaching the target lesion from a second venous access established by a retrograde puncture of the target vein.

NATIVE UPPER ARM SHUNTS

In lesions close to the anastomosis, the brachiocephalic vein is punctured in a retrograde fashion at a far proximal site, i.e., downstream from the target lesion. If the lesion is located close to the trunk (more proximally), the brachiocephalic vein is punctured close to the anastomosis. A double access is often advisable in thromboses of upper arm shunts, whereby a retrograde puncture can be made first in the thrombosed vein to perform partial thrombectomy on one segment to be complemented by a thrombectomy of the rest of the thrombus from a second antegrade access.

Ipsilateral puncture of the internal jugular vein with retrograde probing of the target lesion has been considered an alternative access to the brachiocephalic vein.

IMPLANTED SHUNTS

In PTFE-implant shunts, the puncture site in the loop depends on whether the stenosis is located in the arterial (retrograde) or venous portion of the anastomosis or in the draining veins of the upper arm. A diagnostic puncture made according to the micropuncture technique described earlier can usually be enlarged and used for the intervention.

In loop shunts, the apex of the shunt arch is an advantageous puncture site. After the dilator has been inserted into the catheter, the guidewire can be advanced and directed into either the arterial or the venous shunt portion, making it possible to access both arms of the shunt from one site.

In straight grafts, access should be via the implant itself and is best performed in the direction of flow. Two access sites are frequently necessary in all types of shunts, particularly if thrombectomy has been intended, particularly if the thrombus extends close to the arterial site of the graft anastomosis.

CENTRAL VEINS

In lesions of the proximal cephalic and subclavian veins, preferred access is from the arm using the shunt vein. In rare cases, when large balloons or stent devices are used, transfemoral venous access is selected to avoid injury of the shunt veins. Note, however, that a 10F catheter can be inserted into an arm vein safely. Combined cannulation of the femoral and brachial veins is occasionally necessary to achieve continuous monitoring of the stent implants in central veins. In critical locations, stents can be placed over a guidewire forming a loop through the brachial and femoral vein in order to provide support for the transvenous segment and possibly prevent stent embolization into the pulmonary circulation.

ARTERIAL STENOSES

For proximal lesions of the arterial arm of the shunt, access can be achieved either via retrograde brachial artery puncture or—in the case of the upper arm synthetic shunts—by a retrograde transvenous puncture. If the brachial pulse is weak, the micropuncture technique is occasionally appropriate after the stenosis has been located using a pocket Doppler. Transfemoral arterial access for dilatation is only indicated in the unusual case of arterial stenoses of the proximal brachial artery.

SHUNT STENOSES

Since shunt stenoses are frequently the cause of subsequent shunt thromboses, they should be diagnosed and removed promptly. They present as increased venous counterpressure during hemodialysis, increased recirculation, or lengthened hemostasis, or, if the stenosis is located near the anastomosis, as venous collapse due to suction or insufficient arterial flow.

Although shunt stenoses can develop in any venous segment, with Brescia-Cimino shunts they are frequently located at or close to the arteriovenous anastomosis and the puncture segment, while with PTFE-covered shunts they are more frequently located proximal to the venous anastomosis.

The procedure of choice is balloon dilatation (Fig. 13-2). A 5F low-profile catheter should be selected allowing a smooth navigation and tracking of curves. Alternatively, in the afferent

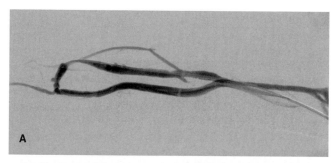

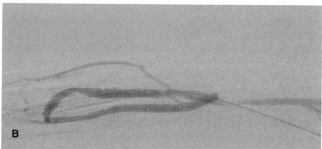

FIGURE 13-2. Venous shunt stenosis in a native forearm fistula. **A:** Stenosis at the anastomosis and a second lesion 1 cm more proximal. Transvenous access. **B:** After balloon dilatation opening of the lesions and improved flow.

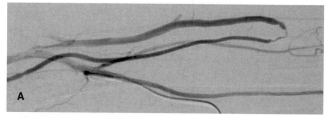

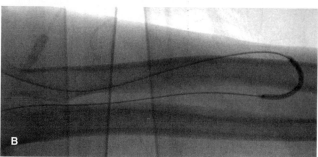

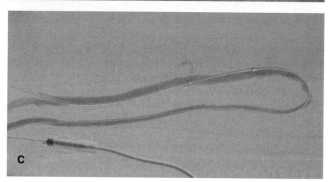

FIGURE 13-3. Arterial stenosis at the anastomosis in a native fistula. **A:** Stenosis at the anastomosis. **B:** PTA balloon both in the artery and across the anastomosis. **C:** After PTA; sufficient widening without dissection.

radial artery, a combination of a catheter with a 0.035-in. hydrophilic guidewire can be used. A 6F sheath is usually sufficient.

Using the retrograde approach to the target lesion prior to introducing the balloon catheter, a catheter and hydrophilic guidewire should pass the lesion first. The guidewire should be placed deep into the artery via the arteriovenous anastomosis. Using this technique, it is possible to dilate distal arterial lesions (Fig. 13-3), stenoses of the anastomosis, and distal venous stenoses. In my own experience, the use of conventional balloon systems is usually sufficient. Special balloon systems with short shafts do not offer any particular advantages.

It is important to note that extremely resistant stenoses are encountered relatively frequently in shunt veins and that they can resist balloon pressures as high as 15 bar and higher. In such cases, high-pressure balloons with an average burst pressure of 20 bar or cutting balloons (BSIC, Boston, MA) are employed.

Other special types of resilient stenoses that can limit the outcome of balloon dilatation. They include collapsing stenoses, which collapse upon themselves immediately after dilatation. Furthermore, increased flow volume can lead to venous dilatation and elongation, which can result in kink stenoses, especially in the proximity of stenotic venous valves. Although these stenoses can be well dilated, they recoil immediately after balloon deflation. They are hardly amenable to a plain balloon percutaneous transluminal angioplasty (PTA); stents may be helpful in the upper arm shunts. Dilatations of central veins may require large balloons, 12 mm to 16 mm in diameter.

During the intervention, 2500 to 5000 U heparin should be administered intravenously. Careful provision should be taken for hemodialysis following the intervention no later than the next day. During hemodialysis, full heparinization is provided but no anticoagulatory treatment is required subsequently.

INDICATIONS FOR INTERVENTION IN STENOSES

Percutaneous intervention of stenotic hemodialysis shunts is always indicated when a stenosis is more than 40% to 50% of the diameter. Sullivan and coworkers reported significant reduction in blood pressure with stenoses >40% diameter,[5,6] which indicates the hemodynamic significance of even moderately sized stenoses. In hemodynamic terms, it is therefore grade shunt stenoses can become significant in the presence of a low peripheral resistance.

Type, length, and location of a stenosis do not predict whether the stenosis will respond to balloon dilatation. Exceptions to this rule are central venous stenoses and long arterial lesions of the supplying lower arm artery, which generally do not respond favorably to balloon dilatation alone.

Whereas stenting is indicated for central stenoses, stenting may not be an alternative in long arterial stenoses. If surgical shortening of the shunt and reimplantation are not possible, then a balloon dilatation must be attempted, regardless of unfavorable prognosis. Interestingly, Beathard et al. were not able to confirm the frequently discussed limitations of PTA in long lesions (>6 cm) or stenoses inside PTFE-covered shunts.[7]

Thus, in most cases, stenoses resistant to dilatation can only be identified during balloon inflations.

RESULTS OF BALLOON DILATATION

The results of plain balloon angioplasty are in most cases technically satisfactory. In large series, the reported success rate ranged between 82% and 94%, and the complication rates ranged from 2% to 6%.[7-10] The long-term results, in contrast, are less convincing. Gmelin and Karnel[10] reported a markedly reduced patency over time, dropping from 75% at 6 months to 34% at 2 years. Glanz et al.[9] reported comparable results. The primary patency reported by Beathard et al.,[7] which they calculated according to the life-table method, was even less favorable. Yet although these results can be regarded as unsatisfactory in comparison with those for other PTA localizations, this is not a reason to reject percutaneous therapy for complicated hemodialysis shunts, because there is no suitable alternative and the results of surgical revision are no better long-term.

In our hospital, although the cases referred for shunt revision represented a negative selection of complicated shunt connections, overall primary patency after percutaneous interventions was 80% after 1 year and 70% after 2 years.[8] This result corresponds to those reported by Keller et al.,[2] who found an overall patency rate of 70% after 1 year, and 60% after 2, whereby surgical reintervention was the standard procedure and the patient population also included well-functioning shunts. It can be concluded that percutaneous therapy improves the overall patency and lifetime even in complicated hemodialysis shunts.

COMPLICATIONS

Complications occur relatively seldom in balloon dilatation of hemodialysis shunts.[8-10] The main complication is venous rupture (Fig. 13-4), which occurs with a frequency of 2%, and—if it happens in larger veins—may be associated with extensive extravasation. Despite the arterialized flow, ruptures of this kind rarely lead to larger hematomas in the veins of the shoulder or upper arm and frequently resolve spontaneously. Treatment consists of a balloon occlusion upstream from the rupture site using the original balloon catheter, which is inflated for several minutes. Occasionally, stent implantation is necessary and may be employed in the upper arm region.

If venous rupture occurs in the veins of the lower arm, it is often associated with the development of a painful hematoma, which in the smaller veins of the lower arm can lead to compression of the vein and subsequent shunt occlusion; careful monitoring and, if necessary, heparinization are indicated here.

In rare cases, venous rupture leads to the development of venous pseudoaneurysms. Serious and flow-reducing dissections can arise and then require stent implantation. If the rupture does not resolve after prolonged PTA and/or stent implantation, implantation of a stent graft, now commercially available, may be an option.

ALTERNATIVE PROCEDURES

As an alternative to balloon dilatation, directional atherectomy has been performed percutaneously. Older atherectomy systems such as the Simpson catheter[11] are no longer commercially available. No data are available on treatment of hemodialysis shunts using the currently available directional atherectomy system (SilverHawk Plaque Excision System, FoxHollow, Redwood City, CA).

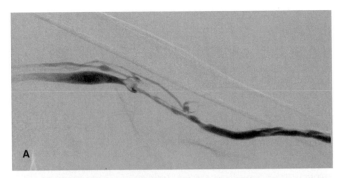

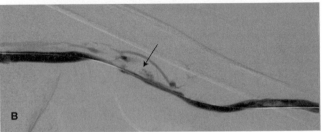

FIGURE 13-4. Venous rupture. **A:** Tight venous stenosis with thrombus attached. **B:** After PTA, the thrombus is gone, but the vein shows a circumscribed rupture (*arrow*) that required prolonged PTA with satifactory outcome (not shown).

The use of metal stents has become more significant, even in stenoses and occlusions of hemodialysis shunts. They are indicated in complicated, central venous stenoses and are described separately.

SHUNT THROMBOSIS

Thrombosis of hemodialysis shunts is the most frequently encountered complication, occurring in 40% to 80% of treated cases.[12] Thrombosis occurs more often in implanted shunts, representing a typical late complication. Brescia-Cimino shunts are less susceptible to thromboses occurring more frequently, during the earlier postoperative stages, but thromboses may also occur late. The extent of the thrombosed portions in implanted shunts almost always involves the entire length of the implant, whereas in native shunts the extent varies greatly, depending on the age of the thrombosis and the course of the collateral veins, often involving only shorter segments. Stenoses of the draining veins and of the supplying tract represent predisposing factors for the development of thromboses. Their development appears also more likely in patients with coagulation disorders, low blood pressure, and probably also erythropoietin therapy.[12]

There are several possible approaches to treating shunt thromboses.

COMBINED RADIOLOGICAL AND SURGICAL THROMBECTOMY

It is often impossible to identify multiple stenoses that are simultaneously present using surgical thrombectomy with Fogarty balloons and concomitant angiographic representation of the shunt. Such stenoses are frequently the cause of the shunt occlusion. Smith et al.[13,14] suggested combined percutaneous and surgical thrombectomy for synthetic shunts.

With this procedure, after surgical opening of the shunt, a Fogarty thrombectomy is first performed. Subsequently, the shunt is visualized via angiography using the customary technique, concomitant thrombi are thrombectomized or dilated in targeted fashion, and stenoses are widened using dilatation.

The use of balloon dilatation to intentionally break up thrombi adhering to the vessel wall, as is frequently the case in lesions close to the arterial anastomosis, has proved to be an additional advantage of this combined strategy. Logistically, the procedure should be performed in the angiography unit because of the advantages offered by imaging; particular attention should be paid to the necessary aseptic conditions.

BALLOON DILATATION

Balloon dilatation of thrombotic shunt occlusions is not generally contraindicated. Its value depends on the local situation.

Not every thrombotic occlusion is accompanied by the development of larger clots. A special form that has been observed involves pluglike, very short thrombi that occlude only the immediate vicinity of the anastomosis. After passing carefully through the occluded segment, a PTA catheter can be brought across. Immediately after dilatation, flow can be restored. However, the PTA catheter should be positioned with the tip placed within the artery such that on dilatation, the thrombus cannot be pressed back into the artery.

Furthermore, although high-grade, long stenoses may be associated with secondary thrombi, these thrombi are often short. In these cases, PTA is also the only means to restore the flow.

Palpation and sonography of the interventional site can provide important clues to identify complex fully thrombosed lesions and to predict success. Thus, in cases with extensive intraluminal thrombus masses, simple balloon dilatation on its own is not a suitable therapy, but tends rather to cause dislocation of thrombus material into the arteries, veins, or lungs.

THROMBOLYSIS

Thrombolysis treatment is used as a percutaneous alternative to surgical thrombectomy, particularly with Brescia-Cimino shunts. For fibrinolysis, urokinase and recombinant plasminogen activator (rtPA) are available for use, as is to a lesser extent streptokinase; the use of all of these has been described previously in hemodialysis shunts. An overall dose of 20 mg rtPA should not be exceeded. Parallel to any lysis therapy, full heparinization should be carried out. Since systemic and transarterial lysis have proved unsuccessful in the treatment of shunt thromboses, there are three options in terms of application technique for lysis therapy:

- Direct injection transcutaneously into the thrombus. Using ultrasound monitoring, the lysis medium is injected into the thrombus using a fine needle and the shunt is clinically observed. Very small quantities of lysis are used (approximately 2 mg rtPA), and the technique is suitable for smaller quantities of thrombus.

- Catheter lysis following percutaneous puncture and mechanical thrombus treatment using catheters and guidewires according to Davis et al.[15] Following retrograde puncture in the venous segment, an angiographic catheter is guided through the occluded segment. Via the catheter, it is injected with up to 150,000 IU of highly concentrated fibrinolytic agent (solution 25,000 IU urokinase per mL). The thrombus is also broken up mechanically using a balloon catheter or dilatator and infused with fibrinolytic agent (by means of the lacing technique). For synthetic shunts, Davis et al. describe a technique in which two catheters are introduced into the shunt from opposite directions, and a fibrinolytic agent is injected into both arms of the shunt simultaneously. Subsequently, 2000 IU urokinase per minute (solution 4000 IU per mL) is injected, up to an overall dose of 150,000 to 250,000 IU, until arterial flow is reestablished, so that in total 300,000 to 500,000 IU urokinase is administered.

- Infiltration lysis using pulsed-spray lysis according to Valji et al.[17] After puncture using the usual technique, the fibrinolytic agent is finely dispersed in small doses at high pressure over a large area via a special pulse-spray catheter with numerous side holes. With this technique, two catheters can be introduced into the graft from opposite directions, as described by Davis et al.[15] A dose of 150,000 IU urokinase (solution 25,000 IU per mL) is administered within 15 to 20 minutes at two pulses per minute. Subsequently, lysis is continued at one pulse per minute up to a total dose of 300,000 IU.

MECHANICAL THROMBECTOMY

Various mechanical thrombectomy systems have been developed as an alternative to lysis therapy. These include:

- Aspiration thrombectomy
- Mechanically accelerated aspiration using rotation, ultrasound, and vibration
- Embolectomy systems such as Fogarty balloons, miniature Dormia basket, or mesh basket
- Hydrodynamic thrombectomy systems

The technically simplest and cheapest method is aspiration thrombectomy, which has also been used in hemodialysis shunts as an additional procedure in lysis therapy.[17] Turmel-Rodrigues has extensively used this technique in hemodialysis shunts.[18] For aspiration, an 8F guiding catheter with a formed tip is used, with which extensive thromboses can be removed, even in curved venous sections.

Various mechanical catheter systems have been employed in experiments and a few clinical settings that perform thrombus maceration with or without subsequent suctioning off of the thrombus material. These include the Amplatz thrombectomy catheter (Microvena Corporation, White Bear Lake, MN) and the Arrow-Trerotola percutaneous thrombolytic device (Arrow International, Reading, PA). The first of these cannot be guided using a guidewire and requires a 7F catheter, whereas the latter is inserted via a 0.025-in. guidewire and introduced into the vascular system via a 7F catheter; it consists of a nitinol basket that rotates on a battery-operated system.

Hydrodynamic thrombectomy is another method that has been described for the removal of fresh thrombotic material and that has already been employed in hemodialysis shunts. Under pressure, saline solution is injected through a narrow lumen, creating a turbulent flow zone around the tip of the catheter. As a consequence of the pressure gradient, the injected fluid immediately leaves the vessel through a large drainage lumen (Venturi effect), macerating and removing the surrounding thrombus material as it does so.

Three different 6F to 7F systems have been used in hemodialysis shunts, namely, the Cordis Hydrolyser system (Cordis Inc., Miami Lakes, FL), the Boston Scientific Oasis system (BSIC Inc., Natick, MA), and the Possis Angiojet system (Possis Medical Inc., Minneapolis, MN). All three systems have been used with good technical success. A randomized study showed the Oasis system to have good results compared with thrombolysis in synthetic grafts.[19]

Our own experience with the Hydrolyser in >50 patients produced a high level of technical success in both Brescia-Cimino shunts and synthetic grafts without any particular risk of venous or arterial embolism.[20]

SPECIAL TECHNICAL DETAILS IN BRESCIA-CIMINO SHUNTS

With Brescia-Cimino fistulas, both the access and the procedure depend on the location of the thrombus. The most favorable access is from a position near the trunk. Arterial embolism is rare. If thrombus formation is found in venous aneurysms, the thrombus can be moved to the thrombectomy system by applying external manual compression, making it possible for the aneurysm to be completely thrombectomized despite the large diameter that would otherwise impair effectiveness.

SPECIAL TECHNICAL DETAILS IN UPPER ARM SHUNTS

In upper arm shunts (Fig. 13-5), it should be taken into account that the thrombus frequently extends up to the anastomosis, so that it can only be securely reached from a retrograde direction. Since there is an increased risk during thrombectomy that portions of the thrombus can be passed arterially, particular care is appropriate. If an arterial embolus is nonetheless found, it can be removed relatively easily using aspiration via the retrograde access.

SPECIAL TECHNICAL DETAILS IN SYNTHETIC SHUNT LOOPS

In synthetic shunt loops, thrombectomy on the venous portion of the shunt should be performed first, to remove the outflow stenosis that is almost always present. After this, the arterial portion of the shunt is probed and a guidewire pushed into the brachial artery. Thrombectomy is then performed over this guidewire. As a rule, a strongly adherent thrombus is found at the arterial anastomosis, which must be removed to prevent early rethrombosis.

An injection of contrast medium into the shunt loop must be avoided at all costs because, if the outflow is not yet free, the pressure created can lead to arterial overflow and thus to passage of thrombi into the brachial artery. Because of the acute

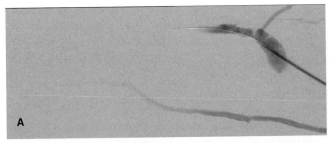

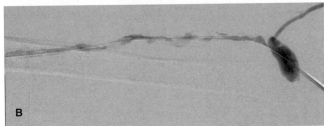

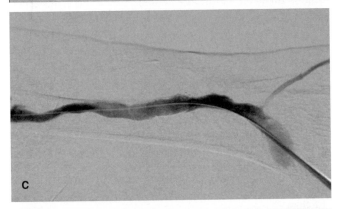

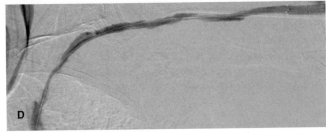

FIGURE 13-5. Upper arm native fistula and thrombosis. **A:** Complete proximal blockage of the upper cephalic vein due to thrombosis and **(B)** long segment stenosis. **C:** Recanalization after mechanical thrombectomy, stenting, and PTA of the proximal segments of the draining vein **(D)**.

angle of the anastomosis, aspiration embolectomy is technically demanding and sometimes impossible. In such cases, surgical thrombectomy should be performed.

COMPLICATIONS

In addition to the usual complications that also occur in PTA, arterial embolism is a possible problem here. Treatment depends on the type of shunt and the local topography (see earlier discussion), but should—if possible—be treated via a percutaneous procedure; aspiration embolectomy is of particular significance.

During thrombectomy, the occlusion material may be displaced into the pulmonary flow, which generally does not become clinically manifest. However, individual cases of clinically symptomatic pulmonary embolisms have been described. No cases of paradoxical embolism are mentioned in this connection in the literature. Because shunt patients frequently develop shunt thromboses or suffer a relapse, care should be taken to prevent more extensive thrombus portions from being pushed in a pulmonary direction.

CHRONIC VENOUS OCCLUSION

Occasionally, there are no early clinical signs of the occlusion of the shunt-draining veins. This is the case particularly when a sufficient collateral venous network is available. Occlusions of this kind usually manifest themselves by delayed shunt flow, increased venous pressure during dialysis, and extended post-dialysis bleeding time.

It is possible to attempt recanalization even in chronic venous occlusions. In our experience, the combination of a guiding catheter with a straight wire and moveable core has proved useful for entry into the occluded segment. If segments to be recanalized are long, success can also be achieved using hydrophilic guidewires or catheters with hydrophilic coating, which facilitate passage through the often strongly stenosed or atrophied venous segments. Balloon dilatation is subsequently carried out in the vein, and a stent may be implanted in the case of a particularly rigid stenosis.

According to our own experience, recanalization of chronic peripheral occlusions is successful in >80% of cases. Although the reocclusion rate is somewhat higher than in stenoses or recent thrombotic occlusions, an attempt is advisable because the procedure has hardly any adverse effects, even if the venous wall is perforated.

Percutaneous recanalization of chronic occlusions in central veins is of particular importance. There is no simple surgical alternative to this procedure, and patients suffer greatly from the often immense venous congestion with elephantiasislike swelling of the extremity. The technical success rate of percutaneous recanalization is high, in our experience, and lies at 80% to 90%. To ensure success, the procedure should be finalized with stent implantation.

STENT IMPLANTATION IN HEMODIALYSIS SHUNTS

The results after surgical or percutaneous revision of complicated hemodialysis shunts are comparable. The reported rates of technical success are 80% to 90%.[7,9] However, certain types of lesion cannot be adequately treated using simple balloon dilatation.[7] Furthermore, the long-term results of balloon dilatation of hemodialysis shunts are limited. Within the first 6 months, a high number of cases suffer relapse.[7,9] This is particularly true for central venous stenoses, which also tend to have shorter reobstruction intervals.[7,9]

There are two separate reasons for the use of stents in hemodialysis shunts

- To improve the technical results in particularly complicated cases
- To improve long-term patency

To date, various stent types have been used in dialysis shunts and in the draining veins. The Wallstent, Gianturco-Rösch, and Palmaz stents are used primarily in central veins, whereas the Strecker stent has been used in peripheral veins.[21] Clinical results are now also available for self-expanding nitinol stents.

TECHNIQUE

Implantation of endoprostheses is possible particularly in the area of the draining veins of hemodialysis shunts that do not serve as puncture sites for hemodialysis. Because the effects of repeated puncture trauma in the stent itself are unknown, implantation should be avoided at the puncture sites of native (Brescia-Cimino) shunts or, if it cannot be avoided, limited to an extremely short distance. In our own patient population, this concerned five of 60 patients (9%). For the same reason, implantation should not be undertaken in PTFE shunts. Stenting the supplying artery should be critically evaluated given the small diameter of the lower arm arteries and should be restricted to special cases.

With regard to the stent characteristics required in veins, it is necessary to distinguish between peripheral and central implantations.

In peripheral veins, arm movement and vein proximity to the skin mean that a stent must be sufficiently flexible to follow the arm movements and, if necessary, to tolerate flexions and extensions over a joint. Furthermore, the stent must resist compression. Since the course of the veins is often tortuous, the stent delivery system must be flexible, and not greater than 7F to 8F. The typical diameter of peripheral veins is 5 mm to 6 mm in lower arm veins and 7 mm to 8 mm in upper arm veins. In ectatic shunt veins, stents with diameters of up to 12 mm may be required in the upper arm.

In central venous stenoses and obstructions, the diameter of the stent is most significant and should be as large as possible. At this location, we prefer stents measuring 14 and 16 mm in diameter.

ACCESS PATHS

Depending on the diameter and type of the stent, insertion instruments of 7F to 10F are necessary. This fact must be taken into consideration when choosing the access. Brachial access should be chosen for implantation that extends into the proximal basilic and cephalic veins, because most stent instruments cannot reach this implantation site from the femoral direction. Stents into subclavian and brachiocephalic veins should be placed transbrachially if the shunt diameter is big enough, as the insertion instruments for large-lumen stents are, at best, 9F.

POSSIBLE COMPLICATIONS

Acute complications from implantation are rare. In our own patient population, acute stent thrombosis occurred in 6% of cases, but could be treated in almost all cases with renewed intervention. Possible causes are an insufficient drainage route or coagulation problems. One complication that should be noted is dislocation of the stent immediately after implantation or during the early course. In our own series, we observed one case in which the stent dislodged into the subclavian vein, but did not embolize systemically. Gray et al. have, however, reported two systemically dislodged stents out of 12 (15%) using the Palmaz stent.[22]

STENT PLACEMENT

Stent geometry and technical problems during implantation must be taken into account to avoid dislocation. If a short stent is chosen and the stent is not implanted exactly in the middle of the often very rigid stenosis, the stenosis may press the stent out of position, after which it will be displaced in the direction in which its longer portion has come to rest. If the stent slips in a central direction, central embolization is a possible consequence.

If the stent design permits a choice of stent length, as is the case with Wallstents or self-expanding nitinol stents, taking the collateral veins into consideration, the longest possible segment should be stented to achieve higher local stability by means of a larger overlap of the stent and the venous wall. If this is not an option, the possibility of the first implant sliding in a peripheral direction should be accepted as a risk, so that a second stent overhanging centrally can be implanted in the bed of the first, improving local fixation by enmeshing the two implants.

Collateral veins bridged by the stent generally remain open. Large veins, however, such as the jugular vein should not be bridged in order to avoid complications in jugular puncture and jugular catheters.

It should be noted that central venous stenoses may grow larger after implantation of self-expanding stents. This is particularly true for very taut stenoses in which the stent is greatly stretched on implantation. If these stenoses expand along their course as a result of stent pressure, the endoprosthesis expands with the lumen and, in the case of Wallstents, becomes shortened as well. As a result, the stenosis may be partially re-exposed and cause restenosis. The same phenomenon may occur in the treatment of occlusions, whereby here partial spontaneous thrombolysis also has a role. For this reason we consider self-expanding stents to be better suited at this location to adapt to the changes of the lesion.

If the stent diameter chosen is too small, this can also lead to direct dislocation.

When, following stent implantation, the stent must be after-dilated using a larger balloon, the afterdilatation must be done with the utmost care to avoid secondary dislocation or damage of the stent by the incompletely refolded balloon.

Quinn et al. reported on permanent peripheral nerves injuries after peripheral implantations of the Gianturco stents.[23] To our knowledge, however, no other reports of this kind of complications have been published.

INDICATIONS

From a technical point of view, stent implantation must be considered in particular cases of stenoses and occlusions of the draining shunt veins if simple PTA is not sufficient. This applies particularly to the following cases:

- Central venous stenosis or occlusion
- Elastic, recollapsing stenoses
- Bent stenoses, which often arise through widening and elongation of the vein in valve regions

- Remodeling of the shunt flow
- Complications of PTA or thrombectomy such as dissection and perforation

Stent implantation reliably maintains functionality in hemodialysis shunts that cannot otherwise be preserved. Stent implantation in puncture site segments should be principally rejected since no data are available on the puncturability of implants. If it is impossible to avoid implantation in puncture site segments, the implanted section is no longer usable as a puncture site, and the implant should thus be kept to a minimum length. A possible indication for this is splinting before aneurysm removal if the venous segment is stenosed.

Restenoses within endoprostheses can be treated percutaneously with no problem; they can best be treated using balloon dilatation. This is particularly true for central venous shunts. In peripheral veins, where diameters are smaller, it is occasionally necessary to perform atherectomy to sufficiently remove the neointima.

RESULTS

Of the available endoprosthesis types, the Wallstent is most often used in hemodialysis shunts, whereas the Wallstent, Rösch Z, and Palmaz stents are most often used in central veins.

In our own patient population of 60 patients, the rate of technical success for stent implantation in hemodialysis shunts is 90%.[24] This corresponds to reports in the literature. Since the indication is basically restricted to those cases where balloon dilatation alone does not provide adequate treatment and giving up the shunt would thus otherwise have been the only other option, these results are satisfactory.

The primary long-term results, however, have not been able to fulfill the expectations placed in them.[23–25] Primary cumulative patency in our own patient population was 56% after 6 months, 48% after 1 year, and 20% after 2 years. This corresponds almost exactly to the results that Beathard reports for balloon dilatation alone.[7] Beathard found in addition, using randomized comparison, no differences in patency rates between implant shunts with stented venous outflow tracts and those with just dilatated venous outflow tracts.[25] The studies published thus far show no reduction in restenosis rate using stent implantation.

One exception to this, however, are central venous lesions, which after simple balloon dilatation demonstrate a very restricted patency, below that of peripheral lesions.[7] The improved cumulative patency achieved in such cases by stent implantation corresponds to that of a general dialysis shunt population.[26] In central venous stents, there is strong proliferation of the neointima. Thus, although this frequently leads to restenoses, it only rarely leads to stent thromboses, so that these can be easily treated by means of repeated PTA. Since surgical revision is very cumbersome and difficult in this location, stent placement is an important and valuable addition in this area.

Overall, renewed intervention (balloon dilatation, atherectomy, stent extension, thrombectomy) generally permits shunt correction, so that even if primary shunt patency is low, the overall functional rate when all renewed interventions are included is a good deal higher. Here, overall function is regarded as the time during which the shunt is available for hemodialysis, regardless of whether reinterventions are carried out during this time or not.

The cumulative overall functional rate in our own patient population was 69% after 2 years, and 64% after 3 years. For central venous stenoses it was even better than this at 91% after 2 and 3 years.[26]

STENT GRAFTS

Stent grafts have played only a minor role up to now in the treatment of insufficient dialysis shunts. They are mainly used to secure rupture sites that cannot be sealed, and seldom to exclude venous aneurysms.

However, their significance may change if it is possible to reduce the restenosis rate using stent grafts. There are first signs of this with the use of expanded PTFE (ePTFE)-coated stent grafts; further developments must be awaited.

FOLLOW-UP TREATMENT

Follow-up treatment consists primarily of ensuring hemostasis at the puncture site. In scarred areas used frequently for puncture, a small subcutaneous purse-string suture has proven useful here.[27] However, this hemostasis only works if no fresh shunt is treated, because otherwise considerable subcutaneous hematomas can arise.

Special follow-up treatment with medication is not required, because good shunt flow is the best prophylaxis against acute restenosis.

SUMMARY

Percutaneous techniques provide starting points in the treatment of almost all possible complications in hemodialysis shunts and are not confined to pure stenoses. They can keep pace with surgical procedures with regard to technical success, long-term results, and complications. Restricted indications do exist, however, in freshly created anastomoses, long arterial lesions, and aneurysms. Shunt infections are treated conservatively or surgically depending on the local findings.

REFERENCES

1. Bell D, Rosenthal J. Arteriovenosus graft life in chronic hemodialysis. A need for prolongation. *Arch Surg.* 1988;123:1169–1172.
2. Keller F, Loewe H, Bauknecht K, et al. Kumulative Funktionsraten von orthotopen Dialysefisteln und Interponaten. *Dtsch Med Wochenschr.* 1988;113:332–336.
3. Beathard GA. Physical examination of AV grafts. *Semin Dialys.* 1992;5:74.
4. Nonnast-Daniel B, Martin R, Lindert O, et al. Colour doppler ultrasound assessment of arteriovenous haemodialysis fistula. *Lancet.* 1992;339:142–145.
5. Sullivan K, Besarab A, Dorell S, et al. The relationship between dialysis graft pressure and stenosis. *Invest Radiol.* 1992;27:352–355.
6. Sullivan K, Besarab A, Bonn J, et al. Haemodynamics of failing dialysis grafts. *Radiology.* 1993;186:867–872.
7. Beathard G. Percutaneous transvenous angioplasty in the treatment of vascular access stenosis. *Kidney Int.* 1992;42:1390–1397.
8. Bohndorf K, Gladziwa U, Kistler D, et al. Rekanalisation von stenosierten oder verschlossenen Hämodialyseshunts. *Fortschr Röntgenstr.* 1993;158:525–531.
9. Glanz S, Gordon D, Butt K, et al. The role of percutaneous angioplasty in the management of chronic hemodialysis fistulas. *Ann Surg.* 1987;206:777–781.
10. Gmelin E, Karnel F. Radiologische Rekanalisation von Venen Gefäßprothesen und Arterien bei insuffizienten Dialysefisteln. *Fortschr Röntgenstr.* 1990;153:432–437.
11. Gray R, Dolmatch B, Buick M. Directional atherectomy treatment for hemodialysis access early results. *J Vasc Intervent Radiol.* 1992;3:497–503.
12. Windus D. Permanent vascular access: a nephrologist's view. Am J Kidney Dis. 1993;21:457–471.
13. Kistler D, Bohndorf K, Günther RW. Kombiniertes chirurgisch-radiologiches Vorgehen beim Verschluss eines Hämodialyseshunts. *Chirurg.* 1990;61:84–86.
14. Smith T, Hunter D, Darca M, et al. Thrombosed synthetic hemodialysis access fistulas. The success of combined thrombectomy and angioplasty: technical note. *AJR Am J Roentgenol.* 1986;147:161–163.
15. Davis G, Dowd C, Bookstein J, et al. Thrombosed dialysis grafts. Efficacy of intrathrombic deposition of concentrated urokinase clot maceration and angioplasty. *AJR Am J Roentgenol.* 1987;149:177–181.
16. Poulain F, Raynaud A, Bourquelet P, et al. Local thrombolysis and thromboaspiration in the treatment of acutely thrombosed arteriovenous hemodialysis fistulas. *Cardiovasc Intervent Radiol.* 1991;14:98–101.
17. Valji K, Bookstein J, Roberts A, et al. Pharmacomechanical thrombolysis and angioplasty in the management of clotted hemodialysis grafts: early and late clinical results. *Radiology.* 1991;178:243–248.
18. Turmel-Rodrigues L, Pengloan J, Rodrigue H, et al. Treatment of failed native arteriovenous fistulae for hemodialysis by interventional radiology. *Kidney Int.* 2000;57(3):1124–1140.
19. Barth KH, Gosnell MR, Palestrant AM, et al. Hydrodynamic thrombectomy system versus pulse-spray thrombolysis for thrombosed hemodialysis grafts: a multicenter prospective randomized comparison. *Radiology.* 2000;217(3):678–684.
20. Vorwerk D, Sohn M, Schürmann K, et al. Hydrodynamic thrombectomy of hemodialysis fistulas. First clinical results. *J Vasc Intervent Radiol.* 1994;5:818-821.
21. Bosnjakovic P, Ivkovic T, Ilic M, et al. Strecker stent in stenotic hemodialysis Brescia-Cimino arteriovenous fistulas. *Cardiovasc Intervent Radiol.* 1992;15:217–220.
22. Gray R, Dolmatch B, Horton K. Metallic stents for hemodialysis access. RSNA 1992 Chicago Paper 195. *Radiology.* 1992;185P:134.
23. Quinn S, Schuman E, Hall L, et al. Venous stenoses in patients who undergo hemodialysis treatment with self-expandable endovascular stents. *Radiology.* 1992;183:499–504.
24. Vorwerk D, Günther RW, Bohndorf K, et al. Follow-up results after stent placement in failing arteriovenous shunts a three-year experiment. *Cardiovasc Intervent Radiol.* 1991;14:285–289.
25. Beathard GA. The use of the Gianturco intravascular stent in stenotic hemodialysis fistulas. *ASAIO Trans.* 1991;37:M 234–235.
26. Haage P, Vorwerk D, Wildberger JE, et al. Percutaneous treatment of thrombosed primary arteriovenous hemodialysis access fistulae. *Kidney Int.* 2000;57(3):1169–1175.
27. Vorwerk D, Konner K, Schurmann K, et al. A simple trick to facilitate bleeding control after percutaneous hemodialysis fistula and graft interventions. *Cardiovasc Intervent Radiol.* 1997;20(2):159–160.

Zubin Irani
John A. Kaufman

CHAPTER **14**

Venous Diseases

Image-guided interventions performed on the venous system of the body encompass a broad anatomic distribution. A practical "how-to" approach to management of these problems is covered in this chapter. Initially some generalities are offered applicable to nearly all procedures, followed by a regional approach to venous disease and interventions. Also covered are the various devices that are placed in the often-normal venous system to aid in patient management.

PATHOLOGY

Venous disease may arise from extrinsic compression. When this is chronic, such as in benign compressive syndromes, intramural intimal hyperplasia develops that further compromises the lumen, which can ultimately occlude from superimposed thrombosis. The specific etiologies and syndromes are described in the relevant sections. Central venous access catheters themselves narrow the lumen, and pericatheter thrombosis causes further narrowing. Otherwise, thrombosis of a normal vein can occur in a systemic procoagulant state.

The luminal narrowing impedes venous outflow, and given time, the body can compensate by developing collateral pathways to help in venous return to the point where the collaterals can be responsible for all the venous return when the main vein becomes occluded by superimposed thrombosis. Thrombus extension into the collaterals compromises venous return, and the acute venous hypertension that develops leads to edema, which, if left untreated, can be fatal in the brain and leads to organ dysfunction in the liver and kidneys. In the extremities, swelling is noted. Over time, this persistent venous hypertension leads to varicose veins and skin ulcerations, especially in the lower extremities. Thus presentations reflect the severity of the lesion and the acuity of its onset, along with the status of collateral pathways.

PRESENTATIONS

Inquire about the presenting complaint. An asymptomatic patient cannot be made to feel any better no matter how abnormal the images appear. Patients complain of swelling and pain in the draining territory of the abnormal vein. Acute onset of symptoms suggests occlusion from thrombosis. Look for edema in the extremities, and if present document the limb circumference. This can be used as an objective marker of improvement. Always examine the arterial pulses as well. Keep in mind the other causes for swelling such as lymphedema and heart failure. Skin changes such as varicosities and prominent collaterals, discolorations, and ulcerations should be sought. The aims here are to review the clinical data, make a diagnosis, and generate a treatment plan.

IMAGING FINDINGS

ULTRASOUND

A normal vein is completely compressible on ultrasound examination (Fig. 14-1), and Doppler interrogation shows respiratory variations and flow augmentation with distal compression. The latter two indicate no obstruction downstream (central) to the probe. The key finding for DVT is to visualize the thrombus within the vein (Fig. 14-2); acute thrombus can be echogenic, isoechoic, or hypoechoic to blood. Thus, this sign is not always present. Thrombus within a vein will prevent that vein from being completely compressed, and this is very diagnostic of thrombus acutely, especially if the compression collapses the artery and not the vein. Other findings include loss of respiratory variations and no flow augmentation on Doppler interrogation; in the absence of any local vein abnormality, the latter two indicate obstruction downstream of the probe.

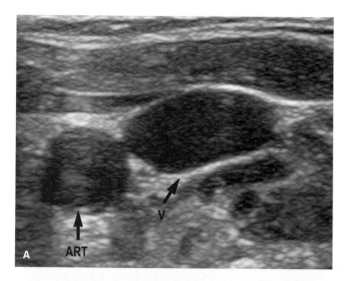

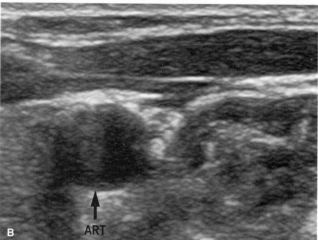

FIGURE 14-1. Effect of compression on normal vein. **A:** No compression on vein (*V*). **B:** With compression. Notice how the normal vein is obliterated. *ART*, artery.

COMPUTED TOMOGRAPHIC SCAN

CT with IV contrast usually shows a narrowed or absent contrast column in the affected vein (Fig. 14-3). A filling defect suggests thrombosis. CT also provides a look at the immediate surrounding tissues, which may show benign or malignant lesions causing compression of the vein.

VENOGRAPHY

Occlusions cause a complete cutoff in the contrast column, whereas stenosis causes a narrowing. Extrinsic compression typically yields a smooth margin at the stenosis; intramural pathology may in addition yield an irregular margin at the stenosis. Acute thrombus is frequently seen as a smooth intraluminal filling defect in more than one view, with occasionally a meniscus. With clot retraction, a "railroad track" sign (Fig. 14-4) is seen, which represents contrast filling between occlusive clot and the vein wall. With chronicity, the vein wall is irregular and narrowed and collateral pathways are demonstrated. Abrupt onset of disease does not give the body a chance to open up collateral channels. Specific findings are discussed in their relevant sections.

TREATMENT

Treatment options include medical therapy, such as anticoagulation, open surgery such as vein bypass, open thrombectomy, and image-guided interventions, discussed later. It is important to have a management plan prior to starting. The steps in image-guided interventions include venous access and performing diagnostic venography. Once a decision to perform an intervention is made, heparin is given (5000 U bolus) and the lesion is crossed with a guidewire. From here a sheath is positioned for angioplasty or stent placement, or, for thrombolysis treatment, an infusion system is introduced over the guidewire. These are discussed in detail.

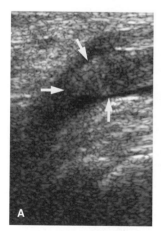
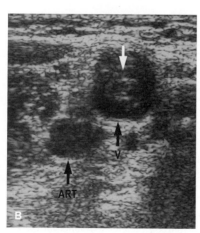
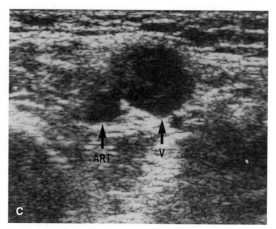

FIGURE 14-2. Ultrasound of deep vein thrombosis (DVT). **A:** Gray-scale long-axis image showing echogenic thrombus (*arrows*) within lumen of common femoral vein. **B:** Cross-sectional image without compression showing echogenic clot (*white arrow*) in the vein (*V*). **C:** Cross-sectional image with compression. Note that the vein (*V*) does not obliterate even though the artery (*ART*) has a reduced caliber. Compare this to Figure 14-1.

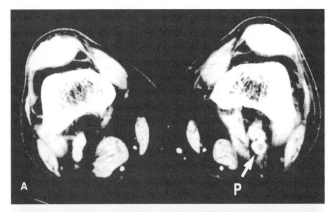

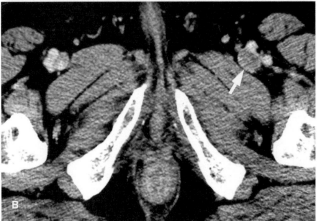

FIGURE 14-3. Computed tomographic image of venous thrombus. **A:** Popliteal vein (*P*). **B:** Common femoral vein (*arrow*). In each case notice the bright rim of contrast surrounding the central hypodense acute thrombus along with the expanded vein diameter.

VENOUS ACCESS (PUNCTURE)

All cases begin with accessing the venous system. Access can be obtained using surface/anatomic landmarks or image guidance, usually ultrasound (Fig. 14-5, Table 14-1). Study the planned vein of access with ultrasound, looking for the vein to be compressible with a hypoechoic lumen and having Doppler flow signal within it. These suggest a patent vein. An incompressible vein with echogenic lumen and no Doppler flow indicates an occluded vein. One can work through an occluded vein, but if this is not possible, then alternative access sites should be used. No matter what the guidance, sterile technique is used and local anesthesia infiltrated in area of access prior to skin incision and access needle introduction.

Either micropuncture (21G) or larger gauge needles can be used to enter the veins, through which guidewires can be passed (Table 14-2). Micropuncture access kits have a 0.018-in. wire, which passes through the needle, and the needle is exchanged out over the 0.018-in. guidewire for an introducer and sheath, which has an inner 3F sheath and an outer 4F or 5F sheath. The outer sheath can accept 0.035- or 0.038-in. guidewires over which it can be exchanged out for a larger diameter sheath or catheter depending on the procedure (Fig. 14-6). The same steps are followed if working through an occlusion. Once the needle tip is confirmed to be within the lumen (thrombus), the guidewire is introduced and advanced through the clotted segment into the patent segment of vein.

Augmentation Maneuvers

In cases where the vein is collapsed, the patient can be asked to perform a Valsalva maneuver or can be placed in an appropriate dependent position to help distend the vein for better

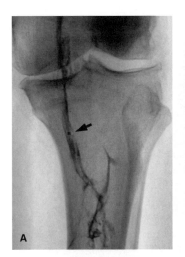
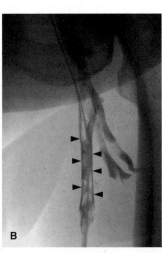
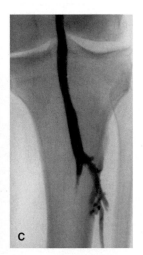
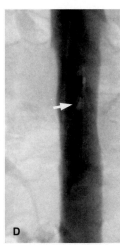

FIGURE 14-4. Thrombolysis in deep vein thrombosis (DVT). This patient had left leg DVT with pulmonary embolism. A jugular approach was used to deploy a filter first and proceed with thrombolysis through the filter from the jugular approach. **A:** Radiopaque tip (*arrow*) of infusion catheter positioned in the popliteal vein. **B:** Venogram at the femoral vein level shows the classic "railroad track" appearance (*arrowheads*) of active clot with arrowheads indicating the contrast on the periphery of the vein with central filling defect representing the thrombus. **C:** Venogram following 48 hours of lytic therapy shows excellent opacification of the popliteal vein [compare to (**A**)]. **D:** Venogram at time of filter retrieval shows a small clot (*arrow*) trapped in the filter. The filter was removed without incident.

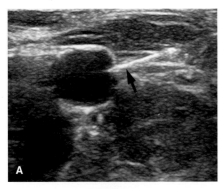
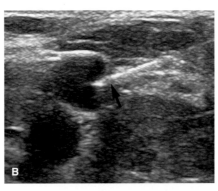
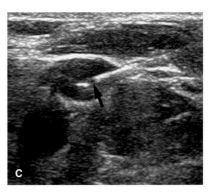

FIGURE 14-5. Ultrasound guided access of vein. **A:** Echogenic needle tip (*arrow*) positioned adjacent to vein wall. **B:** As needle tip is advanced, the vein wall is tented (*arrow*). **C:** Echogenic needle tip is seen within vein lumen (*arrow*). Now the guidewire can be advanced through the needle.

TABLE 14-1. Steps in Ultrasound Guided Venous Puncture (Access)

1. **Examine planned access vein with ultrasound**
   - If one cannot work through thrombosed/occluded vein, consider another access site
2. **Prep and drape site of access vein**
3. **Localize skin entry point over vein access point**
   - Anesthetize skin and make incision large for tools to pass through and blunt dissect soft tissues tract
4. **Enter vein with access needle under ultrasound**
   - Can use syringe with suction to look for blood flashback to confirm vein entry
   - It may be helpful to use a Valsalva maneuver to distend the vein
5. **Pass guidewire via needle into vein**
   - Troubleshoot as needed (Table 14-2)

TABLE 14-2. Troubleshooting Guidewire Difficulties During Venous Access

(A) Guidewire does not pass easily

(Guidewire "coiling up" under fluoroscopy)

1. *Double wall puncture (bevel beyond back wall). Ultrasound may show this.*
   - Pull wire back into needle. Pull needle back into lumen. Readvance guidewire
2. *"Tenting" of front wall. Ultrasound may show this (bevel indenting front wall)*
   - Advance needle until it "pops" into lumen and advance guidewire
3. *Bevel partially in lumen. This can give blood return.*
   - Advance needle marginally and try readvancing guidewire

(B) Resistance after advancing guidewire a short distance

(Guidewire takes unexpected course on fluoroscopy)

1. *Guidewire in side branch (Fluoroscopy reveals unexpected course of guidewire)*
   - Pull back guidewire and redirect under fluoroscopy
2. *Guidewire against unexpected stenosis/occlusion (Fluoroscopy shows guide looping back on itself/deflected into unexpected course)*
   - Advance sheath or catheter over wire and perform venogram to define anatomy/pathology

visualization and cleaner access. For jugular access, a Trendelenburg position is used and the reverse for femoral vein access.

Complications

Complications (Table 14-3) are typically related to inadvertent adjacent structure injury by the needle tip, usually related to poor or no image guidance being used during access.

VENOGRAPHY

This is used to define anatomy or pathology and is the starting diagnostic component of any image-guided procedure. The desired access site is usually "upstream" of the point of interest. Always bear in mind that more than one access site maybe needed to fully define an area of abnormality. Quantitative analysis of the venogram is performed with particular attention to the length of the diseased segment of vein and to the diameter of the normal vein before and after the abnormal segment and of the stenosis, if present. A measuring pigtail catheter or a radiopaque ruler placed in the field of view at the time of imaging can be used to perform quantitative analysis of the images where intervention is planned. With imaging software packages available today, direct measurements can be made. Note is also made of degree of collateral pathway filling. In mild stenosis, manometry (see later section) can be performed to further characterize the hemodynamic severity of the abnormality. In cases where there is a contraindication to using iodinated contrast agents, alternatives include gadolinium or carbon dioxide.

Upper Extremity Veins

Indications are listed in Table 14-4. Upper extremity venography is performed employing the digital subtraction angiography (DSA) imaging technique by hand injection of contrast into the venous system accessed with an 18- to 20-gauge needle or angiocath in the superficial veins on the dorsum of the hand, the cephalic vein, or its tributaries. If injecting via the cephalic system does not yield opacification of all the venous channels of the arm, then flow can be diverted from the

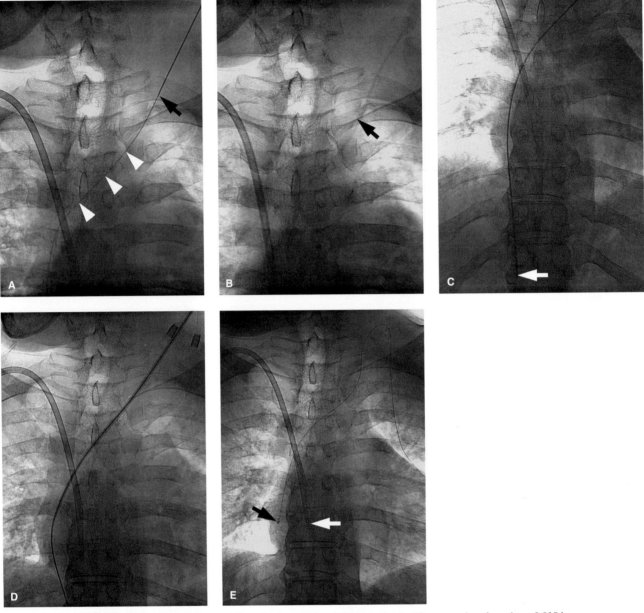

FIGURE 14-6. Steps in central line placement left subclavian vein. **A:** After accessing the vein, a 0.018-in. guidewire (*arrowheads*) passed via micropuncture needle (*arrow*). **B:** Needle is exchanged over wire for the sheath (*arrow*) and microwire removed. **C:** 0.035-in. "J" guidewire is placed via the sheath into IVC (*arrow*). **D:** Sheath is exchanged for the peel-away sheath through which the catheter is advanced into the central venous system. **E:** Note the tips (*arrows*) of both catheters are within high right atrium.

cephalic into the basilic and deeper channels by applying a tourniquet above the elbow. A 20-mLmL saline "chaser" bolus can be used immediately after contrast injection to flush contrast through the veins for better imaging. If the area of

TABLE 14-3. Access Complications

- Hematoma
- Pneumothorax, hemothorax
- Arterial puncture (e.g., carotid artery)
- Neurologic injury (e.g., brachial plexus)

interest is the more central veins (axillary, subclavian, innominate veins), then an antecubital vein or, using ultrasound guidance, the brachial or basilic veins can be accessed. If diagnostic-quality imaging is still not obtained, large-volume injections closer to the point of interest will be needed via a diagnostic (flush type) catheter using a power injector. An 18-gauge IV line will accept a 0.035-in.-diameter guidewire, over which an exchange is made for a "flush" straight or pigtail diagnostic catheter positioned close to the area of interest. Should contrast not flow easily through the axillary-subclavian vein into the brachiocephalic vein, a repeat venogram with the arm elevated is performed to show that there is no mechanical impediment to flow of contrast.

TABLE 14-4. Indications for Arm/Central Venography

To evaluate:
- Anatomy for possible hemodialysis shunt creation
- Anatomy prior to central venous catheter or pacemaker placement
- Suspected upper extremity superficial and/or deep vein thrombosis
- Suspected SVC stenosis/occlusion
- Suspected axillary-subclavian stenosis/occlusion (e.g., Paget-Schrötter syndrome)
- Suspected hemodialysis shunt dysfunction
- Suspected central venous catheter related stenosis/occlusion

Superior Vena Cava

The superior vena cava (SVC) and its innominate tributaries are best visualized by utilizing the DSA imaging technique and performing simultaneous power injections following catheterization with 5F multi-side-hole catheters of the axillary or subclavian veins via ultrasound-guided basilic or brachial vein access. The entire chest and mediastinum are imaged to include collateral circulation. In case of SVC occlusion, the inferior aspect of the occlusion is defined by catheterization into the occluding lesion of the SVC via the right atrium from a femoral route.

Lower Extremity Veins

Indications are listed in Table 14-5. Lower extremity venography is performed employing digital imaging technique by hand injection of contrast after securely accessing the venous system with a 19- to 23-gauge needle or angiocath in the superficial veins on the dorsum of the foot or the superficial vein of the great toe. The patient is placed in a semierect position (45 to 60 degrees) on a tilting radiographic table. To avoid any artifacts from muscular compression, especially at the popliteal vein, and to obtain opacification of the deep and muscular system of the calf, the involved leg is put in a non-weight-bearing position by elevating the uninvolved leg on a box 10 to 20 cm in height. A tourniquet is applied above the ankle and the knee to improve opacification of the deep system, and any compression artifacts from these should be noted. Images are acquired (Table 14-6) along with monitoring for possible flow of contrast from the deep to the superficial system via incompetent perforators after injecting 100 to 150 mL of diluted contrast (half saline, half contrast) and following the contrast column up the leg (ascending venography). The degree of table tilt is adjusted to help control the flow of contrast. Improved opacification of the thigh and pelvic veins can be obtained with a saline "chaser" bolus along with forcible plantar flexion of the foot.

TABLE 14-5. Indications for Ascending Leg Venography

To evaluate:
- Suspected DVT (in patients with nondiagnostic ultrasound)
- Suspected DVT (in patients with high clinical suspicion but negative ultrasound)
- Tumor encasement
- Venous malformations

TABLE 14-6. Images in Ascending Leg Venography

Anatomic Region	Projections
Calf	AP and LAT
Knee	AP and LAT
Thigh	AP & LAO or RAO
Pelvis	AP

Ensure there is overlap so that no segment of the venous system escapes imaging.

AP, anteroposterior; LAT, lateral; LAO, left anterior oblique; RAO, right anterior oblique.

With respect to vein access, warm compresses applied to a dependent foot can help accentuate collapsed veins, whereas applying elastic bandaging 30 to 60 minutes prior to beginning, to a foot that has been elevated for hours, can help reduce swelling. Ultrasound guidance should be used in difficult cases. Rarely, surgical cutdown is needed.

Inferior Vena Cava and Iliac Veins

The inferior vena cava (IVC) is best visualized by utilizing the DSA imaging technique and performing power injection following catheterization of the inferiormost IVC with a multi-side-hole catheter introduced via either the jugular or femoral routes. The common and external iliac veins are best visualized by direct injections of catheters placed in the inferiormost external iliac vein from an ipsilateral femoral access. For bilateral visualization, both femoral veins are accessed and catheterized as mentioned previously and simultaneous power injections performed utilizing the DSA technique.

Complications

Complications include those that are seen with any procedure, such as those related to access, and contrast reactions, including soft-tissue contrast extravasation in extremity venograms.

MANOMETRY

Pressure measurements either side of the stenosis can be used to obtain a pressure gradient; gradients of 3 mm Hg or less are considered normal. Gradients of 5 mm Hg or more are considered significant and, in a symptomatic patient, indicate a need for some intervention. A pressure transducer is connected to a catheter with side holes, and this catheter is positioned on one side of the lesion while pressure readings are recorded. It is then pulled across the lesion to the other side and pressures recorded again. Alternatively, simultaneous readings can be obtained by placing the catheter connected to a transducer inside a sheath that is also connected to a transducer and is one French size larger in diameter than the catheter, and positioning the catheter on one side and the sheath tip on the other side of the lesion. Simultaneous pressures are recorded.

VENOUS STENTING

Table 14-7 shows the indications for venous stenting. Self-expanding stents oversized by at least 15% to 20% relative to the normal vein are ideal for use in the venous system. For stent

TABLE 14-7.   Indications for Venous Stent Placement

- Subclavian and brachiocephalic vein stenoses related to previous indwelling central venous catheters
- Benign and malignant causes of SVC obstruction
- Iliofemoral and IVC vein obstructions
- Recurrent stenosis of subclavian vein following decompressive surgery in patients with Paget-Schrötter syndrome
- Hemodialysis-related venous stenosis
- Budd-Chiari syndrome

SVC, superior vena cava; IVC, inferior vena cava.

diameters up to 14 mm (vein diameters no bigger than 12 mm), 7F-diameter sheaths can be employed to deliver the stents. If larger diameter stent sizes are going to be used, then larger sheath diameters will be needed; consider accessing a larger vein to work from such as the jugular or femoral vein. Some stent options are presented in Table 14-8. Generally, moderate oversizing is of no significant consequence.

Crossing the Lesion

By definition, there is a lumen, albeit narrowed, in a stenosis. If large enough, a "J" tip guidewire should be used to navigate through the stenosis; the "J" shape protects from "digging" into the wall of the vein and potentially perforating out the side of the vein. If the lumen does not allow for this, an angled-tip guidewire will be needed to negotiate the stenosis. Either hydrophilic or nonhydrophilic coated guidewires are acceptable. If the guidewire tip adopts a "J" configuration during manipulations, use this configuration to full advantage to navigate through the stenosis for the reasons just mentioned. Using the guidewire in combination with an angled catheter can be more useful where the stenosis is severe.

With an occlusion, closely examine the venogram for any "nipple" that can be a starting point to begin probing with the guidewire. The authors' preference is to use a hydrophilic-coated angled-tip guidewire, although nonhydrophilic coated guidewires are an acceptable starting point. A guidewire alone does not have enough stiffness to "push through," and so a catheter is used in collaboration to give support to the guidewire to advance through the occlusion. Some patience and lots of persistence may be required as one employs a to-and-fro spinning and pushing motion on the guidewire using

TABLE 14-8.   Some Self-expanding Stent Options for Venous Use

Stent Name	Available Sizes (Diameter)	Delivery Sheath Diameters
SMART (Cordis)	Up to 14 mm	7F
Zilver 518 (Cook)	Up to 10 mm	5F
Zilver 635 (Cook)	Up to 14 mm	6F
Cook Z Stent	15 mm	14F
	20/25/30 mm	16F
	35 mm	16F
	40 mm	18F

the torque device. The guidewire may advance through easily, or it may advance a small distance and begin to buckle over. If this happens, try to advance the catheter up to the guidewire tip and see whether, with the added support of the catheter, the guidewire will advance further. It may be necessary to do this repeatedly until one is through the other side of the occlusion. Throughout this process, keep in mind the expected course of the vein from the venogram; should the guidewire appear to take an unexpected course, it is a good idea to advance the catheter up to the guidewire tip, remove the guidewire, and perform a gentle hand injection of contrast looking for extra-luminal contrast, which will have an amorphous configuration and appear stagnant with poor or slow washout. If this is the case, pull the catheter back to a point where you are confident of being back in the vessel, and try again with the guidewire. This time, look for the guidewire to advance in a different track than before. The guidewire tip has a limited motion while being advanced through the occlusion, but once across the occlusion into a patent segment of vein, the guidewire tip exhibits a more free spinning motion. Once across the lesion, advance the catheter across the occlusion into the patent vein on the other side. If the catheter does not advance easily, try using a hydrophilic-coated catheter or a smaller diameter catheter. For example, exchange a 5F Berenstein for a 4F glide-cath. Usually this advances easily. Remove the guidewire, look for blood return from the patent vein, and confirm this with a venogram. With the catheter across, you are in position to place a suitable guidewire to perform subsequent interventions.

If the starting tools do not appear to be doing the job, exchange for a different guidewire. Try a stiffer or larger diameter guidewire (e.g., 0.038-in. guidewire). If this is unsuccessful, the back end of the guidewire can be used to try and poke a beginning hole into the occluded segment. This involves just a short, sharp jab into the lesion. The region is then probed with the angled guidewire tip. If after trying different combinations and various tools one is still unsuccessful, it may just not be possible to cross the lesion, especially if it has been present for some time. The more chronic the lesion, the tougher the tissue tends to be, and thus the more difficult to cross.

Stent Placement

A sturdy guidewire ("working" wire) is used for subsequent steps. The authors' preference is to use a nonhydrophilic coated wire, such as a Storq, as the slippery nature of the hydrophilic guidewire makes it very easy to unintentionally lose guidewire position and even lose access across the lesion. With the "working" wire in place, the sheath is positioned close to the lesion and a road-map venogram obtained prior to advancing the sheath across the lesion. With a stenosis, the sheath usually passes across with the introducer. However, with a severe stenosis or occlusion, the sheath may not pass easily, and in such cases predilatation angioplasty will be needed. This creates a lumen large enough to pass the sheath across. Usually a 3- to 5-mm-diameter balloon, corresponding to 9F to 15F size, respectively, is sufficient for this step.

From here, the stent is introduced into the sheath and appropriately positioned with the aid of the road-map image obtained, ensuring that the entire lesion is covered and treated. If more than one stent is going to be needed to treat the lesion, ensure that there is overlap of the stents so that the entire lesion is treated with stents. After deployment, the stent is then apposed to the vein wall by an angioplasty balloon sized to the diameter of the normal vein, and a follow-up venogram obtained. Study the images to make sure the diseased segment has been treated, that the lumen caliber is >50% of normal, and that there is reduced collateral filling; if manometric readings were done beforehand, obtain follow-up readings. A larger angioplasty balloon can be used to augment the lumen caliber following stent placement. Also, look for filling defects from thrombus formation within the treated segment of vein. This is discussed next.

Complications

Access site bleeding can be controlled by aggressive and prolonged compression. Vein rupture is discussed in a later subsection. Always maintain guidewire access across the lesion, as this can easily allow one to place a covered stent across the rupture to seal over the point of leakage. The steps are the same as for stent placement, with the proviso that the sheath sizes required will be larger and an exchange for a larger sheath will be required. Should there be thrombus at the site of intervention, this fresh clot will respond to directed pulse-spray thrombolysis with adjunctive angioplasty to macerate and clear the clot.

Undersizing can lead to a free-floating stent within the venous system. Self-expanding stents cannot be stretched to a larger diameter with a balloon, and if there is guidewire access through the stent, another larger diameter stent will need to be placed within the free-floating stent to secure the stent. If the stent has migrated or embolized centrally, the stent can then be collapsed and pulled out via sheaths that typically are oversized by 2F to 5F sizes relative to the delivery sheath size, using standard foreign-body retrieval maneuvers with one or more snare devices to grasp the stent at different points. It cannot be overstated that maintaining guidewire access throughout all this is of paramount importance.

Postprocedure Care

Patients are placed on an antiplatelet agent for 6 to 8 weeks. If stent placement is done on the heels of thrombolysis, oral anticoagulation is also commenced, as for treatment of any deep venous thrombosis.

ANGIOPLASTY

The steps are the same as for stent placement, with the difference being, instead of introducing a stent the angioplasty balloon is positioned correctly prior to inflating the balloon (Fig. 14-7). Make sure the balloon is not within the sheath prior to inflating. Inflating inside the sheath doesn't help dilate the stenotic vein. The balloon diameter should match the vein diameter, and upsizing by 1 to 2 mm used if there is no response. If the lesion persists despite angioplasty with >50% stenosis, this indicates elastic recoil of the lesion and is a poor indicator for long-term patency, and stent placement may be considered.

Complications

Vein rupture (Fig. 14-8) is diagnosed on follow-up venogram in which contrast extravasation is present and can be treated by balloon tamponade, in which prolonged inflation (at least 2 minutes) of the angioplasty balloon is performed against the site of contrast extravasation. This may need to be repeated as often as needed if follow-up venograms continue to show extravasation. A covered stent can also be placed across the site of extravasation to treat the rupture if balloon tamponade is not working, and the steps for this are the same as for any stent placement. In sizing the stent, make sure it is oversized by at least 2 mm in diameter to get a good seal at the site of rupture.

VENOUS THROMBOLYSIS

Indications for thrombolysis are presented in Table 14-9. Ensure that there is no contraindication to thrombolysis (see Table 14-10). Thrombolysis is best applied to acute thrombus with onset of symptoms within the past 14 days. The aim is to re-establish flow quickly, and mechanical thrombectomy can be performed prior to commencing thrombolysis. Preoperative blood work includes PT, PTT, fibrinogen levels, hematocrit, and platelet counts.

Crossing the Lesion

The steps involved are going to be similar to the other procedures (see the section on venous stenting); define the anatomy/pathology and this will require venous access and a

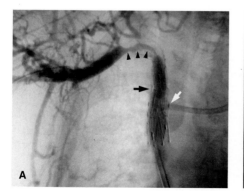
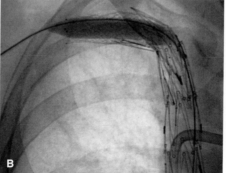
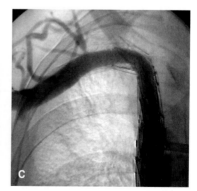

FIGURE 14-7. **A:** This patient has had venous stenosis treated with stent placement. A Z stent (*arrow*) is present more centrally with a dialysis catheter (*white arrow*) placed through its wide interstices. The subclavian vein shows in-stent restenosis (*arrowheads*) with considerable collateral filling. **B:** Angioplasty alone was performed, and follow-up venogram **C:** shows a much improved venographic result with reduced collateral pathway filling.

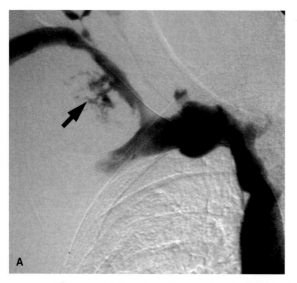

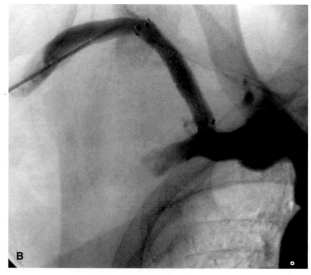

FIGURE 14-8. Complication of angioplasty. **A:** Venogram showing contrast extravasation (*arrow*) into soft tissues indicating vein rupture following angioplasty. **B:** A covered stent was placed across the site of rupture, with follow-up venogram showing no contrast extravasation.

venogram, cross the lesion using road-map image guidance as described earlier. Usually, the guidewire passes effortlessly through acute soft thrombus.

Administering Thrombolysis

Study the venogram to determine the length of vein that needs treatment. Place the infusion system across the lesion so that entire lesion will be bathed in thrombolytic. The infusion system can be composed of using just one catheter with multiple side holes for infusion, or multiple catheter systems in a coaxial fashion (two or three can be utilized) to bathe a longer segment of thrombus (Fig. 14-9). This is better than treating short segments of the thrombus in overlapping fashion by repo-

sitioning the catheter with each follow up venogram until the entire thrombus is treated. Once in position, intrathrombotic

TABLE 14-10. Some Contraindications to Thrombolysis

Ongoing or recent bleeding
• Active internal bleeding
• Recent GI bleed
At risk for precipitating bleeding
• Recent stroke (within 6 months)
• Recent major surgery including biopsy (within 14 days)
• Known coagulopathy
• Recent trauma
Situations where bleeding can be devastating
• Intracerebral neoplasm
• Pregnancy
Known allergy to thrombolytics
Severe uncontrolled hypertension (diastolic >110 mm Hg)
Bacterial endocarditis

TABLE 14-9. Indications for Thrombolysis

• No contraindication to thrombolysis **and**
• Acute DVT (<14 days symptom duration)

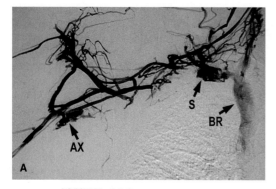

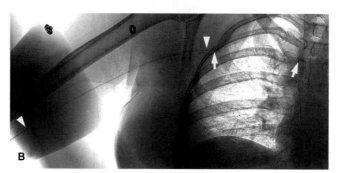

FIGURE 14-9. **A:** Venogram showing upper extremity thrombosis. Segments of the axillary (*AX*) and subclavian (*S*) veins are seen. Notice the collateral channels draining via the neck to return contrast into the brachiocephalic vein (*BR*). **B:** This long segment of venous thrombosis required a coaxial setup with outer 5F and inner 3F infusion catheters so that the entire length of thrombus could be infused with the thrombolytic agent. (*Arrows*) Infusion span on the 3F catheter; (*arrowheads*) the same on the 5F catheter.

lacing using "pulse spray" technique is performed. This involves administering a dose of thrombolytic agent (Table 14-11) in small, short, sharp "pulses" directly into the thrombus. The dose is drawn up in a small syringe (1 to 3 mL), and every 30 seconds a small volume of 0.1 mL or so is "pulsed" into the thrombus. This has the advantage of directly "lacing" the thrombus with the agent, and the "pulsing" theoretically has some mechanical action to cause channels in the thrombus to increase the surface area within the thrombus for the thrombolytic to take effect. The infusion system (Table 14-12) is securely fastened to the patient to maintain position of the infusion system within the thrombus. The thrombolytic infusion is commenced at the chosen rate. Subtherapeutic anticoagulation with a heparin infusion at 500 U per hour following a 2500-U bolus is simultaneously started to prevent further thrombus from forming. Aim for a PTT of 1.5 to 2.0 times normal. If an extremity is being treated, this is elevated above the level of the heart to help with venous return.

The patient is admitted to a step-down or intensive care unit to be closely monitored for complications. Intravenous punctures and intramuscular injections are avoided.

Follow-up

The infusion system is injected with contrast every 6 to 12 hours to assess for response. Thrombolysis should be stopped if clearance is achieved (>90% thrombus burden cleared), a complication develops, or there is no change in venographic appearance after considerable lysis time. This is a point of diminishing returns, which refers to a time frame beyond which continued thrombolysis only increases risk of bleeding complications with minimal further clot lysis. Rarely is lysis carried out beyond 72 hours; usually, it is stopped at the 48-hour point.

During any of the checks, some maneuvers can be used to mechanically reduce the clot burden and further help pharmacologic thrombectomy. The mechanical thrombectomy methods

TABLE 14-11. Some Agents and Suggested Dose Ranges

Thrombolytic Agent	Half-life	Dose Ranges [Lacing Dose in Brackets]
Reteplase	15 min	0.5–1.0 U/hr [2–5 U]
rtPA	5 min	0.5–1.0 mg/hr [5–10 mg]

TABLE 14-12. Possible Infusion Systems

1. Single catheter (3F or 5F) with infusion side holes
   - The side holes span various distances to cover lesions of various lengths. Choose the length with the best match
2. Coaxial systems using multiple catheter combinations
   - 5F infusion catheter with coaxial 3F infusion catheter
   - Triaxial system (outer sheath 5F or 6F, with coaxial inner 5F infusion catheter and 3F infusion catheter). Lytic can be spread over longer span using such systems
   - Total dose is split between number of catheters

No matter which system is employed, patient must be in a closely monitored setting so developing complications can be detected early and managed appropriately.

macerate the thrombus and physically remove the clot from the vein. There are various devices on the market for this. Alternatively, an angioplasty balloon can be inflated within the thrombus to macerate the clot and the inflated balloon can be advanced to push some of the thrombus out of the vein. Size the balloon diameter to be no larger than the vein. To do this, over a guidewire, the infusion system is exchanged out and a sheath is placed that will accept the balloon. If this sheath is going to have a larger diameter than the infusion system, plan to use the infusion system through this sheath; otherwise a hematoma will develop at the access site. Through the sheath a road-map image is obtained to guide balloon positioning. Regular catheters can also be used; if a pigtail catheter can be formed, this is rotated aggressively within the clot. The spinning end of the pigtail scours the thrombus and may also fragment it into smaller pieces. A guidewire can be placed tip-to-tip within the pigtail to offer some robustness to obtain maximum effect.

If during the thrombolysis treatment there are findings to suggest pulmonary embolism, the authors have a low threshold to place a temporary vena cava filtration device in either the IVC for lower extremity lysis, or the SVC for upper extremity lysis. If an underlying lesion is revealed, this will need definitive treatment such as open surgery, angioplasty, or stent placement.

Fibrinogen levels can be measured to follow the systemic effect of the lytic agent, and if this falls below 50% of its initial value or is <100 mg per dL, there is risk of bleeding complication and the lytic dose is decreased, usually halved, until the fibrinogen level returns to a level >100 mg per dL. This practice is not used at the authors' institution.

Choice of agent is operator or institution dependent. Get comfortable with one or two agents. Following lysis, therapeutic anticoagulation with a vitamin K antagonist is commenced as for any DVT treatment. And a quick point of note is that if one is going to perform stent placement immediately after the thrombolytic treatment, use a new access site to minimize chances of infection.

Results

Early results suggested that systemic IV thrombolysis (streptokinase) had better results for treating DVT than systemic IV anticoagulation (heparin).[1] Catheter-directed thrombolysis into the thrombus has better efficacy compared with systemic administration of the lytic agent.[2,3] This also results in lower doses being used with lower complications. Although the majority of the reports are on the use of urokinase, some early results of use of other agents suggests that the outcomes are essentially no different from one thrombolytic agent to another.[4-7] Success rates in achieving >50% clot clearance range from 79% to 100%.[4,8] See the "Outcomes" subsection in the section on iliac and femoral venous disease for specific results.

Complications

The main complications include bleeding and embolization; in the venous system, this results in pulmonary embolism. For iliofemoral thrombolysis, the pulmonary embolism (PE) rate in patients who did not receive an IVC filter is on the order of 1%, whereas in those who did have an IVC filter placed, no PE was reported.[4,8] Bleeding complications (6% to 25%) were commonest at the access site, followed by retroperitoneal bleeds.[4,5,8,9] Kasirajian et al.[10] employed mechanical thrombectomy devices to debulk the thrombus burden prior to thrombolytic administration and reported using far less thrombolytic agent, with no significant bleeding complications. With shorter infusion times and lower thrombolytic doses, it is likely that complication rates will be decreased.[11,12]

AXILLARY-SUBCLAVIAN (UPPER EXTREMITY) VENOUS DISEASE

PRESENTATIONS

Etiologies for axillary-subclavian vein disease are listed in Table 14-13. Patients complain of pain and swelling in the ipsilateral upper extremity, and in addition, females may notice breast swelling. Look for a history of central venous catheter placement, malignancy, radiation treatment, dialysis fistulas, and hypercoagulable states. PE from an upper-extremity DVT is uncommon. In the absence of any local cause, a procoagulant state should be sought. Paget-von Schrötter syndrome typically presents in a young patient with axillary-subclavian thrombosis involving the dominant extremity (Table 14-14).

IMAGING FINDINGS

Ultrasound

Ultrasound is used to confirm suspected DVT.

TABLE 14-13. Causes of Axillary and Subclavian Stenosis/Occlusion

Extramural
- Musculoskeletal structures (e.g., Paget-Schrötter)
- Neoplasms (including lymphadenopathy)

Intramural (intimal hyperplasia/thickening)
- Catheter related (lines, pacemaker leads)
- Outflow veins of dialysis fistulas
- Radiation changes

Intraluminal (thrombosis)
- Superimposed on above causes
- Systemic hypercoagulable state (factor V lidin, deficiency of protein C, S, and antithrombin III, malignancy)

TABLE 14-14. Features of Paget-Schrötter Syndrome

Also known as thoracic outlet syndrome (venous form) and effort thrombosis of the subclavian vein

A compressive syndrome of the axillary-subclavian vein between first rib and subclavius tendon/costoclavicular ligament (but can be in subacromial space or from pectoralis minor impingement)
- Chronic intimal injury results from shoulder activity leading to hyperplasia, luminal narrowing, sluggish flow, and ultimately thrombosis and occlusion.

Clinical findings
- Males 2 times more commonly affected
- Age 20s to 40s
- Right side more commonly involved than left
- Accounts for about 5% of upper-extremity thrombosis

CT Scan

A CT scan is obtained if the clinical picture is not typical for thoracic outlet compressive syndrome or catheter-related complication. An IV contrast-enhanced CT of the neck and chest should be reviewed for level of occlusion and presence of collaterals, and for clues to etiology such as cervical ribs, bony exostosis, hypertrophied muscles, or soft tissue masses that may suggest malignancies.

Venography

This may show occlusion or stenosis that usually has an irregular appearance as the vein courses behind the clavicle and over the first rib in thoracic outlet syndrome. Important collaterals are listed in Table 14-15, and their presence will indicate an underlying chronic process (Fig. 14-10).

TREATMENT DETAILS

Central venous catheters will comprise the majority of cases. Catheter placement itself narrows the venous lumen, and pericatheter thrombus formation further reduces the lumen caliber. It can provoke intimal hyperplasia, which progresses to narrow down the venous lumen around the catheter. Once this reaches a critical point, the flows are reduced and thrombus

TABLE 14-15. Key Collateral Pathways in Stenosis/Occlusion of Upper Extremity Veins

Axillo-subclavian lesion
Muscular/superficial veins around shoulder
- These drain via jugular, brachiocephalic or azygos systems back to SVC

Brachiocephalic vein lesion
- Ipsilateral jugular veins into head and neck channels into contralateral jugular and brachiocephalic veins

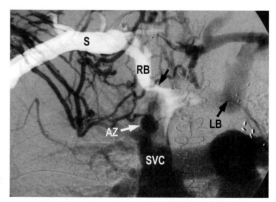

FIGURE 14-10. Collateral pathways in central venous disease. This is a late-phase image that has been remasked. Collateral drainage via midline channels into the contralateral brachiocephalic (*LB*) vein and also drainage into the superior vena cava (*SVC*) via the azygos vein (*AZ*) are shown. Both the collateral pathways return blood central to the stenosis (*black arrow*) of the right brachiocephalic vein (*RB*). *S*, subclavian vein.

formation occurs, occluding the vein. The catheter traverses the axillary-subclavian vein with the tip (the functional aspect of the catheter) being in the larger, more central veins such as the SVC or even in the upper right atrium. If the catheter is functioning, it is kept in situ and anticoagulation is attempted with heparin and a vitamin K antagonist aiming for an international normalized ratio (INR) in the 2 to 3 range, to prevent thrombus propagation into collateral channels that are critical to the patient at this point. This treatment also protects against possible PE. If there is a contraindication to anticoagulation, catheter removal will be needed. Once the catheter is removed, a luminal channel corresponding to the size of the catheter diameter is now available for blood flow. Most patients will respond to catheter removal. If other access sites are available, one can use these to replace the catheter so patient management can continue. In the few who still have persistent arm swelling, thrombolysis should be attempted. Should there be concerns for pulmonary embolism from an upper-extremity source, an SVC filter can be placed in patients who cannot be anticoagulated. Also remember, stenosis may be related to catheter placement that may have occurred some time in the past, and such patients have a relatively durable response to angioplasty.[13]

In Paget-Schrötter syndrome (Figs. 14-11 and 14-12) the aims of management are to perform thrombolysis to restore a lumen and remove the DVT as a prelude to the definitive treatment, which is surgical decompression of the vein. **Stent placement is not recommended primarily,** as the extrinsic compression can pinch off the stent, compressing and possibly fracturing it

(Fig. 14-13). Once the patient has had decompressive surgery and recurrent symptoms or stenosis develop, then angioplasty or stent placement can be done.

Patients with arteriovenous fistula (AVF) have high flows through these veins, which helps keep the treated segment of vein patent. In the absence of an AVF, stent placement overall does not provide durable patency rates because of the relatively low flows in these veins. However, in patients with a limited prognosis such as from malignancy, palliative stenting should be performed.

If PE from upper-extremity thrombus is a concern, and a SVC filter is needed, plan to use an optional filter (see the later section).

Axillary-subclavian Thrombolysis

The preferred access by the authors is the ipsilateral arm venous system, the other choices being the femoral vein or the contralateral internal jugular vein or upper-extremity veins. If DVT extends into the axillary and upper arm veins, plan to access a patent segment of brachial or basilic vein as this will allow the entire thrombosed segment to be treated and restore inflow into the axillary-subclavian vein. Perform an upper-extremity venogram. Using this as a road map, a hydrophilic-coated guidewire should cross the acute DVT relatively effortlessly. Once the thrombus is crossed, a single infusion catheter with infusion side holes of appropriate length is positioned to treat the entire thrombosed segment of vein. Confirm appropriate position with a venogram through the infusion system.

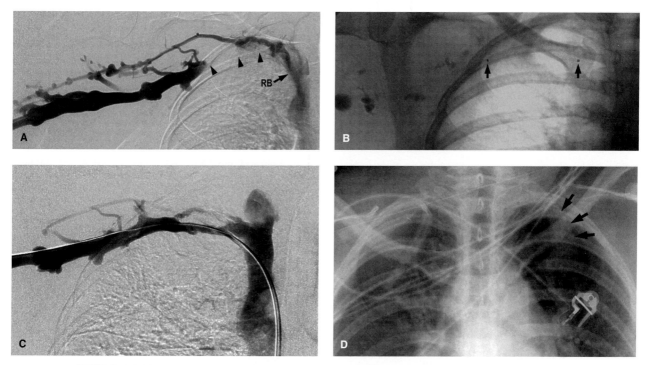

FIGURE 14-11. Paget-Schrötter syndrome right subclavian vein. **A:** Ipsilateral arm access used for venography showing occluded segment of subclavian vein (*arrowheads*) with contrast filling of the right brachiocephalic vein (*RB*) via collaterals. **B:** Arrows indicate the radiopaque ends of the infusion length on the 5F infusion catheter that was used for thrombolysis. **C:** 38 hours into lysis therapy, a moderate-sized channel has opened up with much improved clinical and venographic appearance. **D:** The first rib was resected on the right a few days later (*arrows*, left first rib for comparison).

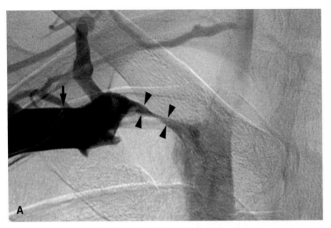 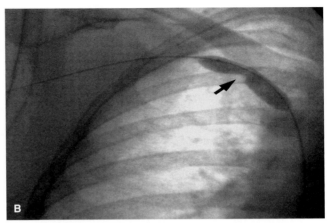

FIGURE 14-12. **A:** Venogram obtained with catheter placement (*arrow*) close to the stenosis revealing a severe stenosis (*arrowheads*) in this patient with subclavian vein compression syndrome. Thrombolysis treatment was carried out to restore a larger flow lumen and the patient then taken to surgery for decompression. **B:** Intraoperative angioplasty of the vein was performed after rib resection. Note the waist in the balloon (*arrow*) at the site of venous stenosis.

Pulse-spray intrathrombotic lacing can be performed prior to thrombolytic infusion. As the clot responds to treatment, a shorter infusion length should be used to treat just the diseased segment of vein. During follow-up venograms, mechanical thrombectomy can be tried (see the section on venous thrombolysis). Once clinical improvement is achieved along with improved venographic appearance (restoration of flow within the axillary-subclavian vein), thrombolysis is stopped and plans made to address the underlying etiology definitely.

Axillary-subclavian Stent Placement

Stent diameters required typically range from 7 to 14 mm. Because of the small size of the arm veins, arm access is not used if sheaths >7F in size are going to be utilized. The authors prefer to access the femoral vein in such cases and advance the needed tools into the axillary-subclavian veins from this

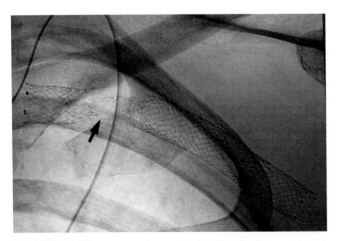

FIGURE 14-13. Fractured stent. Notice that the fracture (*arrow*) has occurred at the point where the stent crosses over the inner aspect of the first rib. This is why stent placement for Paget-Schrötter syndrome without doing surgical decompression is not recommended.

location. Make sure that not only the sheath but also the stent delivery system is of adequate length to reach the diseased segment of vein. If this is not possible, then evaluate an ipsilateral or contralateral internal jugular vein approach (Fig. 14-14). This is not ideal, as one has to negotiate some sharp curves from the jugular into the subclavian vein. Similar technical considerations apply even if one is performing angioplasty alone. The steps otherwise are discussed in the section on venous access. If stent placement is going to cover the internal jugular vein orifice, the authors prefer to use a Cook Z-stent (Cook Inc., Bloomington, IN) as the large interstices can allow for catheter placement through the stent (Fig. 14-7) via the internal jugular vein route and so preserve this option for venous access. This requires larger sheaths, and the femoral vein approach will be needed. If the lesion is already crossed via an arm access, the access can be converted to a femoral route as described in the section on SVC stent placement (Fig. 14-15). This obviates the need to cross the lesion twice, and the arm access can be used to perform road-mapping venograms.

In stenosis caused by benign etiology such as previous central venous catheters, angioplasty should be tried.[13] If there is recoil of >50%, this suggests a tendency of the stenosis to recur and thrombose. In the absence of high flows (such as in patients having hemodialysis fistulas), stents will also tend to thrombose. Stent placement should only be done after repeated failure of angioplasty or if there is significant elastic recoil, as discussed earlier.

OUTCOMES

Using a combined approach of image-guided thrombolysis, surgical decompression, and follow-up angioplasty or stent placement for benign compressive etiologies, especially Paget-Schrötter syndrome, long-term patency is excellent.[15] Results from occlusions from other etiologies treated with thrombolysis and oral anticoagulation appear good with little added long-term benefit by angioplasty and stent placement,[16] with restenosis rates in this location approaching 45% at 1 year with stent placement.[17]

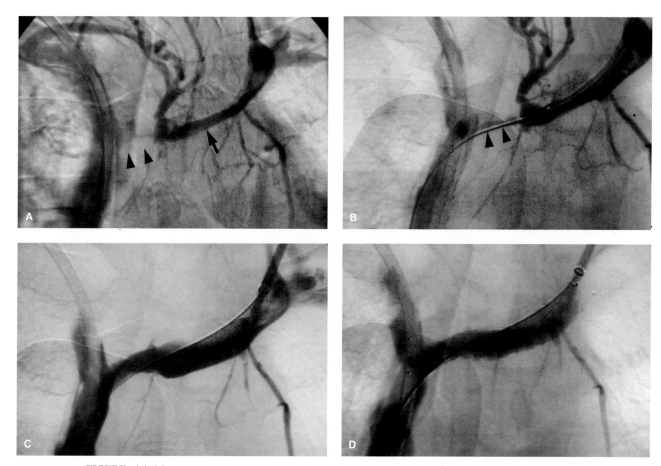

FIGURE 14-14. Recanalization of occluded left brachiocephalic vein. The right internal jugular (IJ) already has a dialysis catheter. The left IJ was accessed. **A:** The micropuncture access sheath was used to perform a diagnostic venogram showing occlusion (*arrowheads*) of the brachiocephalic vein (*arrow*) and midline collaterals returning flow to the contralateral subclavian vein. **B:** The occlusion is crossed using a glidewire (*arrowheads*) and angled glide catheter. At this point the access could have been converted to a femoral approach. In this case we elected to proceed via the IJ approach. **C:** Follow-up venogram is performed via the sheath following angioplasty of the vein. **D:** A 14-mm-diameter stent is placed with good angiographic result.

SUPERIOR VENA CAVA DISEASE

PRESENTATIONS

Etiologies are listed in Table 14-16. Patients develop SVC syndrome, in which edema develops in the draining bed (head and neck structures and upper extremities). Left untreated, severe edema involving the larynx and brain can be fatal. Patients can complain of headaches, facial swelling, and visual disturbances. The azygos vein is an important collateral, and lesions in the SVC below the azygos are better tolerated.

IMAGING FINDINGS

Ultrasound

Ultrasound has no direct role in imaging the SVC. SVC patency can be inferred if the jugular and axillary veins show respiratory variations and flow augmentation on Doppler interrogation.

CT Scan

This is obtained in suspected SVC syndrome and will show SVC occlusion manifested as no contrast channel in the SVC along with collateral filling. Adjacent compression by a soft tissue mass is typical in malignant etiologies involving the mediastinum. A central venous catheter may also be seen.

Venography

Central venography is performed as described in an earlier section. The authors prefer upstream access to the SVC from bilateral upper extremities. Important collateral channels are listed in Table 14-17. SVC occlusion or stenosis is demonstrated, along with collateral channels that will either empty into the SVC below the lesion (if lesion is above the azygos) or into the IVC (if lesion is below the azygos). The lesion may extend into the brachiocephalic veins. Injection via an existing central venous catheter will not be helpful, especially if the catheter tip is beyond the lesion.

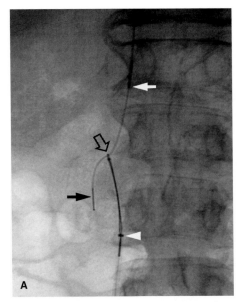
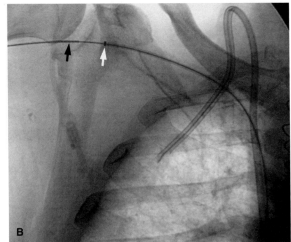

FIGURE 14-15. Converting upper extremity access so that intervention can be done from femoral vein after crossing a lesion. **A:** The diagnostic catheter (*white arrow*) and exchange length guidewire (*black arrow*) are positioned in the inferior vena cava from the upper extremity, and the guidewire is snared (*open arrow*) and pulled through the sheath (*arrowhead*) that is introduced from the femoral vein. **B:** At this point both ends of the guidewire are external to the patient, and these ends are held taut as the sheath (with introducer inside it) is advanced into subclavian vein. *Black arrow*, catheter in subclavian vein; *white arrow*, sheath tip in subclavian vein.

TABLE 14-16. Causes of SVC Syndrome (Stenosis/Occlusion)

Extramural (compression on SVC)
- Malignancy related
  - Thoracic tumors (lung cancer, lymphomas, sarcomas, metastasis)
  - Post radiation
  - Mediastinal (primary fibrosing mediastinitis)
  - Vascular (aortic aneurysm, brachiocephalic aneurysm)
  - Infections (tuberculosis, histoplasmosis)

Intramural
- Intimal thickening from injury
  - Catheters
  - Trauma

SVC, superior vena cava.

TABLE 14-17. Key Collateral Pathways in SVC Stenosis/Occlusion

Lesion above azygos vein
- Superior intercostal branches into azygos/hemiazygos systems. The left brachiocephalic vein can be part of this pathway

Lesion below azygos
- Azygos/hemiazygos systems via lumbars into iliac veins/IVC

SVC completely involved
- Superficial chest wall, internal thoracic and lateral thoracic veins into iliac veins/IVC

SVC, superior vena cava; IVC, inferior vena cava.

TREATMENT DETAILS[18–22]

External beam radiation therapy is the primary treatment for SVC syndrome caused by thoracic malignancy, usually from bronchogenic carcinoma. However, this takes 2 to 4 weeks for symptom relief and recurrence is seen in 10% to 32%. Stent placement is successful with symptom relief within 72 hours. Average survival of these patients is 7 months. Furthermore, there is no time to try thrombolysis, which may take 24 to 48 hours, especially if patients are severely symptomatic.

Lesions of benign etiology are treated on their merits. Angioplasty should be tried and stent placement reserved for recurrent or recalcitrant lesions. For lesions of benign etiology in a young patient, the authors favor repeated angioplasty and deferring stent placement for recalcitrant lesions.

If a central venous catheter is the cause of luminal compromise, anticoagulation alone is often sufficient. This also prevents thrombus propagation and possible PE. If there is a contraindication to anticoagulation, catheter repositioning or removal may be necessary. Most patients will respond to catheter removal, and in the few who still have persistent arm swelling, thrombolysis may be beneficial (see the subsection on SVC thrombolysis). If stent placement is needed, one can pull back the central venous catheter, place a stent, and then reposition the catheter through the stent.

A key point in SVC procedures is to be aware that below the azygos, the SVC is enveloped by the pericardium, and perforations in this location can cause cardiac tamponade. Also, stents protruding into the right atrium can be potential triggers for arrhythmias.

Superior Vena Cava Stent Placement

Refer to the section on venous stenting. Some further technical points are offered here for the SVC. Stent diameters typically can range from 15 to 25 mm. The stent of choice by the authors is the Cook Z-stent (Cook Inc., Bloomington, IN). Note the sheath sizes required for the Cook Z-stent (Cook Inc., Bloomington, IN) (Table 14-8). Access and intervention can be done from the jugular route; lesions low in the SVC are better crossed from an upstream access such as the jugular route. Arm access is usually not sufficient for intervention as the sheath diameters required are typically large and better suited to being placed from the larger jugular or femoral veins (Fig. 14-16). If one is using a stent other than a Cook Z-stent (Cook Inc., Bloomington, IN), then a 14-mm stent can be placed using a 6F or 7F sheath, which can allow for interventions via an arm approach. If one is more comfortable working from the femoral route for doing interventions, one can convert the jugular route to the femoral route. Use an exchange-length guidewire for this step; if one has crossed with a regular-length guidewire, advance a catheter over the guidewire into the IVC and exchange out the guidewire for the exchange-length guidewire. After crossing the SVC from above, position the guidewire tip within the IVC. Now access the common femoral vein and place the sheath for the intervention into the IVC. Snare the guidewire tip and pull it out via the sheath in the femoral vein. Advance a catheter from below over the snared guidewire across the lesion. Now remove this guidewire and introduce a new guidewire into the catheter from the femoral route and position the guidewire tip in the subclavian vein. Use a sturdy guidewire, as this will be the working wire such as a Storq wire (Cordis Corp., Miami, FL). The catheter is removed and the sheath is advanced and positioned

beyond the lesion. Now one is in position to introduce and deploy the stent. When working from the femoral route, ensure that the sheath is long enough to reach the SVC; in a person of average height, a 60-cm-long sheath is usually adequate.

One point of note when placing stents is to consider using a stent with large interstices such as a Cook Z-stent (Cook Inc., Bloomington, IN) if stent placement is going to cover the ostium of any collaterals or tributaries (e.g., left brachiocephalic vein). The wide interstices can allow for central venous line placement through the stent if needed in the future. Also, if stent placement is needed close to the atrium because of lesion location, minimize the amount of stent in the atrium and oversize the stent by an extra 2 to 5 mm to reduce any subsequent migration into the atrium. Arrhythmias encountered during stent placement are accordingly treated.

SVC Thrombolysis

The steps are as for any thrombolysis (see the section on venous thrombolysis). Access sites may be the arm or the jugular veins. If, however, a functioning central venous catheter is already in place in the SVC, this can be used for the thrombolysis infusion. Perform a venogram through this catheter to define the upper margin of the occlusion; this may require pulling the catheter's tip back so the tip is "upstream" of the occlusion. This maneuver itself will restore some flow through the SVC. Begin infusing the thrombolytic agent via the catheter. If the catheter is nonfunctioning, pull it back and leave it in the venous system (to tamponade the catheter access site) and use a new access site for thrombolysis. The other steps are as for any thrombolysis case.

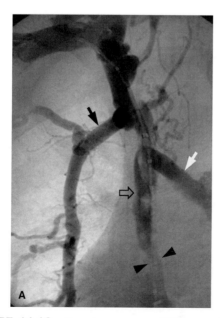
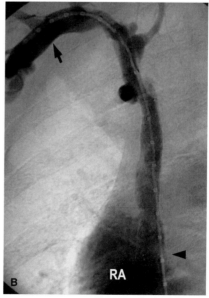

FIGURE 14-16. Superior vena cava (SVC) stent for catheter-related SVC stenosis presenting with facial swelling. **A:** Left anterior oblique projection diagnostic venogram performed via right common femoral vein approach with measuring pigtail catheter positioned through SVC stenosis and into right subclavian vein. Note the collaterals including the prominent internal mammary vein (*black arrow*) and azygos vein (*white arrow*) filling. The stenosis (*arrowheads*) is low in the SVC (*open arrow*) near the right atrium. **B:** Following stent placement, which extends a short distance into the right atrium (*arrowhead*), there is preferential flow via the SVC and no noticeable filling of the collateral channels. *RA,* right atrium; *arrow,* subclavian vein.

OUTCOMES[21,22]

Stent placement is technically highly successful (>95%). Failure to place a stent is due to inability to cross the occlusion. For occlusions of malignant etiology, primary patency rates of 85% to 100% at 3 months and secondary patency rates of 93% to 100% are reported. For lesions of benign etiology, respective patency rates are 77% to 91% at 12 months and 85% at 17 months.

ILIAC AND FEMORAL (LOWER EXTREMITY) VENOUS DISEASE

PRESENTATIONS

Etiologies for iliofemoral disease are listed in Table 14-18. Patients complain of pain and swelling in the ipsilateral leg. Acutely, if limb swelling is severe, this can compromise arterial supply to the leg, from either arterial spasm or tissue engorgement that raises compartment pressures to above arterial levels. This is phlegmasia cerulea dolens: a severely swollen, painful, cyanotic extremity without pulses. The risk of gangrene is high, and some of these patients end up with some form of amputation. This needs emergent surgical consultation for fasciotomy for decompression.

Not only will long-standing iliofemoral vein disease present with pain and swelling, but superimposed will be changes of long-standing venous hypertension including varicose veins, skin pigmentation, and ulcerations.

May-Thurner syndrome presents with left leg DVT in a young female. Its features are listed in Table 14-19. Bilateral iliofemoral DVT should trigger a search for IVC or retroperitoneal etiologies (see the section on IVC disease).

IMAGING FINDINGS

Ultrasound

Ultrasound (US) is used to look for suspected DVT. It has a limited ability to evaluate the pelvic veins and IVC. Bilateral DVT should trigger a search for a more central problem, especially with the IVC. Patent lower-extremity veins but with a reduced

TABLE 14-18. Some Causes of Iliofemoral Vein Stenosis/Occlusion

Extramural compression (from adjacent structure pathology)
- Vascular (iliac artery aneurysms, May-Thurner syndrome)
- Lymphadenopathy (neoplastic)
- Uterus (pregnancy, tumors)
- Gastrointestinal/genitourinary (tumors)
- Retroperitoneum (retroperitoneal fibrosis, sarcomas)
Intramural (Intimal thickening/injury)
- Chronic DVT changes (probably commonest)
- Radiation changes
- Trauma
Intraluminal (thrombosis/DVT)
- Superimposed on above causes
- Systemic hypercoagulant state

DVT, deep vein thrombosis.

TABLE 14-19. Features of May-Thurner Syndrome

Also known as Cockett syndrome, it is an iliac vein compression syndrome
Compression of left common iliac vein between right common iliac artery and the spine
- The intimal injury leads to webs and spurs leading to venous stenosis/occlusion
Clinical findings
- Female 3 times commoner than males
- Age 20s to 40s
- Left lower extremity DVT in otherwise normal patient
Venographic findings
- 3 venographic stages
- Asymptomatic compression (no collaterals and no gradient)
- Intraluminal defects (webs, spurs); usually asymptomatic
- Thrombosis
Management
- Good results with thrombolysis of DVT followed by self-expanding stent placement

DVT, deep vein thrombosis.

or lack of flow augmentation or respiratory variations suggest a more central problem.

CT Scan

A IV contrast-enhanced CT not only shows the status of the venous lumen but also gives information about the surrounding soft tissues, and can show soft tissue masses of malignancies, aneurysmal compression, and organomegaly. This should be obtained if the lower-extremity ultrasound shows no DVT, or bilateral DVT.

Venography

Ascending leg venography (Fig. 14-17) is performed if the diagnosis is unclear after US (Table 14-5). Otherwise venography is performed from either the jugular or the popliteal approach as part of the intervention being performed. Important collateral channels are listed in Table 14-20. Venography may show findings of occlusion from DVT. Once this has been cleared, stenosis of the ilio-femoral veins or webs or focal spurs may be present within the vein lumen. Findings of DVT are discussed in the earlier section on imaging findings.

TREATMENT DETAILS[23–28]

Acute DVT treated with catheter-directed thrombolysis may have better patency rates, lower venous valvular incompetency rates, and improved quality of life compared to anticoagulation alone for DVT management. Iliac stents have good patency rates as long as infrainguinal veins, the inflow veins, are patent; this provides good blood flow into the stent helping to keep it patent (analogous to arteriovenous fistula creation during open surgery).

Patients with May-Thurner syndrome have a good outcome overall if the acute DVT is treated with thrombolysis and iliac vein stenosis is treated with stent placement.

Stent placement below the inguinal ligament is not recommended; also, in the setting of poor inflow, such as no femoral vein inflow, there is a higher chance that the stent will thrombose.

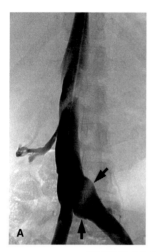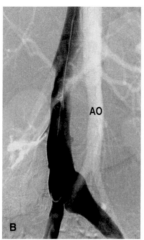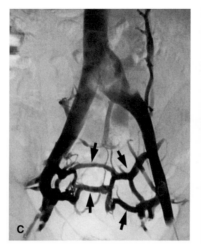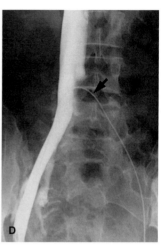

FIGURE 14-17.   Venography in May-Thurner syndrome. **A,B:** Images from cavography performed via right internal jugular approach for filter placement with imaging carried out until aortic (*AO*) filling was seen. In **(A)** note the lucent band (*arrows*) across the left common iliac vein, which with remasking **(B)** corresponds to the crossing of the right common iliac artery over the iliac vein. **C:** A different case showing left common iliac vein impression with cross pelvic collateral channels (*arrows*) filling from left external iliac vein injection. **D:** Note the up and over placement of the catheter (*arrow*) to perform a right iliac venogram and the absence of collateral filling. Manometry was performed and revealed no significant gradient across the left common iliac vein.

TABLE 14-20.   Key Collateral Pathways in Iliofemoral Stenosis/Occlusions

Ascending lumbar veins/vertebral venous plexus
• Into SVC via azygos/hemiazygos venous system
Trans pelvic pathway
• Cross midline collaterals into contralateral iliac system
Veins of abdominal wall
• Into axillary and subclavian veins

SVC, superior vena cava.

In such cases aggressive anticoagulation with antiplatelet agents and vitamin K antagonists may be the only option available to the patient.

Iliofemoral Thrombolysis

The aim here is to clear out the thrombus down to at least the level of popliteals, if not lower. If the popliteal is accessed, the point of access will be the lowest level of lysis. The steps in thrombolysis are discussed in an earlier section. Some further technical points of consideration regarding iliofemoral thrombolysis are offered here. Access options include the jugular veins, contralateral femoral vein, and ipsilateral popliteal vein. If an IVC filter is going to be placed, the jugular route is preferred (Fig. 14-4); otherwise the popliteal route to the thrombus is the authors' preference, as this approach is antegrade and one is not "fighting" the valves in trying to advance guidewires and catheters. If using the jugular route, be mindful to use tools of adequate length to reach the popliteal vein. Study the venographic images to delineate the upper limit of the clot. This guides the length of the infusion system that will be needed. Single infusion catheters with infusion side holes spanning 20 cm are available. For longer distances, coaxial

systems will be needed. Aim to treat the entire thrombus burden by placing the superior and inferior limits of the infusion system across the entire thrombosis. Follow-up venography is performed as described in the section on venous thrombolysis. Be prepared to perform mechanical thrombectomy to reduce the clot burden and facilitate lysis (see the earlier section). During the course of treatment, if pulmonary embolism develops, manifested by tachycardia and dropping oxygen saturations, be prepared to insert a temporary IVC filter (see the later section on vena cava filtration devices). Successful thrombolysis may reveal an underlying lesion such as a stenosis, and luminal caliber can be restored with stent placement.

Iliofemoral Stent Placement

Stent diameters will range from 8 to 16 mm. See the section on venous stenting. Some further technical points are offered here (Fig. 14-18). If stent placement is being done on the heels of thrombolysis, the authors prefer to use a fresh access site to minimize risk of infection, as the site used for lysis will most likely be 36 to 48 hours old and possibly colonized, especially with patients in an ICU setting. An antibiotic to cover skin organisms is given, and if the same access must be used, then a fresh (new) sheath is used.

In other circumstances, the authors prefer the jugular route as this gives slightly better purchase to cross lesions, especially occlusions. Be sure that the tools, including the sheath and stent delivery system, are of sufficient length to reach the diseased segment of vein.

OUTCOMES[23–28]

Antiplatelet agent is commenced along with oral anticoagulation for 3 to 6 months. Outcomes for iliofemoral stent placement show 50% to 85% primary patency rate with secondary patency rates of 90% to 100%. Improved patency was seen in

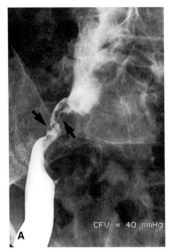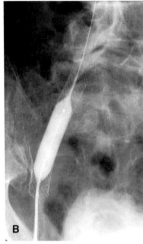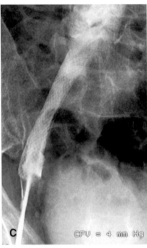

FIGURE 14-18.   This patient with known bladder carcinoma presented with acute right leg swelling. **A:** Diagnostic venogram via right femoral vein approach shows severe stenosis with an irregular appearance (*arrows*) compatible with neoplastic involvement of the vein. **B:** This segment of vein was treated with stent placement; note the use of an angioplasty balloon to help open up the vein and to oppose the stent against the vein wall. Follow-up venogram **(C)** shows no stenosis and brisk flow through the treated segment of vein. Pressures in the right external iliac vein also dropped from 40 mm Hg to 4 mm Hg following treatment.

right iliac vein stenosis, in the absence of malignancy and if a stent was placed (i.e., stent placement is better than angioplasty alone). Iliac vein stents do well if there is good inflow from the femoral veins. Late reocclusion of stents is uncommon. For DVT thrombolysis, patency rates at 1 year for iliofemoral DVT and femoropopliteal DVT were 64% and 47%, respectively.[27] These rates are improved if an underlying lesion is found and a stent placed; the majority of such cases are due to iliac compression syndrome (e.g., May-Thurner).

INFERIOR VENA CAVA DISEASE

PRESENTATIONS

Etiologies are listed in Table 14-21. The IVC syndrome comprises severe bilateral lower extremity pain and swelling, and in males scrotal edema. Ascites may also develop if the intrahepatic segment of the IVC is affected. In long standing disease there will be pain and swelling along with sequelae of chronic venous hypertension including varicose veins, skin pigmentation and ulcerations.

IMAGING FINDINGS

Ultrasound

Ultrasound may show bilateral lower extremity DVT.

CT Scan

An IV contrast-enhanced CT will show stenosis or occlusion; the IVC appears collapsed in extrinsic disease but enlarged with intraluminal pathology. In addition, surrounding soft-tissue abnormalities such as malignant masses, organomegaly, or abdominal aortic aneurysm may be present. Thrombus in a normal-caliber IVC is seen as a filling defect, and this can

TABLE 14-21.   Causes of IVC Occlusion (Majority Involve Infrarenal Segment)

Intraluminal
- Thrombosis (local factors or systemic disease)
  - Tumor extension (by direct invasion, intraluminal extension)
  - Extension of iliofemoral thrombus
  - IVC filter
  - Indwelling lines (catheters)
  - Hypercoagulable states
  - Others (trauma, idiopathic)

Intramural
- Membranous webs
- Resolved thrombus with mural thickening

Extramural compression
- Liver (hepatomegaly, hepatic mass)
- Vascular (abdominal aortic aneurysm, right renal artery, right common iliac artery)
- Vertebral column pathology (spurs, tumors)
- Uterus (pregnancy)
- Retroperitoneal disease (sarcomas, hematomas, retroperitoneal fibrosis)
- Ascites

IVC, inferior vena cava.

commonly be traced down into the iliofemoral veins. If thrombus is present, try to differentiate tumor thrombus from bland thrombus; the former may show contrast enhancement, and one may be able to follow it to its origin, such as the kidneys in renal cell carcinoma. This is an important point, as stent placement is not indicated for tumor thrombus. Review the CT to study the relationship of the affected segment to the renal veins; plan on using a Cook Z-stent (Cook Inc., Bloomington, IN) if treating the stenotic segment requires covering the renal vein ostium with stents.

Venography

Important collateral channels are listed in Table 14-22 (Fig. 14-19). A diagnostic catheter is positioned inferior and near to the abnormal segment. If the injection is performed well away from the abnormal segment, in the setting of good collateral pathways, the contrast may flow away via collaterals and the IVC itself may not be well visualized. IVC occlusion or stenosis is demonstrated; look for any collateral filling.

TREATMENT DETAILS

Because of excellent long-term results with stent placement,[29,30] this should be the aim when dealing with symptomatic patients with a stenotic or compressed vein. If the intrahepatic segment of the IVC is affected, one should inquire if the patient is a liver transplant candidate; stent placement within the intrahepatic segment of the IVC in transplant candidates can adversely affect transplant surgical technique. This

TABLE 14-22. Key Collateral Pathways in IVC Stenosis/Occlusions

---

Ascending lumbar venous plexus/vertebral venous plexus
• Carries blood via azygos/hemiazygos systems to SVC
Abdominal wall veins
• Blood from pelvis/iliac veins enters these veins (inferior epigastric, circumflex iliac, superficial epigastric) and via internal thoracic and lateral thoracic veins drains into subclavian and axillary veins, respectively.
Inferior mesenteric vein (IMV)
• Via hemorrhoidal plexus, into IMV, which drains into portal system. This is a systemic-to-portal pathway.

IVC, inferior vena cava; SVC, superior vena cava.

should be discussed with the liver transplant surgeons prior to beginning.

IVC Stent Placement

Read the section on venous stent placement. Further specific technical points are offered here. The femoral route is used to get access to the IVC. Ultrasound guidance can be used, or if there is a palpable femoral pulse, one can introduce the access needle medial to the pulse, as the common femoral vein is medial to the common femoral artery.

For the IVC, typical stent diameters required range from 15- to 30-mm diameters. This typically means using a Cook Z-stent (Cook Inc., Bloomington, IN), as other self-expanding stents are not available in these large sizes (Fig. 14-20). In long-standing cases, it may be difficult to identify the location of the IVC when multiple collaterals have developed. In such cases, look for a "nipple" to begin probing. Otherwise, begin crossing where one would expect the IVC to be located, and once across, advance a sheath and perform serial dilations beginning with a small-diameter balloon such as 6 to 8 mm. Increase diameters by 1 to 2 mm at a time. If one encounters a great deal of resistance with these small-diameter balloons, it may indicate that this channel is not the true IVC; pull back the sheath and guidewire and try crossing in a different location. If the lesion involves the IVC near the confluence of the common iliac veins, place stents in both common iliac veins and extend the stents into the inferior aspect of the IVC. This will require bilateral common femoral vein access.

IVC Thrombolysis

The reader is referred to the earlier sections on venous thrombolysis and iliofemoral thrombolysis. IVC thrombolysis is indicated for acute DVT <14 days old, and for patients with phlegmasia cerulea dolens. Usually the thrombus extends into

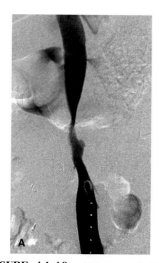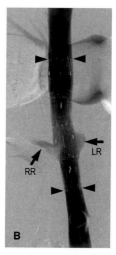

FIGURE 14-19. IVC stent. **A:** Diagnostic venogram from right femoral approach shows severe stenosis in IVC close to level of renal veins. **B:** The orifices of the left (*LR*) and right (*RR*) renal veins were covered in treating this with Z stent placement (*arrowheads*, upper and lower extent of the stent). Given the large interstices, there is relatively little concern over impeding renal vein outflow. A transhepatic intrajugular portosystemic shunt in the liver is seen projecting faintly over the Z stent.

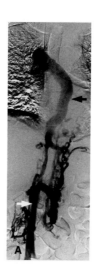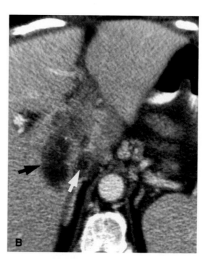

FIGURE 14-20. Collaterals in IVC occlusion. **A:** Venogram showing IVC (*white arrow*) occlusion in its suprarenal (intrahepatic) segment with the azygos vein (*arrow*) returning flow to the heart via the SVC. **B:** CT image shows a malignancy (*arrow*) in the caudate lobe of the liver causing the occlusion. Notice the small size of the IVC (*white arrow*), along with its low-attenuation lumen indicating long-standing thrombosis.

the iliofemoral veins, and in this setting, the technique is as for iliofemoral thrombolysis with the infusion system extended to include the IVC.

If the thrombus is limited to above the femoral veins, access either common femoral vein; if the thrombus extends into the iliac veins, then the ipsilateral common femoral vein is accessed. Following successful thrombolysis if there is a stenosis, which requires stent placement, and if both femoral veins have been used for the thrombolysis, then the authors prefer to use the jugular route to place a stent.

If IVC filter placement may be required, possibly in the suprarenal IVC if there is no room to place a filter in the infrarenal IVC because of the presence of thrombus, plan to use an optional filter.

OUTCOMES[29,30]

Overall IVC stents do well, with primary patency rates at 19 months for IVC stent placement of 80%; this rises to 87% for primary-assisted patency.

VENA CAVA FILTRATION

A filter is an intravascular device designed to trap embolic particles and so prevent pulmonary embolism (PE). As these devices are not involved with the body's hemostatic mechanisms, they do not promote thrombolysis or prevent new thrombus formation. If thrombosis has already occurred within the body, thrombus propagation needs to be halted and embolism prevented. Anticoagulants thus are still the first-line treatment option in thromboembolic disease.

DEVICES

Filters (Table 14-23) are grouped as permanent, optional, or temporary. Permanent filters are not designed for removal or repositioning. Filters that can be removed or repositioned include optional filters and temporary filters. Optional filters have design elements that allow for their removal or repositioning. These filters, however, **do not have to be removed** and can be left in situ to function as permanent filters. Temporary filters by definition **must be removed** or repositioned. These are for temporary use and are advantageous if removal, which is effected via a tether attached to them that exits the skin from the insertion site or is buried subcutaneously, is going to be definite.

PERMANENT FILTRATION AND FILTER PLACEMENT IN THE INFERIOR VENA CAVA

Indications

In thromboembolism management, filters are used when anticoagulation cannot be used. Two patient groups emerge: one in which the thrombus formation event has already occurred manifested as either DVT or PE, and the other in which the thrombus formation event is very likely to happen given the clinical scenario. Table 14-24 summarizes the indications.

TABLE 14-23. Some IVC Filters

Type of Filter	Implant Route	Max Allowable IVC Diameter (mm)	Delivery System Size (OD (F))	Max Implant Time before Retrieval	Retrieval Route
			Filter Characteristics		
PERMANENT FILTERS					
Bird's Nest[C]	Fem/IJ	40	13.8	NA	NA
TrapEase[J]	Fem/IJ	30	8.5	NA	NA
Vena Tech LP[N]	Fem/IJ	28 (35 in Europe)	9		NA	NA
Vena Tech LGM[N]	Fem/IJ	28	12.9	NA	NA
12F Greenfield[s]	Fem/IJ	28	15	NA	NA
OPTIONAL (RETRIEVABLE) FILTERS					
Gunther Tulip[C]	Fem/IJ	30	10	NS	IJ
OptEase[J]	Fem/IJ	30	8.5	NS	Fem
Recovery[B]	Fem	28	9	NS	IJ (with recovery cone)

Fem, femoral vein; IJ, internal jugular vein; OD, outer diameter; NA, not applicable; NS, not specified on the FDA approval letter.

C, Cook, Inc., Bloomington, IN.

B, C.R. Bard, Murray Hill, NJ.

J, Cordis Endovascular, Johnson & Johnson, Warren, NJ.

S, Boston Scientific, Natick, MA.

N, Braun Medical, Inc., Bethlehem, PA.

TABLE 14-24. IVCF Indications

(A) PATIENTS WITH PROVEN DVT AND/OR PE

Anticoagulation cannot be used ("classic" indications)

1. Complications while on anticoagulation (e.g., GI bleeding)
2. Failure of anticoagulation (e.g., DVT propagation, recurrent PE, patient noncompliance)
3. Contraindication to anticoagulation (e.g., allergy to medication)

ADJUNCTIVE USE ("RELATIVE" INDICATIONS)

1. Decreased cardiopulmonary reserve (any further PE may not be tolerated)
2. Tremendous thrombus burden (may be source of large, fatal PE)

(B) PATIENTS WITHOUT PROVEN DVT AND/OR PE ("PROPHYLACTIC" INDICATIONS)

Patients in high risk state for forming DVT/PE **and** anticoagulation (prophylactic in this case) cannot be used

---

DVT, deep venous thrombosis; PE, pulmonary embolism.

The main goal of management is to prevent mortality from PE. Some device options include VenaTech (B. Braun Med Inc., Bethlehem, PA), TrapEase (Cordis Corp., Miami, FL), and the Bird's Nest (Cook Inc., Bloomington, IN) filter. Typically this is done if it is likely that long-term anticoagulation use will not be possible for medical reasons or patient factors, such as noncompliance.

Contraindications

For IVC filter placement, contraindications are very uncommon and include an inability to access the IVC to place the filter and no room in the IVC for filter placement, such as with total IVC thrombosis. Ongoing sepsis should not preclude filter placement.

Preoperative Workup and Planning

Review the clinical data to determine which group of filters to use (see the later section on filters) and examine the patient to determine what access site is available for use. It is good to match the access site to the filter required. Any available imaging should be reviewed, such as an abdominal CT scan, to get some information relating to possible variant IVC anatomy. In a morbidly obese patient, where the fluoroscopy table weight limit is exceeded, plan to use IVUS guidance for placement.

Intraoperative Details

The goal is to place the filter within the infrarenal IVC as close to the renal veins as possible to minimize the potential dead space above the filter should filter occlusion occur. IVC anatomy thus needs to be defined, and this requires an IVC venogram.

ACCESS. Except for the Recovery filter (Bard, Tempe, AZ), which can only be placed via the femoral route, all filters can be placed from the femoral or jugular routes. In addition, the TrapEase (Cordis Corp., Miami, FL) and Simon Nitinol (Bard,

Tempe, AZ) filters can be placed via subclavian and antecubital veins in part because of the flexible nitinol alloy used for their construction. The access technique is described in an earlier section. Keep in mind that a direct translumbar access to the IVC can be employed (see the later subsection).

INFERIOR VENA CAVA VENOGRAM. Using DSA technique, injection parameters of 15 to 25 mL per second for 2 seconds are used with filming at 4 to 6 frames per second in suspended respiration in AP projection. Images should include some portion of the common iliac veins and the renal veins. Catheters that allow for such injection rates should be used; the authors typically use a 5F pigtail catheter positioned in the most inferior portion of the IVC just above the iliac vein confluence. Iodinated contrast is used, and if this is contraindicated, gadolinium chelates, 15 to 20 mL per second for 2 seconds or carbon dioxide 30 to 50 mL by hand injection is used.

The aim is to determine size and patency of the IVC along with anatomy of the IVC and renal veins. Table 14-25 lists the anatomic variations that can be seen.

FILTER PLACEMENT. Unopacified blood inflow into the IVC from the renal veins appears as radiolucent "streaming" in the IVC contrast column (Fig. 14-21). There may be some flash filling of contrast into the renal veins, which makes their identification easier. This inflow of the renal veins is noted relative to some fixed reference point such as a specific disc level or vertebral body of the spine. Having determined this spot, the pigtail catheter is exchanged over a guidewire and under fluoroscopic guidance for the filter delivery sheath, which is advanced just beyond the chosen reference point. The filter is then introduced and advanced to the tip of the sheath. Adjustments are made to the system so that the constrained filter is in the desired location and the filter is deployed (as per the manufacturers instructions). The delivery apparatus is removed from the sheath and follow up cavography is performed via the sheath using the same injection and filming parameters as before to document filter position within the IVC. Alternatively, a spot image can also be obtained.

Table 14-25 lists some alternate filter placement strategies tailored to meet some variant situations (Figs. 14-22 and 14-23).

Results

Decousus[31,32] showed that when compared to anticoagulation alone, filters do reduce PE. In this study in which permanent filters were used, filters did *not* increase the rates of postthrombotic syndrome (see Table 14-26).

Complications[33,34]

An incompletely opened filter usually is of no consequence and can be due to thrombus. The filter legs appear clustered or crossed. A cavogram should be performed to better delineate this. The patient can be asked to cough, and if this does not help, the filter can be gently manipulated with an angled catheter. If this does not work, and there is concern over migration of the filter, a second filter can be placed superior to the filter. If the first filter was placed via a femoral route,

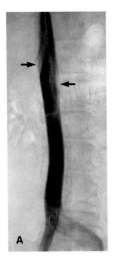
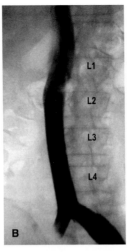
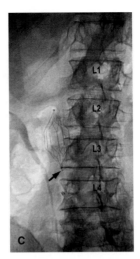

FIGURE 14-21.   Inferior vena cava (IVC) filter placement. **A:** IVC venogram performed via right internal jugular approach. Catheter was positioned at the common iliac vein confluence. Inflow of unopacified blood from the renal veins (*arrows*) appears as lucent streaming in the IVC contrast column. **B:** Pre filter placement cavogram via left femoral vein (right was filled with clot) showing mixing of unopacified blood from the renal veins into the contrast column creating a change in density in the IVC contrast. This is noted to occur at the upper end plate of L2. This bony landmark is used as a guide to deploy a filter in the infrarenal IVC (below the upper end plate of L2). **C:** An OptEase filter was placed in this case. Notice the hook (*arrow*) on the lower aspect of the filter for potential retrieval via a femoral approach.

TABLE 14-25.   Filter Placement Strategies in Various Scenarios

Scenario Encountered	Possible Strategies
Thrombus in IVC	1. Suprarenal filter (if no room in infrarenal IVC), or 2. Infrarenal filter, above clot.
Duplicated IVC	1. One infrarenal filter in each IVC, or 2. Suprarenal filter.
Accessory IVC (small IVC forming venous ring from level of iliac veins to renal veins)	1. Place filter in main IVC and embolize the accessory IVC with coils.
Circumaortic left renal vein (forming venous ring from normal renal vein via hilum into inferior aspect of infrarenal IVC)	1. If room permits place filter below IVC opening of circumaortic vein, or 2. Suprarenal filter.
Retro aortic renal vein (single left renal vein that empties lower in IVC)	1. Infrarenal IVC filter below vein orifice if there is room, or 2. Filter in each iliac vein.
Mega-Cava (IVC diameter >28 mm)	1. Place a bird's nest filter in infrarenal IVC, or 2. One filter in each common iliac vein.
Pregnant woman	1. Suprarenal filter
SVC filter needed (points to keep in mind)	• Keep apex of filter out of RA • Position legs of filter above azygos if possible • Avoid bird's nest filter (components will prolapse into RA)

IVC, inferior vena cava; RA, right atrium.

then a jugular approach will be needed for the second filter placement.

The filter delivery sheath can become kinked, especially if the access route involves a tortuous path, such as from the left jugular or left iliac route. If a kink is noticed, *do not* push on the filter; this can cause the filter to perforate and be pushed out of the sheath. Try to advance the filter and the sheath as a unit so that the kinked portion of the sheath is advanced into a

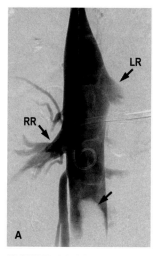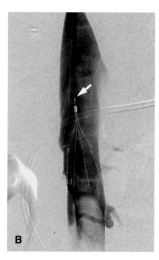

FIGURE 14-22. Thrombus in inferior vena cava (IVC). **A:** Venogram shows large tongue of thrombus (*arrow*) in the IVC approaching the renal veins (*LR*, left renal vein; *RR*, right renal vein). **B:** There is enough room in the infrarenal IVC, however, to place a filter above the clot but below the renal veins. A tulip filter is placed here. Note the hook (*arrow*) on the upper aspect for potential retrieval later on.

straight segment of vein, and recommence filter deployment. If this is unsuccessful, try pulling back on the sheath and filter as a unit to straighten out the sheath. If a new kink develops, pull the system back to the skin access site, leaving as much of the empty sheath within the venous system as possible. Cut the sheath so that the filter is removed and advance a guidewire into the empty exposed portion of the sheath, which is then exchanged out for a different filter with a more flexible design, such as a Simon nitinol (Bard, Tempe, AZ) filter. As a last resort, use a different access site.

Guidewire entrapment[35,36] of the "J" portion of the guidewire tip can occur during deployment of an over-the-wire

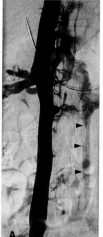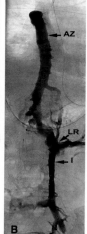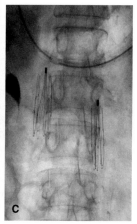

FIGURE 14-23. Duplicated inferior vena cava (IVC). **A:** Cavogram via right femoral approach shows some filling of a left-sided structure (*arrowheads*). The left femoral vein was accessed and venogram performed (**B**) showing a left IVC (*I*) that continues into the azygos vein (*AZ*). IVC filters were placed in each IVC (**C**) below the renal veins. In this case VenaTech filters were placed. *LR*, left renal vein.

TABLE 14-26. IVC Filter Placement Results

Outcome	Frequency
Successful placement	99%
Postfilter PE (filter failure)	5%
IVC occlusion (thrombosis)	5%
Symptomatic access site thrombosis	2%

IVC, inferior vena cava; PE, pulmonary embolism.

filter such as the Greenfield, or if a guidewire is advanced unknowingly during line placement into the IVC. Increased resistance to pulling back on the wire is the first clue to entrapment. Do not pull harder, as this will only make the entrapment worse. Advance a catheter over the guidewire to the point of entrapment and then advance both guidewire and catheter as a unit to free up the guidewire of the filter. The guidewire is then removed via the catheter so that the "J" portion is protected from the filter by the catheter. Be aware that such maneuvers may cause filter migration.

Filter failure (new or recurrent PE; remember that filters are designed to prevent PE), filter migration, filter fracture, and filter occlusion (remember that filters are supposed to trap clots) do occur. In filter failure, the PE source may be the lower or the upper extremities and may be due to a filter that is partially opened, malpositioned, migrated, or fractured. Remember that the desired treatment for any thromboembolic event is anticoagulation, and this is commenced in the absence of any contraindication. If anticoagulants still cannot be used, a second filter will be needed, above the existing filter if either there is clot in the filter or there is no room below the filter. In the setting of a well-positioned, structurally normal filter, place an SVC filter if an upper extremity source is present, or a second IVC filter if a lower extremity source is present (new DVT, or DVT progression). If no source is evident, assume a lower-extremity source and place a second IVC filter. Filter migration may be inferiorly into iliac veins, or superiorly into RA or PA. Asymptomatic filter occlusions require no further treatment. Otherwise commence pharmacologic thrombolysis-anticoagulation in the absence of any contraindications, or mechanical thrombectomy to restore some channel of flow if there are contraindications to former options. If thrombus extends above the filter, a second filter above it will be needed, in either the infrarenal or the suprarenal IVC. A second filter will be needed where filter fracture compromises filter function. Penetration or migration into soft tissues of a filter fragment or portion of a filter needs surgical removal only if symptoms are confirmed to be arising from that filter fragment. Table 14-27 summarizes these and their management.

TEMPORARY INFERIOR VENA CAVA FILTRATION (FILTER RETRIEVAL)

Temporary IVC filtration involves placing a removable IVC filter (optional or temporary kind) and then removing this device some time later. The ability to remove such IVC filters has introduced temporary IVC filtration as a further management option in thromboembolic disease.

TABLE 14-27. Complications and Management

Complication	Management Options
Filter occlusion (no intervention in asymptomatic patient)	• Pharmacologic thrombolysis/anticoagulation • Mechanical thrombolysis (especially if AC contraindicated) to restore flow • Suprarenal IVC filter
Filter migration inferiorly into iliac veins	• Place second filter above in IVC
Filter migration superiorly into RA/PA	• If possible attempt percutaneous filter retrieval/repositioning or • Consult cardiac surgery for removal
Filter failure	• Place second filter below 1st if there is room, or • Suprarenal IVC filter, or • SVC filter (if upper extremity source)

AC, anticoagulation; IVC, inferior vena cava; RA, right atrium; PA. pulmonary artery.

Indications

REMOVABLE FILTER PLACEMENT. Removable IVC filters (IVCFs) should be used when it is known that anticoagulation use, although not possible now, will be so in the near future, yet IVC filtration is needed now for protection against PE. Such a strategy offers patients the short-term benefits of IVC filtration and potentially avoids some of its long-term sequelae. This temporary time period of filtration should correspond with the time that anticoagulation use is not possible.

As before, two patient groups are apparent: those with DVT/PE and those without. These filters are ideally suited for "prophylactic" uses where patients have not formed DVT/PE but are at high risk of doing so and anticoagulation cannot be used for prophylaxis. Because of their potential short-term use, IVC filtration with such devices can also be used as an adjunct to anticoagulation in some clinical settings where PE risk is deemed to be high. Such "relative" indications were listed in Table 14-24. Optional filters can also be used in the "classic" indications, especially as they can be left in situ to function as permanent devices, and indeed arguments have been made to use optional filters in all indications for IVC filtration.[37,38]

REMOVABLE FILTER RETRIEVAL. IVCF removal is performed when the patient has an optional filter and IVC filtration is no longer needed to protect against PE, either because anticoagulation use is now possible, or because the patient is no longer at high risk for developing thromboembolic disease. No definite criteria exist at this time. A working framework is presented in Table 14-28, which summarizes the clinical settings where IVCF removal is appropriate and reflects the protocol used at our institution. Patients who did not have documented DVT/PE will be on prophylactic doses of anticoagulation. In these patients, the authors obtain an ultrasound of the legs to look for DVT; if present, filter removal is deferred until the patient is adequately treated with therapeutic doses of anticoagulation.

TABLE 14-28. DVT/PE Management and IVCF Removal

Indication for Filter Placement	Clinical Status	IVCF Removal Appropriate
+ DVT/PE	TAC	Yes
+ DVT/PE	S/P lysis/ thrombectomy and TAC	Yes
+ DVT/PE	TAC complication/ failure	No
No DVT/PE	Resolution of high-risk state and no new DVT	Yes
No DVT/PE	PAC while in continued high-risk state and no new DVT	Yes
No DVT/PE	New DVT (on US study)	No (unless on therapeutic AC)

DVT, deep vein thrombosis; PE, pulmonary embolism; IVCF, inferior vena cava filter; TAC, therapeutic anticoagulation (prophylactic anticoagulation is inadequate treatment of known DVT/PE); PAC, prophylactic anticoagulation; US, ultrasound.

The time frame within which optional filters should be removed is another factor for consideration. The longer a filter remains in the body, the more embedded or incorporated into the vein wall it becomes, from endothelial ingrowth into the filter. This is critical for optional filters if removal is planned. Filter repositioning is a strategy that is used to prolong IVC filtration using these devices, as collapsing the filter into a sheath and redeploying it in a different location within the IVC minimizes the effect of endothelial ingrowth. On the FDA approval letter for these optional devices, none of the filters had an implantation time specified beyond which retrieval should not be performed. The clinically applicable implantation times are based on manufacturer recommendations, local practice, and the literature. At the time of publication, at our institution, it is recommended that the Tulip and OptEase filters be retrieved within 4 weeks of implantation and the recovery filter within 3 months. Given the reported exceptions to this in the literature[39] and the ongoing trials to evaluate longer implantation times, the timing (and criteria) for when IVCF removal should be performed will continue to evolve.

Preoperative Workup and Planning

Determine the particular filter type that was placed from the reports or by review of filter placement images to ensure that the filter is a retrievable type; this will guide the access site that will be needed. Make sure that that access site is indeed available for use (Table 14-23). Also, review the clinical data to determine that criteria for IVCF removal are present (Table 14-28). During the consent process, advise patients that filter removal might not be possible. Also, check the ultrasound results to make sure that there is no new DVT in patients who did not have DVT/PE to begin with (see the previous subsection).

Intraoperative Details

If no filter placement images are available for review, fluoroscope the abdomen to confirm that the filter is a retrievable type. Then prepare the appropriate access site.

ACCESS. Prepare the appropriate access site for the filter (Table 14-23 and the earlier section on venous access).

IVC VENOGRAM. This is described in the earlier section on venography. Some further technical points are offered. When using the jugular route, the authors' preference is to pass an angled-tip guidewire through the filter into the inferior portion of the IVC and advance a 5F pigtail catheter over this, through the filter, into the IVC inferior to the filter. The catheter is positioned just inferior to the filter for cavography. Study the images for any thrombus within the filter (Fig. 14-24), and if present assess the volume of thrombus relative to the filter volume. Look for any filter protrusion beyond the contrast column of the IVC. Also, try and get a sense of the direction of filter tilt (if present); this may require oblique views. Although no strict criteria are defined for any of these parameters to guide filter retrieval, the authors proceed with filter removal if the thrombus volume represents 25% or less of the filter volume, and although tilted, the filter's hook or nose is not embedded in the vein wall. With respect to filter protrusion, the authors are mindful not to proceed too aggressively with removal to avoid IVC injury. Keep in mind that optional filters can be left in situ to function as permanent filters and do not absolutely have to be removed.

TULIP (COOK INC., BLOOMINGTON, IN) FILTER REMOVAL. The diagnostic catheter is exchanged out over an angled guidewire for a 10F sheath, which is positioned about 3 to 5 cm superior to the filter's hook. A snaring device is used to capture the hook; an angled catheter maybe needed to direct the snare if the filter is tilted. While holding the snare, the sheath is advanced to collapse the filter (the filter is not pulled into the

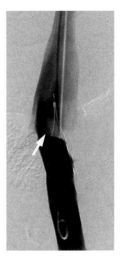

FIGURE 14-24.   This patient presented for filter removal. Venogram of the IVC shows clot (*arrow*) within the filter. This filter was not retrieved and was left in situ as a permanent filter.

sheath). Once the filter is removed, a follow-up venogram is performed via the sheath to look for any stenosis or leak (Fig. 14-25).

OPTEASE (CORDIS ENDOVASCULAR, JOHNSON AND JOHNSON, WARREN, NJ) FILTER REMOVAL. The diagnostic catheter is exchanged out over an angled guidewire for a 10F sheath, which is positioned about 3 to 5 cm inferior to the filter's hook. A snaring device is used to capture the hook; an angled catheter maybe needed to direct the snare if the filter is tilted. While holding the snare, the sheath is advanced to the hook and the filter is pulled into the sheath. Once the filter is removed, a follow-up venogram is performed via the sheath to look for any stenosis or leak.

RECOVERY (C.R. BARD, MURRAY HILL, NJ) FILTER REMOVAL. This has its own retrieval kit, the key component being the retrieval device (cone). This is a cone-shaped grasping device with adherent polyurethane membrane attached to the cone. This also is an over-the-wire system. The diagnostic catheter is exchanged out over an angled guidewire for the sheath included within the kit. The sheath is positioned 3 to 5 cm superior to the filter's nose (no hook on this filter). The retrieval cone is advanced over the wire through the sheath. The sheath keeps the cone in a constrained configuration. The cone is opened by advancing it out of the sheath and then positioned over the filter nose. To capture the filter, the cone is collapsed (closed) by advancing the sheath over the cone. The filter is then removed by pulling it into the sheath. A follow-up cavogram is obtained via the sheath.

Outcomes[40–44]

Table 14-29 summarizes some of the known experience with optional filter usage to date. Even though these filters are placed with the intent to remove them, not all filters were removed, because patients did not meet retrieval criteria, or because a trapped thrombus or incorporation into the IVC wall precluded removal. No long-term prospective data are

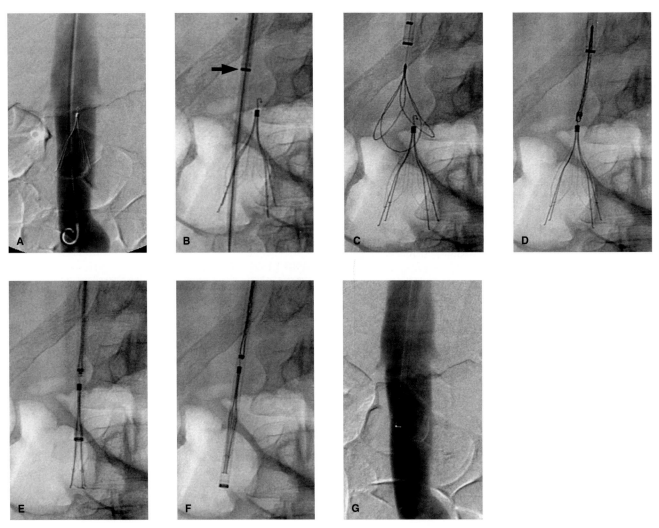

FIGURE 14-25. Steps in Tulip filter removal. **A:** Inferior vena cava (IVC) venogram via right internal jugular approach. Note that the pigtail catheter is placed through filter and just inferior to it. **B:** The radiopaque tip (*arrow*) of a 10F sheath is positioned just above the filter hook. **C:** A snare is positioned at the hook and is then used to capture the hook (**D**). The sheath is advanced all the way over the entire filter to collapse the filter (**E**) and free it from the caval wall. Once completely inside the sheath (**F**) the filter is pulled out. **G:** A follow-up cavogram obtained via the sheath shows no IVC stenosis or contrast extravasation. In this particular case, the patient had an allergy to iodinated contrast, and gadolinium was the contrast agent used.

available for performance characteristics of these filters, either on rates of recurrent PE following retrieval, or on how these filters function as permanent filters with respect to parameters such as rates of recurrent PE and caval occlusion rates. No data are available for incidence of filter retrieval–related IVC injury requiring intervention. With newer filter designs and results of ongoing trials on the horizon, temporary filtration will continue to redefine its role in thromboembolism management.

CENTRAL VENOUS ACCESS DEVICES

Long-term (>3 weeks) venous access devices include tunneled lines (TLs) and ports. Image-guided placement of these devices is cheaper and safer.[45–47]

INDICATIONS

Central veins offer large volumes and flows compared to their small peripheral counterparts, which allows them to tolerate some of the more toxic medications that would thrombose the peripheral veins. Also, a peripheral vein access site will need to be discontinued and a new site accessed at least once a week, which is not ideal when long-term IV access is needed. Table 14-30 lists some of the indications. TLs are useful for blood volume exchanges and frequent or continuous infusions. Ports are useful for intermittent use such as intermittent infusions and blood draws, which will be required over the span of many months. Ports, being completely subcutaneous, provide better cosmesis and require relatively less maintenance.

TABLE 14-29.   Optional Filter Experience to Date

Parameter	Tulip[a]	OptEase[b]	Recovery[c]
	Optional Filter		
Placement success	100%	100%	100%
Retrieval candidates	69%–83%	78%	75%
Retrieval attempted	76%–84%	21/21	24/24
Retrieval success	76%–98%	100%	100%
Max implant time	475 days (39)	48 days	161 days

[a] Kaufman JA, Nutting CW, Smouse HR, et al. Gunther Tulip Filter retrievability multicenter study: final report [Abstract no. 54]. Presented at the 29th annual scientific meeting of Society of Interventional Radiology, March 2004, Phoenix, AZ; Given MF, et al. Retrievable Gunther Tulip Filter: experience in 41 patients. *Radiology (RSNA suppl)* 2002;225(p):642; and Millward SF, Oliva VL, Bell SD, et al. Gunther Tulip retrievable vena caval filter: results from the registry of the Canadian Interventional Radiology Association. *J Vasc Intervent Radiol.* 2001; 12:1053–1058.

[b]Oliva VL, Soulez G, Szatmari F, et al. The Cordis Jonas permanent/retrievable vena cava filter retrieval time extension study [Abstract No. 55]. Presented at the 29th annual scientific meeting of Society of Interventional Radiology, March 2004, Phoenix, AZ.

[c]Asch M. Initial experience in humans with a new retrievable IVC filter. *Radiology.* 2002;225:835–844.

TABLE 14-30.   Some Clinical Examples of Central Venous Access Indications

- Hemodialysis
- Chemotherapy
- Bone marrow transplant protocols
- Total parenteral nutrition
- Plasmapheresis, leukopheresis
- Blood sampling

CONTRAINDICATIONS

These usually include circumstances where device infection risk is high such as with ongoing sepsis/bacteremia or cellulitis/dermatitis at the insertion site.

DEVICE OPTIONS

For hemodialysis and apheresis, catheters that yield high flows (400 to 450 mL per minute) are needed and large-bore (13.5F and up) dual-lumen catheters are used. Usually they have staggered tips with side holes added to allow for high flows. So-called maintenance lines, which are needed for blood draws, medications, parenteral nutrition, and the like, do not require high flows, and smaller caliber catheters are used for this purpose, usually 12F and less in diameter. Ports also come with many options, the main ones being single or dual lumens (chambers) and low or normal profile. The silicone membrane on the ports is designed for use with 20- to 22-gauge noncoring access needles for up to 2000 to 3000 accesses. Table 14-31 lists some further features of these devices.

TABLE 14-31.   Varied Features of Central Access Devices

TUNNELED LINES

Materials	Silicone or polyurethane
Sizes	3F–14.5F
Lumens	1–3
Tips	Staggered or split, valved or valveless
Cuffs	With or without silver impregnation

PORTS

Chambers (lumens/reservoirs)	Single or dual
Profile	Regular or low

DEVICE PLACEMENT

Access Sites [48–51]

Commonly used sites (Table 14-32) include the internal and external jugular and subclavian veins. Collaterals can also be used for access if they communicate with the central venous system. The authors prefer the internal jugular veins to the subclavian veins because of their larger diameter and higher flow rates; unilateral jugular vein stenosis or occlusion is relatively well tolerated because of the rich collaterals in the head and neck region. The one possible exception is in patients who have had a craniotomy, as catheter placement itself can cause luminal compromise and elevated intracranial venous pressures and subsequently intracranial bleeding. The subclavian vein approach might be preferred in this subgroup of patients.

Venous access is performed as for any case using ultrasound guidance. With internal jugular access, a low approach is chosen, either between the heads of SCM or posterior to this muscle to avoid an intramuscular track. Ultrasound guidance may not be possible if the IVC is being accessed; here fluoroscopic guidance is used. IVC puncture is made at L3 level, after placing a catheter, guidewire, or snare into the IVC via the femoral vein to act as a target (Fig. 14-26). Use a needle long enough to reach the IVC.

In patients with renal failure, particular attention must be given to preserving the upper-extremity veins including the subclavian vein, especially if such patients are going to have a hemodialysis shunt placed. Stenosis or occlusion of the subclavian vein resulting from catheter placement can limit hemodialysis management options in such patients. It may be necessary to deliberately work through a thrombosed vein (e.g., internal jugular vein); with the catheter tip high in the

TABLE 14-32.   Various Access Options for Catheter Placement

- Internal jugular veins (right over left as less curves)
- External jugular veins
- Subclavian veins
- Large collateral veins communicating directly with central veins
- Femoral veins
- IVC (via translumbar or transhepatic approach)

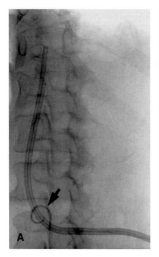 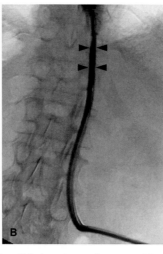

FIGURE 14-26. A: Translumbar dialysis catheter placement. Note the pigtail catheter (*arrow*) positioned in the IVC used as target for fluoroscopic guided IVC access. **B:** This patient presented 3 years later with catheter dysfunction. Catheter check reveals a narrow tubular contrast-filled lumen (*arrowheads*) no wider than the catheter itself, indicating a fibrin sheath around the catheter extending to the right atrium. The catheter was exchanged over a wire for a sheath through which angioplasty was performed.

RA, adequate catheter function can be obtained without compromising other veins.

Tunneled Lines

Tunnel creation and adjusting catheter lengths so that the catheter cuff and catheter tip are in the required locations are essential steps when placing central venous access devices.

CREATING A TUNNEL. Tunneling is the process of creating a track within which the portion of the catheter with the cuff is placed. This tunnel within the subcutaneous fat extends from the venotomy site to the skin exit dermatotomy. For jugular and subclavian access, this will typically be on the upper anterior chest wall, for femoral access within the thigh or lower abdominal wall, and within the flank for IVC access. Most kits will have a tunneling device, which is a long metal or plastic rod that has a blunt tip on one end and a serrated tip on the other for catheter attachment. As the blunt tip is pushed into one end of the tunnel and advanced and pulled out the other end, the catheter follows through the tunnel. Depending on the catheter type being placed, tunneling can be done from the skin exit dermatotomy to the venotomy site or vice-versa, the later being referred to as "back-tunneling." The length should be such that the cuff is at least 2 cm from the skin exit site to decrease the infection rate[52]; usually a tunnel of at least 5 cm is needed. This length is also accounted for in the final required catheter length measurement.

CATHETER LENGTH DETERMINATIONS. The positions of the catheter tip and the cuff will determine how long the catheter needs to be. The intravenous component extends from the venotomy site to the location of the catheter tip (usually high RA) and is measured using a guidewire by placing the

guidewire tip at the desired spot and bending or clamping the wire at the venotomy site. Usually a sheath is used for guidewire placement and the length of the sheath hub is subtracted from this distance. The cuff site is then chosen, and then the skin exit site. Depending on the type of catheter, different strategies are employed for subsequent total length determination.

Catheters not designed to have their lengths altered come in a choice of lengths. To determine which length will be needed, the required IV length is measured and a tunnel length of at least 5 cm is added to determine what "tip-to-cuff" length of catheter is needed. Now fashion a tunnel of sufficient length so that the catheter cuff will be at least 2 cm from the skin exit site. To help with this, the wire (intravenous) length is marked of from the catheter tip and the remaining catheter length placed on the skin from the venotomy site to guide tunnel length and the skin exit site.

TLs used for maintenance come in lengths that are generally longer than needed and the extra redundancy is supposed to be cut off. After obtaining access and measuring the IV component, catheters that are cut to the appropriate length at their tip have their cuff site chosen, which guides the skin exit site. The catheter is then pulled through the tunnel from the skin exit site toward the venotomy site and the cuff appropriately positioned. The measured IV length is added to the catheter from the venotomy site and the catheter cut at the desired distance prior to placement within the central venous system. TLs that are cut at their back end before attaching the hubs typically have a valved tip to prevent back flow of blood into the catheter tip, and the tip is placed into the venous system first at the desired location. The remainder of the catheter is then laid on the patient's skin to decide on the skin exit site such that the cuff will be at least 2 cm away from the skin exit site. After the skin exit site and tunnel is prepared, the TL is tunneled from the venotomy site to the skin exit site ("back tunneled"). Now the back end of the catheter is cut and the catheter hubs attached.

Tables 14-33, 14-34, and 14-35 describe the steps for different device placements. Some technical points are offered. Make sure the vein puncture site dermatotomy (venotomy) is big enough to allow passage of the peel-away sheath for placement of the catheter. Also, perform thorough blunt and deep dissection of the tissues here so that no fibrous strands remain that can kink the catheter. Try to avoid breast tissue, the axilla, and superficial veins when making the skin exit dermatotomy. The tunnel track should have a gentle curve so that the catheter does not kink. The cuff on these TLs should be within the tunnel at least 2 cm in from the skin exit site, and when tunneling the device through the subcutaneous track, make sure the tip of the tunneler is pointed away from the ribs. When placing TLs from the jugular route, the catheter tip should be high in the right atrium, which results in decreased catheter malfunction. Femoral access catheter tips are placed in the infrarenal IVC, whereas translumbar or transhepatic TLs have their tips just beyond the IVC-RA junction into the RA.

After placement, all TLs are flushed and secured in place; if using sutures, make sure the sutures do not kink the catheter.

Ports

Tables 14-36 and 14-37 list the steps in port placement. A dose of IV antibiotic is given to cover skin organisms prior to commencing. In placing anchoring sutures, take bites through the deep

TABLE 14-33. Tunneled Catheter Placement (Cutting to Length at the Back End)

Access vein (Table 14-1)
- Have 0.035-in. guidewire placed into venous system

Dilate and place introducer sheath into venous system
- Introducer sheath and dilators usually included in kit

Place catheter into venous system
- Position tip at desired location (e.g., high right atrium)

Create tunnel
- Measure and make tunnel of required length (this is done by laying catheter on chest and choosing length so that cuff will be within tunnel)
- Anesthetize this tract/length (from venotomy site incision to skin exit site) and make skin incision at this exit site
- Make exit site in a comfortable location for patient

Pull catheter through tunnel
- Use a "tunneling" device (usually included in kit) to bring catheter from venotomy site, through tunnel and out via skin exit site

Cut catheter at back end
- Cut catheter to a convenient/manageable length

Attach hubs, flush and secure device

TABLE 14-34. Tunneled Catheter Placement (Cutting to Length at Catheter Tip)

Vein accessed (as for any case)

Create tunnel
- Lay catheter on patient's chest and decide on cuff location
- Make skin exit site at least 2 cm inferior to the selected cuff location
- Anesthetize track from skin exit site to venotomy site

Pull catheter through tunnel
- Use "tunneling" device (usually included in kit) to pull catheter from skin exit site toward the venotomy site
- Position cuff at desired location 2 cm away from skin exit site

Measure desired intravenous length
- Aim for catheter tip in high right atrium
- Use guidewire (position wire tip, usually through sheath, at desired location and clamp wire at sheath hub. Pull out wire and measure distance from wire tip to clamp; subtract length of sheath hub. Starting at the venotomy site, add this length to the catheter and cut the catheter at this length)

Place catheter into central venous system
- Use introducer sheath (usually in kit) for this step. One may need to dilate tract prior to placing introducer sheath

Flush and secure catheter

TABLE 14-35. Tunneled Catheters with Fixed Lengths

Vein accessed (as for any case)

Measure desired intravenous length
- Aim for catheter tip in high RA
- Use guidewire (position wire tip, usually through sheath, at desired location and clamp wire at sheath hub. Pull out wire and measure distance from wire tip to clamp; subtract length of sheath hub)

Create tunnel of appropriate length
- Choose desired cuff location on patient (ideally some distance inferior to clavicle). Measure the distance from this site to the venotomy site and add it to intravenous measurement (this gives the "tip-to-cuff" distance). Ask for catheter with this distance (note: total length is longer than "tip-to-cuff" length).
- The intravenous length is then subtracted from *total* catheter length to determine required tunnel length.
- Skin exit site is chosen and tunnel tract anesthetized and skin exit incision made.

Pull catheter through tunnel
- Use "tunneling" device (usually included in kit) to pull catheter from skin exit site toward the venotomy site. Position cuff at chosen location.

Place catheter into central venous system
- Use introducer sheath (usually in kit) for this step. One may need to dilate tract prior to placing introducer sheath.

Flush and secure catheter

TABLE 14-36. Chest Port Placement

Access vein as for any case

Create subcutaneous pocket
- Choose location comfortable for patient
- Anesthetize pocket site
- Make skin incision over pocket large enough to accept port
- Use blunt dissection to create subcutaneous space (pocket) of adequate size to accept port
- Place 3-O vicryl anchoring sutures inside pocket through deep fascia

Create tunnel
- Anesthetize site of tunnel linking pocket with venotomy site

Measure required length of catheter (Table 10-37)

Place port/catheter into patient, secure and flush port

Close pocket with subcutaneous-layer and skin-layer sutures

fascia. This helps stabilize the port. The pocket is closed in two layers, the subcuticular layer with interrupted absorbable sutures such as 3-O vicryl. The skin can be closed with interrupted sutures, or a running subcuticular suture with 4-O suture.

POSTOPERATIVE CARE

The goal is to prevent infection and maintain catheter patency and function. Aseptic technique is used when using the catheters. Table 14-38 lists the maintenance protocols used at our institution.

COMPLICATIONS

A discussion of some of the complications (Table 14-39) is presented here. Infection and malfunction are key issues.

Infections[53–56]

Infection related to the TL skin exit site (within 2 cm of the exit site) responds in most cases to antibiotic therapy and local wound care. Tunnel infection itself (>2 cm from the exit site) does not respond as well to antibiotics, and catheter removal is necessary in 75% of cases. Catheter-related sepsis, presenting as fever and bacteremia, requires blood cultures from the catheter and a peripheral site. The diagnosis is made if there is a 10-fold increase in colony count from the catheter site.

TABLE 14-37. Suggested Methods for Catheter Measurements

1. Place catheter intravenously first
   - Position tip at desired location (high right atrium)
   - Tunnel catheter back from venotomy site to pocket
   - Cut catheter to desired length at pocket, connect to port, and place port into pocket over anchoring sutures
2. Connect catheter to port first
   - Place port in pocket
   - Tunnel catheter to venous access site
   - Measure desired intravenous length (wire as in Table 14-5)
   - Cut to length and place catheter intravenously
3. Place wire into central veins with tip at desired location first
   - "Back-tunnel" wire toward pocket (e.g., using Hawkins needle)
   - Measure required length off wire and cut catheter to this length
   - From venotomy site, retrieve wire back out from tunnel (maintaining venous access) and place introducer sheath into venous system
   - Connect catheter to port, place port into pocket
   - Tunnel catheter to venotomy site and place catheter into venous system

TABLE 14-38. Catheter Maintenance

Catheter Type	Standard Flush (mL of Heparin Solution Indicated)	Frequency
TLs (nonvalved)	Adults: 5 mL, 10 U/mL Peds: 3 mL, 10 U/mL	Each day, and pre and post blood draws and medication administration
TLs (valved)	5 mL NS	Each week, and pre and post blood draws and medication administration
TLs (dialysis/ apheresis)	1000 U/mL heparin, total mL as per marked on catheter	Per treating service.
Ports	Adults: 5 mL, 100 U/mL Peds: 3 mL, 100 U/mL	Each month, and pre and post blood draws and medication administration

NS = Normal Saline

Antibiotics are given and device removal is needed. Septic thrombophlebitis requires antibiotics and catheter removal.

Port infections can be similarly addressed and managed. In addition, infection related to the pocket needs further mention. Any fevers, bacteremia, fluctuance, or wound dehiscence with exudate requires the removal of the port and complete drainage of pus from the pocket. The cavity is then allowed to heal by secondary intent, which requires packing the cavity with gauze, and this is changed on a daily basis while IV antibiotic therapy is administered. As the cavity granulates and heals, the gauze packing is progressively diminished over several days, until healing is complete. Catheter-related bacteremia without pocket infection can be managed in 80% with antibiotics, but recurrence is high unless the port is removed. If incision ery-

TABLE 14-39. Complications of Central Venous Catheters

INTRAOPERATIVE
- Access related (Table 14-3)
- Hemopericardium
- Arrhythmia
- Air embolus
- Catheter kink/malposition

POSTOPERATIVE
- Infection (catheter tip, tunnel or pocket, skin exit site, septic thrombophlebitis)
- Catheter dysfunction (thrombosis, kink, leakage, fragmentation, tip migration)
- Venous occlusion

thema is present, antibiotics are commenced. If any exudate fails to respond with 72 hours, then the port should be removed.

Catheter Malfunction

Catheter malfunction may arise from catheter occlusion usually from clot formation within it.[57] This responds well to thrombolytic infusion into the catheter (Table 14-40).[58] A fibrin sheath typically allows for forward flushes but not for aspiration via the catheter. A venogram performed via the catheter will reveal poor washout of the contrast and possible filling of a tubular space immediately surrounding the catheter (Fig. 14-26). This can extend back to the venotomy site. Treatment options include angioplasty of this fibrin sheath by exchanging out the venous access catheter over a guidewire and introducing a sheath via which a balloon catheter can be advanced for angioplasty. Also, snugly snaring the catheter shaft and pulling the snare down along the catheter shaft will also remove the sheath. This requires femoral vein access to introduce the snare via a vascular sheath. If there is no other demonstrable abnormality such as catheter kink, tip malposition, or venous stenosis, then the catheter is exchanged over a wire for a new catheter.

Pericatheter thrombus formation (Fig. 14-27) in the central veins is symptomatic in 30% of cases.[59] This may occur at anytime.

TABLE 14-40. Catheter Thrombosis Management

Prophylaxis
- Low-dose warfarin (Coumadin) 1 mg/day
- Lytic infusion UK 5000 U (weekly for TLs, monthly for ports)

Established catheter dysfunction
- Our protocol is tPA infused into catheter at total of 1 mg/hr for total of 4 hr
- If two lumens are present, total dose is split so each lumen gets 0.5 mg/hr

If catheter dysfunction persists, then catheter venogram needed looking for some other structural cause such as catheter kink, fibrin sheath.

Adapted from Lowell JA, Bothe A. Central venous catheter related thrombosis. *Surgical Oncol Clin N Am.* 1995;4:479–491, and Bern MM, Lokich JJ, Wallach ST, et al. Very low doses of warfarin can prevent thrombosis in central venous catheters: a randomized prospective trial. *Ann Intern Med.* 1990;112:423–428.

Table 14-41 lists some risk factors for this occurring, and the earlier section on treatment of axillary-subclavian venous disease discusses management. It should be noted that catheter removal might not yield patent central veins for future use (even though the patient is asymptomatic).

Catheter tip migration into an unacceptable vascular location can occur at any time; this may be detected incidentally on a radiograph, or catheter malfunction may occur. Repositioning is possible with forceful injection of saline into the catheter or snaring the catheter and pulling it out from this unwanted location. If the problem is because of incorrect catheter length, this will need to be addressed, usually by replacing the device.

Immediate (Periprocedural) Complications

If there is persistent bleeding from the insertion site, look for and correct any coagulopathy and apply local compression; gel foam or topical thrombin can be placed in the tunnel. Bleeding from the port pocket site requires the pocket to be reopened and hemostasis secured with a cautery device or ligature of the culprit vessel. Hematoma here can lead to infection or an inaccessible port.

A pneumothorax (Ptx) is dealt with on its merits. cardiorespiratory status is evaluated, along with serial chest x-rays every 4 to 6 hours. A chest tube should be placed for tension Ptx, increasing size of Ptx, dyspnea at rest, falling oxygen saturations, and large Ptx.

Preventing it from happening is the best treatment for air embolism by having patients in the Trendelenburg position and performing the Valsalva maneuver during catheter introduction into the venous system. Air in the central venous system acts like an embolus and can cause cardiopulmonary arrest. A "sucking" sound while introducing the catheter may be the first clue that this is occurring, and "bubbling lucencies" are visualized under fluoroscopy in the heart and pulmonary arteries. Turn the patient left side down so air accumulates in the RA appendage. Aspirate out as much air as possible via the catheter if it is already in place or by introducing a 5F to 7F pigtail catheter into the air pocket (Table 14-42).

If an arterial puncture is recognized during the initial access puncture with the small-gauge needle, pull the needle out and hold compression until bleeding stops. If, however, it is not recognized until the end, and the catheter is already in the arterial system, leave the catheter in place, heparinize the patient, and consult surgery. In the subclavian artery, a covered stent can be placed to seal up the hole of the catheter.

Arrhythmias usually are the result of the guidewire tip stimulating the myocardium. As soon as it is recognized during the case, pull the guidewire tip out of the heart. For this reason, it is best to have the guidewire tip within the IVC if possible or in the SVC. If this does not reverse the arrhythmia, then treat the rhythm on its merits.

Early (within 30 Days) Complications

Sepsis, pericatheter thrombosis, catheter leakage, and catheter tip migration are discussed elsewhere in this section.

Late (after 30 Days) Complications

Catheter fragmentation and embolization are managed using standard techniques for foreign-body retrieval. Repair kits are available to try and repair leaks, but if this is unsuccessful, then exchange over a guidewire will be needed. The authors prefer to place a 0.038-in. diameter hydrophilic-coated guidewire into each of the lumens, and, after freeing the cuff from the soft tissues using blunt dissection, the catheter is exchanged back for a new catheter, which is advanced over the two guidewires.

For ports, migration or inversion of the reservoir may occur if the pockets created are larger than the port itself, and catheter-port separation and septum failure leads to extravasation. In these cases, the port needs to be removed. See the following section.

DEVICE REMOVAL

Most TLs can be removed at the bedside (Table 14-43). Should the catheter break, and this usually occurs at the site of the cuff, the catheter rides superiorly within the tunnel. Apply pressure over the catheter to reduce chances of air embolism and bleeding, cut down over the cuff, dissect the cuff free, and remove the remainder of the catheter. With port removals, if possible try to work through the incision made for port placement, and remember to cut loose the anchoring sutures.

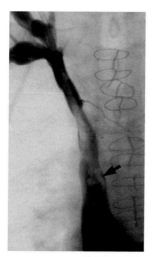

FIGURE 14-27. Tubular filling defects (*arrow*) present around the catheter tip, indicating pericatheter thrombus.

TABLE 14-41. Risk Factors for Central Venous Thrombosis

- Left-sided catheter placement
- Subclavian placement
- Multiple catheters
- High position of catheter tip in SVC
- Hypercoagulable states

SVC, superior vena cava.

TABLE 14-42. Tips for Dealing with Air Embolism

1. Roll patient right side up decubitus (keeps air in right atrium)
2. Place catheter/sheath into right atrium and aspirate vigorously

TABLE 14-43. Device Removal

TUNNELED LINES

- Aseptic preparation of site, local anesthetic into exit site extending into tunnel up to cuff
- Dissect free cuff from surrounding tissues
- Pull catheter out of patient; this may require some vigorous force in some patients

PORTS

- Aseptic preparation of site, local anesthetic into prior incision and pocket
- Open incision and dissect tissues down to neck of port, identify catheter and clamp it.
- Incise capsule around port and dissect free port from pocket; anchoring sutures may need to be cut.
- Pull out port and attached catheter. Secure hemostasis.
- Close up in layers same as when putting in port.

REFERENCES

1. Dotter CT, Rosch J, Seaman AJ. Selective clot lysis with low dose streptokinase. *Radiology.* 1974;111:31–37.
2. Comerota AJ, Aldridge SC, Cohen G, et al. Thrombolytic therapy for deep venous thrombosis: a clinical review. *Can J Surg.* 1992;26:630–637.
3. Comerota AJ, Aldridge SC, Cohen G, et al. A strategy of aggressive regional therapy for acute iliofemoral venous thrombectomy or catheter directed therapy. *J Vasc Surg.* 1994;20:244–254.
4. Grossman C, McPherson S. Safety and efficacy of catheter directed thrombolysis for iliofemoral venous thrombosis. *AJR Am J Roentgenol.* 1999;172:667–672.
5. Ouriel K, Katzen B, Mewissen MW, et al. Reteplase in the treatment of acute arterial and venous occlusion: a pilot study. *J Vasc Intervent Radiol.* 2000;11:849–854.
6. Castenda F, Swischuk JC, Brady TM, et al. Initial results using reteplase for acute deep venous thrombosis [abstract no. 198]. Presented at the 26th annual scientific meeting of SCVIR, March 2001, San Antonio, TX.
7. Chang R, Cannon RO, Chen CC, et al. Daily catheter directed single dosing of t-PA in treatment of acute deep venous thrombosis of the lower extremity. *J Vasc Intervent Radiol.* 2001;12:247–252.
8. Mewissen MW, Seabrook GR, Meissner MH, et al. Catheter directed thrombolysis for the lower extremity deep venous thrombosis: report of a national multicenter registry. *Radiology.* 1999;211:39–49.
9. Sembe CP, Dake DD. Catheter directed venous thrombolysis. *Semin Intervent Radiol.* 1994;11:388–395.
10. Kasirajian K, Gray B, Ouriel K. Percutaneous angio-jet thrombectomy in the management of extremity deep venous thrombosis. *J Vasc Intervent Radiol.* 2001;12:179–185.
11. Valji K. Evolving strategies for thrombolytic therapy of peripheral vascular occlusion. *J Vasc Intervent Radiol.* 2001;12:179–185.
12. Horne MK 3rd, Mayo DJ, Cannon RO, et al. Intraclot recombinant tissue plasminogen activator in the treatment of deep venous thrombosis of lower and upper extremities. *Am J Med.* 2000;108:251–255.
13. Lakin PC. Venous thrombolysis and stenting. In: Baum S, Pentecost MJ, eds. *Abram's Angiography.* Vol 3. Boston: Little, Brown and Company, 1997;1046–1058.
14. Sheeran SR, Hallisey MJ, Murphy TP, et al. Local thrombolytic treatment as part of a multidisciplinary approach to acute subclavian vein thrombosis (Paget-Schroetter syndrome). *J Vasc Intervent Radiol.* 1997;8:253–260.
15. Kreienberg PB, Chang BB, Darling RC, et al. Long term results in patients treated with thrombolysis, thoracic inlet decompression, and subclavian vein stenting for Paget-Schroetter syndrome. *J Vasc Surg.* 2001;33:S100–S105.
16. Beygui RE, Olcott C, Dalman RL. Subclavian vein thrombosis: outcome analysis based on etiology and modality of treatment. *Ann Vasc Surg* 1997;11:247–255.
17. Kaufman J, Lee M. Upper extremity, neck and central thoracic veins. In: *The Requisites: Vascular and Interventional Radiology.* St. Louis, MO:Mosby, 2004:163–193.
18. Escalante CP. Causes and management of superior vena cava syndrome. *Oncology.* 1993;7:61–68.
19. Ostler PJ. Superior vena cava obstruction: a modern management strategy. *Clin Oncol.* 1997;9:83–89.
20. Perez CA, Presant CA, Van Amburg AL. Management of superior vena cava syndrome. *Semin Oncol.* 1978;5:123–134.
21. Nicholson AA, Ettles DF, Arnold A, et al. Treatment of malignant SVC obstruction: metal stent or radiation therapy. *J Vasc Intervent Radiol.* 1997;8:781–788.
22. Kee ST, Kinoshita L, Razavi MK, et al. SCV syndrome: treatment with catheter directed thrombolysis and endovascular stent placement. *Radiology.* 1998;206:187–193.

23. Nazarian GK, Bjarnason H, Dietz, Jr., CA, et al. Iliofemoral venous stenosis: effectiveness of treatment with metallic endovascular stents. *Radiology.* 1996;200:193–199.
24. Semba CP, Dake MD. Iliofemoral deep venous thrombosis: aggressive therapy with catheter directed thrombolysis. *Radiology.* 1994;191:487–494.
25. Patel Nilesh H, Stookey Kenneth R, Ketcham Douglas B, et al. Endovascular management of acute extensive iliofemoral deep venous thrombosis caused by May-Thurner syndrome. *J Vasc Intervent Radiol.* 2000;11:1297–1302.
26. O'Sullivan GJ, Semba CP, Bittner CA, et al. Endovascular management of iliac vein compression (May-Thurner syndrome). *J Vasc Intervent Radiol.* 2000;11:823–836.
27. Mewissen MW, Seabrook GR, Meissner MH, et al. Catheter directed thrombolysis for the lower extremity deep venous thrombosis: report of a national multicenter registry. *Radiology.* 1999;211:39–49.
28. Grossman C, McPherson S. Safety and efficacy of catheter directed thrombolysis for iliofemoral venous thrombosis. *AJR Am J Roentgenol.* 1999;172:667–672.
29. Razavi MK, Hansch EC, Kee ST, et al. Chronically occluded inferior vena cav: endovascular treatment. *Radiology.* 2000;214:133–138.
30. Petersen BD, Uchida BT. Long-term results of treatment of benign central venous obstructions unrelated to dialysis with expandable Z stents. *J Vasc Intervent Radiol.* 1999;10:757–766.
31. Decousus H, Leizorovicz A, Parent F, et al. The Prévention du Risque d'Embolie Pulmonaire par Interruption Cave Study Group. A clinical trial of vena cava filters in prevention of PE in patients with proximal DVT. *N Eng J Med.* 1998;338:409–415.
32. The PREPIC Study Group. Eight-year follow-up of patients with permanent vena cava filters in the prevention of pulmonary embolism The PREPIC (Prevention du risqué d'embolie pulmonaire par interruption cave) Randomised study. *Circulation.* 2005;112:416–422.
33. Athanasoulis C, Kaufman J, Halpern E, et al. Inferior vena cava filters: review of a 26 year single center clinical experience. *Radiology.* 2000;216:54–66.
34. Ray CJ, Kaufman J. Complications of Inferior vena cava filters. *Abdom Imaging.* 1996;21: 368–374.
35. Kaufman J, Thomas J, Geller S, et al. Guidewire entrapment by inferior vena cava filters: in vitro evaluation. *Radiology.* 1996;198:71–76.
36. Stavropoulos SW, Itkin M, Trerotola SO. In vitro study of guidewire entrapment in currently available inferior vena cava filters. *J Vasc Intervent Radiol.* 2003;14:905–910.
37. Millward S. Buy time! Temporary filters. Plenary session presentation at the 29th annual scientific meeting of Society of Interventional Radiology, March 2004, Phoenix, AZ.
38. Ivanovic V, Bjarnason H, Johnson CM, et al. Retrievable IVC filter placement: indications and outcomes [Abstract no. 59]. Presented at the 29th annual scientific meeting of Society of Interventional Radiology, March 2004, Phoenix, AZ.
39. Kachura J. Inferior vena cava filter retrieval after 475 days [letter]. *J Vasc Intervent Radiol.* 2005;16:1156–1158.
40. Kaufman JA, Nutting CW, Smouse HR, et al. Gunther Tulip Filter retrievability multicenter study: final report [Abstract no. 54]. Presented at the 29th annual scientific meeting of Society of Interventional Radiology, March 2004, Phoenix, AZ.
41. Given MF, Lyon SM, Foster A, et al. Retrievable Gunther Tulip Filter: experience in 41 patients. *Radiology (RSNA suppl)* 2002;225(p):642.
42. Millward SF, Oliva VL, Bell SD, et al. Gunther Tulip retrievable vena caval filter: results from the registry of the Canadian Interventional Radiology Association. *J Vasc Intervent Radiol.* 2001;12:1053–1058.
43. Oliva VL, Soulez G, Szatmari F, et al. The Cordis Jonas permanent/retrievable vena cava filter retrieval time extension study [Abstract No. 55]. Presented at the 29th annual scientific meeting of Society of Interventional Radiology, March 2004, Phoenix, AZ.
44. Asch M. Initial experience in humans with a new retrievable IVC filter. *Radiology.* 2002;225:835–844.
45. Ahmad I, Ray CE. Radiologic placement of venous access ports. *Semin Intervent Radiol.* 1998;15:259–272.
46. McBride KD, Fischer R, Warnock N, et al. A comparative analysis of radiological and surgical placement of central venous catheters. *Cardiovasc Intervent Radiol.* 1997;20:17–22.
47. Noh HM, Kaufman J, Fan CM, et al. Radiological approach to central venous catheters: cost analysis. *Semin Intervent Radiol.* 1998;15:335–340.
48. Andrews JC. Percutaneous placement of a Hickman catheter with use of an intercostals vein for access. *J Vasc Intervent Radiol.* 1994;5:859–861.
49. Bertoglio S, Di Somma C, Meszaros P, et al. Long term femoral vein central venous access in cancer patients. *Eur J Surg Oncol.* 1996;22:162–165.
50. Kaufman JA, Greenfield AL, Fitzpatrick GF. Transhepatic cannulation of the inferior vena cava. *J Vasc Intervent Radiol.* 1991;2:331–334.
51. Lund GB, Treotola SO, Scheel PJ. Percutaneous translumbar inferior vena cava cannulation for hemodialysis. *Am J Kidney Dis.* 1995;25:732–737.
52. Hayward SR, Ledgerwood AM, Lucas CE. The fate of 100 prolonged venous access devices. *Am Surg.* 1990;56:515–519.
53. Mauro MA. Delayed complications of venous access. *J Vasc Intervent Radiol.* 1998;1(3):158–167.
54. Owens CA, Yaghimai B, Warner D. Complications of central venous catheterizations. *Semin Intervent Radiol.* 1998;15:341–355.
55. Dickinson GM, Bisno AL. Infections associated with indwelling devices: concepts of pathogenesis: infections associated with intravascular devices. *Antimicrob Agents Chemother.* 1989;33:597–601.
56. Early TF, Gregory RT, Wheeler JR, et al. Increased infection rates in double lumen versus single lumen Hickman catheters in cancer patients. *South Med J.* 1990;83:34–36.
57. Hoch JR. Management of the complications of long term venous access. *Semin Vasc Surg.* 1997;10:135–143.
58. Lawson M, Bottino JC, Hurtubise MR, et al. The use of urokinase to restore the patency of occluded central venous access catheters. *Am J Intraven Ther Clin Nutr.* 1992;5:29–32.
59. Lowell JA, Bothe A. Central venous catheter related thrombosis. *Surgical Oncol Clin N Am.* 1995;4:479–491.
60. Bern MM, Lokich JJ, Wallach ST, et al. Very low doses of warfarin can prevent thrombosis in central venous catheters: a randomized prospective trial. *Ann Intern Med.* 1990; 112: 423–428.

Haresh G. Mehta
Stephan Windecker
Bernhard Meier

CHAPTER **15**

Foreign Bodies

Since the first endovascular catheterization performed by Werner Forssmann[1] on himself, techniques have moved with rapid strides. To improve accessibility and torquability, the caliber of catheters has been declining. This is conducive to kinking, knotting, and possible breakage and embolization. Catheter fragments, guidewires, or vena cava filters used to be the predominant embolized foreign bodies. Intravascular stents, coils, pacemaker electrodes, and closure devices have been additions to the armamentarium, but have also been added to the woes of the vascular interventionist. These devices have become responsible for increasing numbers of arterial embolizations, although venous embolizations still outnumber arterial embolizations.

Complications associated with detachment or fragmentation of endovascular devices, albeit rare, can have grave implications, necessitating removal in nearly all situations. Surgical removal of foreign bodies carries the risks of surgery and anesthesia. Percutaneous retrieval obviates these risks and is usually safe. The first percutaneous removal of an embolized intravascular foreign body was reported four decades ago.[2] Since then percutaneous techniques have matured to their present status.[3–8]

With proliferation of catheter-based techniques, unforeseen complications may occur, and an unprepared mind could add to the risks; thus retrieval techniques are an important component of the curriculum for the training of interventionalists. Each embolization is different and requires an adaptation and refinement of interventional techniques for retrieval. This chapter provides a comprehensive review of intravascular foreign body retrieval.

DO ALL FOREIGN BODIES NEED REMOVAL?

Depending on the location of the foreign bodies in the circulation, they can be broadly classified as follows:

Foreign bodies in the venous circulation:
1. Central veins
2. Peripheral veins
3. Special locations (right atrium and ventricle, pulmonary arteries, and segmental branches)

Foreign bodies in the arterial circulation:
1. Aorta
2. Coronary arteries
3. Cerebral arteries
4. Peripheral arteries

The retrieval decision is individualized, depending on the merits and the risks involved in each case. The localization and size of the foreign body is one of the main factors to be considered with regard to the necessity and means of removal.

Complications of embolizations (Table 15-1) may occur immediately following embolization or months later. They include arrhythmias, perforation, clotting, and infection (sepsis, endocarditis). Bacterial contamination of foreign bodies has been reported in up to 50% within 48 hours; however, infectious complications resulting from bacteremia are much more rare.[9] Fatal complications such as injury of the large vessels (tear or rupture of large veins), perforation of the aorta or heart with resulting hemopericardium, tear or damage of the heart valves, embolization into vital structures such as the brain, heart, or major vessels, myocardial infarction, or death

TABLE 15-1.   Complications of Foreign Body Embolizations

MINOR

Pain
Arrhythmias
Thrombosis of peripheral vessels
Localized infection

MAJOR OR FATAL

Unstable arrhythmias
Rupture of large vessels
Perforation of cardiac chambers
Cardiac tamponade
Limb or coronary ischemia
Embolization to vital structures
Sepsis and endocarditis

---

occur rarely.[10,11] However, in some studies death rates up to 24% and 60% have been reported.[12,13]

Most foreign bodies need removal (Table 15-2). In only a few cases, the particularly low risk derived from foreign body residence in the vasculature does not justify the risk of attempting retrieval.[11]

Foreign bodies lost in the peripheral circulation, for instance, can be left alone unless they have a propensity to develop infection, thrombosis, or embolize. If despite the use of available imaging modalities, embolized foreign bodies cannot be localized, the search must be abandoned. This is usually the case with faintly radiopaque foreign bodies lost in the circulation. In these instances, the decision as to long-term anticoagulation will depend on the estimated risk of thromboembolism. Antibiotic therapy is not recommended because it is ineffective. Persistent pain represents an indication for removal of low-risk foreign bodies.

Catheter fragments, devices, guidewires, valve fragments, etc., located in the heart require early removal to avert the high risk of thrombus formation, perforation, arrhythmias, endocarditis, distal ischemia, etc. Similarly, lost intracoronary stents must be retrieved if at all possible. Foreign bodies localized in the large vessels always need to be extracted, as migration of such foreign bodies or occlusion of the large vessels is a possibility harboring disastrous consequences. Foreign bodies, being the source for pulmonary or arterial emboli, also require retrieval.

Percutaneous retrieval obviates the need for surgery and is safer and simpler to perform.[14] Complications of percutaneous retrieval can be injury to the vessel wall (tears, ruptures, and

TABLE 15-2.   Indications for Removal

RELATIVE (LOW-RISK STATES) INDICATIONS

Pain
Thrombosis
Crosstalk interference between pacemaker and ICD electrodes

ABSOLUTE (HIGH-RISK STATES) INDICATIONS

Active infection, sepsis, or endocarditis
High risk of perforation or arrhythmia
High risk of embolization into vital structure (heart, brain)
Foreign body entrapped in a cardiac chamber or large vessel

---

rarely perforation) and perforation and tearing of heart valves and chambers leading to hemopericardium. Clot and air embolism rarely do occur. Emergency surgery may become necessary in selected cases such as failed retrieval of a lost stent in the left main stem, lost septal closure devices, Greenfield filters, or bullet wounds.

SOURCES OF FOREIGN BODY EMBOLIZATION

The most common source of foreign body embolization is an iatrogenic complication (Table 15-3). Noniatrogenic foreign bodies represent a minority of cases resulting from missile injuries (bullets, splinters) and accidental or purposeful needle sticks. Initially, foreign bodies mainly involved the right side of the heart as a result of severed catheter fragments inserted intravenously. Subsequently, with the advent of angiography and catheter-based therapies, arterial embolizations have also become a significant hazard.[7]

Indwelling catheters such as Hickman catheters are used frequently for infusing long-term antibiotics, anticoagulation, chemotherapy, or nutrition, especially to cancer-afflicted individuals. Their use in the intensive care setting along with monitoring catheters is common. Hence these catheters represent the commonest source of foreign body embolisms. Other commonly retrieved items from the vascular system include wires, catheter fragments, malpositioned or migrated stents, coils, and caval filters.[15–23] Fragments of these devices migrate unpredictably, and interventionalists are regularly called upon to tackle these problems. The migratory fragments generally lodge distally at bifurcations, or they wedge in narrow vessels. A host of factors determine their path and localization. Route of entry, position of the patient at the time of the detachment, the length, shape, material, and stiffness of the object, and the flow patterns within the vessel and its course play a role, as well as presence and absence of valves and orifice size in relation to the size of the object. Venous foreign bodies commonly lodge

TABLE 15-3.   Types of Iatrogenic Intravascular Foreign Bodies

- Fragments of:
  - Diagnostic catheters
  - Balloon catheters
  - Swan-Ganz Thermodilution catheters
  - Valvuloplasty balloons
  - Intra-aortic balloon pump
  - Guidewires (or coatings of wires)
  - Introducer sheaths
  - Pacemaker electrodes
  - Puncture needles
- Stents
- Vascular prostheses
- Valves and rings
- Embolization coils
- Closure devices
- Vena cava filters

in the superior vena cava, right ventricle, or pulmonary artery. Long catheter fragments introduced into the subclavian or jugular veins frequently get stuck in the right ventricle while one end of the catheter is still retained in the vein itself. In contrast, short catheter fragments tend to migrate into the periphery of a pulmonary artery. Arterial foreign bodies may cause spasms, thrombotic vessel occlusions, or infarctions. Within the coronary artery circulation, foreign bodies generally migrate downstream. However, during attempts to retrieve guidewires, balloon catheter tips, or improperly deployed stents, the foreign body might be displaced retrogradely and migrate anywhere into the peripheral circulation. In the presence of an intracardiac shunt, a venous foreign body may become arterial and vice versa.[24] Such a situation should be kept in mind, as this would influence the method of retrieval and may even include repair of the anomaly in one setting.

With expanding indications of pacing and use of newer devices such as implantable cardioverter defibrillators (ICD), biventricular pacemakers, and percutaneous prosthetic valves, device-related problems (infection, dislocation, fracture, etc.) are of increasing importance to the interventionist and call for special extraction devices and techniques.[25]

AVOIDANCE OF EMBOLIZATION

Preferable to treatment for any problem are preventive measures. As has been discussed the majority of foreign body embolizations are iatrogenic and are potentially avoidable by simple attention to safety of techniques, proper selection of material, and standardization of procedures.

Most mishaps are due to inexperience, inattentiveness, improper handling, and inadequate diagnostics during positioning or faulty material.[26] An anxious patient further complicates things. This can be easily avoided by explaining the procedure to the patient, allaying his fears, and, in case the patient is still irritable, employing adequate sedation. It is needless to add that the physician must be skilled and experienced. In case of a trainee, close supervision is mandatory.

1. Accidental failure to secure the extravascular end of guidewires and catheters can lead to vascular embolization. This can be averted by ensuring exit of the guidewire from the distal end of the catheter and emphasizing the importance of fixing the position of the guidewire outside the body. The fellow and the nursing personnel play an important role in alerting the primary operator about this.
2. To minimize injury and encourage early mobilization, the calibers of vascular sheaths and catheters are decreasing. In addition to aiding access to remote locations such as the pulmonary wedge position, the catheters are highly flexible. Excessive torquing and manipulation of these catheters frequently lead to kinking, knotting, and even breakage. Care has to be taken to avoid excessive torquing, and use of a guidewire in the lumen when excessive torquing is anticipated can often avert this problem.
3. Using the Seldinger technique, a guidewire is introduced through a needle. The sharp end of the needle can shear off the guidewire being pulled back and a fragment of the guidewire can embolize. A septal puncture needle inserted through a protective sheath in the femoral vein

can perforate or even sever the sheath, thereby having a propensity not only to injure the vein but also to cause device embolization. Ensuring fluoroscopic guidance throughout the period of advancement can prevent this complication.
4. Hand-crimping of bare coronary stents on balloons was common in the 1990s. Improper crimping of stents before introduction into the guiding catheter is a common source of foreign bodies, and special attention to confirm correct crimping of stents needs to be taken. This complication has substantially decreased with the almost invariable use of premounted stents.
5. The advent of closure devices for PDA (patent ductus arteriosus), ASD (atrial septal defect), or VSD (ventricular septal defect) has added to the pool of foreign bodies. Their risk of embolization is due to a variety of reasons such as improper placement, incorrect sizing, wrong patient selection, and slipping off the delivery cable. The devices are loaded onto a delivery cable and tightened using a screw or other mechanisms. While pushing the delivery cable through a snugly fitting sheath, the screw can inadvertently loosen and cause embolization. Checking the screw or fixation joint under fluoroscopy prior to extruding the device out of the vascular sheath can reduce the risk of potentially life-threatening complications.
6. For procedures requiring small surgical incisions, such as pacemaker cardioverter defibrillator implantations, maintenance of proper instrument and swab count is helpful to prevent accidental loss of objects.

Once a foreign body is embolized, the next step is to localize and decide on retrieval methods, if any. The subsequent sections delve into general measures of detection, instrumentation, and retrieval methods. The last part of the chapter deals with specific instances encountered, and any special investigation, instrumentation, and technique used is highlighted.

TOOLS FOR FOREIGN BODY LOCALIZATION

Precise localization of the foreign body is of paramount importance, as this guides subsequent strategies such as decision for retrieval, mode of retrieval, and choice of devices to be used. Most of the materials used for manufacturing catheters, intravascular stents, and other devices are radiopaque and are thus detectable by conventional fluoroscopy provided sufficient spatial and contrast resolution. Retrievals are always carried out under fluoroscopic guidance. Biplane fluoroscopy is preferable over monoplane because it can obtain two simultaneous orthogonal projections, allowing better spatial orientation. It also facilitates proper topographic localization of the foreign body without having to move the camera as with monoplane equipment. Monoplane equipment is more time consuming to use, but also efficacious, and the absence of biplane equipment will not significantly hamper foreign body retrieval. Contrast-medium angiography can supplement fluoroscopy by delineation of neighboring vessels or heart chambers, and detect hitherto missed information such as formation of a fistula, cardiac tamponade, or a shunt by a protruding or eroding missile embolus. It can be used as a road-map guide during catheter removal of the foreign body.

The new-generation stents with thinner struts are less radiopaque and are difficult to localize with conventional fluoroscopy. This problem can be further compounded in obese patients. In case of incorrect placement or embolization of such stents, intravascular ultrasound (IVUS) is helpful, but a rough idea of the site of foreign body loss is necessary. IVUS has also been used for localization of embolized prosthetic valve fragments.[27]

Transthoracic and transesophageal echocardiography can provide invaluable information before and during catheter removal of foreign bodies. It allows for localization of weakly radiopaque foreign bodies entrapped in cardiac chambers as well as in neighboring structures (e.g., large veins, pulmonary artery, and aorta). Furthermore, it identifies thrombus superimposed on foreign bodies, which may be of importance during removal of pacemaker electrodes or catheter fragments. Its utility is also immeasurable in detection of cardiac tamponade secondary to myocardial or vessel perforation due to a dislodged foreign body. Echocardiography adds more information than conventional fluoroscopy, as once a foreign body is detected within the cardiac silhouette, echocardiography can pinpoint the exact location of the foreign body right ventricular outflow tract embedded in the myocardium, proximity to the coronary arteries, and so forth. This then aids the interventionist in further decision making, such as planning a coronary angiography prior to attempting retrieval, and also selecting the mode (surgical vs. medical) of retrieval. One can also do the retrieval under echocardiographic guidance, thereby attenuating blind operative trauma and procedure time. While using echocardiography, the operator should be aware that pericardial calcifications, fibrosis, and so forth can also cause reverberations mimicking foreign bodies. In this scenario the determination of the probable site of localization by conventional radiography may help the cause.

Magnetic resonance imaging (MRI), computed tomography (CT), and 3D echocardiography have added to the investigational pool for detection of difficult-to-see lost devices. Like echocardiography, CT scan and MRI have a specific role in precisely localizing the foreign body (e.g., embedded end of a guidewire missed by conventional radiography). Use of contrast medium adds further information as regards patency of the distal vessel. These highly advanced techniques have limitations such as availability in small centers, practicality of use in emergency situations, and slow acquisition rates in moving targets. Despite all the currently available imaging modalities, some foreign bodies are too small and radiolucent to be detected in the peripheral circulation. Most of these can be safely left alone in the absence of any complication.[11]

ACCESS ROUTES

The majority of the retrievals are performed via the femoral route with occasional use of upper-extremity venous access in cases of thrombosis of the inferior vena cava or other central

veins. In venous accesses, a double-wire technique[22] can be used. In this, two guidewires are placed in the same vein. Over one of the wires a vascular sheath is inserted, and the other lies parallel, acting as a safety wire. This aids in maintaining access for completion of retrieval or if angiography is required, even when one vascular sheath is pulled out with the foreign body. Alternatively, bilateral femoral routes can be used. This is especially useful for problems of knotting of catheters and also the coaxial snare technique (see later discussion).

DEVICES AND TECHNIQUES FOR FOREIGN BODY RETRIEVAL

Since the first description of percutaneous foreign body retrieval there has been considerable progress in techniques and instrumentation. Earlier devices included use of guidewires, pigtail catheters, etc. The earliest and only available retrieval device during the time of description by Dotter et al.[15] was the Curry snare.[28] Newer devices used include the wire loop snare, retrieval basket, grasping forceps, tip-deflecting wire, pincher devices, oversize sheaths or catheters, and balloon catheters.[15,17,18,22,29–32] Each operator cherishes a individual selection of devices as each device has its pros and cons. However, loop snares are the most commonly used devices. No quick-fix solution is recommended for a particular case, and the choice of device and technique is left to the imagination and expertise of the interventionist.

Following is a brief description of some of the commercially available devices.

DOTTER RETRIEVAL BASKET

The Dotter retrieval basket (Fig. 15-1) consists of a flexible, onion-shaped wire mesh, which is constrained within a guiding sheath and assumes its shape on delivery from the sheath. The device is available in different sizes and can be introduced through an appropriately sized vascular introducer sheath, which is first navigated past the foreign body. The basket is advanced, opened, and pulled back to trap parts of the foreign body, preferably a loose end, within its mesh. As soon as the foreign body is trapped, the guiding sheath is used to fix the foreign body against the distal basket tip, and both are retrieved as a unit. Slight kinking of the tip of the basket, or the catheter it is attached to, may be required to catch foreign bodies in difficult locations.

SNARE CATHETERS

Snare catheters (Figs. 15-2 A,B) consist of a radiopaque nitinol coated loop, which can be collapsed within the catheter shaft and assumes its shape coaxial to the vessel lumen on delivery.[33] The snare diameter varies from 2 to 7 mm (Microsnare, "Microvena") to 5 to 35 mm (Amplatz Goose Neck Snare,

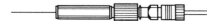 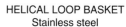

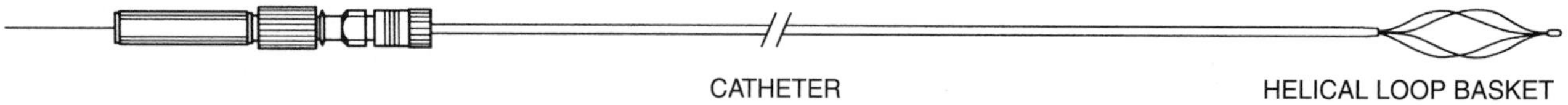

CATHETER
Radiopaque tetrafluoroethylene with metal Luer lock fitting

HELICAL LOOP BASKET
Stainless steel

FIGURE 15-1. Dotter intravascular retrieval set (courtesy of Cook Cardiology).

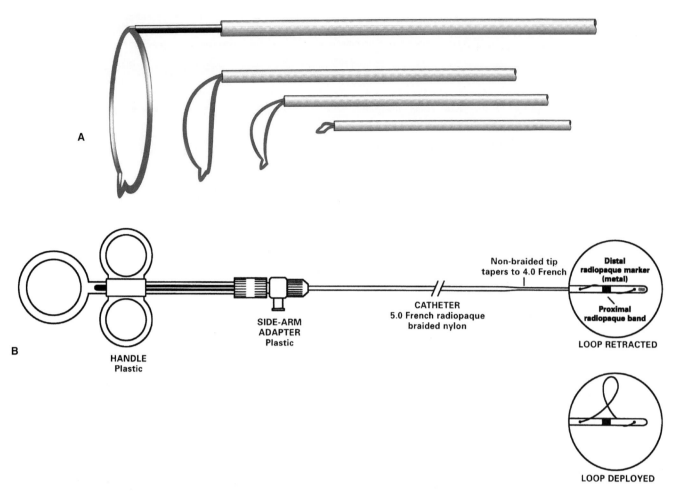

FIGURE 15-2. **A:** Amplatz gooseneck snares (courtesy of Microvena Corp.). **B:** Welter retrieval loop catheter (courtesy of Cook Cardiology).

"Microvena"). The chosen snare size should roughly correspond to the size of the vessel harboring the foreign body. Once the foreign body is entrapped into the snare, the loop is closed by retraction of the snare against the catheter shaft, which is then extracted. Small coronary snares are best introduced over a guidewire close to the foreign body, and once the foreign body is trapped, the complete assembly (guidewire, snare, and foreign body) is removed as a unit. Large loop catheters are stiffer and therefore can be introduced and navigated without a guidewire. An inexpensive snare can be constructed in the catheterization laboratory by folding a common guidewire in the middle and advancing it into a sheath long enough to reach the foreign body. Alternatively, a guidewire may be reintroduced about 10 cm into the tip of a carrier catheter. Pulling in the proximal end of the wire catches the object by the tightening the loop. Finally, a guidewire may be led around the foreign body using, for instance, a left Judkins coronary catheter. The end of the wire is then caught with, for example, a Dotter basket and exteriorized. Both ends are fed through a sheath long enough to reach the object to snare it. The disadvantage of indigenously manufactured snares is that they usually open parallel to the vessel axis. This speaks in favor of preshaped perpendicularly aligned nitinol gooseneck snares. Other advantages of these instruments—their predefined loop diameter and the shape-memory properties of nitinol—facilitate foreign object retrieval in nearly all vascular areas. Furthermore, by manipulation of the external end, variable force can be transmitted to the nitinol snare depending on the need for compressibility of the foreign body.

RETRIEVAL FORCEPS

Miniature retrieval forceps (Fig. 15-3) are suitable for retrieval of fragmented pieces of guidewire fragments and coronary stents.[18] They consist of a small 3F catheter system, which can be introduced through a guiding catheter and then advanced into the peripheral vessels or coronary arteries. A flexible coil is attached to the proximal end to minimize trauma to the vessel wall. Adjacent to the coil is the forceps, which is usually closed. Manipulation at the external catheter end allows for opening the forceps and thereby catching a foreign body. As soon as the foreign body is firmly grasped, the assembly is retrieved into the guiding catheter. These forceps can also be used to deliver embolization coils (for, e.g., coil closure of the PDA and fistulas) and ironically may be responsible for inappropriate location of the misplaced coils. As compared to

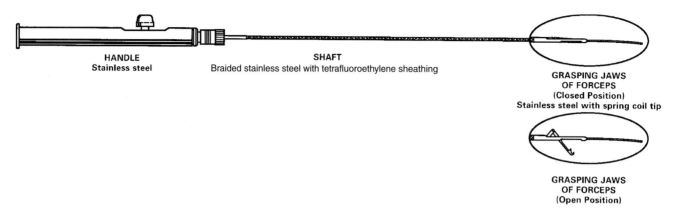

FIGURE 15-3.   Vascular retrieval forceps (courtesy of Cook Cardiology).

snares, forceps can be dangerous, as the edges can grasp the vessel or chamber wall neighboring the foreign body. They require extreme caution when being used.

CATHETERIZATION LABORATORY MISHAPS

Since the majority of the foreign bodies encountered in the venous and arterial circulation require similar modes of retrieval, only instances where specific methods are needed for investigations or retrieval are pointed out separately. The remainder of the description in the following section of the chapter pertains to the entire circulation. This section deals with actual day-to-day problems encountered in the catheterization laboratory and the possible solutions that have been attempted to solve them with preventive and therapeutic hints at every step. This is by no means a comprehensive review of all possible methods of retrieval, and in fact can be used as building blocks by student interventionists to help them develop their own strategies.

VASCULAR STENTS

Stent embolization occurs in 1% to 2% of stent implantation procedures.[33,34] Manually crimped stents have a distinct advantage with regard to production cost. The same balloon can be used for pre- and postdilatation as well as for stent delivery. Manual crimping, however, carries a markedly increased risk of stent embolization as compared with premounted stents (1.04% vs. 0.27% per stent, $p < 0.01$).[11] Other factors predisposing to stent loss are poor guiding catheter or guidewire support, extreme tortuosity, and extensive calcification. Attention to technical details can be helpful in avoiding these complications. Self-crimped stents must be mounted firmly and free of loose struts onto the balloon catheter. Injury to the balloon catheter should be avoided, as a leaking balloon leads to insufficient stent expansion and inadvertent air embolism. During stent delivery, at least two sites of resistance are encountered: first, the connection of the "Y" connector at the distal end of the guiding catheter, and second, the proximal tip of the catheter that engages the coronary ostium. Each site of resistance may dislocate the stent from the balloon catheter. This can be circumvented by widely opening the "Y" connector, eliminating both the risk of stent slippage

and air embolization (suction effect). Aligning the catheter tip coaxially to the coronary artery facilitates stent delivery through the tip of the guiding catheter by reducing friction and bending forces. Proper selection of guiding catheters and extra support guidewires also aid in smoother delivery of stents to the desired location. Smaller caliber, softer tipped catheters can be deeply intubated into the coronary artery with little propensity for trauma. Smaller bore catheters inserted into larger caliber catheters can provide support to stent delivery. Use of the "buddy" (double) wire technique has also reduced the risk of stent loss by providing extra support for precise stent delivery. Stent loss has been largely eliminated with the use of modern premounted stents.

Stents are usually rigid and are often difficult to retrieve. One must weigh the risks associated with the retrieval maneuver, such as permanent vascular wall trauma, against the benefit to the patient from the retrieval procedure. Flexible stents such as the Wallstent can be easily compressed with the snare, elongated, and percutaneously retrieved,[21,35] whereas the old-generation Palmaz Schatz stents were rigid and would most of the time need to be deployed at an innocent site,[36] for instance by pressing the stent against the wall underneath another stent (see later discussion).

Methods of Retrieval

The following case scenarios describe the most frequent problems and their solutions encountered during coronary stent implantation (Table 15-4).

- In patients with extensive tortuosity of the aorta and with increased intracoronary resistance (calcified plaque, dissection, etc.), an attempt to implant the stent in the desired position can result in dislocation of the entire delivery system including the guidewire, balloon, stent, and guiding catheter from the coronary artery into the ascending aorta or at times into the left ventricle. In this situation the entire delivery system should be withdrawn beyond the aortic arch to prevent embolization into the cerebrovascular tree (Table 15-4). In the descending aorta, the stent-balloon assembly is carefully retracted into the guiding catheter to prevent stent loss.[37]
- An unexpanded stent may slip off the balloon catheter during advancement or withdrawal of the stent-balloon

TABLE 15-4. Nonsurgical Methods of Stent Retrieval

Withdrawal of the entire delivery system with the guide catheter in toto

Use of low-profile balloon catheters:
- Implantation of stent at site of stent loss
- Withdrawal of stent hanging on the balloon shaft
- Pushing a stent to the desired location on the partially inflated balloon
- Crushing an unexpanded stent by another stent

Double-wire technique of withdrawal

Use of microsnares and forceps

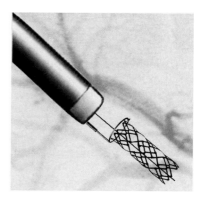

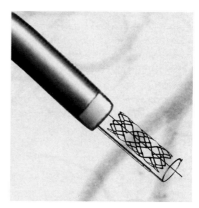

FIGURE 15-4. Stent retrieval using the Amplatz gooseneck snare. **A:** Proximal grab technique. **B:** Distal grab technique.

assembly. The first measure should be to advance the guidewire as far distal into the coronary artery as possible, ensuring that the entry into the coronary artery and through the slipped stent is maintained at all the times. As a next step, the delivery balloon should be replaced with the lowest profile balloon available, which is cautiously advanced over the guidewire through the unexpanded stent (Table 15-4). Once the balloon is successfully maneuvered through the stent, one can choose among three options. One is to implant the stent at its current position, with subsequent introduction of appropriately sized balloons to achieve the desired stent size. This ensures no further stent embolization at the cost of implanting the stent at an unplanned location. Alternatively, a small, low-profile balloon can be placed distal to the stent and then inflated. This prevents distal embolization of the stent, which floats free on the balloon shaft proximal to the inflated balloon. The assembly with the balloon and guiding catheter can be pulled out over the guidewire and removed. Pulling the balloon or the stent into the guiding catheter should be avoided. This method is associated with a small risk of endothelial denudation and perforation of the coronary artery. The small balloon may also be placed centrally in the stent and inflated at <1 bar. This leads to slight "dog boning" on both sides of the stent without opening the stent. The stent may be retrieved in this fashion into the guiding catheter in most instances and can be reused and implanted at the desired location. Alternatively, the third option would be to partially inflate the 1.5-mm balloon inside the stent and push them forward as a unit to the desired location for implantation there. This is the most difficult of the options. In case of failure to retrieve the stent, an alternative approach would be to pass a guidewire alongside the unexpanded stent and crush the unexpanded stent against the vessel wall using another stent deployed alongside, without comprising the coronary flow.

- Another method of stent retrieval consists of the delivery of a second guidewire into the coronary artery. The second guidewire should be manipulated through one of the stent struts avoiding the central lumen.[38] The two guidewires are then twisted around each other with the help of a single common torquer. The twirled guidewires will secure the embolized stent, allowing for retraction of the stent from the coronary artery without tilting.

- Finally, specially designed coronary microsnares (Microsnare 2 to 7 mm, "Microvena" Inc.) (Figs. 15-4 A,B)[33] are the most frequently used devices for stent retrieval and should

be indispensable tools in every catheterization laboratory. This device has a closed, retractile wire loop of variable diameter made of nitinol. A second guidewire is placed with the tip distal to the embolized stent. An exchange catheter is inserted over the second wire, and the microsnare is advanced through the exchange catheter. Retraction of the exchange catheter allows the shape-memory alloy nitinol to retain its predefined loop vertical to the vessel axis. Careful manipulation of the loop by means of an external torquer allows slipping the loop around the guidewire and stent. By retraction of the snare against the exchange catheter, the loop will be tightened, which secures the stent. The whole assembly consisting of snare catheter, guidewire, and stent is then retrieved in toto from the coronary artery tree. At times the snare holds the stent at an angle, and since stents are not foldable, they may be difficult to pull out through the percutaneous route; in such situations a coaxial snare technique needs to be employed. This has been explained in detail in the section on catheter fragments.

Stents are also being used in peripheral, renal, and carotid arteries. Stentlike are also used in the venous circulation, such as vena cava filters, or stents for vena cava thrombosis or stenosis, especially in irradiated patients. They additionally have expanded indications such as use in congenital heart diseases (e.g., peripheral pulmonary artery stenosis, coarctation) and a variety of noncardiac indications (hepatobiliary). The principles and instrumentation for retrieval are similar in all of these scenarios vascular beds.

GUIDEWIRE FRAGMENTS

Coronary guidewires are made up of three components: (a) a tapered steel core, (b) a string of platinum wire or ribbon wound in a tight coil around the steel core, and (c) a forming ribbon that extends between the tip of the core and the distal tip of the wire. A wire trapped in a chronic occlusion can break or uncoil when attempts are made to forcibly torque or pull it out. Since the wire has a coating and a ribboned structure, the length of the lost guidewire is highly variable. In some instances the wire can extend all along the course of the aorta, and extraction may be cumbersome or impossible at times.

The incidence of guidewire fragments left behind is approximately 0.2%.[24] The decision to retrieve guidewire fragments is influenced by their size, length, and localization. Small fragments localized in a chronic total occlusion or the distal coronary artery tree can be left in place. In contrast, long wire fragments with extension into the aorta, the potential for distal migration, or risk for thrombotic complication in proximal coronary arteries constitute absolute indications for retrieval. Infection of embolized coating material usually represents an indication for retrieval, but since the coating is flimsy and may be difficult to visualize, percutaneous retrieval may be impossible. In such cases, surgical intervention may be required.

Methods of Retrieval

Embolized guidewire fragments can be tackled in the following ways:

- If unwinding of a coronary guidewire is recognized early, no further attempts to manipulate the wire should be made. Instead the guiding catheter is aligned with the coronary ostium and a balloon is gently advanced over the wire. Following this the whole assembly, that is, guiding catheter, balloon catheter, and disrupted guidewire, is withdrawn en bloc.
- Severed guidewire fragments, which extend into the aortic root, can be removed by twisting them around a pigtail or Amplatz-type catheter, which is then retrieved.
- Coronary microsnares are suited for guidewire fragments localized within the coronary artery tree.

Retrieval maneuvers for any kind of guidewire are cumbersome, as especially the coronary wires are flimsy and difficult to snare, and they tend to further unwind on snaring. There is also a significant risk for re-embolization or further fragmentation. They also can become embedded in the vessel wall or can be endothelialized; in some of these instances they are better left in situ, as the risk of retrieval may exceed the benefit. A case report documents a 14-year follow-up of a retained uncomplicated wire in the pulmonary arteries.[39] On the other hand, attempts to extract such impacted long fragments have been successfully made.[40] To summarize, most guidewire fragments need extraction, and every attempt must be made to safely do so.

INTRAVASCULAR CATHETER–RELATED PROBLEMS

Kinking

The increasing utilization of central venous catheters, flow-directed catheters, and various angiographic catheters is associated with complications such as breaking and knotting of catheters. This typically occurs as a result of excessive torquing of catheters as encountered during floating of a Swan-Ganz catheter from the femoral route or maneuvering catheters through tortuous vessels.[41] Small catheters and those with a thin and soft wall construction are predisposed to kinking and breaking.

METHODS OF RETRIEVAL. In case of kinking, the catheter should be first pulled back into a larger vessel (i.e., aorta, vena cava) and subsequently straightened by advancing a guidewire or unbending it across a side branch. Once kinking has occurred, catheters tend to kink at the same site again and may have to be replaced.

Knotting

Knotting of devices is a rare occurrence, which is associated with significant morbidity. It is one of the foreign body retrieval situations where the surgical approach is common. It was first reported by Johansson et al.[42] The Swan-Ganz catheter is the commonest culprit catheter for knotting because of its soft walls and its use without fluoroscopy. Other culprit devices include pacemaker electrodes, guidewires, and low-caliber angiography catheters negotiating tortuous vessels and needing excessive torque for difficult coronary intubations.

METHODS OF RETRIEVAL. What appears as a knotted catheter is frequently only a row of catheter loops, which may be untwisted by careful rotation maneuvers in the direction opposite to the previously applied torque. In case of a real catheter knot, however, further pulling must be avoided to prevent tightening of the knot. If one encounters more than one knot, a rule is to unknot the distal one first and the following ones in sequence from distal to proximal. The first measure to unknot a catheter is by means of a guidewire. In case of a tight knot, however, this method rarely succeeds, and the next step is the introduction of special hook-shaped catheters (i.e., sidewinder catheter) (Fig. 15-5) from either the ipsilateral or contralateral site to allow for further manipulation. This catheter can often be negotiated through the loop of the knot[43] or hooked at the knot[44] to exert traction to open the loop. Occasionally, an angioplasty balloon may be utilized. This balloon catheter is passed through the knot and then inflated, saddling the loop, which results in loosening expansion of the knot.[45]

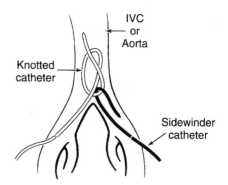

FIGURE 15-5. Untying of a knot using a sidewinder catheter. *IVC,* inferior vena cava.

If a knot in a catheter cannot be opened, the knot size is reduced by tension on the catheter, to a minimal size. This may then allow retrieval of the knotted catheter in a sufficiently sized vascular access site sheath. Occasionally, a surgical incision at the puncture site may be necessary to avoid injury to the vessel wall.

Loose knots in subclavian or jugular catheters may be untied by the femoral approach. A knotted catheter in the subclavian vein is associated with a small risk of hemothorax. Such a catheter should be untied or removed with the use of deflecting wires or grasping forceps via the femoral approach. From the groin, it may have to be removed surgically.

Surgical removal of knotted catheters is utilized for failed percutaneous unknotting, large knots with multiple loops, or if the knot becomes fixed.

Knots should never be left in situ, as the risk of thrombosis is high.

Catheter Fragments

Catheter fragments constitute 0.2% to 1% of cases of central venous insertions.[46,47] To retrieve broken catheter fragments with one end lodged at the puncture site of the vessel, one should refrain from percutaneous intervention. A surgical retrieval under local anesthesia may be easier and safer approach. For embolized catheter fragments, an attempt at percutaneous retrieval should precede surgical intervention. Instruments used include retrieval basket, loop snare, grasping forceps, hook-shaped catheters, and deflecting wires.

METHODS OF RETRIEVAL. For fragments with free ends, the easiest method of retrieval is by using a snare loop (Fig. 15-6) or a retrieval basket. Special retrieval baskets (Meditech, Watertown, MA) are available for use in children and small vessels in adults.

If no free end of the catheter fragment lies in the vessel lumen, then one needs to adapt a three-pronged strategy. (a) The fragment is engaged with a deflecting catheter or wire via the femoral approach. (b) The fragment is dragged down into the femoral area with continuous rotation of the catheter in one direction. This maneuver usually frees at least one end of the fragment and prevents further embolization of the fragment. (c) Once the fragment end is accessible, a loop snare or a basket is used from the contralateral or

ipsilateral approach to grasp the free end of the fragment and retrieve it.

Alternatively, a retrieval forceps can be employed via the femoral approach to grasp the middle of the fragment to remove it. Caution is necessary to avoid any damage to the vessel wall. Another maneuver involves gently bringing the fragment down to the puncture site with a deflecting wire, securing the catheter with one hand by compression above the inguinal region, and using a small clamp to grasp the catheter fragment and remove it via the puncture site.

COAXIAL SNARE TECHNIQUE. The loop snare technique is one of the most frequently used techniques for foreign body retrieval and has evolved to become the method of choice. The diameter of the loop snare is adjusted depending on the diameter of the vessel trapping the foreign body, and the position of the foreign body in the three-dimensional vessel determines the angulations of the snare to be employed. The snare can also be directed by using additional catheters. In the case of large foreign bodies, however, the simple snare technique may result in folding or angulation of the entrapped foreign body and then necessitate the use of larger caliber sheaths for percutaneous withdrawal. However, because these large-lumen access sheaths and rigid entrapped foreign bodies may become precursors for traumatic injury to the vessel wall and also lead to life-threatening hemorrhage or other serious complications involving the access site, they must be approached with utmost care, even by experienced interventionists. To overcome these problems to a great extent, the coaxial snare technique is employed.

The coaxial snare technique is a modification of the previously described loop snare technique.[22,23,35,48] This technique involves grasping of the foreign body with the help of a regular loop snare. The snare is placed beyond the object, tightened, and slowly retracted into a larger vessel (for example, the inferior vena cava). Snaring may result in formation of an obtuse angle between the object and the snare axis (Fig. 15-7A). A second puncture, usually contralateral, is made, and through that an angiographic catheter and a guidewire are passed. The lumen of the foreign body is located, which is then crossed with the guidewire (Fig. 15-7B). A vascular sheath dilator is then threaded over the guidewire to tightly coaxially fix the foreign body, which is then retrieved (Fig. 15-7C). The placement of a guidewire through the center of the object not only allows its rapid capture with a loop snare but also greatly reduces the angle between

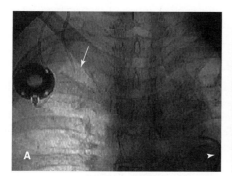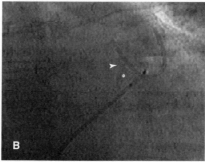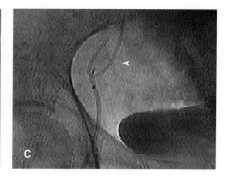

FIGURE 15-6. Free catheter fragment snaring. **A:** Proximal end of the Hickman catheter in the right subclavian vein (*arrow*) and the free-floating catheter fragment (*arrow head*). **B:** the loop snare capturing the free-floating catheter fragment in the pulmonary artery (*arrow head*). **C:** Removal of the catheter fragment percutaneously from the right femoral vein (*arrow head*).

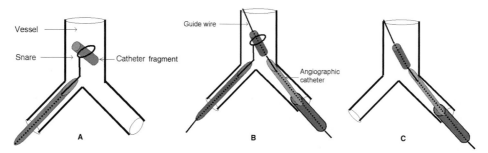

FIGURE 15-7. Coaxial snare technique. **A:** The loop snare captures the catheter fragment at an angle. **B:** Realignment of the catheter using another guidewire through the fragment introduced via an angiographic catheter through the contralateral side. **C:** Removal of the catheter fragment percutaneously after realignment.

the object and the snare axis. The engagement of a dilator with the end of a fragmented catheter eliminates the shoulder between the guidewire and the catheter. However, it is sometimes very difficult to locate the lumen (patency is often impaired in a chronically indwelling fragment) of a free-floating fragment within a greater patulous space.

For retrieval of an intravascular foreign body using the coaxial snare technique, the minimum inner diameter of the vascular sheath should be greater than the sum of the outer diameter of the foreign body and the catheter used with the loop snare. In order to minimize the profile of the retrieval system for large-bore intravascular foreign objects, the use of a coaxial system using dual vascular access is preferred. In this technique, one access is for the snare and the other access is for the angiographic catheter and the guidewire over which a vascular sheath dilator is threaded after aligning the object, which now needs a smaller caliber sheath for withdrawal. This prevents traumatic sequelae associated with retrieval of rigid objects and large-bore catheter fragments.

SHUNT CLOSURE DEVICES

Percutaneous devices are increasingly used to close shunts such as atrial and ventricular septal defects as well as patent ductus arteriosus and patent foramen ovale in case of paradoxical embolism. The devices are positioned across the atrial or ventricular septum or the ductus and released after confirmation of appropriate position. Most percutaneous closure devices consist of two umbrellas interconnected by a waist of variable size. In case of an atrial septal defect or patent foramen ovale, the device is positioned by release of the left-sided umbrella in the left atrium, followed by tension against the septum and subsequent release of the right-sided umbrella in the right atrium, with the interconnecting waist serving as a strut across the septal defect. The device is passively locked by the differential size and counter tension of the umbrellas relative to the septal defect. The procedure is associated with a small but definite risk of device embolization. Most commonly the devices embolize from left to right into the right atrium, the right ventricle, or the pulmonary artery. However, embolization into left-sided cavities can occur. These relatively large foreign bodies have to be retrieved to avoid thrombus formation at the embolization site.

Methods of Retrieval

The devices are usually extracted by use of a snare, a forceps, or a Dotter retrieval basket. However, because of their relative large size, it may become difficult to withdraw the crumpled device into an intravascular sheath. It can perhaps be removed directly through the skin without a sheath by gentle pulling in case of a vein. Devices pulled back into a peripheral artery may require a surgical cutdown for final removal.

Pfammatter et al. reported an interesting case of an embolized Amplatzer patent ductus arteriosus occluder.[49] It was percutaneously retrieved and successfully repositioned at its desired location without actual removal of the device from the circulation. A 14/12-mm Amplatzer device screwed onto the delivery cable, had accidentally unscrewed during delivery of the aortic end, and had embolized into the descending aorta (Fig. 15-8A). The angle of the device precluded reattachment to the delivery cable. The waist of the device was snared with a 20-mm Amplatz microsnare from the venous access through the delivery sheath (Fig. 15-8B). By multiple manipulations the device was aligned along the sheath. Using a contralateral venous puncture, a 4-mm Amplatz microsnare was advanced through the Judkins right coronary catheter and the screw of the device could be snared (Fig. 15-8C). Traction on the small Amplatz snare could pull the device back into the desired location into the ductus (Fig. 15-8D). After confirming the correct position by aortography both the snares were removed (Fig. 15-8E).

This could constitute another mode of management of an embolization with definitive treatment.

OTHER FOREIGN BODIES

Other foreign bodies that need retrieval include missile emboli (bullets). The largest series was reported in 1979.[50] Most of the earlier reports were on surgical retrieval. Kaushik et al.[51] reported percutaneous retrieval of a bullet embolus from the right side of the heart using a Dotter retrieval basket. As a rule, free-floating missiles should be percutaneously retrieved, and embedded bullets may need surgical removal or can be left alone, though one series reported a 25% complication rate of left-alone intravascular projectiles.[52] Large foreign bodies such as expanded peripheral stents or vena cava filters can be

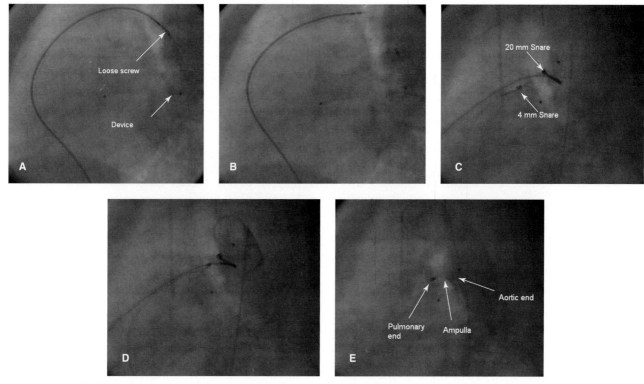

FIGURE 15-8. 14/12-mm Amplatzer PDA Occluder. **A:** A loose screw of the device prior to release. **B:** Device lost in the descending aorta (*arrows*). **C:** Waist of the device held by a 20-mm Amplatzer microsnare and screw of the device held by a 4-mm Amplatzer microsnare. **D:** Device pulled back into the ampulla. **E:** Device repositioned in the PDA and snares removed. Position confirmed with a contrast injection into the descending aorta confirming the PDA occlusion. PDA—patent ductus arteriosus.

brought as close as possible to the access site. Commonly they will need a surgical cutdown for final extraction. Other foreign bodies such as embolization coils or prosthetic valve fragments can be retrieved using similar principles.

SUMMARY

Success rates of judicious percutaneous foreign body retrieval attempts have been around 95%. Complications are few and include distal embolization, transient arrhythmias, and perforations. Death is also a rare possibility. A need for conversion to surgical means is rare. Percutaneous foreign body retrieval is highly effective, minimally invasive, safe, and generally atraumatic. With the availability of newer devices and the possibility of safer techniques, percutaneous retrieval will become faster and more cost effective. Hence, initial attempts at foreign body removal should primarily be percutaneous. Only compelling indications should prompt a surgical option.

Patience, willingness to learn, and sound application of safety techniques should all but preclude foreign body embolization. In the event of inadvertent embolization, knowledge of the experiences presented in this chapter combined with creativity, adaptability, and imagination should permit safe and speedy percutaneous removal in a majority of cases. One must remember that each embolization is unique, and no single technique is universally applicable to all intravascular foreign bodies.

REFERENCES

1. Forssmann W. Die Sondierung des rechten Herzens. *Klin Wochenschr.* 1929;8:2085.
2. Thomas J, Sinclair-Smith B, Bloomfield D, et al. Non-surgical retrieval of a broken segment of steel spring guide from right atrium and inferior vena cava. *Circulation.* 1964;30:106–108.
3. Fisher RG, Ferreyro R. Evaluation of current techniques for nonsurgical removal of intravascular iatrogenic foreign bodies. *AJR Am J Roentgenol.* 1978;130:541–548.
4. Mahon T, Lawrence D Sr. Technical report: an injection technique for repositioning subclavian catheters. *Clin Radiol.* 1991;44:197–198.
5. Roizental M, Hartnell GG. The misplaced central venous catheter: a long loop technique for repositioning. *J Vasc Intervent Radiol.* 1995;6:263–265.
6. Haskal Z, Leen V, Thomas-Hawkins C, et al. Transvenous removal of fibrin sheaths from tunneled hemodialysis catheter. *J Vasc Intervent Radiol.* 1996;7:513–517.
7. Gabelmann A, Kramer S, Gorich J. Percutaneous retrieval of lost or misplaced intravascular objects. *AJR Am J Roentgenol.* 2001;176:1509–1513.
8. Bessoud B, de Baere, T, Kuoch, V, et al. Experience at a single institution with endovascular treatment of mechanical complications caused by implanted central venous access devices in pediatric and adult patients. *AJR Am J Roentgenol.* 2003;180:527–532.
9. Druskin MS, Siegel DD. Bacterial contamination of indwelling intravenous polyethylene catheter. *JAMA.* 1963;185:966–970.
10. Turner DD, Sommers SC. Accidental passage of a polyethylene catheter from cubital vein to right atrium: report of a fatal case. *N Engl J Med.* 1954;251:744–745.
11. Eggebrecht H, Haude M, von Birgelen C, et al. Nonsurgical retrieval of embolized coronary stents. *Cathet Cardiovasc Intervent.* 2000;51:432–440.
12. Bernhardt LC, Wegner GP, Mendenhall JT. Intravenous catheter embolization of the pulmonary artery. *Chest.* 1970;57:329–332.
13. Richardson JD, Grover FL, Trinkle JK. Intravenous catheter emboli: experience with 20 cases and collective review. *Am J Surg.* 1974;128:722–727.
14. Kadir S, Athanasoulis CA. Percutaneous retrieval of intravascular foreign bodies. In: Athanasoulis CA, Green RE, Pfister RC, et al., eds. *Interventional Radiology.* 1982:379–390.
15. Dotter CT, Roesch J, Bilbao MK. Transluminal extraction of catheter and guide fragments from the heart and great vessels: 29 collected cases. *AJR Am J Roentgenol.* 1971;111:467–472.
16. Bloomfield DA. The nonsurgical retrieval of intracardiac foreign bodies: an international survey. *Cathet Cardiovasc Diagn.* 1978;4:1–14.
17. Uflacker R, Lima S, Melichar AC. Intravascular foreign bodies: percutaneous retrieval. *Radiology.* 1986;160:731–735.

18. Selby JB, Tegtmeyer CJ, Bittner GM. Experience with new retrieval forceps for foreign body removal in the vascular, urinary and biliary systems. *Radiology.* 1990;176:535–538.

19. Dondeliger RF, Lepontre B, Kurdziel JC. Percutaneous vascular foreign body retrieval: experience of an 11-year period. *Eur J Radiol.* 1991;12:4–10.

20. Siegel EL, Robertson EF. Percutaneous transfemoral retrieval of a free-floating titanium Greenfield filter with an Amplatz gooseneck snare. *J Vasc Intervent Radiol.* 1993;4: 565–568.

21. Cekirge S, Weiss JP, Foster RG, et al. Percutaneous retrieval of foreign bodies: experience with the nitinol gooseneck snare. *J Vasc Intervent Radiol.* 1993;4:805–810.

22. Egglin TKP, Dickey KW, Rosenblatt M, et al. Retrieval of intravascular foreign bodies: experience in 32 cases. *AJR Am J Roentgenol.* 1995;164:1259–1264.

23. Hartnell GG, Jordan SJ. Percutaneous removal of a misplaced Palmaz stent with a coaxial snare technique. *J Vasc Intervent Radiol.* 1995;6:799–801.

24. Hartzler GO, Rutherford BD, McConahay DR. Retained percutaneous transluminal coronary angioplasty equipment components and their management. *Am J Cardiol.* 1987;60:1260–1264.

25. Byrd CL. Management of implant complications. In: Ellenbogen KA, Kay GN, Wlikoff BL, eds. *Clinical Cardiac Pacing.* 2nd ed. Philadelphia: WB Saunders, 2000.

26. Vlietstra R. Retrieval of foreign bodies. In: Uretzky BF, ed. *Cardiac Catheterization.* Malden, UK: Blackwell, 1997:604–615.

27. Miller SF, McCowan TC, Eidt JF, et al. Embolization of a prosthetic mitral valve leaflet: localization with intravascular US. *J Vasc Intervent Radiol.* 1991;2:375–378.

28. Curry JL. Recovery of detached intravascular catheter or guide wire fragments. *AJR Am J Roentgenol.* 1969;105:894–896.

29. Nemcek AA Jr, Vogelzang RL. Modified use of the tip-deflecting wire in manipulation of foreign bodies. *AJR Am J Roentgenol.* 1987;149:777–779.

30. Boren SR, Dotter CT, McKinney M, et al. Percutaneous removal of ureteral stents. *Radiology.* 1984;152:230–231.

31. Park JH, Yoon DY, Han JK, et al. Retrieval of intravascular foreign bodies with the snare and catheter capture technique. *J Vasc Intervent Radiol.* 1992;3:581–582.

32. Katske FA, Celis P. Technique for removal of migrated double-J ureteral stent. *Urology.* 1991;37:579.

33. Elsner M, Pfeifer A, Kasper W. Intracoronary loss of balloon mounted stents: successful retrieval with a 2mm-Microsnare device. *Cathet Cardiovasc Diagn.* 1996;39:271–276.

34. Schatz RA, Baim DS, Leon M, et al. Clinical experience of Palmaz-Schatz coronary stent. Initial results of a multicenter study. *Circulation.* 1991;83:148–161.

35. Sanchez RB, Roberts AC, Valji K, et al. Wallstent misplacement during transjugular placement of an intrahepatic portosystemic shunt: retrieval with a loop snare. *AJR Am J Roentgenol.* 1992;159:129–130.

36. Kamalesh M, Stokes K, Burger AJ. Transoesophageal echocardiography assisted retrieval of embolized inferior vena cava stent. *Cathet Cardiovasc Diagn.* 1994;33:178–180.

37. Iyer S, Roubin GS. Nonsurgical management of retained intracoronary products following coronary interventions. In: Roubin GS, Califf RM, O'Neill WW, eds. *Interventional Cardiovascular Medicine.* New York: Churchill Livingstone, 1994.

38. Veldhuijzen FLMJ, Bonnier HJRM, Michels R, et al. Retrieval of undeployed stents from the right coronary artery: report of two cases. *Cathet Cardiovasc Diagn.* 1993;30:245–248.

39. Reynen, K. 14-year follow-up of central embolization by a guide wire. *N Engl J Med.* 1993;329(13):970–971.

40. Farrell AG, Parikh SR, Darragh RK, et al. Retrieval of "old" foreign bodies from the cardiovascular system in children. *Cathet Cardiovasc Diagn.* 1998;44:212–216.

41. Cho SR, Tisando J, Beachley MC, et al. Percutaneous unknotting of intravascular catheters and retrieval of catheter fragments. *AJR Am J Roentgenol.* 1983;141:397–402.

42. Johansson L, Malmstrom G, Ugglia LG. Intracardiac knotting of the catheter in heart catheterization. *J Thorac Surg.* 1954;27(6):605–607.

43. Chinichian A, Liebeskind A, Zingesser LH, et al. Knotting of an 8-French "headhunter catheter" and its successful removal. *Radiology.* 1972;104(2):282.

44. Thomas HA, Sievers RE. Nonsurgical reduction of arterial catheter knots. *AJR Am J Roentgenol.* 1979;132(6):1018–1019.

45. Tan C, Bristow PJ, Segal, P, et al. A technique to remove knotted pulmonary artery catheters. *Anaesth Intensive Care.* 1997;25(2):160–162.

46. Klotz HP, Schopke W, Kohler A, et al. Catheter fracture: a rare complication of totally implantable subclavian venous access devices. *J Surg Oncol.* 1996;62:222–225.

47. Kock HJ, Pietsch M, Krause U, et al. Implantable vascular access systems: experience in 1500 patients with totally implanted central venous port systems. *World J Surg.* 1998;22:12–16.

48. Cekirge S, Foster RG, Weiss JP, et al. Percutaneous removal of an embolized Wallstent during a transjugular intrahepatic portosystemic shunt procedure. *J Vasc Intervent Radiol.* 1993;4:559–560.

49. Pfammatter JP, Meier B. Successful repositioning of an Amplatzer duct occluder immediately after inadvertent embolization in the descending aorta. *Cathet Cardiovasc Intervent.* 2003;59(1):83–85.

50. Mattox, KL, Beall, AC, Jr., Ennix, CL, et al. Intravascular migratory bullets. *Am J Surg.* 1979;137(2):192–195.

51. Kaushik, VS, Mandal, AK. Non-surgical retrieval of a bullet embolus from the right heart. *Cathet Cardiovasc Intervent.* 1999;47(1):55–57.

52. Shannon FL, McCrosky BL, Moore EE, et al. Venous bullet embolism: rationale for mandatory extraction. *J Trauma.* 1987;27:1118–1122.

INDEX

Page numbers followed by *f* indicate figures; those followed by *t* indicate tables.